TOXICOLOGY OF THE EYE

THIRD EDITION

TOXICOLOGY
OF THE EYE

Effects on the Eyes and Visual System from
Chemicals, Drugs, Metals and Minerals,
Plants, Toxins and Venoms; also,
Systemic Side Effects from Eye Medications

By

W. MORTON GRANT, M.D.

David Glendenning Cogan Professor of Ophthalmology, Emeritus
Harvard University Medical School
Howe Laboratory of Ophthalmology
Massachusetts Eye and Ear Infirmary

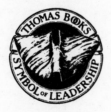

CHARLES C THOMAS • PUBLISHER
Springfield • Illinois • U.S.A.

Published and Distributed Throughout the World by

CHARLES C THOMAS • PUBLISHER
2600 South First Street
Springfield, Illinois 62717

© *1986 by* CHARLES C THOMAS • PUBLISHER

ISBN 0-398-05184-4

Library of Congress Catalog Card Number: 85-17366

With THOMAS BOOKS *careful attention is given to all details of manufacturing and design. It is the Publisher's desire to present books that are satisfactory as to their physical qualities and artistic possibilities and appropriate for their particular use.* THOMAS BOOKS *will be true to those laws of quality that assure a good name and good will.*

Printed in the United States of America
SC-R-3

Library of Congress Cataloging-in-Publication Data

Grant, W. Morton (Walter Morton), 1915–
    Toxicology of the eye.

    Bibliography: p.
    Includes index.
    1. Eye—Diseases and defects. 2. Toxicology.
I. Title. [DNLM: 1. Eye Injuries—chemically induced.
2. Vision Disorders—chemically induced. WW 100 G763t]
RE901.T67G73   1986   617.7'1   85-17366
ISBN 0-398-05184-4

PREFACE TO THE THIRD EDITION

Since the original edition of this book was prepared in the early 1960s, and the Second Edition in the early 1970s, a great deal of new material has become available, and has been incorporated in this new edition. To make room for this new material, portions of the older text that are still of some importance have been condensed, and portions that seem to be of least current interest have not been carried forward to the new edition. However, the new INDEX tells the reader when old eye toxicity information can still be found by referring back to the Second Edition.

For most bibliographic references, a space-saving system of superscript letters and numbers has been used as in previous editions, but the number of references has become so great, and so rapidly growing, that for some subjects the old system has become unwieldy. In such cases, authors' names have been used in the text, with alphabetical bibliographies corresponding, in a familiar manner.

The number of bibliographic references has now grown to more than 7000, approximately 40 percent of which are new since the Second Edition. The number of substances covered is more than 2800. The titles of most references are now given in English, in keeping with a current trend in abstract systems. The amount of cross-referencing in the INDEX has steadily increased, both as to synonyms and to lists of substances responsible for specific types of toxic effects.

PREFACE TO SECOND EDITION

During approximately ten years since preparation of the First Edition, nearly as many new reports have been published concerning drugs, chemicals, venoms, and plants involving the eyes as were found in all the literature of the previous one hundred years.

The purpose of the Second Edition is to bring together this accumulated information and to make it conveniently available to the people who may have need of it.

An introductory part (Section I) has been added in this edition, providing an outline of toxic effects systematized according to signs, symptoms, and sites of action. This is intended to help if one wishes to review the types of substances and modes of action that may produce a given effect. Mechanisms of action are included when known.

The largest portion of this edition (Section II) provides, as in the First Edition, a compendium of information and source references, plus occasional original observations, indexed alphabetically by names of substances. Increased attention has been given to observations on intraocular pressure, and also to non-ocular effects of drugs that are used in ophthalmology.

To save space, I have confined to the Index the numerical toxicity ratings of chemicals for which I have found no information on ocular toxicity other than the twenty-four-hour ratings from standard external tests on rabbit eyes.

The Bibliography of numbered references for these ratings and for the whole text immediately follows the Index.

PREFACE TO FIRST EDITION

The purpose of this book is to present a synopsis of what we know about substances which have toxic properties injurious to the eyes, disturbing to vision, or affecting the eyes in other unwanted ways.

The information which is summarized in this book represents what has been published in approximately the last one hundred years, plus a moderate number of previously unpublished observations. Approximately 1,600 substances are covered, with previously unpublished observations on more than two hundred.

The information is presented in simple form, alphabetically by substances, as in an encyclopedia. To make it easy to locate information also from signs or symptoms, or according to origins or occupations, extensive cross-referencing is provided in the Index.

An effort has been made to examine the material critically, and to present data and references accurately, in most instances from original publications, and in certain instances according to results of retesting in the laboratory.

References are given to the sources of information for all substances discussed. Those sources which are referred to several times are generally listed in the Bibliography, just preceding the Index, and are indicated in the text by superscript numbers. References pertaining to single substances are given immediately following the discussion of each substance, and are indicated in the text by superscript letters.

Intentionally in this book the weaknesses and deficiencies of our knowledge are made quite evident, so that anyone having an opportunity to make further observations may easily see where the need is for more complete and accurate information.

In the same vein, in the interests of research and investigation, attention is called to unsolved problems of mechanism of injurious action and to conditions for which specific treatments are lacking, yet by scientific methods could conceivably be developed.

ACKNOWLEDGMENTS

Experimental work by the author was supported by the United States Office of Scientific Research and Development during World War II, and by research grant B-103 from The National Institutes of Health, United States Public Health Service from 1951 to 1960.

In preparation of the First Edition, the author gave thanks to Charles J. Snyder, former librarian of the Howe Library of Ophthalmology, and to those others who helped in the laboratory and literary research, in particular Harold L. Kern, Sc.D., Helen Pentz Nardin, Myra Rolston, Elizabeth Cushing Kolm, and Hellen L. Crewe.

In preparation of the Second Edition, the author was especially grateful to Joann S. Perkins and Audrey Melanson, who, in addition to assisting in the research, typed and retyped all the material of which the book was composed.

Now, in preparing the Third Edition, the author especially thanks Patricia Fitzgerald for transforming the new handwritten text, via word-processor, to type-script ready for publication, with the assistance of Cheryl Morrison, and the technical guidance of P. John Anderson, Ph.D. Thanks are also due Chris Nims and Kathleen Kennedy of the Howe Library, for help in obtaining publications from distant and unusual sources.

The whole undertaking of the Third Edition has been made feasible by kind and understanding support from Mr. Edward V. French and Mrs. Catherine L. French, and from the Ophthalmic Staff of the Massachusetts Eye and Ear Infirmary.

W.M.G.

CONTENTS

TOXICOLOGY OF THE EYE

INTRODUCTORY OUTLINE OF TOXIC EFFECTS INVOLVING THE EYES OR VISION

Contents

This first chapter provides an outline of toxic disturbances of the eyes or vision produced either by direct contact or by systemic routes. Lists are given in the INDEX naming substances that have caused each of the various disturbances. A more detailed description of properties and effects of responsible chemicals, drugs, plant substances, toxins, and venoms is given in Chapter II, supported by bibliographic references. A review of the gross and microscopic pathology of the eye relating to toxic effects of some of the drugs has been published in a convenient synopsis by R.C. and B.J. Tripathi in 1982.[373]

A. DISTURBANCES OF CORNEA AND CONJUNCTIVA

Contents

---

1. Local Action on Cornea and Conjunctiva, Immediate Effects

Accidental splashing or squirting of substances into contact with the eyes is the commonest cause of toxic eye injuries. Some substances produce serious injury or pain almost immediately. Others produce superficial reversible damage, and others induce injury that may appear unimpressive at first, but becomes progressively worse after a latent period. It is important to recognize these different types of toxic action, because of their bearing on prognosis and treatment. The following discussions will stress these differences.

a. Caustic Chemicals, Immediate Injuries

Rapid, deep penetrating injuries of cornea, conjunctiva, sclera, and even lens and iris are most notoriously produced by alkalies and acids. (Detailed descriptions are given in Chapter II.) Injuries produced by alkalies and acids are principally a result of extreme change of the pH within the tissues. This has very rapid, almost immediate, action on the tissues which can be prevented or minimized only by very rapid emergency action. Some physical changes in the tissues are immediately evident, such as dissolution of epithelium and mottled clouding of corneal stroma from alkalies, or coagulation of epithelium by acids, but many other changes appear later, including edema, loss of mucopolysaccharide from the corneal stroma, further opacification and vascularization and degeneration of the cornea. Research is being aimed toward reversing the initial physicochemical changes and toward anticipating and preventing the secondary changes. At present, the main principle in initial treatment has been prolonged irrigation with water or saline solution to remove excess alkali or acid, hoping that this might interrupt the process.

There is a paradox to be noted, that the most serious chemical burns may produce little pain, because severe chemical injury destroys the sensory nerves of the cornea and renders the cornea anesthetic; whereas injuries that are relatively slight, superficial, and reversible, involving principally the corneal epithelium, may cause great discomfort, apparently by exposing corneal nerve endings to irritation rather than destroying them.

b. Solvent Splashes, Immediate Effects

A splash of a chemically inert solvent usually causes immediate stinging and smarting pain, and it may cause loss of some or all of the corneal epithelium, particularly if it is a good fat solvent. Even if all the epithelium is lost from the cornea as a result of splash of ordinary organic solvents, it generally regenerates in a few days without residual permanent damage. While the epithelium is missing, the corneal stroma may be slightly swollen and the posterior surface of the cornea may appear wrinkled.

Most organic solvents that are employed mainly for their physical solvent properties have no strongly acidic or alkaline character, and have little or no tendency to react chemically with tissues. Fortunately, many organic solvent splashes are well tolerated by the eye. Descriptions of the properties of individual solvents can be found in Chapter II. Ratings from tests on rabbit eyes can be found in the INDEX.

The first aid treatment of solvent splashes is immediate irrigation with water. Since these substances do not bind chemically with tissues and are readily eliminated by the irrigation, it seems that a brief irrigation, for a minute or two, should suffice. The very prolonged irrigations that have been recommended for acid and alkali burns should not be necessary.

c. Detergent or Surfactant Splashes

Contamination of the eye with surfactants and detergents presents a complex problem that is discussed in more detail in Chapter II under *Surfactants*. A great many of these substances are listed there in cationic, anionic, and nonionic categories, pointing out some related differences in type and severity of injury. It is noteworthy that there are practical differences and species differences in the dangers to the eyes presented by these substances. Some detergents that are used industrially and in the household rarely cause serious eye injuries in the people using them, though tests on rabbit eyes commonly show serious results. Some surfactants, such as ordinary soap, cause immediate stinging or burning with little or no injury. Other surfactants have produced corneal edema and loss of corneal epithelium with no warning discomfort, as described in Chapter II, particularly under *Ointments*. Some surfactants have delayed effects after a latent period, which will be described below.

In first aid treatment of eyes contaminated by surfactant or detergent liquids or powders immediate irrigation with water is appropriate. How long this irrigation should be continued has not been established, and this seems to deserve experimental investigation.

d. Lacrimators (tear gases), Immediate Effects

In the INDEX under "Lacrimator" is a list of substances that at low concentration in air have the special property of causing immediate stinging and smarting sensation in the eyes, with tearing. The lacrimogenic sensation is produced by selective stimulation of sensory nerve endings in the cornea, but with certain exceptions there is very little organized information on relationship of lacrimogenic discomfort and physical or chemical properties of the lacrimators. Substances that have the most intense lacrimatory action tend to be very reactive chemically, and may stimulate the nerve endings through specific chemical mechanisms.

Most of these chemically reactive substances which produce stinging and lacrimation without evident injury to the cornea at *low* concentration can, at *high* concentrations, cause severe damage and opacification of the cornea. These severe reactions are described in Chapter II under *Tear gas weapons,* and under the individual names of the *tear gases.*

In examining the mechanisms of action of lacrimatory agents on the eye, the first problem is to explain the stimulatory effect on the sensory nerve endings of the cornea. The second problem is to explain the injurious actions at higher concentrations. What relation one may have to the other is unknown, but it is clear that injury to the cornea and conjunctiva is quite independent of stimulatory effect on nerve endings. Investigators have so far been much more intrigued with trying to explain how lacrimators may stimulate the sensory nerve endings than with explaining the basis for serious injury.

Bacq has pointed out that representative lacrimatory agents as well as nonlacrimatory vesicants react with sulfhydryl groups and reduce the activity of sulfhydryl-dependent enzymes.[a] Mackworth reported having tested several lacrimators *in vitro* for inhibitory effect on a variety of enzymes.[f] Mackworth reported that lacrimators which he tested were selectively toxic to sulfhydryl or thiol enzymes, whereas enzymes such as cytochrome oxidase and lactic dehydrogenase, which were known to be insensitive to thiol reagents in general, were also insensitive to lacrimators. Mackworth hypothesized that lacrimators acted *in vivo* by combining with sulfhydryl (thiol) enzymes, but reported no actual tests on eyes or eye tissues. Dixon similarly concluded that lacrimator action was due to reaction with sulfhydryl enzymes, and that this involved either a positive halogen or a carbon-carbon double bond which was made reactive by neighboring ketone, ester, aldehyde, nitro, or other groups.[c,d] Dixon also indicated that the site of action must be in the corneal nerve endings, and noted that similar molar concentrations were required for stimulating the nerve endings as required for poisoning enzymes. Dixon acknowledged that the relationship between sulfhydryl groups in the nerve ending and the production of nerve impulses was unknown. Dixon also called attention to the fact that lacrimators were strong inhibitors of cell respiration and glycolysis, and that on the skin they could cause vesication if in sufficient concentration. Peters, reviewing the subject in 1963, pointed out difficulties in the concept of lacrimatory action being based on reaction with sulfhydryl groups in the nerve endings.[g] One problem was that most of the inhibitions of sulfhydryl enzymes by lacrimators had been found to be essentially irreversible, whereas the stinging sensation induced by low concentrations of lacrimators obviously and characteristically disappears when exposure of the eye to the lacrimator is terminated. Peters commented in 1963, "If it is an -SH group in the eye with which the lachrymator combines to produce the irritation, where is this -SH group in the eye? Is it the nerve itself or is it some sensitive nerve ending? Since the lachrymatory effect wears off, the combination could not be irreversible unless there can be some rapid regeneration of the group in question."

Fleckenstein in a series of biochemical studies on lacrimators confirmed that they were very active inhibitors of cellular respiration, often more effective than cyanide. However, concentrations of lacrimators necessary to interfere with tissue metabolism or respiration *in vitro* were often several hundred times greater than the concentrations in air that would produce distinct discomfort of the eye. As a possible escape from this dilemma, Fleckenstein postulated that there might be an adsorptive and selective concentrating effect in the superficial layers of the corneal epithelium and nerve endings to produce a locally higher concentration of lacrimator than in the surrounding air. Fleckenstein postulated that the concentrated lacrimatory agent caused depolarization of the nerves and drop of the resting membrane potential by local inhibition of oxidation.[e]

Castro studied the inhibition of cholinesterase by several alkylating agents, including some lacrimators, and obtained evidence of an inhibitory effect that involved reaction through some group other than sulfhydryl, and which was reversible *in vitro*.[b] Although there was no direct evidence that cholinesterase itself was involved in lacrimatory action in the cornea, the demonstration that a lacrimator, such as chloroacetophenone, could have an inhibitory action on an enzyme through reaction with groups other than sulfhydryl, and that this type of reaction was reversible, seemed to provide a new possibility for explaining the transitory nature of the sensory response when the eye is exposed to a lacrimator. Inhibition of cholinesterase itself in the cornea can hardly be involved in the lacrimogenic action, since some strong lacrimators (bromoacetone and chloropicrin) do not inactivate cholinesterase, and powerful anticholinesterase drugs, such as echothiophate, produce no lacrimatory sensory stimulation when applied to the cornea.

Treatment is not ordinarily required for the lacrimatory action, since it is self-limited when exposure is discontinued. Potentially it could be suppressed by local anesthesia. When treatment is needed after exposure to lacrimogenic substances, it is for corneal and conjunctival injury which may be produced by concentrations greater than those that are simply lacrimogenic. No specific antidotes or effective countermeasures are known at present. (This aspect of lacrimators is discussed in Chapter II under *Tear Gas Weapons* and *Chloroacetophenone*.)

a. Bacq ZM: Thiol-binding substances. *EXPERIENTIA* 2:349–354, 1946. (French)
b. Castro JA: Effect of alkylating agents on human plasma cholinesterase. *BIOCHEM PHARMACOL* 17:295–303, 1968.
c. Dixon M: Reactions of lachrymators with enzymes and proteins. *BIOCHEM J* 42:xxvi–xxvii, 1948.
d. Dixon M, Needham DM: Biochemical research on chemical warfare agents. *NATURE* 158:432–438, 1946.
e. Fleckenstein A: Adsorptive concentration of substances with mucous membrane irritating action in the respiratory tract. *EXPERIENTIA* (Suppl. 13):117–125, 1967. (German)
f. Mackworth JF: The inhibition of thiol enzymes by lachrymators. *BIOCHEM J* 42:82–90, 1948.
g. Peters RA: *Biochemical Lesions and Lethal Synthesis.* New York, Macmillan, 1963.

2. Local Action on Cornea and Conjunctiva, Delayed Effects

a. Corneal Epithelial Edema, after Latent Period

In the INDEX under "*Corneal epithelial edema (painless), with delayed onset of haloes, from local action*" is a list of chemicals, mostly amines, which in vapor form, after several hours of exposure, induce swelling of the corneal epithelial cells. People exposed to this effect may then see colored haloes about lights because of diffraction effects from the myriads of swollen cells.

This peculiar reaction to the vapors of these substances has in most cases occurred in workmen who have been exposed for several hours to concentrations of the vapors that were not unduly unpleasant at the time of exposure, and they have usually noted no disturbance of the eye during the working day, but in the evening ȯn the way home from work they have seen colored haloes around lights. Usually there has been no discomfort such as results from death or loss of epithelial cells, and the condition has been spontaneously reversible, sometimes by the next day, and at least within a couple of days. The mechanism by which these substances produce reversible corneal epithelial edema with a delay in onset after exposure is unknown.

With excessive exposure, it is possible to develop eye discomfort or pain as a result of more severe injury of the epithelial cells, as will be discussed in following paragraphs.

No special treatment except avoidance of excessive concentrations appears indicated, since the condition has characteristically been spontaneously reversible.

b. *Corneal Epithelial Injury, after Latent Period*

In the INDEX under "*Corneal epithelial injury (painful), with delayed onset, from local action*" is a list of chemicals, drugs, and plant materials which have the striking feature of a delay or latent period before onset of symptoms. (Details are given in Chapter II.) These substances cause injury, with death or loss of corneal epithelial cells and associated discomfort several hours after exposure. (It is notable that some of these substances at lower levels cause only epithelial edema with haloes, but without pain, as described in preceding paragraphs.) When exposure causes delayed onset of discomfort, it appears to be similar to the reaction to excessive exposure to ultraviolet (in so-called ultraviolet keratitis, sun lamp keratitis, snow blindness, or welders' flash), and analogous to the delayed reaction of the skin in sunburn. Typically, during exposure these substances cause essentially no discomfort or irritation, but several hours later the eyes may develop a sensation of burning and irritation, with conjunctival hyperemia, tearing, photophobia or discomfort from bright light, blurred vision, and a defensive blepharospasm or closure of the eyelids. At this stage the eyes may be difficult to examine without first applying a drop of local anesthetic. Ophthalmoscopically the cornea shows fine optical irregularity, accounting for subjective blurring of vision and reduced visual acuity. When inspected with a flashlight, the cornea may appear slightly hazy, and the reflection of the light from the surface may appear finely irregular, making the corneal surface seem lusterless. Characteristically the surface lacks its normal shiny smoothness and distinct reflecting properties. When examined with a slit-lamp biomicroscope, the surface may be seen speckled with fine gray dots, representing abnormal or dead epithelial cells, and these stain readily if tested with fluorescein. The subsequent course is variable, depending on the severity of exposure. In the mildest cases the epithelium heals spontaneously, returning to normal in a day or two. In more severe cases the fine speckling of epithelial damage that is evident early at the time of onset of symptoms may progress, and the whole epithelium may be lost, requiring a longer time to regenerate. In the most extreme cases the damaging action can involve the corneal stroma and endothelium as well as epithelium, and the stroma may undergo swelling with wrinkling of the posterior surface, infiltration with inflammatory cells, invasion by interstitial vessels and fibrous tissue, finally permanent scarring, vascularization, and opacity. Such extreme reactions are rare, but have been seen particularly with *dimethyl sulfate* and *mustard gas.*

The mechanisms by which substances produce injury with delayed onset can at present only be guessed at. Most fundamentally it appears that these substances must interfere with biological processes such as by inhibiting an enzyme, altering nucleic acid of the cell nuclei, or denaturing other proteins, so that after a time the affected cell can no longer survive. Some of the substances with these injurious effects of delayed onset are recognizable as alkylating agents. Mustard gas has been shown to form a persistent and disturbing cross linkage between strands of DNA in the nucleus, and colchicine is also well known to interfere in mitotic processes. Hydrogen sulfide is poisonous, particularly to metal-dependent enzymes. Osmic acid is a fixative that has specific reactivities with cell components. Presumably these various actions are incompatible with the normal biological processes of the cell.

c. Corneal Epithelial Vacuoles

Vacuoles in the corneal epithelium which develop after chronic exposure to the vapors of a small number of chemicals are quite special and different from edema or injury of corneal epithelial cells such as discussed in the foregoing paragraphs. In the case of vacuoles, the surface reflex (reflection of the light from the surface) of the cornea is quite lustrous, smooth, and undisturbed by the presence of vacuoles within the epithelium, whereas both edema and keratitis epithelialis render the surface finely but distinctly irregular and also lusterless. By slit-lamp biomicroscope, when vacuoles are present in the corneal epithelium, they are seen with ordinary (10 to 20 times) magnification as spherical, shiny, colorless spheres that look like tiny gas bubbles within the epithelium, but except for occasional and inconstant tiny gray flecks at the surface, the surrounding epithelium appears entirely normal. (In epithelial edema the epithelium has diffuse ground-glass sort of fine optical irregularity made up of myriads of swollen epithelial cells; in keratitis epithelialis the surface of the epithelium is stippled with many gray specks or dots presumably representing damaged or dead epithelial cells.) Usually symptoms from corneal epithelial vacuoles are slight or absent.

In human beings, corneal epithelial vacuoles have been produced by *n-butanol, xylene* and probably *nitronaphthalene.* They have not been produced in rabbits or guinea pigs, but have been produced in cats with *n-butanol, ethyl acetate, methyl acetate, toluene,* and *xylene.* These substances are described further in Chapter II; see INDEX.

d. Corneal and Conjunctival Discoloration from Vapors or Dusts

Brown discoloration of the conjunctiva and cornea in the palpebral fissure from exposure to dusts or vapors has been observed principally in manufacture of *aniline* and *hydroquinone,* which entails also exposure to the oxidation product *benzoquinone.* A different type of discoloration consisting of dark granules in the palpebral conjunctiva hidden under the upper lid at the upper border of the tarsus has been produced by chronic exposure to mineral dust containing *iron,* resembling the discoloration in the same location produced by certain *eye cosmetics,* such as *mascaras,* after they have been used for long periods on the lid margins. (The individual substances are described further in Chapter II; see INDEX.)

e. Late Corneal Scarring and Distortion from Vapors or Dusts

Scarring and distortion of the cornea have been severe problems which have disabled workmen many years after chronic industrial exposure in manufacture of *aniline* and *hydroquinone.* Also scarring and distortion of the cornea in many cases developed years after severe exposure to *mustard gas* in World War I, somewhat analogous to the late effects of *hydroquinone* exposure. In the case of the *mustard gas* injuries, the corneal distortions were frequently accompanied by peculiar varicose distortions of blood vessels in the conjunctiva near the limbus or in blood vessels that had invaded the injured cornea. (See INDEX and Chapter II.)

3. Systemic Actions, Effects on Cornea and Conjunctiva

a. Corneal Epithelial Deposits from Systemic Substances

Chronic systemic administration of several drugs produces deposits in the corneal epithelium that are visible with the slit-lamp biomicroscope. Of the drugs identified and listed in the INDEX under *"Corneal epithelial deposits,"* at least *amiodarone, amodiaquine, chloroquine, hydroxychloroquine, monobenzone, perhexiline,* and *tilorone* appear to produce corneal lipidosis or phospholipidosis. (See INDEX for *Lipidosis.*)

The deposits generally have appeared as very fine granules scattered throughout the epithelium, most often gray, but sometimes yellowish or brownish, particularly in patients taking *chloroquine* or *chlorpromazine.* In most instances the deposits have not appreciably interfered with vision, but they have been known to diffract light entering the eye and produce an appearance of haloes around lights. This has been noted especially in the case of *mepacrine.* The deposits of most of these substances have gradually disappeared from the cornea if the medications have been discontinued, and they apparently have done no harm while present.

Patterns which the deposits may form include whorls, bow-ties, and cat's whiskers. The condition has been called thesaurismosis and cornea verticillata.

b. Corneal Stromal Deposits from Systemic Substances

Corneal stromal discoloration is well known from deposits of the metals, *copper, gold, mercury,* and *silver,* while finely granular stromal deposits have been attributed to *chlorpromazine, clofazimine, indomethacin,* and probably *methotrimeprazine.* None appear to have harmed the cornea.

c. Lacrimation, Burning or Itching Sensation from Systemic Substances

In the INDEX under this heading is a list of drugs and chemicals which when given systemically can produce ocular discomfort without keratitis or other visible evidence of eye disturbance.

d. Corneal, Conjunctival Inflammation, sometimes with Dermatitis, from Systemic Substances

In the INDEX under this heading is a list of drugs, chemicals, and plants which when taken systemically can cause keratitis, conjunctivitis, and sometimes dermatitis. While the mechanism in most cases is not known, it seems noteworthy that the systemic substances that cause this kind of ocular inflammation are mostly different from systemic substances that produce corneal epithelial deposits. They appear to overlap with systemic substances that cause corneal opacities only in the cases of *chlorpropamide, isotretinoin, phthalofyne,* and *practolol.*

e. Photosensitized Keratitis from Systemic Substances

Exposure to light can induce keratitis in animals that have ingested *ammi majus seeds, hypericum, methoxsalen, phenothiazine,* and probably *lantana.* The same photo-sensitized keratitis can be induced in human beings by *methoxsalen* systemically. There is discomfort from injury of the corneal epithelium, but recovery on discontinuing exposure. Similar light-induced reactions can occur in human beings whose eyes are exposed externally to *proflavin* or *pitch fumes.*

f. Corneal Epithelial Vacuoles from Systemic Drugs

Vacuoles in the corneal epithelium like those produced by vapor of *n-butanol* have been induced in humans by systemic *nicothiazone* and *thiacetazone.*

d. Corneal Endothelial Injury by Systemic Chemicals in Animals

Corneal edema in animals resulted from inhalation of *1,2-dibromoethane, 1,2-dichloroethane, 1,2-dichloroethylene,* and *methylhydrazine.* Dogs and other canine animals are most susceptible to injury of the endothelium and development of edema of the cornea from inhalation of these substances. Particularly *dichloroethane* has a remarkably selective toxic effect on the corneal endothelium, causing acute degeneration and consequent development of bluish edema and swelling of the cornea several hours after inhalation or systemic administration in dogs. The species specificity appears to relate to how easily the *dichloroethane* gets from the blood stream to the aqueous humor. Injury of the endothelium and corneal edema can be produced in species other than the canine animals if dichloroethane is introduced directly into the aqueous humor in comparable concentration. Human beings have so far been fortunate in escaping this type of toxic effect.

B. DISTURBANCES OF LENS, IRIS, AND ANTERIOR CHAMBER

Contents

Notable reviews of toxic effects on the lens, with many references, have been published by Koch* and by Kuck, both in 1977.**

1. Cataracts from Systemic Substances

In the INDEX under "Cataract (opacity of lens substance) from systemic drugs or chemicals" is a list of more than 80 substances that are believed to have caused cataracts, approximately one third of them in humans and two thirds in animals. (This list does not include another dozen substances that cause acute transient white clouding of the lens in small rodents owing to drying of the anterior segment under the influence of substances that prevent blinking or normal wetting of the anterior surface of the eye by tears.) (This list of cataractogenic substances also does not include substances which produce deposits or discoloration in the lens without opacification of lens substance itself.)

The fact that at least twice as many substances are known to cause cataracts in animals than in humans can be partially explained on the basis that many more drugs and chemicals are tested in animals, and often at very much higher dosage in experimental animals than in human beings. There is another important difference — the age at the time of exposure. Cataracts can be induced much more readily in younger animals than in older, and for this reason young animals are nearly always

---

*Koch HR: Lens. *Arzneimittelnebenwirkungen am Auge.* 49–82, 1977. Edited by Hockwin O, Koch HR. Gustav Fischer: Stuttgart-New York. (German)

**Kuck JFR Jr: Drugs influencing the lens. pp. 433–523, in Dikstein.[299]

used in studies of cataractogenic agents, whereas human beings tend not to be exposed to drugs until they are older.

Several categories of toxic cataracts can be recognized and will be outlined in the following paragraphs. More factual details and bibliographic information on each of the substances are to be found in Chapter II under their individual names (see INDEX).

a. Sugar cataracts

These are produced by *galactose, xylose,* and *glucose. Galactose* has been the prime example and the subject of extensive investigation. *Galactose* and *xylose* administered in large amounts to animals, and *glucose* in excess, as in severe diabetes with persistent severe hyperglycemia, can produce sugar cataract. The mechanism consists in easy entry of the sugar into the lens, where it is converted to a sugar alcohol, which is trapped in the lens because the sugar alcohol does not have the proper solubility characteristics to get out. When the sugar alcohols accumulate in the lens, they appear not to be toxic to the lens, but rather they act osmotically, attracting water and causing excessive hydration of the lens, with swelling of cells and lakes of fluid between cells, producing localized changes in refractive index, scattering of light, and a ground-glass appearance. Secondarily, potassium, amino acids, and other constituents leak out of the lens, metabolic processes are affected, and sodium chloride and more water enter the lens, causing further swelling, disruption of nerve fibers, and changes in lens proteins, producing irreversible cataract.

b. Diabetes with cataract

This can be induced by poisoning animals with *alloxan* or *streptozotocin.* Severe persistent hyperglycemia from injury to the pancreas may lead to sugar cataracts by the mechanism already described, but at least in the case of *alloxan,* which is poisonous to many ocular tissues besides the lens, it has been seriously questioned whether it is the hyperglycemia or a direct toxic effect of the *alloxan* on the lens that is responsible for the cataractogenesis.

c. Radiomimetic toxic cataracts

These have been produced by several of the chemicals and drugs that have antimitotic actions, presumably due to effects on the nuclei of the cells of the lens analogous to the effects produced by radiation. This type of cataract appears to have been induced by *busulfan, dibromomannitol, dimethylaminostyrylquinoline, iodoacetate, nitrogen mustards, tretamine,* and *triaziquone,* the majority of which are recognizable as antineoplastic antimitotic agents. As in development of radiation-type lens opacities, the most actively mitotic cells at the equator of the lens show the most obvious morphologic changes. These cells gradually become opaque and are gradually pushed posteriorly by fibers that are formed later in more natural manner, resulting eventually in opacities both at the lens equator and at the posterior pole of the lens.

If poisoning has been severe and many cells injured, a more diffuse death of cells and gradually more diffuse cataract develops.

d. Protein disturbance and enzyme inhibition cataracts

This is obviously a vague and ill-defined category, but may include *chlorophenylalanine,* an antimetabolite that interferes with phenylalanine metabolism and may interfere with formation of lens proteins. Similarly *phenylhydrazopropionitrile,* a cataractogenic osteolathyrogen, may interfere with the formation of lens proteins and the growth of the lens. Also *mimosine* is known to interfere with enzyme action and protein metabolism. *Dichloronitroaniline* produces changes in the collagen of the cornea and may also affect the proteins of the lens. *Naphthalene* and the related chemicals *decahydronaphthalene, naphthol, naphthoquinone,* and *tetrahydronaphthalene* may work through conversion to *naphthoquinone,* which has been shown to react with lens proteins. *Naphthoquinone* can also inhibit NaK-ATPase, interfere with the cation pump of the lens and with lens glycolysis, and can produce vacuoles and swelling of the lens. Finally, *dinitro-o-cresol* and *dinitrophenol,* which are known particularly to uncouple oxidative phosphorylation, presumably are toxic to the lens on this basis. However, beyond that supposition the mechanism of the cataractogenic action of these last two substances is still obscure.

e. Cataracts associated with disturbances of skin and hair

These have been produced in human beings particularly by *triparanol* and by *bis-phenylisopropylpiperazine,* and in animals by *clomiphene* (a chemical relative of *triparanol*), and by *thallium,* as well as by *triparanol.* While this clinical relationship has so far shed practically no light on the biochemical mechanism, it has called attention to the embryologic ectodermal origin of the crystalline lens, suggesting that the toxic reactions of skin and hair and of the crystalline lens may in these particular instances represent fundamentally parallel processes.

f. Corticosteroid cataracts

These are typically posterior subcapsular, and have been produced by a variety of glucocorticoids used medically for long periods either systemically or applied to the surface of the eye. This category may include the corticosteroid derivatives *dichlorisone* and *methyldichlorisone,* which have also been reported to produce cataracts in human beings during chronic systemic administration.

g. Actinic or photosensitization cataracts

These have been reported in animals exposed to intense illumination after administration of *hematoporphyrin* or *methoxsalen.* In development of senile cataracts there is suspicion of a toxic mechanism involving light and the formation of hydrogen peroxide and free radicals in the aqueous humor, with oxidative effects on the lens. (See INDEX for *Hydrogen peroxide.*)

h. Metal chelators and cataracts

These seem to be circumstantially related in the cases of *deferoxamine, dithizone,* and *pyrithione.* Since these substances also produce severe disturbances in other portions of the eyes of the animals in which they produce cataracts, it seems possible that the cataractogenesis may be secondary to the disturbances of the other portions of the eye, rather than due to direct action on the lens.

i. Keratitis with cataract

In rats this has been produced by near-lethal doses of medications used in treatment of human diabetes, *carbutamide, chloropropamide,* and *tolbutamide,* but not in human beings.

j. Acute reversible white clouding of the lens

In rats and mice this is not a toxic action on the lens, but is secondary to exposure and dehydration of the front of the eye when blinking is stopped. This phenomenon has been thoroughly reviewed by Koch in 1977. (See reference at the beginning of this section on the Lens.)

2. Lens Nuclear Sclerosis

A peculiar gradual change in refractive power of the nucleus of the lens, without opacification, has given an ophthalmoscopic and slit-lamp appearance of a lens within a lens in subprimate animals (dogs, rabbits, pigs, guinea pigs, and rats) after chronic administration of *dimethyl sulfoxide.* This has not as yet been encountered in human beings. (For details, see INDEX for *Dimethyl sulfoxide.*)

3. Myopia, Acute Transient

In the INDEX under "*Myopia, acute transient, from systemic drugs in humans*" more than 20 drugs are listed as having caused a peculiar acute transient myopia in one or more patients. This myopia has *not* been attributable to cholinergic or parasympathomimetic contraction of the ciliary muscle with spasm of accommodation for near. In no case has the myopia been relieved by applying atropine or other anticholinergic drugs. Furthermore none of the substances listed has sufficient cholinergic activity to cause a contraction of the ciliary muscle. Also, in association with this type of myopia there has been no constriction of the pupil such as might be expected if a cholinergic or parasympathomimetic mechanism were involved.

There has been a remarkable uniformity in the characteristics of the acute transient myopic reaction to these substances, despite the fact that they represent a considerable diversity of pharmacologic types. None of these substances induces myopia frequently or regularly. It occurs only as a rare, apparently idiosyncratic reaction. Most characteristically the patients who have experienced the peculiar myopic reaction have a history of having taken the drug previously without notable side effects, but when they have taken the same drug again weeks or months later they have noticed within a few hours or a few days that their vision of distant objects has become blurred.

In nearly all cases it has been demonstrated that visual acuity could be promptly restored to normal by use of lenses which corrected for several diopters of myopia. In nearly all cases that have been reported, medication has been suspected to be the cause of the myopia, and the medication has been stopped. Then the myopia has disappeared spontaneously within a few days. Practically all the patients who have had this type of reaction have been nonglaucomatous. Several patients who have experienced this reaction in association with use of diuretic agents have been women in the first few months of pregnancy with excessive water retention. Generally the patients have been young or middle-aged adults, and characteristically not old people with nuclear sclerosis or cataracts. No other common features seem to have been recognized to identify the type of patient who may be predisposed to this particular reaction.

Reviews of the literature with numerous references have been provided by Dralands and Garvin (1972)[301] and by Schroeder and Schwarzer (1978).[b]

The mechanism of the acute idiosyncratic transient myopia is incompletely explained. There have been atypical instances in response to *acetazolamide* in which the intraocular pressure has become very low or has become temporarily elevated, but disturbance of intraocular pressure is not a characteristic. There have also been atypical instances associated with noticeable shallowing of the anterior chamber in response to *acetazolamide* and *sulfanilamide,* but in most cases the depth of the anterior chamber has not been noticeably altered. In very rare instances, cells and slight flare have been seen in the aqueous humor.

In several cases the ophthalmoscopic appearance of the posterior pole of the eye has suggested to the observer that there was retinal edema, but in these cases the visual acuity was correctable to normal with appropriate spectacle lenses, and in most cases there has been no suspicion of retinal edema. The validity of the impression of retinal edema from ophthalmoscopic examination is difficult to judge.

One of the best pieces of evidence to implicate the crystalline lens in the acute myopic reaction has been presented in the case of a woman with unilateral aphakia, having no lens in one eye, but a normal lens in the other eye. She experienced a typical acute myopic reaction to *dichlorphenamide* only in the eye that had the crystalline lens present, no change in the aphakic eye. The same phenomenon has been reported with *phenformin* in another unilaterally aphakic patient. (As a rule, case reports of idiosyncratic acute transient myopia have described patients with lenses normally present in both eyes, and have indicated essentially equal degree of myopia induced in both eyes.)

Another very instructive case implicating the crystalline lens has been reported in association with transient myopic reaction to *chlorthalidone* in which studies with ultrasound showed that during the transient myopia the crystalline lens was abnormally thick, the anterior chamber was slightly shallowed, but the distance from the lens to the posterior wall of the eye was not affected.

Other ultrasound measurements, by Bovino and Marcus (1982), on a patient with acute transient myopia from a combination of drugs showed no significant changes in lens thickness, but shallowing of the anterior chamber.[a] They postulated that there might have been edema of the ciliary body to explain these findings.

An ultrasound study of Schroeder and Schwarzer on a patient with bilateral acute transient myopia from a combination of sulphonamide and corticosteroid drugs, showed not only thickening of the lenses but also shallowing of the anterior chambers, which was complicated by angle-closure glaucoma.[b]

Although there has been diversity in the ultrasound findings as to whether there is thickening or forward movement of the lens, there appears now to be general agreement that it is in the lens that an explanation for the change in refraction must be sought. Possibly transitory abnormal hydration causes change in refraction without change in transparency, as may happen in unregulated diabetes. As yet no ultrasound studies of the ciliary body have been made to determine whether there may be edema there as some have speculated. The variety of types of drugs that have been implicated, the rarity of the reaction, and the common history of previous exposure to the same drug without side effects suggest that some type of sensitizing process may be involved.

As a rule the myopic reaction has been completely spontaneously reversible and no permanent changes in the lenses have been recorded. In some instances the reaction has been induced two or three times by resuming use of the drug, either by chance or by design, and in one case five separate episodes of reversible myopia were induced by *tetracycline*. What would happen ultimately if a patient persisted in taking a drug that induced this myopic reaction is at present unknown.

a. Bovino JA, Marcus DF: The mechanism of transient myopia induced by sulfonamide therapy. *AM J OPHTHALMOL* 94:99–102, 1982.
b. Schroeder W, Schwarzer J: Transient myopia with angle closure glaucoma. *KLIN MONATSBL AUGENHEILKD* 172:762–766, 1978.

4. Lens Deposits and Discoloration

Discoloration of the lens by *copper, iron, mercury,* or *silver* is seen just beneath the anterior capsule. It is blue-green in the case of *copper,* rust yellow or brown in the case of *iron,* rosy brown or pink from *mercury,* and grayish blue from *silver.* These discolorations no doubt represent actual deposits of the metals, as insoluble salts or in combination with proteins. The colored deposits are observed with the slit-lamp biomicroscope, and are significant mainly as an aid in diagnosis. As a rule they do not interfere with vision, nor do they of themselves lead to formation of cataracts.

Deposition of fine yellowish or brownish granules are seen beneath the anterior lens capsule in people who have been taking large amount of *chlorpromazine* over long periods, and possibly in a few patients who have taken *thiothixene*. The significance seems to be similar to that of the fine deposits of metals. The deposits are rarely sufficient to interfere with vision, and apparently not likely to lead to formation of cataracts.

Each of these substances that produce fine deposits beneath the anterior lens capsule can also produce fine deposits in the most posterior layers of the cornea and sometimes in the conjunctiva, but they are most readily detectable in the lens.

C. POSTERIOR SEGMENT AND VISUAL PATHWAYS

Contents

1. Morphologic Changes from Toxic Substances Taken Systemically

Morphologic changes include abnormalities diagnosed clinically, as well as those detected microscopically.

a. Ciliary Body Edema, Inflammation, or Degeneration

Reactions of this sort have been produced in animals by systemic administration of *colchicine, ergot, naphthalene, naphthol,* and *urethane.* (See INDEX.)

b. Retinal Edema

Under "Retinal edema" in the INDEX is a list of nearly 30 substances that have been reported to cause edema of the retina in animals and human beings when taken systemically. No generalization has been arrived at concerning the mechanism.

c. Retinal Hemorrhages

According to the list under "Retinal hemorrhages" in the INDEX many toxic substances in considerable variety have been involved. Retinal hemorrhages have been diagnosed several times more frequently in human beings than in animals, possibly because of more frequent ophthalmoscopic examination in humans. A small proportion of the substances involved are recognizable as potential causes of blood dyscrasias or clotting abnormalities, but for most the mechanism responsible for retinal hemorrhage is not clear.

d. Retinal Vessel Narrowing

Optic nerve atrophy from any cause is characteristically accompanied by narrowing of arteries on and about the disc, but a small list of substances (in the INDEX under "Retinal vessel narrowing") can cause retinal arteries to narrow acutely. The most classic example is *quinine,* which can cause acute narrowing of the arteries in a few days after poisoning, even while vision is improving. The mechanism is not yet known, but in optic atrophy it has been supposed that reduced nutritional demand by the tissues may lead to narrowing of the vessels.

e. Maculopathy

In human beings, maculopathy has been suspected as a side effect of some 20 systemically absorbed substances, as listed under "Maculopathy" in the INDEX. It is noteworthy that in most instances the diagnosis has been rather tenuous (indicated by question-marks in the list), usually based on suspected slightly abnormal ophthalmoscopic appearance of the macula, with or without some other-wise unexplained subnormality of visual acuity. In only a few instances has fluorescein angiography or the frequency and distinctiveness established the diagnosis securely.

In patients taking *phenothiazine derivatives,* deposits of lipofuschin have caused brownish discoloration of the macula without reducing vision significantly, according to Meier-Ruge (1977).[356, 357]

Topical *epinephrine* in aphakic eyes can produce cystic maculopathy, and there has been suspicion that *dipivefrin* may also. (See INDEX) However, when the lens is present in human eyes it appears to be an effective barrier to diffusion of drugs and chemicals from the anterior segment to the posterior pole of the eye. Apart from instances of very severe chemical damage of the anterior segment, as by sodium hydroxide, there appear to be no proven cases of maculopathy from contact of drugs or chemicals with the cornea when the crystalline lens has been present.

f. Retinal Ganglion Cell Damage by Systemic Substances

In practically all instances this diagnosis has been made by microscopic examination of the retina. In the list of approximately 19 substances under this heading in the INDEX only about a third have affected human beings, and these have been drugs in most instances (*arsanilic acid, chloramphemicol, ethylhydrocupreine, methanol, quinine, thallium, vincristine,* and *carbon dioxide*). Among the substances shown to be toxic to retinal ganglion cells in animals, six are of plant origin (*ammi majus seeds, aspidium, cinchona derivatives, ergot, locoweed, Swainsona plants*). No doubt damage of retinal ganglion cells would also be found, if looked for, in poisoning by the numerous additional substances that cause optic nerve atrophy (see INDEX), since death of optic nerve fibers ultimately leads to death of ganglion cells.

The retinal ganglion cells presumably can be poisoned and damaged directly, but they also show morphologic changes and disappear when their nerve fibers are killed. Death of retinal ganglion cells is associated with optic atrophy from any cause, such as from excessive elevation of intracranial pressure, from elevation of intraocular pressure, or from optic neuritis, as well as from primary toxic effects on the ganglion cells themselves.

g. Retinal Photoreceptor Damage by Systemic Substances

A long list of substances is to be found under this heading in the INDEX, but poisoning of photoreceptors in human beings accounts for only about one sixth of the list (i.e. *cardiac glycosides, chloramphenicol, digitalis, digitoxin, furmethonol, quinine*). In animals the larger number presumably is associated with more experimental testing and larger doses.

The diagnosis of photoreceptor damage may be based on changes in the electroretinogram and on histology. Some substances affect also the retinal pigment epithelium. Some cause changes in other portions of the visual system. The actions of each of the substances listed are described in Chapter II.

h. Retinal Pigment Epithelial Changes from Systemic Drugs and Chemicals

In the INDEX is a long list of substances which affect the retinal pigment epithelium when absorbed systemically. Changes in the pigment epithelium may be determined histologically, or they may be evident clinically. Ophthalmoscopy may show changes in the retinal pigment. Fluorescence of the choroid in fluorescein angiography may show up abnormalities in the retinal pigment. The standing potential determined by electrooculography may indicate change in the retinal pigment epithelium. Often changes in the retinal photoreceptors are associated with abnormalities of the pigment epithelium. Reviews of mechanisms of toxic retinopathies affecting the retinal pigment epithelium have been published by Meier-Ruge,[356, 357] and by Zinn and Marmor.[389] Details concerning the substances listed in the INDEX are to be found in Chapter II of this book.

i. Retinal Dots or Flecks from Substances Taken Systemically

Several substances can give rise to tiny yellow or white dots in the fundi visible by ophthalmoscopy. Glistening yellow or gold specks can be produced in human eyes by *canthaxanthin*. White flecks in human eyes can be produced by *methoxyflurane, 2-naphthol, 2-naphthyl benzoate, talc,* and *tamoxifen,* and in animal eyes by *dibutyl oxalate* and *quinoline*. The substance seen after administration of *methoxyflurane* or *dibutyl oxalate* (possibly also after *2-naphthol* and *2-naphthyl benzoate*) are inert calcium oxalate crystals. *Talc* emboli in retinal vessels are seen after intravenous injection of talc. (For descriptions of each substance, see the INDEX.)

j. Retinal Lipidosis

Microscopically a number of substances (see INDEX) have produced lipidosis of the retina in addition to other tissues, but study of the functional significance is needed.

k. Choroidal Edema, Exudate, and Detachment, from Systemic Substances

In animals, reactions of this type can be produced by administering *diethyldithiocarbamate, diquat, dithizone, epinephrine, iodate, naphthalene, oxygen,* and *pyrithione,* (also by subconjunctival injection of *deferoxamine*). Related choroidal degenerative changes in animals have also been ascribed to *cobalt salts, mercuric chloride, P1727,* and *thioridazine*. No comparable reactions seem to have been described in human beings. (For descriptions of the above substances, see INDEX.)

l. Tapetal Disturbances from Systemic Substances, in Animals

The tapetum in certain animals has been affected by experimental administration of *diethyldithiocarbamate, dithizone, edetate, ethambutol, ethylenediamine derivatives, hydroxychloroquine, imidazo quinazoline, oxypertine,* and *pyrithione*. Most of these substances can chelate metals. Zinc is an important element in the tapetum. An interaction is thought to be important. (For descriptions of the individual substances, see the INDEX.)

m. Papilledema from Systemic Substances

In the INDEX under this heading is a list of more than 40 substances which have been reported to have produced papilledema when taken systemically. In nearly all instances the papilledema has been diagnosed in human beings. Three of the substances listed (*p-dichlorobenzene; helichrysum; hexachlorophene*) have been reported to cause papilledema in dogs.

Papilledema can occur as an accompaniment of optic neuritis, or as a manifestation of elevation of intracranial pressure. The usual basis for the diagnosis is a characteristic elevated swollen and congested appearance of the optic nervehead seen with the ophthalmoscope. Edema of the nervehead is found histologically.

Central scotoma is commonly detected in cases of optic neuritis or retrobulbar neuritis, but central scotomas characteristically do not appear when drugs and chemicals cause elevation of intracranial pressure and papilledema appears secondarily. Patients with papilledema from increased intracranial pressure may have repeated transient momentary dimmings or obscurations of vision. They also may have weakness or paralysis of the lateral rectus muscles from partial or complete sixth nerve palsy, presumably due to pressure on these nerves.

Increased cerebrospinal fluid pressure in the absence of brain tumor or other brain disease has been called "Pseudotumor cerebri" and "Benign intracranial hypertension." In many cases this condition occurs without known cause. Reviews and collections of cases are available.[a-c]

Substances that most clearly raise cerebrospinal fluid pressure and cause papilledema are *corticosteroids, nalidixic acid, tetracycline,* and *vitamin A.*

Certain exceptional substances cause edema of the brain substance itself ("status spongiosus") with brain swelling that may damage visual pathways or the visual cortex. These substances tend not to raise cerebrospinal fluid pressure, and may cause compression of the ventricles, rather than dilation.

   a. Hierons R: Papilloedema not needing surgery. *TRANS OPHTHALMOL SOC UK* 89:147–157, 1969.
   b. Katzman B, Lu LW, et al: Pseudotumor cerebri: An observation and review. *ANN OPHTHALMOL* 13:887–892, 1981.
   c. VanDyk HJL, Swan KC: Drug induced pseudotumor cerebri. In Leopold IH (Ed.): SYMPOSIUM ON OCULAR THERAPY. St. Louis, Mosby, 1969, vol. 4, ch. 9.
   d. Wall M, Hart WM Jr, Burde RM: Visual field defects in idiopathic intracranial hypertension. *AM J OPHTHALMOL* 96:654–669, 1983.

n. *Optic Neuropathy, or Optic Neuritis from Systemic Substances*

The INDEX provides a long list of substances which are believed to have caused optic neuropathy or neuritis after systemic absorption. In most instances the diagnosis has been made in human beings, usually on the basis of clinical observations of reduction of vision associated with ophthalmoscopically visible changes in the optic nerve head, particularly hyperemia with variable amounts of edema. Symmetrical involvement of the two eyes is particularly characteristic. For a small proportion of the substances listed, the diagnosis has been supported by histologic evidence. Several of the substances listed have also been observed to produce optic atrophy, which has been interpreted as confirmatory evidence of toxic action on the optic nerves. However, this evidence is not conclusive. The finding of optic atrophy does not establish whether the primary site of toxic action was at the ganglion cell, on the visible portion of the nerve fibers, on the retrobulbar portion of the nerve fibers, or upon their blood supply.

In some cases of toxic optic neuropathy the prime site of action is just behind the globe, so-called "Retrobulbar neuritis", described further in following paragraphs.

Certain substances affect the optic nerves further back, for unknown reasons. The *chiasm* is a peculiarly favored site of action of *chloramphenicol, ethambutol, hexachlorophene,* and *vincristine* in human beings, and of *ethambutol, helichrysum, stypandra imbricata, tellurium,* and *triethyl tin* in animals.

The *lateral geniculate bodies* and *optic tracts* are among the sites of action of *clioquinol* and *hexachlorophene* in human beings, and of *hexanedione* and *tellurium* in animals. (See the INDEX for more information on the individual substances.)

Little is known of the mechanism of action of must substances that cause toxic optic neuropathy. A comparison with substances that are known to cause *peripheral neuropathy* is intriguing, but shows both similarities and dissimilarities.

The following substances have been reported to cause both toxic *optic neuropathy* and *peripheral neuropathy,* but not necessarily in the same animals or patients: *acrylamide, carbon disulfide, chloramphenicol, clioquinol, dinitrobenzene, dinitrochlorobenzene, dinitrotoluene, disulfiram, isoniazid, perhexilene, thallium,* and *vincristine.*

Peripheral neuropathy, but not optic neuropathy, is caused by *tricresyl phosphate.* The degree to which the hexacarbons (*n-hexane* and related compounds), which are well known for their peripheral neurotoxicity, may also affect the visual system needs more investigation.

In clinical diagnosis of toxic optic neuritis, non-toxic causes of optic nerve involvement should be kept in mind. When the unqualified term "optic neuritis" is used, it most often refers to a manifestation of multiple sclerosis.

o. Retrobulbar neuritis, from Systemic Substances

Retrobulbar neuritis is an optic neuritis in which there is selective involvement of the fibers in the optic nerve from the papillomacula bundle, characteristically producing central scotoma. The site of involvement seems mainly to be posterior to the optic nervehead and may produce no ophthalmoscopically visible abnormalities, but in some instances this diagnosis is made when there is visible hyperemia and edema of the nervehead in conjunction with central scotoma.

In the INDEX, under "Retrobulbar neuritis" is a list of substances believed to cause this condition.

In many cases the diagnosis of retrobulbar neuritis has been based on a finding of central scotoma with reduction of visual acuity and disturbance of central color vision, but without localizing clues. Often the disturbance of vision has been reversible and there have been no confirmatory findings to support the diagnosis. However, in some cases the condition has not been completely reversible and later appearance of pallor of the temporal portion of the optic nervehead or partial optic atrophy has been taken as supportive evidence for the diagnosis. In a relatively few instances the diagnosis of retrobulbar neuritis has been confirmed histologically either in human beings or experimental animals.

It is quite possible that further study will show that some of the substances that have been assumed to affect central vision by producing retrobulbar neuritis may instead have their primary site of action in the photosensitive portion of the central retina, as appears to be the case at least for some of the *cardiac glycosides.*

The diagnosis of retrobulbar neuritis has been made clinically only in human beings, mainly because of the reliance on visual field examination in the diagnosis.

p. Optic Nerve Atrophy (Optic Atrophy)

Optic atrophy can result from retinal ganglion cell injury, optic neuritis, and retrobulbar neuritis. It can also result from injury of the optic nerve from prolonged elevation of intracranial pressure accompanied by papilledema, such as has been produced particularly by *ethylene glycol, triethyl tin,* and *lead poisoning* in children. More often optic atrophy is produced by glaucoma, brain tumors, and demyelinating diseases than by intoxications.

Optic atrophy is diagnosed clinically by an abnormally white or pale appearance of the optic nervehead, with decrease in the number of fine blood vessels on the optic disc. Histologically there is disappearance of nerve fibers and disappearance of ganglion cells in the retina. The nerve fibers may be replaced by glial tissue in the optic nervehead. If optic neuritis has preceded optic atrophy, the clinical appearance of the optic nervehead may include indistinctness of the disc margins from glial and fibrous tissue, narrowing of the vessels, with white lines ensheathing the retinal vessels on and close to the disc.

A list of substances that can cause "optic nerve atrophy" is provided in the INDEX.

One of the conditions which, unless thought of, may be mistaken for toxic optic nerve atrophy is "Leber's hereditary optic atrophy", which can present and behave in a manner resembling toxic optic neuropathy in young people. Some investigators have, in fact, hypothesized that Leber's optic atrophy itself may represent a genetic inability to detoxicate *cyamide* normally.

2. Functional Changes in Retina and Visual Pathways from Substances Taken Systemically

a. Electroretinogram Alteration

Significant disturbance of the ERG is evidence that specifically identifiable portions of the retina have been affected other than the ganglion cells and optic nerve fibers. Some substances, such as the *cardiac glycosides* and *trimethadione,* seem to cause this sort of disturbance in a reversible manner without inducing morphologic changes, but a larger number of substances that alter the ERG appear to produce microscopically or even clinically evident damage. Such is the case with the *aminophenoxyalkanes, copper, iodate, iodoacetate, iron,* and *piperidylchlorophenothiazine.*

When a disturbance of the ERG is detected, it does not necessarily mean that the substance under investigation has toxic effects solely on the light-sensitive and contiguous portions of the retina, although it does seem to be good evidence that this is one of its sites of toxic action. Several substances that have caused disturbances of the ERG have been shown to have toxic actions also on other portions of the visual pathways. For instance, *carbon disulfide* and *ethambutol* have been well known to cause retrobulbar or optic neuritis, which in some cases has led to optic atrophy. Also both *methanol* and *quinine* have repeatedly been shown to cause atrophy of the optic nerve fibers and retinal ganglion cells. In *methanol* and *quinine* poisoning, the ERG may be undisturbed at the acute onset of loss of vision, but be affected secondarily at a later stage.

In the case of the *digitalis-related cardiac glycosides,* detection of changes in the ERG has provided additional reason for considering that disturbances of central visual acuity and color perception by these drugs may well be attributable to a toxic functional disturbance within the retina, rather than a manifestation of some sort of retrobulbar neuritis as was often supposed.

Lists of substances that affect the ERG are given in the INDEX under "Electroretinogram altered, by systemic drugs or chemicals", and under "Electroretinogram altered, by intravitreal substances".

The ERG is valuable in identifying specific sites of toxic effects within the retina, and in evaluating concentrations of substances within the vitreous humor which may be disturbing to the retina.

The ERG is additionally valuable when correlated with Electrooculograms (EOG) and Visual evoked (cortical) responses (VER). The EOG reflects the corneo-retinal potential, and provides information particularly concerning the retinal pigment epithelium. The VER can evaluate the quality of transmission from retina to visual cortex when the ERG is normal.

b. *Central Scotoma*

Under this heading in the INDEX is a list of substances that are reported to cause central or cecocentral scotomas in human beings. If this list is compared with the list of substances suspected of causing retrobulbar neuritis, it will be evident that most of the substances listed under *Retrobulbar Neuritis* are also included here. This is explained by the fact that a clinical presumptive diagnosis of retrobulbar neuritis has often been based simply on a finding of bilateral central scotomas and lack of other localizing evidence. Some of the same substances can be found listed among those suspected of producing optic neuritis, which is likely to be the diagnosis when hyperemia and edema of the optic nervehead is seen in association with central scotomas. These generally are presumptive diagnoses which time may show to have been unwarranted.

There is evidence pointing to an intraretinal site of action in the case of the *cardiac glycosides,* and there is obvious disturbance of retinal pigment epithelium in *chloroquine* poisoning when it has severely reduced central vision. The site of action of several other substances is open to question.

c. *Peripheral Visual Field Constriction*

Under this heading in the INDEX is a list of substances that have been reported to cause visual field constriction in human beings when absorbed systemically. There is still little known about why some substances cause constriction of the field and other substances produce central scotomas, as discussed in preceding paragraphs.

No doubt the anatomical sites of action of the toxic substances, whether at the level of retina, optic nerve, or cerebral cortex determines whether central or peripheral vision is affected. In the cases of *quinine* and its relatives and *tryparsamide* the action appears to be on the optic nerves and retinal ganglion cells, whereas *piperidylchlorophenothiazine* and *iodate* affect the outer layers of the retina and pigment epithelium.

It is intriguing that several substances best known for inducing central scotoma or producing retrobulbar neuritis also have been observed to produce constriction of the peripheral visual fields. This includes *chloramphenicol, chlorodinitrobenzene, ethambutol, methanol,* and *pheniprazine.* Apparently these substances may sometimes affect peripheral portions of the visual system as well as the papillomacular bundle, with which they are more commonly associated.

Methylmercury compounds are most notorious for causing narrowing of the visual fields by damaging the cerebral cortex, rather than by any known action on the optic nerves or retina.

Explanations in biochemical terms for these toxic effects and various sites of action have scarcely been speculated upon.

3. Posterior Segment Changes from Substances Injected Intravitreally

a. ERG Alteration from Intravitreal Injection

In the INDEX under this heading is given a list of substances tested in animal eyes, and found to alter the ERG.

b. Retinal Structural Changes from Intravitreal Injection

Substances tested in animal eyes and found to alter retinal structure include the substances referred to above as causing alteration of the ERG and in addition: *amphotericin B, cephalothin, colchicine, colloidal carbon, miconazole, ornithine, phenylhydrazine, streptomycin, trypsin, urea, vancomycin,* and *vincristine.* (The ERG may also be found altered by these substances, if tested.)

c. Vitreous Body Degeneration from Intravitreal Injection

In animal eyes, the vitreous body has been found to undergo degeneration when injected with a list of substances under this heading in the INDEX. Accompanying *uveitis* has been noted particularly with *bacterial endotoxin, bradykinin, FMLP, gentamicin, polyethylene sulfonic acid,* and *urokinase.* In some instances vitreous body degeneration and uveitis have led to retinal detachment.

D. VISUAL EFFECTS OF UNCERTAIN ORIGIN

These are effects of substances absorbed systemically, and include visual hallucinations, photophobia from seeming excessive brightness, flashing or flickering lights, alteration of the flicker fusion threshold, and disturbances of color vision.

Lists of some of the substances that are responsible are provided in the INDEX under "Visual hallucinations", "Photophobia", and "Color vision alteration".

E. INTRAOCULAR PRESSURE DISTURBANCES

Prolonged large elevations of intraocular pressure in human beings are a potential complication of chronic local or systemic administration of *corticosteroids,* and a complication of chemical injury of the eye by *ammonia, calcium hydroxide,* and *formaldehyde.* Glaucoma induced in this way can cause serious loss of vision. (Mechanisms are discussed in Chapter II.)

Furthermore, acute angle-closure glaucoma and chronic open-angle glaucoma can be induced in predisposed eyes by substances that have *anticholinergic* properties and dilate the pupils or paralyze the ciliary muscle. (The mechanisms are discussed in Chapter II under "Anticholinergics".)

In human eyes, subconjunctival injection of *vasodilators,* such as *bamethan, isoxsuprine, tolazoline,* and *triaziquone,* can cause a transient small rise of intraocular pressure, especially in glaucomatous eyes, though systemically administered vasodilators have little or no effect on intraocular pressure.

In rabbit eyes, the intraocular pressure is generally more responsive to topical irritants than is the human eye. The rabbit eye, for instance responds much more than the human eye to *prostaglandins* and the substances that cause their release. Although topical tests and pressure measurements on rabbit eyes are of limited value for predicting the effect of the test substances on intraocular pressure in human beings, this sort of test can be used to give an indirect indication of the irritancy, injuriousness, or pain-producing properties of test substances. Such a test, based on change in intraocular pressure, was developed and evaluated by Ballantyne in 1977.[276] Substances found in this test to give large transient pressure rises in rabbits' eyes included *tear gases, ammonia, sodium dichloroisocyanurate,* and *crystal violet.* Surprisingly, the tear gas *dibenz (b.f):4-oxazepine* caused less rise in intraocular pressure in rabbits than in man.

In rabbits, acid and alkali burns cause a biphasic pressure rise, an immediate phase from shrinkage of the globe, and a more prolonged phase from release of prostaglandins, which can be blocked with indomethacin. (See INDEX for *acids.*)

Fine particulate material introduced into the anterior chamber can obstruct aqueous outflow and raise intraocular pressure without invoking a toxic mechanism. Such substances include *calcium carbonate, cotton, India ink, iron hydroxide, Laminaria digitata,* and *talc.*

In human beings a number of substances topically or systemically can lower the intraocular pressure, but the pressure is very rarely lowered so much as to be of any significant danger to the eye. (Rare exceptions are noted under *Myopia, acute transient;* see INDEX.) When intraocular pressure is reduced by a drug or chemical, the prime interest is whether it may be exploited in treatment of glaucoma. Toxicologic interest is directed at whether such substances have accompanying adverse effects that interfere with therapeutic use. Pressure-lowering substances that have been successful in treatment of glaucoma, with acceptably low adverse side effects include cholinergic miotics, carbonic anhydrase inhibitors, beta-adrenergic blocking agents, epinephrine, and hypertonic osmotic agents. The cardiac glycosides are an example of drugs which can reduce intraocular pressure, but for this purpose would have to be used in such amounts systemically or topically that adverse side effects would be excessive.

More pressure-reducing substances are listed in the INDEX under *Intraocular pressure reduction, by systemic substances.*

F. EYE AND LID MOVEMENT DISTURBANCES

Lists of substances which cause these disturbances are given in the INDEX under the following headings:

Nystagmus, Oculogyric crisis and head-neck syndrome, Extraocular muscle weakness or paralysis, Ptosis of eyelids, Lid retraction

G. EYELASH, EYEBROW, AND ORBITAL DISTURBANCES

Whitening of the eyelashes and eyebrows (poliosis) has been attributed to *amodiaquine, bis-(phenylisopropyl)piperazine, chloroquine, hydroxychloroquine, nitrofurfurylidenamino- guanidine,* and *triparanol.*

Alopecia of eyelids or eyebrows has been attributed to *actinomycin D, thallium, triparanol,* and *vitamin A.*

Exophthalmos has been reported in human beings from *corticosteroids, lithium carbonate,* and *vitamin A,* and in animals from *acetonitrile, aminocaproic acid, mephenytoin, organic cyanides, propyl thiouracil,* and *vitamin A.*

H. TERATOGENESIS

Substances taken during pregnancy which can cause abnormalities of the eyes or other portions of the visual system are listed in the INDEX under *Teratogenesis, ocular, from systemic drugs or chemicals.* In most instances, ocular teratogenesis has been diagnosed in animals, but at least nine substances have been reported to have been responsible for ocular teratogenesis in human beings.

The possibility of *teratogenesis from drugs used to treat eye diseases* is a worry when patients have to be treated during pregnancy. So far there is little positive information to serve as a guide. Antineoplastic drugs fortunately are rarely re- quired. Among drugs used in chronic treatment of glaucoma, such as miotics (pilocarpine, carbachol, echothiophate, demecarium, physostigmine), topical beta- adrenergic blockers (e.g. timolol), epinephrine, and carbonic anhydrase inhibitors (e.g. acetazolamide, methazolamide), none appear so far to have been shown to cause fetal abnormalities, except that a limb abnormality has been reported in small rodents from acetazolamide given during pregnancy. Michael Van Buskirk reported in a personal communication in May 1985 that Fraunfelder's National Registry[312] had so far not received reports of teratogenesis in human beings from the drugs mentioned above used in treatment of glaucoma.

CHAPTER II

ENCYCLOPEDIA OF CHEMICALS, DRUGS, PLANTS, TOXINS, AND VENOMS, AND THEIR EFFECTS ON THE EYES OR VISION; ALSO, DRUGS USED IN TREATING EYE DISEASES, AND THEIR GENERAL SIDE EFFECTS

A-200 Pyrinate is a liquid pediculocide shampoo which has caused acute pain and temporary loss of corneal epithelium in many patients, mostly children, when the shampoo has run down from the scalp into the eyes. The eyes have been contaminated when the hair has been rinsed with water after the material has been applied for treatment of head lice.[a,b] Typically, extensive loss of corneal epithelium has resulted, but the corneal stroma has remained clear, and the eyes healed completely in two days. As late as 1980 similar eye injuries in children were being observed from this medicated shampoo in Australia and the United States.

Tests on rabbits have substantiated the toxic effect on the cornea. Testing of several of the ingredients listed on the label led to a conclusion that the most toxic component probably was a surfactant or detergent in the shampoo.[a]

    a. Reinecke RD, Kinder RSL: Corneal toxicity of the pediculocide A-200 pyrinate. *ARCH OPHTHALMOL* 68:36, 1962.

    b. Walton DS: Personal communication, 1969.

Acacia extract has been used in animal experiments to produce toxic non-necrotizing inflammation of the eye. The preparation of the extract from the flowers of *Acacia baileyana*, and the biomicroscopic and histologic reactions to surface and intracorneal administration in rabbits and guinea pigs have been described in detail.[a]

    a. Aronson SB, Yamamoto EA, et al: Mechanisms of the host response in the eye. *ARCH OPHTHALMOL* 78:384–396, 1967.

Acacia thorn, with the tip broken off and retained in the ciliary body, has caused severe recurrent iridocyclitis in one case. Excision of a piece of ciliary body containing the foreign body relieved the inflammation. Residual secondary glaucoma due to peripheral anterior synechias was subsequently relieved by a filtering operation.[a] (Compare *Aloe barb.*)

    a. Paufique L, Hugonnier R: Recurrent iridocyclitis from an acacia thorn in the ciliary body. *BULL SOC OPHTALMOL FRANCE* 66:547–549, 1966. (French)

Acebutolol, a beta-adrenergic blocking drug, given orally may have caused microscopic punctate lesions of the conjunctiva in the palpebral fissure and abnormal Schirmer test results, but no seriously harmful effects during 18 months of clinical observation.[a]

a. Wagner C, Fillastre JP, et al: Prolonged treatment with acebutolol. *NOUV PRESSE MED* 7:725–730, 1978. (French)

Acetaldehyde vapor irritation of the human eye is detectable at 50 ppm in air and becomes excessive for chronic industrial exposure above 200 ppm. Higher concentration and extended exposure may injure the corneal epithelium, causing persistent lacrimation, photophobia, and foreign body sensation.[a,217] A splash of liquid acetaldehyde can be expected to cause painful but superficial injury of the cornea, with rapid healing; the liquid evaporates so rapidly at body temperature that contact is brief and self-limited.[165]

a. Halbertsma KTA: Injury of the cornea in using acetone. *ZENTRALBL GES OPHTHAL-MOL* 18:48, 1927. (German)
b. Gofmekler VA: Experimental observation of the reflex effect of acetaldehyde upon human organism. *CESK HYG* 12:369–375, 1967.

Acetaminophen (paracetamol), an analgesic and antipyretic, is without known ocular side effects, with the exception that in genetically very special mice it can cause irreversible opacification of the anterior portion of the lens when a large dose is given intraperitoneally.[a,b]

a. Shichi H, Gaasterland DE, et al: Ah locus: Genetic differences in susceptibility to cataracts induced by acetaminophen. *SCIENCE* 200:539–541, 1978.
b. Shichi H, Nebert DW: Drug metabolism in ocular tissues. *MONOGR PHARMACOL PHYSIOLOGY* 5:333–363, 1980.

Acetarsone (acetarsol, Spirocid, Stovarsol) has been used in treatment of syphilis. Acetarsol, similar to other derivatives of *arsanilic acid,* has caused optic neuritis and optic atrophy. The greatest danger is said to have attended intravenous injection.[d] Typically, when the eyes were affected, the visual fields contracted and vision became poor in dim illumination. In one unusual case, retrobulbar neuritis with central scotoma for colors, rather than the typical constriction of the fields, occurred after twenty days of treatment, but returned to normal in six weeks after the medication was stopped.[b] In children under treatment with acetarsol for congenital syphilis, the treatment is said to have commonly led to encephalopathy, poor vision from optic neuritis, optic atrophy, and nystagmus.[194]

Acetylarsan (i.e. acetarsol diethylamine salt) can also produce acute optic neuritis. Formerly many patients were treated with the drug without ocular complications, but, particularly in those having poor renal function and in those given the drug intravenously, in many instances a rapid narrowing of the visual fields and reduction in visual acuity occurred. At the onset no distinctive ophthalmosopic changes were seen, but in some cases the optic nerveheads later became partially or totally atrophic. Prognosis was especially bad in cases of sudden onset of blindness.[a,e,f] In those having slow onset of visual disturbance it was possible sometimes to avoid blindness by stopping the drug promptly.

Dimercaprol administered as an antidote following contraction of visual fields by acetarsol is reported to have resulted in improvement within two months.[c] (See also, *Arsenicals, organic* in INDEX.)

a. Mukherjee BB, Ghose SK: Sudden blindness following injections of diethylamine acetarsol solution. *J INDIAN MED ASSOC* 30:292–293, 1958.
b. Nida: Acute bilateral retrobulbar neuritis in the course of intensive treatment with Stovarsol. *BULL MEM SOC FR OPHTALMOL* 44:557–560, 1931. (French)
c. Oehninger C, Barrios RR, Gomez Haedo CA: Optic neuritis caused by arsenicals. Treatment with BAL. *BR J OPHTHALMOL* 39:422–427, 1955.
d. Sezary A, Barbe A: Study of some cases of arsenical optic neuritis. *BULL SOC MED HOP PARIS*, III, 48:1617–1621, 1932. (French)
e. Shukla BR, Ahufa OP, Paul SD: Arsenical optic atrophy. *ALL-INDIA OPHTHALMOL SOC* 12:15–18, 1964.
f. Stroobants C, Schepens C: Acetylarsan and its adverse effects on the visual apparatus. *ANN OCULIST* (*Paris*) 176:519–537, 1939. (French)
g. Tissot-Daguette M: Visual troubles after injection of acetylarsan. *ARCH OPHTALMOL* (*Paris*) 51:17–32, 1934. (French)

Acetazolamide (Diamox), a carbonic anhydrase inhibitor, has been used since 1954 in treatment of glaucoma, also as a diuretic. Side effects on the eye will be discussed first, then the systemic side effects that are encountered when acetazolamide is used in treatment of glaucoma or as a diuretic, administered orally in either case.

Side effects of acetazolamide on the eye are rare. The principal one is *acute transient myopia*. Although acute myopia occurs in very low incidence, descriptions of one or more cases have been published by numerous authors (Andreani; Arentsen; Back; Boureau; Cirstiansson; Galin; Giessmann; Gohar; Gortz; Halpern; Kroning; Muirhead, and a few others tabularized by Watillon). Except in these rare patients, acetazolamide generally has no effect on refraction (Sbordone). It is mysterious what is different or special about those rare individuals who develop acute myopia, as it is also mysterious in the case of many other drugs that cause a similar reaction in rare individuals. (See the INDEX for *Myopia, acute transient.*)

Patients who have an idiosyncratic myopic reaction to acetazolamide have most characteristically been non-glaucomatous women in the last months of pregnancy, having water retention but no toxemia. Characteristically the patient has developed from 1 to 8 diopters of myopia within four hours to five days after starting to take acetazolamide at the rate of 250 mg per day. Usually there has been a history of taking the same medicine briefly previously without side effects, and the acute myopia has developed when the patient resumed medication after an interval. The myopia is not attributable to spasm of the ciliary muscle, because it has not been relieved by atropine (Andreani). However, careful measurements have shown that systemically administered acetazolamide may slightly but significantly deepen the anterior chamber, at least in glaucomatous patients. In some cases the myopia has developed without measurable change in the depth of the anterior chamber (Galin). An alteration of the hydration of the lens with change in refractive power in the lens could account for the transient myopia. In all cases when the drug has been discontinued the vision has returned to normal within two days.

A small proportion of reported cases of acute myopia from acetazolamide have been more complicated. In one patient the intraocular pressure was found to be very low and a flare was noted in the aqueous humor in both eyes (Cristiansson). In another case, 4.5 diopters of myopia developed in a man in the course of several hours after a standard dose of acetazolamide, and his anterior chambers became very shallow, with elevation of the pressure in both eyes to 40 mm Hg. His pressure returned to normal under treatment with pilocarpine, and four days later the vision was normal, the anterior chambers were of normal depth, and there was no evidence of glaucoma (Arentsen). In another case, myopia developed in association with transient flattening of the anterior chamber, but without elevation of the pressure (Kronning). By contrast a man who had been under treatment with acetazolamide and salt-free diet had such lowering of intraocular pressure that the posterior surface of the cornea became wrinkled, yet the anterior chamber remained deep. In this case, the blood potassium was found to be subnormal, and within a day after the potassium deficit was corrected the condition of the eye improved (Giessmann). Another patient with transitory myopia after acetazolamide was found to have perimacular retinal edema for several days. However, in this case, as in most of the others, the visual acuity could be restored to normal with correcting lenses (Muirhead).

In glaucomatous patients under treatment with miotic eyedrops it is conceivable that acute myopia from acetazolamide may be masked by the accommodation induced by the miotic, and therefore the mechanism might go undetected in such cases. In patients treated with timolol instead of miotics one would not expect such a masking of myopia from acetazolamide, since timolol does not induce accommodation. However, it would be rare for a glaucomatous patient to be advanced to treatment with acetazolamide without having first been advanced to miotic treatment.

The lenses of patients treated with acetazolamide formerly were feared to be in some jeopardy from reduced formation of aqueous humor, the source of metabolic essentials for the lens, but since no increase in frequency of development of cataract has been detected under the influence of acetazolamide, the lens seems to have ceased to be a concern. In rabbits, Bisantis has found mitotic activity of lens epithelium to be reduced for several days after very large doses of acetazolamide, but this effect has been attributed to secondary acidosis, and has been reversible.

Corneal thickness after cataract extraction has been undesirably increased by administration of acetazolamide to patients with central corneal guttae preoperatively, but not in patients with normal corneas (Nielson).

Retinal functions appear unaffected by acetazolamide according to routine clinical testing, but Stanescu has reported an increase in the b-wave of the ERG in 15 volunteers, and Missotten has reported a decrease in the dark component of the standing potential of the human eye. Yonemura also has reported rapid decrease in standing potential of human and monkey eyes after intravenous acetazolamide. This effect may be at least partially related to the action of acetazolamide on the ciliary body, associated with reduction of formation of aqueous humor.

Systemic side effects of acetazolamide range from very common to rare. They include paresthesias, malaise syndrome, gastrointestinal distress, urolithiasis, uric acid retention, blood dyscrasias, teratogenesis in animals, and miscellaneous. Most have been described in greater detail in previous reviews (Epstein; Grant; Watillon), and are updated in less detail here.

Paresthesias, a tingling or feeling of pins and needles in the hands, face, and feet are most common, but generally not so unpleasant or long-lasting as to cause the patient to discontinue treatment.

Malaise syndrome consisting of fatigue, anorexia, loss of weight, depression, and often loss of libido (Wallace), appears to be the most common side effect of acetazolamide (and methazolamide) causing patients to discontinue treatment (Epstein). Acidosis is well recognized to be induced by acetazolamide (Andreani; Arrentsen; Cowan; Gamm; Goodfield; Hill; Maisey; Patton), and patients suffering from the malaise syndrome have been found to be more acidotic than other patients, sometimes associated with excessively high blood levels of the drug (Alm; Epstein). Treating the acidosis with sodium bicarbonate (Epstein), or sodium acetate (Arrigg), and adjusting the drug dosage (Alm; Berson), can help dramatically in relieving this condition.

Patients with renal insufficiency or disease affecting the urinary tract are especially susceptible to excessive blood levels of acetazolamide and serious acidosis (Goodfield; Maisey).

Salicylate-acetazolamide interaction in patients taking both aspirin and acetazolamide, particularly in the presence of renal disease, can develop more serious acidosis than is produced by the same dosage of each drug alone (Anderson; Hill). This interaction-induced acidosis can also be serious in patients with normal kidneys (Cowan).

The role of potassium has also been studied in patients with systemic symptoms, as in the malaise syndrome, because increased urinary excretion of potassium is known to occur in early weeks of acetazolamide treatment, but a new steady state is soon reached with the potassium level still within the normal range, not requiring supplementation. However, patients taking chlorothiazide drugs in addition to actazolamide tend to lose more potassium, and may require potassium supplementation. Management of this aspect should be based on blood chemistry measurements (Berson; Critchlow; Epstein; Grant).

Gastrointestinal distress seems not particularly related to degree of systemic acidosis, but to be from a local irritative action which may be reduced by taking acetazolamide with food, using a slow-release form of medication, or taking an antacid supplement (Epstein).

Urolithiasis, the production of kidney stones, often accompanied by renal colic, has been reported many times in patients taking acetazolamide (Abeshouse; Barraquer; Charron; Constant; Davies; Gill; Glushien; Gordon; Kass; Kondo; MacKenzie; Orchard; Parfitt; Pepys; Persky; Rodriquez-Gonzales; Rubenstein; Shah; Yates-Bell). A controlled statistical study by Kass has shown that the incidence of stones was 11 to 15 times higher than normal during chronic treatment with acetazolamide. A reduction in citrate excretion in the urine under the influence of acetazolamide is an explanation for precipitation of calcium stones (Abeshouse; Constant; Gordon; Shah). However, urinary stones are apparently not often analyzed, and other kinds of stones and other mechanisms may be involved. Instances have been reported of crystalluria apparently involving the drug itself (Glushien; Orchard).

Uric acid retention has led to elevated blood urate and acute gouty arthritis in several patients being treated with acetazolamide (Ayvazian; Ferry; Frascarelli).

Blood dyscrasias occur rarely in patients taking acetazolamide, but probably are the most life-threatening complication. Cases have been reported in the following categories: (1) Thrombocytopenia (Bertino; Fowler; McIlvanie; Reisner), (2) Agranulocytosis (Arora; Englund; Hoffman; Pearson), (3) Agranulocytosis and thrombocytopenia (Underwood), (4) Aplastic anemia (Lubeck; Rentiers; Wisch). Most of these case reports have been reviewed in detail by Grant (1973), with the following tentative conclusion. "Since it appears that most instances of blood dyscrasias from acetazolamide have been of the type that has occurred acutely as a result of an immunologic sensitivity reaction, one could not expect to predict this complication even if blood studies were done week by week for long periods in advance. The cases characterized by slow onset have been so rare in comparison with the large numbers of patients treated with carbonic anhydrase inhibitors that it does not seem warranted to put the great number of patients receiving these drugs routinely through periodic blood testing."

Respiratory difficulties may be increased by acetazolamide in patients with chronic obstructive lung disease. This has been reviewed by Block.

Osteomalacia with demineralization of the skeleton from chronic treatment with acetazolamide has occurred particularly in patients simultaneously taking anticonvulsants (Mallette; Matsuda).

Skin rashes are not uncommon, but seem to have received little attention, probably because they usually go away when acetazolamide is stopped (Spring).

Hair loss from the scalp has been reported by Aminlari, and rare excess growth of hair by Weiss.

Teratogenesis has been reported in small experimental animals, particularly affecting the limbs (Biddle; Layton; Maren; Vickers), but in human beings teratogenesis from acetazolamide has not yet been recognized, nor ruled out.

Abeshouse BS, Applefeld W: Citrate metabolism in urolithiasis. *SINAI HOSP J* 5:73–85, 1956.

Alm A, Berggren L, et al: Monitoring acetazolamide treatment. *ACTA OPHTHALMOL* 60:24–34, 1982.

Aminlari A: Falling scalp hairs. *GLAUCOMA* 6:41–42, 1984.

Anderson CJ, Kaufman PL, Sturn RJ: Toxicity of combined therapy with carbonic anhydrase inhibitors and aspirin. *AM J OPHTHALMOL* 86:516–519, 1978.

Andreani D, Lepri G: Observations on transitory myopia from treatment with acetazolamide. *ANN OTTALMOL CLIN OCUL* 87:713–720, 1961. (Italian)

Arentsen IS: A case of acute myopia with glaucoma from ingestion of Diamox. *ARCH CHILENOS OFTALMOL* 13:82–84, 1956. (Spanish)

Arora YC: Agranulocytosis following acetazolamide therapy. *NEW YORK STATE MED J* 59:1119–1120, 1959.

Arrigg CA, Epstein DL, et al: The influence of supplemental sodium acetate on carbonic anhydrase inhibitor-induced side effects. *ARCH OPHTHALMOL* 99:1969–1972, 1981.

Ayvazian JH, Ayvazia LF: A study of the hyperuricemia induced by hydrochlorothiazide and acetazolamide. *J CLIN INVEST* 40:1961–1966, 1961.

Back M: Transient myopia after use of acetazolamide. *ARCH OPHTHALMOL* 55:546–547, 1956.

Barraquer J, Escribano J: Renal colic in the course of treatment with acetazolamide. *REV CLIN ESP* 64:310–313, 1957. (Spanish)

Berson FG, Epstein DL: Carbonic anhydrase inhibitors: Management of side effects. *PERSPECTIVES IN OPHTHALMOLOGY* 4:91–95, 1980.

Bertino JR, Rodman T, Myerson RM: Thrombocytopenia and renal lesions associated with acetazolamide therapy. *ARCH INT MED* 99:1006–1008, 1957.

Biddle FG: Teratogenesis of acetazolamide in the CBA/J and SWV strains of mice. *TERATOLOGY* 11:31–46, 1975.

Bisantis C, Giraldi JP, Pezzi PP: Morphologic and functional modifications in the lens in the course of induced metabolic acidosis. *BOLL OCULIST* 53:143–151, 1974. (Italian)

Block ER, Rostand RA: Carbonic anhydrase inhibition in glaucoma: hazard or benefit for the chronic lunger. *SURVEY OPHTHALMOL* 23:169–172, 1978.

Boureau M: Acute myopia induced by acetazolamide. *ANN OCULIST* 194:627–630, 1961. (French)

Charron RC, Feldman F: Acetazolamide therapy with renal complications. *CAN J OPHTHALMOL* 9:282–284, 1974.

Cowan RA, Hartnell GG, et al: Metabolic acidosis induced by carbonic anhydrase inhibitors and salicylates in patients with normal renal function. *BR MED J* 289:347–348, 1984.

Critchlow AS, Freeborn SF, Roddie RA: Potassium supplements during treatment of glaucoma with acetazolamide. *BR MED J* 289:21, 1984.

Cristiansson J: Transient myopia after the administration of Diamox. *ACTA OPHTHALMOL* 36:356–357, 1958.

Davies DW: Acetazolamide therapy with renal complications. *BR MED J* 1:214–215, 1959.

Englund DW: Fatal pancytopenia and acetazolamide therapy. *J AM MED ASSOC* 210:2282, 1969.

Epstein DL, Grant WM: Carbonic anhydrase inhibitor side effects. *ARCH OPHTHALMOL* 95:1378–1382, 1977.

Epstein DL, Grant WM: Management of carbonic anhydrase inhibitor side effects. In *SYMPOSIUM ON OCULAR THERAPY*. Edited by I.H. Leopold and R.P. Burns. John Wiley and Sons 11:51–64, 1979.

Ferry AP, Lichtig M: Gouty arthritis as a complication of acetazolamide (Diamox) therapy for glaucoma. *CAN J OPHTHALMOL* 4:145–147, 1969.

Fowler WM: Personal communication quoted by Hoffman.

Frascarelli R, Lucidi E, Cozzali G: The influence of sulfonamide diuretics on the urinary excretion of uric acid and on the uric acid level. *MINERVA MED* 51:1954–1961, 1960. (Italian)

Galin MA, Baras I, Zweifach P: Diamox-induced myopia. *AM J OPHTHALMOL* 54:237–239, 1962.

Gamm E: Origination of side effects of acetazolamide. *GLAUCOMA* 6:60–63, 1984.

Giessmann HG: Acute ocular hypotony. *KLIN MONATSBL AUGENHEILKD* 134:890–892, 1959. (German)

Gill WB, Vermuelen CW: Causation of stones by two co-acting agents, Diamox and operative insult on urinary tract. *J UROL* 88:103, 1962.

Glushien AS, Fisher ER: Renal lesions of sulfonamide type after treatment with acetazolmide. *J AM MED ASSOC* 160:204–206, 1956.

Gohar MA, Tadros MA: Transient myopia after acetazolamide therapy. *BULL OPHTHALMOL SOC EGYPT* 52:367–369, 1959.

Goodfield M, Davis J, Jeffcoate W: Acetazolamide and symptomatic metabolic acidosis in mild renal failure. *BR MED J* 284:422, 1982.

Gordon EE, Sheps SG: Effect of acetazolamide on citrate excretion and formation of renal calculi. *N ENGL J MED* 256:1215, 1957.

Gortz H: On transitory myopia after Diamox. *KLIN MONATSBL AUGENHEILKD* 137:21–25, 1960. (German)

Grant WM: Antiglaucoma drugs: Problems with carbonic anhydrase inhibitors. In: *SYMPOSIUM ON OCULAR THERAPY.* Ed by IH Leopold. St. Louis, CV Mosby 6:19–39, 1973.

Halpern AE, Kulvin MM: Transient myopia during treatment with carbonic anhydrase inhibitors. *AM J OPHTHALMOL* 48:534–435, 1959.

Hill JB: Salicylate intoxication. *N ENGL J MED* 288:1110–1113, 1973.

Hoffman FG, Zimmerman SL, Reese JD: Fatal agranulocytosis associated with acetazolamide. *N ENGL J MED* 262:242, 1960.

Kass MA, Kolker AE, et al: Acetazolamide and urolithiasis. *OPHTHALMOLOGY* 88:261–265, 1981.

Kondo T, Matsuo M, Takahashi Y: Urolithiasis during treatment of carbonic anhydrase inhibitors. *FOLIA OPHTHALMOL JPN* 19:576–584, 1968.

Kristinsson A: Fatal reaction to acetazolamide. *BR J OPHTHALMOL* 51:348–349, 1967.

Kronning E: Transient myopia following the use of acetazolamide. *ACTA OPHTHALMOL* 35:478–484, 1957.

Layton WM Jr: Teratogenic action of acetazolamide in golden hamsters. *TERATOLOGY* 4:95, 1971.

Lubeck MJ: Aplastic anemia following acetazolamide therapy. *AM J OPHTHALMOL* 69:684–685, 1970.

MacKenzie AR: Acetazolamide-induced renal stone. *J UROL* 84:453–455, 1960.

Maisey DN, Brown RD: Acetazolamide and symptomatic metabolic acidosis in mild renal failure. *BR MED J* 283:1527–1528, 1981.

Mallette LE: Anticonvulsants, acetazolamide and osteomalacia. *N ENGL J MED* 293:668, 1975.

Maren TH: Teratology and carbonic anhydrase inhibition. *ARCH OPHTHALMOL* 85:1–2, 1971.

Matsuda I, et al: Renal tubular acidosis and skeletal demineralization in patients on long-term anticonvulsant therapy. *J PEDIATR* 87:202–205, 1975.

Missotten L, Van Tornout I, et al: The effect of beta blocking drugs and carboxyanhydrase inhibitors on the standing potential of the eye. *BULL SOC BELGE OPHTALMOL* 191:65–68, 1980.

Muirhead JF, Scheie HG: Transient myopia after acetazolamide. *ARCH OPHTHALMOL* 63:315–318, 1960.

Orchard RT, Taylor DJE, Parkins RA: Sulphonamide crystalluria with acetazolamide. *BR MED J* 2:646, 1972.

Parfitt AM: Acetazolamide and sodium bicarbonate induced nephrocalcinosis and nephrolithiasis. *ARCH INTERN MED* 124:736–740, 1969.

Parfitt AM: Acetazolamide and renal stone formation. *LANCET* 2:153, 1970.

Patton RD, Berkowitz R, et al: Hypothermia and profound acidosis due to benign prostatic hyperplasia. *J UROL* 105:547–548, 1971.

Pearson JR: Agranulocytosis following Diamox therapy. *J AM MED ASSOC* 157:339–341, 1955.

Pepys MB: Acetazolamide and renal stone formation. *LANCET* 1:837, 1970.

Persky L, Chambers D, Potts A: Calculus formation and ureteral colic following acetazolamide (Diamox) therapy. *J AM MED ASSOC* 161:1625–1626, 1956.

Reisner EH Jr, Morgan MI: Thrombocytopenia following acetazolamide (Diamox) therapy. *J AM MED ASSOC* 160:206–207, 1956.

Rentiers PK, Johnston AC, Bushard N: Severe aplastic anemia as a complication of acetazolamide therapy. *CAN J OPHTHALMOL* 5:337–342, 1970.

Rodriguez-Gonzales A: Renal lithiasis resulting from use of inhibitors of carbonic anhydrase in ophthalmology. *ARCH SOC OFTALMOL HISP-AM* 26:232, 1966. (Spanish)

Rubenstein MA, Bucy JG: Acetazolamide-induced renal calculi. *J UROL* 114:610–612, 1975.

Sbordone G: Ocular refraction and Diamox. *ARCH OTTALMOL* 62:257–260, 1958. (Italian)

Shah A, Constant MA, Becker B: Urinary excretion of citrate in humans following administration of acetazolamide (Diamox). *ARCH OPHTHALMOL* 59:536–540, 1958.

Spring M: Skin eruptions following the use of Diamox. *ANN ALLERGY* 14:41–43, 1956.

Stanescu B, Michels J: The effects of acetazolamide on the human electroretinogram. *INVEST OPHTHALMOL* 14:935–937, 1975.

Tellone CI, Baldwin J, Sofia RD: Teratogenic activity in the mouse after oral administration of acetazolamide. *DRUG CHEM TOXIKOL* 3:83–98, 1980.

Underwood LD: Fatal bone marrow depression after treatment with acetazolamide (Diamox). *J AM MED ASSOC* 161:1477, 1956.

Vickers TH: Acetazolamide dysmelia in rats. *BR J EXP PATHOL* 53:5–21, 1972.

Wallace TR, Fraunfelder FT, et al: Decreased libido — a side effect of carbonic anhydrase inhibitor. *ANN OPHTHALMOL* 11:1563–1566, 1979.

Watillon M, Robe-Vanwijk A: Chapter 10 in Michiels (1972).[359]

Weiss IS: Hirsutism after chronic administration of acetazolamide. *AM J OPHTHALMOL* 78:327–328, 1974.

Wisch N, Fischbein FI, et al: Aplastic anemia resulting from the use of carbonic anhydrase inhibitors. *AM J OPHTHALMOL* 75:130–132, 1973.

Yates-Bell JG: Renal colic and anuria from acetazolamide. *BR MED J* 2:1392–1393, 1958.

Yonemura D: Susceptibility of the standing potential of the eye to acetazolamide and its clinical application. *FOLIA OPHTHALMOL JPN* 29:408–415, 1978.

Acetic acid in its most concentrated form, *glacial acetic acid,* causes devastating injury when applied to the eyes of rabbits,[225] and in human beings it has caused permanent opacification of the cornea.[a, d] In two patients accidental application of acetic acid followed very quickly by irrigation with water resulted in immediate corneal opacification. The corneas cleared sufficiently in a few days to reveal severe iritis and small pupils fixed by posterior synechias. Regeneration of the epithelium took many months, but corneal anesthesia and opacity were permanent.[d]

After a spatter of boiling glacial acetic acid struck one eye, a patient that I know of was more fortunate. After the eye was irrigated with water the cornea appeared slightly hazy but was reported not to stain with fluorescein, and vision was 20/20. Two days later the lids were more swollen, and adjacent to the limbus in the lower nasal quadrant there was edema of the cornea and whitish opacification of the adjacent conjunctiva, with vision reduced to 20/70, but the anterior chamber remained clear. Five days after the injury the patient had photophobia, hyperemia of the conjunctiva, and a few inflammatory cells on the back surface of the cornea at the site of the burn. During the next month the inflammation subsided and vision improved to 20/25. Mild corneal scarring persisted near the limbus at the site of the burn. Treatment had consisted of antibiotic ointment until the photophobia and inflammatory cells in the anterior chamber appeared; then atropine and topical corticosteroids were added.

It is interesting to note that the severity of injury by acetic acid, and also by *acetic anhydride,* which forms acetic acid on reaction with water, may not be so evident immediately following injury as it is a day or two later.

Acetic acid may also be encountered at 4% to 10% concentration in ordinary *vinegar,* and at 80% in *essence of vinegar.* A splash of ordinary vinegar in the eye causes immediate pain and conjunctival hyperemia, sometimes with injury of the corneal epithelium. Cases have been reported in which residual corneal nebula has followed a splash of vinegar, but in some reports it has not been stated clearly whether the essence or the more dilute form was involved.[249] In one case vinegar specified to contain 6% to 10% acetic acid caused considerable inflammation when splashed in a woman's eye, but the eye recovered with only small faint corneal opacity. Another young woman who fainted when vinegar of the same concentration was thrown in her face developed permanent moderate corneal opacification with recurrences of inflammation of the eye.[153]

Tests of diluted acetic acid on animal eyes have given varied results. A 1% solution is reported to have caused considerable inflammation and permanent opacity in rabbits,[153] but a drop of 2% solution applied and washed off within a minute caused no permanent damage.[101] In guinea pigs a 6% to 9% solution was found to cause only transient loss of epithelium.[153] In comparison with other diluted acids on excised cattle cornea, I found diluted acetic acid not to have exceptional ability to penetrate, or to denature the cornea.[79]

Intravitreal injection of 0.5% acetic acid (0.5 ml in human eyes, 0.3 ml in rabbits) has been performed by Mortada in treatment of persistent vitreous hemorrhages after an attempt at aspiration, reporting that the vitreous body became liquified in a week or two, without "bad effects" in human beings, or damage to the retina, choroid, optic disc, or lens in rabbits.[b]

Replacement of the aqueous humor in rabbits by 7% acetic acid caused corneal edema and death of lens epithelial cells in the pupillary area, then hyperplasia of adjacent cells.[e]

The vapor of acetic acid is irritating to the eyes and nose, causing lacrimation and hyperemia.[56] Examination of five workers exposed for seven to twelve years to unusually high concentrations of vapor (0.2 to 0.65 mg/liter of air) showed much conjunctival hyperemia and congestion of the pharynx, but no lesions of the corneas.[c]

a. Kaminisij D: Case of bilateral burning of the eyes with acetic acid. *ZENTRALBL GES OPHTHALMOL* 31:437, 1934. (German)
b. Mortada A: Chemical vitrectomy. *ANN OPHTHALMOL* 14:465–469, 1982.
c. Parmeggiani L, Sassi C: On the dangers for health caused by acetic acid in production of cellulose. *MED LAV* 45:319–323, 1954. (Italian)
d. Shafto CM: Two cases of acetic acid burns of the cornea. *BR J OPHTHALMOL* 34:559–562, 1950.

e. Weinsieder A, Briggs R, et al: Induction of mitosis in ocular tissue by chemotoxic agents. *EXP EYE RES* 20:33–44, 1975.

Acetic anhydride reacts with water to form acetic acid. Both liquid and vapor are irritating and necrotizing to tissues, capable of causing severe damage to the eye. Contamination of the eye by even small amounts of liquid causes immediate burning discomfort, and this characteristically is followed some hours later by increasing severity of reaction, with corneal and conjunctival edema. Interstitial corneal opacity may develop in subsequent days owing to progressive infiltration.[81] In mild cases this can be completely reversible,[81] but has been known to go to permanent opacification.[165] In most instances when the eyes have been promptly irrigated with water following exposure, recovery has been complete in a few days.[165]

The eyes of workers in a factory have been exposed to a mixture of vapors of acetic anhydride and acetic acid as a result of an accident, causing all to have intense sensation of burning of the eyes, photophobia, lacrimation, accompanied by much irritation of the nose and respiratory tract. Loss of corneal epithelium occurred in one or both eyes of twelve of the exposed workers, and they had intense conjunctival inflammation and damage of the mucosa of the nose and pharynx. However, the eyes healed promptly and all recovered completely.[a]

a. Capellini A, Sartorelli E: Episode of combined poisoning by acetic anhydride and acetic acid. *MED LAV* 58:108–112, 1967. (Italian)

Acetone at high vapor concentrations (above 1000 ppm) causes some sensation of burning of the eyes and irritation of the respiratory tract.[372] Experimentally at uncomfortably high concentrations it can cause corneal epithelial and conjunctival injury in animals, but at concentrations which are acceptable to human beings, the vapor is not dangerous to the eye. In only one instance has corneal epithelial injury in human beings been reported in association with exposure to acetone vapor, and in this instance a considerable amount of acetaldehyde was also present and was thought to be responsible.[b]

Prolonged contact of liquid acetone with the human eye has been reported in a single instance to have caused deep damage of the cornea with permanent opacity. In this unusual case the acetone contained considerable cellulose acetate which formed a cast over the surface of the eye, and this cast had to be removed manually.[a] A second patient having the same accident recovered corneal clarity.

Splash of a drop of liquid acetone on the human eye causes immediate stinging sensation, but, especially if it is washed out promptly, it causes injury only to the epithelium, characterized by the presence of microscopic gray dots and foreign-body sensation. Usually healing is complete in a day or two.[81,165]

Several drops squirted on the eyes of anesthetized rabbits and washed away two minutes later with water caused temporary edema and irregularity of the corneal epithelium and grayness of the stroma, but the eyes recovered completely in two to five days.[81] Corneal epithelial alkaline phophatase is found to be activated 7 to 28 days after exposure of rabbit eyes to acetone.[h]

Experiments have been done to determine the feasibility of using acetone on the outer surface of the cornea to remove or remodel cyanoacrylate tissue adhesive of the type used medically to close corneal perforations or attach contact lenses.[g] Rubbing the corneas of rabbits for several minutes with a cotton swab soaked with acetone was found to cause the epithelium to come off. The adhesive also came off. The eyes returned entirely to normal in four to six days. However, further experiments showed that acetone should not be allowed to enter the anterior chamber through any wound or hole in the cornea, because when acetone was injected experimentally into the anterior chamber it caused iritis and clouding and necrosis of the cornea.[g]

Occasionally people have had their lids glued shut with cyanoacrylate cement, and it has been found that acetone applied with a cotton-tipped applicator is effective in releasing the cement.[f] An effort is made not to allow the solvent to run into the conjunctival sac, but, as the above observations show, contact with the cornea itself should cause only transient disturbance of the epithelium, with prompt recovery.[g]

There is no substantial evidence of injury of the optic nerve or of induction of cataract by acetone. In one instance a transitory central scotoma resulted from exposure to vapors composed mostly of methanol plus 5% acetone; the intoxication is more reasonably attributable to the methanol.[e] In another instance a young man who had been spray-painting was found to have mature cataract in one eye and very early lens abnormality in the other eye, and the speculation was offered that acetone might be responsible; however, there was no good evidence to incriminate acetone.[d] In several recorded instances of systemic intoxication no known ocular complications have occurred.[c]

a. Gomer JJ: Corneal opacities from pure acetone. *GRAEFES ARCH OPHTHALMOL* 150:622–644, 1950. (German)
b. Halbertsma KTA: Corneal injury from use of acetone. *ZENTRALBL GES OPHTHALMOL* 18:48, 1927. (German)
c. Harris LC, Jackson RH: Acute acetone poisoning caused by setting fluid for immobilizing casts. *BR MED J* 4792:1024–1026, 1952.
d. Mayou MC: Cataract in an acetone worker. *PROC R SOC MED* 25:475, 1932.
e. Weill MG: Severe ocular disturbance from inhalation of impure acetone. *BULL SOC FRANC OPHTALMOL* 47:412–414, 1934. (French)
f. Mindlin AM: Acetone used as a solvent in accidental tarsorrhaphy. *AM J OPHTHALMOL* 83:136–137, 1977.
g. Turss U, Turss R, Refojo MF: Removal of isobutyl cyanoacrylate adhesive from the cornea with acetone. *AM J OPHTHALMOL* 70:725–728, 1970.
h. Bolkova A, Cejkova J: Changes in alkaline and acid phosphatases of the rabbit cornea following experimental exposure to ethanol and acetone. *GRAEFES ARCH OPHTHALMOL* 220:96–99, 1983.

Acetonitrile (methyl cyanide), tested on rabbit eyes by application of a drop, has caused superficial reversible injury like that caused by acetone; graded 5 on a scale of 1 to 10 after twenty-four hours.[223] Administered by intramuscular injection of 0.05 to 0.1 ml daily to prepubertal rabbits, acetonitrile has caused exophthalmos, appearing between the fourteenth and sixtieth day after the beginning of the injections. The degree of exophthalmos is proportional to the degree of thyroid hyperplasia, and is hastened and increased by thyroidectomy. This exophthalmos can be prevented by administration of iodine, by feeding fresh vegetables instead of alfalfa, hay, or oats, and by removing the superior cervical ganglion.[a]

a. Marine D, Rosen SH, Cipra A: Further studies on the exophthalmos in rabbits, produced by methyl cyanide. *PROC SOC EXP BIOL MED* 30:649–651, 1933.

Acetophenazine maleate (Tindal), an antianxiety agent, has caused blurring of vision with dryness of the mouth in less than 5 percent of patients. The blurring is reversible, and it has been presumed to be due to anticholinergic interference with accommodation.[a-d]

a. Darling HF: Acetophenazine (Tindal) and thiopropazate (Dartal) in ambulatory psychoneurotic patients. *AM J PSYCHIATRY* 118:358–359, 1961.
b. Darling HF: The treatment of ambulatory adolescent schizophrenia with acetophenazine. *AM J PSYCHIATRY* 120:68–69, 1963.
c. Witton K, Hermann HT: Clinical experiences with acetophenazine in the elderly psychotic. *DIS NERV SYST* 24:314–318, 1963.
d. Honigfeld G, Rosenblum M, et al: *J AM GERIATR SOC* 8:57–72, 1965.

Acetophenone (phenyl methyl ketone, Hypnone) is only slightly soluble in water (less than 1%). Tested by application to rabbit eyes, the pure liquid caused rather severe initial reaction, graded 8 on a scale of 1 to 10, an effect said to be similar to that of pure butyl alcohol.[27,222] However, in rabbits in which the eyes were briefly irrigated with water two minutes after application of pure acetophenone, there was no more than transient optical irregularity of the corneal epithelium, with no opacity, and the eyes returned to normal by the next day.[81] Application of two drops of saturated aqueous solution of acetophenone to eyes of rabbits caused discomfort despite prior application of local anesthetic drops. However, these eyes were entirely normal within half an hour, and remained normal indefinitely, although no treatment was applied.[81]

Acetyl bromide and **acetyl chloride** are fuming, volatile liquids, producing vapors which are very irritating to the eyes. The liquids react violently with water and presumably could cause severe ocular damage if splashed on the eye. However, in one instance of corneal burn, recovery is reported to have been complete in forty-eight hours.[165]

Acetylcholine chloride is a parasympathomimetic agent that has been used parenterally as a vasodilator in attempts to relieve occlusion of the retinal arteries and to treat toxic optic neuropathies. Side effects from these uses have been systemic rather than ocular, though lacrimation and miosis may be induced. Acetylcholine has been more widely used for inducing miosis during intraocular surgery. For this purpose a sterile solution is introduced directly into the anterior chamber of the patient's eye, usually in the form of the commercial preparation "Miochol", a 1% solution in a 5% solution of mannitol, put into solution immediately before use. Observations on patients have so far shown no evidences of damage to the corneal endothelium. Similarly, rabbit and cat corneas have shown no injury when evaluated by specular and electron microscopy, and by measurement of swelling.[1,366] In dogs, 1% concentration is tolerated without adverse effect, but 2% and 4% solutions have caused immediate clouding of the aqueous humor, a sign of irritation of the iris,[c,f,j] or of breakdown of the blood-aqueous barrier in the ciliary body.[d] Commercial Miochol is slightly hypertonic compared to aqueous humor, and when introduced into the anterior chamber in patients has occasionally induced acute but transient white clouding of the anterior layers of the lens.[g,i] In rabbits, both Miochol and 1% acetylcholine chloride dissolved in physiologic salt solution have similarly caused acute transient opacity of the lens when placed in the anterior chamber,[i,k] but 1% acetylcholine dissolved in distilled water has not.[k] Accordingly, it was concluded that hypertonicity, rather than drug toxicity, accounted for the clouding of the lens.[k] Paradoxically, the water content of the opacified lenses was reported to have increased slightly.[i]

An entirely different problem was encountered in a small group of patients in whom Miochol was used after it had been inadvertently contaminated by exposure to *ethylene oxide* gas.[h] Rubber-stoppered glass vials of Miochol that were left over unused and unopened from previous operations had their exterior surfaces subjected to resterilization without realization that ethylene oxide would permeate the rubber stoppers and by reaction with the aqueous contents would form products toxic to the eye. (The reaction products are discussed under *Ethylene oxide* — see INDEX.) Severe ocular inflammation resulted, with, in varying degrees, corneal edema and opacity, lens opacities, retinal vascular changes, and optic atrophy. In rabbits the same type of material similarly induced ocular inflammation and corneal edema.[h]

Systemic reactions to 1% acetylcholine chloride placed in the anterior chamber during cataract surgery have been reported in several cases, characterized by systemic hypotension, bradycardia, and sometimes difficulty in breathing.[a,b,e]

a. Babinski M, Smith B, Wickerham EP: Hypotension and bradycardia following intraocular acetylcholine injection. *ARCH OPHTHALMOL* 94:675–676, 1976.

b. Brinkley JR Jr, Henrick A: Vascular hypotension and bradycardia following intraocular injection of acetylcholine during cataract surgery. *AM J OPHTHALMOL* 97:40–42, 1984.

c. Catford GV, Millis E: Clinical experience in the intraocular use of acetylcholine. *BR J OPHTHALMOL* 51:183–187, 1967.

d. Cole DF: Site of breakdown of the blood aqueous barrier under the influence of vasodilator drugs. *EXP EYE RES* 19:591–607, 1974.

e. Gombos GM: Systemic reactions following intraocular acetycholine instillation. *ANN OPHTHALMOL* 14:529–530, 1982.

f. Harley RD, Mishler JE: Acetylcholine in cataract surgery. *BR J OPHTHALMOL* 50:429–433, 1966.

g. Lazar M, Rosen N, Nemet P: Miochol induced transient cataract. *ANN OPHTHALMOL* 9:1142–1143, 1977.

h. Leibowitz HM: Unexpected problems with intraocular acetylcholine. Page 109 in Fraunfelder (1979).[311]

i. Mester U, Stein HJ, Koch HR: Experimental lens opacities in rabbits induced by intraocular application of acetylcholine. *OPHTHALMIC RES* 9:99–105, 1977.

j. Rizzuti AB: Acetylcholine in surgery of the lens, iris and cornea. *AM J OPHTHALMOL* 63:484–487, 1967.

k. Rosen N, Lazar M: The mechanism of the Miochol lens opacity. *AM J OPHTHALMOL* 86:570–571, 1978.

l. Vaughn ED, Hull DS, Green K: Effect of intraocular miotics on corneal endothelium. *ARCH OPHTHALMOL* 96:1897–1901, 1978. Page 109 in Fraunfelder (1979).[311]

Acetylcysteine (Mucomyst) is a derivative of the naturally occurring amino acid L-cysteine, used medically to reduce the viscosity of secretions in the respiratory tract,[4] and as a collagenase inhibitor.

Eyedrops containing 20% acetylcysteine at pH 7 have been applied several times a day for two months to the eyes of patients with keratoconjunctivitis sicca as a potential treatment. The patients noted some stinging, but examination by slit-lamp and by staining with fluorescein and rose bengal showed no adverse effects, and some improvement in amount of filaments and mucous shreds.[a,b] Although adequately tolerated when applied as drops to alkali-burned corneas (as a collagenase inhibitor), a 20% solution was severely damaging when injected into the corneal stroma.[c,e] In rabbits receiving drops, corneal epithelial wound healing was not retarded.[d] Also see *Treatment of Chemical Burns.*

a. Absolon MJ, Brown CA: Acetylcysteine in keratoconjunctivitis sicca. *BR J OPHTHALMOL* 52:310–316, 1968.

b. Messner K, Leibowitz HM: Acetylcysteine treatment of keratitis sicca. *ARCH OPHTHALMOL* 86:357–359, 1971.

c. Obenberger J, Cejkova J: Corneal damage following intracorneal injection of N-acetyl-L-cysteine. *GRAEFES ARCH OPHTHALMOL* 185:171–175, 1972.

d. Petroutsos G, Guimaraer R, et al: Effect of acetylcystein on epithelial would healing. *OPHTHALMIC RES* 14:241–248, 1982.

e. Sugar A, Waltman SR: Corneal toxicity of collagenase inhibitors. *INVEST OPHTHALMOL* 12:779–782, 1973.

Acetyldigitoxin is one of several cardiac glycosides related to digitalis that affect vision, usually reversibly. Acetyldigitoxin has been said to have a particular propensity to cause yellow vision when given in overdosage, more readily than other preparations related to digitalis.[a] In one case, after fourteen days of treatment with acetyldigitoxin everything seemed to be surrounded by a white halo and in the evening everything looked hazy, but after the dosage was reduced, the symptoms slowly disappeared.[b] (See also *Cardiac glycosides.*)

a. Crouch RB, Hejtmancik MR, Herrmann GR: Seeing yellow cautions heart drug overdosage. *SCI NEWS LETTER,* Nov 5, 1955, p. 300.

b. Meyler L (Ed): *Side effects of drugs,* 4th ed, NY EXCERPTA MED FOUNDATION, 1963, p. 88.

Acetylene tetrabromide tested by application to eyes of rabbits is reported to cause pain, but only slight irritation of the conjunctiva and superficial injury of the cornea, much as other chemically inert organic solvents.[a]

a. Hollingsworth RL, Rowe VK, Oyen F: Toxicity of acetylene tetrabromide determined on experimental animals. *AM IND HYG ASSOC J* 24:28–35, 1963.

Acetyl ethyl tetramethyl tetralin (AETT), formerly used as musk fragrance in cosmetics and soaps, can cause blue discoloration of the eyes (sclera), brain and peripheral nerves of rats, with demyelination in both central and peripheral nervous systems when chronically administered.[a] The optic nerves and tracts are relatively faintly discolored, and no disturbance of vision has been noted. Limb weakness and ataxia have been most evident. Human beings have probably not been affected.[378]

a. Spencer PS, Sterman AB, et al: Neurotoxic fragrance produces ceroid and myelin disease. *SCIENCE* 204:633–635, 1979.

Acidic lake water, presumably resulting from "acid rain" from industrial emission of sulfur and nitrogen oxides into the air, has been tested on human and rabbit eyes to determine whether it should be of concern to swimmers. Exposure of eyes of human volunteers for 5 minutes and rabbits for 15 minutes to pH 4.6 or pH 6.3 lake water had no injurious effect discernible by slit-lamp, fluorescein staining, or histology.[a] In rabbits, application of acidic lake water to one eye, and near-neutral lake water to the other eye, 15 minutes a day for 7 days produced no consistent significantly different effects.[b]

a. Basu PK, Avaria M, Hasany SM: Effects of acidic lake water on the eye. *CAN J OPHTHALMOL* 17:74–78, 1982.
b. Basu PK, Avaria M, et al: Ocular effects of water from acidic lakes. *CAN J OPHTHALMOL* 19:134–141, 1984.

Acids have a reputation that they cause less severe damage than alkalies, but this applies mainly to weak or dilute acids, for instance to concentrations of mineral acids of 10% or less in water. Splash contact of concentrated strong acids, such as sulfuric, hydrochloric, nitric, phosphoric, and chromic acids, and liquid sulfur dioxide, can prove as severely and devastatingly injurious to the eye as splashes of strong alkalies. (The characteristic effects of individual acids are described elsewhere under their individual names.) (See INDEX.)

In tests on normal rabbit eyes, acids are found significantly injurious only when the pH is as low as 2.5 or lower. Applied to human eyes, solutions from pH 7 down to pH 2 induce an increasingly strong stinging sensation, but on brief contact cause no damage. For example, dilutions of sulfuric acid applied as a drop to a normal human eye evoked the following responses: 0.0001 M (pH 4.0) felt like distilled water; 0.001 M (pH 3.0) felt only slightly different from distilled water; 0.01 M (pH 2.1) caused moderate immediate smarting and tearing, lasting only 10 to 15 seconds; 0.03 M (pH 1.75) caused immediate strong smarting (like soap), with a slight burning sensation persisting for about an hour, but with no influence on vision and no residual injury evident clinically. However, scanning electron microscopy has shown changes in the surface of the corneal epithelium from contact with acid more dilute than 0.0001 M.[a]

Experiments in which acids have been tested on rabbit eyes after removal of the protective epithelium have shown that certain anions which are known to be protein precipitants may cause appreciable injury to the corneal stroma at pH values above 2.5.[d] For instance, appreciable injury has been produced by irrigating denuded rabbit corneas with *trichloroacetate* solutions up to pH 3, with *metaphosphate* or *sulfosalicylate* solutions up to pH 5.5 or 6, and with *picrate, tungstate,* and *tannate* solutions up to pH 9. Normally, however, the corneal epithelium offers sufficient protection so that injuries would be rarely encountered unless the pH were 2.0 or less. Measurement of the pH of the aqueous humor of rabbit eyes after application of acid has shown a greater change in eyes with abraded corneal epithelium, demonstrating the protective role of the epithelium.[e,f]

In the mildest acid burns of the eye observed clinically after contact with a small amount of dilute acid, the corneal epithelium develops slight turbidity or superficial erosion, and the surface of the conjunctiva becomes slightly dull. Hyperemia, chemosis and small ecchymoses appear in the conjunctiva. With more severe exposure, the epithelium of both cornea and conjunctiva immediately become opaque and white, or in case of burns from nitric or chromic acids may become yellow or brown. The necrotic epithelium comes loose or disintegrates in the next day or two, leaving a clear corneal stroma and hyperemic, somewhat hemorrhagic, chemotic conjunctiva.

In mild burns the epithelium regenerates rapidly and the eye recovers completely. In more severe burns, after the epithelium is sloughed, the corneal stroma may have a grayish ground-glass appearance, yet be clear enough to permit examination of iris and lens. Since only slight turbidity of the corneal stroma may be evident the first day or two, even in cases in which eventually the cornea becomes totally opaque or perforates, it is sometimes difficult at the outset to judge the depth and severity of injury. This is especially true of burns from liquid sulfur dioxide.

Early indications of very severe injury are complete anesthesia of the cornea and pallor and ischemia of surrounding tissues from thrombosis of conjunctival and episcleral blood vessels. Severe iritis also suggests severe injury, and opacification of the lens indicates very deep penetration. In the most severe burns from concentrated acids the severity of damage may be quite obvious from the start. Yet in some severe injuries the axial portions of the corneal stroma may retain considerable clarity for a week or two while cells and blood vessels slowly invade from the periphery. Ultimately the whole cornea may become deeply vascularized and opaque, or in the worst cases the cornea may soften and the whole stroma may slough, leaving nothing but a clear, bulging Descemet's membrane, or the globe may perforate with loss of most of the ocular contents. The acids most likely to cause such devastating injury are the concentrated mineral acids, especially sulfuric acid.

Rates of penetration of whole cornea by acids *in vitro,* according to my own testing of a series of acids at 0.1 M concentration adjusted to pH 1 and pH 2, differ considerably from one acid to another, probably largely related to differences in lipid solubility. For instance, *sulfurous acid* penetrates many times more rapidly than hydrochloric, phosphoric, or sulfuric acids under these conditions.[79] However, at higher concentrations and lower pH there likely would be less difference in the penetrability of the various acids because of destruction of the epithelium.

Comparing the denaturing effect of seventeen different acids by measuring their inhibitory effect on the normal swelling properties of pieces of rabbit cornea in distilled water, I found that 0.1 M solutions of the various acids adjusted to pH 2 had a wide range of different denaturing effectiveness, but the relationship of this action to clinical or histologic evidences of acid injury is not yet clear.[79]

Numerous experimental studies of acid burns of the eye have been reported since 1840.[253] Most have consisted of clinical or histological descriptions of changes produced in animal eyes by application of various acids. It has been established in studies on hydrochloric acid that there is no early loss of metachromatic staining or of hexosamine from the cornea, and in this respect acid burns differ fundamentally from alkali burns, in which there is a rapid loss. A decrease of metachromatic staining and decrease of hexosamine do occur later in acid burns in scarred areas.[d] More recent detailed histologic studies have shown the damage caused by common mineral acids at 10 N concentration to be essentially alike.[k] Concentrated sulfuric acid injury of rabbit cornea has been shown to result in poor adhesion of regenerated epithelium due to altered persistent basement membrane and stromal edema from endothelial damage.[h]

Other recent studies have included demonstration that oxygen uptake by the cornea is reduced after acid injury,[c] and that the number of leucocytes in the aqueous humor in rabbits is proportional to the severity of acid burn.[g] Also, decrease in concentration of lactate, pyruvate, and glucose has been shown in the aqueous humor and cornea of acid burned rabbit eyes, but the levels may subsequently return to normal, even in the presence of corneal ulceration.[j]

The intraocular pressure in rabbit eyes rises rapidly when 2 N hydrochloric acid is applied,[b] and since this can occur postmortem or post-enucleation as well as *in vivo,* it is attributed to immediate shrinkage of the globe.[i] In live rabbits a secondary phase of elevation of intraocular pressure for as long as 3 hours is observed,[b,i] and this has been shown to be caused by prostaglandins released within the eye.[i] It can be prevented by pretreatment with indomethacin.

In treatment of acid burns of the eye, irrigation with water remains first choice. Most important is the speed with which irrigation can be started.

(For more information on specific acids, see the INDEX, particularly for *Hydrochloric acid, Hydrofluoric acid, Sulfur dioxide,* and *Sulfuric acid.*)

a. Brewitt H, Honegger H: Early morphological changes of the corneal epithelium after burning with hydrochloric acid. *OPHTHALMOLOGICA* 178:327–336, 1979.

b. Chiang TS, Moorman LR, Thomas RP: Ocular hypertensive response following acid and alkali burns in rabbits. *INVEST OPHTHALMOL* 10:270–273, 1971.

c. Flynn WJ, Mauger TF, Hill RM: Corneal burns: A quantitative comparison of acid and base. *ACTA OPHTHALMOL* 62:542–548, 1984.

d. Friedenwald JS, Hughes WF, Herrmann H: Acid burns of the eye. *ARCH OPHTHALMOL* 35:98–108, 1946.

e. Graupner OK: Importance of the corneal epithelium to the alteration of the pH in the anterior chamber of the rabbit eye after experimental burning with acid. *GRAEFES ARCH OPHTHALMOL* 181:65–70, 1970. (German)

f. Graupner OK, Kalman EV, LePetit GF: The importance of the buffer properties of cornea and aqueous humor for the protection of the eye from burns. *GRAEFES ARCH OPHTHALMOL* 182:351–356, 1971. (German)

g. Graupner OK, Hausmann CM, Kalman EV: The leucocyte content of the aqueous humor of the rabbit eye after experimental burning with acid or alkali. *GRAEFES ARCH OPHTHALMOL* 184:202–207, 1972. (German)

h. Hirst LW, Fogle JA, et al: Corneal epithelial regeneration and adhesion following acid burns in the rhesus monkey. *INVEST OPHTHALMOL VIS SCI* 23:764–773, 1982.

i. Paterson CA, Eakins KE, et al: The ocular hypertensive response following experimental acid burns in the rabbit eye. *INVEST OPHTHALMOL VIS SCI* 18:67–74, 1979.
j. Turss R, Klenn B: Metabolite changes and ulceration of the cornea. *KLIN MONATSBL AUGENHEILKD* 173:214–220, 1978. (German)
k. Vrabec F, Obenberger J: Ring-shaped acid burns of the rabbit cornea. *GRAEFES ARCH OPHTHALMOL* 201:79–88, 1976.

Aconite and **Aconitine,** formerly used to reduce blood pressure, are violent poisons. Poisoning is said to have produced parasthesias (especially in the face), confusion, headache, blurring of vision, and diplopia.[142] Transient blurring of vision has also been described as accompanied by yellowish-green vision, mydriasis, and cycloplegia.[b] There appears to be no known instance of injury to the optic nerve. Experiments in dogs indicated that mydriasis from aconitine resulted from subnormal oxygen levels in the oculomotor nucleus secondary to ventricular fibrillation and reduced cardiac output.[a]

a. Binnion PF, McFarland RJ: Relationship between cardiac massage and pupil size in cardiac arrest in dogs. *CARDIOVASC RES* 3:247–251, 1968.
b. Fuhner H: Medicinal aconite poisoning. *SAMML VERGIFTUNGSF* 2:1–4, 1931.

Acridine (dibenzopyridine; 10-azaanthracene) is irritating to the skin and mucous membranes, especially to the nose, causing sneezing. Administered systemically to rabbits, acridine has been reported to induce localized edema in the nerve fiber layer of the retina, but the dose, time or consistency of response were not specified, and no related effect has been reported for human beings.[131] The effect on rabbit retina was reported to be much less than that from quinoline.[131]

Acriflavine, a diaminoacridine dye, has had some use as a germicide in treatment of wounds. Dust or particles of acriflavine transferred on the hands to the eyes cause considerable ocular irritation.[258] In rabbits the corneal stroma is injured by acriflavine as by other cationic dyes.[81,123] Injection into the cornea or irrigation of the cornea after removing epithelium causes definite injury at 1:10,000 dilution in water and total opacification and vascularization at 1:200.[123]

Acrolein (2-propenal) is irritating to the skin and mucous membranes. The vapor causes a burning sensation in the eyes at low concentration and is violently irritant and lacrimatory at high concentrations.[218] Acrolein has been employed as a lacrimogenic warning agent in methyl chloride refrigerant, and as a component of military poison gases.[171] In World War I, it was used as a tear gas under the name Papite.[b]

For human beings exposure to 5.5 ppm of acrolein in air is intolerable in the first minute. Exposure to 1 ppm induces lacrimation and becomes intolerable in four to five minutes.[b,d,218]

In relation to smog the recommendation has been made that acrolein should not be allowed to exceed 0.01 ppm in air to prevent sensations of eye irritation.[32]

Champeix and Catilina described skin contact with liquid acrolein as causing irritation, erythema, and edema, and a splash in the eye as causing blepharocon-

junctivitis, lid edema, fibrinous or purulent discharge, and corneal injury, which
they say may be deep and longlasting. They indicate severe damage is possible as
from alkali burns, but do not indicate the source of the information.[b] McLaughlin
reported an injury of the cornea by acrolein to have healed in forty-eight hours, but
did not described the nature of the injury.[165]

Experimental studies in animals have shown that 2 to 8 ppm in air for four hours
or 0.6 ppm in air for four hours daily for thirty days caused in rabbits no clinically
evident damage to the eyes, with no increase in thickness of the cornea, no delay in
regeneration of test wounds of the corneal epithelium, no recognizable histopathology,
and in the corneal epithelium no decrease in activity of a series of enzymes.[114, 172] At
12 ppm in air, acrolein causes severe eye irritation in rats.[c]

a. Albin TB: In Smith CW (Ed): *Acrolein*, NY, John Wiley & Sons, 1962.
b. Champeix J, Catilina P: *Poisonings by acrolein.* Paris, Masson, 1967. (French)
c. Murphy SD, Davis HV, Zaratzian VL: Biochemical effect in rats from irritating air
    contaminants. *TOXICOL APPL PHARMACOL* 6:520–528, 1964.
d. Pattle RE, Collumbine H: Toxicity of some atmospheric pollutants. *BR MED J* 2:913–916,
    1956.

Acrylamide is neurotoxic and can be absorbed through the skin, mucous membranes,
and lungs as well as the gastrointestinal tract. Systemic poisoning by acrylamide
causes peripheral neuropathy and midbrain disturbances, but so far no disturbances
of vision or eyes have been reported among human victims of systemic poisoning.[a-c]
Experimentally, however, Schaumburg and Spencer produced early distal degeneration in the optic tracts of rats in which they had induced peripheral neuropathy with
acrylamide.[g] Also, Merigan et al, from experiments on monkeys, thought that, "the
visual system is an important target of acrylamide poisoning." Their experiments
showed early in poisoning an increase in thresholds for visual acuity and flicker
fusion, with prolonged latency of pattern-evoked cortical potentials.[e] Clinical examinations of eye movements, ocular media, and fundi were normal, and they suspected
that the changes in vision were therefore attributable to changes induced in the
visual pathways. Visual acuity only partially recovered after administration of
acrylamide was discontinued.

Acute testing of solutions of acrylamide on the eyes of rabbits has shown that a
10% aqueous solution causes immediate slight pain and conjunctival irritation, but
no corneal injury, and the eyes are all normal in twenty-four hours. A 40% aqueous
solution allowed to remain in contact for only thirty seconds caused more pain but
no greater injury. When 40% solution was applied and not washed off, superficial
corneal injury resulted, but healed completely within twenty-four hours.[d]

When an aqueous solution containing 3% acrylamide plus a very small concentration of persulfate was injected into the vitreous humor of rabbits' eyes, it polymerized
to a clear gel with physical properties resembling the vitreous, and produced mild
iritis during the first three days after injection, but this quickly subsided. Two out of
ten eyes injected developed opacities in the posterior layers of the lens, and three
eyes developed vitreous opacities, but in the other seven the polyacrylamide remained
clear and appeared well tolerated during three months of observation.[f]

a. Auld RB, Bedwell SF: Peripheral neuropathy with sympathetic overactivity from industrial contact with acrylamide. *CAN MED ASSOC J* 96:652–654, 1967.

b. Garland TO, Patterson MWH: Six cases of acrylamide poisoning. *BR MED J* 2:134–138, 1967.

c. Hopkins AP, Gilliatt RW: Acrylamide poisoning. *BR MED J* 2:417, 1967.

d. McCollister DD, Oyen F, Rowe VK: Toxicology of acrylamide. *TOXICOL APPL PHARMACOL* 6:172–181, 1964.

e. Merigan WH, Barkdoll E, Maurissen JPJ: Acrylamide-induced visual impairment in primates. *TOXICOL APPL PHARMACOL* 62:342–345, 1982.

f. Muller-Jensen K, Kohler H: Trial of vitreous humor substitution by polyacrylamide. *BER DTSCH OPHTHALMOL GESELLSCH* 68:181–184, 1968. (German)

g. Schaumburg HH, Spencer PS: Environmental hydrocarbons produce degeneration in cat hypothalamus and optic tract. *SCIENCE* 199:199, 1978.

Acrylic acid is a corrosive liquid with an acrid odor, but it is not a lacrimator, despite the fact pointed out by Dixon that some esters of acrylic acid are lacrimators.[42] It has been supposed that lacrimogenic stimulation of corneal nerves depends on a specific reaction with sulfhydryl groups in the cornea, and that the double bond between carbons in acrylic acid is less activated for this specific reaction by a simple carboxyl group than by carboxylic ester groups.[42] (See also *Ethyl acrylate* and *Methyl acrylate*. Other esters are listed in the INDEX as *Acrylic acid, . . . ester.*)

Concentrated "glacial" acrylic acid tested by application to rabbit eyes with special attention to degree of corneal damage caused injury graded 9 on a scale with the maximum of 10.[228]

Acrylonitrile (vinyl cyanide) is a very poisonous volatile liquid. Its vapor at concentrations which are dangerous to inhale causes irritation of the nose and eyes. The liquid is strongly irritating to human skin, but when applied as a single drop to a rabbit cornea, it has caused only a transient disturbance without corneal opacification.[a]

a. McOmie WA: Comparative toxicity of methacrylonitrile and acrylonitrile. *J IND HYG* 31:113–115, 1949.

Actaea rubra (red baneberry) is one of several plants said to contain *protoanemonin*, which is a contact irritant to the eyes and skin, and severely irritant to the gastrointestinal tract. An experimental ingestion of the berries reported in 1903 has been quoted as having resulted in a display of visual hallucinations consisting of blue-colored objects and dancing sparks in addition to the gastrointestinal effects.[43]

Actinomycin D (meractinomycin; dactinomycin), an antineoplastic, is administered intravenously and may cause toxic effects on the skin with temporary loss of scalp hair and eyebrows.[4]

In rabbits, injection of actinomycin either into the lens or into the vitreous body has caused a severe intraocular reaction of both anterior and posterior segments, with opacification of the lens and the cornea.[b]

In bullfrogs, intraperitoneal injection of actinomycin D interferes with healing of experimental wounds in the epithelium of the lens. It is believed that actinomycin D blocks the normal process of healing by suppressing RNA and DNA manufacture in the epithelial cells, inhibiting their mitosis and migration.[a]

In cats, injection into the anterior chamber has caused acute fibrinous iritis, corneal edema and bullous keratopathy, with necrosis of the lens epithelium in the pupillary area.[c,d] In subsequent weeks the central lens epithelium could regenerate, associated with transient increased cellularity of the germinative zone.

In goldfish, intraocular injection reduced incorporation of precursors into RNA in the retina and optic tectum.[e]

a. Rothstein H, Fortin J, Bagchi M: Influence of actinomycin D upon repair of lenticular injuries. *EXP EYE RES* 6:292–296, 1967.
b. Zeller EA, Schoch D, Andujar E: On the enzymology of the refractory media of the eye. *AM J OPHTHALMOL* 61:1364–1371, 1966.
c. Betrix AF: Tolerence to antimitotics introduced into the anterior chamber of the cat eye. *OPHTHALMOLOGICA* 170:199–200, 1975.
d. Betrix AF: Tolerance to antimitotics introduced into the anterior chamber of the cat eye. *GRAEFES ARCH OPHTHALMOL* 189:265–279, 281–296, 1974.
e. Ingoglia NA, Grafstein B, McEwen BS: Effect of actinomycin D on labeled material in the retina and optic tectum of goldfish after intraocular injection of tritiated RNA precursors. *J NEUROCHEM* 23:681–687, 1974.

Acyclovir, an antiviral, has been tested as a 3% ophthalmic ointment, and clinically has evidenced low toxicity, with only occasional stinging.[a] In rabbits, it has not interfered with healing of corneal wounds.[b] Injected into the vitreous body it is toxic to the retina, but a dose of 80 mcg/0.1 ml is tolerable.[c]

a. Collum LMT, Benedict-Smith A, Hillary IB: Randomized double-blind trial of acyclovir and idoxuridine in dendritic corneal ulceration. *BR J OPHTHALMOL* 64:766–769, 1980.
b. Lass JH, Pavan-Langston D, Park NH: Acyclovir and corneal wound healing. *AM J OPHTHALMOL* 88:102–108, 1979.
c. Pulido JS, Palacio M, et al: Toxicity of intravitreal antiviral drugs. *OPHTHAL SURG* 15:666–669, 1984.

Agrostemma seed (corn cockle seed, Agrostemma githago) contains a saponin known as *agrostemmin* or *githagin,* which has been demonstrated to be hemolytic and irritating to the cornea and conjunctiva. Agrostemma seeds have been placed in the conjunctival sac by patients with the intention of inducing keratoconjunctivitis.[a] To be effective for this purpose, the outer hull of the seeds must be removed or cut. (See also *Saponins.*)

a. Roberg M: Conjunctivitis from corn cockle seeds. *KLIN MONATSBL AUGENHEILKD* 116:425–426, 1950. (German)

Air may be left as a bubble inside the eye after intraocular surgery. How well this air is tolerated in contact with the cornea compared with artificial irrigating solutions has been examined experimentally in animal and human eyes. Conclusions have varied depending upon the species tested, and upon whether corneal swelling or a count of corneal endothelial cells has been the basis for comparison. In patients who have undergone cataract extraction a significantly greater loss of corneal endothelial cells has been reported when air was left in the anterior chamber instead of "balanced saline solution",[a] yet measurements of the thickness of the corneas after operation showed less unwanted temporary increase in thickness.[d] Air in eyes of cats has caused a decrease in the number of endothelial cells,[e] and damage has been seen microscopically in the corneal endothelium of rabbits eyes,[a, e] yet air has been shown to interfere less with the corneal deturgescence mechanism than artificial solutions in rabbit and pig eyes, as in human eyes.[a, b]

Hyperbaric air has been tested in animal experiments as a conceivable means of retarding corneal vascularization after chemical burns, but has been disappointing.[c]

a. Eiferman RA, Wilkins EL: The effect of air on human corneal endothelium. *AM J OPHTHALMOL* 92:328–331, 1981.
b. Harris RE, Hassard DTR: Corneal effects of intraocular air. *CAN J OPHTHALMOL* 13:262–264, 1978.
c. Kaiser RJ, Klopp DW: Hyperbaric air and corneal vascularization. *ANN OPHTHALMOL* 5:44–47, 1973.
d. Norn MS: Corneal thickness after cataract extraction with air in the anterior chamber. *ACTA OPHTHALMOL* 53:747–750, 1975.
e. Olson RJ: Air and the corneal endothelium. *ARCH OPHTHALMOL* 98:1283–1284, 1980.

Alcohol (ethanol, ethyl alcohol) has a variety of effects on the eyes and on vision, to be outlined under the following headings: (1) Direct contact of alcohol with the eye; (2) Alcohol vapor exposure; (3) Alcohol injections into the orbit; (4) Acute alcohol intoxication; (5) Chronic alcoholism; (6) Fetal alcohol syndrome.

(1) Direct contact of alcohol with the eye, such as by a splash on a human eye, causes immediate burning and stinging discomfort with reflex closure of the lids. This acute pain quickly passes, but a foreign-body type of discomfort may be experienced for a day or two, then complete recovery.[34,165,225,249] A drop full-strength on rabbit eyes causes reversible injury graded only 3 on a scale of 10 after 24 hours.[27,222] Application of 70% alcohol to rabbit corneas injures and temporarily loosens the corneal epithelium, but recovery is complete (Hood[330]; MacRae[350]). Splashes of whiskey, brandy, gin, or vodka containing 40 to 50% alcohol on human eyes also cause immediate smarting, but injury is superficial and discomfort and hyperemia are transitory. On rabbits, 50% causes a mild reaction graded 20 on a scale of 100.[123]

Under anesthesia, more prolonged contact is possible. Irrigation of the surface of the eye with 3 to 10% alcohol for several minutes has not been reported to cause injury. In a study of treatment of dye stains of the cornea with alcohol it has been reported that 50 to 100% alcohol could be held in contact with the cornea for at least a minute without causing permanent opacity (Comberg 1928; Sedan 1940). However, repeated applications (7 drops) of 40 to 80% alcohol to rabbit eyes over an unspecified but presumably longer time caused loss of corneal epithelium and endothelium, followed by hemorrhages in the conjunctiva, and infiltration and vascularization of the corneal stroma (Meyerratken 1954).

Replacement of the aqueous humor in rabbits by 50 to 70% alcohol has caused corneal edema and death of lens epithelial cells in the pupillary area (Weinsieder 1975).

It has been determined experimentally that the concentration of alcohol in corneas from severely intoxicated postmortem donors is not high enough to present a significant hazard to eyes receiving corneal transplants (Basu 1983).

Shaving lotions, colognes, and perfumes commonly contain 50 to 90% alcohol, and usually the effect of a splash is the effect of the alcohol, but rarely a more severe reaction with slow recovery may occur, suggesting that some other unidentified component may be responsible.

(2) Alcohol vapor exposure at sufficiently high concentration may cause prompt stinging and watering of the eyes, but there appear to be no reports of eye injury from industrial exposure to alcohol vapors. Human volunteers exposed to alcohol vapor have observed at concentration of 0.7 to 1% vapor in air the smell of alcohol was at first almost unbearable, although less unpleasant later, and that the eyes began to burn with increasing intensity after several minutes (Loewy 1918). This discomfort continued for the remainder of the exposure, which lasted for more than an hour, but no subsequent disturbance of the eyes was noted. A vapor concentration of 0.25% had no notable effect on the eyes.

(3) Alcohol injections into the orbit have been used for many years for long-lasting relief of severe ocular or neuralgic pain. Mostly retrobulbar injections have been used as an alternative to enucleation of blind painful eyes, but with proper technique they can be used without excessive danger with seeing eyes (Michels 1973). A comprehensive review has been provided by Lebrun, with analysis of results in 133 blind patients (Lebrun 1971). In another series of 75 patients, the principal complications were temporary blepharoptosis or external ophthalmoplegia (Olurin 1978). An injection to block an infraorbital nerve in treatment of tic douloureux in one case was accompanied by sudden loss of vision on that side, maybe due to accidental embolization (Markham 1973).

(4) Acute alcohol intoxication and its effects on vision and eye movements have been studied in people who have overdosed themselves with alcoholic beverages and in volunteers who have been given alcohol under scientifically controlled experimental conditions. Many years ago, before clear distinctions between ethanol and methanol when writing about "alcohol," very likely there were cases of blindness attributed to ethanol that were actually caused by methanol. (See INDEX for *Methanol.*) Proven acute reduction of visual acuity by ethanol has been rare, but five cases were accepted by Walsh as authentic examples of temporary blindness from ethanol, without possibility of confusion with methanol. In one of these cases the pupils were widely dilated and unreactive to light, but in the other cases the pupils were normally reactive to light and convergence. The fundi were normal in all. In each case the vision returned within a few days.[255] Another instance of temporary blindness has been reported by Sorensen (1977) associated with lactic acidosis in a diabetic patient from a combination of ethanol and phenformin. Some years ago,

acute administration of alcohol was said not to affect visual acuity, visual fields, or color vision (Colson 1940; King 1943; Powell 1938; Verriest 1965). However, more recent evidence indicates change in color vision which may be transient (Russell 1980); more attention has been given to the effect of chronic alcoholism on color vision. Also, it has been reported that acutely administered alcohol can affect the rate of recovery from exposure to bright or dazzling light (Adams 1978; Sekuler 1977; Tiburtius 1966).

Acute alcohol administration has been shown to modify the ERG in rabbits, monkeys, and human beings (Bernhard 1973; Jacobson 1969; Knave 1974; Levett 1980; Manfredini 1968; Skoog 1975; VanNorren 1977[387]). Effect on the c-wave analogous to effect on the standing potential of the eye has suggested an influence on the retinal pigment epithelial cells (Knave 1974; Skoog 1975). Alcohol appears to retard dark adaptation of retinal cone cells (VanNorren 1977[387]). Visually evoked cortical responses have been reported by some investigators to be slowed by acutely administered alcohol (Erwin 1981; Muller 1967), but not by other investigators (Jensen 1984). The influence on critical fusion frequency has also been examined (Granger 1968).

In relation to automobile driving and performance of demanding manual tasks there has been considerable interest in the influence of acutely administered alcohol on the function of the eyes. Gramberg-Danielsen (1965) concluded that no significant effects on the sensory aspects of vision were involved, but that vision and performance could be affected by nystagmus, poorly controlled eye movements and diplopia. Many studies have now been carried out on the effects on eye movements. Nystagmus has been studied by Aschan (1958), Howells (1956), Murphree (1966), Philipszoon (1968)[197], and others. In normal adult human beings it is reported that a minimum of 50 ml of alcohol is required to induce nystagmus (Howells 1956). The nystagmus is accentuated by changing direction of gaze and changing position of the head (Aschan 1958). Disturbance of the vestibular system and nystagmus may persist after blood alcohol levels have dropped. Murphree (1966) has reported that alcohol nystagmus may be aggravated by other substances present in bourbon and vodka.

Acute alcohol effects on binocular vision, stereopsis, convergence, and phorias have been examined by Hogan (1983), Modugno (1967), and Wilson (1983), showing the possibility of causing esophoria, temporary convergent strabismus, and diplopia. Abnormalities that would impair performance of many tasks that involve vision have been reported with a blood alcohol concentration of 0.05% (Wilson 1983).

Acute effects of alcohol on following or pursuit movements of the eye seem to have received the greatest attention (Baloh 1979; Bittencourt 1981; Flom 1976; Jantti 1983; Levett 1980; Stern 1976; Wilkinson 1974). Conclusions expressed by Wilkinson (1974), which seem to be representative, are that eye movements are profoundly affected by alcohol, saccadic movements are slowed within 30 to 60 minutes of ingestion of alcohol, smooth following movements are impaired and replaced by inefficient and jerky movements, thereby reducing visual acuity through temporary loss of macular fixation. However, doll's-head eye movements may remain normal. Derangement of saccadic and smooth pursuit movements appears to be attributable to disturbance of cerebral function, whereas doll's-head movement depends on mid-brain or brain stem function.

Reduction of intraocular pressure as a result of acute administration of alcohol is the subject of numerous publications, but since it may be considered a pharmacologic, or even a therapeutic effect in glaucoma[85, 191], rather than a harmful or toxic effect, it will not be further considered here. The amount of reduction of intraocular pressure caused by alcohol is not harmful to the eye.

(5) Chronic alcoholism is well known to cause "toxic amblyopia" in some patients. This amblyopia has commonly been associated with peripheral neuritis. Characteristically, onset of clouding of vision is bilateral, coming on gradually with a papillomacula scotoma in the form of a horizontal oval, at first best detectable with red and green test objects. The peripheral field usually remains normal. Temporal pallor of the nervehead may be observed, but there are no other characteristic abnormalities of the fundi (Uhthoff 1931[247]; Walsh 1957[255]).

Histologically a circumscribed interstitial inflammatory process has been observed in the optic nerve, causing degenerative changes in the papillomacula bundle of nerve fibers in both central and peripheral directions, ultimately affecting the associated ganglion cells of the retina.

Extensive clinical studies by Carroll and others have shown that correction of deficiencies of B vitamins if initiated early enough can cause complete recovery of vision and relief of peripheral neuritis, even though the intake of alcohol and tobacco is not altered (Carroll 1938, 1943; Quatermass 1958; Victor 1960; Walsh 1957[255]).

Alcohol amblyopia has been reviewed and discussed by Dunphy (1969) from a historical viewpoint, with special interest in the controversies that have existed concerning the relationship of alcohol amblyopia to tobacco amblyopia. Some authors distinguish these conditions; others refer to "tobacco-alcohol amblyopia," or to "alcohol-tobacco amblyopia," expressing the thought that most affected individuals usually both drink and smoke. (See INDEX for *Tobacco smoking* for discussion of tobacco as an independent cause of amblyopia.)

The belief that alcohol amblyopia is mainly a vitamin deficiency condition is supported not only by the favorable effect of B-vitamins, but by observations that the condition has become rare in countries where foods, particularly bread, have been enriched with added vitamins. An interest in the possible role of zinc in several other types of amblyopia has led Bechetoille and colleagues (1983, 1983) to investigate zinc in the retrobulbar neuropathy (tobacco-alcohol amblyopia) of chronic alcoholics, revealing in 52 patients subnormal amounts of zinc in their plasma and red blood cells. Administration of zinc sulfate by mouth to 8 such patients for a month had questionable effect in a comparison with control patients not given zinc. Van Lith and Henke (1979) have expressed the opinion that vitamin deficiency is a major factor affecting the optic nerve fibers, but that there are also toxic effects on the retina itself.

Disturbance of color vision in chronic alcoholism earlier reported by Fialkow and others (1966) has been substantiated by Francq (1979), Sakuma (1973), and Swinson (1972), sometimes with undisturbed visual acuity, and tending to disappear after abstinence from alcohol. Disturbance of both photopic and scotopic electroretinographic values have been studied in old chronic alcoholics with or without amblyopia or alcoholic cirrhosis (Mirgain 1983).

A new clinical finding in "tobacco-alcohol amblyopia" has been reported by Frisen (1983) in the form of a transient dilation and tortuosity of vessels in the arcuate nerve fiber area in 8 patients. Frisen has proposed that these vessel changes are specific indicators of an early phase of the disease.

Eye movements seem to have been of much less interest in chronic alcoholism than in acute alcoholic intoxication, but Costin and colleagues (1980) have reported 4 rare cases of chronic alcoholic patients who developed oscillopsia (illusory movement of the environment) with downbeat nystagmus, associated with ataxia of gait and cerebellar atrophy.

(6) Fetal alcohol syndrome is the name given to a collection of characteristic malformations that have been found in the infants and children of mothers who drank alcohol during pregnancy. Series of cases of eye abnormalities have been reported by Altman (1976), Fried (1976), Jones (1973), and Miller (1981). The subject has been well reviewed by Miller (1981). Most common has been horizontal shortness of the palpebral fissure due principally to an abnormally large distance between the medial canthi. Also common are ptosis and strabismus, either convergent or divergent. High myopia, amblyopia, and pale optic discs have also been reported. These ocular abnormalities typically have been associated with facial anomalies, subnormal weight, delayed growth, and mental retardation.

Adams AJ, Brown B, et al: Marijuana, alcohol, and combined drug effects on the time course of glare recovery. *PSYCHOPHARMACOLOGY* 56:81–86, 1978.

Altman B: Fetal alcohol syndrome. *J PEDIATR OPHTHALMOL* 13:255–258, 1976.

Aschan G: Different types of alcoholic nystagmus. *ACTA OTOLARYNGOL* (Suppl. 140):69, 1958.

Baloh RW, Sharma S, et al: Effect of alcohol and marijuana on eye movements. *AVIAT SPACE ENVIRON MED* 50:18–23, 1979.

Basu PK, Avaria M, et al: Ethanol concentrations in the eye. *CAN J OPHTHALMOL* 18:206–207, 1983.

Bechetoille A, Allain P, et al: Alterations of blood concentrations of zinc, lead, and the activity of ALA-dehydratase in the course of alcohol-tobacco optic neuropathies. *J FR OPHTALMOL* 6:231–235, 1983. (French)

Bechetoille A, Ebran JM, et al: Therapeutic effect of zinc sulfate on the central scotoma of alcohol-tobacco optic neuropathies. *J FR OPHTALMOL* 6:237–242, 1983. (French)

Bernhard CG, Knaol B, Persson HE: Differential effects of ethyl alcohol on retinal functions. *ACTA PHYSIOL SCAND* 88:373–381, 1973.

Bittencourt P, Wade P, et al: Blood alcohol and eye movement. *LANCET* 2:981, 1980.

Brecher GA, Hartman AP, Leonard DD: Effect of alcohol in binocular vision. *AM J OPHTHALMOL* 39:44–51, 1955.

Carroll FD, Goodhart R: Acute alcoholic amaurosis. *ARCH OPHTHALMOL* 20:797–803, 1938.

Carroll FD: The etiology and treatment of tobacco-alcohol amblyopia. *TRANS AM OPHTHALMOL SOC* 41:385–431, 1943.

Colson ZW: The effect of alcohol on vision. *J AM MED ASSOC* 115:1525–1527, 1940.

Comberg: Demonstration concerning the question of acid-alcohol effect in dye burns of the eye. *KLIN MONATSBL AUGENHEILKD* 80:685–686, 1928. (German)

Costin JA, Smith JL, et al: Alcohol downbeat nystagmus. *ANN OPHTHALMOL* 12:1127–1131, 1980.

Dunphy E: Alcohol and tobacco amblyopia. *AM J OPHTHALMOL* 68:569–578, 1969.

Erwin CW, Linnoila M: Effect of ethyl alcohol on visual evoked potentials. *ALCOHOL CLIN EXP RES* 5:49–55, 1981.

Fialkow PJ, Thuline HC, Fenster L: Lack of association between cirrhosis and the common types of color blindness. *N ENGL J MED* 275:584–587, 1966.

Flam MC, Brown B, et al: Alcohol and marijuana effects on ocular tracking. *AM J OPTOM PHYSIOL OPT* 53:764–773, 1976.

Francq P, Pierart P, Verriest G: Results of color vision testing in alcoholics and in the mentally ill. *BULL SOC BELGE OPHTALMOL* 186:73–86, 1979. (French)

Fried RI, Ravin JG: Fetal alcohol syndrome. *J PEDIATR OPHTHALMOL* 15:394–395, 1978.

Frisen L: Fundus changes in acute malnutritional optic neuropathy. *ARCH OPHTHALMOL* 101:577–579, 1983.

Gramberg-Danielsen B: Ophthalmological findings after the use of alcohol. *ZBL VERKEHRSMED* 11:129–134, 1965.

Granger GW, Hisako Ikeda: Drugs and visual thresholds. In Herxheimer, A. (Ed.): *DRUGS AND SENSORY FUNCTIONS.* Boston, Little, 1968, pp. 229–244.

Hogan RE, Linfield PB: The effects of moderate doses of ethanol on heterophoria and other aspects of binocular vision. *OPHTHALMIC PHYSIOL OPT* 3:21–31, 1983.

Howells DE: Nystagmus as a physical sign in alcoholic intoxication. *BR MED J* 1:1405–1406, 1956.

Jacobson JH, Hirose T, Stokes PE: Changes in human ERG induced by intravenous alcohol. *OPHTHALMOLOGICA ADDIT AD* 158:669–677, 1969.

Jantti V, Lang AH, et al: Acute effects of intravenously given alcohol on saccadic eye movements and subjective evaluations of intoxication. *PSYCHOPHARMACOLOGY* 79:251–255, 1983.

Jensen OL, Krogh E: Visual evoked responses and alcohol intoxication. *ACTA OPHTHALMOL* 62:651–657, 1984.

Jones KI, Smith DW: Recognition of the fetal alcohol syndrome in early infancy. *LANCET* 2:999–1001, 1973.

King AR: Tunnel vision. *QUART J STUD ALCOHOL* 4:362–367, 1943–1944.

Knave B, Persson HE, Nilsson SE: A comparative study on the effects of barbiturates and ethyl alcohol on retinal functions. *ACTA OPHTHALMOL* 52:254–259, 1974.

Lebrun G: Thirty four years of retrobulbar alcohol injections. *BULL SOC BELGE OPHTALMOL* 158:475–501, 1971.

Levett J, Jaeger R: Effects of alcohol on retinal potentials, eye movements, accommodation, and the pupillary light reflex. Pages 87–100 in Merigan and Weiss.[358]

Loewy A, Heide Rvd: On respiratory absorption of ethyl alcohol. *BIOCHEM Z* 86:125–175, 1918. (German)

Manfredini V, Trimarchi F: The influence of ethyl alcohol on the electroretinogram. *ANN OTTALMOL* 94:155–160, 1968. (Italian)

Markham JW: Sudden loss of vision following alcohol block of the infraorbital nerve. *J NEUROSURG* 38:655–657, 1973.

Meyerratken E: Experimental investigations of alcohol injury of the cornea. *KLIN MONATSBL AUGENHEILKD* 125:21–30, 1954. (German)

Michels RG, Maumenee AE: Retrobulbar alcohol injection in seeing eyes. *TRANS AM ACAD OPHTHALMOL OTOL* 77:164–167, 1973.

Miller M, Israel J, Cuttone J: Fetal alcohol syndrome. *J PEDIATR OPHTHALMOL* 18:6–15, 1981.

Mirgain C, Malbrel C, et al: Electroretinogram and alcoholism. *BULL SOC OPTALMOL FRANCE* 83:1425–1435, 1983. (French)

Modugno GC, Moschini GB: Variations in stereoscopic perception in relation to ingestion of alcohol. *BOLL OCULIST* 46:377–383, 1967. (Italian)

Muller W, Haase E: The behavior of cortical response under the influence of alcohol. *GRAEFES ARCH OPHTHALMOL* 173:108–113, 1967. (German)

Murphree HB, Price LM, Greenberg LA: Effect of congeners in alcoholic beverages on the incidence of nystagmus. *QUART J STUD ALCOHOL* 27:201–213, 1966.

Olurin O, Osuntokun O: Complications of retrobulbar alcohol injections. *ANN OPHTHALMOL* 10:474–476, 1978.

Powell WH, Jr: Ocular manifestations of alcohol and a consideration of individual variations in 7 cases studied. *J AVIAT MED* 9:97–103, 1938.

Quatermass M: Amblyopia due to ethyl alcohol. *BR J OPHTHALMOL* 42:628–631, 1958.

Russell RM, Carney EA, et al: Acute ethanol administration causes transient impairment of blue-yellow color vision. *ALCOHOL CLIN EXP RES* 4:396–399, 1980.

Sakuma Y: Studies on color vision anomalies in subjects with alcoholism. *ANN OPHTHALMOL* 5:1277–1292, 1973.

Sedan J: On alcohol treatment of corneal injuries from colored pencils. *ANN OCULIST (Paris)* 177:65–77, 1940. (French)

Sekuler R, MacArthur RD: Alcohol retards viscual recovery from glare by hampering target aquisition. *NATURE* 270:428–429, 1977.

Skoog KO, Textorius O, Nilsson SEG: Effects of ethyl alcohol on the directly recorded standing potential of the human eye. *ACTA OPHTHALMOL* 53:710–720, 1975.

Sorensen PN: Transitory blindness during ethanol and phenethylbiguanide induced lactic acidosis in a subject with diabetes. *ACTA OPHTHALMOL* 55:177–182, 1977.

Stern J, Beideman L, Chen SC: Effect of alcohol on visual search and motor performance. *ADVERSE EFF ENVIRON CHEM PSYCHOTROPIC DRUGS* 2:53–68, 1976.

Swinson RP: Colour vision defects in alcoholism. *BR J PHYSIOL OPT* 27:43–50, 1972.

Tiburtius H, Wojahan H, Glass F: On change in the readaptation time of the human eye after foveal dazzle under the influence of alcohol. *GRAEFES ARCH OPHTHALMOL* 169:318–327, 1966. (German)

Van Lith GHM, Henkes HE: Low vision in alcohol abuse. *DOC OPHTHALMOL* 46:333–338, 1979.

Verriest G, Laplasse D: New data concerning the influence of ethyl alcohol on human visual thresholds. *EXP EYE RES* 4:95–101, 1965.

Victor M, Mancall EL, Dreyfus PM: Deficiency amblyopia in the alcoholic patient. *ARCH OPHTHALMOL* 64:1–33, 1960.

Weinsieder A, Briggs R, et al: Induction of mitosis in ocular tissue by chemotoxic agents. *EXP EYE RES* 20:33–44, 1975.

Wilkinson IMS, Kime R, Purnell M: Alcohol and human eye movement. *BRAIN* 97:785–792, 1974.

Wilson G, Mitchell R: The effect of alcohol on the visual and ocular motor systems. *AUST J OPHTHALMOL* 11:315–319, 1983.

Zuschlag HG: Alcohol-induced disturbances of visual functions. *KLIN MONATSBL AUGENHEILKD* 147:595–600, 1965. (German)

Alcoholic essences and extracts normally contain ethyl alcohol, but on occasion have been adulterated by substitution of methyl alcohol (methanol). Essences adulterated with methyl alcohol have caused numerous severe poisonings with optic neuritis and optic atrophy.[a,153] (In the case of Jamaica ginger, there has also been poisoning from adulteration with *tricresyl phosphate,* causing the so-called ginger or Jake paralysis, but no eye disturbance.)

   a. Harlan: Blindness and death from drinking essence of ginger, peppermint, etc., due to
        methyl alcohol. *OPHTHAL REC* 84:1901.

Aldrin, an insecticide, deranges the ERG and VER when given intraperitoneally in mice.[290]

Alkalies (bases) are substances which dissociate in water to yield an excess of hydroxyl ions, producing a pH above 7. In general the higher the pH, the greater the danger to the eye. The commonest alkalies are *calcium hydroxide* (lime), *sodium hydroxide* (lye), and *ammonium hydroxide* (ammonia). Besides the inorganic alkalies, there are many organic amines which are sufficiently alkaline to be injurious on contact with the eye.

   Here we will compare the properties of the common alkalies with one another, but will provide more detailed and specific descriptions of each of the alkalies elsewhere under their individual names. (See the INDEX.) We will describe treatment of alkali burns elsewhere in a chapter entitled "Treatment of Chemical Burns of the Eye." (See the INDEX.)

   A comprehensive review of alkali burns of the eye was published by Hughes in 1946.[c] He concluded that the severity of the damage to the eye is less dependent upon the character of the cation than upon the concentration of the alkali, the duration of the exposure, and the pH of the solution. Earlier experimental studies by Friedenwald, Hughes, and Herrmann had established that in the case of a solution containing sodium as the principal cation, when the alkalinity was increased above pH 11.5 the severity of injury to the corneal stroma increased sharply.[a]

   Subsequent tests of numerous other alkalies on rabbit corneas from which the corneal epithelium had been removed established a general rule, applicable to cations which are not injurious at neutrality, that solutions having alkalinity as high as pH 11 cause only slight and reversible injury to the corneal stroma on brief (10 minute) exposure.[89] Injuriousness increases greatly between pH 11 and pH 12, probably most steeply at pH 11.5. At pH 12 and higher, severe injury of the cornea with opacification can be induced by all alkalies.[89] Certain cations cause greater immediate opacification of the stroma than do others, but the ultimate degree of damage is governed solely by the hydroxyl ion concentration.

   When the corneal epithelium is present, conditions are more complex, and greater differences in the character of injury of the eye by different alkalies are notable even at equal pH. Variations in manner and rate of penetration through the epithelial barrier account for certain differences recognizable clinically in burns by calcium hydroxide, sodium hydroxide, and ammonium hydroxide. For instance, in patients, calcium hydroxide most commonly causes superficial opacification of the cornea, whereas sodium hydroxide commonly induces pearly opacification of deeper layers of the stroma, and ammonium hydroxide tends to cause the deepest injury, with edema and wrinkling of the posterior surface of the cornea, also iritis and even cataract.

These clinical differences are in part explicable by differences in rate of penetration which have been demonstrated experimentally in animal eyes, enucleated eyes, and in excised corneas.[81] Measurements comparing solutions of similar concentration and alkalinity have shown that the rates of penetration through excised beef corneas with epithelium present can be graded from slowest to fastest in the following order: *calcium hydroxide, tetraethylammonium hydroxide, barium hydroxide, strontium hydroxide, lithium hydroxide, potassium hydroxide, sodium hydroxide*, and *ammonium hydroxide*. Removal of the epithelium increases the rate of penetration three or four fold, making it essentially equal for all of the alkalies except ammonia, which continues to be fastest.

The differences in rate with which alkalies have been observed to penetrate the cornea may have the following basis. Ammonium hydroxide penetrates most rapidly, not only because it diffuses fastest through the corneal stroma, but also because it is exceptionally injurious to the epithelium. Possibly this is attributable to the fact that in alkaline solutions ammonia molecules are present in equilibrium with ammonium ions and ammonium hydroxide, and that ammonia is fat-soluble and may therefore penetrate especially well into and through fatty cellular barriers. Injury to epithelial cells may be accomplished by all alkalies by saponification of the fatty components of the cells at high pH levels. However, most alkalies lack the advantages of fat solubility and high mobility of ammonia to permeate layers of cells. Calcium hydroxide appears to be at a particular disadvantage compared to both ammonium and sodium hydroxides, because the soaps of calcium formed by saponification of fats generally are relatively insoluble, and can form precipitates which may hinder penetration.

In the corneal stroma the injurious effect of high pH has been found to involve temporary binding of the alkali cations to corneal mucoproteins and collagen, increasing steeply as the pH is raised above 11.5.[89, 90] Binding of cations at high pH appears to be an essential part of the injury process, but subsequent removal of the cations from combination with corneal mucoproteins and collagen does not appear to influence the severity of injury.

Reaction of alkalies with corneal stroma at high pH causes rapid loss of corneal mucoprotein, which is demonstrable by chemical analysis and metachromatic staining.[b, 89] For instance, much of the hexosamine of the cornea is lost within the first twenty-four hours after exposure to 0.05N sodium hydroxide.[b] Only alkalies appear to cause a great loss of mucoprotein within the first twenty-four hours after injury, although a slow and relatively slight loss does occur in association with corneal edema and infiltration of inflammatory cells induced by injury of other types, such as by injection of turpentine into the stroma, or mechanical removal of the corneal epithelium.[b]

Hughes, in his comprehensive review and analysis of alkali burns, has outlined the principal clinical and histologic features as follows.[b] In the acute stage there is sloughing of the corneal epithelium, necrosis of cells of the corneal stroma and endothelium, loss of corneal mucoid, edema of the corneal stroma and the ciliary processes, ischemic necrosis and edema of the conjunctiva and limbal region of the sclera, and infiltration of inflammatory cells into the cornea and iris. There is a strong tendency for corneal infiltration and degeneration to develop one to three weeks after injury.

Poor results are particularly likely to result from destruction of the corneal endothelium with resulting corneal edema, from secondary infection with infiltration and ulceration, and from iritis and secondary glaucoma. In the reparative stage, when injury has not been excessively severe, there is a tendency to subsidence of edema, regeneration of epithelium, clearing of corneal opacification, regeneration of endothelium, and disappearance of iritis. Late complications in severe burns consist of persistent edema, vascularization of the cornea, fibrous tissue scarring of the cornea, growth of vessels throughout the cornea, permanent opacity, staphyloma, cataract, and symblepharon.[c]

The role of injury to blood vessels in alkali burns, as well as in other chemical injuries of the eye, remains obscure. In alkali and other chemical burns, the blood vessels of the conjunctiva and episclera may be seen by slit-lamp biomicroscope to be thrombosed immediately after exposure. The significance of the resultant limbal ischemia to the cornea has been subject of much speculation. Commonly the degree of injury of episcleral tissues parallels the degree of injury of the cornea, and many observers have assumed that limbal ischemia is severely detrimental to the cornea. However, Pfister et al (1971) have described producing in rabbits a severe sodium hydroxide burn limited to the conjunctiva and anterior sclera, avoiding the cornea, and this caused no visible injury to the cornea.[d] It did cause necrosis and atrophy of the underlying ciliary body, with consequent hypotony.

Since 1968 much has been learned of mechanisms of alkali injury of the eye, mostly from experiments with sodium hydroxide in animal eyes. Generally, it seems to be assumed the same mechanisms are involved in injuries of the eye by other alkalies. Reviews by Lemp (1974),[c] Pfister (1983),[e] Ralph and Slansky (1974),[f] Reim and Schmidt-Martens (1982),[g] and Wright (1982)[h] are especially instructive. In the period since 1968 it was recognized that in severe burns there was release of collagenase enzymes from cells surrounding the burn. It was at first thought that these collagenases came from epithelial cells, but subsequently it has appeared that polymorphonuclear leukocytes infiltrating the damaged region were a more important source. The collagenases did not attack corneal collagen that had a normal protective sheath of mucopolysaccharide, but when the sheath was damaged by an alkali the collagenases could degrade the corneal collagen, leading to melting or ulceration of the stroma, formation of Descemetoceles and perforation of the cornea. This phase of breakdown generally became evident 3 days to a week or more after a severe alkali burn had occurred.

Working toward repairing alkali damage to the stroma, surviving keratocytes tried to form new collagen, but a decrease in available ascorbate, which resulted from injury to the main source of ascorbate in the ciliary body, appeared to be one limiting factor in formation of new collagen. It also appeared possible that deficiency of ascorbate might render the cornea susceptible to injury by oxygen free radicals. In severely damaged untreated eyes, inflammatory destruction and ulceration could prevail for weeks or months, ending at worst in corneal perforation, or at best in dense vascular invasion and opaque scarring. The scientific development of treatments designed to limit breakdown and encourage repair is described in the chapter "Treatment of Chemical Burns of the Eye." (See the INDEX.)

The intraocular pressure can be acutely disturbed in both alkali and acid burns of the eye. When the coats of the eye are exposed to sufficiently high or sufficiently low pH to be chemically damaging, an immediate shrinkage takes place which can raise the intraocular pressure to a high peak, but this is short-lasting. A secondary phase of pressure elevation, particularly in rabbits, can be produced by prostaglandin release. At a still later stage, seen particularly in patients, glaucoma may be produced by obstruction of the aqueous outflow system by inflammation or synechias. In some cases, hypotony may result from alkali damage to the ciliary body and consequent reduced formation of aqueous humor.

Cataracts can be produced by the most serious alkali burns, especially by rapidly penetrating ammonia. When cataract sufficient to interfere with vision occurs in alkali burns the rest of the eye usually is hopelessly damaged.

Chorioretinal injury has been described as a consequence of severe alkali burns, particularly by sodium hydroxide. (See INDEX for *Sodium hydroxide.*)

Differences between burns from alkalies and burns from acids are obvious clinically and experimentally. The characteristic deeper penetrating injury of alkalies and a tendency to superficial injury by acids may be explained partially by differences in ability to penetrate the cornea and partially by the nature of the chemical reactions induced in the corneal stroma. Alkalies applied to the epithelial surface of the cornea reach the anterior chamber much more rapidly than acids. When the epithelium is removed, the acids penetrate at about the same rate as the alkalies, indicating that the epithelium is the principal barrier to penetration.

Another fundamental difference in the nature of interaction of acids and alkalies with the cornea is evident in the rate at which the pH of the tissue returns toward neutrality during irrigation with water or saline following acid or alkali burn. By testing the surface of the cornea or conjunctiva with indicator paper, it is readily demonstrable in animals and in patients that during irrigation of the surface of the eye with water or saline, neutrality is much more rapidly approached after acid burn than after alkali burn. In the case of alkali burns, free alkali appears to be regenerated by slow dissociation of cation from combination with corneal proteins sufficient to keep the pH above normal during fifteen or twenty minutes of irrigation.[81,89]

a. Friedenwald JS, Hughes WF, Herrmann H: Acid-base tolerance of the cornea. *ARCH OPHTHALMOL* 31:279–283, 1944.
b. Hughes WF: Alkali burns of the eye. *ARCH OPHTHALMOL* 35:423–449, 1946; and 36:189–214, 1946.
c. Lemp MA: Cornea and sclera. *ARCH OPHTHALMOL* 92:158–170, 1974.
d. Pfister RR, McCulley JP, et al: Collagenase activity of intact corneal epithelium in peripheral alkali burns. *ARCH OPHTHALMOL* 86:309–313, 1971.
e. Pfister RR: Chemical injuries of the eye. *OPHTHALMOLOGY* 90:1246–1253, 1983.
f. Ralph RA, Slansky HH: Therapy of chemical burns. *INT OPHTHALMOL CLIN* 14:171–191, 1974.

g. Reim M, Schmidt-Martens FW: Management of burns. *KLIN MONATSBL AUGEN-HEILKD* 181:1–9, 1982.

h. Wright P: The chemically injured eye. *TRANS OPHTHALMOL SOC UK* 102:85–87, 1982.

Allopurinol (Zyloprim, Zyloric) is a xanthine oxidase inhibitor used in gout. Literature from a manufacturer has mentioned "a few reports of cataract," but the unpublished details upon which this cautionary statement was based consisted of a study of patients who were elderly and had had no eye examination prior to treatment with the drug. The incidence of cataract in the treated patients was said to be not significantly greater than in the general population of the same age group. However, more suggestive observations have been accumulating. A woman in her twenties who was known to have clear lenses developed bilateral posterior subcapsular lens opacities after she had taken allopurinol for 18 months.[g] Vision remained 20/20, and after the drug was discontinued the opacities did not progress during the next 2 years. In 1982 Lerman used phosphorence spectroscopy to demonstrate proteinbound allopurinol in cataracts from three men who had been taking this medication,[e] and Fraunfelder reported that his National Registry had received reports of 24 previously unpublished cases in which patients mostly between ages 50 and 65 had developed cataracts, after taking allopurinol for more than a year in most cases.[b] Histology disclosed nothing specific or pathognomic about these cataracts. Eleven of the lenses studied by Fraunfelder were examined by Lerman, who reported in 1984 that they contained bound allopurinol, whereas 4 non-cataractous human lenses postmortem did not, although the donors had been taking allopurinol.[f] Lerman postulated on the basis of irradiation experiments in vitro and in rats that ultraviolet promoted reaction of allopurinol with the lens, tending to increase susceptibility to development of cataract, and suggested protective glasses for patients taking allopurinol.

Impressive clinical evidence against a positive association of allopurinol and cataracts was reported in 1984 by Jick and Brandt on the basis of systematic surveys of several hundreds of patients.[c]

Attempts to produce cataracts in rabbits by feeding allopurinol at a dosage approximately twice the human dosage for 8 months were unsuccessful.[g]

Two patients receiving allopurinol in treatment of gout have developed macular lesions. Both were unilateral. One was a small exudate reducing vision temporarily to 20/40. The other was a disciform hemorrhagic lesion that developed acutely in the macula and regressed considerably after use of this drug was discontinued.[d,h] Both could well have been coincidental, since the same types of disturbance occur sporadically in patients without medications.

Toxic epidermal necrolysis with pseudomembranous conjunctivitis and ulceration of lids, conjunctivae and both corneas has been reported in one patient after taking allopurinol for 3 weeks.[a]

a. Bennett TO, Sugar J, Sakgal S: Ocular manifestations of toxic epidermal necrolysis associated with allopurinol use. *ARCH OPHTHALMOL* 95:1362–1364, 1977.

b. Fraunfelder FT, Hanna C, et al: Cataracts associated with allopurinol therapy. *AM J OPHTHALMOL* 94:137–140, 1982.

c. Jick H, Brandt DE: Allopurinol and cataracts. *AM J OPHTHALMOL* 98:355–358, 1984.

d. Laval J: Allopurinol and macular lesions. *ARCH OPHTHALMOL* 80:415, 1968.

e. Lerman S, Megaw JM, Gardner K: Allopurinol therapy and cataractogenesis in humans. *AM J OPHTHALMOL* 94:141–146, 1982.

f. Lerman S, Megaw J, Fraunfelder FT: Further studies on allopurinol therapy and human cataracts. *AM J OPHTHALMOL* 97:205–209, 1984.

g. March WF, Goren S, Shoch D: Action of allopurinol on the lens. *SYMPOSIUM ON OCULAR THERAPY* 7:83–95, 1974, edited by I.H. Leopold. C.V. Mosby, St. Louis, 1974.

h. Pinnas G: Possible association between macular lesions and allopurinol. *ARCH OPHTHALMOL* 79:786–787, 1968.

Alloxan is a sulfhydryl poison that has been used as an antineoplastic agent and has held great interest for study of toxic effects on the eye. In experimental animals it is severely injurious if applied to the eye or injected into the vitreous body, and if given systemically it produces cataract and severe toxic changes in the retina. It also has teratogenic action.

Injurious action of alloxan on the cornea in animals has been studied both by injection into the anterior chamber and by application to the outer surface. Injection of alloxan into the anterior chamber in rabbits has been repeatedly observed to injure the endothelium of the cornea, causing edema of the cornea and producing opacification and vascularization of the stroma of the cornea.[a-d,m,q,2,221] This has been utilized as a method of injuring the cornea for use in other experiments concerned principally with mechanism of vascularization and with both medical and surgical treatments intended to suppress scarring and vascularization of injured corneas or of corneal grafts. However, the use of alloxan by injection into the anterior chamber has been criticized as being unsatisfactory for obtaining uniform corneal vascularization, and furthermore that the corneal injury is complicated by development of secondary glaucoma.[d]

To obviate some of these difficulties, several investigators have applied alloxan externally to the eyes in rabbits and guinea pigs, sometimes restricting the area of exposure by means of a glass cup or tube,[e,g,h,r,w] or by limited removal of epithelium.[zb] This method of application also destroys the endothelium of the cornea, causing edema and vascularization of the stroma. Besides being more convenient, the external application avoids the severe plastic iritis that is caused by injection into the anterior chamber. Occasionally calcific plaques have appeared at a late stage after severe corneal injury.[r,za]

Histological studies provide evidence of direct perpendicular penetration, with little tangential diffusion along stromal lamellae.[zb]

Biochemical studies on corneas exposed to alloxan have led to the suggestion that an initial effect is an alteration of nicotine adenine dinucleotide which leads to failure of the dehydrogenase system, evident as striking inhibition of lactic acid dehydrogenase in all layers of the cornea within thirty minutes after exposure to alloxan.[g,h]

Parenteral administration of alloxan to rabbits and rats produces diabetes through injurious action on the pancreas; cataracts develop several weeks later.[i,j,n,s,y,u,v,z] The development of cataracts appears not to be secondary to the diabetes or the height of blood sugar concentration, though development of cataract can be interfered with, or prevented, by high fat diets.[s,u] In the aqueous humor the concentration of amino acids and their uptake by the lens are reduced by systemic alloxan poisoning, but this, according to studies by Reddy and Kinsey, appears to be secondary to the diabetes and not due to a toxic effect of alloxan either on the epithelium of the ciliary body or the lens.[t] However, Bernat and Bombicki have reported that in rats in which cataracts are induced, the concentration of amino acids in both lens and chamber fluid has been reduced without reduction of concentration in the blood. This also occurred when cataracts were produced by galactose and naphthalene as well as by alloxan.[12] Considering the toxic properties of alloxan, it seems likely that the effect of this chemical on the lens and particularly on mitotic activity in the lens should be more significant for the development of cataracts than the indirect effects of the diabetes and its associated metabolic derangements.

Changes in the retina have been sought repeatedly in animals made diabetic by parenterally administered alloxan, in the hopes of obtaining an experimental model of the diabetic retinopathy, which is a great therapeutic problem in human diabetes. In 1966 Toussaint published a table listing the numerous reports of experiments by others, mostly negative, but occasionally describing retinal hemorrhages, exudate, or tortuosity of retinal vessels, but not reporting vascular changes such as are characteristic of human diabetic retinopathy.[x] Later, a histologic study of dogs that had alloxan diabetes, with cataracts, and with non-proliferative diabetic retinopathy comparable to that of man, showed after 5 years a breakdown of the blood-retinal barrier, with horseradish peroxidase tracer around retinal blood vessels, appearing to have permeated endothelial junctions.

Numerous biochemical studies have been published on retinas from animals with alloxan diabetes, assuming the changes to be a manifestation of the diabetes. References to investigations in which interest has been primarily in the effects of diabetes and in which alloxan was utilized merely as a means of inducing diabetes are mostly omitted from the bibliography at the end of this section. However, representative publications by Futterman and Hollenberg concerning biochemical and histological changes in alloxan diabetes are listed in the bibliography to give background information on those aspects.[f,k]

Direct toxic effects of alloxan on the retina, rather than secondary changes from diabetes, have been claimed by Manuelli in interpreting electron microscopic findings in albino rats after administering alloxan intraperitoneally.[o] Also studies on rabbit retina in vitro have shown alloxan to be capable of inhibiting oxidative phosphorylation in retinal mitochondria.[p]

There seem to have been no reports of injury of human eyes by alloxan.

Teratogenic effects of alloxan in mice have been observed, including anomalies of the lens and iris.[1]

a. Ashton N, Cook C, Langham M: Effect of cortisone on vascularization and opacification of the cornea induced by alloxan. *BR J OPHTHALMOL* 35:718, 1951.
b. Baily CC, Baily OT, Leech RS: Alloxan diabetes with diabetic complications. *N ENGL J MED* 230:533–536, 1944.
c. Collin HB: Corneal lymphatics in alloxan vascularized rabbit eyes. *INVEST OPHTHALMOL* 5:1–13, 1966.

d. Ey RC, Hughes WF, et al: Prevention of corneal vascularization. *AM J OPHTHALMOL* 66:1118–1131, 1968.

e. Faure J-P, Kim YZ: Observations on the effects of alloxan on the cornea of the guinea-pig. *ARCH OPHTALMOL (Paris)* 26:677–686, 1966; and 27:513–520, 1967. (French)

f. Futterman S, Sturtevant R, Kupfer C: Effect of alloxan diabetes on the fatty acid composition of the retina. *INVEST OPHTHALMOL* 8:542–544, 1969.

g. Graymore C, Ashton N, McCormick A: Alloxan and lactic acid dehydrogenase activity of the cornea. *BR J OPHTHALMOL* 52:677–681, 1968.

h. Graymore C, McCormick A: Induction of corneal vascularization with alloxan. *BR J OPHTHALMOL* 52:138–140, 1968.

i. Grimes P, vonSallman L: Lens epithelium proliferation in sugar cataracts. *INVEST OPHTHALMOL* 7:535–543, 1968.

j. Hammar H: *ACTA OPHTHALMOL* 43:61–74, 442–453, 543–556, 1965.

k. Hollenberg MJ, Nayyar RP, Burt WL: Histochemical and electron microscopic studies of the retinal pigment epithelium in the normal and diabetic rat. *CAN J OPHTHALMOL* 3:65–76, 1968.

l. Koskenoja M: Alloxan diabetes in the pregnant mouse. *ACTA OPHTHALMOL* (Suppl 68) 11–84, 1961.

m. Langham M: Observations on the growth of blood vessels into the cornea. *BR J OPHTHALMOL* 37:210, 1953.

n. Lerman S: Metabolic pathways in experimental diabetic cataract. *INVEST OPHTHALMOL* 1:507–512, 1962.

o. Manuelli G: Retinal ultrastructural alterations induced by alloxan in the rat. *RASS ITAL OTTALMOL* 33:62–70, 1964. (Italian)

p. Matsuda H: Oxidative phosphorylation in the retinal mitochondria from alloxan diabetic rabbits. *ACTA SOC OPHTHALMOL JPN* 73:131–142, 1969; *FOLIA OPHTHALMOL JPN* 20:393–394, 1969.

q. McCoy GA, Leopold IH: Steroid treatment of alloxan-induced corneal opacification and vascularization. *AM J OPHTHALMOL* 49:906–908, 1960.

r. Obenberger J: Calcification in corneas with alloxan-induced vascularization. *AM J OPHTHALMOL* 68:113–119, 1969.

s. Patterson JW, Patterson ME, et al: Lens assays on diabetic and galactosemic rats receiving diets that modify cataract development. *INVEST OPHTHALMOL* 4:98–103, 1965.

t. Reddy DVN, Kinsey VE, Nathorst-Windahl G: Comparison of amino acid transport in ocular structures of rabbits made diabetic by alloxan and pancreatectomy. *INVEST OPHTHALMOL* 5:166–169, 1966.

u. Schrader KE: Blood sugar curves and lens opacities after administration of alloxan to rats. *BER DTSCH OPHTHALMOL GESELLSCH* 65:299–303, 1963. (German)

v. Schimizu S: Studies of aqueous humor dynamics in Pco₂ and pH on the experimental diabetes of rabbits. *ACTA SOC OPHTHALMOL JPN* 73:1379–1388, 1969.

w. Sugiura S, Matsuda H: Electron microscopic studies on the cornea: neovascularization. *ACTA SOC OPHTHALMOL JPN* 73:1208–1221, 1969.

x. Toussaint D: Retinal lesions in the course of alloxan diabetes in rats. *BULL SOC BELGE OPHTALMOL* 143:648–657, 1966. (French)

y. vonSallmann L, Caravaggio L, et al: Morphological study of alloxan-induced cataract. *ARCH OPHTHALMOL* 59:55–67, 1958.

z. Waters JW: Biochemical and clinical changes in the rabbit lens during alloxan diabetes. *BIOCHEM J* 46:575–578, 1950.

za. Obenberger J, Babicky A: Pentration of radioactive calcium into the aqueous and cornea of normal and alloxan-treated rabbits. *AM J OPHTHALMOL* 70:1003–1005, 1970.

zb. Vrabec F, Smelser GK, Ozanics V: Rabbit cornea damage induced by alloxan. *OPHTHAL-MIC RES* 8:262–275, 1976.

zc. Wallow IHL, Engerman RL: Permeability and patency of retinal blood vessels in experimental diabetes. *INVEST OPHTHALMOL VIS SCI* 16:447–461, 1977.

zd. Varma SD, Reddy VN: Phospholipid composition of aqueous humor, plasma and lens in normal and alloxan diabetic rabbits. *EXP EYE RES* 13:120–125, 1972.

Allyl alcohol on the skin has a delayed effect, causing aching beginning several hours after contact, followed by blistering. The liquid tested on rabbit eyes by application of a drop caused moderately severe reaction consisting of conjunctival edema and hyperemia with transient clouding of the cornea, graded 5 on a scale of 10 at twenty-four hours.[27] The corneal opacities disappeared within forty-eight hours, and the eyes were completely normal within a week.[a] Accidental splashes of liquid in human eyes similarly have produced moderately severe reactions, usually with prompt healing, but in one exceptional case healing took several days.[165]

The vapors of allyl alcohol in air are irritating to the nose and eyes. In human beings irritation of the nose begins at 10 to 15 ppm and irritation of eyes is noticeable at 5 ppm.[a,b] Men exposed to the vapors industrially complain of lacrimation, retrobulbar pain, photophobia, and some blurring of vision,[a] presumably secondary to corneal epithelial edema or keratitis epithelialis. Symptoms persist for as long as twenty-four to forty-eight hours following exposure. As a rule recovery from vapor exposure is complete.

On the basis of animal tests for systemic toxicity, Torkelson has recommended that industrially the average concentration in air should not exceed 2 ppm, and that the concentration always be kept below 5 ppm, in other words below the concentration at which irritation of the eyes is noticeable.[d]

Exposure of rabbits to 1,000 ppm in air until death in three to four hours resulted in hemorrhages in the eyes of one rabbit and histologic changes in retinal ganglion cells, but severe damage and hemorrhages were found in practically all body tissues.[b] The ERG in mice is reported to be almost completely abolished 3 hours after intraperitoneal injection of 100 mg/kg.[e]

An allegation has been reiterated in the literature that accommodation of the eyes for near is impaired by vapors of allyl alcohol; however, this appears to be based on no other evidence than incidental mention in 1891 that one worker had a feeling of farsightedness all day each time he worked with allyl alcohol; there were no actual measurements of accommodation, and no confirmation has appeared in nearly a century since then.[c]

a. Dunlap MK, Kodama JK, et al: The toxicity of allyl alcohol. *ARCH IND HEALTH* 18:303–311, 1958.

b. McCord CP: Toxicity of allyl alcohol. *J AM MED ASSOC* 98:2269–2270, 1932.

c. Miessner: Concerning the effect of allyl alcohol. *BER KLIN WSCHR* 28:819–822, 1891. (German)

d. Torkelson TR, Wolf MA, et al: Vapor toxicity of allyl alcohol as determined on laboratory animals. *AM IND HYG ASSOC J* 20:224–229, 1959.

e. Gauri KK, Hellner KA: Retinotropic activity of omegahydroxyhexylpyridone-2 in methanol and allyl alcohol injury. *DOC OPHTHALMOL PROC SERIES* 13:35–340, 1977.

Allyl amines have been tested by dropping on rabbit eyes. *Monoallyl amine* was extremely irritating. *Diallyl amine* was severely irritating. *Triallyl amine* was mildly irritating.[a, 228]

Tests of the vapors on human subjects established that *monoallyl amine* at 14 ppm caused intolerable irritation of eyes and respiratory tract.[a]

Diallyl amine even at 70 ppm did not cause severe respiratory or eye irritation.

Triallyl amine at 50 to 100 ppm caused increasing irritation, coughing, nausea and headache.

In general the allyl amines irritated the nose and throat at lower concentrations than were irritant to the eyes. The vapors are so unpleasant that it is unlikely human beings would voluntarily submit to systemically dangerous concentrations.

a. Hine CH, Kodama JK, et al: The toxicity of allylamines. *ARCH ENVIRON HEALTH* 1:343–352, 1960.

Allyl bromide vapor is irritating to the eyes and respiratory passages.[171]

3-Allyl catechol and **4-allyl catechol** tested by injection of 0.05 M aqueous solution into rabbit's corneas caused moderately severe damage.[123]

Allyl chloride is damaging to the skin, but application of a drop to a rabbit's eye has caused only mild transient injury, graded 2 on a scale of 1 to 10.[223] Possibly the eye escaped greater injury because of the low boiling point and rapid evaporation of allyl chloride. The vapor itself causes irritation of the eyes and respiratory passages. In human beings, eye irritation occurs between 50 and 100 ppm, and overexposure has been followed by eye pain and photophobia.[372]

Allyl cyanide given subcutaneously to albino rats at a dose of 100–120 mg/kg caused transient clouding of the corneas, but 200 mg/kg caused perforating ulceration of the corneas and anterior subcapsular cataracts.[a]

a. Dobrynina VV, Larionov LN: Eye damage from allyl cyanide. *FARMAKOL TOKSIKOL (Moscow)* 33:628–630, 1970. (Russian)

Allyl dibromide in one instance is reported to have caused poisoning from inhalation of its vapors. Acute onset of weakness, vomiting, and trembling of the hands was accompanied by watering of the eyes and blurring of vision with difficulty in reading. Two hours later, left convergent strabismus and impaired accommodation were noted, also slight bilateral peripapillary edema, but normal pupillary reactions to light. (No measurements of accommodation or visual acuity were reported.) In twelve hours the patient was essentially back to normal except for slight effort in reading.[a]

a. Mockel W, Seusing J: Intoxication with allyl dibromide. *ARCH TOXIKOL* 15:195–196, 1955. (German)

Allyl glycerol ether tested by application of a drop to a rabbit's eye caused moderate reversible injury, graded 44 on a scale of 0 to 100.[116]

Allyl glycidyl ether (1, 2-epoxy-3-allyloxypropane) causes severe but reversible corneal damage when dropped on a rabbit's eye. High vapor concentration produces corneal opacities in rats. Low vapor concentrations produce such severe eye and respiratory irritation that this serves as adequate warning against dangerous exposures.[115]

Allylglycine inhibits cerebral glutamic acid decarboxylase, and when given intravenously to baboons causes a succession of conjugate deviation of the eyes, turning of head and neck, horizontal nystagmus, and epileptic seizure, with myoclonus beginning in peri-orbital muscles.[a]

a. Meldrum PS, Horton RW, Brierley JB: Epileptic brain damage in adolescent baboons following seizures induced by allylglycine. *BRAIN* 97:407–417, 1974.

Allylisothiocyanate (allylisosulfocyanate, volatile oil of mustard) is a liquid having a very pungent irritating odor. It is present in black mustard seed and in horseradish. It has been used in dog repellent sprays, one of which is named "Ridz."[b] It has also been added to certain plastic glues or cements to discourage "glue sniffing." The vapor is lacrimogenic and can cause keratitis which interferes with vision. According to Flury and Zernik, in some instances recovery has been slow, taking weeks.[61] (See also *Mustard oil.*)

The irritating and lacrimogenic effects of allyl isothiocyanate have been considered probably related to the reactivity of this compound with sulfhydryl groups of nerve endings, but apparently no attempt has yet been made to identify this reaction specifically in the cornea.[a]

a. Bacq ZM: Thiol-depriving substances. *EXPERIENTIA* 2:349–354, 1946. (French)
b. King MJ: Personal communication, 1969.
c. Verhulst HL, Crotty JJ: Glue-sniffing deterrent. *NATL CLEARINGHOUSE FOR POISON CONTROL CENTERS BULL* 4–5, Nov.–Dec. 1969.

Allyl propyl disulfide, along with *diallyl disulfide* and *propenyl sulfenic acid* (see INDEX), is said to be one of the principal volatile substances in onion which irritate the eyes and cause lacrimation. The maximum concentration of vapor in air advised for industrial conditions is 2 to 3 ppm.[a]

a. Feiner B, Burke WJ, Baliff J: An industrial hygiene survey of an onion dehydrating plant. *J IND HYG* 28:278, 1946.

Allyl thiourea tested by injection of 0.05 M aqueous solution into the cornea of a rabbit has caused minor injury, graded 18 on a scale of 0 to 100.[123]

Aloe barb from a shrub in Northern Africa and Southern France is reported to have produced severe iridocyclitis in several cases when it penetrated the eye. Sedan and Rouher in 1956 gathered observations from other ophthalmologists and reported four of their own cases in which the barb accidentally perforated the sclera. Several mm of the barbs broke off and were retained in the sclera extending into the vitreous body. This produced a severe anterior and posterior uveitis with hypotony and great reduction of vision. Symptoms as a rule did not develop until many hours after the injury. Some eyes were lost from this type of injury and others took many months to recover. The authors suspected a toxin, but experiments on rabbits produced relatively slight reaction. Clinically it was judged not to be an infection, and some response to treatment with corticosteroids was observed.[a] (Compare *Acacia thorn.*)

a. Sedan J, Rouher F: Ocular wounds from aloe barbs. *ANN OCULIST (Paris)* 189:619–627, 1956. (French)

Alum (aluminum potassium sulfate, or aluminum ammonium sulfate) at one time was used as eyedrops as a 1% aqueous solution in the treatment of trachoma. Eyes contaminated with alum of unstated concentration and given first aid irrigation with water have been reported normal in a day or two.[165]

Aluminum metal in the form of small particles has been observed many times as an intraocular foreign body in patients and in animals. Generally these particles have been nonirritating and well tolerated. In human eyes, aluminum foreign bodies in the posterior segment, on the retina or close to it have been reported in several cases to have been well tolerated for long periods.[d,g,h,k,136] There has been little evidence of toxicity, the particles gradually changing to a white powder and disappearing in two or three years, leaving only a slight "imprint." Knave, presenting a review of the literature and a clinical study of sixty-eight human eyes with intraocular metallic foreign bodies, has reported that with aluminum the ERG became altered only after a long time and that the toxicity appeared to be low.[136] Experimentally in rabbits introduction of aluminum particles into the posterior segment, according to Fontana, has produced very little reaction when the particles were in the vitreous.[a] Savin also reported the same benign course as in human eyes, but in rabbits he observed a low-grade uveal inflammation with posterior synechias and partial atrophy of the iris. In both rabbit and human eyes when the particles had been in contact with the retina, the same characteristic local necrotic "imprints" have been noted in the fundus at the site of absorbed aluminum particles. In rabbits small opacities in the lenses and pigmentation of the fundus have been described, but in human eyes no cataract has been observed, except when the lens has been injured mechanically, none when aluminum has simply been in proximity to the lens.[a,c,h,136]

A case reported by May seems to have indicated greater damage to the retina. A patient who was seen twelve years after injury with a foreign body that penetrated the lens and caused traumatic cataract was observed to have large areas of destruction and pigmentation in the retina, also atrophic and whitish appearance in the iris adjacent to a particle of aluminum in the anterior chamber, but whether the injury in the posterior segment was traumatic or toxic was not entirely clear.[e]

Also exceptional toxicity has been shown by aluminum alloys containing 90% copper which were practically as toxic as copper itself, but alloys with low copper content were essentially as nontoxic as aluminum itself.[j]

Aluminum metal particles in the anterior chamber and on the iris have several times been described in patients remaining at least for several years without inflammation or evident injurious effect, except occasionally slight depigmentation of adjacent iris.[b,c] In one patient the iris has been described as becoming atrophic and whitish adjacent to a particle of aluminum.[e]

In rabbits aluminum particles in the anterior chamber have also been tolerated with very little reaction.[a,c]

In the human cornea, particles of metallic aluminum have been tolerated without reaction, remaining shiny and without corneal infiltration for long periods.[b,c] In a case observed by Sherman, a boy had many very fine particles of metallic aluminum driven into his corneal stroma by an explosion which resulted when he mixed potassium chlorate, sulfur, and powdered aluminum. Because of the known low toxicity of aluminum and because of the considerable mechanical damage that would have to be done to the cornea in attempting to remove them, the particles were left in the cornea undisturbed. Five years later the aluminum particles appeared by slit-lamp biomicroscopy to be exactly as they appeared soon after the explosion, with no inflammatory reaction. Only a few particles were in the pupillary area, and vision was not affected.[i]

a. Fontana G: Behavior of the tissues of the eye in the presence of intraocular metallic fragments. *RASS ITAL OTTALMOL* 7:695–720, 1938. (Italian)

b. Fricke E: Aluminum in the eye. *KLIN MONATSBL AUGENHEILKD* 74:209–213, 1925. (German)

c. Jess A: On the behavior of aluminum in the eye. *KLIN MONATSBL AUGENHEILKD* 72:133–136, 1924. (German)

d. Marisi F: On the long-term behavior of intraocular fragments of aluminum. *BOLL OCULIST* 29:661–675, 1950. (Italian)

e. May W: Intraocular fragment of aluminum alloy tolerated for 12 years. *BR J OPHTHALMOL* 41:574–575, 1957.

f. Mielke S: On injuries of the eyes by metallic foreign bodies. *DTSCH MED WSCHR* 67:350, 1941. (German)

g. Savin LH: The effect of aluminum and its alloys on human and rabbit eyes. *PROC R SOC MED* 38:471–472, 1945.

h. Savin LH: The effect of aluminum and its alloys on the eye. *BR J OPHTHALMOL* 31:449–503, 1947.

i. Sherman AG: Metallic particles in the cornea. *J AM MED ASSOC* 186:282, 1963, and personal communication Feb. 1968.

j. Tanzariello R: Experimental study of the tolerance of the eye to intraocular aluminum and some of its modern industrial alloys. *RASS ITAL OTTALMOL* 16:199–223, 1947. (Italian)

k. Vignalou P: Intraocular foreign body (from explosion of a military shell) perfectly tolerated for six years. *ANN OCULIST (Paris)* 184:270, 1951. (French)

Aluminum alkyls are organic aluminum compounds that are highly reactive and dangerous because of spontaneous burning in air. Irritation of the eyes has been noted in patients who have been exposed. Severe irritation of the conjunctivae and respiratory tract has been observed in mice exposed to the fumes of *aluminum triisobutyl, aluminum diethylmonochloride,* and *aluminum diisobutylmonochloride,* but the eyes were not examined in detail.[a,b]

   a. Bonari R: Burns caused by organic metal compounds and toxicity of their fumes and vapors in industry (aluminium alkyls). *MED LAV* 57:188–194, 1966. (*EXCERPTA MED* (Sect 2C), 20:1467, 1967).
   b. Bonari R, Martini E: Toxicity of the fumes of metallo-organic compounds. *MED LAV* 58:290–296, 1967. (Italian)

Aluminum chloride (aluminum trichloride) is encountered in two different forms. The anhydrous form is a very acidic solid which fumes in moist air and reacts violently with water to release strongly acid hydrogen chloride. The anhydrous salt is caustic and irritating to the eyes and skin, but in only one out of five instances of industrial corneal burns has healing been delayed beyond two days.[165] (For other form, see *Aluminum chloride hexahydrate.*)

Aluminum chloride hexahydrate (aluminum oxychloride) is the other form of aluminum chloride. This is a nonfuming water-soluble crystalline substance, available in U.S.P. grade, used principally as a deodorant and antiperspirant, usually as 10% to 25% solution, sometimes as a spray. Such sprays or solutions have many times accidentally contacted the eyes, sometimes causing slight transient disturbance of the corneal epithelium, but no serious or persistent injury has been reported from aluminum chloride hexahydrate. Testing under extreme conditions of applying 100 mg of crystals to the cornea of a rabbit after applying a local anesthetic eyedrop caused immediate blepharospasm, despite the local anesthetic. When the crystals were allowed to remain until washed away by the tears, they caused transient epithelial damage, and a persistent faint nebula in the corneal stroma.[81]

Aluminum poisoning from systemic absorption has been considered a possibility in patients given large amounts of aluminum hydroxide by mouth, especially in uremic patients being treated by dialysis. Rats poisoned by administering aluminum hydroxide intraperitoneally, or aluminum chloride or sulfate in their drinking water, developed a curious syndrome of periorbital bleeding, lethargy and death.[a] Thinning of the corneal and conjunctival epithelium was associated with the periorbital bleeding. Nothing like this has been reported in patients. The experimental poisoning procedure seems significantly different from clinical oral administration of aluminum hydroxide.

   a. Berlyne GM, Ben Ari J, et al: Aluminum toxicity in rats. *LANCET* 1:564–568, 1972.

Amanita aureola, a mushroom, has been suspected in one case of having caused poisoning with prolonged but reversible paralysis of convergence and accommodation.[a]

a. Baquis G, Aiello F, et al: Paralysis of accommodation and convergence due to probable poisoning by Amanita aureola. *ANN OTTALMOL CLIN OCUL* 104:133–137, 1978. (Italian)

Amanita muscaria, a poisonous mushroom, according to a comprehensive review by Waser in 1967, causes salivation, perspiration, nausea, bradycardia, and mydriasis. According to this review, one to four mushrooms cause euphoria, a sense of lightness, colored visions, and visual hallucinations. Although muscarine is a constituent of these mushrooms, there is no constriction of the pupils in this poisoning. Instead there is mydriasis, which is thought to be a sympathetic effect from action on the CNS. *Muscimol,* and to a minor degree, *ibotenic acid* are believed to be the constituents largely responsible.[257] No persistent ocular disturbances have been reported.

Amanita phalloides is a very poisonous mushroom, causing death in some instances, but unlike *Amanita muscaria,* having no uniform side effect on the eyes. In some cases miosis, and in some cases mydriasis have been noted, and rarely blindness, but no permanent ocular injury.[153, 225] Characteristically, some hours after ingestion there is a sudden acute onset of gastrointestinal disturbance and general collapse, which may be accompanied by tetanic convulsions.[194] Strabismus has been known to occur and histologic alterations of the eye muscles, as well as those of the diaphragm and tongue, have been described.[b]

A series of twelve cases of poisoning observed by Bock and associates included description of edematous swelling of the brain with punctate hemorrhages, and mention of occasional miosis, diplopia, and impairment of vision. These were presumed to be secondary to disturbances of the cranial nerves.[a]

a. Bock HE, Neith H, et al: Amanita phalloides poisoning. *DTSCH MED WSCHR* 89:1617–1622, 1964. (German)
b. Schmidt MB: On the pathologic-anatomic changes after mushroom poisoning. FESTSCHRIFT FUR GASSER, Berlin Springer, 1917. (German)

Amantadine hydrochloride (Symmetrel), an antiviral drug which has also been used in control of parkinsonism, has had no definite or well-defined ocular toxic effect. Literature from the manufacturer has said that "occasional blurred vision" has been reported at high dosage. In a letter to the editor one patient is described who had normal eyes and normal vision before taking this drug, but after taking 200 mg daily for tremor had decrease in visual acuity overnight to 20/70 right, 20/200 left.[a] Ophthalmic and neurologic examinations were otherwise negative. After the medication was discontinued, vision gradually returned to normal in several weeks. Bilateral retrobulbar neuritis was considered a possibility. In dogs and monkeys no abnormalities of the eyes were found ophthalmoscopically or histologically after chronic administration at doses 13 to 33 times the human dose during six months to two years, although a number of pharmacologic functional effects were observed that did not evidently involve the eyes.[b]

Fraunfelder's National Registry has received reports of rare visual hallucinations, and 3 reports of superficial punctate keratitis which disappeared in a few days.[312]

a. Pearlman JT, Kadish AH, Ramseyer JC: Vision loss associated with amantidine hydrochloride use. *J AM MED ASSOC* 237:1200, 1977; *ARCH NEUROL* 34:199–200, 1977.

b. Vernier VG, Harmon JB, et al: The toxicologic and pharmacologic properties of amantadine hydrochloride. *TOXICOL APPL PHARMACOL* 15:642–665, 1969.

Amikacin sulfate (Amikin), an aminoglycoside antibacterial, has been tested for toxicity in rabbits upon intravitreal injection. Nelsen et al injecting 0.1 ml of solutions containing varying amounts found that 0.5 mg produced no signs of toxicity or alteration of the ERG, but 0.75 mg or more caused retinal degeneration which was evident histologically, and 3 to 6 mg produced lens opacities in 24 hours, developing to mature cataracts in 2 to 3 weeks.[a] Testing in owl monkeys in the same manner by Bennett et al showed that 0.5 mg produced no signs of toxicity.[280]

In rabbits, when vitrectomy was performed and amikacin was used in the infusion fluid, Stainer et al found that 0.01 mg/ml could be used with no toxic effect on the retina, but 0.02 to 0.05 mg/ml extinguished the ERG and produced histologic abnormalities in the retina.[380]

a. Nelsen P, Peyman GA, Bennett TO: BB-K8: A new aminoglycoside for intravitreal injection in bacterial endophthalmitis. *AM J OPHTHALMOL* 78:82–89, 1974.

Amines are alkaline organic compounds, many of which are either irritating or damaging on contact with the eye. The volatile aliphatic amines, particularly the *methyl, ethyl,* and *propyl* or *isopropyl amines,* in vapor form are irritating to the eyes, causing burning discomfort, and at high concentrations causing destruction of the epithelium in experimental animal eyes. Injuriousness appears to be closely related to alkalinity. The aliphatic amines have strong ammonia-like odor, and like ammonia the amines tend to be fat soluble, which may favor their absorption by the corneal epithelium.

Neutralization of amines by addition of acid to form neutral salts changes them in the same manner as ammonia is changed by neutralization. Volatility is greatly reduced, and tests of neutral aqueous solutions on animal eyes show that the toxicity is also greatly reduced.

Apart from the simple aliphatic amines just discussed are other types of amines of more complex structure having toxic properties of a different sort. Certain *polyamines,* both aliphatic and aromatic (e.g., *diethylenetriamine, toluenediamine, p-phenylenediamine*), have notorious sensitizing properties. A group of *2-chloroethylamines* are extremely injurious to the eye, even in neutral solution, owing to their alkylating properties. *Cyclic imines* (ethylenimine, propylene imine) have similar serious injurious effects.

Edema of the epithelium of the cornea, generally without pain, has been produced by amine vapors, causing colored haloes to be seen around lights, usually in the evening, after industrial exposure to the vapors of various amines, including *diethylamine, diisopropylamine, dimethylamine, ethylenediamine, N-ethylmorpholine, N-ethylpiperidine, N-methylmorpholine, morpholine, tert-octylamine, tetramethylbutanediamine, tetramethyl ethylenediamine,* as described by Dernehl (1966),[40] Mastromatteo (1965),[164] Mellerio (1966),[170] and Munn (1967),[363] among others. This phenomenon has been reviewed by Jones and Kipling (1972), with their own observations on industrial vapors of *morpholine* and its derivatives.[a] Because workers commonly complained of blue vision, gray vision or haloes, they proposed the term "glaucopsia" for this symptom. Typically, vision has become misty and haloes have appeared several hours after workmen have been exposed to the vapors of these amines at concentrations too low to cause discomfort or disability during several hours of exposure. Generally the edema of the corneal epithelium, which is principally responsible for the disturbance of vision, clears spontaneously by the next day, but after exceptionally intense exposures the edema and blurring have taken several days to clear and have been accompanied by photophobia and discomfort from roughness of the corneal surface.

As described elsewhere under *Fish*, amines from decomposing fish have also been suspected as a cause of keratitis like this.

Corneal epithelial disturbance in animals have been produced by exposure to vapors of *butyl amine, diethyl amine, diisopropylamine,* and *ethyl amine;* and by instillation of the liquids *dimethylamine, N-ethyl morpholine, N-ethyl piperidine, N-methyl morpholine,* and *tetramethylenediamine.*

Dilated pupil and paralysis of accommodation, both spontaneously reversible, have occurred in people exposed to vapors of *tetramethylbutanediamine.*

Further information and bibliographic sources are available for each of the above amines by referring to the INDEX.

a. Jones WT, Kipling MD: Glaucopsia—blue-gray vision. *BR J IND MED* 29:480–481, 1972.

p-Aminoacetophenone has been tested in 0.02 M aqueous solution at pH 6.5 by dropping for ten minutes on rabbit corneas from which the epithelium had been removed. No significant corneal opacity resulted, and recovery was complete within five days.[81]

a-**Aminoadipic acid,** an analogue of glutamic acid, injected into the vitreous body of rats causes selective acute degeneration of the Muller cells, without producing morphologic changes in other elements of the retina, providing a scientific tool for study of Muller cell functions.[c] Subcutaneous injection in 9-day old rats also produced specific acute morphologic changes in the Muller cells, but these changes were gone in 24 hours.[b] In adult rabbits, intravitreal injection to damage the Muller cells caused selective changes in the ERG, increase in c-wave, extinction of b-wave, and increase in a-wave.[d] In most animal experiments a DL racemic mixture was used, but studies on chick embryo retina showed that there were differences in the morpholic changes produced by the D and the L isomers, the D form affecting glial cells, and the L form affecting both glia and neurons.[a]

a. Casper DS, Reif-Lehrer L: Effects of *a*-aminoadipate isomers on the morphology of the isolated chick embryo retina. *INVEST OPHTHALMOL VIS SCI* 24:1480–1488, 1983.
b. Karlsen RL, Pedersen OO, et al: Toxic effects of DL-*a*-aminoadipic acid on Mueller cells from rats in vivo and cultured cerebral astrocytes. *EXP EYE RES* 35:305–311, 1982.
c. Pedersen OO, Karlsen RL: Destruction of Muller cells in the adult rat by intravitreal injection of D,L aminoadipic acid. *EXP EYE RES* 28:569–575, 1979.
d. Welinder E, Textorius O, Nilsson SEG: Effects of intravitreally injected DL-*a*-aminoadipic acid on the c-wave of the D.C. recorded electroretinogram in albino rabbits. *INVEST OPHTHALMOL VIS SCI* 23:240–245, 1982.

2-Aminobutane acetate, an agent used to protect fruits and vegetables from rotting, has had no known effect on the eyes except to produce slight mydriasis in dogs fed high doses, probably due to sympathomimetic activity.[a]

a. Worth HM, Anderson RD: Safety evaluation of 2-aminobutane. *TOXICOL APPL PHARMACOL* 12:314, 1968.

2-Amino-4-n-butylaniline was found to be injurious to the cornea of rabbit eyes when 0.1 to 0.5 ml of 1% to 10% solution was applied. Swelling of the lids and inflammatory discharge were described, but the severity of injury and degree of recovery were not stated.[a]

a. Pollock JJ, Payne BJ, et al: *TOXICOL APPL PHARMACOL* 12:302, 1968.

4-Aminobutyric acid (gamma-aminobutyric acid, GABA), a compound found normally in the brain and involved in synaptic transmission, has been tested by systemic administration to immature chickens with a deficient blood-brain barrier, and has been found to alter the ERG as well as visual evoked responses.[a]

Direct electrophoretic application of 4-aminobutyric acid to ganglion cells of the retina had an inhibitory effect, similar to dopamine hydrochloride, on spontaneous and lightdriven activity of ganglion cells. The effect was readily reversible.[b]

a. Kramer SZ, Sherman PA, Seifter J: Effects of gammaaminobutyric acid (GABA) and sodium L-glutamate on the visual system and EEG of chicks. *INT J NEUROPHARMACOL* 6:463–472, 1967.
b. Straschill M, Perwein J: *PFLEUGER ARCH* 312:42–54, 1969. (*CHEM ABSTR* 72:2038, 1970.)

Aminocaproic acid (epsilon aminocaproic acid, 6-aminohexanoic acid, Amicar, Epsicapron), hemostatic, when given intravenously to cats has sympathomimetic effects, including dilated pupils and exophthalmos.[a] When given chronically by mouth it occasionally causes nasal congestion and conjunctival hyperemia.[b]

a. Cummings JR, Welter AN: Cardiovascular studies on aminocaproic acid. *TOXICOL APPL PHARMACOL* 9:57–69, 1966.
b. Today's drugs: Epsilon aminocaproic acid. *BR MED J* 2:725–726, 1967.

2-Aminoethoxyethanol tested by application of a drop to rabbit eyes was very severely injurious, similar to other strongly basic amines and alkalies.[222]

Aminoethylethanolamine tested by application of a drop to a rabbit's eye caused injury similar to that caused by acetone.[222]

N-Aminoethylmorpholine tested by application of a drop to a rabbit's eye was as severely damaging as concentrated ammonium hydroxide.[222]

4-Amino-2-hydroxytoluene applied to rabbit eyes produced only a mild conjunctival reaction.[347]

6-Aminonicotinamide, an antimetabolite of nicotinamide, inhibits the pentose phosphate shunt and induces glial alterations that secondarily cause axonal changes in rat optic nerves.[a] It is also teratogenic, causing eye defects in rats.[b]

Given systemically to human beings, it has produced blepharoconjunctivitis.[333]

   a. Meyer-Konig E: Ultrastructure of glial and axonal damage by 6-amino-nicotinamide (6-An) in the optic nerve of the rat. *ACTA NEUROPATHOL* 26:115–126, 1973. (German)
   b. Sandor S, Amels D, Checiu M: 6-Aminonicotinamide-induced eye defects in rats. *REV ROUM MEP SER MORPHOL* 24:311–323, 1978.

Aminophenazone (amidopyrine, aminopyrine, Pyramidon), an antipyretic and analgesic, rarely affects the eyes. Aminophenazone has been one of many drugs that have caused in rare individuals acute transient myopia, unaffected by cycloplegic drops, and with no abnormality discoverable by ophthalmoscope or slit-lamp.[a] (See INDEX for *Myopia, acute transient.*)

   a. Brancato R, Campana G: A case of transitory myopia after administration of amino-phenazone. *ARCH OTTALMOL* 68:503–507, 1964. (Italian)

Aminophenoxy alkanes are compounds of pharmacologic interest because of schistosomicidal activity, and of toxicologic significance because they have been found in some instances to impair vision.

Diaminodiphenoxypentane (1,5-bis[p-aminophenoxy] pentane; 1,5-di[p-amino-phenoxy] pentane; MB968A) is the aminophenoxyalkane that so far has been the subject of most investigations for toxic effects on the retina in experimental animals. When fed to monkeys, dogs, and cats, it has caused loss of vision and dilation of the pupils with almost complete loss of reaction to light.[f] Within a week the retinal vessels have appeared constricted and the optic discs pale. In about two months a gradually developing disturbance of the retinal pigment has produced an appearance resembling retinitis pigmentosa. Detailed histologic examination has demonstrated loss of visual cells and destruction of the outer nuclear layer, degeneration of the pigment epithelium, destruction of the outer limiting membrane, and migration of pigment into the retina. The bipolar cells, ganglion cells, and optic nerve were, however, relatively unaffected.[b]

In rabbits that have been given diaminodiphenoxypentane intravenously, irreversible damage is done to the retina. Electron microscopic observations by Orzalesi, Grignolo, and associates have suggested that the retinal pigment epithelium may be injured primarily, but the visual cells are affected practically simultaneously, with morphologic changes evident within thirty hours, consisting of choroidal reaction, fibrinous exudation, and macrophage migration. Rhodospin resynthesis is impaired.[j,m,94] The irreversibly damaged neuroepithelium of the rabbit retina has been found by Reading and Sorsby to have abnormally high total sulfhydryl content, and they have suggested that this may reflect denaturation of a specific protein.[207]

The ERG in rabbits poisoned with diaminodiphenoxypentane has been reported by Arden and Fojas to be altered in amplitude and form. Even at smaller doses that do not affect the ERG, they have found alteration of the corneal standing potential.

The findings indicated specific effect on biochemical reactions involved in synthesis of rhodopsin.[a] Reading has shown this biochemically.[m]

Diaminodiphenoxyheptane is another aminophenoxy alkane that has been a particular subject of investigation for its toxic effect on the retina. Sung and associates in 1957 reported that the pupils of dogs became dilated within twenty-four hours after this drug was administered orally.[l] Glocklin and Potts examined the effect of this compound on retinal biochemistry *in vitro*, finding that it reduced the incorporation of radioactive phosphorous into organic phosphates in the retinal pigment epithelium, but did not interfere with this process in the retina itself, suggesting to them that the compound had a specific inhibitory effect in the pigment epithelium, probably acting at an enzyme or cell membrane level.[g]

Testing of a large number of aminophenoxyalkanes of varied structure by oral or parenteral administration to cats and rabbits has revealed that many are toxic to the retina.[c,e,i,k]

Many diaminodiphenoxyalkanes were tested for retinotoxicity in rabbits by Sorsby and Nakajima in 1958.[k] The original publication should be consulted for identification of the various derivatives that were found to be injurious to the retina.[k] Compounds in which p-aminophenoxy groups are attached to both ends of alkane chains ranging from one to ten carbons have caused impaired vision. Also certain compounds in which the alkane chain was replaced by branched or unsaturated chains or by rings have had similar toxic effect.

The most extensive testing of aminophenoxyalkanes, especially derivatives of p-aminophenoxy pentane for retinotoxic effects was carried out by Collins and associates from 1958 through 1967. Though some generalizations have been made concerning relations of chemical structure and retinotoxicity among these compounds, the number and variety of compounds tested has been so great that the original publications should be consulted.[c,f]

1-(p-Aminophenoxy-5-phthalimido) pentane (MB2948A) deserves special mention here. It has shown relatively slight retinotoxic effect in cats but, according to Collins, has been reported by McFadzean to have reduced the visual fields in three patients when used in 1961 in treatment of schistosomiasis.[e]

1,5-(p-Aminophenyl) pentane (MB2562) also is of special interest because it has proved to be retinotoxic in cats, though it lacks the ether linkage of the typically retinotoxic p-aminophenoxy compounds.[c]

4,4'-Diaminodiphenylmethane, though similarly lacking the ether linkage of the aminophenoxyalkanes, has also had severe retinotoxic effects in animals. (See INDEX for additional information.)

Several simpler related compounds that were tested by Sorsby and Nakajima and found *not* to be damaging when administered parenterally to rabbits included the following: *p-aminophenol, p-anisidine, p-phenethidine,* and *p-aminophenoxybutane*.[k] (Topical application of *p-* or *m-aminophenol* caused slight conjunctival reaction in rabbits.)[347]

a. Arden GB, Fojas MR: The mode of action of diaminophenoxyalkanes and related compounds on the retina. *VISION RES* 2:163–174, 1962.

b. Ashton N: Degeneration of the retina due to 1,5-bis(p-aminophenoxy) pentane dihydrochloride. *J PATH BACT* 74:103–112, 1957.

c. Collins RF, Davis M, et al: The schistosomicidal and toxic effects of some di)p-aminophenoxy) alkanes and related monoamines. *BR J PHARMACOL* 13:238–243, 1958.

d. Collins RF, Davis M, et al: The schistosomicidal and toxic effects of some N-(p-aminophenoxyalkyl) amides. *BR J PHARMACOL* 14:467–475, 1959.

e. Collins RF, Cox VA, et al: The antischistosomal and retinotoxic effects of some nuclear-substituted aminophenoxyalkanes. *BR J PHARMACOL* 29:248–258, 1967.

f. Edge ND, Mason DFJ, et al: The pharmacological effects of certain diaminodiphenoxy alkanes. *NATURE* 178:806–807, 1956.

g. Glocklin VS, Potts AM: The metabolism of retinal pigment cell epithelium. *INVEST OPHTHALMOL* 1:111–116, 1962.

h. Goodwin LG, Richards WHG, Udall V: The toxicity of diaminophenoxyalkanes. *BR J PHARMACOL* 12:468–474, 1957.

i. Nakajima A: The effect of aminophenoxy alkanes on the rabbit ERG. *OPHTHALMOLOGICA* 136:332–344, 1958.

j. Orzalesi N, Grignolo A, et al: A study on the fine structure and the rhodopsin cycle of the rabbit retina in experimental degeneration induced by diaminodiphenoxypentane. *EXP EYE RES* 6:376–382, 1967.

k. Sorsby A, Nakajima A: Experimental degeneration of the retina. *BR J OPHTHALMOL* 42:563–570, 1958.

l. Sung CY, Chang HY, et al: The toxicity and pharmacological actions of p,p'-diaminodiphenoxyheptane, a compound with schistosomicidal activity. *YOAHSUEH HSUEH PAO* 5:208–217, 1957. (*CHEM ABSTR* 55:25039, 1961.)

m. Reading HW: Effects of a retinotoxic phenoxyalkane on the visual cycle in rabbit retinae. *BIOCHEM PHARMACOL* 19:1307–1313, 1970.

Aminophylline (theophylline-ethylenediamine, theophyllamine), a smooth muscle relaxant, myocardial stimulant, and diuretic[171] when administered orally is said to be without significant influence on the ocular pressure in glaucomatous patients;[a] but if given intravenously it has been reported to cause transient rapid reduction of ocular pressure in glaucoma.[b] It apparently has had no significant toxic effects on the eye.

a. Smeral L, Rehak S, Juran J: Combination of tonography with loading tests for early diagnosis of glaucoma. *CESK OFTALMOL* 20:289–293, 1964; *ZENTRALBL GES OPHTHALMOL* 95:114, 1965. (German)

b. De Michele T, Serafini A: Effect of aminophylline on the tension of the eye. *ANN OTTALMOL CLIN OCUL* 90:245–249, 1964. (Italian)

β-Aminopropionitrile (3-aminopropionitrile) has been tested for toxic actions on the eye in relation to osteolathyrism. (See INDEX for *Lathyrism.*)

In vitro in ox cornea it has inhibited incorporation of radioactive sulfate into the acid mucopolysaccharides, but has caused no elution of mucopolysaccharides or collagen.[g] It had no effect on consumption of oxygen, binding of radioactive phosphorous, or formation of lactic acid.[g]

In animal tissues, β-aminopropionitrile interferes with cross-linking of collagen.[b] In rats it causes corneal collagen fibers to be abnormally small and disorganized.[a] In rabbits it has caused full-thickness corneal wounds to heal with abnormally low tensile strength.[c]

These properties of the compound have been exploited experimentally with therapeutic aims. It has been applied to alkali-burned rabbit eyes to interfere with shrinkage of conjunctiva in the process of scarring.[d] It has been applied to rabbit eyes after radial keratotomy to prevent regression of refraction.[f] It has been given to rabbits to interfere with vitreous proliferation after posterior penetrating wounds.[e] In each of these therapeutic applications it has been reported effective.

a. Bettelheim FA, Wang TJY: Lathyritic cornea. *EXP EYE RES* 19:511–519, 1974.
b. Brettschneider I, Praus R: Effect of lathyrogens on glycosaminoglycans of bovine cornea *in vitro. OPHTHALMIC RES* 1:220–227, 1970.
c. Denlinger D, Keates RH: Effect of β-aminopropionitrile on corneal wound strength. *ANN OPHTHALMOL* 16:625–627, 1984.
d. Moorhead LC: Inhibition of collagen cross-linkage: A new approach to ocular scarring. *CURR EYE RES* 1:77–83, 1981.
e. Moorhead LC: Effects of β-aminopropionitrile after posterior penetrating injury in the rabbit. *AM J OPHTHALMOL* 95:97–109, 1983.
f. Moorhead LC, Carroll J, et al: Effects of topical treatment with β-aminopropionitrile after radial keratotomy in the rabbit. *ARCH OPHTHALMOL* 102:304–307, 1984.
g. Praus R, Brettschneider I: Effect of lathyrogens on the cornea. *CESK OFTALMOL* 21:244–248, 1965; 22:249–255, 1966.

Aminotriazole (3-amino-1H-1,2,4-triazole; Amizol; Amitrol) a herbicide and cotton-defoliant has been found to produce cataracts in young rabbits, and to reduce the catalase activity of the lens.[a] The loss of catalase can cause a 2 to 3 fold increase in hydrogen peroxide in aqueous and vitreous humors, without change in glutathione peroxidase, glutathione, or ascorbate concentration.[b,c] However, excessive hydrogen peroxide inhibits lens superoxide dismutase, which may render the lens vulnerable to superoxide ions or hydroxyl radicals.[c]

In incubated human and animal lenses addition of aminotriazole has been shown to enhance yellowing or browning of the lens nucleus during exposure to ultraviolet.[e,f] The coloration is attributed to formation of a fluorogen like that associated with aging and development of nuclear sclerosis and presbyopia in human beings. Under experimental conditions in which aminotriazole causes decrease in lens glutathione it has been supposed that loss of this scavenger of free radicals leaves the lens abnormally unprotected from free radicals generated by ultraviolet irradiation.[e,f]

a. Bhuyan KC, Bhuyan DK, Katzin HM: Amizol-induced cataract and inhibition of lens catalase in rabbit. *OPHTHALMIC RES* 5:236–247, 1973.
b. Bhuyan KC, Bhuyan DK, Turtz AI: Aminotriazole. Effect on the ocular tissues in rabbit. *IRCS LIBR COMPEND* 2:1594, 1974.
c. Bhuyan KC, Bhuyan DK: Regulation of hydrogen peroxide in eye humors. *BIOCHEM BIOPHYS ACTA* 497:641–651, 1977; 542:28–38, 1978.
d. Bhuyan KC, Bhuyan DK: Mechanism of cataractogenesis induced by 3-amino-1H-1,2,4-triazole. *BIOCHEM CLIN ASPECTS OXYGEN* (Proc Symp 1978) 785–809. Ed. by WS and H Caughey. Academic: New York, NY 1979

e. Lerman S, Kuck JF, et al: Acceleration of an aging parameter (Fluorogen) in the ocular lens. *ANN OPHTHALMOL* 8:558–562, 1976.

f. Lerman S, Kuck FJ, et al: Induction, acceleration and prevention (in vitro) of an aging parameter in the ocular lens. *OPHTHALMIC RES* 8:213–226, 1976.

Amiodarone (Cordarone, Atlansil, Trangorex), a coronary vasodilator related to Benziodarone, produces deposits in the corneal epithelium in patients after they have taken this medication daily for one to four months, eventually occurring in practically all patients. The deposits resemble very closely those produced by chloroquine. No difficulties have been experienced from these deposits apart from an appearance of haloes around lights or fogging of vision in a very small proportion of patients. The deposits have regularly disappeared in a few months when medication has been stopped, and there have been no aftereffects. The deposits have been described as consisting of myriads of fine yellowish dots in the corneal epithelium, sometimes condensed in a line and sometimes in arborescent pattern, predominantly in the palpebral fissure.

Since 1968 many series of cases have been published. Most are listed in the accompanying bibliography, but only publications containing something specially noteworthy will be cited in the text.

Extensive clinical studies have usually revealed no abnormalities of the eyes other than keratopathy that could be definitely considered attributable to the drug. These studies have included measurements of intraocular pressure, visual fields, flicker fusion frequency, color vision, absolute light sensitivity (dark adaptation), ERG, EOG, fluorescein angiography, and ophthalmoscopy (Babel; Deodati; Francois; Watillon).

The first histologic study of corneal deposits in a patient who had been treated with amiodarone was reported by Toussaint and Pohl, who found the deposits to consist of lysosomal inclusions, probably of lipofuscins, in the cytoplasm of the cells. They thought that this finding was more likely a product of altered cellular metabolism than a deposit of the drug or its metabolites.[g] (Later studies classified the condition as "lipidosis", or "phospholipidosis". See bibliography. Also see INDEX for *Lipidosis.*) Similar findings were reported by Verin and by Brini. D'Amico found in biopsy material membranous lamellar intralysosomal deposits in corneal and conjunctival epithelium, and in the lens epithelium. Ghosk and McCulloch in two post-mortem eyes also found these bodies, which they likened to myelin, but they were present not only in the cornea, conjunctiva and lens, but also in iris, ciliary body, retina and choroid. Clinically no ocular abnormalities had been evident in these patients other than the common amiodarone keratopathy.

After deposits in the lens were found in the above studies, a very careful clinical search by Flach and colleagues revealed in the lenses of 7 out of 14 patients taking the drug "tiny white-yellow punctate, anterior subcapsular deposits that clustered within the pupillary aperture." They resembled the deposits that are associated with chlorpromazine, and did not interfere with vision. Dahl also had suspected anterior subcapsular lens opacities from amiodarone, associated with typical keratopathy, in a patient age 42 whom he had examined closely before and five months after starting this medication.

Experimentally in rats, Bockhardt and colleagues succeeded in producing corneal epithelial inclusions by administering amiodarone topically, but not by giving it orally. Liposomal inclusions were also induced in the rats' retinal pigment epithelium, retinal ganglion and Muller's cells, and in the ciliary epithelium and iris.

The findings in human and rat retinas raise the question whether there is some related but undiscovered disturbance of retinal functions.

Alzner E: Corneal deposits from amiodarone treatment. *KLIN MONATSBL AUGEN-HEILKD* 185:333–334, 1984. (German)

Babel J, Stangos N: Iatrogenic ocular lesions; effect of a new medication for angina pectoris. *OPHTHALMOLOGICA* 161:115–117, 1970; *ARCH OPHTALMOL (Paris)* 30:197–208, 1970. (French)

Babel J, Stangos N: The action of amiodarone on the eye. *SCHWEIZ MED WSCHR* 120:220–223, 1972. (French)

Babel J, Leuenberger PM: Ultrastructural changes in the cornea after administration of certain drugs. *BER DTSCH OPHTHAL GESELLSCH* 71:18–23, 1972. (German)

Bockhardt H, Drenckhahn D, Lullmann-Rauch R: Amiodarone-induced lipidosis-like alterations in ocular tissues of rats. *GRAEFES ARCH OPHTHALMOL* 207:91–96, 1978.

Bonamour G, Bonnet M, Bouattour M: Corneal lesions in the course of treatment with amiodarone. *BULL SOC OPHTALMOL FRANCE* 70:534–538, 1970. (French)

Brini A, Porte A, Flament J: Corneal lesions from cordarone (amiodarone). *BULL SOC OPHTALMOL FRANCE* 72:83–87, 1972. (French)

Bronner A, Payeur G: Corneal ulceration after prolonged treatment with amiodarone. *BULL SOC OPHTALMOL FRANCE* 70:927–929, 1970. (French)

Chew E, Ghosh M, McCulloch C: Amiodarone-induced cornea verticillata. *CAN J OPHTHALMOL* 17:96–99, 1982.

D'Amico DJ, Kenyon KR, Ruskin JN: Amiodarone keratopathy. Drug-induced lipid storage disease. *ARCH OPHTHALMOL* 99:257–261, 1981.

Dahl A: Personal communication, March 1981.

Darleguy P, Blade J, Gacon R, Riu R: Ocular reverberation in the course of treatment with cordarone. *BULL SOC OPHTALMOL FRANCE* 71:82–92, 1971. (French)

DeCarvalha CA, Betinjane AJ: Cornea verticillata—amiodarone. *REV BRAS OFTALMOL* 35:485–488, 1976. (Portuguese)

Deodati F, Bec P, Cuq G, Vergnes R: Corneal thesaurismosis in treatment with amiodarone hydrochloride. *BULL SOC OFTALMOL FRANCE* 69:967–973, 1969. (French)

Feiler-Ofry V, Lazar M, et al: Amiodarone keratopathy. *OPHTHALMOLOGICA* 180:257–261, 1980.

Flach AJ, Dolan BJ, et al: Amiodarone-induced lens opacities. *ARCH OPHTHALMOL* 101:1554–1556, 1983.

Flach AJ, Peterson JS, Dolan BJ: Anterior subcapsular cataracts. *ANN OPHTHALMOL* 17:78–80, 1985.

Francois J: Cornea verticillata. *BULL SOC BELGE OPHTALMOL* 150:656–670, 1968. (French)

Francois J: Cornea verticillata. *DOC OPHTHALMOL* 27:235–250, 1969.

Ghosh M, McCulloch C: Amiodarone-induced ultrastructural changes in human eyes. *CAN J OPHTHALMOL* 19:178–186, 1984.

Harris L, McKenna WJ, et al: Side effects and possible complications of amiodarone use. *AM HEART J* 106:916–923, 1983.

Hurlez C, et al: Cutaneous and ocular complications of recent coronary dilator agents. *BULL ACAD NATL MED (Paris)* 155:671–679, 1971.

Ingram DV, Jaggarao NSV, Chamberlain DA: Ocular changes resulting from therapy with amiodarone. *BR J OPHTHALMOL* 66:676–679, 1982.

Ingram DV: Ocular effects in long-term amiodarone therapy. *AM HEART J* 106:902–905, 1983.

Kaplan LJ, Cappaert WE: Amiodarone keratopathy. Correlation to dosage and duration. *ARCH OPHTHALMOL* 100:601–602, 1982.

Kaplan LJ, Cappaert WE: Amiodarone-induced corneal deposits. *ANN OPHTHALMOL* 16:762–766, 1984.

Kingele TG, Alves LE, Rose EP: Amiodarone keratopathy. *ANN OPHTHALMOL* 16:1172–1176, 1984.

Leyder A: Disturbance of the cornea in the course of treatment with amiodarone (Thesis, Nancy, 1969). (French)

Mascarell EV: Corneal ulcer appearing during treatment with amiodarone. *REV ESP OTONEUROOFTALMOL NEUROCIR* 32:127–130, 1974. (Spanish)

Miglior M: Keratopathy from amiodarone. *ANN OTTALMOL CLIN OCUL* 101:67–74, 1975. (Italian)

Miller HA: Keratopathy following treatment with Cordarone. *BULL SOC OPHTALMOL FRANCE* 12:1059–1065, 1969. (French)

Moreau P-G, Pichon P: Corneal lesions from amiodarone. *BULL SOC OPHTALMOL FRANCE* 70:538–543, 1970. (French)

Nielsen CE, Andreasen F, Bjerregaard P: Amiodarone induced cornea verticillata. *ACTA OPHTHALMOL* 61:474–480, 1983.

Peyresblanques J: Keratopathy from cordarone. *BULL SOC OPHTALMOL FRANCE* 69:973–977, 1969. (French)

Pochulu AM: Corneal thesaurismosis from Cordarone (Thesis, Bordeaux, 1970): *ARCH OPHTALMOL (Paris)* 31:455–456, 1971. (French)

Thilges V: Cordarone, cause of micro-deposits in the corneal epithelium resembling those from chloroquine. *ANN OCULIST (Paris)* 203:151–157, 1970.

Thilges V: Corneal thesaurismosis from cordarone. *ANN OCULIST (Paris)* 206:385–392, 1973. (French)

Toussaint D, Pohl S: Histologic and ultrastructural aspects of the corneal deposits caused by amiodarone hydrochloride. *BULL SOC BELGE OPHTALMOL* 153:675–686, 1969. (French)

Verin P, Blanquet P, Gendre P, et al: Current knowledge about the medication-induced corneal thesaurismosis from cordarone. *BULL SOC BELGE OPHTALMOL* 160:591–600, 1972. (French)

Verin P, Sekkat A: A new drug-induced eye disease: amiodarone thesaurismosis. *KLIN MONATSBL AUGENHEILKD* 162:675–680, 1973. (German)

Watillon M, Lavergne G, Weekers JF: Corneal lesions in the course of treatment with cordarone (amiodarone hydrochloride). *BULL SOC BELGE OPHTALMOL* 150:715–726, 1968. (French)

Watillon M, Robe-Vanwyck A: IX. Cardiovascular drugs. The noxious effects of systemic medications on the visual apparatus (J Michiels, ed). *BULL SOC BELGE OPHTALMOL* 160:185–192, 1972. (French)

Wilson FW, Schmitt TE, Grayson M: Amiodarone-induced cornea verticillata. *ANN OPHTHALMOL* 12:657–660, 1980.

Amitriptyline (Elavil), an antidepressant and tranquilizing drug, frequently causes the pupil to dilate slightly and interferes with accommodation for near because of atropine-like anticholinergic action.[244] This effect has been accentuated in cases of accidental poisoning in children.[e] Visual hallucinations are reported to have been produced in three cases.[b] In a case of acute overdosage (225 mg) a patient in light coma had temporary complete oculomotor paresis, unresponsive to caloric stimulation or doll's head maneuvers.[d]

Precipitation of angle-closure glaucoma in predisposed elderly individuals with shallow anterior chambers and narrow angles might logically be feared from use of amitriptyline, because it has a slight anticholinergic mydriatic effect. An estimate by Lowe of the incidence of this type of glaucoma indicated it might not be more than one per thousand users of the drug, with no conclusive evidence that the drug was responsible or that the incidence was greater than for spontaneous occurrence of this type of glaucoma in a comparable population.[c] Specific cases in which amitriptyline has been suspected, but not proven, to have contributed to glaucoma in eyes with shallow anterior chambers have been briefly described by Rosselet and Fagioni.[210]

In cats, amitriptyline has been found to become highly concentrated in the uvea after intravenous injection, but the functional or toxicologic significance of this is not known yet.[a] Experimental evidences of effects on retinal function and on the visual cortex have been obtained in cats by Heiss and associates, but the significance of this too is yet to be learned.[105, 106]

In mice, amitriptyline is one of many drugs that produces a rapid but reversible clouding of the lens, if the eyes are allowed to remain open and unprotected from evaporation.[261]

a. Cassano GB, Sjostrand SE, et al: Eye distribution of chlorpromazine, amitriptyline, thiopentone and phenobarbitone in the cat. *EXP EYE RES* 7:196–199, 1968.
b. Hudgens RW, Tanna VL, et al: Visual hallucinations with iminodibenzyl antidepressants. *J AM MED ASSOC* 198:81–82, 1966.
c. Lowe RF: Amitriptyline and glaucoma. *MED J AUST* 2:509–510, 1966.
d. Mladinick EK, Carlow TJ: Total gaze paresis in amitriptyline overdose. *NEUROLOGY* 27:695, 1977.
e. Steel CM, O'Duffy J, Brown SS: Clinical effects and treatment of imipramine and amitriptyline poisoning in children. *BR MED J* 2:663–667, 1967.

Ammeline, a herbicide, has been found to cause blindness in chicks when fed for 6 days.[a,b] The a- and b-waves of the ERG disappeared in 3 days, and histologically changes appeared, first in the retinal pigment epithelium, then in the rod and cone outer and inner segments.

a. Takahashi K: Early receptor potential and retinal degeneration. *ACTA SOC OPHTHALMOL JPN* 78:79–92, 1974. (English abstract).
b. Matsubara H, Obara Y: Studies on the biological activity of heterocyclic compounds. *NIPPON NOGEI KAGAKU KAISHI* 52:123–127, 1978. (English abstract).

Ammi majus seeds (bishops weed) when ingested by ducks, geese and cattle causes photosensitization and sunburn. The plant is said to have been used in the Middle East since 2300 BC to treat disorders of pigmentation of the skin in human beings.[c] Psoralens which can be extracted from the plant are in current use in conjunction with long wavelength ultraviolet particularly in treatment of psoriasis and vitiligo. (See further under *Methoxsalen.*)

Ducks and geese exposed to sunlight and fed the seeds develop widely dilated pupils from atrophy of the iris sphincter muscle.[a] They also show keratoconjunctivitis and burning and necrosis of the skin. When photosensitized in this way ducklings have been shown to develop vacuolization of their retinal ganglion cells, and later pigmentary retinopathy with hyperplasia of the retinal pigment epithelium and congestion of vessels at the periphery of the choroid.[b] At this stage there is edema of the optic disc, retina and choroid.

a. Barishak YR, Beemer AM, et al: Histology of the iris in geese and ducks photosensitized by ingestion of Ammi majus seeds. *ACTA OPHTHALMOL* 53:585–590, 1975.

b. Barishak YR, Beemer AM, et al: Histology of the retina and choroid in ducklings photosensitized by feeding Ammi majus seeds. *OPHTHALMIC RES* 8:169–178, 1976.

c. Thompson RC: A Dictionary of Assyrian Botany, 1949.

Ammonia is a colorless gas, having a characteristic strong pungent odor perceptible at concentrations greater than 50 ppm in air.[171] Ammonia is readily liquified under pressure, and liquid ammonia is manufactured in enormous quantities, shipped in steel cylinders or by special truck or railroad tank car, used as a fertilizer, as a refrigerant, and in manufacture of other chemicals. Ammonia is very soluble in water, with which it combines to form ammonium hydroxide. The strongest aqueous solution commonly available contains 28% to 29% ammonia. A 10% solution is also in common use. "Household ammonia" contains 7%.

Gaseous ammonia at concentrations which may be injurious to the eye causes stinging and pain, which induces protective tearing and blepharospasm. As a result, ammonia gas in the air may irritate, but does not injure the eye except under special circumstances of unconsciousness, or forceful blasting of a stream of concentrated gas into the eye before reflex closure of the lids.

Ammonia is slightly irritant to human eyes at a concentration of 140 ppm in air and immediately irritating at 700 ppm.[e,188] Ammonia is especially irritating and damaging to the respiratory tract. The maximum concentration considered safe for eight hour exposure is 100 ppm.[e] Rabbits and guinea pigs exposed for two to three days to concentrations of ammonia in air which were very irritating to the respiratory passages caused no damage to the corneal epithelium detectible by slit-lamp examination or fluorescein staining.[81] However, continuous exposure for several weeks to 470 mg/cu meter caused much irritation of the eyes of dogs and rabbits, and produced opacity over one-fourth to one-half of the cornea in rabbits.[296]

In human beings it is questionable whether chronic exposure to ammonia gas in air has caused anything more than hyperemia of the conjunctiva and lids. In rare instances it has been claimed that keratitis epithelialis was produced by low concentrations of ammonia occurring in sewers and stables. It is more probable that the keratitis epithelialis was actually caused by *hydrogen sulfide.*

In a single instance a fine band-shaped corneal clouding with slight impairment of vision has been ascribed to chronic exposure to ammonia in the air.[v] Only one eye of the patient had significant abnormality, consisting of a band of very fine gray dots superficially in the cornea in a horizontal band across the pupillary area, reducing vision to 0.5 but causing no irritation or other symptoms. The supposed role of ammonia was in no way investigated and was merely a guess.

High concentrations of gaseous ammonia have caused acute corneal injury in accidents in which individuals were trapped where they could not escape, and in which they received severe or even lethal damage to the respiratory tract.[b] Similarly, a forceful blast of concentrated ammonia gas directed into the eyes has been observed to cause serious ocular damage having the same characteristics as injuries produced by splash contact with liquefied ammonia or strong aqueous ammonia.[u,t] This has been substantiated by animal experiment.[81]

Sprays of liquefied ammonia from refrigeration machines or storage tanks and splashes of concentrated aqueous ammonium hydroxide appear to have been among the commonest causes of serious chemical injury of the eye. During the past one-hundred years many descriptive case reports have been published.[f, h, k, p, s, v, 46, 129, 153, 242, 249, 253]

Typically, ammonia tends to cause more corneal endothelial damage, corneal stromal edema, iritis, and lens damage, and less immediate pearly gray or white opacification of the corneal stroma than do other common alkalies such as sodium hydroxide or calcium hydroxide. A great variation in severity of injury is encountered clinically on account of variation in amount, concentration, and duration of exposure of the eye.

The least serious injuries have naturally been associated with low concentration and prompt irrigation. For example, in a case in which one drop of ammonium hydroxide solution of approximately 9% concentration was accidentally applied to a patient's eye, and irrigation with water was started within ten seconds because of immediate severe pain and blepharospasm, the pH of the conjunctiva and cornea was found by testing with indicator paper within three minutes to have returned to normal, yet most of the corneal epithelium was already lost.[81] The next day there was slight corneal edema and wrinkling of the posterior surface, but the eye recovered completely in three or four days.

More severe injury has developed in cases in which there was slightly longer delay in instituting irrigation, or a droplet of more concentrated ammonium hydroxide solution had contacted the eye. In such cases, soon after exposure and first aid treatment the corneal epithelium has characteristically been absent over the lower portions of the cornea, but the stroma has appeared clear. Typically, by the next day the involved portion of the cornea has developed bluish stromal edema with grossly evident wrinkling of the posterior surface, attributable to injury of the endothelium. With a limited area of corneal involvement and no initial opacification and no iritis or injury of the lens, complete recovery has occurred in such cases in the course of a week or two.

In severe injuries, where concentrated ammonium hydroxide solution or liquefied ammonia has splashed into the eye, or following contact with dilute solutions but with delay in first aid irrigation, thrombosis of conjunctival and episcleral vessels, evident on biomicroscopic examination, may early give the eye unnatural pallor and a cooked appearance. However, because of the tendency of the cornea in severe ammonia burns not to show as much immediate opacification as from other common alkalies, the severity of injury may not be evident for several days. Complete anesthesia of the cornea early after exposure to ammonia is taken as a sign of severe injury.[34]

Severe ammonia burns develop all the serious complications caused by strong alkalies in general. (See INDEX for *Alkalies*.) Ammonia has greater tendency than other alkalies to penetrate and damage the iris, and to cause cataract, which in exceptional cases may be evident within a day following ammonia burn of the eye.[j] Iritis may be accompanied by hypopyon or hemorrhages, and there may be extensive loss of pigment from the posterior pigment layer of the iris, and severe glaucoma. Cataract in some cases develops later.

In cases in which atrophy of the iris and cataract occur, the cornea usually is irreparably damaged and ultimately becomes opaque. The following case is an example of such a course.[c] A man was filling carboys with concentrated aqueous ammonium hydroxide and was accidentally squirted in both eyes. His eyes were immediately irrigated with water. Vision was not seriously impaired until about ten days following injury, when vision became worse and cataracts were observed. In about a month the cataracts were mature. By slit-lamp examination, in both eyes the posterior surface of the cornea and anterior surface of the lens were seen to be coated with pigment from degeneration of the iris. The intraocular pressures were between 40 and 50 mm Hg. The corneas were still clear enough at that time so that an uncomplicated, intracapsular cataract extraction was performed in both eyes, and vision of 20/40 was obtained with correcting lenses. However, in the course of the next two months the corneas gradually became almost totally opaque, thickened and vascularized, both deep in the stroma and superficially, reducing vision to hand movements close before the eyes. Hypopyon could be barely discerned in one eye, and the tensions had become subnormal.[c]

A similar case, in which there was severe injury of the iris with detachment of the pigment layer, early complete cataract, but slow development of corneal opacity and vascularization, was reported in detail with histologic examination in 1936 by Kiss.[j]

A third case of similar severity has been observed and treated in a different manner.[c] A spray of liquified ammonia struck both eyes, causing much edema of the corneal stroma and reduction of vision. Twelve days later the corneal edema decreased enough to reveal extensive atrophy of each iris, dense cataracts, hypopyons, and much pigment deposited on the posterior surface of the corneas. After a month the intraocular pressures were found elevated to 40 or 50 mm Hg. Treatment with pilocarpine and acetazolamide was rather ineffectual. After two months, despite continuing glaucoma and a persisting completely white ischemic band encircling both corneas, the corneal thickening decreased and transparency improved, not sufficient, however, to distinguish by gonioscopy whether the glaucoma was due to peripheral anterior synechias or pigment accumulation in the trabecular meshwork, or other cause. The corneas were still completely anesthetic. Paracentesis and evacuation of aqueous humor on two occasions washed considerable pigment loose from the anterior chamber, but did not appear to relieve the glaucoma for more than a day or two. Cataract extraction was postponed with the hope that the eyes might be able to tolerate operation better if the ischemic pericorneal tissues had time to revascularize. Five months after injury, cyclodialysis was performed on each eye because of glaucoma, and one mature cataract was extracted. The corneas remained thick and the deepest layers irregular and opaque. Vision was then counting fingers at a few inches with the better eye.

Acute glaucoma within four hours after severe ammonia burns of the eye has been very well documented in two cases by Highman (1969). The striking features were corneal edema and oval semidilated fixed pupil, suggestive of acute angle-closure glaucoma, but other clinical findings, including gonioscopy, indicated at this time that the angles most likely were open. The intraocular pressures were satisfactorily reduced initially by oral acetazolamide and pilocarpine eyedrops. The damage to the eyes by the ammonia, which had been squirted into the eyes in the course of a robbery, was very severe in both cases, leading later to development of cataracts and progressively increasing edema and opacification of the corneas. Also, glaucoma recurred in both cases, after ten days in one, and after a year in the other. The glaucoma at this later stage was caused in both cases by closure of the angle and formation of peripheral anterior synechias in association with cataract and obstruction of the pupil. Iridectomies and cataract extractions were performed, but chronic glaucoma due to peripheral anterior synechias persisted, requiring continuing use of acetazolamide. In both cases the eyes had been so damaged by the ammonia that they were essentially useless.[h]

These several cases suggest that a typical course for an eye badly damaged by concentrated ammonium hydroxide or liquid ammonia may consist of rapid development of corneal edema and swelling, corneal anesthesia, acute open-angle glaucoma with tension 30 to 50 mm Hg, oval and permanently unreactive pupil. This may be followed by a second stage after some weeks during which there is development of cataract and severe secondary glaucoma attributable either to obstruction of the pupil, with secondary angle-closure and formation of peripheral anterior synechias, or to atrophy of the iris and dissemination of pigment and other decomposition products to obstruct aqueous outflow channels. At this stage one may still be able to see through the cornea well enough to evaluate what is going on in the anterior chamber and to obtain useful vision for the patient by extraction of the cataractous lens, but it seems that generally after this seemingly encouraging phase, there is characteristically a progression of the opacification of the cornea. Scarring and vascularization may become so severe that keratoplasty is impractical, and phthisis with band keratopathy may develop. The treatments employed so far, including corticosteroids, antiglaucoma medications, and surgery, appear to have been ineffectual.

In an apparently less severe case, anterior subcapsular lens opacities similar to Glaukomflecken have been described by McGuinness in a patient who had ammonia thrown in the eye. She had severe damage to the cornea, and discoloration and distortion of the iris, but no elevation of intraocular pressure was detected. The lens opacities did not progress during five months of observation.[m]

Ballantyne has demonstrated that application of 0.1 ml of an ammonia solution as dilute as 1% to eyes of rabbits can evoke a prompt rise of intraocular pressure to 70% above normal.[276]

Experimental studies of ammonia burns have been concerned mostly with evaluating the concentration and time of exposure required to induce injuries in animal eyes, or have been concerned with the ability of ammonia to penetrate into the eye, and with evaluating possible means of treatment. Little has been learned of the mechanism of chemical damage of tissues by ammonia, other than discovery of a rapid loss of mucoid from the cornea, the same as occurs in other strong alkali burns. The histology has been examined in detail.[j,161] One misconception regarding the action of ammonia which has been many times repeated in the literature concerns a supposed dehydrating or water-withdrawing effect, which has never actually been established, nor is there a sound theoretical basis for postulating such an action.

Among studies of penetration of ammonia into the eye, Pichler in 1910 exposed rabbit eyes to 10% ammonium hydroxide solution, and tested the aqueous humor for ammonium ions with Nessler's reagent, finding a very strong reaction in ten minutes, and persistence of ammonium ions in the anterior chamber for at least two hours, but none was discoverable in the vitreous humor.[q] Similarly, Siegrist in 1920 applied ammonium hydroxide solution to rabbit eyes and found that ammonium ions by the same chemical test were first definitely detectable in the aqueous humor in five seconds, with the concentration increasing greatly during the first minute.[r] Neither investigator determined how alkaline the aqueous became. Hoffman in 1922 experimented on rabbit and ox eyes, and found that the aqueous humor of rabbits became alkaline to litmus in ten minutes after 10% aqueous ammonium hydroxide was applied to the cornea.[i]

Because of the chemical evidences of rapid penetration and the clinical evidences of injury of iris and lens in the most severe cases, it has been suggested that surgical paracentesis and release of the aqueous humor from the anterior chamber might be beneficial. In experiments on three rabbits, Siegrist reported obtaining slight benefit by this procedure, but the benefit was so slight that a much larger number of treated and control animals would be needed to establish statistical significance.[r] Furthermore, it has been suggested that repeated paracentesis be employed because of the chemical detection of ammonium ions in the aqueous humor for more than two hours following experimental exposure. An important point ignored in early investigations is that the ammonium ion itself is well tolerated in the anterior chamber, and that it is the hydroxyl ion concentration, or pH, which is significant relative to injury.[g,89]

In rabbits, application of 28.5% ammonium hydroxide to the eyes for two to twenty seconds (before irrigation with water) causes injury ranging from faint permanent corneal nebula to profound corneal opacification and vascularization proportional to the length of exposure, but paracentesis performed 0.5 to 45 minutes after exposure is without benefit to eyes exposed in this manner.[g,89] Measurement of the pH of the aqueous humor removed from these eyes revealed a maximum alkalinity of pH 9.8 at 3.5 minutes after the most severe (20 seconds) exposure. However, no cataract or severe injury of the iris occurred either in paracentesed or untreated eyes, despite devastating corneal damage. This is quite different from what typically occurs in human eyes with severe ammonia burns, in which there is usually a longer period before first-aid irrigation.

In rabbits, it was established that the anterior chamber could be irrigated for several minutes with saline solutions adjusted to pH 10 (with ammonium, sodium, or calcium hydroxide) without causing permanent injury to the iris or lens.[89] Whether the iris and lens may be less subject to injury by elevated pH in rabbits than in human beings has not been determined. The experimental data so far available suggest that paracentesis would be of no significant value in treatment of ammonia-burned eyes unless the exposures were more severe than in the experiments, or the intraocular structures of the human eye should prove to be more vulnerable than those of the animal.[g]

For further discussion of alkali burns and treatment, see INDEX for *Alkalies,* and for *Treatment of Chemical Burns.*

Mixtures of ammonia with hypochlorite produce additional substances that are toxic to the cornea, which may be encountered when household cleaning agents are mixed, also in swimming pool water in low concentration. (See INDEX for *Hypochlorite-ammonia mixtures.*)

b. Caplin M: Ammonia gas poisoning. *LANCET* 2:95–96, 1941.

c. Chandler PA, Johnson L: Personal communications.

e. Clinton M: Toxicological review on ammonia. *AM PETROLEUM INST* 104, 1948.

f. Editorial: Ammonia in the eyes. *BR MED J* 2:430, 1969.

g. Grant WM: Experimental investigation of paracentesis in the treatment of ocular ammonia burns. *ARCH OPHTHALMOL* 44:399–404, 1950.

h. Highman VN: Early rise in intraocular pressure after ammonia burns. *BR MED J* 1:359–360, 1969.

i. Hoffman V: Experiment to test the rapidity of diffusion of ammonia solution in the eye. *ARCH AUGENHEILKD* 91:300–307, 1922. (German)

j. Kiss W: Early injury of the iris and lens in ammonia burn of the eye. *ARCH AUGENHEILKD* 98–105, 1937. (German)

k. Kearsky AK: Autoplastic transplantation of the cornea and conjunctiva in an alkaline burn of the eye. *VESTN OFTALMOL* 79:65–67, 1966. (*ZENTRALBL GES OPHTHALMOL* 97:157, 1966.)

l. Levy DM, Divertie MB, Litzow TJ: Ammonia burns of the face and respiratory tract. *J AM MED ASSOC* 190:873–876, 1964.

m. McGuiness R: Ammonia in the eye. *BR MED J* 1:575, 1969.

n. Osmand AH, Tallents CJ: Ammonia attacks. *BR MED J* 2:740, 1968.

o. Peyresblanques J, Clabe M: Accidents to the eyes in paper manufacture in the Landais region. *ANN OCULIST (Paris)* 199:683–698, 1966. (French)

p. Peyresblanques J, LeGoff J: Burns of the eye by ammonia in agriculture. *BULL SOC OPHTALMOL FRANCE* 68:877–879, 1968. (French)

q. Pichler A: Ammonia burn of the eyes and skin. *Z AUGENHEILKD* 23:279–321, 1910. (German)

r. Siegrist A: Action of concentrated alkali and acid on the eye. *Z AUGENHEILKD* 43:176–194, 1920. (German)

s. Takemoto Y: Complete cure of ocular damage due to ammonia occurring in traffic accidents. *JPN J CLIN OPHTHALMOL* 19:1049–1056, 1965. (*ZENTRALBL GES OPHTHALMOL* 96:151, 1966.)

t. Thies O: Most severe ammonia burn of both eyes. *KLIN MONATSBL AUGENHEILKD* 70:769, 1923. (German)

u. Thies O: A case of the most severe ammonia burn with bilateral development of secondary cataracts and finally blindness. *KLIN MONATSBL AUGENHEILKD* 72:378–382, 1924. (German)

v. Trantas A: Superficial keratitis from ammoniacal vapors. *RECUEIL OPHTALMOL* 31:16–19, 1909. (French)

w. Zucchini G: Concerning an unusual case of hematoma of the corneal stroma secondary to alkali burn. *ANN OTTALMOL CLIN OCUL* 88:161–165, 1962. (Italian)

Ammonium chloride in solution in contact with the eye is well tolerated. Clinically, 5% to 10% aqueous solution has occasionally been used to irrigate the surface of the eye in the treatment of chemical burns, and no injury has been attributed to the treatment.[176]

Experimentally in rabbits, replacement of the aqueous humor with 1% solution of ammonium chloride has caused considerable hyperemia of the iris, but by the next day the eyes were almost normal, and in another day were completely recovered.[a] Replacement of the aqueous humor by 10% ammonium chloride solution is, however, definitely more toxic to the eye than replacement with sodium chloride solution of equivalent tonicity. The 10% ammonium chloride solution has induced immediate "salt cataract" and rise in intraocular pressure. Also, in the next day or two hemorrhages have appeared in the iris and fibrin in the anterior chamber, but soon this reaction has subsided, and ultimately the cornea and lens have been left clear.[81]

Toxicity to the epithelium of the cornea has been demonstrated for several types of ammonium salts in neutral solution under the unusual condition of continuous exposure for several hours. Although neutral solutions of ammonium salts generally have such low toxicity to the cornea that they produce no damage during exposures of several minutes, it has been shown that solutions containing 0.1 M *ammonium chloride, ammonium bicarbonate, ammonium phosphate, ammonium nitrate, ammonium acetate*, or *ammonium lactate* at pH 7 to 7.5 made up of 0.46 osmolar (1.5 times isotonic concentration) by addition of sodium chloride or sucrose and dripped continuously on the eyes of rabbits cause edema of the epithelium of the cornea within 3 to 3.5 hours. This toxic effect on the epithelium of the cornea is shown to be attributable to the ammonium component by the fact that no disturbance of the cornea is induced when *sodium chloride, sodium bicarbonate, sodium phosphate, sodium nitrate, sodium acetate*, or *sodium lactate* is substituted for the corresponding ammonium salts and the solutions are applied by continuous drops in the same manner for longer than three hours. Furthermore, when the tonicity is maintained at 0.46 osmolar and the pH at 7 to 7.5, but the ammonium concentration is varied, the time of onset of edema of the corneal epithelium is affected, the time of onset of edema being shortened to one-half hour with 0.3 M ammonium chloride and lengthened to 6.6 hours with 0.05 M ammonium chloride. Histologically in the eyes of rabbits in which edema of the corneal epithelium has been induced by prolonged exposure to ammonium salts in neutral solution there has been no change in other parts of the cornea but the epithelial cells have shown edema and vacuolization and shrinkage of the nuclei, with loss of intracellular carbohydrate. In some cases the epithelial cells have been lost from the cornea. The toxic effect of prolonged exposure to ammonium salts in neutral solution is attributed to penetration of ammonia in the form NH_3 into the cells.[b] In neutral ammonium salt solutions an equilibrium exists with a very small fraction in the form of ammonia which is lipid soluble and can penetrate walls of cells much more easily than ammonium or sodium ions.[c]

Effects of ammonium chloride on the retina have been demonstrated when rabbits were given 20 to 50 mg/kg via the common carotid artery.[d,e] After a single injection, alterations of the ERG and the histology of the retina were short lasting, but after three daily injections the changes were irreversible. Feeding ammonium chloride for 120 days to rabbits with the liver damaged and the adrenals removed to maintain a high concentration of ammonium ions in the blood caused permanent changes in the ERG and degeneration of the ganglion cell layer of the retina.

a. Grant WM: Experimental investigation of paracentesis in the treatment of ocular ammonia burns. *ARCH OPHTHALMOL* 44:399–404, 1950.
b. Rizzo AA: Rabbit corneal irrigation as a model system for studies on the relative toxicity of bacterial products implicated in periodontal disease. J PERIODONTOL 38:491–499, 1967.
c. Warren KS: Ammonia toxicity and pH. *NATURE* 195:47–49, 1962.
d. Kondo M: Influences of ammonium on the ERG of rabbit. *ACTA SOC OPHTHALMOL JPN* 71:1517–1527, 1968.
e. Ieb QS: Experimental studies on influence of ammonia solution on rabbit retina. *ACTA SOC OPHTHALMOL JPN* 74:341, 349, 1970.

Ammonium sulfamate (Ammate) is a yellow-orange crystalline solid employed principally as a weed killer. Tested by instillation of 0.5 ml of a 4% solution in water in the conjunctival sac of rabbits, it produced no irritation.[a]

a. Ambrose AM: Studies on the physiological effects of sulfamic acid and ammonium sulfamate. *J IND HYG* 43:25–28, 1943.

Ammonium tartrate is rather unstable, either as a solid or in solution, tending to lose ammonia and become more acid, requiring adjustment of the pH to maintain neutrality. A neutral 5% to 10% solution long ago was recommended for irrigation of the surface of the eye to remove incrustations of calcium and other metals from the surface of the cornea.

Solutions of ammonium tartrate, as well as solutions of other ammonium salts, dissolve certain metal salts which are poorly soluble in water by forming complexes with them. The solubilizing action of ammonium tartrate on calcium carbonate, lead carbonate, and copper precipitates has been exploited for dissolving incrustations of these compounds from the cornea of enucleated pig eyes, living rabbit eyes, and eyes of patients.[268] Many observations have been published on the use of this treatment, in many instances applied indiscriminately and illogically where no metal incrustations existed. The rational basis for use of complexing ammonium salts such as ammonium tartrate to solubilize deposits of lime and other metals in the cornea apparently was forgotten during the half century after the introduction of this treatment, and an unfortunate custom developed of treating all sorts of alkali burns of the eye with neutral ammonium tartrate solution, with no evidence that this was of any value, except possibly in removing deposits of lime (calcific deposits).

A careful evaluation of neutral ammonium tartrate solution in treatment of sodium hydroxide burns has been carried out by Geeraets, Aaron, and Guerry on the eyes of rabbits, and has established clearly that this old treatment did not accomplish any better removal of alkali from the tissues than irrigation with water, and did not have any better influence on the clinical course or final results of the injury.[65]

A 10% solution of ammonium tartrate is not completely innocuous. Such a solution at pH 7 applied continuously for thirty minutes to a rabbit's eye after mechanical removal of the epithelium caused no permanent damage, but did cause edema of the cornea lasting several days.[81] Use of a similar solution on patients' eyes following chemical burns seems to have caused no recognized additional injury, but the treatment is painful, especially if the solution has decomposed and is no longer neutral.

Ammonium salts have been replaced by much more efficient chelating agents such as sodium edetate (EDTA) for dissolving calcific corneal opacities and for removal of the metals from the cornea.

Amodiaquine (Amodiaquin, Camoquin) is a quinoline derivative that has been employed in treatment of malaria, arthritis, and lupus erythematosis. Like chloroquine it produces deposits of fine granular material in the corneal epithelium of patients. If examined with inadequate magnification these deposits sometimes have an appearance suggesting edema of the epithelium.[c,e,f] Deposits have been observed also overlying the sclera, but not in the lens or vitreous. Administration of 0.1 to 0.2 g per day for five months to rabbits is reported to have produced slight diffuse corneal clouding, but did not produce the fine granular type of deposits seen in patients. In patients the deposits have been seen to regress in the course of several months after the drug was discontinued.[b,c,e]

An extraordinary acute change in both corneas has been reported in one patient within eighteen days of starting treatment with amodiaquine for chronic discoid lupus erythematosis.[a] A ground-glass haze with streaks of greater opacity in horizontal bands involving epithelium and Bowman's zone was described in both corneas, associated with partial blindness, and discoloration of the skin and white of the eye suggestive of icterus. After amodiaquine was discontinued, the vision became normal in about nine weeks. When the drug was resumed experimentally, all the toxic effects, including the decrease in vision, reappeared. No information was reported on ophthalmoscopy, tensions, or quantitative measurements of the vision in this apparently unique case.

Little has been said about the effect of amodiaquine on the retina. A study has been made of five patients who had no ophthalmoscopic or visual abnormality while under treatment with amodiaquine in doses up to 200 mg per day, but according to electro-oculography they had depression of retinal function within one month after starting treatment, and this returned to normal within two months after stopping amodiaquine.[d]

A particularly instructive case report by Hirst and colleagues describes a man age 34 who took 250 g of amodiaquine hydrochloride during 14 months, and developed yellowish-brown deposits in the epithelium of cornea and conjunctiva, impaired color vision, moderate constriction of visual fields, and unrecordable ERG, but maintained normal visual acuity and normal fundi.[b] Two years after stopping the drug there were some improvements in the corneal deposits, the color vision, and the ERG. Acuity and fundi remained normal. Electron microscopy of biopsy specimens showed in corneal and conjunctival epithelial cells intralysosomal membranes and amorphous inclusions, indicative of drug-induced phospholipidosis. Fewer of these inclusions were present after the medication had been stopped for two years. (For comparable drugs, see INDEX for *Lipidosis.*)

a. Bleil DC: Unusual toxic manifestations to amodiaquin (Camoquin). *ARCH DERMATOL* 77:106–107, 1958.
b. Hirst LW, Sanborn G, et al: Amodiaquine ocular changes. *ARCH OPHTHALMOL* 100:1300–1304, 1982.
c. Maguire A: Amodiaquine hydrochloride. *LANCET* 1:667, 1962.
d. Maguire A, Kolb H: The effect of a synthetic antimalarial (amodiaquine) on the retina. *BR J DERMATOL* 76:471–474, 1964.
e. Marx F, Brech P, Meisner T: Visual disturbances and eye changes accompanying quinoline therapy in rheumatoid arthritis. *KLIN WOCHENSCHR* 38:443–447, 1960. (German)
f. Schloeder FX: Unusual toxic reaction to amodiaquine (camoquin). *ARCH DERMATOL* 84:601–602, 1961. (*SURVEY OPHTHALMOL* 7:430–431, 1962.)

Amoproxan (Mederel, Mexderel), a coronary artery dilator and antiarrythmic, apparently withdrawn from production, produced pellagroid skin changes and several cases of axial optic neuropathy in France.[e] Huriez and Francois reported on 3 patients using this drug who developed dermatitis and large central scotomas, but no abnormality of the ocular fundi except a little temporal pallor of the optic nerves.[a,b,c] Saraux reported two similar cases with dermatologic signs of pellagra and bilateral central scotoma, but normal fundi.[d] Neither Francois nor Saraux reported whether loss of vision was reversible in their patients.[a,d] However, when Huriez described another three cases of light-induced skin erythema and acutely reduced central vision, it was clearly stated that in these patients vision returned to normal in 4 to 6 weeks after the amoproxan was discontinued and vitamin PP was given.[c] In all cases amoproxan had been taken from 5 months to more than a year before the patients were seen for rapidly failing vision.

a. Francois P, Woillez M, et al: A new cause of toxic optic neuritis: amoproxan. *BULL SOC OPHTALMOL FRANCE* 70:665–666, 1970. (French)
b. Huriez C, Francois P, et al: Optic neuritis with regression during dermomucosal reactions to Mederel. *BULL SOC FR DERM SYPH* 78:11–14, 1971. (French)
c. Huriez C, Francois P, et al: Cutaneous and ocular complications of recent coronary dilators. *BULL ACAD NATL MED (PARIS)* 155:671–679, 1971. (French)
d. Saraux H, Cavicchi L: Optic neuritis from amoproxan. *BULL SOC OPHTALMOL FRANCE* 70:664–665, 1970. (French)
e. Texier L, Verin P, et al: Iatrogenic oculocutaneous syndromes. *BORDEAUX MED* 7:1545–1552, 1974. (French)

Amopyroquin (Propoquin), a derivative of 4-aminoquinoline related to chloroquine, has been demonstrated to be toxic to the retina in albino rats and beagle dogs, but not in rhesus monkeys. Degenerative atrophic changes in the retinas in susceptible species were induced during twenty-six weeks of medication, but not within a year in monkeys.[a]

a. Kurtz SM, Kaump DH, et al: The effect of long-term administration of amopyroquin, a 4-aminoquinoline compound, on the retina of pigmented and nonpigmented laboratory animals. *INVEST OPHTHALMOL* 6:420–425, 1967.

Amphetamine (DL-2-methylphenethylamine, β-phenylisopropylamine, Benzedrine) is a synthetic CNS stimulant with adrenergic properties which cause restlessness and insomnia, and in large doses systemically can dilate the pupils and cause slight blurring of near vision. Applied to the eye, amphetamine dilates the pupil and retracts the upper lid, but these actions are prevented by previous depletion of catecholamines such as is brought about by local guanethidine.[a]

Testing for toxicity to the retina has been negative; 10 mg/kg given daily to dogs for three months caused occasional slight ophthalmoscopic appearance of blanching of the fundus, but no histologic change in the retina.[b]

Experimental regeneration of the lens in amphibian eyes is found to be delayed when the animals are placed in a solution containing amphetamine.[c]

Amphetamine given intramuscularly has been claimed to cause elevation of pressure in eyes with primary glaucoma and not in normal eyes, but this claim needs further investigation with careful attention to gonioscopy and comparative observations without amphetamine.[d] In monkeys no elevation of ocular pressure has been found when amphetamine is given systemically unless given in doses so large that a rapid rise of blood pressure is induced, which is reflected in a brief small elevation of ocular pressure.[e]

a. Sneddon JM, Turner P: Structure activity relation of some sympathomimetic amines in the guanethidine-treated human eye. *J PHYSIOL* 192:23P–26P, 1967.
b. Delahunt CS, O'Connor RA, et al: Toxic retinopathy following prolonged treatment with dl (p-trifluoromethyl (phenyl) isopropylamine hydrochloride (P-1727) in experimental animals. *TOXICOL APPL PHARMACOL* 5:298–305, 1963.
c. Restivo Manfridi ML: On the regeneration of the crystalline lens in amphibians. *BULL OCULIST* 46:605–612, 1967. (Italian)
d. Torres Lucena M: Influence of intravenous atropine on the ocular tension of the patient with primary glaucoma. *ARCH SOC OFTALMOL HISP-AM* 6:446, 1946.
e. Beria FE, Dzhalagonia SL: The influence of neurotropic substances on intraocular tension in monkeys. *OFTALMOL ZH* 20:533–537, 1965. (*ZENTRALBL GES OPHTHALMOL* 96:416, 1966.)

Amphotericin B (Fungizone), an antifungal drug, with high systemic toxicity, has been used topically in and about the eye within the limits of its toxicity to eye tissues. On the corneas of rabbits even 0.0025% disrupts the epithelial cells,[285] and 1% causes extensive damage to these cells and markedly delays healing of epithelial defects.[309] When more than 5 mg are injected subconjunctivally, a severe local reaction results with permanent yellow discoloration of the conjunctiva and formation of raised nodules that are slow in resolving.[b] Injected into the anterior chamber in rabbits, 0.5 mg severely damaged the corneal endothelium, but 25 μg or 50 μg did not.[271,341] When injected into the vitreous body in rabbits, some investigators report 5 to 10 μg to be non-toxic,[a] while others have reported inflammation, cataract and retinal detachment and necrosis from as little as 1 or 2 μg.[d] The *methyl ester of amphotericin B* at a concentration of 10 μg/ml in vitrectomy infusion fluid has been reported to be clinically satisfactory, but more than 75 μg/ml was judged excessive.[c]

a. Axelrod AJ, Peyman GA, Apple DJ: Toxicity of intravitreal injection of amphotericin B. *AM J OPHTHALMOL* 76:578–583, 1973.

b. Bell RW, Ritchey JP: Subconjunctival nodules after amphotericin B injection. *ARCH OPHTHALMOL* 90:402–404, 1973.

c. Raichmand M, Peyman Ga, et al: Toxicity and efficacy of vitrectomy fluids. *OPHTHALMIC SURGERY* 11:246–248, 1980.

d. Souri EN, Green WR: Intravitreal amphotericin B toxicity. *AM J OPHTHALMOL* 78:77–81, 1974.

Amyl acetate (isoamylacetate), a volatile solvent, at 300 ppm in air is noticeably irritating to human eyes.[183] At higher concentrations it causes a burning sensation in the eyes and hyperemia of the conjunctiva, but no corneal damage has been observed.[61, 188] Exposure of thirty workers to 20 to 80 mg/liter of air caused initially a sensation of irritation of the eyes to which the workers gradually became accustomed, and examination after chronic exposure showed only hyperemia of the bulbar conjunctiva, and no abnormalities of the cornea, particularly no vacuoles in the corneal epithelium.[g]

Experimentally, several drops of liquid amyl acetate squirted on the eyes of anesthetized rabbits and washed off with water two minutes later caused temporary corneal epithelial injury, but recovery was complete in a day or two.[81] By standardized testing on rabbit eyes, amyl acetate has been graded only 2 (slightly injurious) on a scale of 1 to 10.[228]

In rare instances disturbances of the optic nerve have been reported in association with exposure to amyl acetate. In the first report in 1930 a young man developed blurred vision, headache, and retrobulbar neuritis in one eye, with slight blurring of the papilla, prominence of the veins, and relative central scotoma after exposure to "Duco" spray-painting solvents for about a year. He recovered completely in nineteen days. The paint contained benzene in addition to amyl acetate, but no lead, and little or no methyl, allyl, or amyl alcohol.[a] A group of investigators apparently all from one university in Italy then published additional reports, some of which are quoted here second-hand.[c, e, f] They cited Lund as having described in 1944 a case of bilateral optic atrophy with visual field changes in a worker who had been in an atmosphere saturated with amyl acetate vapors.[e] They themselves in 1968 reported two cases of subatrophy of the optic nerve, primary or descending, in two workers exposed to amyl acetate in splicing cinema film.[b, f] They also reported in 1969 four other cases of subatrophy of the optic nerve in workers in contact with amyl acetate vapors.[b, c] At the same time they said histology of optic nerves of animals poisoned by inhalation of the solvent showed slight degeneration of the nerve fibers and cells, which appeared reduced in volume as part of a clearly atrophic process.[b, c] Other publications from the same group described ERG measurements on guinea pigs, reporting a gradual extinction of the ERG either by exposure to 320 mg/liter of air for 30 minutes a day for 15 days, or to 110 mg/liter of air for 60 minutes a day for 60 days.[b, d] However, after exposures were discontinued, the ERG returned completely to normal in 15 to 45 days, and it was concluded that the changes had been entirely functional and reversible.[b, d]

There seem to have been no reports of disturbances of vision in association with amyl acetate outside of Europe.

a. Goldmann H: A new industrial retrobulbar neuritis. *KLIN MONATSBL AUGENHEILKD* 84:761–762, 1930. (German)

b. Gorgone G, Inserra A, et al: Electroretinographic studies in experimental poisoning with amyl acetate. *ANN OTTALMOL CLIN OCUL* 96:313–319, 1970. (Italian)

c. Inserra A, Malfitano D, Guardabasso B: Ocular pathology of industrial solvents. *FOLIA MED* (Naples) 52:348–361, 1969. (Italian)

d. Inserra A, Gorgone G, et al: Electroretinographic studies in experimental poisoning with amyl acetate. *ANN OTTALMOL CLIN OCUL* 96:321–324, 1970. (Italian)

e. Lund A (1944): cited by Sfogliano et al,[f] and Gorgone et al.[b]

f. Sfogliano C, Fazio C, Parlato G: On two cases of subatrophy of the optic nerve in workers exposed to poisoning by amyl acetate. *BULL SOC MED CHIR CATANIA* 36:113, 1968. (Italian)

g. Valvo A, Spagna C, Parlato G: Ocular pathology of industrial solvents. *ANN OTTALMOL CLIN OCUL* 93:799–807, 1967. (Italian)

Amyl alcohol vapor causes stinging sensation of the eyes and irritation of the respiratory passages, producing lacrimation, and hyperemia of the conjunctiva, but no significant corneal injury. Long ago a disturbance of color vision in a brewer was alleged to have been caused by amyl alcohol, but otherwise there appears to have been no authentic case of visual disturbance from amyl alcohol.[56,143]

Amyl nitrite (iso-amyl nitrite, isopentyl nitrite, Vaporole) is a volatile vasodilator employed in treatment of angina pectoris. Inhalation of small amount of vapor causes flushing of the face, throbbing of the head, and in some individuals and in animals a slight momentary rise in intraocular pressure.[a,h]

A transient decrease in intraocular pressure has been reported in some normal individuals as a consequence of decrease in blood pressure after inhalation of five drops of amyl nitrite.[f] On the other hand, an initial slight rise of about 3 mm Hg lasting several seconds, similar to emotional blushing, has been recorded during tonography.[g] In glaucomatous patients similarly, inhalation of amyl nitrite has occasionally been noted to cause a rise of ocular pressure within the first minute, followed by a decrease and return to original pressure in two to five minutes.[a,i,e] In most of a series of glaucomatous eyes, a brief fall of pressure has been reported associated with a decrease in blood pressure.[c,d] There has been no actual demonstration of danger from amyl nitrite in glaucoma. Amyl nitrite is reported to have been tried and failed as a provocative test agent for angle-closure glaucoma.[b]

Many years ago hallucinations of color and occasional very transient decreases of visual acuity were reported,[153] but there have been no recent observations of such effects.

In external contact with the eye the vapor induces stinging and transient lacrimation. Liquid amyl nitrite tested on normal rabbit eyes causes only slight superficial injury. Similarly, only transient superficial injuries are to be expected from splash contamination of human eyes. However, there are in the literature two instances of severe corneal damage in patients in which liquid amyl nitrite was involved. One case was complicated by lacerations from glass splinters,[j] and in the other case the injury was attributed to free nitric acid which was thought to have been produced by decomposition of the amyl nitrite.[153]

a. Baillart B, Bollack J: On the comparative effect of certain medicinal substances on the ocular tension and the arterial pressure. *ANN OCULIST (Paris)*, 158:641–654, 1921. (French)

b. Becker B: In *Symposium on Glaucoma.* Transactions of the First Conference. Edited by FW Newell. New York, Josiah Macy Jr. Foundation, 1955, page 32.

c. Bramsen T: Amyl nitrite test in glaucoma simplex. *ACTA OPHTHALMOL SUPPL* 125:35, 1975.

d. Cristini G, Pagliarani N: Amyl nitrite test in primary glaucoma. *BR J OPHTHALMOL* 37:741–745, 1953.

e. Cristini G, Pagliarani N: Slit-lamp study of the aqueous veins in simple glaucoma during the amyl nitrite test. *BR J OPHTHALMOL* 39:685–687, 1955.

f. Endo F: On the effect of dropping various medications in the conjunctival sac on the blood circulation, especially on the capillary pressure of the macula lutea of the retina. *ACTA SOC OPHTHALMOL JPN* 39:47–49, 545–575, 1935.

g. Grant WM: Physiological and pharmacological influences upon intraocular pressure. *PHARMACOL REV* 7:143–182, 1955.

h. Kochmann M, Romer P: Experimental contribution concerning pathologic fluid exchange of the eye. *GRAEFES ARCH OPHTHALMOL* 88:528, 1914. (German)

i. Kollner H: Concerning the eye pressure in glaucoma simplex and its relationship to the circulation. *ARCH AUGENHEILKD* 83:135–167, 1918. (German)

j. Stastnick E: Burn of the eye by amyl nitrite. *CESK OFTALMOL* 2:201–203, 1935. (*ZENTRALBL GES OPHTHALMOL* 36:587, 1936.)

Anesthesia, general, is accompanied by characteristic changes in the pupils at different depths of anesthesia. During induction the pupil is dilated; in the stage of narcosis the pupil is constricted but still reacts to light; in the stage of coma, when a dangerous excess of anesthetic has been given, the pupils dilate and are unresponsive to light. The pupils return to normal upon recovery from anesthesia. The pharmacology of general anesthesia relating to the eyes has been reviewed by Duncan and Rhodes, and by Havener.[47, 103]

Rarely brain damage and loss of vision result from general anesthesia, and in these instances asphyxia rather than a toxic effect of the anesthetic is probably to blame. Nitrous oxide has been involved in most instances, but in rare cases brain damage has occurred with ether or chloroform. Unusually slow recovery of consciousness after anesthesia suggests brain damage. Walsh made the observation that when there is loss of vision on recovery of consciousness, the chances of return of vision to normal are less than even.[255] Loss of vision is attributable to damage of the cortex of the brain.

Certain inhalation anesthetics have noteworthy toxic side effects involving the eyes, particularly *trichloroethylene, methoxyflurane,* and *halothane.*

Trichloroethylene, when contaminated by decomposition products, has caused palsies of oculomotor and trigeminal nerves, and optic neuropathy. (For details, see INDEX for *Trichloroethylene.*) Pure trichloroethylene in general anesthesia causes a rise of intraocular pressure to a mean of 17.8 mm Hg from a pre-trichloroethylene mean of 13.6 mm Hg in normal people, associated with a rise in central venous pressure.[a]

Methoxyflurane anesthesia causes flecked retina syndrome due to formation and deposition of oxalate crystals. (For details, see INDEX for *Methoxyflurane.*)

Halothane plus nitrous oxide anesthesia in rabbits lasting 5 to 6 hours is found by Johnson and colleagues to cause degenerative changes in the retinal pigment epithelium and visual cells when concentrations of halothane up to 2.5% are used, but not when 0.5% is used.[b,c] In human beings, Raitta and colleagues have found that in general anesthesia from halothane plus thiopentone and nitrous oxide the a- and b- waves of the ERG are significantly diminished and visual evoked cortical potentials are lowered.[e]

Several volatile anesthetics, including *halothane, methoxyflurane, ethrane, ether,* and *chloroform,* in a study by Van Noren and Dirk on monkey ERG, have been found to retard dark adaptation of the cone cells.[387]

Suppression of tear production and influences of general anesthesia on intraocular pressure have been reviewed by Krupin and Becker.[d]

a. Al-Abrak MH, Samuel JR: Effects of general anesthesia on the intraocular pressure in man. *BR J OPHTHALMOL* 59:107–110, 1975.

b. Johnson NF, Wilson TM, et al: Retinal fine structure after long term anesthesia. *EXP EYE RES* 15:127–139, 1973.

c. Johnson NF, Strang R, et al: Further observations on the retinal fine structure after long-term anesthesia. *EXP EYE RES* 17:73–85, 1973.

d. Krupin T, Becker B: General anesthesia and the eye. *SYMPOSIUM ON OCULAR THERAPY,* vol. 11, ed. by Leopold IH and Burns RP. John Wiley and Sons, New York, pp. 121–126, 1979.

e. Raitta C, Karhunen V, et al: Changes in the electroretinogram and visual evoked potentials during general anesthesia. *GRAEFES ARCH OPHTHALMOL* 211:139–144, 1979.

Anesthetics, local, toxic effects are discussed according to routes of administration, as follows:

1. *Local anesthetics: intraocular*
2. *Local anesthetics: applied to the cornea*
   a. Ocular toxic effects
   b. Systemic toxic effects
3. *Local anesthetics: retrobulbar and dental*
4. *Local anesthetics: spinal*

The pharmacology and side effects of local anesthetics have been reviewed by Ellis[306], Fraunfelder[312], and Havener[47].

1. Local anesthetics: intraocular (anterior chamber or posterior segment of the eye)

a. *Anterior chamber injection of local anesthetics* was investigated in rabbits by Spencer and colleagues, who found different degrees of corneal clouding after 24 hours were produced by different anesthetics, due to varied degrees of injurious effect on the corneal endothelium.[b] The least irritant by this test were dibucaine, tetracaine, procaine, and piperocaine. The more irritant were lidocaine and hexylcaine.

Lidocaine (0.2 ml, 2%) injected into the anterior chamber of a cat by Lincoff et al caused the pupil to dilate immediately and become unresponsive to light.[a] After 12 minutes the pupil of this eye was still dilated, but the pupil of the other eye responded well consensually. By eighteen hours both pupils were normal.

Tetracaine injected into the anterior chamber of a patient caused severe injury. The patient's ophthalmologist injected 1% tetracaine hydrochloride into the lids in preparation for operation on a chalazion, but the patient squeezed his lids tightly during the injection, and shortly thereafter when the lids were separated, the pupil was noted to have become widely dilated. A fine needle tract through the cornea was visible. During the next twenty-four hours the vision became blurred and the cornea developed a bluish appearance, with much edema and much wrinkling of Descemet's membrane. The intraocular pressure became temporarily elevated to about 30 mm Hg. In both eyes the anterior chambers were deep normal. Subsequently, the tension in the injured eye became chronically slightly lower than the tension in the normal eye. Eight months after the injury the cornea still had extensive wrinkling of Descemet's membrane with folds radiating from the original puncture wound, and the epithelium was chronically edematous. Vision in the injured eye was 20/100. Eighteen months after the accident, bullous keratopathy had developed in addition to the permanent wrinkling of Descemet's membrane. At no time had the edema reached the most peripheral portions of the cornea, and presumably on this account, there was no vascularization of the cornea. Because of pain and low vision a penetrating keratoplasty was contemplated. The lens had remained normal and the iris showed only a small patch of atrophy. The pupil remained semidilated and almost immobile from the time of injury.

b. *Posterior segment intraocular injection of local anesthetic* has been reported with lidocaine. Lincoff et al have described three patients in whom inadvertently an injection needle penetrated the sclera and a small amount of lidocaine with epinephrine was injected into the eye.[a] Immediate elevation of intraocular pressure was either sensed by the person making the injection, or was recognized from sudden dilation of the pupil and haziness of the cornea. In two of these cases the vision returned to its previous level by the next day, although in one the vision had been immediately reduced to light perception, and it took several hours for return of pupil and vision to normal. The third case was complicated by development of a dark area in the retina temporally, not easily seen because of cataract, but probably hemorrhage. Scleral buckling was done in this region, but a dense scotoma in the nasal field including fixation was still present two years later. Paracentesis had been done promptly in these cases to relieve the initial elevation of pressure.

Experiments in cats and rabbits showed that intravitreal injection of saline solution without lidocaine or epinephrine could cause a rise of pressure to more than 70 mm Hg, closing the central retinal artery, causing the pupil to dilate and blocking consensual response in the other eye, but this lasted only 5 to 7 minutes even without paracentesis, and the eyes recovered promptly.[a] Injection of epinephrine or hyaluronidase had the same effect, but injection of lidocaine caused dilation of the pupil for at least 50 minutes, and blocked consensual response to light for between

12 and 33 minutes. The ERG was extinguished by lidocaine for a half hour, recovering in 4 hours. No cytological damage was found. It appears from the animal experiments, and from the first two clinical cases, that blockage of retinal function and afferent transmission by lidocaine is temporary, and should not pose a serious toxic threat. The threat of physical trauma from needle penetration of the posterior segment may be more varied.

    a. Lincoff H, Zweifach P, et al: The inadvertent injection of lidocaine into the eye. *OPHTHALMOLOGY* (in press).

    b. Spencer RW, Scheie HS, Dripps RD: Anterior chamber injection in the rabbit as a method for determining irritancy of local anesthetics. *J PHARMACOL EXP THER* 113:421–430, 1955.

2. *Local Anesthetics: applied to the cornea*

a. *Ocular toxic effects.* Local anesthetics applied to the cornea for diagnostic purposes may cause transient stinging, varying in intensity from one anesthetic to another, e.g. more from tetracaine than from proparacaine or benoxinate. Older anesthetics, such as cocaine and tetracaine, also caused irregularity of the surface of the cornea which interfered with visual examination of the inner parts of the eye. Local anesthetics increase the permeability of the corneal epithelium to drugs and chemicals, and render the cornea abnormally susceptible to both physical and chemical injury. Local anesthesia suppresses automatic blinking and allows abnormal drying of the cornea.

Serious toxic keratopathy. Repeated application of local anesthetics following injury of the cornea may seriously delay or prevent regeneration of the epithelium. This may promote a vicious cycle in which an anesthetic agent that was applied to relieve discomfort from toxic or mechanical injury of the corneal epithelium interferes with healing and causes the discomfort to worsen. Under these circumstances, reapplication of the anesthetic provides only brief periods of relief of discomfort and may lead to chronic ulceration of the cornea. It is for this reason that it is quite inadvisable to employ local anesthetics in the treatment of corneal injuries. Local anesthetics should not be prescribed for patient's use, but should be applied only by medical personnel, when necessary to facilitate an adequate examination.

In typical cases of chronic keratopathy resulting from repeated application of local anesthetics, the corneal epithelium first develops a speckled punctate keratitis, then loss of epithelium in the palpebral fissure, with the remaining epithelium heaped up in a gray ridge about a patch of bare stroma. The stroma itself presents a finely granular surface with diffuse gray turbidity and infiltration in its deeper layers. In most cases when the applications of local anesthetic are discontinued, the cornea generally recovers its clarity and smooth surface in the course of several weeks. However, some eyes have developed irreversible vascularized leukomas requiring surgery, sometimes complicated by cataract and glaucoma. During the course of the toxic reaction the lids are usually swollen and the conjunctivae hyperemic. The patient experiences great photophobia and has impaired visual acuity from corneal edema and clouding of the cornea. This may be accompanied by folds in the posterior surface of the cornea and iridocyclitis.

Toxic keratopathy of this sort from repeated application of local anesthetics has been reported many times in the literature, as single cases or series of cases. (The following are reports of this type: Bodereau (1981), Burns (1977), Campinchi (1965), Couderc (1975), Duffin (1984), Eerden (1962), Epstein (1968), Graeber (1961), Henkes (1978), Henrotte (1972), Hilsdorf (1973), Jallet (1980), Judit (1972), Klima (1974), Lagoutte-Descamp (1973), Meyer (1965), Pau (1980), Pouliquen (1980), Schmoger (1953), Sheldon (1971), Tanifuji (1979), Tesinski (1977), Willis (1970).) Cases with especially serious results have been described by Henrotte (1972), Jallet (1980), and Pouliquen (1980).

Various local anesthetics have been responsible, including benoxinate (oxybuprocaine; Novesine), butacaine, cornecaine, lidocaine, proparacaine, and tetracaine. Possibly the most rapid induction of serious keratopathy was caused by application of 0.05% benoxinate hydrochloride approximately every 5 minutes for 48 hours (Jallett). Usually a week or two of less frequent application is responsible.

Clinical examination by endothelial specular microscopy has shown in typical cases loss of $1/3$ to $2/3$ of the corneal endothelial cells, explaining swelling of the corneal stroma and bullous keratopathy (Bodereau). Light and electron microscopy of discs of cornea removed when keratoplasty has been required have provided similar findings (Pouliquen).

Experiments on animals and *in vitro* have established that local anesthetics have toxic effects on corneal epithelium (Steiner), depressing respiration and glycolysis (Herrmann), and interfering with regeneration (Gundersen; Herrmann; Kuchle; Marr; Smelser). Local anesthetics interfere with migration of rat corneal epithelial cells in culture (Burns).

In rabbits, scanning electron microscopy shows after application of an ophthalmic local anesthetic within 15 minutes there is extensive disturbance of the corneal epithelial cells (Brewitt), though in the case of benoxinate recovery may take place in an hour (Harnisch). Electrical resistance measurements *in vitro* have shown increase in permeability of the epithelium correlated with the morphologic changes (Weekers; Burnstein[285]). Ultrastructural changes in rat corneal epithelium have been studied using several different local anesthetics (Leuenberger). Corneal epithelial cultures were destroyed by these drugs (Krejci).

Repeated applications to rabbit eyes have reproduced the clinical appearances of local anesthetic keratopathy (Tanifuji).

Treatment for toxic keratopathy from local anesthetics consists foremost in stopping the use of the anesthetic, protecting the cornea from further injury, and relieving inflammation. Sometimes stopping the use of the anesthetic is not easy because some patients may continue their use surreptitiously. An eye bandage securely applied can be helpful. Several reports speak highly of hydrophilic bandage contact lenses for relief of discomfort and promotion of healing. Topical corticosteroid treatment has also been commended, especially when iridocyclitis accompanies the keratopathy.

b. *Systemic toxic effects from local anesthetics applied to the cornea* have been reported rarely, but two cases have been described in which a drop of benoxinate hydrochloride plus fluorescein (Fluress) applied to each eye for tonometry was followed by sudden collapse within one or a few minutes, with brief tonic-clonic convulsions, then spontaneous recovery. Fraunfelder's National Registry was quoted as having reports of vaso-vagal symptoms in 3 patients, but no seizures (Cohn).

Bodereau X, Baikoff G: Endothelial response to an external topical anesthetic: specular microscopic study. *BULL SOC OPHTALMOL FRANCE* 81:1207–1209, 1981. (French)

Brewitt H, Honegger H: The influence of surface anesthetics on the corneal epithelium. A scanning electron microscopic study. *KLIN MONATSBL AUGENHEILKD* 173:347–354, 1978. (German)

Burns RP, Forster RK, et al: Chronic toxicity of local anesthetics on the cornea. Chapter 3, Leopold IH and Burns RP editors, *SYMPOSIUM ON OCULAR THERAPY,* Vol. 10, New York, John Wiley and Sons, 1977, pp. 31–44.

Campinchi R, Dhermy P, et al: Keratitis from prolonged usage of local anesthetic collyrium. *BULL SOC OPHTHALMOL FRANCE* 65:120–123, 1965. (French)

Cohn HC, Jocson VL: A unique case of grand mal seizures after Fluress. *ANN OPHTHALMOL* 13:1379–1380, 1981.

Couderc JL, Hamard H, et al: Keratitis from prolonged use of anesthetic collyria: three new cases. *BULL SOC OPHTALMOL FRANCE* 75:31–35, 1975. (French)

Duffin RM, Olson RJ: Tetracaine toxicity. *ANN OPHTHALMOL* 16:836–838, 1984.

Eerden vd AAJJ: Changes in corneal epithelium due to local anesthetics. *OPHTHALMOLOGICA* 143:154–162, 1962.

Epstein DL, Paton D: Keratitis from misuse of corneal anesthetics. *N ENGL J MED* 279:396–399, 1968.

Graeber W: Anesthetic injury of the cornea. *KLIN MONATSBL AUGENHEILKD* 136:369–377, 1961. (German)

Gundersen T, Liebmann S: Effects of local anesthetics on regeneration of corneal epithelium. *ARCH OPHTHALMOL* 31:29–33, 1944.

Harnisch JP, Hoffmann F, Dumitrescu L: Side-effects of local anesthetics on the corneal epithelium of the rabbit eye. *GRAEFES ARCH OPHTHALMOL* 197:71–81, 1975.

Heitz R, Jegham H: Adverse effects of local anesthesia in ophthalmology. *BULL SOC OPHTALMOL FRANCE* 73:933–937, 1973. (French)

Henkes HE, Waubke TN: Keratitis from abuse of corneal anesthetics. *BR J OPHTHALMOL* 62:62–65, 1978.

Henrotte J, Weekers JF: Clinical study of corneal lesions from prolonged local application of anesthetics. *ARCH OPHTALMOL (Paris)* 32:449–456, 1972. (French)

Henrotte J, Weekers JF: Corneal lesions from prolonged local application of anesthetics. *BULL SOC BELGE OPHTALMOL* 160:619–629, 1972.

Hermann H, Moses SG, Friedenwald JS: Influence of Pontocaine hydrochloride and chlorobutanol on respiration and glycolysis of cornea. *ARCH OPHTHALMOL* 28:652–660, 1942.

Hilsdorf C, Zenklusen G: Novesin injury of the cornea. *KLIN MONATSBL AUGENHEILKD* 162:525–527, 1973. (German)

Jallet G, Cleirens S, et al: Serious toxic keratopathy from oxybuprocaine of particularly rapid onset. *BULL SOC OPHTALMOL FRANCE* 80:385–387, 1980. (French)

Judit BS: A contribution to the subject of iatrogenic injury in ophthalmic anesthesia. *KLIN MONATSBL AUGENHEILKD* 161:352–356, 1972. (German)

Klima A, Ruckerooa H: Serious damage of the eye by Novesine. *CESK OFTALMOL* 30:375–380, 1974. (English abstract)

Krejci L: Effect of eye drugs on corneal epithelium. Comparative test on tissue culture. *CESK OFTALMOL* 32:163–168, 1976. (English abstract)

Kuchle HJ: On the effect of local anesthetics on regeneration of the corneal epithelium. *KLIN MONATSBL AUGENHEILKD* 126:313–322, 1955. (German)

Lagoutte-Descamp F: Dangers of local anesthetics in ophthalmology. *BULL SOC OPHTALMOL FRANCE* 73:1035–1038, 1973. (French)

Leuenberger PM: Ultrastructural changes in the corneal epithelium after topical anesthesia. *GRAEFES ARCH OPHTHALMOL* 18:73–90, 1973. (German)

Marr WG, Wood R, et al: Effects of topical anesthetics on regeneration of corneal epithelium. *AM J OPHTHALMOL* 43:606–614, 1957.

Mayer HJ: Treatment injury of the eye by topical anesthetics. *DTSCH MED WOCHEN-SCHR* 90:1676–1678, 1965.

Pau H: Anesthetic-induced keratitis. *KLIN MONSTSBL AUGENHEILKD* 176:885–892, 1980. (German)

Pouliquen YJM, Beaumont CC: Topical anesthetics and the cornea. A perpetual danger inspite of reiterated warnings. *BULL SOC OPHTALMOL FRANCE* 80:505–509, 1980.

Schmoger E: Pontocaine injury. *KLIN MONATSBL AUGENHEILKD* 122:527–535, 1953. (German)

Sheldon GM: Misuse of corneal anesthetics. *CAN MED ASSOC J* 104:528, 1971.

Smelser G, Ozanics V: Effect of local anesthetics on cell division and migration following thermal burns of the cornea. *ARCH OPHTHALMOL* 34:271–277, 1945.

Steiner L: Clinical-experimental investigations on the effect of some local anesthetics on the cornea. *KLIN MONATSBL AUGENHEILKD* 148:536–540, 1966. (German)

Tanifuji Y, Kondo T, Kumagai S: Severe keratitis from abuse of corneal anesthetics. *FOLIA OPHTHALMOL JPN* 30:1782, 1979. (English summary)

Tesinsky P, Beran V: Damage of the eyes by improper application of the local anesthetic Novesine. *CESK OFTALMOL* 33:411–415, 1977. (English summary)

Weekers JF: Experimental investigations into the pathogenesis of corneal lesions from anesthetics. *ARCH OPHTALMOL (Paris)* 34:121–132, 1974. (French)

Willis WE, Laibson PR: Corneal complications of topical anesthetic abuse. *CAN J OPHTHALMOL* 5:239–243, 1970.

3. *Local anesthetics: retrobulbar and dental,* without penetration of the ocular globe, can cause both ocular and systemic side effects. (Adverse effects of penetrating and injecting local anesthetics into the globe itself have been reviewed in "*1. Local anesthetics, intraocular.*")

Retrobulbar injection of local anesthetics commonly causes temporary loss of vision by blocking transmission in the optic nerve, but recovery of function is prompt and complete except in extremely rare instances, and in these instances there is a possibility that the optic nerve has been damaged by the needle used for injection rather than by the toxic effect of the local anesthetic. Transient loss of vision is practically routine from retrobulbar injections of local anesthetics.[b,c,e,f,h–j] Hanisch and Fodo, and Doden and Makabe, have particularly published clinical studies of this effect and have provided reviews with extensive bibliographies of earlier observations of reduction of vision by retrobulbar local anesthetics.[b,c] Confirmatory studies in cats have been reported by Pruett, and in rabbits by Sugita.[i,m]

Apart from the ordinary transitory losses of vision from regular retrobulbar local anesthetic injections already mentioned, there have been some extraordinary cases, as follows. Reed and associates described a case in which retrobulbar injection of a mixture of lidocaine and a radiopaque substance, sodium diatrizoate, caused temporary loss of vision and temporary contralateral sixth nerve palsy. By x-ray examination this appeared to be due to inadvertent injection into the sheaths of the optic nerve, with spread up the optic nerve into the intracranial subdural space.[j]

Retrobulbar injection of local anesthetics can cause central nervous system and cardiopulmonary complications. This has been reviewed by Ellis (1976).[306] Grand mal seizures in two cases after retrobulbar bupivicaine have been reported by Meyers et al (1978),[g] and after procaine in one case by Verin (1971).[n] Cardiopulmonary arrest, with incomplete recovery, has been reported in one case after procaine by Verin (1971),[g] and after a mixture of bupivicaine and mepivicaine in one case, with recovery, by Rosenblatt et al (1980).[k] A series of cases of temporary respiratory (not cardiac) arrest after retrobulbar bupivicaine has been described in an editorial by Smith (1982).[1]

Dental injections of local anesthetics have been known to affect the eyes. Hyams (1976) described a patient who had paralysis of right third and fourth cranial nerves for about six weeks, probably from inadvertent intra-arterial injection.[d] Mandibular nerve block injection of local anesthetic caused transient loss of vision, presumably due to inadvertent intra-arterial injection in two cases reported by Blaxter and Britten.[a] In two other instances loss of vision followed injection of procaine for extraction of teeth. In one of these instances severe visual loss was noted within a day following the extraction and there was no subsequent improvement. Ultimately the optic nerves became atrophic and vision was perception of hand movements (Walsh).[255] Hyams reviewed a small number of other cases, which are not included in the following bibliography.[d]

a. Blaxter PL, Britten MJA: Transient amaurosis after mandibular nerve block. *BR MED J* 1:681, 1967.

b. Doden W, Makabe R: Transitory loss of vision after retrobulbar anesthesia. *OPHTHALMOLOGICA ADDIT AD* 158:441–447, 1969. (German)

c. Hanisch J, Fodo V: On transitory amaurosis from retrobulbar and stomatologic local anesthesias. *KLIN MONATSBL AUGENHEILKD* 153:247–252, 1968. (German)

d. Hyam SW: Oculomotor palsy following dental anesthesia. *ARCH OPHTHALMOL* 94:1281–1282, 1976.

e. Kruger KE: Transitory blindness after retrobulbar anesthesia. *KLIN MONATSBL AUGENHEILKD* 149:523–526, 1966. (German)

f. Marx P, Langlois J, Brasseur G: Transitory amaurosis after retrobulbar anesthesia. *BULL SOC OPHTALMOL FRANCE* 79:925–928, 1979. (French)

g. Meyers EF, Ramierz RC, Boniuk I: Grand mal seizures after retrobulbar block. *ARCH OPHTHALMOL* 96:847, 1978.

h. Mishima K, Tsuda T, Sakai T: Effects of retrobulbar anesthesia on the eye. *ACTA SOC OPHTHALMOL JPN* 69:2069–2085, 1965.

i. Pruett RC: The effects of local anesthetics upon optic nerve conduction in the cat. *ARCH OPHTHALMOL* 77:119–123, 1967.

j. Reed JW, MacMillan Jr AS, Lazenby GW: Transient neurologic complications of positive contrast orbitography. *ARCH OPHTHALMOL* 81:508–511, 1969.

k. Rosenblatt RM, May DR, Barsoumian K: Cardiopulmonary arrest after retrobulbar block. *AM J OPHTHALMOL* 90:425–427, 1980.

l. Smith JL: Retrobulbar bupicaine can cause respiratory arrest. *ANN OPHTHALMOL* 14:1005–1006, 1982.

m. Sugita K: The effects of retrobulbar anesthesia upon optic nerve conduction. *ACTA SOC OPHTHALMOL JPN* 73:1830–1840, 1969.

n. Verin P, Yaccoubi M: Accidents of retrobulbar anesthesia. *BULL SOC OPHTHALMOL FRANCE* 71:397–403, 1971. (French)

4. Local anesthetics, spinal and related. Spinal anesthesia induced by injection of local anesthetics has caused palsies of the extraocular muscles.[a–h,255] Most frequently the sixth nerve has been affected, less often the third or fourth nerves. Typically the onset of weakness of extraocular muscles has been preceded by headache for several days. Exceptionally the palsies may become evident within one or two hours after spinal anesthesia, but more commonly they develop three days to three weeks later.[d,255] Recovery has usually occurred spontaneously in three days to three weeks, but exceptionally has taken as long as eighteen months.

Although many cases have been reported, the incidence of palsies of extraocular muscles after spinal anesthesia is low. A low incidence, particularly with lidocaine, is shown by a report by Phillips (1969) on 10,440 patients, of whom only eight had abducens paralysis, and this was temporary in each case.[g]

The mechanism of extraocular muscle paralysis following spinal anesthesia has not been established. In rare cases sixth nerve palsies have been accompanied by papilledema,[h] and retrobulbar neuritis.[b] Loss of vision has been reported developing six weeks after spinal anesthesia in one case and was thought to be due to a chemical meningitis and arachnoiditis from contamination of the anesthetic agent by a detergent solution in which ampules of the drug were stored. The patient died twelve weeks after the injection.[255]

a. Arne JL, Salvaing P, et al: Sixth nerve paralysis after peridural anesthesia. *BULL SOC OPHTALMOL FRANCE* 82:1451–1453, 1982. (French)

b. Bartolozzi SR: External oculomotor paralysis and retrobulbar optic neuritis after spinal anesthesia. *ARCH SOC OFTALMOL HISP-AM* 12:1037–1044, 1952. (Spanish)

c. Bryce-Smith R, Macintosh RR: Sixth nerve palsy after lumbar puncture and spinal analgesia. *BR MED J* 1:275–276, 1951.

d. Faulkner SH: Ocular paralysis following spinal anesthesia. *TRANS OPHTHALMOL SOC UK* 64:234–236, 1944.

e. Greene BA, Berkowitz S, Goldsmith M: The prevention of cranial nerve palsies following spinal anesthesia. *ANESTHESIOLOGY* 15:302–309, 1954.

f. Huismans H: Eye muscle disturbance after spinal anesthesia. *KLIN MONATSBL AUGENHEILKD* 174:735–738, 1979.

g. Phillips OC, Ebner H, et al: Neurologic complications following spinal anesthesia with lidocaine. *ANESTHESIOLOGY* 30:284–289, 1969.

h. Voisin J, Mignot A: Bilateral papilledema accompanying sixth nerve paralysis after spinal anesthesia with Novocaine. *ARCH OPHTALMOL* 6:314, 1946. (French)

Aniline is a weakly basic, oily liquid, colorless when pure, but on exposure to air and light it rapidly oxidizes and becomes brown. Many years ago workers chronically exposed to crude aniline vapors had irritation of the eyes, photophobia, and impairment of vision.[d] They had brownish discoloration of the conjunctiva and cornea in the palpebral fissure, in some instances dense enough to interfere with ophthalmoscopic examination. These disturbances of conjunctiva and cornea seem to have been similar to those caused by quinones in the manufacture of hydroquinone, and it seems quite probable that in the case of aniline the discoloration and irritation of the eyes were also caused by quinone-like oxidation products. (See INDEX for *Quinones.*)

Aniline is readily absorbed from the skin and gastrointestinal tract, causing severe systemic poisoning similar to that caused by nitrobenzene.[252] Under its influence, hemoglobin is converted to methemoglobin, giving the patient a dusky appearance. The vessels of the conjunctiva and retina may appear discolored as though filled with ink, and the ocular fundus may assume a violet color without affecting vision.

In very rare case reports, disturbance of vision has been attributed to systemic poisoning.[c] These reports date from many years ago when diagnostic methods and criteria were somewhat inexact and the aniline was always chemically impure. Uhthoff concluded that aniline rarely had any effect on the optic nerve and that it seldom affected vision.[247] Lewin and Guillery mentioned two cases of narrowing of visual fields and one case of bilateral iritis with amblyopia occurring in aniline workers, but in only one case was evidence presented of systemic aniline poisoning.[153] In this case there was acute poisoning and coma from contact with crude aniline oil, with gradual recovery, but much impairment of vision and constriction of temporal fields, ascertained three weeks after the poisoning. The optic disc margins were slightly indistinct. In two weeks the vision and visual fields returned to normal.[a]

Sattler referred to occasional reports at the turn of the century of transient retrobulbar neuritis with central scotoma attributed to aniline, but in these particular cases dinitrobenzene was more likely the responsible agent.[214] In experimental poisoning of dogs, cats, and rabbits with aniline, Igersheimer never produced pathologic changes in the fundus, except in one cat which died twenty-four hours after injection of 0.5 ml of pure aniline. The pupils had become dilated and unreactive, and he found changes in ganglion cells and inner nuclear layer microscopically.[125]

Two cases of impaired visual acuity were cited by de Schweinitz in connection with aniline, but appear inconclusive because the workers involved were exposed chronically to various coal tar products, not just aniline.[41] Flury and Zernik in a thorough discussion of aniline poisoning mentioned that in the most severe cases when there are disturbances of the central nervous system manifested by disturbance of speech, headache, tinnitus, faintness, fatigue, paresthesias, and pains in the muscles, there may also be photophobia, weakness of vision, and sluggish pupillary reaction,[61] but they did not present original observations on visual effects. A case reported by Veasey in 1898 has often been cited as an example of transient paracentral scotomas and constriction of fields from aniline, but actually the patient was exposed to dyes rather than to aniline.[b]

It seems fair to conclude from the available evidence that it is doubtful that aniline poisoning has a specific effect on the eye, apart from the discoloration of the blood seen in the vessels of conjunctiva and fundus. Industrial instances of conjunctival and corneal discoloration are attributable to accompanying or contaminating quinones.

Several derivatives or relatives of aniline, bearing such names as aniline blue, aniline dyes, and aniline pencils, do not involve aniline itself and are considered under *Dyes and Pencils, indelible.* (See INDEX).

   a. Bocci D: On a case of acute poisoning by aniline oil. *ARCH OTTALMOL* 10:286–293, 1903. (Italian)
   b. Veasey CA: Central amblyopia in a dye worker probably produced by inhalation of the aniline dyes. *AM J OPHTHALMOL* 15:149–152, 1898.
   c. Berger E: Visual disturbances from aniline. *ARCH OPHTHALMOL* 38:396, 1909.
   d. Tyson HH: Aniline pigmentation of the eye. *ARCH OPHTHALMOL* 30:77, 1901.

p-Anisyl chloride (p-methoxybenzyl chloride) is said to yield vapors which have only moderate immediate lacrimogenic effect, but cause more severe reaction of the eyes on prolonged exposure. In an accident in which a bottle of p-anisyl chloride exploded spontaneously, three people cleaning up the debris noted slight irritation of the eyes when they started, but after about four hours suffered an increase in burning sensation and pain.[a] Details of the condition of the eyes have not been published, but it has been implied that they recovered.

   a. Carroll DW: *CHEM ENG NEWS* Aug. 22, 1960, p. 40.

Antazoline (phenazoline, Antistine) is an antihistamine used orally and also in eyedrops (0.5% solution).[171] On rabbit eyes 1.5% solution of antazoline hydrochloride was the maximum concentration that could be applied without causing keratitis epithelialis.[91] In human eyes 0.75% solution between pH 5 and pH 8 was about the maximum suitable for clinical use.[91]

Oral administration of 400 mg antazoline hydrochloride per day for five days to patients with normal eyes caused no change in intraocular pressure or tonographic measurements.[a]

   a. D'Ermo F, Pirodda A: Antihistamimics and the eye. *BOLL OCULIST* 39:715–721, 1960. (Italian)

Anthraquinone is a crystalline solid which has been noted only in experimental animal eyes to cause irritation and inflammation when applied to the eye. Anthraquinone is practically insoluble in water and it is possible that the irritation is due to a mechanical action of the powder rather than to a toxic effect.[53]

Anticholinergic drugs and Parasympatholytic agents block the actions of parasympathetic innervation and cholinergic drugs on the muscles of the iris, ciliary body, and blood vessels of the eye.

In ophthalmology, parasympatholytic agents are commonly employed in eyedrops or ointment for relaxing accommodation, dilating the pupil, and reducing vasodilation when there is inflammation in the anterior segment of the eye. However, paralysis of accommodation and dilation of the pupil may be unwanted side effects in the case of drugs administered systemically for treatment of disturbances of gastrointestinal tract, treatment of hypertension, treatment of allergies, or treatment of parkinsonism.

Parasympatholytic agents have some unpleasant and even dangerous actions on the eyes. Cycloplegia, or paralysis of accommodation, from interference with the normal innervation of the sphincter-like circular fibers of the ciliary muscle causes blurring of vision for near objects in young people, but may cause relatively little inconvenience to old people who are presbyopic and naturally have limited range of accommodation for near. In either case the visual difficulty can be corrected by means of plus lenses and is merely an inconvenience.

On the other hand, blocking parasympathetic innervation to the ciliary muscle can be dangerous to patients having borderline or actual, chronic open-angle glaucoma, because this may cause increase in resistance to escape of aqueous humor from the eye and increase of intraocular pressure.

In normal eyes with adequate channels for outflow of aqueous humor the influence of ciliary muscle tone may be relatively insignificant, and blocking parasympathetic innervation either by systemically or locally administered parasympatholytic agents have little effect on facility of outflow. However, in eyes bordering on glaucomatous or actually glaucomatous, the role of ciliary muscle tone may be more critical, and parasympatholytic agents may cause an unwanted increase in resistance to outflow and an increase in intraocular pressure.

In open-angle glaucoma, application of anticholinergic eyedrops can cause elevation of intraocular pressure with the anterior chamber angle remaining open. Reviews of relevant literature were published in 1968 and 1969.[83,84,85]

The fact that anticholinergic drugs applied in eyedrops have been shown to raise intraocular pressure in some eyes with open-angle glaucoma has caused concern that the many drugs used systemically that have anticholinergic properties might also have adverse effects on the pressure in patients with open-angle glaucoma.

Little actual clinical testing or experimentation was done before 1970 to establish how much danger there might be from systemic use of anticholinergic drugs in patients with open-angle glaucoma. Tests which are mentioned further under *Atropine* (see INDEX) indicate that some patients may be able to use systemic anticholinergic medications without adverse effect, while those whose pressure may be raised can be identified by routine tonometry, and by testing with an anticholinergic eyedrop such as cyclopentolate or tropicamide.

There are so many drugs in common use that have anticholinergic side effects, and so many people with glaucoma, that much more clinical investigation of this relationship is needed. In particular there is need for information on how effective standard miotic antiglaucoma eyedrops may be in opposing the effect of systemic anticholinergic drugs on intraocular pressure.

The size of the pupil normally is regulated largely by the tone and state of parasympathetic innervation of the sphincter muscle of the iris. Interference with parasympathetic innervation leads to mydriasis, or dilation of the pupil. In normal eyes this merely results in admitting more light to the eye and in slightly poorer quality of image than is formed with a small pupil. These effects are relatively trivial in normal eyes.

A much more dangerous effect of dilating the pupils is encountered in eyes having abnormally shallow anterior chambers. Normally the aqueous humor originating behind the iris in the ciliary processes flows forward through the pupil into the anterior chamber to reach the outflow channels of the corneoscleral trabecular meshwork and Schlemm's canal in the angle of the anterior chamber. On the way, the aqueous encounters a slight resistance in passing between the lens surface and iris to reach the pupil, and this causes a slight difference in pressure between the posterior and anterior chambers, billowing the iris slightly forward into convex contour in most eyes.

When the anterior segment is small or when the lens is disproportionately large or its anterior surface is further forward than ordinary, forming a shallow anterior chamber, the pupillary portion of the iris may be unusually closely applied to the anterior surface of the lens. In such eyes the aqueous humor encounters greater than ordinary resistance to flow through the pupil, and an abnormal billowing or forward bulging of the iris may result, sufficient to push the iris into actual contact with the trabecular meshwork, blocking the exit for aqueous humor, and causing the intraocular pressure to rise. This constitutes an attack of angle-closure glaucoma, which may be acute, painful, and extremely dangerous to the eye, requiring immediate emergency treatment.

In general, semidilation of the pupil most favors angle-closure. In semidilation, there is most likely to be enough slack or laxness of the iris, and at the same time enough resistance to flow from posterior to anterior chamber, to cause the iris to bulge forward in the periphery and close the angle. On the other hand if the pupil is widely dilated, particularly if this is accomplished rapidly, the resistance to flow from posterior to anterior chamber may be so reduced from diminished contact between iris and lens that there is little or no tendency to forward bulging or angle-closure.

Symptoms of blurring of vision, colored haloes about lights, or pain in the eye associated with pupillary dilation should raise suspicion of angle-closure glaucoma and call for immediate measurement of intraocular pressure, as well as gonioscopic examination of the angle of the anterior chamber if the pressure is elevated.

Anatomical shallowness of the anterior chamber which predisposes to angle-closure glaucoma may be suspected from simple inspection with a focused beam from a flashlight, or by examination with a slit-lamp biomicroscope, but the true circumstances can be established definitely only by examination utilizing a gonioscopic contact lens. Direct inspection of the angle, and certainty about its condition, can be achieved only by this means.

Treatment of severe acute angle-closure glaucoma, whether induced by parasympatholytic agents or occurring spontaneously, consists of inducing miosis through local application of miotic drugs such as pilocarpine, aided by topical timolol, or by oral or intravenous administration of carbonic anhydrase inhibitors, such as acetazolamide, and hyperosmotic agents, followed promptly by laser iridotomy if the cornea is sufficiently clear. In subacute attacks, less medical treatment is needed before iridotomy.

If no adhesions or synechias have formed between iris and trabecular meshwork as a result of angle-closure, the glaucoma can be cured in almost all cases by iridotomy. Once a hole has been made in the iris to permit unobstructed flow of aqueous humor from posterior chamber to anterior chamber, the pressure differential across the iris is abolished. Consequently the iris is no longer caused to billow or bulge forward in the previous manner, and the tendency for the angle to close is much reduced. Usually when unobstructed communication between posterior and anterior chamber has been provided, the intraocular pressure is no longer affected by the size of the pupil, and anticholinergic or parasympatholytic agents are much less likely to cause closure of the angle or elevation of the pressure.

Systemic intoxication by atropine-like anticholinergic drugs from excessive dosage administered systemically or absorbed following application to the eye is characterized by redness and dryness of the skin, dryness of the mouth, increased body temperature, increased pulse rate, disorientation, and visual hallucinations. The patient usually recovers spontaneously when administration is discontinued.

This systemic poisoning, when sufficiently severe to require treatment, can be counteracted by giving 1 to 2 mg of physostigmine salicylate parenterally, repeated as needed.[a, b]

(For more details of a typical anticholinergic drug, see INDEX for *Atropine*.)

a. Duvoisin RC, Katz R: Reversal of central anticholinergic syndrome in man by physostigmine. *J AM MED ASSOC* 206:1963–1965, 1968.
b. Johnson AL, Hollister LE, Berger PA: The anticholinergic intoxication syndrome: diagnosis and treatment. *J CLIN PSYCHIATRY* 41:313–317, 1981.

Antihistaminics (antihistamine drugs) seldom cause ocular disturbance, but certain compounds, particularly *diphenhydramine* (Benadryl) and *prophenpyridamine* (Trimeton) have atropine-like action and occasionally cause slight dilation of the pupils and impairment of accommodation for near.[a, b] Some antihistaminics also have local anesthetic action when applied in solution to the cornea.[b] *Mepyramine* (Pyrilamine) and *antazoline* applied as 2.5% solutions to eyes of rabbits have caused rapid clouding of the corneal epithelium, local-anesthesia, and transitory swelling of the cornea, with recovery in a few days.[48] For a series of antihistaminics, concentrations which might be considered maximum suitable for topical ophthalmic use range from 0.5% to 1%.[91]

a. Sheldon JM, Lovell Rg, Kiess RD: Observations of the effect of anti-histaminic compounds on the corneal reflex of rabbits. *UNIV HOSP BULL* (*Ann Arbor*) 15:42, 1949.
b. Wyngaarden VB, Seevers MH: Toxic effects of antihistamine drugs. *J AM MED ASSOC* 145:277–282, 1951.

Antimony pentachloride and **antimony trichloride** are irritating and caustic to the skin, and their fumes are strongly irritating to the eyes, face, and mucous membranes of the respiratory tract. Severe burns of the cornea are said to have been caused by exposure to high concentrations of the fumes, and destruction of the cornea and conjunctiva has resulted from contact with a solution of antimony trichloride in hydrochloric acid.[6, 42, 79] In a case in which apparently the eyes were protected by the lids from a spray of such a solution only small superficial injury of the cornea occurred and promptly healed, though there were second degree burns of the skin around the eyes and disturbances of upper respiratory and gastrointestinal tracts.[a]

a. Taylor PJ: Acute intoxication from antimony trichloride. *BR J IND MED* 23:318–321, 1966.

Antimony potassium tartrate (tartar emetic) has been used by intravenous injection mostly in treatment of schistosomiasis and leishmaniasis. One boy who had received twenty-three injections of this drug in treatment of kala-azar suddenly developed bilateral blindness with dilated unreactive pupils. Papilledema was observed associated with acute hydrocephalus and glomerulonephritis. Vision slowly improved enough for the boy to go to school, but the optic nerveheads remained permanently pale.[a]

Three other children when receiving their third course of treatments for bilharziasis all developed optic atrophy without papilledema, with gradual progressive diminution of vision to low levels.[b] Neurologically they were normal otherwise, and no cause was found for the optic atrophy other than the antimony compound.

a. D'Amino D: Observations on a case of sudden bilateral blindness from antimony tartrate in treatment of Kalaazar. *LETT OFTALMOL* 8:474–482, 1931.
b. Kassem A, Hussein HA, et al: Optic atrophy following repeated courses of tartar emetic for the treatment of bilharziasis. *BULL OPHTHALMOL SOC EGYPT* 69:459–463, 1976.

Antiperspirants or deodorants employed in the form of liquids, powders, sprays, and sticks have generally contained an aluminum salt, or occasionally a zinc salt, as the active agent. In spray form the antiperspirants are most likely to reach the eye, sometimes causing a slight transient irritation and fine gray stippling of the corneal epithelial cells visible by biomicroscope.[81] No permanent disturbance has been observed. (See also *Aluminum chloride hexahydrate.*)

Arabinose is a sugar which can be reduced to a sugar alcohol by rat lens aldose reductase. When administered to rats repeatedly intraperitoneally, it produces peripheral cortical cataracts, initially resembling galactose cataracts, but later evolving into equatorial zonular opacities like those produced by xylose.[a]

a. Keller HW, Koch HR, Ohrloff C: Experimental arabinose cataracts in young rats. *OPHTHALMIC RES* 9:205–212, 1977.

Arachidonic acid is a natural precursor of prostaglandins. Applied to rabbit eyes as sodium arachidonate it causes increase in intraocular pressure, constriction of the pupil and increase in proteins in the aqueous humor.[a] (Also see *Prostaglandins.*)

Exploratory studies of intraocular effects of metabolic products of arachidonic acid have been published by Stjernschantz et al,[b] and effects of synthetic lipid hydroperoxide from arachidonic acid on the ERG by Armstrong et al.[274]

a. Bhattacherjee P, Eakins KE: Inhibition of the ocular effects of sodium arachidonate by anti-inflammatory compounds. *PROSTAGLANDINS* 9:175–182, 1975.
b. Stjernschantz J, Sherk T, et al: Intraocular effects of lipoxygenase pathway products in arachidonic acid metabolism. *ACTA OPHTHALMOL* 62:104–111, 1984.

Aramite, a commercial contact miticide for plants, has been found to give electro-retinographic indications of intoxication of retinal photoreceptors when injected into mice,[a] and when applied to the eyeball.[289]

a. Carricabura P, Lacroix R, et al: Electroretinographic study during acute Aramite intoxication of the white mouse. *TOXICOL EUR RES* 2:195–198, 1979.

Araroba (Goa powder, crude chrysarobin) is a brownish dermatologic powder which has often caused severe irritation of eyes and face when handled, attributable to its content of *chrysarobin* and *chrysophanic acid.*[246]

Armazide, a swimming pool algicide consisting of a mixture of alkyl quaternary ammonium salts has been tested at a dilution of 1:80,000 on rabbit eyes and at that high dilution was found to cause no irritation or injury.[a] Undiluted it probably would be damaging to the eye, since at full strength it was moderately irritating on the skin of rabbits.[a] (Compare *Exalgae.*)

a. Antonides HJ, Chacharonis P: Toxicologic studies on Armazide. *TOXICOL APPL PHARMACOL* 4:44–54, 1962.

Arsacetin (sodium acetylarsanilate) has been used in treatment of syphilis. Similar to other derivatives of *arsanilic acid* it has caused blindness from optic neuritis and atrophy in numerous cases. Characteristically it has caused the visual fields rapidly to become narrowed until central vision was lost. Histologically, degeneration of the retinal ganglion cells and nerve fibers have been found, with least damage to the papillomacular bundle, and with no signs of inflammation.[214]

Arsanilic acid (sodium arsanilate, Atoxyl, Soamin, sodium p-aminophenylarsonate) was formerly used in treatment of syphilis and trypanosomiasis. There have been at least fifty reports in the literature on disturbances of vision, and by 1932 sodium arsanilate was known to have caused more than eighty cases of blindness, and was no longer used.[214]

The dose causing blindness was as small as 0.5 g, but on the average was 7 g. Typically it caused progressive constriction of the visual fields, with the fundi appearing normal at first. Constriction progressed until central vision was involved, and subsequently optic atrophy developed.[b] Isolated central scotomas did not occur.[214] The prognosis for vision was very poor once constriction of the fields started.[a,b]

Histology showed degeneration of the retinal ganglion cells and of the fibers of the optic nerve, also changes in the nuclei of the rods in the outer nuclear layer, but the rods themselves and the cones were not abnormal.[a,214]

In animals, similar injuries of ganglion cells and optic nerve were induced.[a,b,214] Arsanilate appeared to have a special affinity for retina and optic nerve. In pigs blinded by arsanilate the visually evoked cortical response was non-recordable, but the ERG remained normal. This was explainable on the basis of atrophy of the optic nerve, which was evident ophthalmoscopically.

However, in cultures of retina in vitro addition of 5×10^{-3} M sodium arsanilate has caused degeneration of the rod cells.[99] (See also *Arsenicals, organic* in INDEX.)

a. Birch-Hirshfeld A, Koster G: Injury of the eye by Atoxyl. *GRAEFES ARCH OPHTHAL-MOL* 76:403, 1910. (German)

b. Igersheimer J, Rothmann A: On the behavior of Atoxyl in the organism. *Z PHYSIOL CHEM* 59:259, 1909. (German)

c. Witzel DA, Smith EL, et al: Arsanilic acid-induced blindness in swine. *AM J VET RES* 37:521–524, 1976.

Arsenic, inorganic, in a variety of forms is irritating and injurious, both by local contact and systemic absorption. Arsenical dusts such as *arsenic trioxide*, encountered in smelting of ores, and *copper acetoarsenite* (Paris green) employed agriculturally, are irritating to the upper respiratory tract and eyes. The conjunctivitis produced by these substances is characterized by itching, burning, and watering of the eyes, with photophobia and sometimes hyperemia and chemosis.[j,51,61,129,188]

In chronic systemic poisoning by inorganic arsenic compounds, a similar conjunctivitis with sensation of irritation and tearing very commonly occurs, possibly due to excretion of arsenic in the tears.[j] Changes in the skin, hair, and nails are characteristic of chronic inorganic arsenic poisoning. Hyperkeratosis of the feet and hands is particularly characteristic, and dry scaling, and deep pigmentation may involve the lids and face as well as the trunk and extremities.[j,129] Pigment spots in the epithelium of both cornea and conjunctiva have been described accompanying melanosis of the skin,[l,129] but the character of these spots has not been determined. Transverse lines appear in the fingernails, and arsenic accumulates in the hair, but the growth of eyebrows and eyelashes is said not to be disturbed.[h,129] Rarely, in acute or chronic poisoning from inorganic arsenic, there has been severe keratitis accompanying conjunctivitis and exfoliative dermatitis. Approximately a dozen cases have been reported.[a,b,g,i]

Systemic poisoning is characterized by gastrointestinal irritation, peripheral neuritis, manifested by paresthesia, hyperesthesia, and burning discomfort in the hands and feet, confusion and weakness, as well as the skin manifestations already described. Whether there may be disturbance of the optic nerve and retina by inorganic arsenic in human beings is uncertain and has at times been denied.[c,214] There is great opportunity for confusion in the literature, since many cases of genuine optic neuritis and optic atrophy have been caused by certain organic compounds of arsenic as described under *Arsenicals, organic,* and in some instances a critical distinction appears not to have been made between *inorganic* and *organic* arsenicals.

Search of the literature produces essentially no reports which might be accepted as valid evidences of injury of the optic nerve by *inorganic* arsenic. Surveys by Igersheimer and Schirmer in 1909 and 1910 disclosed six reports up to that time suggesting such injury,[r,125] but review of these reports shows them to have been vague and inconclusive. Valuable evidence relating to this question was furnished in 1900 by a mass poisoning of several thousand persons in England by beer contaminated with arsenic. Although the recognized signs and symptoms of chronic arsenic poisoning were quite distinct and often very severe, including irritation and "running of the eyes" in more than half of the cases,[q] extensive careful examination revealed no case of optic atrophy.[r]

Since that time, a case of bilateral primary optic atrophy has been ascribed to handling of *copper acetoarsenite,* but the patient had a positive Wassermann test, absent knee jerks, and no definite evidence of arsenic poisoning.[m] Also an instance of a transitory acute blurring of vision in only one eye to 5/18 accompanied by wide dilation of the pupil of that eye, followed by complete recovery in two to three days has been ascribed to taking eight drops of *Fowler's solution* (*potassium arsenite*), but there were no symptoms of arsenic poisoning and the fundi were normal.[d] A brief note has been made of dense central scotomas and optic atrophy in a farmer who had been employing a spray containing arsenic, nicotine, and lead, but there was no conclusive evidence that any one of these substances was responsible.[k]

A claim that a so-called neuroretinitis of extremely vague character in fifty-eight cases was due to arsenic[f] has been refuted on the basis that the only evidence of arsenic poisoning was the presence of an amount of arsenic in the urine which was insignificant when compared to normal controls.[n,214]

More recently, in a survey of patients having peripheral neuropathy associated with urinary arsenic excretion significantly above normal, one patient is said to have had evidence of optic neuritis with a history of transient blindness lasting several days, and mention was made in other cases of dimness of vision or diplopia, but no ophthalmologic details were given.[h] Chronic alcoholism or consumption of illegal whiskey were recognized complicating factors in these patients and could have caused the visual disturbances. In another medical study of forty patients with definite peripheral neuropathy from either acute or chronic inorganic arsenic poisoning, with characteristic numbness, tingling, formication, and pain in upper and lower extremities, the ocular fundi were reported normal in all cases, and no cranial nerves were involved except in one patient who had sixth nerve palsy.[s]

A variety of other ocular disturbances have been ascribed to inorganic arsenic poisoning in isolated reports, such as ptosis, weakness of extraocular and intraocular muscles, and transient narrowing of the visual fields for color, but no substantial evidence is found to establish these as characteristic effects of inorganic arsenic poisoning. Individual reports of retinal pigmentation and retinal vascular abnormalities appear ill-founded.[e,p]

In 1960 one case was reported in which cotton wool patches, scattered small hemorrhages, and dilated capillaries appeared in the central fundi of a man with sinus trouble and asthma who for two years had taken a proprietary medicine said to include Fowler's solution or potassium arsenite in unstated amounts. Five years after arsenical medication was stopped, the patient had a hemorrhage in the vitreous in one eye after hard coughing, and he was found to have dilated venules, microaneurysms, and proliferative vascular retinopathy in both maculas, unchanging during the next year. It was concluded that the cause of the retinal changes was not clear, but that possibly the previous use of arsenic had contributed to its occurrence.[o] However, in this case apart from suggestive hyperkeratosis and detection of arsenic in the hair there was little evidence of poisoning. In 1967 one other case was reported in which vision became reduced because of spots of retinitis with hemorrhages in both eyes after three years of systemic treatment for psoriasis with a medication containing arsenic. (No information was given on what chemical form the arsenic was in, or how much was present.) After the arsenic-containing medication was stopped, the hemorrhages absorbed in two months, leaving spots of degeneration, and vision improved a little. At six months there appeared to be partial optic atrophy. The neuroretinitis was assumed to be attributable to the arsenic medication but there was no other evidence of poisoning.[u]

Experimentally, acute poisoning of rabbits and rats with *sodium arsenite* has caused no retinal degeneration.[231] *Sodium arsenate* administered to dogs and cats in doses sufficient to cause severe chronic poisoning has caused much conjunctivitis, but no abnormality of the pupils or ophthalmoscopically visible abnormalities.[125] *Sodium arsenate* injected into the carotid artery in rabbits in doses that were commonly lethal in one to six days caused no ophthalmoscopically recognizable changes in the retina.[t] However, in one cat poisoned for a month with *arsenate*, Igersheimer reported microscopically demonstrable abnormalities in the ganglion cells and inner nuclear layer.[125]

Experiments on retina surviving in culture *in vitro* has shown *arsenic trioxide* at 5 × 10⁻⁶ M to cause degeneration of the rod cells.[99]

Evidence for any toxic action of inorganic arsenic on the optic nerve is on the whole extremely poor, yet biochemical grounds for such a toxic effect are conceivable. The characteristic peripheral neuritis of arsenic poisoning appears to be closely related to the peripheral neuritis of thiamine deficiency which is encountered in beriberi and chronic alcoholism.[q] Interference with pyruvate oxidation appears to be the basis of both types of neuritis. Nutritional deficiency neuritis has often been associated with retrobulbar optic neuritis under the name of tobacco-alcohol amblyopia, yet in inorganic arsenic poisoning, for reasons unknown, the optic nerve appears rarely if ever to be disturbed.

Injury of the eye from direct gross contact with inorganic arsenic compounds, such as result from a splash or from experimental application, has been reported several times. *Arsenic trioxide* applied and reapplied to rabbit eyes causes discomfort, edema of the lids, corneal injury, and opacity, and when placed in the anterior chamber has local necrotizing action.[53,150]

Tests on rabbit eyes by application to the cornea after removal of the epithelium or by injection into the corneal stroma caused severe injury when 0.08 M *sodium arsenate* or 0.005 M *sodium metarsenite* was employed.[123] In human beings, four cases of very severe ocular burning and scarring have been noted following splash of *sodium arsenate* solution, but in these cases injury was attributed to a great excess of alkali in the solution rather than to the arsenate.[249]

Arsenic pentafluoride and *arsenic trichloride* are especially irritating compounds and are to be found indexed individually. *Arsenic sulfide* in a single instance of an industrial explosion is said to have caused permanent opacification of the cornea.[46] Industrially, injuries by splash of arsenicals has been much rarer than the irritation induced by exposure to arsenical dusts.

a. Bonamour G: Keratoconjunctivitis in severe arsenical poisoning. *ANN OCULIST* (*Paris*) 180:483, 1947. (French)
b. Chan E: Arsenical exfoliative conjunctivitis and keratitis. *NAT MED J CHINA* 28:114, 1942. (*AM J OPHTHALMOL* 25:1145, 1942.)
c. Clarke E: Optic atrophy following the use of arylarsonates in the treatment of syphilis. *TRANS OPHTHALMOL SOC UK* 30:240–251, 1910.
d. Cohn P: Acute arsenic intoxication of eye. *DTSCH MED WOCHENSCHR* 41:1137–1138, 1918. (German)

e. Engelking: Demonstration. *KLIN MONATSBL AUGENHEILKD* 100:620, 1938. (German)

f. Haas HK de: On disturbance of the retina and the optic nerve from arsenic poisoning. *GRAEFES ARCH OPHTHALMOL* 99:16, 1919. (German)

g. Hallum A: Involvement of the cornea in arsenic poisoning. *ARCH OPHTHALMOL* 21:93, 1934.

h. Heyman A, Pfeiffer JB, et al: Peripheral neuropathy caused by arsenical intoxication. *N ENGL J MED* 254:401–409, 1956.

i. Hyde FT: Arsenical exfoliative keratitis. *AM J OPHTHALMOL* 14:611–616, 1931.

j. Leschke E: *Clinical Toxicology.* London, Churchill, 1934.

k. Mayou MS: Industrial toxic amblyopia. *PROC ROY SOC MED* 20:1112, 1927.

l. Meesmann: A case of arsenic melanosis. *KLIN MONATSBL AUGENHEILKD* 64:548, 1920. (German)

m. Moleen GA: Metallic poisons and the nervous system. *AM J MED SCI* 173:883–895, 1913.

n. Petren K, Ramberg L: Comments on the question of the occurrence of an arsenical neuroretinitis (de Haas). *GRAEFES ARCH OPHTHALMOL* 101:257–264, 1920. (German)

o. Prickman L, Hollenhorst R, Ammermann E: Toxic retinopathy. *AM J OPHTHALMOL* 50:64–70, 1960.

p. Reiser: Demonstration. *KLIN MONATSBL AUGENHEILKD* 103:248, 1939. (German)

q. Satterlee HS: The arsenic-poisoning epidemic of 1900. *N ENGL J MED* 263:676–684, 1960.

r. Shirmer O: On optic nerve diseases due to poisoning with organic and inorganic arsenical preparations. *ARCH OPHTHALMOL* 39:456–466, 1910.

s. Chhutani PN, Chawla LS, Sharma TD: Arsenical neuropathy. *NEUROLOGY* 17:269–274, 1967.

t. D'Agostino A, Vecchione L, Tieri O: Further contribution to the study of experimental retinal degeneration. *ARCH OTTALMOL* 66:417–422, 1962. (Italian)

u. Nover A, Koinis G: Arsenical injury of the retina. *KLIN MONATSBL AUGENHEILKD* 150:535–537, 1967. (German)

Arsenicals, organic, are drugs which were employed in the treatment of syphilis and other diseases since the beginning of this century, and have had toxic side effects upon the eyes in a great many cases. Certain of these drugs typically have induced optic neuritis with rapidly constricting visual fields, often progressing to loss of central vision and optic atrophy. Optic neuritis and atrophy have been caused in most cases by the following derivatives of *p-* or *m-arsanilic acid: sodium arsanilate* (Atoxyl, Soamin); *arsacetin* (sodium acetylarsanilate); *acetarsone* (acetarsol, Spirocid, Stovarsol); *Acetylarsan; 3-methylarsacetin* (Orsudan); and *Tryparsamide.* Rare instances have been attributed to *Indarsol, Hectin, Sulfostat,* and *Rhodarson.*

In contrast to arsanilic acid and its derivatives, with their notorious selective toxicity to the retina and optic nerves, the newer and chemically different compounds *Arsphenamine* and *Neoarsphenamine* have not with certainty been demonstrated to have this type of toxicity, and *Marpharsen* has apparently given no indication of damaging optic nerve or retina.

Experimental investigation of the relationship of chemical constitution to injurious effect has indicated that selective toxicity to the retina and optic nerve is associated with the presence of an amino group or a substituted amino group in either the *p-* or *m-* positions relative to the arsenic acid group of arsanilic acid.[a,b]

However, in monkeys it has been possible to produce optic atrophy and blindness by a derivative lacking an amino group, *4-β-(β'-hydroxy)ethoxy-ethoxyphenylarsonic acid.*[b] (Inorganic arsenic is not selectively toxic to the retina and optic nerve. See *Arsenic, inorganic.*)

For further information on individual organic arsenicals see INDEX for *Acetarsone, Acetylarsan, Arsacetin, Arsanilic acid, Arsphenamine, Mapharsen, Neoarsphenamine, Orsudan, Arsanilic acid,* and *Tryparsamide.*

a. Longley BJ, Clausen NM, Tatum AL: Experimental production of primary optic atrophy in monkeys by administration of organic arsenical compounds. *J PHARMACOL* 76:202–206, 1942.
b. Young AG, Loevenhart AS: The relation of chemical constitution of certain organic arsenical compounds to their action on the optic tract. *J PHARMACOL EXP THER* 21:197–198, 1923; and 23:107–126, 1924.

Arsenic trichloride is a fuming liquid, toxic and caustic owing not only to the poisonous nature of arsenic but also to the release of hydrochloric acid in the presence of water. The fumes are a strong respiratory tract irritant, and industrially have been observed to cause blepharospasm, lacrimation and photophobia.[a]

a. Scherling SS, Blondis RR: The effect of chemical warfare agents on the human eye. *MILIT SURG* 96:70–78, 1945.

Arsine (arsenic trihydride) is a very poisonous gas. Death may be caused by a few inhalations. Because of its great systemic toxicity, few observations have been made of the local effects of arsine on the eye, and the gas is not sufficiently irritating to prevent serious poisoning. Persons exposed to poisonous concentrations may be unaware of their exposure until symptoms and signs of systemic poisoning develop several to many hours later.[b] A striking feature is a development of intense orange discoloration of the sclera and skin from blood pigment released by the massive hemolysis induced by arsine.[a,c,d,155]

a. Levinsky WJ, et al: Arsine hemolysis. *ARCH ENVIRON HEALTH* 20:436–440, 1970.
b. Schrenk HH: Arsine. *IND ENG CHEM* 43:141A–142A, 1951.
c. Teitelbaum DT, Arsine poisoning. *ARCH ENVIRON HEALTH* 19:133–143, 1969.
d. Wilkinson SP, McHugh P, et al: Arsine toxicity aboard Asiafreighter. *BR MED J* 2:559–563, 1975.

Arsphenamine (Arsenobenzol; Salvarsan; Arsaminol), formerly used in treatment of syphilis, differs chemically from derivatives of arsanilic acid which cause optic neuritis and atrophy. Arsephenamine appears rarely, if ever, to have caused this type of injury.

It is known to have caused encephalitis with headache, loss of consciousness, convulsions and meningitic symptoms with increased intracranial pressure, resulting in papilledema and paralysis of cranial nerves to the eye muscles and face. Rare instances of neuroretinitis and of retrobulbar neuritis with central or paracentral scotomas have been reported, but these are quite exceptional and may therefore have been attributable to other causes.[c,h] In three cases of visual disturbance discussed by Birch-Hirschfeld, he pointed out that evidence was quite inadequate to inculpate arsphenamine. Similarly in rare and exceptional cases, retinal hemorrhages have been observed.[a,e,f,194]

Another rare side effect consists of transient myopia of several diopters, coming on rapidly and lasting from one day to a month in several cases.[b,d,i,j] More rarely there has been transient paralysis of accommodation.

Exfoliative dermatitis has occasionally occurred, and in a few instances has been associated with conjunctivitis and keratitis.[g,k] In most, but not all cases the eyes have recovered. Occupational exposure to arsphenamine dust has been said to cause blepharospasm and keratitis, but no details are available.[176]

a. Birch-Hirschfeld A, Inouye N: Experimental investigation of the action of Indarsol on the optic nerve and retina. *GRAEFES ARCH OPHTHALMOL* 79:81–95, 1911. (German)
b. Cergueira Falcao E de: Transient spasmodic myopia caused by arsenobenzol. *ANN OCULIST (Paris)* 174:847–853, 1937. (French)
c. Chartina C: Optic neuritis as an effect of lues or of Salvarsan? *ARCH OFTALMOL HISP-AM* 28:257–261, 1928.
d. Dupuy, Dutemps, Perin: Transient spasmodic myopia from arsenobenzol. *BULL SOC FRANC DERM SYPH* 32:394–399, 1925. (French)
e. Horvath V: Hemorrhagic retinitis after Salvarsan. *SZEMESZET* 56:4, 1922. (*ZENTRALBL GES OPHTHALMOL* 9:294, 1923.)
f. Imachi J: Concerning ophthalmia hepatic. *ACTA SOC OPHTHALMOL JPN* 42:2099–2108, and German Summary 143, 1938.
g. Kirby DB: Keratitis exfoliativa complicating dermatitis exfoliativa (Arsphenamine). *ARCH OPHTHALMOL* 2:661–669, 1929.
h. Kogoshima S: On two cases of neuroretintits after Salvarsan injection. *NIPPON GANKAGAKKAI ZASSHI* 18:458–466, 1914. (*JBER OPHTHALMOL* 451:314, 1914.)
i. Paglsit-Durante G: Transitory myopia from arsenebanzol. *BOLL OCULIST* 18:641–645, 1939.
j. Sauferlin H: Severe topical corneal injury in a case of Salvarsandermatitis. *MUNCH MED WOCHENSCHR* II; 1476–1477, 1932. (German)

Ascorbic acid (vitamin C) has been examined for effects on the eye principally in connection with study of its therapeutic use orally and intravenously in reducing ocular pressure in glaucoma. Subconjunctival injections of 1 ml of 10% solution daily for ten days in rabbits caused no significant irritation.[b] Repeated application of 10% solutions of ascorbic acid or sodium ascorbate to the eyes of patients also has caused no injury.[c,d]

In rabbit corneal endothelial cell culture *in vitro* addition of ascorbate had an inhibitory effect on cell growth.[a]

a. Beatrice YJT, Niedra R, Baum JL: Effects of ascorbic acid on cultured rabbit corneal endothelial cells. *INVEST OPHTHALMOL VIS SCI* 19:1471–1476, 1980.
b. Esila R, Liesmaa M, et al: The effect of ascorbic acid on the intraocular pressure and the aqueous humor of the rabbit eye. *ACTA OPHTHALMOL* 44:631–636, 1966.
c. Linner E: The effect of ascorbic acid on intraocular pressure. In Paterson; Miller; Paterson (Eds): *DRUG MECHANISMS IN GLAUCOMA.* London, Churchill, 1966, pp. 153–161.
d. Suzuki Y, Kitazawa Y: The effects of topical administration of ascorbic acid on aqueous

humor dynamics of glaucomatous eyes. *ACTA SOC OPHTHALMOL JPN* 71:57–60, 1967.

Aspartic acid, or sodium aspartate, is a natural nonessential amino acid that can be converted to glutamate *in vivo,* and like glutamate may serve as a neurotransmitter in the outer plexiform layer of the retina, as well as in some cones and ganglion cells.[c] There is a large literature concerning the neurophysiologic roles of aspartate, but discussion here will be limited to the toxicologic aspects. Aspartate, like glutamate, when administered to young rodents in large dosage alters the ERG and causes wide-spread histologically demonstrable injury to the retina.[f] In amphibians, aspartate interferes with protein synthesis by the retina,[a] and suppresses electrical activity of the retina, though leaving the response of photoreceptors unaffected.[e] In monkeys, when sodium aspartate has been infused into the vitreous humor, a striking constriction of retinal vessels has been observed, and fortuitously opacities were observed to develop in the crystalline lens.[b] Cataracts have also been produced in rabbits by the same procedure.[d]

a. Anderson RE, Hollyfield JE, Berner GE: Regional effects of sodium aspartate and sodium glutamate on protein synthesis in the retina. *INVEST OPHTHALMOL VIS SCI* 21:554–562, 1981.
b. Baron WS: Lenticular and fundus changes induced by the intraocular infusion of sodium aspartate. *INVEST OPHTHALMOL* 13:459–462, 1974.
c. Ehinger B: [3H]-D-Aspartate accumulation in the retina of pigeon, guinea pig and rabbit. *EXP EYE RES* 33:381–391, 1981.
d. Hikita K: Experimental cataract of rabbits induced by sodium aspartate. *NIPPON IKA DAIGAKU ZASSHI* 44:73–83, 1977.
e. Sillman AJ, Ito H, Tomita T: Studies on the mass receptor potential of the isolated frog retina. *VISION RES* 9:1435–1442, 1969.
f. Yamada K: Experimental studies on the ERG and EOG of the adult albino rabbits eyes treated with L-Na-aspartate. *ACTA SOC OPHTHALMOL JPN* 73:1952–1967, 1969.

Aspidium (filix mas; male fern; oleoresin aspidium), an anthelmintic containing *filicin* or *filixic acid* as the main active principle, has been used mainly in the treatment of tapeworm infestations in man and animals. It was most widely employed in the nineteenth and early twentieth centuries. Most information about poisoning comes from before 1908.[153,214,247] Little is to be found in recent clinical literature, except a case of poisoning ending in bilateral blindness and optic atrophy in Ethiopia,[a] also a case of optic atrophy in a breast-fed infant whose mother was receiving extract of filix,[e] and a case of suspected toxic effect on the eyes of a mother and fetus in early pregnancy reported by Bonnett and Leopold in 1969.[b] The child in this report, who was seen only at ages nine and twelve years, was found to have consistently subnormal vision (3/10, 5/10 with glasses), associated with fine disseminated pigmentary retinopathy, very constricted visual fields, but normal optic nerveheads and only slightly abnormal ERG, unlike retinitis pigmentosa. Similar but milder abnormalities were found in the mother. The history was obtained that at the second to third months of gestation, the mother had been treated for taenia infestation with aspidium and had been made very sick by it. However, no visual or eye complications had been noted at that time.[b]

Even in the days of widespread medical use of aspidium, the incidence of poisoning and serious visual disturbance was very low, of the order of one out of a thousand patients treated with the medication; and about one out of five to six thousand were blinded by it. On the other hand, in at least half of all patients who showed any significant signs of systemic intoxication, visual disturbance was one of the principal manifestations.[153,214,247]

Reaction to the drug was characterized by headache, faintness, noises in the ears, prostration, diarrhea, vomiting, trembling, convulsions, or coma, and in some instances poisoning was fatal. Involvement of vision was characteristically associated with deep pain in both orbits or upon motion of the globes, sometimes with the appearance of flashes of light or with dilation and paralysis of the pupils and blurred vision.

Typically visual disturbances appeared after several hours of sleep or on the day following administration of the drug, developing rapidly, sometimes to complete blindness. In very rare instances, five to eleven days passed before the loss of vision. Most commonly, visual disturbance followed ingestion of 10 g of the extract, but in exceptional cases blindness was reported after 6 g, and in one case after 3 g. As a rule, both eyes were involved, but usually one was involved to a greater extent than the other. In the majority of cases some vision was recovered at least in one eye, and pemanent bilateral blindness was uncommon. In occasional cases, return to normal occurred even after initial complete blindness in both eyes.

In association with blindness the pupils were always dilated and unreactive, and when blindness was permanent there was always definite optic atrophy. Early after the onset of visual disturbance, the fundus usually appeared normal, but sometimes presented the appearance of retinal edema and blurring of the edges of the optic nervehead with some narrowing of the arteries, but less than in quinine poisoning.[a] Hemorrhages were rarely noted. With permanent blindness, the ophthalmoscopic picture was of optic atrophy, with narrowed, sometimes obliterated, retinal vessels.

Histologic information in this type of poisoning has essentially all come from experimental animals, dogs and rabbits, showing death of retinal ganglion cells and degeneration of optic nerve fibers, but no indication of primary inflammatory process, although endovasculitis and perivasculitis with obliteration of the vessels has been described. Visual disturbance and optic nerve damage is readily induced in animals.[153,214,247] Rosen (1969) has studied such effects in cattle that have eaten male fern.[d]

In studies on experimental animals reported by Georges and associates in 1969, purified *filicin* was used. In dogs daily oral administration of 40 to 80 mg/kg for one month caused progressive loss of vision in five out of twelve animals and complete blindness in two of these. The loss of vision became noticeable after ten to fifteen days of administration of *filicin*. The lenses and fundi continued to appear normal ophthalmoscopically except for slight pallor of the optic nerveheads, but histologically "diffuse spongiosis" was described in the nerve fibers of the optic nerve and brain. The treatment was lethal for five of the twelve animals in the course of a month. In rats the same investigators looked for teratogenic effect and found that *filicin* caused microphthalmia, anophthalmia, abnormalities of the retina and optic nerve fibers, disorganization of the CNS, in addition to many non-ocular abnormalities.[c]

a. Agnello F: Toxic amaurosis from filix mas. *RASS ITAL OTTALMOL* 8:210–221, 1939. (Italian)

b. Bonnett M, Leopold P: Pigmentary pseudoretinopathy acquired by a mother and infant by poisoning in the second month of pregnancy by chloroform extract of male fern. *BULL SOC OPHTALMOL FRANCE* 69:583–586, 1969. (French)

c. Georges A, Gerin Y, Denef J: Study of the toxic effects of purified fern extracts. *X PROC EUROP SOC STUDY DRUG TOXICITY.* AMSTERDAM EXCERPTA MED FOUNDATION 1969, pp. 219–226.

d. Rosen ES, Edgar JT, Smith JLS: Male fern retrobulbar neuropathy in cattle. *TRANS OPHTHALMOL SOC UK* 89:289–299, 1969.

e. Gregersen E: Optic atrophy in a breast-fed infant and treatment of maternal cestode infection with filix. *ACTA OPHTHALMOL* 36:115–119, 1958.

Aspirin (acetylsalicylic acid) is reported to have been used by a patient for self-mutilation by insertion in the lower conjunctival sac. This caused severe ulceration of the conjunctiva and superficial injury of the cornea in one eye, and may have been responsible for severe corneal ulceration and loss of the patient's other eye.[d]

Salicylate poisoning many years ago, before aspirin became popular, was caused almost exclusively by overdosage of *sodium salicylate* employed as an antipyretic and analgesic. When *sodium salicylate* was in common use, it was reported to have caused temporary complete or partial blindness in numerous cases.[q,153,214,247]

Typically, visual disturbances were reported after ingestion of 8 to 20 g of *sodium salicylate* in the course of one to several days. Vision usually faded to complete blindness in the course of several hours. Commonly, but not always, visual disturbances were accompanied by tinnitus or deafness, and sometimes by headache, stupor, or coma. Blindness usually lasted from three to twenty-four hours. Then normal vision gradually returned. Slight functional disturbances occasionally persisted for a week or more.[153]

The cause of the loss of vision has not been firmly established. Occasionally either narrowing or widening of the retinal vessels was described, but more often the ocular fundi appeared normal. The pupils appeared dilated in most cases, but usually continued to react to light. A functional disturbance of the optic nerve was suspected, but the behavior of the pupils suggested that the disturbance might be in the occipital visual cortex. No characteristic change of visual field was recognized, but narrowing of the visual fields was observed infrequently, and in one instance hemianopsia was reported. Defective color perception was found in three cases. Nystagmus has rarely been reported.[153]

Since aspirin has largely replaced *sodium salicylate*, overdosage has caused many severe and sometimes fatal poisonings, especially in children, but descriptions of effects on the eyes or on vision have been very rare. Aspirin taken with carbonic anhydrase inhibitors produces greater acidosis than aspirin alone.

A young girl treated for acidosis and dehydration from aspirin had temporary amaurosis after a period of water retention, hyponatremia and coma. Although the VER regained normal appearance, signs of optic atrophy were noted.[f]

An older patient in twenty-four hours took approximately 35 g of aspirin, 2 to 5 g of acetophenetidin, and less than 200 mg of codeine phosphate, from which the patient became severely intoxicated, and on the second day had severely diminished visual acuity, with mydriasis and diminished pupillary reaction to light in both eyes. Both optic papillas and surrounding retinas were edematous, and large hemorrhagic spots were present in both fundi. Complete optic atrophy ensued in one eye, and partial optic atrophy with ultimate recovery of 9/10 vision in the other eye.[o] The author of this case subsequently mentioned having seen two other patients who had small peripheral retinal hemorrhages while taking aspirin, but the relationship seemed uncertain.[p]

In another case a woman who was in the habit of taking 6 to 30 g of aspirin a day had nausea, vomiting and unsteadiness of gait for which no obvious neurologic basis was discovered. She was ataxic and had difficulty speaking and hearing. She complained of headache and distorted vision, scintillating visual scotomas, and episodes of diplopia without visible abnormalities in the eye. She was then found to have papilledema of as much as 2 diopters, which subsided completely in a few days when the large intake of aspirin was discontinued. However, many of her previous complaints persisted. It was supposed that the papilledema in this case was due to cerebral edema and was related to an electrolyte disturbance.[i]

Aspirin has been reported in rare instances to have caused allergic dermatitis with keratitis and conjunctivitis, but without permanent damage.[r]

Two episodes of acute transitory myopia have been attributed to aspirin.[a,n] (This type of reaction is further discussed under *Myopia, acute transient.* See INDEX.)

In one series of patients who took 16 to 50 g of aspirin the intraocular pressure was temporarily reduced about 10 mm Hg.[s] When the patients recovered from acidosis, the intraocular pressures returned to normal.

Ordinary doses of 0.6 g of aspirin had no significant effect on intraocular pressure in a series of fourteen patients with primary open-angle glaucoma studied by Peczon.[k] There appears to be no danger in use of aspirin in the presence of glaucoma, although in rabbits intravenous administration of 5 to 40 mg/kg was said to raise the pressure.[l]

Tetratogenic effects of *sodium salicylate* have been reported in rats, including anophthalmia, microphthalmia, and exophthalmia in the offspring, apparently governed somewhat by the degree of acidosis induced.[h] An infant with cyclopia was born by a woman who took 3 to 4.5 g of aspirin per day during the first trimester of pregnancy, but a relationship is questionable.[b]

Aspirin administered after traumatic hyphema has been clearly shown to predispose to rebleeding.[e,g,m] Spontaneous hyphema has occurred in association with ingestion of aspirin,[j] but spontaneous hyphema is not rare in the absence of medications. Bilateral subconjunctival hemorrhages have been described in one case after ingestion of 6.5 g of aspirin.[c]

a. Baron A, Michel G, et al: Spasmodic myopia. *BULL SOC OPHTALMOL FRANCE* 67:716–717, 1967. (French)
b. Benaura R, Mangurten HH, Duffell EL: Cyclopia and other anomalies following maternal ingestion of salicylates. *J PEDIATR* 96:1069–1071, 1980.

c. Black RA, Bensinger RE: Bilateral subconjunctival hemorrhage after acetylsalicylic acid overdose. *ANN OPHTHALMOL* 14:1024–1025, 1982.

d. Copenhaver RM: A report of an unusual self-inflicted eye injury. *ARCH OPHTHALMOL* 63:266–272, 1960.

e. Crawford JS: The effect of aspirin on rebleeding in traumatic hyphema. *TRANS AM OPHTHALMOL SOC* 74:357–362, 1976; *AM J OPHTHALMOL* 80:543–545, 1975.

f. Engel R, Lambert JD, Cunningham A: EEG studies of cortical blindness in a case of salicylate poisoning. *NEUROPADIATRIE* 3:377–385, 1972.

g. Ganley JP, Geiger JM, et al: Aspirin and recurrent hyphema after blunt ocular trauma. *AM J OPHTHALMOL* 96:797–801, 1983.

h. Goldman AS, Yakovac WC: Salicylate intoxication and congenital anomalies. *ARCH ENVIRON HEALTH* 8:648–656, 1964.

i. Greer HD III, Ward HP, Corbin KB: Chronic salicylate intoxication in adults. *J AM MED ASSOC* 193:85–88, 1965.

j. Kageler WV, Moake JL, Garcia CA: Spontaneous hyphema associated with ingestion of aspirin and alcohol. *AM J OPHTHALMOL* 82:631–634, 1976.

k. Peczon JD: Personal communication, 1967.

l. Ramos L, Ramos AO, Caldeira JAF: Action of anti-pyretic-analgesic drugs on intraocular pressure in the rabbit. *MED PHARMACOL EXP* 16:350–354, 1967.

m. Romano P: Aspirin and recurrent hyphema after blunt ocular trauma. *AM J OPHTHALMOL* 97:663–664, 1984.

n. Sandford-Smith JH: Transient myopia after aspirin. *BR J OPHTHALMOL* 58:698–700, 1974.

o. Sedan J: Acute hemorrhagic papillitis in the course of a very acute poisoning by aspirin. *BULL SOC OPHTALMOL FRANCE* 58:333–336, 1958. (French)

p. Sedan J: Iatrogenic retinal accidents caused by aspirin. *J REV ESP OTONEURO-OFTALMOL* 27:272–275, 1968. (Spanish)

q. Snell S: A case of blindness resulting from the administration of salicylate of sodium. *TRANS OPHTHALMOL SOC UK* 21:306–308, 1901.

r. Uchida Y: On ocular disturbances due to intoxication with aspirin. *FOLIA OPHTHALMOL ORIENT* 2:38–41, 1935.

s. Varady J, Jahn F: On hypotony in poisoning with salicylic acid preparations. *DTSCH MED WOCHENSCHR* 66:322–323, 1940. (German)   •

Asthmador is a proprietary drug containing *Atropa belladonna* and *Datura stramonium*, whose principal active components are atropine and scopolamine.[d] The preparation is sold in the form of powder or in cigarettes intended to be ignited and the vapor to be inhaled for relief of asthma. Several episodes of poisoning have occurred, mostly in young people, who have ingested one-half to four teaspoons of the powder or have eaten several of the cigarettes. All of the characteristic signs of atropine poisoning have been described, including dilated and unreactive pupils, weakness of accommodation for near, and visual hallucinations. The pulse has been fast, the patient's skin red and dry, and the patients have been severely confused and disoriented. Spontaneous recovery has been the rule.[a-e] Concerning possible treatment, see *Anticholinergic drugs.*

a. Dean ES: Self-induced stramonium intoxication. *J AM MED ASSOC* 185:168–169, 1963.

b. DiGiacomo JN: Toxic effect of stramonium simulating LSD trip. *J AM MED ASSOC* 204:265–267, 1968.

   c. Goldsmith SR, Frank I, Ungerleider JT: *J AM MED ASSOC* 204:169–170, 1968.
   d. Koff M: Poisoning from ingestion of asthma "powders". *J AM MED ASSOC* 198:170, 1966.
   e. Wilcox WP Jr: *N ENGL J MED* 277:1209, 1967.

Atropine; dl-hyoscyamine, an anticholinergic alkaloid from *Atropa belladonna* and *Datura stramonium,* is used most commonly in the form of atropine sulfate.

1. Ocular effects of topical atropine. Atropine dilates the pupil and paralyzes accommodation for near by anticholinergic blocking of parasympathetic innervation to the sphincter muscles of the iris and ciliary body. The paralytic effect may persist for days or weeks, depending on the amount used and the responsiveness of the individual. Topical atropine has long been recognized to be clinically helpful in the treatment of anterior uveitis.

Adverse ocular effects of topical atropine, apart from occasional contact allergy,[e] are practically entirely related to induction of glaucoma. Several different mechanisms can be involved. In certain eyes that have glaucoma secondary to intraocular inflammation but have wide angles with good space between periphery of the iris and the aqueous outflow system of the trabecular meshwork in the outer wall of the angle, atropine can prove beneficial and help reduce intraocular pressure as it helps reduce intraocular inflammation. However, when this therapeutically beneficial effect of atropine is not obtained, atropine can cause elevation of intraocular pressure by one or more of the following mechanisms: (a) With intraocular inflammation in an eye that does not have a wide angle between iris and trabecular meshwork, dilating the pupil with atropine may allow the iris to come in contact with inflammatory exudates on the angle wall, forming peripheral anterior synechias, resulting in chronic synechial glaucoma. (b) In eyes with abnormally narrow angles with or without intraocular inflammation, dilating the pupil may induce angle-closure glaucoma by allowing the iris to come into contact with the trabecular meshwork, blocking the aqueous outflow. (Paradoxically, occasionally in eyes with spontaneous acute angle-closure glaucoma when atropine has been applied because of a mistaken diagnosis, it has occasionally made it easier for aqueous to flow from posterior to anterior chamber through a greatly widened pupil, temporarily relieving the so-called pupillary block mechanism which may have caused the iris to bulge forward against the trabecular meshwork at the start. This mechanism, however, is not to be counted upon therapeutically. Induction of angle-closure glaucoma by atropine in anatomically predisposed eyes is much better known.) (c) In eyes with chronic open-angle glaucoma and without inflammation, the intraocular pressure may be raised by application of atropine, without closing the angle. (Though atropine does not significantly raise the intraocular pressure in nonglaucomatous eyes with wide angles and probably does not cause significant rise of pressure in two out of three eyes with mild primary open-angle glaucoma, in about one out of three a significant rise occurs when cycloplegia is induced by atropine or other anticholinergic drugs. It seems in general the poorer the facility of outflow in open-angle glaucomatous eyes, the greater the likelihood of elevation of intraocular pressure when cycloplegia is induced, suggesting that cycloplegia may act in the opposite sense from miotic eyedrops on the ciliary muscle and interfere with its action on the aqueous outflow system in the angle.)[83,85]

In school children, application of atropine eyedrops daily for nearly five years has had no adverse effect on intraocular pressure, and no other injurious effect.[s] Also the eyes of dogs have been found histologically normal after atropine eyedrops were applied once or twice daily for as long as a year.[r] In rabbits, frequently repeated applications of 1% atropine sulfate for five days gave no evidence of injurious effect and caused no interference with regeneration of the endothelium in eyes in which the corneal endothelium had been abraded.[120] In cats, injection of 0.05 ml of solution containing 0.04 mg atropine sulfate into the anterior caused no significant loss of corneal endothelial cells.[f]

2. Ocular effects of systemically administered atropine. When atropine is given orally or parenterally, its effects on the eyes are essentially the same as when applied directly to the eye, except that the amount reaching the eye is relatively small and the effects accordingly much less. People receiving atropine or related drugs systemically not uncommonly note enlargement of the pupils and weakened accommodation for near, usually associated with unpleasant dryness of the mouth.[70,103,109,177]

Atropine sulfate 0.6 mg injected intramuscularly in eight normal patients has been reported to cause appreciable decrease in accommodation in ten out of sixteen eyes, but to have dilated the pupil in only three of the patients, not more than 1.5 mm in any.[152] The same dosage given three times a day by mouth to six normal patients for seven days caused no subjective blurring of vision or enlargement of the pupil.[o] Intramuscular injection of 0.01 mg/kg in healthy volunteers caused no change in the pupil or intraocular pressure.[d]

Effects on pupil and accommodation are merely nuisances, rather than serious side effects, unless the patient either has abnormally shallow anterior chambers and narrow angles predisposing to angle-closure glaucoma, or has chronic open-angle glaucoma which could theoretically be made worse by cycloplegia. Clinical studies by Lazenby and Reed strongly suggest that administration of atropine orally in ordinary dosage to patients with open-angle glaucoma is unlikely to elevate the intraocular pressure in individuals who have shown no significant rise in pressure when tested by application of eyedrops containing a strong anticholinergic drug, such as cyclopentolate, directly to the eyes.[148] It appears that the simple topical test, which can be done in an hour or two, offers a guide to estimating the risk from systemic atropine or other anticholinergic drugs in patients with open-angle glaucoma. However, even those who do show a rise in pressure from topical testing with cyclopentolate may have no significant aggravation of the glaucoma from the small amount of atropine reaching the eye from ordinary systemic dosage. Standard anti-glaucoma medications may suffice to counteract the effect of systemic atropine. This can be ascertained by routine tonometry.

3. Systemic adverse effects from atropine applied to the eye. Systemic intoxication from atropine eyedrops is very well known both in children and adults. There seems to be considerable variation in individual susceptibility. (A question of whether children with Down's syndrome are particularly susceptible will be discussed later.) Systemic poisoning from atropine eyedrops and ointment has occurred innumerable times and has been the subject of many case reports and reviews.[c,h,i,j,m,p,q]

The most striking feature of the poisoning is psychotic agitated behavior with hallucinations, disorientation, and unawareness of actual surroundings or identity. The patient may be very restless and have visual hallucinations, particularly of insects, typically plucking at or brushing at clothing or bedclothes, showing behavior and personality quite foreign to the patient. Associated characteristic signs of atropine poisoning are fast pulse, dry red skin, and elevated body temperature. Blocking of sweating by atropine mainly accounts for the dryness of the skin and the elevation of temperature.

The poisoning is distressing but rarely fatal, even with large overdoses of atropine,[a] and it is self-limited if the cause is recognized and the atropine medication is discontinued. More prompt relief of the intoxication can be obtained by administering cholinergic drugs, such as physostigmine. (This treatment is described under *Anticholinergic drugs*.)

In children with Down's syndrome there is a legend that atropine eyedrops have greater effect than in normal children. The first published mention seems to have been by McKusick in 1957, who simply asked the question, "What is the basis for the not infrequently fatal idiosyncrasy of mongoloid idiots to agents of the atropine group?", but he gave no evidence or references to support the implication.[k] In response to this remark several groups of investigators who had had considerable experience with monogloid children in special hospitals reported that in their own experience when they had occasionally used atropine as preoperative medication and for dilating pupils, they had not been aware of any special adverse effects.[b,l,n] Controlled comparisons of mydriasis in mongoloid and normal children induced by atropine drops showed that in fact the pupils of the mongoloid children dilated more rapidly.[b,l,n] The greater responsiveness of the pupils was not influenced by giving reserpine.[l] Homatropine eyedrops did not act differently in the two groups.[l] However, hydroxyamphetamine did produce a greater pupillary response in the mongoloids, like atropine. It was postulated by most observers that probably the slightly greater responsiveness was attributable to some anatomical difference in the irides of the mongoloid children. There were no indications in these studies of adverse systemic side effects from the atropine eyedrops, although groups of ten to thirty were tested in the various studies, mostly with 1% atropine sulfate.

A review of the literature on reactivity of the pupil to atropine in Down's syndrome was provided by Harris and Goodman in 1968, and they also determined experimentally that apart from the greater mydriatic response attributed to atropine applied to the eye, children with Down's syndrome had abnormally great cardio-accelerator response to intravenously administered atropine.[g] They did not investigate or compare the effects on the central nervous system.

a. Alexander E, Morris d, Eslick R: Atropine poisoning. *N ENGL J MED* 234:258, 1946.
b. Berg JM, Gillian Brandon MW, Kirman BH: Atropine in mongolism. *LANCET* 2:441–442, 1959.
c. Costello JM, Shannon FT: Drugs and children. *NEW ZEAL MED J* 67:402–405, 1968.
d. Cozanitis DA, Dundee JW, et al: Atropine versus glycopyrrolate. *ANESTHESIA* 34:236–238, 1979.
e. Gallasch G, Schutz R, et al: Side-effects of atropine: Pharmacologic, allergic, pseudo-allergic or toxic reactions? *KLIN MONATSBL AUGENHEILKD* 181:96–99, 1982. (German)

f. Hammer ME, Chenoweth RG: The effect of intraocular dilating solution on cat endothelium. *OPHTHALMIC SURG* 15:585–587, 1984.

g. Harris WS, Goodman RM: Hyper-reactivity to atropine in Down's syndrome. *N ENGL J MED* 279:407–410, 1969.

h. Hoefnagel D: Toxic effects of atropine and hematropine eyedrops in children. *N ENGL J MED* 264:168–171, 1961.

i. Hoffman GM, Gray JR: Accidental atropine poisoning. *PENN MED J* 62:1340–1341, 1959.

j. Lehmann H: Acute atropine poisoning after application as eye drops in glaucoma simplex. *KLIN MONATSBL AUGENHEILKD* 65:112, 1920. (German)

k. McKusick VA: Symposium on inborn errors of metabolism. *AM J MED* 22:676–686, 1957.

l. O'Brien D, Haake MW, Braid B: Atropine sensitivity and serotonin in mongolism. *J DIS CHILD* 100:873–874, 1960.

m. Polson CJ, Tattersall RN: *CLINICAL TOXICOLOGY* 2nd ed. Philadelphia, Lippincott, 1969.

n. Priest JH: Atropine response of the eyes in mongolism. *J DIS CHILD* 100:869–872, 1960.

o. Rider JA, Moeller HC, DeFelice EA: Antisecretory effects of modaline sulfate. *TOXICOL APPL PHARMACOL* 7:438–444, 1965.

p. Sanitato JJ, Burke MJ: Atropine toxicity in identical twins. *ANN OPHTHALMOL* 15:380–382, 1983.

q. Van Deuren H, Misotten L: Atropine intoxication and the acute delirium of the elderly blind patient. *BULL SOC BELGE OPHTALMOL* 186:27–29, 1979.

r. Watanabe C, Miyaura K, et al: Histological findings on ciliary body. *ACTA SOC OPHTHALMOL JPN* 72:1494–1511, 1968.

s. Yamaji R, et al: Study on pseudomyopia. *ACTA SOC OPHTHALMOL JPN* 72:2083–2150, 1968.

AY-9944, a potent experimental inhibitor of cholesterol biosynthesis, has been shown when given to rats to cause lamellar inclusion bodies to accumulate in cells in the eye, especially in retinal ganglion cells and glial cells of the optic nerves.[a] Upon prolonged administration these cells degenerate.

a. Sakuragawa M: Niemann-Pick disease-like inclusions caused by a hypocholesteremic. *INVEST OPHTHALMOL* 15:1022–1027, 1976.

Azathioprine (Imuran), an immunosuppressive drug, has been investigated as an agent to suppress the rejection of corneal grafts. Given parenterally to rabbits, it has been found to interfere with development of normal tensile strength of corneal wounds and to retard healing.[a,b] Teratogenic effects, including malformation of eyes, particularly the lens, have been produced by administering azathioprine to pregnant rabbits.[c]

a. Elliott JH, Leibowitz HM: The influence of immunosuppressive agents upon corneal wound healing. *ARCH OPHTHALMOL* 76:334–337, 1966.

b. Francois J, Feher J: The effect of azathioprine and chlorpromazine on corneal regeneration. *EXP EYE RES* 14:69–72, 1972.

c. Tuchmann-Duplessis H, Mercier-Parot L: Dissociation of antitumor and teratogenic properties of a purine antimetabolite, azathioprine. *C R SOC BIOL* 159:2290–2294, 1965. (*CHEM ABSTR* 65:6079, 1966.)

5-Aziridino-2,4-dinitrobenzamide has caused cataracts in rats.

Cobb LM: Toxicity of the selective antitumor agent 5-aziridino-2,4-dinitrobenzamide in rats. *TOXICOL APPL PHARMACOL* 17:231–238, 1970.

Azoester, an agent known to oxidize glutathione in red blood cells, has been shown to do the same in rat lenses, and also to reduce lens ATP content and adversely affect lens cation transport and permeability.[a]

a. Epstein DL, Kinoshita JH: Effect of methyl phenyldiazenecarboxylate (azoester) on lens membrane function. *EXP EYE RES* 10:228–236, 1970.

BA6650, an experimental sympathomimetic agent, given orally to dogs for 2 weeks caused corneal opacities, hypopyon, anterior synechias, and hypotony.[a]

a. Steffen GR, Henderson JD, et al: Ocular toxicity in beagle dogs with an experimental fluoromethane sulfonanilide sympathomimetic agent. *DRUG CHEM TOXICOL* 3:165–172, 1980.

Bacitracin, an antibacterial, applied to de-epithelialized corneas at a concentration of 10,000 units/ml interfered with healing, but 500 units/ml did not.[368] In the anterior chamber of enucleated rabbit eyes, 2,000 to 6,000 units/ml caused swelling of the corneas.[293]

Bacterial endotoxins prepared from *Escherichi coli* and *Shigella flexneri* injected into rabbits' corneas can cause serious keratitis, scarring and vascularization.[b] Intravitreal injection in rabbits and chickens can produce endophthalmitis with cellular infiltration, breakdown of the blood-aqueous barrier, uveitis, and cataract.[a,c] The endotoxins have been utilized in experimental studies of ocular inflammatory and antiinflammatory mechanism.[a,b,d] (Compare *Proteases from bacteria*.)

a. Bhattacherjee P, Butler JM: Responses of the sympathetically denervated rabbit eye to intravitreal or intravenous injection of *Shigella* endotoxin. *EXP EYE RES* 28:611–614, 1979.
b. Howers EL, Cruse VK, Kwok MT: Mononuclear cells in the corneal response to endotoxin. *INVEST OPHTHALMOL VIS SCI* 22:494–501, 1982.
c. Shimizu M: Experimental cataract caused by bacterial endotoxin. *FOLIA OPHTHALMOL JPN* 29:562, 1978. (English summary)
d. Stetz DE, Bito LZ: The insensitivity of the chicken eye to the inflammatory effects of x-rays in contrast to other inflammatory agents. *INVEST OPHTHALMOL VIS SCI* 17:412–419, 1978.

Bacterial exotoxin prepared from *Pseudomonas aeruginosa* injected into the corneas of rabbits kills epithelial, endothelial, and stromal cells, resulting in necrosis of the cornea.[a] Exotoxin neutralized by specific antitoxin does not have this severe effect. (Compare *Bacterial endotoxins, Collagenase,* and *Proteases from bacteria*.)

a. Iglewski BH, Burns RP, Gipson IK: Pathogenesis of corneal damage from Pseudomonas exotoxin. *INVEST OPHTHALMOL VIS SCI* 16:73–76, 1977.

Bamethan (Butylsympathol, Buty-nor-sympatol, Vasculate, Bupatol), a peripheral vasodilator, when injected subconjunctivally causes much redness and swelling, and may elevate the ocular pressure several mm Hg, reaching a maximum in one to two hours and subsiding within three to six hours. The pressure is raised more in open-angle glaucomatous than in normal eyes, and this has been the basis of a test for glaucoma.[a]

a. Leydhecker W: A new stress test for diagnosis of glaucoma. *KLIN MONATSBL AUGENHEILKD* 123:568–577, 1953. (German)

Barbiturates (barbituric acid derivatives employed as sedatives and hypnotics) include a very large number of drugs that vary mostly in duration and intensity of action. Poisoning affecting the eyes has been reported, mainly from *barbital* and *phenobarbital.*

There appears to be no constant or characteristic effect upon the pupils in either acute or chronic poisoning, although hippus with sluggish reaction to light is said to be common.[e,24] Mydriasis and miosis occur with about equal frequency.[q]

The eyelids may give a clue in detecting people who have become habitual users or have become dependent upon barbiturates. Bilateral ptosis is characteristic, and blepharoclonus, consisting of a rapid fluttering of the eyelids, can be induced by tapping the glabella area, increasing with repeated tapping, different from the normal individual who responds with a few blinks only at the start of tapping.[f,j]

Disturbance of eye movement has been among the most common neurologic findings in both acute and chronic barbiturate poisoning.[24] Nystagmus, both horizontal and vertical, weakness of convergence, as well as weakness of vertical gaze and of individual extraocular muscles have many times been noted.[g,o,p,y,24,255] Nystagmus presumably represents a functional disturbance in most instances, since it is transitory. Transient nystagmus has, for instance, been induced without causing organic damage by administration of *amobarbital.*[a] Similar effects are seen in patients during induction of anesthesia by means of shorter-acting barbiturates. *Pentobarbital* given intravenously to rabbits commonly causes nystagmus as anesthesia is being induced.[81] Smooth tracking eye movements are interfered with,[k,r] and the convergence mechanism is temporarily impaired by barbiturates in normal people.[t,u,za,zc]

Bilateral blindness or subnormal vision has been reported in several patients during recovery from coma induced by *barbital.*[v,x,y,z] Generally these patients have had no distinctive abnormalities of the fundus, but one person had central scotomas with slight constriction of the fields and appeared to have slight neuroretinitis with papilledema.[z] Recovery in all instances has apparently been complete within a week or two, except in one case noted by Lewin and Guillery in 1913 in which a man accustomed to taking large amounts of *barbital* awoke one morning blind in both eyes, and subsequently developed optic atrophy.[153]

Transient loss of vision following coma has also been reported in several cases of acute poisoning by *phenobarbital.*[d,i,s,w,194,255] In some of these cases the fundi have been normal despite complete blindness.[194] In other cases the ophthalmoscopic findings have included contraction of the retinal arteries,[d,194] increased pressure in the retinal arteries,[j] and in one case papillitis.[194] As a rule, vision has been recovered in one to two weeks following poisoning by *phenobarbital* or *barbital*, but in one case vision improved only to 2/10.[i] In rare instances transient disturbances of color vision, xanthopsia, and chloropsia have been noted in the period of recovery from coma.[h,v]

It is difficult from the literature on either *barbital* or *phenobarbital* to ascertain the basis of the impairment of vision. Some reports indicate normal fundi and normal pupillary reaction to light, suggesting an effect at a high level in the central nervous system, but other reports describe abnormalities of the fundi with sluggish pupillary response to light. These reports seem to indicate that barbiturates may affect vision at various levels.

A revealing investigation has been carried out by determining the effect of unilateral intracarotid injection of *amytal* on the visual field in man, with the result that homolateral ocular blindness was produced, not associated with contralateral hemianopia, indicating that functional blockage can occur at the level of the retina.[zb]

The critical thresholds of flicker fusion and two-flash fusion are depressed by barbiturates, but this is regarded as a measure of general depressant effect on the central nervous system, rather than a specific effect on vision.[b,n,za]

ERGs in animals, in excised eyes and retinas, have shown increase in the a- and b-waves under the influence of barbiturates.[c,l,m,zd] Also, the c-wave and the standing potential are affected.[zm] It seems likely that barbiturates affect both the neuroretina and the pigment epithelium of the retina.

In the presence of glaucoma, use of barbiturates appears to present no special hazard, since ordinary doses of moderate- to long-acting derivatives either have no effect on ocular pressure or tend to reduce it, and the shorter-acting used as general anesthetics have greater tendency to reduce the pressure. There appears to be no report of elevation of pressure in human eyes by barbiturates.

With average doses of barbiturates, sensitization and dermatitis may develop, in some instances associated with dermatitis of the lids and conjunctivitis.[214] In one case the conjunctival reaction has led to symblepharon.[x] Bullae of the conjunctivae have been associated with profound coma.[ze]

a. Bender MB, Brown CA: The character of the nystagmus induced by amytal in chronic alcoholics. *AM J OPHTHALMOL* 31:825–828, 1948.

b. Besser GM, Duncan C: The time course of action of single dose of diazepam, chlorpromazine and some barbiturates as measured by auditory flutter fusion and visual flicker fusion thresholds in man. *BR J PHARMACOL* 30:341–348, 1967.

c. Bornschein H, Hanitzsch R, Lutzow AV: Demonstration of the barbiturate effect on excised retina of warm-blooded animals. *EXPERIENTIA (Basel)* 22:98–99, 1966. (German)

d. Carillo R, Malbran J, Chichilnisky S: Barbiturate optic neuritis. *ARCH OFTALMOL B AIR* 13:370–380, 1938.

e. Carlson VR: Individual pupillary reactions to certain centrally acting drugs in man. *J PHARMACOL EXP THER* 121:501–506, 1957.

f. Committee on Alcoholism and Addiction and Council on Mental Health: Dependence on Barbiturates and other sedative drugs. *J AM MED ASSOC* 193:673–677, 1965.

g. Edis RH, et al: Vertical gaze palsy in barbiturate intoxication. *BR MED J* 1:144, 1977.

h. Euziere J, Vidal J, et al: Barbiturate coma with transitory xanthopsia following. *REV OTOL* 12:344–346, 1934.

i. Franceschetti A, Doret M: Amaurosis after acute barbiturate poisoning. *REV OTO-NEUROOPHTALMOL* 19:91–92, 1947. (French)

j. Hamburger E: Identification and treatment of barbiturate abusers. *J AM MED ASSOC* 193:143–144, 1965.

k. Holzman PS, Levy DL, et al: Smooth pursuit eye movements, and diazepam, CPZ, and secobarbital. *PSYCHOPHARMACOLOGIA* 44:111–115, 1975.

l. Honda Y, Nagata M: Some observations of the effects of barbiturates upon the electroretinogram of rabbits. *OPHTHALMIC RES* 4:129–136, 1972/73.

m. Knave B, Persson HE, Nilsson SEG: A comparative study on the effects of barbiturate and ethyl alcohol on retinal functions. *ACTA OPHTHALMOL* 52:254–259, 1974.

n. Kopell BS, Noble EP, Silver J: The effect of thiamylal and methamphetamine on the two-flash fusion threshold. *LIFE SCI* 4:2211–2214, 1965.

o. Korbsch H: On disturbances of vertical eye movements in Veronal and Medinal poisoning. *ARCH PSYCHIATR* 72:473–477, 1924. (German)

p. Lessell S, Wolf PA, Chronley D: Prolonged vertical nystagmus after pentobarbital sodium administration. *AM J OPHTHALMOL* 80:151–152, 1975.

q. Levin M: Eye disturbances in bromide intoxication. *AM J OPHTHALMOL* 50:478–483, 1960.

r. Norris H: The time course of barbiturate action in man investigated by measurement of smooth tracking eye movement. *BR J PHARMACOL* 33:117–128, 1968.

s. Oppenheim H: Infirmation on Veronal poisoning and functional forms of visual disturbance. *DTSCH Z NERVENHEILKD* 57:1, 1917. (German)

t. Rashbass C: Barbiturate nystagmus and the mechanism of visual fixation. *NATURE* 183:897, 1958.

u. Rashbass C, Westheimer G: Barbiturates and eye vergence. *NATURE* 191:833–834, 1961.

v. Rivet L, Sambron J: Transient toxic amaurosis followed by chloropsia after barbiturate coma treated by strychnine. *BULL SOC MED HOP PARIS* 50:17–19, 1934. (French)

w. Rivet L, Magitot A, Bouree J: A new case of transitory amaurosis after barbiturate coma treated with strychnine. *BULL SOC MED HOP PARIS* 52:583–586, 1936. (French)

x. Roth JH: Luminal poisoning with conjunctival residue. *AM J OPHTHALMOL* 9:533–534, 1926.

y. Steindorff K: Eye disturbances in poisoning by Veronal and related sleep medications. *DTSCH MED WOCHENSCHR* 51:1565–1567, 1925. (German)

z. Terrien F: Neuroretinitis and amblyopia after ingestion of Veronal. *ARCH OPHTALMOL* (*Paris*) 41:204–206, 1924. (French)

za. Turner P: Effect of a mixture of dexamphetamine and amylobarbitone on critical flicker fusion frequency. *J PHARMACOL* 17:388–389, 1965.

zb. Waltregny A, Lambert JL, Petrov V: Visual field and intracarotid sodium amytal in man. *ACTA NEUROL BELGE* 72:416–420, 1972. (French)

zc. Westheimer G: Amphetamine, barbiturates, and accommodation convergence. *ARCH OPHTHALMOL* 70:830–836, 1963.

zd. Wundsch L: Experimental study of the problem of retinal ischemia. *GRAEFES ARCH OPHTHALMOL* 197:241–253, 1975.

ze. Yatzidis H: Bullous lesions in acute barbiturate poisoning. *J AM MED ASSOC* 217:211, 1971.

Barium hydroxide (barium hydrate, caustic baryta) and **Barium oxide** (calcined baryta) dissolve in water to give strongly alkaline solutions. They closely resembles calcium hydroxide in their damaging action on the eye. Rabbit eyes are severely injured and the corneas rendered opaque by a solution at pH 12, but below pH 11 only slight and reversible injury is induced.[a, 46, 89, 90]

   a. Gerard G: Prognosis of chemical burns of the eye; especially of burns by baryta. *CLIN OPHTALMOL* 15:251–268, 1926. (French)

Barium chloride, a readily soluble salt, has been tested in neutral 0.08 to 0.1 M solution on rabbit eyes by injection into the cornea or by dropping for ten minutes on the eye after the corneal epithelium was removed to facilitate penetration. Under these conditions barium chloride caused no opacification of the cornea, but did cause considerable iritis, which subsided in a few days.[81, 90, 123]

Barium sulfate is used as a radiopaque contrast medium for gastrointestinal x-ray examinations and as a weighting substance in some golf balls. Its use in the gastrointestinal tract rarely causes intoxication, but there is a unique report of rapid development of bilateral retrobulbar neuritis with central scotomas in a seventy-year-old man after ingestion of 125 g. The central scotomas cleared and vision returned to normal in three or four weeks. It was postulated that the material was impure, possibly containing barium sulfide or carbonate.[a]

A fine suspension of barium sulfate injected experimentally into the anterior chamber of eyes of rabbits attracts many leukocytes, causes much hyperemia of the iris, dilation of perilimbal vessels, and clouding and vascularization of the cornea. The barium sulfate particles later become encapsulated by fibrin and endothelial cells.[150]

The conjunctiva and eyelids of children have in several instances become injected accidentally with barium sulfate which was squirted under very high pressure from the centers of certain makes of golf balls, which the children had cut into. X-ray diffraction and electron probe examination have been employed to identify barium sulfate in the extraocular tissues. Barium sulfate in the center of the golf balls commonly has been mixed with other substances, such as zinc sulfide. Fortunately this material deposited in the conjunctiva and lids is reported to have been remarkably inert, causing little injury, with mainly a macrophage reaction evident microscopically.[b,c] (See *Golf balls* in INDEX for comparison of other chemical injuries from this source.)

   a. Garraud, LeRoux: Bilateral retrobulbar optic neuritis following ingestion of barium sulfate. *ARCH OPHTALMOL* 492–494, 1920. (French)
   b. Johnson FB, Zimmermann LE: Barium sulfate and zinc sulfide deposits resulting from golf-ball injury to the conjunctiva and eyelid. *AM J CLIN PATHOL* 44:533–538, 1965.
   c. Penner R: The liquid center golf ball. *ARCH OPHTHALMOL* 75:68–71, 1966.

Battery explosions occur when automobile storage batteries with lead plates and sulfuric acid generate hydrogen which is ignited by a spark or flame.[a–e] Several series of serious injuries have been reported, mainly involving severe blast trauma, which may damage all portions of the eye. In many instances sulfuric acid burns of conjunctiva and cornea have been described, but generally the acid burns have been less serious than the physical injuries. In general, epithelium lost in this type of accident has regenerated, suggesting that a spray of acid, rather than a gross splash, may be involved.

a. Davidorf FH: Battery explosions: a hazard to health. *J AM MED ASSOC* 223:1509, 1973.

b. Holenkamp TLR, Becker B: Ocular injuries from automobile batteries. *TRANS AM ACAD OPHTHALMOL OTOL* 83:805–810, 1977.

c. Minatoya HK: Eye injuries from exploding car batteries. *ARCH OPHTHALMOL* 96:477–481, 1978.

d. Moore AT, Cheng H, Boase DL: Eye injuries from car battery explosions. *BR J OPHTHALMOL* 66:141–144, 1982.

e. Siebert S: Ocular trauma from lead-acid vehicle battery explosions. *AUST J OPHTHALMOL* 10:53–61, 1982.

Bee stings of the eye have been especially well discussed by Lewin and Guillery in 1913[153], by Young in 1931[p], and by Kranning who in 1955 surveyed fifty-seven publications on the subject to that time.[h]

Toxic and damaging effects on the anterior segment in human beings and in experimental animals will be discussed first, then disturbances of the retina and optic nerve. (*Wasp stings* are described separately—see INDEX.)

The most serious reactions of the anterior segment of the eye from bee stings have been encountered in cases in which the stinger entered the cornea; this has been the subject of most of the publications.[k] The victim suffers much pain and photophobia, associated with clouding and swelling of the cornea, iritis, hypopyon, and mixed conjunctival and ciliary injection. The lens has been known to develop small gray opacities on the anterior surface even when not mechanically injured by the sting. During the height of the reaction the cornea may become heavily infiltrated at the site of the sting. Thereafter, the inflammatory reaction gradually subsides, but the area of the cornea surrounding the sting has commonly been left permanently clouded and vascularized. However, there have been cases of initial severe reaction and opacification of the cornea but subsequent gradual complete clearing and a recovery of normal vision, even though the stinger remained in the cornea.[f,j] From clinical observations on cases such as these, and from experiments on rabbits, Strebel concluded that once the toxic material was gone from the bee sting, the stinger became completely inert and could be left in the anterior chamber or cornea without concern.[m,n]

In one case a wasp sting remained inert in a patient's lens for at least 28 years.[b]

Bee sting of the ciliary body has also been reported to cause initial severe corneal opacity which gradually cleared in several months. In one instance bee sting of the ciliary body caused partial depigmentation of the iris, although there was no associated iridocylitis, cataract, or glaucoma.[i]

In another unusual instance in which the stinger entered the sclera rather than the cornea, a posterior and equatorial subcapsular cataract resulted, although the stinger was removed within two minutes. The injury of the lens in this case may have been induced mechanically by the barb itself, as evidenced by a localized peripheral opacity. The eye was otherwise undisturbed except for semidilation of the pupil and appearance of a few fine pigmented corneal precipitates.[h]

Experiments on rabbits have shown that the venom associated with the bee sting is responsible for the severe inflammatory reaction. The toxic components of bee venom have been described by Smolin and Wong.[l] Studies of bee stings in the corneas of rabbits showed that for the severity of the ensuing reaction it was unimportant whether the sting itself remained in the cornea. If Descemet's membrane was not perforated, the lens remained normal; but with all the poison remaining in the cornea there was an especially severe purulent keratitis.

In experimental animals, a severe inflammatory reaction with purulent secretion has developed, as in patients. Clouding of the cornea, purulent infiltration, and loss of epithelium occurred at the site of sting, and hypopyon appeared with white flecks on the lens capsule. In two or three weeks the reaction subsided and the cornea cleared to a variable degree, with the stinger seeming to cause no further irritation, although it remained in place. The most severely affected animals developed permanent leukomatous opacity and posterior synechias.

The posterior segment of the eye in human beings, particularly the retina and optic nerve, has been affected in several cases of bee sting, but peculiarly complications in the posterior segment in most instances have not been associated with bee stings of the eye, but with stings of the lid or elsewhere on the head.

An unusual combination of anterior segment injury and narrowing of visual field has been reported by Szeghy in a man who had a corneoscleral bee sting which led to depigmentation and distortion of the iris in the region of the sting, associated with cycloplegia, slight opacity of the lens, and diffuse haze in the vitreous. The pupil did not lose its reactivity to miotic drugs. The visual acuity was only slightly impaired and the fundus of the eye continued to appear normal, but the visual field in the injured eye was observed to become concentrically narrowed.[o]

The optic nerve and surrounding retina have been affected by stings outside of the eye in the following cases. Loss of vision in one eye has been described by Walsh and Hoyt in a boy who had been stung on the upper lid several years before he was seen by these authors. They found optic atrophy, narrowing of the arterioles, and extensive sheathing of the veins which they concluded had been caused by a papillitis secondary to the bee sting.[256]

In another case a bee sting on the temple was followed in two weeks by optic neuritis on the same side, with very slight blurring of vision, papilledema of one diopter, engorgement of the capillaries, and a few small hemorrhages on and about the optic nerve head. These abnormalities cleared in two to three months and were considered an allergic manifestation.[e] Another patient was stung on the head by a bee and had encephalopathy associated with bilateral papilledema of one diopter and retinal venous engorgement, but normal visual acuity nine days after being stung. The eyes gradually returned to normal. This was considered probably an anaphylactoid or hypersensitivity response.[d] Another patient was stung on the upper lid and developed local pain and swelling with vision reduced to about 5/10 in twenty-four hours, gradually recovering in the course of several weeks nearly to normal, but with residual temporal pallor of the nerveheads and relative central scotoma.[g]

An elderly patient had bilateral rapid loss of vision with optic disc swelling within 24 hours of receiving multiple bee stings.[a] (See INDEX for *Wasp stings*.)

a. Breen LA, Burde RM, Mendelsohn GE: Beesting papillitis. *J CLIN NEUROOPHTHAL-MOL* 3:97–100, 1983.
b. Gilboa M, Gdal-on M, Zonis S: Bee and wasp stings of the eye. *BR J OPHTHALMOL* 6:662–664, 1977.
c. Goddard SJ: Bee stings through the cornea. *MED J AUST* 1:530–531, 1959.
d. Goldstein NP, Rucker CW, Klass DW: Encephalopathy and papilledema after bee sting. *J AM MED ASSOC* 188:1083–1084, 1964.
e. Goldstein NP, Rucker CW, Woltman HW: Neuritis occurring after insect stings. *J AM MED ASSOC* 173:1727–1730, 1960.
f. Khachaturova NK: Bee sting of the cornea. *VESTN OFTALMOL* 73:17–19, 1960.
g. Konstas P, Nikolinakos G: Retrobulbar neuritis after bee sting. *SOC OPHTALMOL GRECE NORD* 14:144–146, 1965.
h. Kranning HD: Scleral injury by bee sting and posterior stellate cataract. *KLIN MONATSBL AUGENHEILKD* 126:750–753, 1955. (German)
i. Lundsgaard KKK: Transitory depigmentation of the iris in sequel to a bee's sting on the eyeball. *ACTA OPHTHALMOL* 6:181–183, 1928.
j. Milrud PA: Clinical picture and features peculiar to the treatment of cornea bee stings. *VESTN OFTALMOL* 74:85–86, 1961.
k. Singh G: Bee sting of the cornea. *ANN OPHTHALMOL* 16:320–322, 1984.
l. Smolin G, Wong I: Bee stings of the cornea. *ANN OPHTHALMOL* 14:324–343, 1982.
m. Strebel J: On insect-sting injuries of the eye and on tolerence of a bee sting sticking in the cornea-anterior chamber for more than twenty years. *OPHTHALMOLOGICA* 120:16–19, 1950. (German)
n. Strebel J: Bee and wasp-sting injuries of the eye. *KLIN MONATSBL AUGENHEILKD* 86:657–662, 1931. (German)
o. Szeghy G, Papai IC, Vas Z: Information on eye injuries by bee stings. *OPHTHAL-MOLOGICA* 146:74–82, 1963. (German)
p. Young CA: Bee sting of the cornea with case report. *AM J OPHTHALMOL* 14:208–216, 1931.

Beer with 5% alcohol content has been tested on untreated glaucomatous patients and normal volunteers by administering 1 liter within one-half hour; this has been found only occasionally to cause inconsequential small transient rise of ocular pressure during about fifteen minutes. More commonly it has reduced ocular pressure during several hours, particularly in glaucomatous patients.[a,b] The same effect is obtained by alcohol in other forms given either orally or intravenously.

a. Peczon JD, Grant WM: Glaucoma, alcohol, and intraocular pressure. *ARCH OPHTHAL-MOL* 73:495–501, 1965.
b. Ricklefs G, Gossmann K: The influence of television on intraocular pressure. *KLIN MONATSBL AUGENHEILKD* 153:400–403, 1968. (German)

Befunolol, an adrenergic beta-blocking drug, has been examined experimentally in Japan for possible adverse action on the retina because of incorporation into mela-nin granules of the uvea, although so far no clinical counterpart has been recognized.

Honda et al (1981),[a] according to Matsuda (1983),[b] reported effects of befunolol *in vitro* on the rabbit's ERG, and Yamashita et al (1981),[c] also according to Matsuda et al (1983),[b] reported that the subconjunctival injection of the drug caused whitish retinal opacity, flat elevation of the retina, and morphologic changes in the retinal pigment epithelium. Matsuda et al (1983),[b] found that phagocytosis by the pigment epithelium of chick embryo in culture could be inhibited by concentrations of befunolol such as might be found in the retina after application of eyedrops to rabbits. Other beta-blockers, *timolol* and *propranolol* also had inhibitory effects.

   a. Honda Y, Kawano S, Nego A: Toxic effect of befunolol, a betaadrenergic blocking agent on the *in vitro* retinal preparation of adult albino rabbits. *ACTA SOC OPHTHALMOL JPN* 85:780–783, 1981.
   b. Matsuda H, Yoshimura N, et al: The retinal toxicity of befunolol and other adrenergic beta-blocking agents. *ACTA OPHTHALMOL* 61:343–352, 1983.
   c. Yamashita H, Hiramatsu K, Uyama M: Effects of beta-adrenergic blocker on ocular structure. *ACTA SOC OPHTHALMOL JPN* 56:83–94, 1981.

Benoxaprofen (Opren) is a non-steroid antiflammatory agent, a member of the propionic group which includes *ibuprofen*. In one case a woman under treatment for rheumatoid arthritis gradually developed central scotomas, attributed to toxic optic neuropathy, with significant improvement after the medication was discontinued.[a] The optic discs looked normal throughout.

   a. Dodd MJ, Griffiths ID, et al: Toxic optic neuropathy caused by benoxaprofen. *BR MED J* 283:193–194, 1981.

Bentonite, a natural aluminum silicate clay, has been held to blame for an extremely severe and protracted keratitis and anterior uveitis in a young dental assistant.[a] It was suspected that a tooth polishing compound had been thrown against the patient's eye by a spinning rubber polishing cup, and had become embedded in the cornea. Bentonite was the only component of the polishing compound that produced a reaction similar to that in the patient when injected into the corneal stroma in rabbits. Oddly, the polishing compound that contained the bentonite produced no significant reaction when it was injected into rabbit eyes.

   a. Austin PS, Doughman DJ: Reaction to intraocular penetration of bentonite. *AM J OPHTHALMOL* 89:719–723, 1980.

Benzalkonium chloride (Zephiran), a quaternary ammonium wetting agent or cationic surfactant, composed of a mixture of alkylbenzyldimethylammonium chlorides, has been widely used as a pharmaceutical preservative in eyedrops. For this application benzalkonium has been used at a dilution of 1:3,000 or 1:4,000 (0.033% or 0.025%), which increases the permeability of the cornea, usually without inducing clinically detectable injury. At this dilution, a single drop applied to the human eye causes no sensation or indication of irritation or injury, but application three or four times daily for two to eight weeks has been noted in some patients to cause a "sandy" sensation which disappeared rapidly when the drops were discontinued.[k] Perhaps this is related to instability of the tear film induced by benzalkonium.[n] Regeneration of epithelium following corneal abrasion (in rabbits) is retarded by repeated application of this same concentration.[h] Use in conjunction with soft contact lenses has presented a special problem of toxicity to the human cornea, not from eyedrops, but from soaking.[c]

At a dilution of 1:1,000 (or 0.1% concentration) of benzalkonium chloride, a drop applied to the human eye causes mild discomfort which persists for two or three hours as a slight, scratchy, foreign-body type sensation. Slit-lamp examination within ninety seconds shows fine gray dots of keratitis epithelialis in the corneal epithelium.[k,81] Within ten minutes a gray haze may be seen in the corneal surface, and superficial desquamation of conjunctival epithelium may follow, in the form of sticky clumps or strands.[k,300] The superficial irritation and disturbance disappear in a day or less. The same concentration applied to rabbit eyes as a drop two or three times a day for one to three months has caused thickening and roughening of the corneal epithelium, with superficial vascularization, but no deeper damage.[a] Cats blink and lacrimate at concentrations that produce no symptoms in rabbits, but both cats and rabbits show corneal epithelial injury by 0.001% and 0.01% solutions when examined by scanning electronmicroscopy.[i,m]

Studies on rabbit corneas have shown that at low concentrations there is increase in permeability,[f,l] and change in the electric potential.[e] A threshold for interference with oxygen uptake has been established at 0.01% concentration.[b]

In rabbit eyes severe injury of the endothelium and much swelling and grayness of the cornea have been induced by irrigation of the outer surface with 0.1% solution for fifteen minutes,[81] or by replacement of the aqueous humor with 0.25% to 0.5% solutions. Damage to the corneal endothelium is a serious concern when benzalkonium is used in solutions introduced within the eye.[d,g,j] The threshold for rabbit endothelial injury, has been found to be approximately 0.0001%. The endothelium may not be injured by intermittent application of as much as 0.1% to the outer surface of the cornea,[h] but it is injured by application 5 times a day for a week.[314]

When higher concentrations of benzalkonium are applied to the outer surface, acute damage of the epithelium and endothelium is extensive and severe. A drop of 2% or 10% solution can cause very serious damage to the whole cornea.[c,316] The corneas of rabbit eyes have become blue and swollen, then completely opaque and vascularized,[81] but one human eye is known to have slowly recovered from such an exposure. In monkeys, application of 10% benzalkonium chloride solution immediately causes much edema and erythema of the conjunctiva and clouding of the cornea. Swelling of the tissues is maximum at one day, beginning to subside on the second day. From the seventh to the eighteenth days, opacity of the cornea gradually clears and the conjunctiva appears normal. By the twenty-first day there is residual slight corneal epithelial hyperplasia and some blood vessel pannus.[a]

a. Burstein NL: Preservation cytotoxic threshold for benzalkonium chloride and chlorhexidine digluconate in cat and rabbit corneas. *INVEST OPHTHALMOL VIS SCI* 19:308–313, 1980.
b. Burton GD, Hill RM: Aerobic responses of the cornea to ophthalmic preservatives, measured *in vivo. INVEST OPHTHALMOL VIS SCI* 21:842–845, 1981.
c. Gasset AR: Benzalkonium chloride toxicity to the human cornea. *AM J OPHTHALMOL* 84:169–171, 1977.

d. Green K, Hull DS, et al: Rabbit endothelial response to ophthalmic preservatives. *ARCH OPHTHALMOL* 95:2218–2221, 1977.

e. Green K, Tonjum AM: The effect of benzalkonium chloride on the electro-potential of the rabbit cornea. *ACTA OPHTHALMOL* 53:348–357, 1975.

f. Keller N, Moore D, et al: Increased corneal permeability induced by the dual effects of transient tear film acidification and exposure to benzalkonium chloride. *EXP EYE RES* 30:203–210, 1980.

g. Lavine JB, Binder PS, Wickham MG: Antimicrobials and the corneal endothelium. *ANN OPHTHALMOL* 11:1517–1528, 1979.

h. Leopold IH: Local toxic effect of detergents on ocular structures. *ARCH OPHTHALMOL* 34:99–102, 1945.

i. Maudgal PC, Cornelis H, Missotten L: Effects of commercial ophthalmic drugs on rabbit corneal epithelium. A scanning electronmicroscope study. *GRAEFES ARCH OPHTHALMOL* 216:191–203, 1981.

j. Maurice D, Perlman M: Permanent destruction of the corneal endothelium in rabbits. *INVEST OPHTHALMOL VIS SCI* 16:646–649, 1977.

k. Swan KC: Reactivity of the ocular tissues to wetting agents. *AM J OPHTHALMOL* 27:1118–1122, 1944.

l. Tonjum AM: Permeability of the rabbit corneal epithelium to horseradish peroxidase after the influence of benzalkonium chloride. *ACTA OPHTHALMOL* 53:335–347, 1975.

m. Tonjum AM: Effects of benzalkonium chloride upon the corneal epithelium studied with scanning electron microscopy. *ACTA OPHTHALMOL* 53:358–366, 1975.

n. Wilson WS, Duncan AJ, Jay JL: Effect of benzalkonium on the stability of the precorneal tear film in rabbit and man. *BR J OPHTHALMOL* 59:667–669, 1975.

Benzene (benzol), an unsaturated six-carbon ring compound (not to be confused with "benzine" which is composed of aliphatic petroleum hydrocarbons), has a specific toxic effect on blood formation, causing aplastic anemia and tendency to hemorrhage. Occasionally hemorrhages in the retina and in the conjunctiva are found in systemic poisoning by benzene. In rare instances neuroretinal edema and papilledema have been described accompanying the retinal hemorrhages.[a, d, 255]

It has not been established that benzene can induce retrobulbar neuritis or optic neuritis, but the possibility has been suggested in connection with the six following rare cases.

In case 1, a man appeared to be acutely intoxicated from inhaling benzene vapors, and two days later almost completely lost his vision from retrobulbar neuritis, which progressed to partial atrophy.[c]

In case 2, reduced vision and congestion of the optic nerveheads were associated with evidences of chronic benezene poisoning with anemia. Partial optic atrophy developed in one eye, and vision was permanently impaired.[6]

In case 3, bilateral optic atrophy developed after intermittent industrial exposure to a mixture of benzene, carbon disulfide, and touene, but there was no evidence of poisoning other than the ocular disturbance, and the cause of this was uncertain.[f]

In cases 4 and 5, the patients each developed symptoms of retrobulbar neuritis in one eye after chronic exposure to vapors of benzene mixed with several other common solvents, including various acetate esters used in spray painting.[b, e] There was no hematologic evidence of benzene poisoning. There was some suspicion of the other solvents, e.g., see *Amyl acetate.*

In case 6, a girl had severe decrease in central vision due to scotomas in both eyes after working eight to nine hours a day for fifteen months exposed to the vapors of a mixture composed mainly of trichloroethylene with 8% dichloroethane and only 0.5% benzene.[g] Several months later she showed temporal atrophy of the nervehead, but extensive neurologic studies were otherwise negative.

It appears that only in the first two of these six cases was there reasonably close association between benzene poisoning and optic neuritis. In one of these cases the poisoning was acute, and in the other it was chronic.

Experimentally, administration of benzene to rabbits has been found to cause no abnormality in the eyes detectable ophthalmoscopically.[37]

The local effects of benzene vapor or liquid on the eye are slight. Only at very high vapor concentrations, higher than would be safe for systemic absorption, is there any smarting sensation in the eye.[81] Keratitis has been ascribed to industrial contact with benzene vapor, but most likely was caused by other solvents, which were present at the same time. Benzene vapor exposed to photo-oxidation with ozone and nitrogen dioxide, as in formation of smog, yields little eye irritance, in contrast to derivatives of benzene that have carbon side chains of benzylic type.[110]

Droplet contamination of the eye by benzene causes moderate burning sensation, but only slight transient injury of the epithelial cells, and the eye recovers rapidly.[35,165,265] Benzene tested on rabbit eyes caused only slight transient injury,[h] grade 3 on a scale of 10.[228]

Cataracts have developed in 50 percent of rats exposed to benzene vapor 50 ppm in air for more than 600 hours.[180]

a. Albrecht: Chronic benzene poisoning with a course resembling a brain tumor. *MSCHR PSYCHIAT* 82:108–112, 1932. (German)
b. Goldmann, H: A new industrial retrobulbar neuritis. *KLIN MONATSBL AUGENHEILKD* 84:761, 1954. (German)
c. Perlia: Acute retrobulbar neuritis after breathing benzene vapors. *KLIN MONATSBL AUGENHEILKD* 67:109–110, 1921. (German)
d. Renard, Cavigneaux et al: Do changes in the fundus of the eye follow changes in the blood in benzene poisoning? *ARCH MAL PROF* 11:38–43, 1950. (French)
e. Schirmer R: A contribution on chronic poisoning by nirocellulose lacquer. *KLIN MONATSBL AUGENHEILKD* 123:449–454, 1953.
f. Schutz H: Optic nerve atrophy from benzene poisoning. *KLIN MONATSBL AUGENHEILKD* 106:706, 1941.
g. Tabacchi G, Corsico R, Gallenelli R: Retrobulbar neuritis from suspected chronic poisoning by trichloroethylene. *ANN OTTALMOL CLIN OCUL* 92:787–792, 1966. (Italian)
h. Wolf MA, Rowe VK, McCollistser DD: Toxicological studies of certain alkylated benzenes and benzene. *ARCH IND HEALTH* 14:387–397, 1956.

Benzenethiol (phenyl mercaptan, thiophenol) tested by application of a drop to rabbit eyes caused severe irritation, moderate redness, and chemosis of the conjunctiva for three or four days, gradually subsiding with return of conjunctiva to normal in ten to sixteen days.[55] The corneas developed opacities which gradually increased during two to three weeks, becoming opalescent and obscuring details of pupil and iris. However, in the course of two months the eyes recovered.

Peculiarly, the eyes of rabbits which were flushed with water after application of benzenethiol had more severe injury, with opalescent opacity of the corneas lasting several weeks, and requiring three to four months to clear. On the other hand, flushing the eyes with 0.5% silver nitrate solution immediately after application of benzenethiol, followed by copious irrigation with water to remove the precipitated silverthiol compound, gave good protection and reduced the severity of injury to slight conjunctival inflammation and relatively small transient, diffuse corneal opacification.[55]

Benzoic acid, usually as *sodium benzoate,* an antifungal agent in pharmaceuticals and foods, shows large species differences in its systemic toxicity, cats being particularly prone to poisoning. One experimental study on brown rabbits has produced histologic evidence of toxicity to the retina.[a] A 4% solution of sodium benzoate (1 ml/kg) was injected intravenously daily, and the animals were killed with a gas embolus after 12 hours to 3 days. Histologically, exudative detachment of the retinal neuroepithelium from the pigment epithelium was found. The toxic action appeared to have been predominantly on the layer of rods and cones, without appreciable involvement of the other layers. Acid mucopolysaccharides appeared to be increased in the rod and cone layer, but also irregularly in other parts of the retina.

  a. DeCrecchio G, Menna F, et al: Experimental retinal degeneration. *ANN OTTALMOL CLIN OCUL* 103:311–322, 1977. (Italian)

1,2-Benzopyrene has been employed for the experimental production of tumors of the rat conjunctiva.[a] It has been observed to cause violent uveitis when injected intraocularly in oil solution in animal eyes.[b]

  a. Gandolfi C, Tanzi B: Experimental production of tumors of the eye with 1,2-benzopyrene. *BOLL SOC ITAL BIOL SPER* 16:685–686, 1941. (Chem Abstr 41:1748.)
  b. Moro F: Research on the effect of benzopyrene injected in the anterior chamber, and in the vitreous chamber of eye of the rat. *ATTI CONG SOC ITAL OTTAL* 37:173–189, 1948. (Italian)

Benzoyl peroxide (Lucidol) applied experimentally to animal eyes produces superficial opacities in the cornea and inflammation of the conjunctiva according to one investigator,[b] but according to another no injury results from single application of a 93% pure powder or a 50% paste in dimethyl phthalate to rabbit eyes.[a]

  a. Kuchle WJ: Investigations into the eye-injuring effect of organic peroxides. *Z ARBEITS-MED ARBEITSCHUTZ* 8:25–31, 1958.
  b. Oettel H: Health risk from synthetics? *ARCH EXP PATH PHARMAKOL* 232:77–132, 1957.

Benztropine mesylate, (Benzatropine methanesulfonate, Cogentin) is an anticholinergic, antiparkinsonism drug which commonly causes blurring of vision from mydriasis and cycloplegia, reaching a maximum cumulative effect during several days of repeated oral doses. Inconvenience from weakness of accommodation for near has most often been noticed by the young people who have been under treatment with this drug to counteract the extrapyramidal side effects of psychotropic phenothiazine derivative drugs. In these patients the inconvenience can sometimes be alleviated by administering weak long-acting anticholinesterase miotic drops such as 0.06% echothiophate iodide once every two or three days.

Benzyl alcohol is commonly used as a preservative in sterile solutions for intramuscular or intravenous use, particularly in multiple-dose containers, as permitted by the U.S. Pharmacopeia. However, intraocular use of such solutions is injurious to the eye, and should be carefully avoided.

The danger has been pointed out by Roberto Quesada Guardia (personal communication, 1968), who observed that intraocular use of sodium chloride solution preserved with 2% benzyl alcohol during cataract surgery and peripheral iridectomy caused severe striate keratopathy, progressing to chronic edema of the cornea, with vesicles, bullae, and dirty pigmented appearance of the endothelium. In such eyes the pupils did not respond normally to miotics or mydriatics, indicating that the iris was also affected. The corneas very slowly cleared. This unusual complication of otherwise uncomplicated surgery was traced to sterile saline solution that had been used to irrigate the anterior chamber and that had no statement on the label concerning a preservative, but on analysis was found to contain 2% benzyl alcohol. In tests in rabbit eyes, I have confirmed that this solution is toxic. When the aqueous humor was replaced in one eye with pure sterile 0.9% sodium chloride solution and in the other eye was replaced with the same solution plus 2% benzyl alcohol, no toxic effect was produced by the plain saline solution, but the eyes with benzyl alcohol solution rapidly developed evidence of injury of the endothelium, with much bluish swelling of the cornea. Also the irides in the eyes with benzyl alcohol solution became hyperemic and had poorly reactive pupils. The corneal edema in rabbits disappeared more rapidly than in the human patients, clearing partially in one week and completely in two weeks.

Perfusing the anterior chamber of enucleated rabbit eyes with 0.18% benzyl alcohol was observed by Coles (1975) to change the appearance of corneal endothelial cells, and to cause the corneas to swell.[293]

It seems very important to avoid the accident of using solutions preserved with benzyl alcohol during intraocular surgery. Labels should bear a warning to this effect. The U.S. Pharmacopeia (17th edition) states "ophthalmic solutions that are used during surgery must be sterile, and should contain no preservative." If there is any doubt about the possibility of benzyl alcohol being present in solutions of sodium chloride in the eye operating room, a simple test consists of administering a drop of the solution to the conjunctival sac of a normal volunteer. If 2% benzyl alcohol is present, the solution causes immediate smarting like soap solution, but the effect of external application is brief and without injury to the eye. When pure 0.9% sodium chloride solution (without benzyl alcohol) is applied in the same manner, it causes no discomfort at all.

Full strength benzyl alcohol, not aqueous solution, tested by application of a drop to rabbits' eyes appears to have moderate potential injurious effect, rated 8 on a scale of 1 to 10.[222,225] No direct ocular injury from external contact has been reported in human beings, but one death and one case of serious illness with delirium and visual disturbances were supposed to have been caused by absorption of benzyl alcohol from an impure preparation of benzyl benzoate which was employed in massaging the skin.[a] There appears to be no other report of such toxicity, although both substances have been commonly applied to the skin.

> a. Jaulmes P: A case of poisoning by impure benzyl benzoate (containing benzyl alcohol). *TRAV SOC PHARM MONTPELLIER* 6:47–50, 1946–1947. (Chem Abstr 42:5561.)

Benzyl chloride (alpha-chlorotoluene) vapors are intensely irritating to all mucous membranes, particularly to the eye. Unbearable eye irritation in human beings is produced by 31 ppm in air.[61] Cats exposed to 2 mg/liter of air showed immediate irritation, and after exposure for 7.5 hours to this concentration, turbidity of the cornea was noted the next day.[188] Guinea pigs have shown remarkably less irritation of the eyes than cats.[188]

Lohs has pointed out that the lacrimogenic effect is made still stronger by addition of a nitro group to benzyl chloride, as in *o-nitrobenzylchloride*.[155]

Benzyl nitrite has been tested as a vapor and found not to irritate human eyes at a concentration of 0.2 ppm in air, but after photooxidation in the presence of ozone and nitrogen dioxide definite eye irritancy results; this is probably due to formation of *peroxybenzoyl nitrate*.[68]

Beryllium is encountered industrially in various compounds and as a lightweight strong metal. Inhalation of beryllium metal dust has caused severe disease of the lungs, but experimental introduction of the powdered metal into the corneas of rabbits has caused only slight clouding of the surrounding cornea, and after two months the metal was still visible as fine glistening particles, apparently well tolerated. There appear to be no reports of reactions of human eyes to beryllium metal.

Compounds of beryllium have caused acute and chronic reactions in the lungs and superficial tissues varying according to the reactivity and concentration of the individual compounds and the site of contact.[j] *Beryllium chloride, fluoride, nitrate,* and *sulfate,* which are acidic salts, cause acute irritation of the skin, eyes, and respiratory tract when human beings and animals are exposed to dusts of these compounds.[b,252] Ocular irritation from industrial exposure has not been serious, consisting of conjunctivitis, but scarcely ever involving the cornea. The hyperemia of the conjunctiva and edema of the lids which result from exposure to dust or direct contamination by particles are said to cause rather persistent burning sensation and photophobia, but recovery is usually complete in five to ten days. In instances of hypersensitivity, individuals may be so prone to recurrences of irritation that a change of occupation is necessary.[b]

Experimentally, exposures of animals to dust of beryllium sulfate with median particle size of 4 microns at a concentration of 88 mg/cu m of air for six hours daily caused conjunctivitis in guinea pigs and dogs, and in many animals caused corneal ulceration and vascularization. In some animals exposed in this manner for eleven days, a mild uveitis with purulent exudates in the anterior chamber was observed.[e]

Experimental injection of aqueous solutions of *beryllium sulfate* or *beryllium fluoride* of unspecified concentration into the cornea of rabbits has caused diffuse clouding within an hour, subsequently progressing to leukoma and permanent scarring.[b] Similar experiments using *beryllium citrate,* which is soluble but less dissociated and less acidic, caused only small permanent nebulas.[b] Beryllium compounds which are less soluble and not acidic, such as *beryllium oxide, hydroxide,* and *carbonate,* are not immediately irritating like the acidic compounds, but upon inhalation as dust are capable of causing severe disease of the lungs after long latent periods.[252] Experimental introduction of *beryllium carbonate* powder into the cornea of rabbits caused very little reaction for several months, but after six months, when most of the powder had disappeared, a local vascularized granulomatous reaction developed, accompanied by indolent corneal ulceration. Histologically, masses of epithelioid cells and a few giant cells were found.[b]

In the skin, granulomatous reaction has been observed following injuries from fragments of fluorescent lamps, which formerly were lined with insoluble compounds of beryllium, silicon, and other elements.[252] (The use of beryllium in fluorescent lamps is said to have discontinued in 1949.) Two cases of laceration of the eye by broken pieces of fluorescent lamp have been reported, and the ensuing reaction has been assumed to be due to the presence of beryllium, but in neither case was evidence presented to establish that beryllium was actually present.[c, d]

Experimentally, tests of pure soluble beryllium salts have been somewhat complicated by their acidity and by confusion of acid injury with beryllium toxicity. The problem has been symplified by testing solutions of *beryllium sulfate and nitrate which have been sufficiently neutralized* to remove the possibility of injury from low pH alone. Application of 0.05 to 0.1 M *beryllium sulfate* or *nitrate* solutions at pH 5 to pH 6 for ten minutes to normal rabbit eyes caused no injury.[81, 90] By contrast, the same solutions applied to rabbit corneas from which the epithelium had been removed by scraping caused complete permanent corneal opacification, often with extensive necrosis and perforation. (Scraped but unexposed control eyes healed rapidly and completely.)

The corneas which were exposed to the beryllium-containing solutions appeared at first only slightly bluish and hazy, but in several days became progressively densely clouded. Experimental treatment of such eyes was investigated by applying substances immediately after exposure which were expected to bind or chelate beryllium. Treatment with 0.1 M *aurin tricarboxylate* prevented necrosis of the cornea, but left the tissue stained red and opaque by the insoluble lake formed from the reaction of the dye with beryllium. Neutral 0.1 to 0.5 M *sodium sulfosalicylate* solution definitely reduced the injurious effect of beryllium and prevented much of the corneal opacification. On the other hand, neutral 0.03 to 0.1 M *sodium edetate* solution was disappointing, having only slight therapeutic value.[81, 90]

In chronic systemic beryllium poisoning, which may develop years after exposure, there may be clinical resemblance to Boeck's sarcoid. Rarely this may be accompanied by calcification of the cornea in the form of band keratopathy such as develops in hypercalcemia from various causes.[a]

a. Cogan DG, Albright F, Bartter FC: Hypercalcemia and band keratopathy. *ARCH OPHTHALMOL* 40:624–638, 1948.

b. Ferraris de Gaspare PF: Experimental investigation of eye lesions from beryllium. *BOLL OCULIST* 31:337–346, 1952. (Italian)

c. Flynn G, Raiford M: Beryllium and corneal healing. *ARCH OPHTHALMOL* 51:89–90, 1954.

d. Rizzuti AB: Beryllium granulomas of the anterior ocular structures. *NEW YORK J MED* 51:1065–1067, 1951.

e. Scott JK: Pathologic anatomy of acute experimental beryllium poisoning. *ARCH PATH* 45:354–359, 1948.

Bicycloheptadiene dibromide, an alkylating agent, has great tendency to induce sensitization, having caused severe asthma in three chemists, with fatal poisoning in two. All had skin rash but only minor eye involvement consisting of conjunctivitis associated with rhinitis early after exposure, but one of the patients who died had pancytopenia with several large hemorrhages in the fundus of each eye, also hemorrhages in the central nervous system and lungs.[a]

a. Murray JF, Fink A: Toxicity from certain brominated alkylating agents. *ARCH ENVIRON HEALTH* 5:5–11, 1962.

Bile in contact with the cornea causes epithelial injury. Most observations of this injury have been from experiments on rabbits, but in one instance a nurse had corneal epithelial injury when she splashed bile in her eyes from a biliary duct T-tube.[a] In another case a fisherman was observed to have sustained corneal injury from a squirt of fish bile in the eye.[153] The situation was complicated in this patient by treatment with a lead solution. Permanent corneal opacification resulted, but this may have been caused mainly by the lead treatment.

In experimental injuries induced by applying fish, ox, or hog bile to rabbit eyes, the corneas have not become permanently opacified.[a,c,e,153] Either ox bile or 1% solution of sodium glycocholate applied to rabbit corneas causes diffuse punctate stainability by fluorescein, but does not remove the epithelium completely, and recovery is prompt.[b] When applied with rubbing with an applicator stick the removal is more extensive, and the recovery slower.[330]

Biblical stories tell of fish bile having been used to remove white opacities from the eyes, and the suggestion has been made that the opacities may have been calcific deposits like band keratopathy, and that the fish bile acted as a surfactant and chelating agent to remove the epithelium and the calcific deposits.[d]

Experimental intraocular injection of bile in rabbits is seriously damaging, causing cataract, degeneration of retina and choroid, and hypertrophy of the iris and ciliary processes. Rabbits that have been killed by subcutaneous injection of bile are said to have shown retinal degeneration at death.[153] (See also *Bilirubin*).

a. Adams JD: Drug induced lupus erythematosis: a case report. *AUSTRALASIAN J DERM* 19:31–32, 1978.

b. Friedenwald JS, Hughes WF, Herrmann H: Acid base tolerance of the cornea. *ARCH OPHTHALMOL* 31:279–283, 1944.

c. Stassi M: Action of bile on the eye. *BULL SOC ITAL BIOL* 21:19–21, 1946. (Chem Abstr 40:7392, 1946.)

d. Sudarsky RD: Tobit and chelating agents. *AM J OPHTHALMOL* 57:963–967, 1964.

e. Verhoeff FH, Friedenwald JS: Injury to the cornea and conjunctiva due to fish bile. *AM J OPHTHALMOL* 5:857–858, 1922.

Bilirubin is the principal pigment of bile, and is present in low concentration in blood serum. Bilirubin has been shown to be severely injurious to the retina when injected intraocularly, and it has been held responsible for loss of vision in patients with intraocular hemorrhages. Kahan and associates in 1968 identified unesterified bilirubin in intraocular fluids in fourteen patients with intraocular hemorrhages.[a] They correlated disappearance of the ERG and loss of vision with yellow staining of the retinas by bilirubin, which was observed when the eyes were enucleated. They also demonstrated that repeated injection of bilirubin into the vitreous humor in rabbits caused similar loss of ERG.

Lewin and Guillery had already in 1913 reported in their book on toxicology of the eye that bile injected subcutaneously in rabbits caused retinal degeneration, evident at death, and that when bile was injected directly into the eye, it caused degeneration of the retina and choroid, hypertrophy of the iris and ciliary processes, and development of cataract.[153]

Kahan and associates noted that in jaundice the intraocular concentration of bilirubin apparently is never as high as from intraocular hemorrhages and is not enough to poison the retina.[a] Bilirubin can be found in the vitreous humor of premature infants, but apparently not enough to be injurious.[b]

a. Kahan A, Malnasi S, et al: Bilirubin retinopathy. *BR J OPHTHALMOL* 52:808–817, 1968.

b. Kurzel RB, Heinrikson RL: On the presence of bilirubin in the ocular humors of premature infants. *INVEST OPHTHALMOL* 15:509–512, 1976.

Bis(dimethoxythiophosphoryl) disulfide has been found very irritating to the eye, causing inflammation and corneal opacity when applied to eyes of rabbits.[a]

a. Wenzel KD, Dedek W: Isolation and identification of eye-irritating by-products of dimethoate synthesis. *Z CHEM* 11:461–462, 1971.

Bis(2-ethylhexyl)hydrogen phosphite, a corrosion inhibitor and antioxidant, when dropped on rabbit eyes causes immediate inflammatory response, with return to normal in a few days.[a]

a. Joffe MH, Gongwer LE, Punte CL: Studies on the acute and subacute toxicity of bis(2-ethylhexyl)hydrogen phosphite. *ARCH IND HEALTH* 18:464–469, 1958.

1,2-Bis(ethylsulfonyl)-1,2-dichloroethylene was kept from commercial development as a fungicide for seeds because of the severity of its injurious effect on the eye, causing irreversible penetrating damage to rabbit corneas.[a]

a. Morrow RW: Eye injury potential. *CHEM ENG NEWS* June 28, 1976, page 3.

Bismuth compounds have been employed medically in several forms, mainly in treatment of syphilis. Disturbance of vision in systemic poisoning by bismuth has apparently been reported in only one instance. A patient poisoned by taking 8 g of *bismuth subnitrate,* temporarily had foggy vision on the second day of poisoning.[153] The eye has very rarely been affected, although fine white crystals appeared in the corneal epithelium of one patient, and on discontinuation of the treatment the white particles gradually disappeared. Bismuth was detectable chemically in scrapings from the cornea, but it was not proved that the crystals were composed of bismuth.[a] Possibly this was similar to a condition encountered in severe experimental poisoning of dogs by daily subcutaneous injections of *bismuth subnitrate.* This treatment induced irritation of the eyes and lacrimation, then development of white opacities in the upper two-thirds of the corneas.[153]

There appear to have been no injuries from external contact of the eye with bismuth compounds, and experimentally in rabbit eyes no toxicity to the cornea has been noted except in the case of strongly acidic salts such as *bismuth trinitrate,* which causes an acid-type burn of the epithelium. This salt loses its injuriousness if it is neutralized before application to the cornea.[81]

a. Fischer FP: Secondary bismuthiasis of the cornea. *ANN OCULIST (Paris)* 183:615, 1950.

Bismuth pentafluoride is a crystalline solid which is violently reactive to water and highly toxic and irritating to the skin, eyes, and respiratory tract.[171]

Bisphenol A (4,4'-isopropylidenediphenol), used in manufacture of epoxy resins, has been reported when tested as 5% solution in dimethylsulfoxide or propylene glycol to cause "severe injury" to the eye.[a]

a. Bisphenol A (Hygienic Guide Series). *AM IND HYG ASSOC J* 28:301–304, 1967.

1,4-Bis-(phenylisopropyl)-piperazine (1,4-bis-[3-phenylprop-2-yl]-piperazine; Diphenazine; Quietidin), a tranquilizer, has caused photosensitized dermatitis and a reversible depigmentation of the hair and eyebrows. When used daily during two months to several years, it has produced cataracts in numerous patients.[a,b,d,e,f] Early change in the lenses has consisted of glittering punctate and foamy posterior subcapsular and anterior radial cortical opacities, not progressing in some patients; but in numerous patients the cataracts have developed rapidly, interfering with vision and requiring cataract extraction.[c] The eyes have been normal otherwise after removal of the cataracts. Histology of the cataracts has shown them to be like ordinary senile cataracts except for granular material in the cortex staining blue with hematoxylin.[b] Apparently in most, if not all cases, the development of cataracts was preceded by skin disturbances. The mechanism is to be worked out. Administration of the drug to rats for as long a six months has been unsuccessful in producing changes in the lenses.[e,f]

a. Mezey P: The significance of piperazine derivatives in the pathogenesis of cataract. *KLIN MONATSBL AUGENHEILKD* 151:885–887, 1967. (German)
b. Radnot M, Varga M: Histologic structure of the cataract caused by piperazine (derivative). *ANN OCULIST (Paris)* 202:325–329, 1969. (French)

c. Radnot M, Varga M: Operation for cataract caused by piperazine. *AN INST BARRAQUER* 9:122–126, 1969. (French)

d. Soos S, Jakab J: Further data to the problem of the iatrogen effect of Quietidin. *ORVIL HETIL* 109:1549–1550, 1968.

e. Varga M, Jobbagyi P: Cataracts from tranquilizers. *ANN OCULIST* (*Paris*) 201:769–770, 1968. (French)

f. Varga M, Jobbaghi P, et al: Photodermatitis and cataract. *OPHTHALMOLOGICA ADDIT AD* 158:477–480, 1969.

Bis(tri-n-butyltin) oxide (TBTO, Lastanox, Hollicide, Biomet, Fungiban) is widely used in agriculture and industry as a bactericide, fungicide, and insecticide. Tests in 1969 on Lastanox in water to give a concentration of 2% of the tin compound caused rapid ulceration of rabbit corneas, perforation in two out of twelve, total permanent opacity in eleven out of twelve, and severe symblepharon, after 0.03 ml was applied. Hemorrhages in the iris and hypopyon were found histologically, and there were severe signs of systemic poisoning. Even at a dilution corresponding to 0.2% of the tin compound, very severe injury of rabbit eyes was produced, with permanent extensive vascularization and corneal scarring.[a]

There seems to be no published account of human eye injury, but, in a letter, Ian Schiller described a patient who touched the medial canthus of one eye, and apparently contaminated it with the fungicide and paint which he was mixing.[b] Fortunately, the eye itself was not involved, but the skin and conjunctiva of the medial portions of the lids underwent a considerable inflammatory reaction, taking 3 or 4 days to become quiet under treatment with topical corticosteroid.

No specific antidote or treatment is known. (See also *Organotin compounds*).

a. Pelikan Z: Effects of bis(tri-n-butyltin) oxide on the eyes of rabbits. *BR J IND MED* 26:165–170, 1969.

b. Schiller I: Personal communication, 1982.

Blackberry thorn has been described in one case to have penetrated the cornea and to have remained protruding into the anterior chamber for 12 years, with the eye remaining quiet, but cataractous.[a]

a. Albers EC: Blackberry thorn in the anterior chamber of the eye for twelve years. *ARCH OPHTHALMOL* 25:662–663, 1941.

Blasticidin-S (Blaes-M), an antimicrobial, has been used as an agricultural chemical in Japan. The dust has proved irritating to the eyes of workers.[a,b] Tests on rabbit eyes have shown the smallest amount to cause conjunctivitis is 1 μg, and the minimum to cause keratitis is 20 μg. It is found more toxic in the form of an emulsion than as a solution or powder. When sufficient blasticidin is applied to the eye, a pseudo-membranous conjunctivitis with superficial keratitis and hyperemia of the iris develops in five hours, but the eyes recover in ten days. The reaction is said to be similar in rabbits and human beings. In rabbits, irrigation with water or saline solution one minute after start of exposure has not prevented keratitis.[d] Addition of calcium salts was found to reduce the irritation of the eyes of workers and guinea pigs.[e]

a. Ohoka R, Shiozaki H: Ocular lesion due to agricultural medicine. *JPN J CLIN OPHTHALMOL* 19:937–941, 1965.

b. Ojima M: Ocular lesion by Blasticidin (agricultural medicine). *JPN J CLIN OPHTHALMOL* 18:813–823, 1964.

c. Ooka R, et al: Agricultural chemicals, Blasticidin and the eye. *OPHTHALMOLOGY (Tokyo)* 9:166–175, 1967.

d. Shiozaki H: Studies on the ocular toxicity of Blasticidin-S. *JPN J CLIN OPHTHALMOL* 21:111–122, 1967.

e. Sugimoto T: Reduction of eye irritation caused by blasticidin S. *KURUME IGAKKAI ZASSHI* 41:103–113, 1978.

Bleomycin sulfate (Blenoxane), an antineoplastic and antibiotic, produces cataracts in newborn white rats after intraperitoneal injection.[a] Cataracts appear at 14 to 16 days and progress to become nearly complete. If the drug is not administered until 10 or more days after birth, no cataracts are produced.

For use in intravitreal infusion fluid a concentration of 10 μg/ml, or 15 μg/ml for single injection, has been reported non-toxic to the retina.[277,369]

a. Edwards GA, Bernardino VB, et al: Cataracts in bleomycin-treated rats. *AM J OPHTHALMOL* 80:538–542, 1975.

Boric acid or **borate salts** have been employed medically as eye washes and as lotions and dressings on the skin without inducing local injury. However, there have been numerous instances of systemic poisoning, and death has resulted in several instances. Ocular involvement appears to have been rare, although Lewin and Guillery in 1913 said that many instances of disturbances of vision had been observed in patients who had been poisoned by boric acid used as a wash or dressing for wounds.[153]

These disturbances were said not only to be hallucinations of vision, but also decrease of visual acuity to half normal, plus diplopia lasting for more than two weeks. In only one case was boric acid suspected of causing optic neuritis, and in this case the situation was complicated by the presence of syphilis and incipient dementia. The patient had blurring of vision for seven days with pale and blurred optic papillas after ingesting 80 g of boric acid in the course of five weeks.[153]

(No further reports of visual disturbances from boric acid were found after 1913, although numerous additional poisonings have occurred.)

Boron hydride disulfide, a dimer of a complicated boron-hydrogen-sulfur mercapto compound, has been found to cause cataract in 3 to 4 hours in mice, as well as in mouse, rat and rabbit lenses in culture, but the monomer did not have this effect.[a] A comprehensive biochemical study of the mechanism led to a conclusion that the disulfide compound reacted with the sulfhydryl group of Na-KATPase in the epithelium of the lens, inactivating this enzyme, interfering with cation pump activity, and causing leakage of Na and K, increased hydration, and opacification.

a. Fukui HN, Iwata S, et al: Cataractogenic effects of a boron hydride disulfide compound. *INVEST OPHTHALMOL VIS SCI* 16:654–657, 1977.

Boron oxide (boric anhydride; boron trioxide) tested on rabbit eyes in the form of a dust has been found to cause almost immediate irritation. However, this substance appears to pose no practical eye problem as an atmospheric contaminant.[a]

a. Wilding JL, Smith WJ, et al: The toxicity of boron oxide. *AM IND HYG ASSOC J* 20:284–289, 1959.

Boron tribromide is a liquid which fumes in moist air and is severely corrosive to the eye. In one instance it has caused severe localized scarring of cornea and conjunctiva.[81] A sealed flask containing boron tribromide and metallic mercury exploded in a chemist's hand. His vision immediately became foggy, but he felt no pain in his eyes, and no irrigation of the eyes was carried out for at least half an hour. Two or three hours later, the corneal epithelium appeared gray and the conjunctiva pale.

By microscopic examination very little circulation was evident in the blood vessels of the conjunctiva near the limbus in one eye. Subsequently the less injured eye gradually returned to normal, but in the worse eye the corneal endothelium became brownish, granular, and rough appearing, and Descemet's membrane became wrinkled. Soon the endothelium was hidden by stromal infiltration and edema in the lower half of the cornea. Later this area became permanently opaque and vascularized, but the pupillary area of the cornea remained clear. The severely injured cornea was hypesthetic from the start, but the slightly injured cornea had normal sensation.

Botulism is the poisoning caused by eating food contaminated with the toxin of *Clostridium botulinum.*[f] (The properties of *botulinus toxin* itself are described in a subsequent section.) In botulism, illness generally begins within twenty-four hours, with dryness of the mouth, and thirst. This may be followed by nausea, constipation, and urinary retention, but disturbance of the gastrointestinal tract may be slight, and there is no fever. In severe cases the muscles of the throat are paralyzed, affecting swallowing and altering the voice. Paralysis of the diaphragm or extremities is relatively rare. Occasionally noises in the ears and impairment of hearing have been reported. When death results, it is from respiratory failure.

Most characteristic of botulism is onset of paralysis of intraocular and extraocular muscles within one to three days, causing pupillary dilatation, impairment of accommodation, ptosis, and diplopia. Many cases of internal and external ophthalmoplegia have been reported.[a,e,i,l,p,s,24,177,194,214,247,255] Oculography has shown quivering movements of the eyes when gaze is shifted from one object to another.[d] Analysis of ophthalmic signs in 1,100 cases of botulism with 10 per cent mortality has shown that disturbance of accommodation may be the earliest and only ophthalmic sign in mild cases, and that dilated fixed pupils are seen mainly in the severe cases.[f] Complete recovery from the palsies of internal and external ocular muscles may require as long as nine months, but usually is complete.

Several series of case reports indicate that ocular signs and symptoms tend to predominate in botulism involving particularly type B toxin.[e,i,l,p,s]

Belladonna or atropine poisoning is occasionally confused with botulism when the pupils are seen to be widely dilated and unreactive to light.[c] However, in botulism the paralysis of pupils and accommodation differs from that in atropine poisoning; in botulism the pupils and ciliary muscle respond normally to topical pilocarpine.[214] Furthermore, in botulism the body temperature is not elevated and the skin is not red, in contrast to atropine poisoning, which causes redness and dryness of the skin, and fever.

Subnormal production of tears for one to two months has been noted in three out of four recently reported cases of botulism with dilated fixed pupils, poor accommodation, weakness of lateral gaze, and ptosis.[h] The eyes in such cases may become dry and irritated from lack of tears. Corneal and conjunctival hypesthesia has been reported in one case supposedly secondary to injury of the trigeminal nucleus.[a]

The vision in most instances is not affected in botulism except by the mydriasis and the disturbance of accommodation. However, in rare instances hyperemia of the optic papillas and engorgement of the retinal vessels have been described,[a,o] and in three reports optic neuritis has been diagnosed,[a,n] with central scotomas in one and retinal hemorrhages in another.[247] In two of these cases optic atrophy developed.[n,247] A critical review of the literature and thorough study of another patient has led one investigator to conclude that botulism can cause reduction of visual acuity, narrowing of visual field, and impairment of retinal adaptation and color sensitivity, in addition to causing motor disturbances.[t]

In one well-studied, fatal case, microscopic examination showed lymphocytic retrobulbar infiltration of the optic nerve, but none in the retina, and no degeneration of nerve fibers or retinal ganglion cells.[a] In other fatal human cases and after experimental poisoning of animals there have been found degenerative changes and hemorrhages in the ocular motor nuclei, also in the optic nerve and tract, in the chiasm, retina, choroid, and ciliary body.[a,k,m,q,r,24,214] As will be discussed subsequently under the heading of *Botulinus toxin*, many of these findings do not appear to be explainable as direct effects of the toxin.

However, in treatment, internal and external ophthalmoplegia are reported to have been relieved by intravenous administration of Botulinus antitoxin.[g] Guanidine hydrochloride has had some beneficial effect on the eye disturbances.[b,i]

a. Bar A: Eye changes in botulism. *KLIN MONATSBL AUGENHEILKD* 72:675–682, 1924. (German)
b. Cherington M, Ryan DW: Botulism and guanidine. *N ENGL J MED* 278:931–933, 1968.
c. Eichner ER, Gunsolus JM, Powers JF: "Belladonna" poisoning confused with botulism. *J AM MED ASSOC* 201:695–696, 1967.
d. Hedges TR, Jones A, et al: Botulin ophthalmoplegia. *ARCH OPHTHALMOL* 101:211–213, 1983.
e. Henry C, Moulin M, et al: Concerning twelve cases of ambulatory botulism. *BULL SOC OPHTALMOL FRANCE* 70:296–301, 1970. (French)
f. Januszkiewicz J, Pachowska-Onichimowska D: Ophthalmic signs in botulismus. *POL TYG LEK* 19:428–430, 1964. (*ZENTRALBL GES OPHTHALMOL* 93:216, 1965.)
g. Kochler GD: On treatment of meat poisoning with botulism serum. *DTSCH MED WOCHENSCHR* 1:283–284, 1934, 1934. (German)
h. Koenig MG, Drutz DJ, et al: Type B botulism in man. *AM J MED* 42:208–219, 1967.
i. Konig H, Gassman HB, Jenzer G: Ocular involvement in benign botulism B. *AM J OPHTHALMOL* 80:430–432, 1975.

j. Lamanna C: The most poisonous poison. *SCIENCE* 130:763–772, 1959.

k. Lenz: Anatomical investigation in a case of botulism with ophthalmoplegia. *Z NEUR* 92:221, 1924. (German)

l. Peyresblanques J, SainVal C, et al: Concerning a familial occurrence of botulism with elevated serum level. *BULL SOC OPHTALMOL FRANCE* 78:961–963, 1978. (French)

m. Romer, Stein: Experimental contribution to the question of the site and nature of paresis of accommodation in botulism. *GRAEFES ARCH OPHTHALMOL* 58:291, 1094. (German)

n. Rousseau R, Hermann P: Optic atrophy with blindness from botulism. *ANN OCULIST* (*Paris*) 181:380, 1948; (*BULL SOC OPHTALMOL* (*Paris*) 125, 1948.) (French)

o. Ruge: A case of papilloretinitis in botulism. *KLIN MONATSBL AUGENHEILKD* 4:408, 1902.

p. Sheelo B: A case of botulism of type B. *OPHTHALMOLOGICA* 172:211–214, 1976. (German)

q. Swab CM: The status of food poisoning in relation to ophthalmology. *AM J OPHTHAL-MOL* 12:949–958, 1929.

r. Swab CM, Gerald HF: The ophthalmic lesions of botulism; additional notes and research. *BR J OPHTHALMOL* 17:129–144, 1933.

s. Terranova W, Palumbo JN, Breman JG: Ocular findings in botulism type B. *J AM MED ASSOC* 241:475–477, 1979.

t. Zanen J, Meunier A: Ocular sensorial deficits in botulism. *BULL SOC FRANC OPHTALMOL* 75:316–332, 1962. (French)

Botulinus toxin is produced by *Clostridium botulinum,* which may grow in improperly preserved foods and causes a type of food poisoning known clinically as *botulism,* as described in the foregoing section. The botulinus toxin has been purified and extensively studied. It is known to act strictly at terminal ends of cholinergic autonomic nerves and at neuromuscular junctions, and is believed to have no direct toxic effect on the central nervous system.[f,i]

Experimental intraocular injection has caused paralysis of cholinergic nerves of the ciliary body for more than six months without interference with neighboring adrenergic nerves.[e] The basis of paralysis is interference with release of acetylcholine from the terminal ends of the nerves, without interference with the responsiveness of the muscular receptor to acetylcholine or to pilocarpine. Sensory nerves are unaffected.[a,e,f,i]

Injection of botulinus toxin into the vitreous humor, or intravenously in lethal doses, has caused no electrical potential changes in the optic nerve or visual cortex in rabbits, yet study of isolated rabbit retinas exposed to the toxin has indicated interference with presynaptic cholinergic endings early in the visual pathway.[c,d] Intravitreal toxin produced no significant change in intraocular pressure, ophthalmoscopy, ERG, or light microscopy of the retina.[j] It seems as though there is a barrier to the toxin between vitreous humor and retina *in vivo.*[d]

Botulinus A toxin has been injected in small amount into the extraocular muscles of monkeys and in human patients for treatment of strabismus or nystagmus, without any systemic effects or changes in pupils or accommodation.[b,g,h]

Studies on the pure toxin appear to explain internal and external ophthalmoplegia observed in botulism on the basis of interference at the neuromuscular junction, but do not explain lesions which have been found in the ocular motor nuclei, nor the exceptional instances of optic neuritis or papilloretinitis to be found described under *Botulism*. Botulinus antitoxin appears to be effective against the toxin only in a prophylactic sense, and does not stop or reverse effects of the toxin already initiated.[i] (See also *Botulism*.)

a. Ambache N: A further survey of the action of Clostridium botulinum toxin upon different types of autonomic nerve fibre. *J PHYSIOL* 113:1–17, 1951.

b. Crone JA, de Jong, et: Treatment of nystagmus by injection of botulinus toxin into the eye muscles. *KLIN MONATSBL AUGENHEILKD* 184:216–217, 1984.

c. Dawson WM: Botulinum intoxication of rabbit retina. *ASSOC RES VIS OPHTHALMOL ABSTRACTS* p. 92, 1973.

d. Honda Y, Dawson WM: Botulinum intoxication of isolated retinas. *OPHTHALMIC RES* 72:108–117, 1975.

e. Kupfer C: Selective block of synaptic transmission in ciliary ganglion of type A botulinus toxin in rabbits. *PROC SOC EXP BIOL* 99:474–476, 1958.

f. Lamana C: The most poisonous poison. *SCIENCE* 130:763–772, 1959.

g. Scott AB: Botulinum toxin injection into extraocular muscles as an alternative to strabismus surgery. *OPHTHALMOLOGY* 87:1044–1049, 1980; *J PEDIATR OPHTHALMOLOGY* 17:21–25, 1980.

h. Scott AB: Botulinum toxin injection of eye muscles to correct strabismus. *TRANS AM OPHTHALMOL SOC* 79:734–770, 1981.

i. Stevenson JW: Bacterial neurotoxins. *AM J MED SCI* 235:317–336, 1958.

j. Wienkers K, Helveston EM, et al: Botulinum toxin injection into rabbit vitreous. *OPHTHALMIC SURGERY* 15:310–314, 1984.

Bracken fern (Pteris aquilina) fed to sheep has caused degeneration of retinal rods and cones and outer nuclear layer, most severely in the tapetal region, without apparently affecting the pigment epithelium or inner retinal layer.[a] This has been called "Bright blindness". Affected sheep have no conjunctivitis, keratitis, or cataract, but have permanent blindness in both eyes associated with retinal degeneration and increased reflection from the tapetum lucidum.[b-e]

a. Barnett KC, Watson WA: Bright blindness in sheep. *RES VET SCI* 11:289, 1970.

b. Barnett KC, Blakemore WF, Mason J: Bracken retinopathy in sheep. *TRANS OPHTHALMOL SOC UK* 92:741–744, 1972.

c. Sweasey D, Patterson DSP, Terlecki S: Lactate dehydrogenase (LDH) isoenzymes in the retina of the sheep and changes associated with progressive retinal degeneration (bright blindness). *EXP EYE RES* 12:60–69, 1971.

d. Terlecki S, et al: Absence of simple genetic factors in progressive retinal degeneration (bright blindness) in sheep. *BR VET J* 129:45–48, 1973.

e. Watson WA, Barnett KC, Terlecki S: Progressive retinal degeneration (bright blindness) in sheep: A review. *VET REC* 91:665, 1972.

Bradykinin injected into the vitreous body in rabbits has caused hyalitis and subcapsular changes in the lens.[a] Injected into the anterior chamber, it has caused inflammation, miosis, and breakdown of the blood-aqueous barrier, affecting the ciliary body especially.[284,292]

a. Zeller EA, Shoch D, Andujar E: On the enzymology of the refractory media of the eye. *AM J OPHTHALMOL* 61:1364–1371, 1966.
b. Butler JM, Hammond B: Neurogenic responses of the eye to injury. *TRANS OPHTHAL-MOL SOC UK* 97:668–674, 1977.

Brake fluid, automobile, generally has been composed of alcohols, glycols, and a lubricant, such as castor oil. It has been common experience for brake-fluid to squirt into the eye of automobile mechanics, causing severe smarting and burning sensation. The corneal epithelium is usually injured by the brake fluid, but not the deeper parts of the cornea, and healing as a rule is prompt. Discomfort may persist for some hours or even a day or two while the epithelium is healing, and it is important during this time not to allow the patient the use of topical anesthetics, but to depend on rest and systemic analgesics.[81]

Brayera (Kosso, Hagenia abyssinica), used as a tapeworm remedy in Ethiopia, has been known to cause bilateral optic atrophy.[a]

a. Roko L: Eye complications in poisoning caused by "Kosso" (Hagenia abyssinica). *ETHIOP MED J* 71:11–16, 1969.

Brinolase, a proteolytic enzyme, has been compared with α-chymotrypsin in rabbits and monkeys for facilitating extraction of the lens. It was found similarly effective at concentrations below those that were damaging to the cornea. Higher concentrations injured the endothelium and caused perforations of the cornea.[a,b]

a. Prompitak A, Chisholm L: Brinolase for lens extraction in cynomolgus monkey. *CAN J OPHTHALMOL* 9:360–362, 1974.
b. Hull DS, Bowman K, Green K: Effect of brinolase on corneal endothelium. *CAN J OPHTHALMOL* 11:82–86, 1976

Brilliant green is a basic cationic dye, closely related to Malachite green. It has been employed topically on the skin as an antiseptic, but in contact with the eye is severely injurious.[250,251] In one instance an attempt to treat conjunctivitis with 1% solution of this dye resulted in destructive keratitis with hypopyon and terminated in bilateral blindness due to corneal opacification.[a] Experimentally in rabbit eyes the dye is severely injurious. (See also *Dyes, cationic.*)

a. Kruckels H: On Brilliant green injury of the eye. *KLIN MONATSBL AUGENHEILKD* 106:571–574, 1941. (German)

Bromate is commonly employed in the form of *potassium bromate* as the neutralizing agent in the cold-wave process for waving the hair. The bromate acts as an oxidizing agent after the application of ammonium thioglycolate. No clinical injury has been traced to potassium bromate, and after irrigation of the surface of rabbit eyes for four minutes with a saturated solution of this compound, I have found no injury.[81] (Compare *Hair-waving preparations.*)

In rabbits, intravenous bromate was said by Sorsby to have an effect like *iodate* on the retina, but Cima could not substantiate this. (See *Iodate* for references.)

Bromides, usually in the form of *potassium bromide* or *sodium bromide,* formerly were employed as sedatives and antiepileptic drugs. The most frequent side effects of bromide medication were dermatitis and urticaria, with occasional blepharitis and conjunctivitis.[f,153] There seems, however, to have been no valid report of keratitis associated with the dermatitis and conjunctivitis.

No direct injurious action of bromides on the optic nerve or retina has been established, but visual hallucinations and disturbances of color vision have been occasionally noted.[a,b,c,153,247] Instances in which edema or pallor of the optic nervehead have been ascribed to poisoning by bromides have been so rare that it seems more likely that some coincidental disease rather than bromidism was responsible.[d,e,153,247] However, compounds containing bromide and used as sleep medications appear to have caused retrobulbar neuritis. See *Bromisoval* and *Carbromal.*

In a survey of eye disturbances in seventy cases of bromide intoxication in 1960, Levin found in addition to frequent mydriasis, that occasional patients complained of disturbances of the apparent color of objects, blurring or indistinctness of vision, apparent movement or wiggling, and change in the apparent size of objects. Visual hallucinations were common. Photophobia and diplopia were rare. The basis of the symptoms was not established by actual measurement of visual acuity, color sense, or fields. Objective findings in this series of patients were confined to pupillary disturbances. Paresis of accommodation in company with mydriasis was considered as a possible basis for blurring of vision and occasional micropsia, but no actual measurements of accommodation were reported. Owing to the mental condition of severely intoxicated patients, quantitative evaluation of vision is of course difficult.[c]

a. Barbour RF, Pilkington F, Sargent W: Bromide intoxication. *BR MED J* 2:957–960, 1936.
b. Doane JC, Weiner JG: Bromide intoxication. *MED J REC* 134:585–588, 1931.
c. Levin M: Eye disturbances in bromide intoxication. *AM J OPHTHALMOL* 50:478–483, 1960.
d. Rubel: Potassium bromide amaurosis. *RECUEIL OPHTALMOL* 7:113, 1885. (German)
e. Sharpe JC: Bromide intoxication. *J AM MED ASSOC* 102:1462–1465, 1934.
f. Washburne AC: Bromism, a review of the more recent literature and analysis of 16 new cases. *WISCONSIN MED J* 33:746–750, 1934.

Bromisovalum (Bromisoval, Bromurea, Bromural, Isoval) is a sedative and hypnotic drug. A comprehensive review and study of neurologic symptoms in sixty-five patients having chronic bromisovalum poisoning indicated the predominant symptom to be cerebellar ataxia and dysarthria with tremor and abnormal tendon reflexes, commonly accompanied by abnormalities of the pupil and nystagmus.[b,c] The pupils were found sometimes constricted and sometimes enlarged with considerable variability, less commonly unequal. Reduced reaction of the pupils to light was noted in 40 per cent of cases. Nystagmus was observed in about one third of the cases, generally horizontal, uncommonly vertical, usually disappearing in a few days after bromisovalum was discontinued. In a few cases subjective diplopia was noted and in others temporary heterophoria or weakness of convergence. In two patients reduction of visual acuity occurred with only partial recovery, remaining in the range of 0.2 to 0.67 with permanent pallor of the temporal portions of the optic nerveheads. In another patient, separately reported, after daily use for a year, bromisovalum was suspected of causing bilateral reduction of vision with central scotoma and temporal pallor of the optic nerveheads. Recovery was incomplete.[a]

a. Sattler CH: Bromural and Adalin poisoning of the eyes. *KLIN MONATSBL AUGEN-HEILKD* 70:149–152, 1923. (German)

b. Harenko A: Irreversible cerebello-bulbar syndrome as the sequela of bromisovalum poisoning. *ANN MED INTERN FENN* 56:29–36, 1967.

c. Harenko A: Neurologic findings in chronic bromisovalum poisoning. *ANN MED INTERN FENN* 57:181–188, 1967.

Bromoacetate administered as *sodium bromoacetate* to rabbits causes retinal degeneration similar ophthalmoscopically and histologically to that induced by iodoacetate. The visual cells of the central retina are most vulnerable, but all layers of the retina usually degenerate within a week after poisoning. *In vitro* bromoacetate and iodoacetate inhibit retinal respiration and glycolysis.[a,157,231]

a. Lucas DR, Newhouse JP, Davery JB: Experimental degeneration of the retina. *BR J OPHTHALMOL* 41:313–316, 1957.

Bromoacetone has been used as a tear gas. Permanent dense opacification of the cornea has resulted from splashing liquid bromoacetone on the eye.[a] Relatively minor injury has occurred in a case in which only a few fine droplets came in contact with the eye. Spots of gray opacity and necrosis appeared in the corneal epithelium, but in a few days the damaged areas were replaced by normal epithelium and the eye recovered completely.[81] (Also see *Tear gas weapons* and *Lacrimatory action.*)

a. Heinsius E: On severe injury of the cornea from concentrated tear gas (Bromoacetone). *Z AUGENHEILKD* 90:266–273, 1936. (German)

2-Bromoacetophenone (phenacyl bromide) is a solid which gives off lacrimogenic vapors similar to those of chloroacetophenone. Like many other lacrimators, bromoacetophenone has been shown to have a powerful inhibitory effect on thiol or sulfhydryl enzymes.[155,160] (See also *Lacrimators.*)

In vitro 0.005 to 0.05 mM bromoacetophenone has caused histologic and metabolic changes in rabbit retina, producing selective destruction of rod cells at the lowest concentration. However, no retinal injury or disturbance of vision from poisoning of the retina has been known in human beings, or in rabbits and rats that have been given 80 percent of a minimal lethal dose intravenously.[99,157,231]

α-Bromobenzylcyanide vapors are strongly lacrimatory. At high concentration bromobenzylcyanide is damaging to the cornea, but causes less permanent injury than the common tear gas chloroacetophenone.

The changes induced in rabbit eyes experimentally and in one human eye have been examined and described in detail.[161] Characteristically the corneal corpuscles become swollen and brownish during the first twenty-four hours. This is followed by infiltration of the cornea by macrophages, a loss of normal endothelial reflex, and appearance of fine irregularity in the endothelium. The stroma tends to recover without vascularization unless the limbus is severely involved. The cornea may ultimately be quite clear, but many minute excrescences visible by slit-lamp biomicroscope persist on the posterior surface of the cornea.[161]

Bromocriptine mesylate, a prolactin enzyme inhibitor, has been associated with development of bitemporal hemianopsia when used to induce pregnancy in patients with pituitary adenomas.[b,e] On the contrary, in the absence of pregnancy, bromocriptine treatment of pituitary prolactinoma has brought about dramatic improvement of visual fields.[a]

Bromocriptine produced a small amount of myopia in one patient, unrelieved by a cycloplegic, but relieved by stopping bromocriptine.[c] In normal volunteers, bromocriptine caused a small decrease in intraocular pressure without affecting the pupils.[d]

a. Grimson BS, Bowman ZL: Rapid decompression of anterior intracranial visual pathways with bromocriptine. *ARCH OPHTHALMOL* 101:604–606, 1983.

b. Lamberts SW, et al: Transient bitemporal hemianopsia during pregnancy after treatment of galactorrhea-amenorrhea syndrome with bromocriptine. *J CLIN ENDOCRINOL METAB* 44:180–184, 1977.

c. Manor RS, Dickerman Z, Llaron Z: Myopia during bromocriptine treatment. *LANCET* 1:102, 1981.

d. Mekki QA, Hassan SM, Turner P: Bromocriptine lowers intraocular pressure without affecting blood pressure. *LANCET* 1:1250–1251, 1983.

e. Van Dalen JTW, Grese EL: Rapid deterioration of visual fields during bromocriptine-induced pregnancy in a patient with a pituitary adenoma. *BR J OPHTHALMOL* 61:729–733, 1977.

5-Bromo-2′-deoxyuridine (broxuridine), an experimental antiviral drug, has been found to produce congenital, reversible cataracts in the offspring when fed to pregnant rats.[a,c,d] In chick embryo retinas in culture it interfered with melanogenesis, and caused extensive malformations.[b,e]

a. Fujita K, Chiyoda K, Johita H: BUDR (5-bromo-2′-deoxyuridine) and experimental fetal cataract. *J SAITAMA MED SCHOOL* 4:375–377, 1978. (English summary)

b. Garcia RI, Werner I, Szabo G: Effect of 5-bromo-2′-deoxy-uridine on growth and differentiation of cultured embryonic retinal pigment cells. *IN VITRO* 15:779–788, 1979.

c. Gasset AR, Itoi M, Ishil Y: Experimental BrdU congenital cataracts. *INVEST OPHTHALMOL* 14:145–148, 1975.

d. Itoi M: 5-Bromo-2′-deoxyuridine and experimental congenital cataract. *ACTA SOC OPHTHALMOL JPN* 77:1962–1963, 1973.

e. Mayerson P, Moscona AA: Malformation of embryonic neural retina elicited by BrdU. *DIFFERENTIATION* 13:173–184, 1979.

Bromomethyl ethyl ketone is a strongly lacrimatory substance which has been used in tear gas cartridges. In at least one instance, when a high concentration of this material struck the eye at short range, permanent blindness from corneal necrosis and scarring resulted. (See also *Tear gas weapons* and *Lacrimatory action.*)

  a. Schmidt R: Unusual consequence of an injury by concentrated tear gas. *BER DTSCH OPHTHALMOL GES* 51:449–450, 1936. (German)

alpha-Bromotoluene (benzyl bromide, Cyclite) is a liquid which gives off strongly lacrimogenic vapors despite a high boiling point.[61]

Bromoxylene (brominated xylol, T–Stoff) is a substance which has been used in warfare as tear gas. Its vapors cause long-lasting irritation.[61] (See also *Xylyl bromides.*)

Broxyquinoline (Broxykinolin; 5,7-dibromo-8-quinolinol; 5,7-dibromo-8-hydroxy-quinoline), a drug used as an intestinal antiseptic, was thought to be the cause of neurological symptoms like those in demyelinating disease and of progressive optic atrophy in a boy with acute gastroenteritis, to whom a total of 40 g was given in 27 days. His gait became ataxic and he developed optic atrophy in one eye. After the medication was stopped, some of the neurological abnormalities disappeared within a few months, but the optic atrophy became worse and the boy became completely blind in three months.[b] One or two other cases of optic neuropathy have been suspected.[294] A case has been reported in which oral self-medication during 3 years with nearly 1800 g of a mixture of broxyquinoline, broxaldine, and related compounds, but no chloroquine, was followed by progressive irreversible bull's eye maculopathy, central scotoma, and partial optic atrophy in both eyes.[a] (See also *Quinoline derivatives.*)

  a. Bonin P, Passot M: Toxic maculopathy from abuse of derivatives of hydroxyquinoline. *BULL SOC OPHTALMOL FRANCE* 84:131–136, 1984. (French)
  b. Strandvik B, Zetterstrom R: Amaurosis after broxyquinoline. *LANCET* 1:922–923, 1968.

Brucine is an alkaloid obtained from Strychnos nux-vomica. Similar to strychnine, it is bitter tasting and very poisonous. Rather vague visual effects have been ascribed to it. It has been said to cause weakness of vision as though seeing through fog, along with tinnitus and headache. Purely subjective experiences have been reported by Lewin and Guillery from trial on themselves; it was their impression that brucine sensitized discrimination of light and color differences, and increased visual field for colors.[153]

Bufotenine (N,N-dimethylserotonin; 5-hydroxy-N,N-dimethyl-tryptamine), a natural supposedly hallucinogenic substance, was reported by Fabing and Hawkins in 1956 to have been used in experiments in human beings in which intravenous injections of 4 to 16 mg were given within three minutes and caused immediate mydriasis, nystagmus, and colored visual hallucinations, but these effects were all gone within minutes.[a] However, Holmstedt and Lindgren in 1967 found that volunteers could take doses of as much as 100 mg orally or by inhalation with no effect on the CNS or on the pupils.[b]

  a. Fabing HD, Hawkins JR: Intravenous bufotenine injection in the human being. *SCIENCE* 123:886–887, 1956.
  b. Holmstedt B, Lindgren J: Chemical constituents and pharmacology of South American snuffs. In Efron, D.H. (Ed.): *Ethnopharmacologic Search for Psychoactive Drugs* (1967), U.S. P.H. Publication No. 1645.

Burdock burs (from the plant *Lappa vulgaris*) have both sharp, stiff bristles and delicate, clinging hairs which may get caught in the palpebral conjunctiva, particularly over the tarsus, and cause irritation and injury of the cornea as the lids and eye move. This may be accompanied by considerable inflammation and corneal ulceration.

The sharp bristle or bract has been known to become embedded in the cornea and to cause persistent ulceration and scarring.[b,129] More commonly, irritation is caused by slender pointed and barbed hairs, which are present in tufts on the burdock seed and which are freed in the late summer at the time of ripening of the fruit and opening of the pod. Typically these hairs become embedded in the conjunctiva and cause swelling and formation of nodules, especially in the upper fornix. This may be accompanied by formation of a pseudomembrane on the conjunctiva of the upper lid, and erosions of the cornea.

The hairs may be removed with forceps under the biomicroscope, but it is difficult to remove all, and sometimes the conjunctiva has to be excised. In the excised tissue the hairs are demonstrable and are found to be surrounded by granulation tissue with inflammatory and giant cells.[a] In only one case in the literature has there been penetration into the globe (Stargardt 1921), and in that instance two plant hairs were found in the iris, but their type was not well identified.[a]

Concerning whether the irritation and granuloma formation in the conjunctiva is attributable to a toxic substance, two experimental investigations have been made. In one (Gredstedt 1928), an oily extract of barbs of burdock was put in the anterior chamber of rabbits, but the inflammation induced was not distinctly different from that caused by the oil alone.[a]

A second investigation on rabbits showed that when the hairs from the seeds were introduced into the conjunctival sac they induced an inflammatory reaction similar to that in human beings, although the hairs did not penetrate into the globe. An oil extract of the hairs had no irritant effect when applied to the eye or injected subconjunctivally or into the cornea, but sterile aqueous extracts did cause considerable reaction when injected superficially into the cornea, inducing diffuse clouding of the whole cornea, with inflammation of the conjunctiva and vascularization of the cornea. The cornea was found to become edematous, with nodular opacities in the deepest layers and erosion of the epithelium. By microscopy, many inflammatory cells were found in the cornea and the anterior chamber. The hairs themselves lost many of their irritant properties when extracted with water, but the aqueous extract retained its irritant properties while standing for at least four weeks.[a]

It appears that the irritant effects of hairs and bristles from Burdock bur are to be attributed partly to mechanical effect and partly to toxic action.[a]

    a. Bruhn AM: Clinical and experimental investigations concerning eye injuries by bur-
        dock hairs. *KLIN MONATSBL AUGENHEILKD* 101:730–741, 1938. (German)
    b. Havener WH, Falls HF, McReynolds WU: Burdock bur ophthalmia. *ARCH OPHTHAL-
        MOL* 53:260–263, 1955.
    c. Breed FB, Kuwabara T: Burdock ophthalmia. *ARCH OPHTHALMOL* 75:16–20, 1966.

Busulfan (Myleran; 1,4-butanediol dimethanesulfonate), an antineoplastic, produces cataracts in human beings and experimental animals.[a,f,g,h] In rats it has been shown to injure the lens epithelium by interfering with production of lens nucleic acid during mitosis.[a-e] In human beings the cataract is mainly posterior subcapsular with scattered punctate cortical opacities.[h] Histologically, the human cataract is somewhat different from that of the rat, with evidence of migration of epithelial cells from the equatorial region to the posterior pole.[h]

One patient under chronic treatment with busulfan has had not only cataracts but also the sicca syndrome.[j]

Several patients have been treated with busulfan during pregnancy. From these pregnancies, one infant had microphthalmos. One had retinal degeneration. Busulfan is probably toxic to the fetal retina.[i]

a. DelPianto E, Bozzoni F, Valesini GA: Cataract from busulfan and the sufhydryl content of lenses having such cataracts. *BOLL OCULIST* 37:40–49, 1958. (Italian)

b. Soloman C, Light AE, DeBeer EJ: Cataracts produced in rats by 1,4-dimethane-sulfonoxybutane (Myleran). *ARCH OPHTHALMOL* 54:850–852, 1955.

c. Grimes P, von Sallmann L, Frichette A: Influence of Myleran on cell proliferation in the lens epithelium. *INVEST OPHTHALMOL* 3:566–576, 1965.

d. Hammar H, Brolin SW: The fluorescence of the eye lens in rats with Myleran cataract. *ACTA OPHTHALMOL* 37:344–349, 1959.

e. Light AE: Additional observations on the effects of busulfan on cataract formation, duration of anesthesia, and reproduction in rats. *TOXICOL APPL PHARMACOL* 10:459–466, 1967.

f. Podos SM, Canellos GP: Lens changes in chronic granulocytic leukemia. *AM J OPHTHALMOL* 68:500–504, 1969.

g. Ravindranathan MP, Paul VJ, Kuriakose ET: Cataract after busulphan treatment. *BR MED J* 1:218–219, 1972.

h. Hamming NA, Apple DJ, Goldberg MF: Histopathology and ultrastructure of busulfan-induced cataract. *GRAEFES ARCH OPHTHALMOL* 200:139–147, 1976. (German)

i. Saraux H, LeFrancois A: Degenerative retinal conditions after treatment of the mother with busulfan during pregnancy. *KLIN MONATSBL AUGENHEILKD* 170:818–820, 1977. (German)

j. Sidi Y, Douer D, Pinkhas J: Sicca syndrome in a patient with toxic reaction to busulfan. *J AM MED ASSOC* 238:1951, 1977.

1,3-Butadiene is a gas employed in manufacture of synthetic rubber. A concentration of 8,000 ppm in air produces no symptoms in human beings.[a] Dogs and rabbits exposed experimentally to as much as 6,700 ppm 7.5 hours a day for 8 months have developed no histologically demonstrable abnormality in any part of the eyes.[a] However, when exposed to photo-oxidation with ozone and nitrogen dioxide, as in formation of smog, 1,3-butadiene is an outstandingly potent precursor of products that are irritating to the human eye, producing both formaldehyde and acrolein.[110]

a. Carpenter CP, Shaffer CB, et al: Studies on the inhalation of 1:3 butadiene. *J IND HYG TOXIC* 26:69–78, 1944.

Butane is an essentially nontoxic petroleum gas which causes no disturbance of the eye, even when injected into the anterior chamber experimentally in rabbits, disappearing spontaneously from the eye in two to four days.[81] Butane is used in some cigarette lighters, and one person's experience suggested that a spray on the eye (pre-ignition) repeatedly caused transient blurring of vision.[a]

  a. Hallett IH: Another hazard of smoking? LANCET 1:141, 1970.

1,3-Butanediol (1,3-butylene glycol) tested by application of a drop to rabbits' corneas caused no persisting injury.[225] A tiny drop applied to the human eye causes immediate severe stinging, but irrigation with water brings rapid complete relief.[81]

n-Butanol (n-butyl alcohol) vapor has a characteristic but not unpleasant smell; it is not lacrimatory, but causes slight sensation of irritation of the eye noticeable at 50 ppm in air.[183] Chronic exposure to concentrations above 50 to 200 ppm causes objectionable irritation of human eyes.[f,g]

Circumstantial evidence points to butyl alcohol vapor as a cause of a special vacuolar keratopathy in human beings.[a,c,d] In cases in which suspicion has been directed most strongly to butyl alcohol, slit-lamp biomicroscopy has shown many very fine transparent vacuoles which look like tiny bubbles of gas in the epithelial layers of otherwise normal corneas. The vacuoles are seen best by retroillumination. In some patients vacuolar keratopathy causes no complaints, but in the most severely affected it has been associated with pain and tearing, characteristically most marked on first opening the eyes in the morning. Vision is generally unaffected, and the vacuoles disappear within a few days when exposure to solvents is discontinued.

Butyl alcohol appears to have been the solvent most commonly present in the industrial situations where this special keratopathy has been observed. Experimentally, however, although vapors of pure butyl alcohol at high concentration have been shown to cause small readily healing defects in the epithelium of rabbit cornea, these vapors have not induced typical vacuoles either in rabbit or cat eyes.[81,230] Furthermore, exposure of mice, guinea pigs, rabbits, and dogs to the vapor of butanol alone, or mixed with diacetone alcohol and ethyl alcohol has been unsuccessful in reproducing the conditions seen in human beings.[a]

Liquid n-butyl alcohol tested by applying a drop to rabbit eyes caused moderate temporary injury, graded 7 on a scale of 1 to 10 after twenty-four hours.[225] In 0.5 M aqueous solution butyl alcohol has been found to be one of the most effective substances for loosening the corneal epithelium from the stroma of excised cattle corneas.[b] A saturated aqueous solution also loosens the epithelium from excised human cornea.[81] The relationship of this effect to vapor-induced vacuolar keratopathy is not known.

A saturated aqueous solution has been given intravenously to many patients in volumes up to 300 ml per day for reducing postoperative pain, for ocular conditions in sixty-eight patients, without note of any untoward effect on the eyes or central nervous system.[h]

(Further discussion of vacuolar keratopathy from solvents is to be found under *Solvent vapors*).

  a. Cogan DG, Grant WM: An unusual type of keratitis associated with exposure to n-butyl alcohol (butanol). *ARCH OPHTHALMOL* 35:106–109, 1945.
  b. Hermann H, Hickman FH: The adhesion of epithelium to stroma. *BULL JOHNS HOPKINS HOSP* 82:182–207, 1948.

c. Jaeger W: Injury of the cornea by butyl alcohol. *GRAEFES ARCH OPHTHALMOL* 156:480–483, 1955. (German)

d. Kruger E: Eye disturbances in using nitrocellulose lacquers in the straw hat industry. *ARCH GEWERBEPATH* 3:798–807, 1932. (German)

e. Schmid E: Concerning the corneal disturbance of furniture polishers. *KLIN MONATSBL AUGENHEILKD* 130:110–115, 1957. (German)

f. Sterner JH, Crouch HC, et al: A ten year old study of butyl alcohol exposure. *AM IND HYG ASSOC QUART* 10:53–59, 1949.

g. Tabershaw IR, Fahy JP, Skinner JB: Industrial exposure to butanol. *J IND HYG* 26:328, 1944.

h. Welt B: n-Butanol: its use in control of postoperative pain in otorhinolaryngological surgery. *ARCH OTOLARYNG* 52:549–564, 1950.

2-Butoxyethanol (butyl Cellosolve; ethyleneglycolmonobutylether), an industrial solvent, has caused mild eye and nose irritation in workmen exposed to its vapors.[a, 151] Tests of the liquid by dropping on rabbit eyes induces reddening and swelling of the conjunctiva with slight clouding of the corneal epithelium. The degree of injury judged twenty-four hours after the application of a single drop has been graded 4 on a scale of 1 to 10.[a, 27] Rabbit eyes in contact with the liquid for eight minutes before irrigation with water have recovered completely in four days.[81]

On excised beef corneas, butyl Cellosolve has an effect similar to butyl alcohol, reducing the adhesion of eplithelium to stroma,[107] but in the corneas of human beings exposed to the vapors no vacuolar keratitis has yet been described like that induced by the vapor of butyl alcohol.

a. Carpenter CP, Pozzani UC, et al: The toxicity of butyl Cellosolve solvent. *ARCH IND HEALTH* 14:114–130, 1956.

Butyl acetate has no notable systemic toxicity to the eyes, but its vapor causes irritation of the eyes and nose, first noticeable to human beings at a concentration of 300 ppm in air,[183] and objectionable at 3,300 ppm; higher concentrations cause tearing and hyperemia of the conjunctiva.[61, 188]

Exposure of albino rabbits to 500 ppm for twenty days and to 1,000 ppm for four days, and exposure of guinea pigs to 500 ppm for ten days, and 1000 ppm for four days, caused no corneal or conjunctival injury detectable by slit-lamp biomicroscopy, and corneal sensation was not altered.[81]

Results of other tests of butyl acetate vapor on animal eyes have been complicated by an admixture of butyl alcohol, and it is uncertain whether damage to the corneal epilthelium reported to occur at high concentration was caused by the butyl acetate or the butyl alcohol.[230] A similar equivocal situation is encountered in a report of several cases of vacuolar keratopathy among workers exposed to a mixture of vapors of butyl acetate and isobutyl alcohol.[a] (See also *Solvent vapors.*)

Application of the liquid to rabbit eyes caused superficial reversible injury, graded 5 on a scale of 1 to 10.[226]

a. Busing KH: Eye injuries from butylacetate plus isobutyl alcohol in a cable works. *ZENTRALBL ARBEITSMED* 2:13–14, 1952. (German)

n-Butyl amine is a volatile liquid having an odor similar to ammonia. The vapor is only mildly irritating to the eyes,[a] but the liquid tested on experimental animal eyes is as severely injurious as ammonium hydroxide. The injurious effect seems to be attributable to the alkalinity of butyl amine, since as with other amines its damaging effect on the cornea is prevented if it is neutralized with acid before testing.[107,222]

  a. Hanzlik PJ: Toxicity and actions of the normal butylamines. *J PHARMACOL EXP THER* 20:435, 1923.

Butylated hydroxytoluene, an anti-oxidant food additive, when tested for teratogenic properties is reported to have produced anophthalmia in offspring in rats, but not in mice.[a]

  a. Johnson AR: A re-examination of the possible teratogenic effects of butylated hydroxytoluene (BHT). *FOOD COSMET TOXICOL* 3:371–375, 1965.

Butyl digol applied as a 10% solution in water to rabbit eyes is reported to cause a 30% rise in intraocular pressure.[276]

n-Butyl formate at high vapor concentrations is strongly irritant to the eyes. In animals exposed to 4,000 ppm, irritation of eyes and respiratory passages was evident. Men exposed to 10,000 ppm had so much ocular discomfort that they could not keep their eyes open, and conditions became unbearable after a few breaths.[61]

t-Butyl hydroperoxide, used as a catalyst in polymerization reactions. tested as a 75% solution in dimethylphthalate by application of two drops to rabbit eyes, caused injury graded 5 on a scale of 0 to 7.[a] A drop of 35% solution in propylene glycol caused a reaction graded between 46 and 79 on a scale of 0 to 100, persisting at least a week.[59] A 7% solution in the same solvent was the maximum which could be tolerated without significant irritation. Washing the eyes with water within four seconds after application of the test substance prevented injury in all cases.[59]

In rabbit corneas exposed *in vitro* to 1 or 2.5 mM t-butyl hydroperoxide the glutathione in the endothelial cells was oxidized and the cells were destroyed.[b]

  a. Kuchle HJ: Investigations of the eye injuring effects of organic peroxides. *ZENTRALBL ARBEITSMED* 8:25–31, 1958. (German)
  b. Whikehart DR, Edelhauser HF: Glutathione in rabbit corneal endothelia. *INVEST OPHTHALMOL VIS SCI* 17:455–464, 1978.

t-Butyl peracetate tested as 50% solution in dimethyl phthalate by application of two drops to rabbit eyes caused injury graded 3 on a scale of 0 to 7.[a]

  a. Kuchle (1958) see *t-Butyl hydroperoxide.*

t-Butyl perbenzoate tested as 50% solution in dimethyl phthalate by application of two drops to rabbit eyes caused slight injury, graded 1 on a scale of 0 to 7.[a]

  a. Kuchle (1958) see *t-Butyl hydroperoxide.*

Butyl trimethylammonium bromide has been tested in 0.1 M neutral aqueous solution on rabbit eyes by irrigation for ten minutes, both with and without the epithelium present; transient miosis and salivation resulted, but no significant corneal injury.[80,81]

1,4-Butynediol liberated into the air of working areas during the synthesis of poly(vinylpyrrolidinone) has been reported to be severely irritating to the eyes and to penetrate the skin and cause severe irritation.[a]

    a. Stasenkova KP, Kochetkova: Toxicological characteristics of new commercial chemicals used in production of poly(vinylpyrrolidinone). *CHEM ABSTR* 62:12366d, 1965.

Butyraldehyde (butylaldehyde) has been tested for irritant effect on human eyes at vapor concentrations in air such as might occur in smog, and has been found nonirritant.[218] The liquid applied as a drop to rabbit eyes proved to be rather damaging, graded 8 on a scale of 1 to 10 after twenty-four hours.[225] However, in six instances of industrial corneal injury from butyraldehyde recovery is said to have been prompt and complete.[165]

Cactus of the *prickly pear* variety (*Opuntia microdasys*) in one eye of a patient caused keratoconjunctivitis associated with a barbed bristle in the palpebral conjunctiva. Removal brought rapid healing.[a] Either a toxic or a mechanical mechanism could be postulated.

    a. Whiting DA, Bristow JH: Dermatitis and keratoconjunctivitis caused by a prickly pear (*Opuntia microdasys*). *S AFR MED J* 49:1445–1448, 1975.

Cadmium chloride applied as a 0.05 to 0.1M aqueous solution to rabbit eyes for ten minutes after mechanical removal of the corneal epithelium to facilitate penetration has caused total opacification and scarring of the cornea. The severity of reaction was not reduced by irrigation of the eyes with 0.03 M sodium EDTA solution (pH 8) immediately after the exposure.[81]

    Tested on perfused bullfrog retina, low concentrations depressed rod photoreceptor potentials, but not those of cones.[a]

    a. Fox DA, Sillman AJ: Heavy metals affect rod, but not cone, photoreceptors. *SCIENCE* 206:78–80, 1979.

Cadmium metal gives off fumes when burned or heated strongly, as in welding, and inhalation can cause poisoning, but smarting of the eyes occurs relatively infrequently, and no injury to the eyes of human beings from fumes has been reported. However cadmium metal implanted experimentally in rabbit eyes has proved very toxic, causing severe purulent intraocular inflammation and cataract.[340]

Cadmium sulfide (cadmium yellow) is an insoluble pigment which has been introduced by tatooing into normal and scarred corneas of rabbits and patients, producing permanent coloration of the cornea, but no irritation.[199]

Caffeine is an alkaloid present in tea and coffee. In 1896 de Schweinitz conjectured on disturbances of vision which might be caused by caffeine, but his clinical examples were quite vague.[41] There appears to be no good evidence of toxic effect of caffeine on vision.[255] However, in one instance bilateral papillitis has been attributed to treatment with *Caffergot,* a medication containing caffeine, as well as *ergotamine,* but it would be hard to know where to place the blame.[d]

Experimentally in normal people it has been reported that coffee produces a rise in the electro-oculogram (EOG) potential, and this has been interpreted as evidence of stimulation of the blood flow in chorio-retinal vessels, presumably a beneficial effect.[e]

Caffeine has been used in a provocative test for glaucoma. A large test dose given orally (0.4 g caffeine or 45 g coffee) causes a significant rise in ocular pressure in some glaucomatous eyes, but it is not a reliable test.[b] The possibility of adverse effect from ordinary dietary consumption of caffeine in glaucoma has been considered many times and the literature has been reviewed.[a] Experimentally, in 210 open-angle glaucomatous eyes thorough testing of ocular pressure before and after intravenous injection of 0.3 g of pure caffeine in a small amount of water showed that only in a few cases did this raise the pressure more than 5 or 6 mm Hg.[a] The maximum was reached between thirty and sixty minutes. and the pressure returned to original levels within sixty to ninety minutes. The rise of pressure tended to be greatest in eyes with tension already elevated before testing. The results of these and other tests support the belief that a cup or two of coffee is safely tolerated in the great majority of cases of glaucoma.

Teratogenic influence upon the developing fetal rat lens has been ascribed to caffeine.[c]

a. Graeber W: On the effect of caffeine on the intraocular pressure in surgically or medically managed chronic simple glaucoma. *KLIN MONATSBL AUGENHEILKD* 152:357–365, 1968. (German)

b. Leydhecker W: Influence of coffee upon ocular tension. *AM J OPHTHALMOL* 39:700–704, 1955.

c. Pitel M, Lerman S: Further studies on the effects of intrauterine vasoconstrictors on the fetal rat lens. *AM J OPHTHALMOL* 58:464–470, 1964.

d. Gupta DR, et al: Bilateral papillitis associated with Caffergot therapy. *NEUROLOGY* 22:793–797, 1972.

e. Muller W, Hasse E, et al: The behavior of the EOG after coffee intake. *KLIN MONTASBL AUGENHEILKD* 162:379–383, 1973. (German)

Calcium carbide is a solid which reacts rapidly with water, liberating acetylene and forming calcium hydroxide. In several instances burns of the eye resulting in opacity and scarring have been caused by contact with particles of calcium carbide or with strongly alkaline residues from its reaction with water.[46] The clinical character of the burns is the same as those produced by calcium hydroxide.[a, 34] If particles of calcium carbide are removed promptly, healing may be rapid.[165] (Compare *Calcium hydroxide.*)

a. Heinsius E: On calcific crystalline deposits in the conjunctiva after a carbide burn. *KLIN MONATSBL AUGENHEILKD* 115:673–676, 1949. (German)

Calcium carbonate (chalk) has no toxic effect when applied to the surface of rabbit eyes.[81] Injecting 8 mg of calcium carbonate powder of 35μ maximum particle size into the anterior chamber of rabbits causes a moderate rise of intraocular pressure lasting less than twenty-four hours, more likely owing to physical obstruction of aqueous outflow than to a toxic effect.[a] Excessive oral calcium carbonate in chronic renal failure can produce hypercalcemia and band keratopathy.[b]

a. Priestley BS, Pecori-Giraldi J, Valvo A: Experimental glaucoma from Laminaria digitata. *BOLL OCULIST* 47:652–668, 1968. (Italian)
b. Ginsburg DS, Kaplan EL, Katz AI: Hypercalcemia after oral calcium carbonate therapy in patients on chronic haemodialysis. *LANCET* 1:1271–1274, 1973.

Calcium chloride is a neutral, water-soluble salt which in solution is essentially innocuous, but solid particles have been known to cause transient irritation and superficial injury without permanent damage.[a] Application of 2% to 10% solution to rabbit eyes after removal of the corneal eplithelium, or injection into the corneal stroma, causes no permanent damage.[46,81,89,123]

a. Gat L, Nagy L: Lesions of the conjunctiva and cornea self-inflicted with calcium chloride. *OPHTHALMOLOGICA* 138:406–412, 1959. (German)

Calcium hydroxide (calcium hydrate, slaked lime, hydrated lime) is a white powdered or granular solid which is used in making mortar, plaster, cement, and whitewash. Calcium hydroxide is not very soluble in water; to dissolve 1 g requires approximately 600 ml of water at room temperature, but a strongly alkaline solution of pH 12.4 results. Calcium hydroxide in various forms is one of the commonest causes of severe chemical burns of the eye, most commonly known as "lime burns". At least 130 articles have been published presenting original observations on lime burns of the eye, mostly in patients. The subject has been reviewed and discussed at length in several comprehensive texts on eye burns.[33,34,46,129,153,249]

Lime burns present many of the features common to burns with all strong alkalies, as described elsewhere under *Alkalies.* However, certain special properties of calcium hydroxide give lime burns some distinctive characteristics.

Most commonly lime burns of the eye are caused by a splash of a thick, moist, pasty material (plaster, mortar, or cement), less commonly by a splash of milky fluid (whitewash) and rarely by a clear solution of calcium hydroxide (lime water).

The result in almost all cases is that there is a particulate paste in contact with the cornea and conjunctiva tending to adhere and to dissolve slowly, forming strongly alkaline calcium hydroxide solution. Because of the low solubility of semisolid or solid deposits of calcium hydroxide, irrigation with tears and water is less effective in removing calcium hydroxide than in removing the usual simple solutions or soluble particles of most other alkalies.

Special efforts must be made to remove the deposits promptly in order to avoid prolonged exposure of the eye to a continuing source of calcium hydroxide from the reservoir of solid material. Vigorous irrigation dislodges some particles mechanically. Pulsatile irrigation may be advantageous.[k] For complete cleansing it may be necessary to double evert the lids and swab or brush material from the fornices. This procedure is facilitated by application of a local anesthetic and by use of a solution of 0.01 to 0.05 M disodium edetate (EDTA) at pH 4.6 to 7, for irrigation to aid in loosening and dissolving the solid. (See also *Edetate*)

Calcium hydroxide has chemical properties which influence in special ways the manner in which this alkali penetrates and damages the cornea. The injurious action of calcium hydroxide on the stroma of the cornea, tested in the absence of the epithelium, is governed exclusively by the hydroxyl ion concentration, the same as for all other alkalies tested. In the range pH 11 to pH 12, injurious effect and amount of chemical interaction with the cornea increases greatly.[89] At this high pH the calcium ions react with the corneal mucoproteins and collagen, causing loss of some of the mucoprotein from the cornea. Measurements in rabbit corneas burned by calcium hydroxide by Teterwak have shown the normal content to start to decrease within an hour after exposure, reaching a minimum after one day, beginning recovery after six days, but remaining subnormal for months.[t]

In its direct effect on bare corneal stroma, calcium hydroxide appears not to differ from other alkalies, except that it induces a greater immediate opacification in the stroma of certain species than do the common monovalent alkalies. (Immediate whitening of the corneal stroma by calcium hydroxide is much more evident in cattle and rabbit corneas than in human.[89])

Clinically, the features which principally distinguish lime burns from other alkali burns are associated with the epithelium and relatively slow penetration of calcium hydroxide. Calcium hydroxide, is slower in breaking down and penetrating the epithelial barrier than are most other alkalies, especially the monovalent ones. It may be that saponification of epithelial lipids is involved in a breakdown of the epithelial barrier by alkalies, and that in the case of calcium hydroxide, the soaps which result are insoluble calcium soaps which themselves may interfere with penetration.

Mild lime burns in patients typically cause a frosted or groundglass type of opacity located very superficially approximately at the level of Bowman's membrane, resembling band keratopathy of hypercalcemia in its biomicroscopic appearance. This type of opacity is observable immediately after lime burn in human eyes, but does not seem to occur in experimental animals. It is frequently seen in patients with considerable loss of epithelium but no underlying opacity of the stroma. This thin lamina or veil of opacity may be covered by the corneal epithelium when it regenerates, retaining a close resemblance to calcific band keratopathy. The overlying epithelium has to be removed before the deposit can be dissolved by edetate (EDTA) solution.[e,f,237]

In lime burns of greater severity, usually from protracted contact rather than from brief exposure, evidence of penetration and opacification in the stroma deeper than Bowman's membrane is found by slit-lamp biomicroscopic examination. Pearly grayness in the corneal stroma itself is not due to deposition of calcium, and is not amenable to clearing by means of calcium-dissolving agents such as sodium edetate. Stromal opacification by calcium hydroxide occurs immediately at pH 12 or higher and is associated with a loosening of the mucoid from other components of the cornea so that it is lost from the cornea in a few hours.

Corneas severely burned by calcium hydroxide (and many other caustic chemicals) typically are anesthetic for many days after the injury; this is presumed to be due to damage of corneal nerves. A systematic clinical study by Simkova, in which corneal nerves were studied biomicroscopically with vital staining by methylene blue in fifty-nine patients after calcium hydroxide burns, substantiated that there were degenerative changes in the nerves and that thirty days might be required for reappearance of normal nerve fibers following the injury.[s]

Measurement of the calcium content of corneas from experimentally exposed rabbit eyes have demonstrated that the calcium content can drop to normal spontaneously within a few hours or can be lowered to normal by treatment with edetate, with no change in the degree of opacity of the corneal stroma. Additional evidence that the opacity of the stroma is not attributable to a high calcium content is the fact that by bathing the cornea with *calcium chloride* solution the calcium content can be raised experimentally to the same levels as found immediately after lime burns, yet no opacification or injury results. Formerly it was thought that calcium hydroxide precipitated the mucoid in the cornea,[a,h] but Kern and I have shown this not to be so.[89]

There are only two conditions in which an excess of calcium in the cornea is directly associated with opacity; one is the precipitation of a thin lamina of calcific material at Bowman's membrane, occuring in mild lime burns, and in band keratopathy of hypercalcemia or chronic uveitis; the other is the formation of plaques of dense secondary calcification which occur late after severe burns, frequently in rabbit eyes and occasionally in human eyes. The diffuse or mottled pearly gray of the stroma of the cornea which is evident in moderately severe as well as very severe burns is not due to the continuing presence of calcium, but, as in the case of burns by other alkalies such as sodium hydroxide, is due to some fundamental derangement or denaturation of corneal structure which cannot be reversed by treatment with any calcium-extracting agent, or for that matter by any known means.

Histological and histochemical studies of calcium hydroxide-burned corneas, mostly experimental in rabbits, by Chakyrov, Heinc, Klima, and Uglova have provided descriptions of the tissue changes.[b,i,j,u]

In the most severe calcium hydroxide burns, the corneal stroma becomes and remains totally opaque grayish-white. Many of the late complications described under *Alkalies* may occur, as in other strong alkali burns, with the exception that calcium hydroxide does not have great tendency to penetrate like *ammonium hydroxide* into the eye or to damage iris and lens.

Glaucoma as a complication of calcium hydroxide burns of the eye has generally gone unrecognized until Heydenreich reported fifteen cases in which severely injured eyes with gray corneas developed elevated intraocular pressure.[112] In half the cases the onset was within a few hours and was responsive to treatment with miotics. In the other cases the onset was six to twelve weeks later, with gradually increasing pressure, some requiring multiple operations for control. In general, these eyes were so badly damaged that the visual outcome was very poor. It was supposed, based largely on experiments on rabbits with *sodium hydroxide*, that the glaucoma in the later stages was due to scarring and obstruction of aqueous outflow channels. Related studies by Heydenreich on rabbits with glaucoma secondary to cauterization with heat or *sodium hydroxide* indicated that if hypotony were induced by surgery, this too could have adverse effect, tending to favor vascularization and ulceration of burned corneas.[113]

In treatment of lime burns of the eye many nonspecific measures have been advised and tried, as well as numerous measure specifically aimed at removing calcium from the cornea. The treatments designed to extract calcium have, of course, been predicated upon a belief that excess calcium in the cornea after exposure to calcium hydroxide is responsible for opacity, but this is not true, except in the special cases already mentioned in which there is a fine ground-glass lamina at Bowman's membrane, or in late secondary calcification. Efforts to extract calcium are appropriate only in these two circumstances.

Among the many calcium-extracting agents which have been investigated and employed in the last sixty years are hydrochloric acid, ammonium chloride, ammonium acetate, ammonium tartrate, sodium citrate, acetic acid, sugar solution, reverse iontophoresis, and sodium edetate. The last has proved the least irritating and most effective.

For first aid treatment of lime-burned eyes, it is recommended that the eye be washed with running water as quickly as possible, aiming to remove solid and semisolid material from the conjunctival sac as well as from the cornea. A 0.01 to 0.05 M (0.3% to 1.5%) solution of sodium edetate at pH 4.6 to 7 is helpful as an irrigant to loosen masses of adherent lime from the tissues, but promptness in starting irrigation is the most important consideration, and the first water at hand should be employed. After cleansing of the surface of the globe and the fornices of the conjunctival sac has been accomplished with water or saline, if the cornea is observed by slit-lamp to have a finely granular ground-glass film of opacity at the level of Bowman's membrane, this may be removed by irrigation with the above mentioned edetate solution for fifteen minutes.[e, 185]

Experimental evaluations of use of sodium edetate solutions have shown that after exposure to calcium hydroxide more calcium is removed from rabbits' eyes by irrigation with this type of solution than by sodium chloride solution; but unless greater than 1% disodium edetate was used, the clinical results were not superior to those from sodium chloride solution, according to observations by Lohse and Giesecke. A 10% concentration of sodium edetate was found to be injurious.[156]

Experiments by Glasmacher on excised animal corneas have shown that 2.5% solution of sodium edetate at pH 4.68 is much more effective in extracting calcium than sodium edetate at pH 7, and also more effective than water or ascorbic acid. Glasmacher has pointed out that the weak acidity of pH 4.68 solution appeared to favor release of calcium from the cornea enough to outweigh some weakening of chelating action of edetate by the lower pH.[69]

A wide variety of other medical and surgical treatments have been tried in experimental animals and in patients. In rabbits, measurements of the pH of the surface and the pH of the aqueous humor have been used as a basis for comparisons of various treatments.[d, 1, 58] Comparisons of disodium edetate, ascorbic acid, and trometamol-ascorbic acid solutions have shown the last to have an advantage as a neutralizing agent.[d] Results comparing treatment with vasodilators and treatment with vasoconstrictors showed no advantage over treatment with antibiotics alone.[16, 17] Subconjunctival injections of the rabbit's blood or blood serum after symmetrical exposure of the eyes to calcium hydroxide appeared to have favorable influence on the outcome in experiments by Sallai and associates.[213] The same has been recommended for human beings by some authors.[m]

Early surgical treatment of eyes burned with calcium hydroxide has been recommended by a number of authors. Alberth and associates, in a series of publications culminating in a monograph in 1968 based on rabbit experiments and clinical observations, have supported a thesis that lamellar keratoplasty done in the first day or two is beneficial in severely burned eyes.[3] This procedure appears to be based on a concept of a depot of some toxic material in the anterior layers of the cornea which the lamellar keratoplasty is intended to eliminate.

Clinical observations on series of patients with calcium hydroxide burns of the eye in which a variety of treatments were used have been published with reviews of the literature and expression of personal preferences and opinions, agreeing only on the importance of getting first aid irrigation of the eyes started as quickly as possible.[p–r,235] Use of sodium edetate irrigation has been favored on the basis of clinical observations by Gundorova, Oksala, Oosterhuis, Praus, Ricklefs, and Stagni,[g,m,o,q,r,185,235] while it has been discontinued by Puglisi-Duranti.[p]

In the case of disodium edetate treatment there has been an interesting fortuitous development. Originally it was intended that irrigation with this solution would be used once as a first-aid help in removing residual calcium hydroxide and calcific deposits from the cornea and conjunctival sac, but in some cases the solution was used repeatedly, sometimes for days, and it appeared that results were improved. It now appears that part of the problem in alkali-injured corneas is release and activation of collagenase from injured cells, and that edetate (either sodium or calcium) is an inhibitor of this injurious enzyme.[o] Thus the substance may act in two disimilar but desirable ways. (More is said in the section on *Alkalies.*)

a. Braun G, Haurowitz F: Experimental histologic and therapeutic investigations in lime burn of the cornea. *KLIN MONATSBL AUGENHEILKD* 70:157–165, 1923. (German)

b. Chakyrov E, Uglova T: Cytochemical studies of the lipids of the cornea from burning by calcium hydroxide. *C R ACAD BULGARE SCI* 16:853–856, 1963. (Chem Abstr 61:7543, 1964.)

c. D'arrigo P, Genovesi E: Current means of treatment of burns of the eye by lime. *ANN OTTALMOL CLIN OCUL* 92:1349–1357, 1966. (Italian)

d. Feller K, Graupner: The pH in the anterior chamber of the rabbit eye after experimental burning with calcium hydroxide and the influence on it of various buffer substances. *GRAEFES ARCH OPHTHALMOL* 173:71–77, 1967. (German)

e. Grant WM: A new treatment for calcific corneal opacities. *ARCH OPHTHALMOL* 48:681–685, 1952.

f. Grant WM: Chemical burns of the eye: emergency treatment. *MED CLIN N AM* 36:1215–1222, 1952.

g. Gundorova RA, Lenkevich MM, Tartakovskaya AI: Treatment of lime burns of the cornea with EDTA. *VESTN OPHTHALMOL* 80: 42–45, 1967.

h. Haurowitz F, Braun G: On lime burn of the cornea. *HOPPE SEYLER Z PHYSIOL CHEM* 123:79–89, 1922.

i. Heine A, Malinsky J, Kubena K: Changes of the corneal ultrastructure after lime burns in rabbits. *CESK OFTALMOL* 25:6–9, 1969.

j. Klima M: Lime burn of the eye. *CESK OFTALMOL* 18:339, 1962; and 19:397–402, 1963. (*ZENTRALBL GES OPHTHALMOL* 91:178, 1964.)

k. Laux U, Roth HW: Intensive irrigation of the eye in lime burns by means of a pulsating water stream. *KLIN MONATSBL AUGENHEILKD* 165:664–669, 1974. (German)

l. Oancea I, Vasinca M: The pH of the corneo-conjunctival surface in lime burns. *OFTALMOLOGIA (Buc)* 11:17–22, 1967.

m. Oksala A: Ethylenediaminetetraacetic acid in treatment of injuries of the eye by lime. *KLIN MONATSBL AUGENHEILKD* 125: 99–102, 1954. (German)

n. Pezzi PP, Grenge R: Subconjunctival autohemotherapy in corneo-conjunctival burns by lime. *BOLL OCULIST* 51:153–158, 1972. (Italian)

o. Praus R, Brettschneider I, Krejci L: Ethylenediamine tetraacetate: Its release from hydrophilic gel contact lenses, intraocular penetration and effect on calcium in the cornea after lime burns. *OPHTHALMIC RES* 8:161–168, 1976.

p. Puglisi-Duranti G, Luongo E: Local and general treatment of severe corneo-conjunctival burns by lime. *BOLL OCULIST* 44:461–475, 1965. (Italian)

q. Ricklefs G: Lime burns in children in the years 1948–1967. *BER DTSCH OPHTHALMOL GESELLSCH* 69:432–436, 1969. (German)

r. Ricklefs G, Gossmann K: Report on 250 lime burns from the years 1948–1967. *KLIN MONATSBL AUGENHEILKD* 153:59–67, 1968. (German)

s. Simkova M: Reaction of corneal nerves to chemical burns. *CESK OFTAL* 22:381–384, 1966. (Chem Abstr 65:20739, 1966.)

t. Teterwak J: Acid mucopolysaccharides in the cornea damaged by calcium hydroxide. *KLIN OCZNA* 39:543–548, 1969.

u. Uglova TG: Histochemical study of the distribution of calcium and lipids in corneal burns caused by calcium hydroxide. *Histochem Cytochim Lipides Simp Int Histol 5th Sofia* 1963, pp 517–519. (Chem Abstr 69:17720g, 1968.)

Calcium hypochlorite is usually a whitish, granular powder, having a strong odor of chlorine. Agitation of the powder creates a dust which is irritating to the nose and respiratory tract. At high concentrations the eyes are also irritated. Particles in contact with the eye cause local injury of the epithelium, but if promptly washed away cause no permanent damage.[81]

Experimental application of 5% aqueous solution of calcium hypochlorite, pH 11.5, to the eyes of rabbits for thirty seconds, followed by irrigation with water, caused superficial loss of epithelium from corneas and conjunctivas, but within a day the corneas healed and the conjunctivae were normal except for slight residual hyperemia.[81]

A single case has been reported in which calcium hypochlorite purportedly caused a fourth nerve palsy, but this can scarcely be considered a characteristic toxic effect of this chemical, since the palsy was believed to have resulted from hemorrhage in the nucleus of the fourth nerve, probably caused by elevation of blood pressure.[a] (See also *Hypochlorites.*)

a. Rehsteiner K: Fourth nerve paralysis from poisoning with chlorinated lime. *SCHWEIZ MED WOCHENSCHR* II:1128–1129, 1929. (German)

Calcium oxlate is a very insoluble inert solid having no injurious effect on contact with the eye.[81] It has been shown not to be irritating to rabbit eyes when applied as a

0.15% suspension.[a,81] Instances of injury of the eye by juices of certain plants have been incorrectly attributed to calcium oxalate, without adequate evidence. Irritation of the eye by plants of the genus *Dieffenbachia* are probably caused by a toxic protein, not by calcium oxalate. (See INDEX for *Dieffenbachia plants.*)

Calcium oxalate crystals in the retina, lens, and aqueous humor have been reported a number of times as products of degeneration in these tissues, but the calcium oxalate crystals have not given evidence of toxicity. Ascorbic acid has been one probable source of these crystals. (See INDEX for *Oxalosis.* Also see *Dibutyl Oxalate* and *Methoxyflurane* as other sources.)

    a. Manno JE, Fochtman FW, et al: Toxicitiy of plants of the genus Dieffenbachia. *TOXIC APPL PHARMACOL* 12:405, 1967.

Calcium oxide (quicklime) is a granular or lumpy solid which reacts with water, evolving heat and forming calcium hydroxide. Burns of the eye caused by particles of calcium oxide are severe and of the same nature as those caused by calcium hydroxide.

Calcium sulfate (plaster of paris) is nearly neutral and inert. Applied experimentally to rabbit eyes it has been found innocuous.[81] One report of four cases of severe injuries of the eye from contact with plaster of unspecified type attributes the injuries to calcium sulfate,[249] but this must be an error.

Intraocular penetration of particles of calcium sulfate is reported in one rare case in which a practice grenade made of plaster blasted fine particles through a man's cornea and was demonstrable as fine white granules on the posterior surface of the cornea and in the aqueous humor. They were chemically identified when paracentesis and irrigation of the anterior chamber were done. The eye returned to normal after surgical treatment.[a] It seems possible that these particles would have done no harm if left in the anterior chamber.

    a. Payrau P, Raynaud G: Lesions of the cornea from a blast: microscopic perforating foreign bodies; posterior velvety rings. *ANN OCULIST* 198:1057–1074, 1965. (French)

Calcium superphosphate (monobasic calcium phosphate) is a solid which partially hydrolyzes in water to form a strongly acidic solution. It has been alleged that certain cases of ocular irritation and corneal burns caused by contact with fertilizers were attributable either to free phosphoric acid or to phosphoric acid liberated from superphosphate in the fertilizer.[34,153,242] Particles of calcium superphosphate characteristically appeared to cause localized bluish-white corneal opacities which eventually cleared.[153]

Camphor administered medically in excessive doses of 0.06 to 4 g is said to have caused flickering, darkening, or veiling of vision accompanied noises in the ears, weakness, and sometimes convulsions. All visual effects have been transitory.[153]

An instance of industrial exposure to camphor vapors resulted in several cases of superficial keratitis with temporary loss of corneal epithelium, but formaldehyde and acetic acid were also present and may have contributed to the injuries.[a]

a. Matsuoka Y: Chemical injury of the cornea in a camphor factory. *ACTA SOC OPHTHALMOL JPN* 39: 1803–1809, 1935.

Cannabis (marihuana, Indian hemp, hashish) induces disturbances of vision which have always been transient, and presumably arise in the central nervous system, although in some cases functional disturbance of retina and optic nerve has been suggested. Most characteristic are visual hallucinations and abnormalities of color perception. It has often been said that with central excitation there is mydriasis and occasionally some impairment of accommodation for near.[153,214,247,255]

However, careful studies of the response of the pupils have shown that smoking marihuana either has no influence on the size of the pupil, or causes slight constriction.[a,b,d,g,h] It causes the conjunctival vessels to dilate, about maximum at fifteen minutes.[h]

There is little to be said regarding toxic effects on the eye, but much has been written concerning pharmacologic actions, studied mainly using the principal active constituents, the tetrahydrocannabinols. The principal ophthalmologic interest has been in the possibility of exploiting some constituents to reduce intraocular pressure in glaucoma. The problems in this application have so far not been one of toxicity, but of inefficacy.[b-g]

a. Brown B, Adams AJ, et al: Pupil size after use of marijuana and alcohol. *AM J OPHTHALMOL* 83:350–354, 1977.
b. Dawson WW: Cannabis and eye function. *INVEST OPHTHALMOL* 15:243–245, 1976.
c. Dawson WW, Jimenez-Antillon CF, et al: Marijuana and vision—after ten years' use in Costa Rica. *INVEST OPHTHALMOL VIS SCI* 16:689–699, 1977.
d. Green K: Marijuana and the eye. *INVEST OPHTHALMOL* 14:261–263, 1975.
e. Green K, Sobel RE, et al: Subchronic ocular and systemic toxicity of topically applied Δ9-tetrahydrocannabinol. *ANNALS OPHTHALMOL* 13:1219–1222, 1981.
f. Green K, Roth M: Ocular effects of topical administration of delta-9-tetrahydrocannabinol in man. *ARCH OPHTHALMOL* 100: 265–267, 1982.
g. Heppler RS, Frank IM, Ungerleider JT: Pupillary constriction after marijuana smoking. *AM J OPHTHALMOL* 74:1185–1190, 1972.
h. Weil AT, Zinberg NE, Nelson JM: Clinical and psychological effects of marihuana in man. *SCIENCE* 162:1234–1242, 1968.

Cantharides (Spanish fly, blistering beetle, *Cantharis vesicatoria*) contains an active principle, *cantharidin,* which is irritant and vesicant to the skin, and in contact with human or rabbit eyes causes conjunctivitis, keratitis, and iritis, with much edema of the lids.[a,c,150,153,252,253] Experimentally injected into the anterior chamber of rabbits, cantharides causes fibrinous exudate, hyperemia, accumulation of leukocytes, and extensive necrosis. The intraocular pressure is lowered, presumably because of injury of the ciliary body.[150]

Cantharone liquid is a preparation for treatment of warts, containing 0.7% *cantharidin* in a vehicle of acetone and collodion. It has been found safe to apply to warts on the skin of the lids up to the eyelashes, but would presumably be too irritating to apply to the inner side of the lid margin.[b] It has been tested by applying a small drop to the corneas of rabbits and did not give permanent stromal change visible with the slit-lamp.[b]

 a. Kowalewski R: Action of cantharides. *DTSCH MED WOCHENSCHR* 15:1908; and Ophthalmic Year Book, 5:285, 1908.
 b. Bock RH: Treatment of palpebral warts with cantharon. *AM J OPHTHALMOL* 60:529–530, 1965.
 c. Brinchmann Hansen O: Cantharides (Spanish fly). *NOR-TIDSSKR NORLAEGEFOREN* 98:1141–1143, 1157, 1978. (English summary)

Canthaxanthin (β,β-carotene-4,4'-dione; Food Orange 8; Orobronze; component of Bronzactive and Phenoro), an internationally accepted food color, is also taken orally to produce temporary yellow coloration of the skin, imitating sun-tan (but with particularly distinctive yellowing of the palms of the hands). Cortin and Corriveau discovered that this practice in some people could cause the appearance of many fine glistening yellow or gold particles in their retinas, mainly around the macula depression. These photographed well, and appeared to be in all layers of the retina, but predominantly in the superficial layers.[a] Some have been seen overlying retinal vessels.[d] This retinal condition was found in 6 out of 51 people who took canthaxanthin for skin coloring.[b] In a series of three publications (1982–1984) Cortin and colleagues described studies on 14 patients with this condition.[a,b,c] They found its occurrence was related to dose, and slightly to age. Extensive studies showed no visual functional impairment. Among the 14 patients, 2 or 3 might be considered glaucoma suspects, 3 had evidence of old retinal focal epitheliopathy, some had also taken β-carotene, but the majority had no special feature that might be considered a predisposing factor. (See INDEX for possible effect of β-carotene on the retina.)

 a. Cortin P, Corriveau LA, et al: Gold sequin maculopathy. *CAN J OPHTHALMOL* 17:103–106, 1982. (French)
 b. Boudreault G, Cortin P, et al: Canthaxanthin retinopathy. 1. Study of 51 consumers. *CAN J OPHTHALMOL* 18:325–328, 1983. (French)
 c. Cortin P, Boudreault G, et al: Canthaxanthin retinopathy. 2. Predisposing factors. *CAN J OPHTHALMOL* 19:215–219, 1984. (French)
 d. Saraux H, Laroche L: Gold sequin maculopathy after taking canthaxanthine. *BULL SOC OPHTALMOL FRANCE* 83:1273–1275, 1983. (French)

Capreomycin, an antibiotic, in prolonged administration to animals has appeared to cause injury of hearing and possibly development of cataracts in two out of twenty-four dogs, but not in cats.[a] There has apparently been no indication of cataractogenesis in human beings, though there have been occasional complaints from patients of transient flickering or temporary whiteness or black-outs of vision.[298,312]

 a. Wells JS, Harris PN, et al: The toxicity of capreomycin in laboratory animals. *ANN NY ACAD SCI* 135:960–973, 1966.

Capsaicin is a pungent irritant substance from *Capsicum* (Hungarian red pepper). On the eyes of rats 50 μg/ml has caused obvious pain and blepharospasm. The blood vessels of the conjunctivae and lids became abnormally permeable to Evans blue dye injected intravenously. Application of local anesthetic prevented pain, but did not alter the vascular reaction.[130]

This irritating effect on the eyes has been utilized in pressurized dog-repellent sprays which incorporate capsaicin. One boy accidentally had his eyes sprayed with this material. His eyes immediately smarted, teared, and became red, but were normal by the next day. Treatment had consisted only of irrigating with water, then mineral oil.[d]

Intravitreal injection of capsaicin in rabbits causes miosis and breakdown of the blood-aqueous barrier. This response can be blocked by pretreatment with tetrodotoxin or a "substance P" antagonist.[a]

Besides its obvious irritating effect, capsaicin has a second, remarkably different and seemingly paradoxical effect. When given systemically to rodents, it temporarily blocks their nociceptive sensory nerves, probably by depleting them of substance P.[b,c,e,f] The eyes of animals pre-treated in this manner do not react normally to painful chemical stimuli, such as topical nitrogen mustard, or intracameral formaldehyde or capsaicin. These eyes do not develop miosis, hyperemia of the iris, or elevation of intraocular pressure in the way the eyes of untreated animals do.

a. Bynke G, Hakanson R, Horig J: Ocular responses evoked by capsaicin and prostaglandin E₂ are inhibited by a substance P antagonist. *EXPERIENTIA* 39:996–998, 1983.

b. Bynke G: Capsaicin pretreatment prevents disruption of the bloodaqueous barrier in the rabbit eye. *INVEST OPHTHALMOL VIS SCI* 24:744–748, 1983.

c. Camras CB, Bito LZ: The pathophysiological effects of nitrogen mustard on the rabbit eye. *INVEST OPHTHALMOL Vis Sci* 19:423–428, 1980.

d. Drinker CK: Personal communication, 1975.

e. Szolcsanyi J, Jancso-Gabor A, Joo F: Functional and fine structural characteristics of the sensory neuron blocking effect of capsaicin. *NAUNYN-SCHMIEDEBERGS PHARMACOL* 287:157–169, 1975.

f. Tervo K: Effect of prolonged and neonatal capsaicin treatments on the substance P immunoreactive nerves in the rabbit eye and spinal cord. *ACTA OPHTHALMOL* 59:737–746, 1981.

Captopril (Capoten), an antihypertensive, is reported in one case to have produced severe necrotizing blepharitis as a first sign of agranulocytosis.[a]

a. Wizemann A: Necrotizing blepharitis following captopril-induced agranulocytosis. *KLIN MONATSBL AUGENHEILKD* 182:82–85, 1983. (German)

Carbachol (Carcholin, Miostat) is a cholinergic miotic drug used in eyedrops in treatment of glaucoma. Tests of 0.01% solution introduced into the anterior chamber of eyes of rabbits, cats, and human beings have shown no significant irritating or injurious action, but prompt miotic effect.[a,b,366] However, the manufacturer of Miostat has supplied a warning with the product that there has been occasional corneal edema after use of this preparation in the anterior chamber in patients.

a. Beasley H, Borgmann AR, et al: Carbachol in cataract surgery. *ARCH OPHTHALMOL* 80:39–41, 1968.

   b. Vaughn ED, Hull DS, Green K: Effect of intraocular miotics on corneal endothelium. *ARCH OPHTHALMOL* 96:1897–1901, 1978.

Carbamazepine (Tegretol), an anticonvulsant and analgesic, has occasionally affected eye movements, variously producing diplopia, difficulty in convergence, and oculogyric crises.[a,b,c,e,f] Large doses have caused temporary complete external ophthalmoplegia in one case,[d] and nystagmus with ataxia in others.[e,298,312]

   a. Henry EV: Oculogyric crisis and carbamazepine. *ARCH NEUROL* 37:326, 1980.
   b. Livingston S, Villamater C, et al: Use of carbamazepine in epilepsy. *J AM MED ASSOC* 200:204–208, 1967.
   c. Lorge M: Clinical experiences with a new anti-epileptic, Tegretol. *SCHWEIZ MED WOCHENSCHR* 93:1042–1047, 1963.
   d. Mullally WJ: Carbamazepine-induced ophthalmoplegia. *ARCH NEUROL* 39:64, 1982.
   e. Warot P, Arnott G, et al: Acute ataxia following massive ingestion of carbamazepine. *LILLE MED* 12: 601–604, 1967. (Excerpta Med (Sec IIC), 21:948, 1968.)
   f. Umeda Y: Transitory convergence disorders in Tegretol intoxication. *ACTA SOC OPHTHALMOL JPN* 80: 222, 1976. (English summary.)

Carbaryl (Sevin; Arylam; 1-naphthyl-N-methylcarbamate), a cholinesterase inhibitor insecticide, is rapidly hydrolyzed by warm-blooded animals, and appears to have caused no eye disturbance except in one case of suicidal poisoning in which disturbance of vision was complained of but not explained.[b] Atropine rather than cholinesterase reactivators is appropriate for treatment of poisoning by this substance.[a,b] Splash contact of an insecticide liquid containing both carbaryl and dimethoate in one patient on two different occasions caused transient injury of the corneal epithelium and much swelling of the lids, but recovery was rapid and complete. This suggests that carbaryl is not particularly dangerous to the eye.[c]

   However, in mice intraperitoneal carbaryl has produced disturbances in the ERG.[289]

   a. Best EM, Murray BL: Observations on workers exposed to Sevin insecticide. *J OCCUP MED* 4:507–517, 1962.
   b. Farago A: Fatal, suicidal case of Sevin (1-naphthyl-N-methyl-carbamate) poisoning. *ARCH TOXIKOL* 24:309–315, 1969.
   c. Haley W: Personal communication, 1968.

Carbarsone (N-carbamylarsanilic acid), an antiamebic, is closely related to drugs which have caused optic neuritis and atrophy, but carbarsone apparently has not caused this kind of toxic side effect.[171]

Carbenoxolone, a glucocorticoid, used to accelerate healing of gastric ulcers, appears prone to cause electrolyte disturbances, especially sodium retention. In one patient this was associated with rise of blood pressure, severe headache, left homonymous hemianopia, bizarre visual hallucinations, all of which disappeared within 48 hours when the drug was stopped, and were interpreted as hemiplegic migraine precipitated by carbenoxolone.[a] Another patient had rise of blood pressure, severe headache, and decrease in vision associated with papilledema and retinal hemorrhages, attributed to hypertensive retinopathy from this drug.[a]

a. Davies GJ, Rhodes J, Calcraft BJ: Complications of carbenoxolone therapy. *BR MED J* 2:400–402, 1974.

Carbon, when pure, has no toxic effect. As superficial foreign bodies, *carbon black* and *graphite* may be slightly irritating mechanically and may cause discoloration of lids and conjunctivae, but they are chemically inert.[215] However, graphite-containing pencil lead fragments buried in the conjunctiva may cause low-grade granulomatous reaction for many years.[d] *Soot* and *charcoal,* contain irritating chemicals in addition to carbon. *Soot* is said on chronic exposure to cause corneal epithelial hyperplasia and eczematous inflammation of the lids.[215] Experimental intravenous injection of pure carbon suspensions in rabbits produces no ocular inflammation, although carbon particles are deposited within the blood vessels.[a,141,176] Small quantities of carbon suspensions in the form of *graphite* or *India ink* injected into the anterior chamber of rabbits is mostly taken up by leukocytes and by the corneal endothelium, producing essentially no signs of inflammation.[150] Large quantities may obstruct aqueous outflow mechanically.[81] *India ink* injected into the posterior chamber is taken up by ciliary epithelial cells, inciting swelling and proliferation of the non-pigmented epithelium, and increase in lysosomal enzyme activity.[c]

Intravitreal injection of a colloidal suspension of 20-nm carbon particles in rabbits has induced macrophages and glial cells, in particular Muller cells, to penetrate the internal limiting membrane to remove the foreign carbon particles, producing epiretinal membranes, and causing retinal detachments in some animals.[a]

Carbon black used as a pigment in eye cosmetics, particularly liquid eye liners and mascara, has produced black pigmentation of the palpebral conjunctiva at the upper tarsal border after regular application to the lid margins for at least two years. The conjunctiva of the lower lid is less involved. Although there is lymphocytic infiltration and the pigment is taken up by macrophages, the deposits cause essentially no symptoms. (See also *Eye cosmetics.*)

Charcoal may be slightly more irritating than purer forms of carbon in the eye. Explosions of gas generators in which charcoal was undergoing combustion in the presence of steam has blasted particles into the skin of the face and lids, where they produce a peculiar discoloration. When some of these fine particles have been embedded in the cornea and conjunctiva, there has been inflammation of the anterior segment lasting two to three weeks while some of the particles were sloughed. Particles that have remained as long as two months usually have been retained permanently without further inflammation, causing only punctate purplish-black discoloration.[b]

a. Algvere P, Kock E: Experimental epiretinal membranes induced by intravitreal carbon particles. *AM J OPHTHALMOL* 96:345–353, 1983.
b. Kinnas JS: Corneal and conjunctival xylanthracosis caused by carbon-gas from generators. *BR J OPHTHALMOL* 51:622–626, 1967.
c. Mizuno K, Hayasaka S: Changes of lysosomal enzymes in the ciliary epithelium by foreign bodies. *EXP EYE RES* 31:691–698, 1980.

  d. Offret H, Saraux H, et al: Orbital foreign body of "graphite". *J FR OPHTALMOL*
     1:615–616, 1978. (French)
  e. Persichetti C: Experimental studies on the behavior of the eye in the presence of
     intravenous injections of animal carbon. *BOLL OCULIST* 18:373–389, 1939. (Italian)

Carbon dioxide is an odorless gas, forming a very weak acid, carbonic acid, in water
solution. This has no caustic effect. Carbon dioxide at high concentration in air
causes a stinging sensation in the eyes, nose, and throat. Carbonated beverages, such
as beer, if splashed in the eye, cause a very brief stinging sensation and momentary
local vasodilation, but no injury. Carbon dioxide gas injected into rabbit eyes is
absorbed within an hour, also without injuring the eye.[81,345]

Dry ice, the solid, low temperature form of carbon dioxide, contacting the eye
externally in the form of fine particles was decided in 1967 in a medicolegal case in
Germany not likely to be responsible for serious adverse effect.[c]

Asphyxiation with carbon dioxide is said to have induced temporary proptosis
and mydriasis in very rare instances, also to have caused yellow vision, with transient blindness in one case.[129,153] Severe damage of the CNS and retinal ganglion
cells has been reported.[b]

Detailed case reports have been made of two men who suddenly became unconscious in a well, presumably from excessive carbon dioxide, one being exposed for
five minutes, and the other for only one minute. Repeated eye examinations were
made in the course of two years beginning six weeks after the exposures. Constriction of visual fields, enlargement of blindspots, photophobia, loss of convergence
and accommodation, deficient dark adaptation, headache, insomnia, and personality changes were observed.[a] A supposition that some of these persistent abnormalities were due to damage to retinal ganglion cells and central nervous system was
supported by histologic examinations of another patient who was thought to have
been exposed to a high concentration of carbon dioxide for ten minutes and had
remained in profound coma in a decerebrate state, apparently blind, and died in
eleven months. The retinas showed atrophy and gliosis with loss of all ganglion
cells.[b]

Intraocular pressure is raised briefly and slightly in human eyes by inhalation of
10% carbon dioxide.[193]

  a. Freedman A, Sevel D: The cerebro-ocular effects of carbon dioxide poisoning. *ARCH
     OPHTHALMOL* 76:59–65, 1966.

Carbon disulfide (carbon bisulfide) is a highly volatile liquid. Poisoning from the
vapor has occurred particularly in the rubber and rayon industries. Acute exposure
to high concentrations produces inebriation and unconsciousness, but very rarely
has any persistent abnormality followed a single acute exposure.[194] Chronic exposure during several months caused a type of poisoning which was common and well
recognized in the mid-nineteenth century, but had already become less common by
the beginning of the twentieth century, owing presumably to improved industrial
hygiene.[153,247] Concentrations of 160 to 800 ppm were known to have caused poisoning in the course of a few months.[176] No significant evidence of disturbance of the
eyes during a similar period was found in industries where the concentrations of

carbon disulfide in the air was kept below 30 ppm.[a,s] By 1980 the official Threshold Limit Value for carbon disulfide had been reduced to 20 ppm in the United States and Great Britain, and to 10 ppm in Finnland.

The extensive older literature which accumulated on the subject indicated that chronic poisoning affected different portions of the nervous system at the same time, inducing quite varied signs and symptoms, both peripheral and central. Peripheral sensory neuritis with paresthesias and pain, mostly in the legs, was common.[194] Peripheral tendon reflexes were impaired, and the legs were sometimes weak, but typically carbon disulfide did not cause gross muscle palsies or ataxia. An effect on the brain was manifested by excitement, insomnia, and psychic disturbance.[194]

One of the most characteristic consequences of severe chronic poisoning 40 or 50 years ago was a disturbance of vision suggestive of retrobulbar neuritis, characterized by central scotoma, decreased visual acuity, impaired recognition of red and green, but rarely, complete permanent blindness.[m,zc,zd,153,247] Pallor of the temporal portion of the optic nerveheads corresponding to the papillomacula nerve fibers was occasioinally observed, and, exceptionally, more extensive atrophy of the optic nerve.[153,247] Teleky in his book on toxicology provided a partial review of case reports of retrobulbar neuritis attributed to carbon disulfide.[239] Xanthopsia and slight constriction of the fields have also been observed in accompaniment with central scotoma.[r,33] Reaction of the pupils to light and accommodation was poor in some cases, but this could have been secondary to impaired visual acuity. Nystagmus and diplopia have also been observed,[153] but cranial nerves other than the optic nerve have rarely been affected.[24]

Some thirty to forty years ago there were several surveys of workers in industries where moderate concentrations of carbon disulfide existed. The results of these surveys have not given a uniform picture. Vigliani found polyneuritis of the lower extremities far more common than retrobulbar neuritis.[zc] Surveys by Lewey and by McDonald indicated that the corneal reflex was most commonly depressed and that enlargement of the blindspot and nystagmus were particularly common.[j,l] Teleky believed from firsthand experience that reduction of the corneal reflex was the first sign of toxic action in workers exposed industrially to carbon disulfide vapor.[239]

Although retrobulbar neuritis from carbon disulfide has become rare in recent decades, Savic reports that the pupillary reaction to light has frequently been disturbed.[t] Vervelskaya has observed that dark adaptation is commonly abnormal after several years of industrial exposure to carbon disulfide and that this may be a diagnostic indicator of chronic poisoning.[zb]

Surveys of large numbers of people exposed industrially to carbon disulfide in the 1960's and 1970's, mainly in artificial silk factories, put much emphasis on examination of the retinal arteries and on measurement of the pressure in them by ophthalmodynamometry.[k,t,za,zb] After careful study, Savic has reported that, despite exposure of workers to unusually high concentrations of carbon disulfide for several years, the pressure in the central retinal arteries has not been significantly affected.[t]

In a book devoted to toxicology of carbon disulfide published in 1967, edited by Brieger and Teisinger,[b] several chapters by various authors have included observations on ocular effects. Nesswetha reviewed the records of thirty-three patients in Germany who had been certified officially as having carbon disulfide poisoning, and found that only two had optic neuritis, while fifteen had polyneuritis.[n] Hotta and colleagues reporting on examination of 757 workers in Japanese viscose rayon plants indicated that small round retinal hemorrhages were found in sixty who had been exposed for more than five years, with the incidence greatest after ten to twenty-five years. Retinal microaneurysms were found in 135 out of 241 workers exposed for many years.[f,g]

The finding of microaneurysms and dot hemorrhages in the fundi of workers in Japan stimulated a series of investigations in other countries, and led to international collaborative studies.[d,o,p,v,x,y,z] These have confirmed that in Japan and Yugoslavia these vascular retinopathies occur in similar manner and frequency increasing with both duration and intensity of exposure to carbon disulfide, but in Finnland these changes have not occurred, for reasons unknown.[p,y,z]

The retinal microaneurysms by fluorescein angiography appeared different from those of diabetes, more like senile changes.[i] There has been no neovascularization as in diabetes, but there have been suspicions of associated slight abnormalities of carbohydrate metabolism. There is also concern that systemic vasculopathy may accompany the retinal vasculopathy. Effects on vision, if any, have been slight.[q]

Experimental studies in animals have as yet shed little light on the mechanism of poisoning. Acute poisoning of rabbits and mice has been reported to cause degenerative changes in the ganglion cells of the retina and in the optic nerve, also an immediate drop in the b-potential of the electroretinogram.[c,w] Mice deficient in thiamine showed damage of the optic nerve earlier than did those on normal diet.[h]

In rabbits daily intramuscular administration of carbon disulfide during three weeks by Hockwin and Savic produced no ocular abnormalities detectable by ophthalmoscope or slit-lamp biomicroscope, but did reduce the ATP content of the retina and modified the activities of enzymes in the lenses.[e,u] No clinical evidence of injury of the lens has been reported.

Exposures of white rats for ten to sixty minutes a day for forty-eight days to concentrations between 1,500 and 5,000 mg/cu m of air have failed to produce histologically detectable lesions in the retina or optic nerves.[t]

a. Barthelemy HL: Ten years experience with industrial hygiene in connection with the manufacture of viscose rayon. *J IND HYG* 21:141, 1939.

b. Brieger H, Teisinger J, (Eds.): Toxicology of Carbon Disulphide. Amsterdam, Excerpta Med. Foundation, 1967.

c. Caffi M, Bettaglio M, Pasotti C: Contribution to knowledge of experimental carbon disulfide poisoning. *RASS ITAL OTTALMOL* 31:49–60, 1966. (Italian)

d. Goto S, Sugimoto K, et al: Retinal microaneurysms in carbon disulfide workers in Yugoslavia. *PRAC LEK* 24:66–70, 1972.

e. Hockwin O, Savic S: On the reversibility of biochemical changes in the lens and retina of rabbit eyes caused by carbon disulfide poisoning. *GRAEFES ARCH OPHTHALMOL* 175:7–12, 1968. (German)

f. Hotta R, Goto S: A fluorescein angiographic study on microangiopathia sulfocarbonica. *ACTA SOC OPHTHALMOL JPN* 74:1463–1467, 1970.

g. Hotta R, Sugimoto K, Goto S: Retinopathia sulfocarbonica and its natural history. *ACTA SOC OPHTHALMOL JPN* 76:1561–1566, 1972.

h. Ide T: Histopathological studies on retina, optic nerve and arachnoidal membrane of mouse exposed to carbon disulfide poisoning. *ACTA SOC OPHTHALMOL JPN* 62A:85–108, 1958.

i. Karai I, Sugimoto K, Goto S: A case comparison study of carbon disulfide retinopathy and diabetic retinopathy using fluorescein fundus angiography. *ACTA OPHTHALMOL* 61:1074–1086, 1983.

j. Lewey FH: Survey of carbon disulfide and hydrogen sulfide hazards in the viscose rayon industry. Bull 46, Pennsylvanis Dept. Labor and Industry, 1938.

k. Maugeri U, Cavalleri A, Visconti E: Ophthalmodynamography in work-related carbon disulfide poisoning. *MED LAV* 57:739–740, 1966. (Italian)

l. McDonald R: Carbon disulfide poisoning. *ARCH OPHTHALMOL* 20:839–845, 1938.

m. Nectoux R, Gallois RA: Four cases of retrobulbar neuritis from carbon disulfide. *BULL SOC OPHTALMOL PARIS* 9:750–756, 1931. (French)

n. Nesswetha L, Nesswetha W: The clinical evaluation of compensated carbon disulphide intoxications in the German Federal Republic since 1948. Pages 214–216 in Brieger and Teisinger.[b]

o. Raitta C, Tolonen M, Nureminen M: Microcirculation of ocular fundus in viscose rayon workers exposed to carbon disulfide. *GRAEFES ARCH OPHTHALMOL* 191:151–164, 1974.

p. Raitta C, Tolonen M: Microcirculation of the eye in workers exposed to carbon disulfide. Pages 73–86 in Merigan and Weiss (1980).[358]

q. Raitta C, Teir H, et al: Impaired color discrimination among viscose rayon workers exposed to carbon disulfide. *J OCCUP MED* 23:189–192, 1981.

r. Roger H, Roger J: Carbon disulfide poisoning. *ANN MED PSYCHOL* 1:1–17, 1950. (French)

s. Rubin HH, Arieff AJ: Carbon disulfide and hydrogen sulfide; clinical study of chronic low grade exposures. *J IND HYG* 27:123–129, 1945.

t. Savic SM: Influence of carbon disulfide on the eye. *ARCH ENVIRON HEALTH* 14:325–326, 1967.

u. Savic S, Hockwin O: Biochemical changes in the rabbit eye in poisoning with organic solvents. *OPHTHALMOLOGICA ADDIT AD* 158:359–363, 1969. (German)

v. Savic S: Ophthalmologic and angiographic findings in workers who have been exposed to carbon disulfide. *KLIN MONATSBL AUGENHEILKD* 180:90–91, 1982. (German)

w. Seto Y: Experimental studies on the influences of carbon disulfide on the electro-retinogram. *ACTA SOC OPHTHALMOL JPN* 62B:951–961, 1958.

x. Sugimoto K, Goto S, Hotta R: Studies on chronic carbon disulfide poisoning; a 5 year follow up study on retinopathy. *INT ARCH OCCUP ENVIRON HEALTH* 37:233–248, 1976.

y. Sugimoto K, Taniguchi H, et al: Ocular fundus photography of workers exposed to carbon disulfide. *INT ARCH OCCUP ENVIRON HEALTH* 39:97–101, 1977.

z. Sugimoto K, Goto S: Retinopathy in chronic carbon disulfide exposure. Pages 55–71 in Merigan and Weiss (1980).[358]

za. Szymankowa G: Observations on the influence of CS_2 on the visual system in workers of a synthetic fiber plant. *KLIN OCZNA* 38:41–44, 1968.

zb. Vervelskaya VM: The importance of adaptometry in the early diagnosis of chronic carbon disulfide poisoning. *VESTN OFTALMOL* 80:59–61, 1967.

zc. Vigliani EC: Clinical observations on carbon disulfide intoxication in Italy. *IND MED SURG* 19:240–242, 1950.

zd. Von Krudener H: On blinding by Atoxyl, methanol, carbon disulfide and Filix mas. *Z AUGENHEILKD* 16:47–53, 1906. (German)

Carbon monoxide is a colorless, odorless, nonirritating gas, a product of incomplete combustion. Carbon monoxide may cause severe neurologic disturbances, and has caused many deaths. However, disturbances which occur in individuals who remain conscious appear to be entirely transient and functional. In these cases, when the carbon monoxide is removed from the blood stream, abnormal signs and symptoms disappear. However, when exposure to carbon monoxide is severe enough to produce unconsciousness, permanent damage to the central nervous system may result, varying in severity in proportion to the duration and depth of coma. Clinically and experimentally, general brain edema and increased intracranial pressure with extensive damage of brain tissue have frequently been observed. Disturbances of the eyes and vision from carbon monoxide have several times been well reviewed.[153,214,247,255]

Carbon monoxide at levels encountered in tobacco smoke has been suspected to impair night-time vision.[p] (See INDEX for *Tobacco smoking.*) In rats, chronic prenatal exposure to similar concentrations has been shown to affect visual evoked cortical potentials.[h]

Mild transient ocular disturbances may be produced by chronic exposure to low concentrations of carbon monoxide such as induce headache, general depression or nausea without unconsciousness. A number of well documented cases of subacute poisoning, mostly from malfunctioning gas heaters, have been reported in which the principal abnormal physical findings have been discovered by ophthalmoscopy. Retinopathy has been observed in these cases, consisting of flame-shaped hemorrhages in the nerve fiber layer of the retina, and sometimes cotton-wool exudates, with a tendency to tortuosity of the veins, but with normal or mildly edematous optic discs, and normal visual acuity and fields.[d,f,u,w,y,zf,153,247] In such cases exposures to carbon monoxide typically have been of at least 12 hours duration, but in some cases have been intermittent for weeks at concentrations inducing flulike symptoms, but too low to produce coma. However, the same findings can occur in patients who have had a period of coma. As a rule the retinopathy has gradually cleared after exposure to carbon monoxide has been stopped. Ferguson et al (1985) reported an exceptionally severe case.[zk]

Severe visual disturbances occur as a consequence of acute poisoning in which there has been a period of unconsciousness. When a patient slowly recovers following a period of coma lasting from 30 minutes to several days, it may be discovered at once that he is blind, but in a considerable number of instances, when consciousness was first regained, it seemed that vision was normal, only to have it become markedly diminished during the next few days. The size and reactivity of the pupils furnish significant information on the neurologic level of the visual disturbances which may remain after consciousness is regained. During coma the size of the pupils is not characteristically abnormal, but the pupils do not react to light. After recovery from coma in the majority of cases of residual loss of vision the pupils have regained reactivity to light despite subjective blindness, indicating that the residual neurologic disturbance is at a level higher than the lateral geniculate bodies, and may well be cortical.

The types of visual disturbance which have been reported may be grouped symptomatically as follows: (a) amaurosis or hemianopsia, (b) constriction of visual fields, and (c) visual abnormalities associated with optic nerve disturbances.

In the group in which amaurosis is cortical in origin, the pupillary response to light is preserved despite complete inability to perceive light.[b,i,k,o,q] In these cases partial recovery of vision is usual, and complete recovery may take place in a few hours, days, or weeks. The course of recovery and the nature of the residua, sometimes including impairment of mentality,[b,j,zg,q] attest to the high level of the neurologic disturbance. Visual hallucinations,[e] and visual agnosia,[u] have been noted. In a few cases homonymous hemianopsia has been observed.[k,l,v,153] In company with hemianopsia, the central vision has been good in some cases and poor in others. Visual failure of probable cortical origin has been particularly well illustrated in one report of three cases by Garland and Pearce (1967).[m]

One patient was totally blind after recovering from coma, but had normal reactive pupils and normal fundi; vision became normal in seventeen days. The second patient was essentially blind at first, but gradually recovered normal vision in four weeks. The third patient had gradual return of vision to normal after seeing only hand movements.

A fourth case, described by Duncan and Gumpert (1983), illustrates recurrent episodes of cortical blindness, possibly associated with preexisting critical cerebral blood supply, and apparent benefit from treatment with dopamine to increase cerebral blood flow.[g] In this case a young man with a history of childhood migraine and transitory blindness had decrease in vision to light perception immediately after 10 minutes of coma from carbon monoxide, then, after oxygen treatment, return of vision to normal within 20 hours, but a recurrence of severe visual impairment several days later. After treatment with dopamine, infused intravenously to raise the blood pressure, vision and EEG gradually returned to normal, and remained normal when the treatment was discontinued.

Visual agnosia has been particularly notable in association with the cortical blindness in some cases, and in one young man many months after acute carbon monoxide poisoning profound visual form agnosia was the main residual problem.[c]

Permanent homonymous hemianopsia after acute carbon monoxide poisoning and coma in an elderly patient has been associated with subnormal carotid artery circulation on the affected side, suggesting that asymmetry of blood supply may be a factor in determining the relative vulnerability of the two sides of the brain.[zi]

Constriction of the visual fields after acute exposure and coma has been described in rare instances.[a,j,za,153] The fundi have been normal in each case. In two instances, the fields gradually enlarged, and in one instance persistent constriction was demonstrable principally by means of colored test objects. In one case complete recovery occurred despite initial nearly complete blindness.[a] On the contrary, in the case of a man who had been in coma, the visual fields became increasingly constricted during four weeks following the exposure, and this was associated with development of color blindness and eventually amaurosis.[za] The site of the disturbance in these rare cases of constriction of the visual fields has not been established.

Optic neuritis has been diagnosed several times in patients with various visual disturbances following exposure to carbon monoxide, but in most instances, the evidence to implicate carbon monoxide has not been conclusive. In some cases, involvement of the optic nerve has been inferred from absence of pupillary response to light, although no abnormalities were seen in the fundus.

The occurrence of optic nerve disturbances in carbon monoxide poisoning seems best substantiated in the following case. A man who had been in coma for four to five days following inhalation of carbon monoxide was completely blind without abnormality of the fundus on regaining consciousness, but a year later when a small amount of vision had returned, had bilateral optic atrophy and signs of former juxtapapillary hemorrhages.[w]

In other instances in which the diagnosis of optic neuritis has been made, the relationship to carbon monoxide poisoning has been more indefinite. Thus, in one case, bilateral marked reduction of vision, binasal hemianopsia, and papilledema, which went on to optic atrophy, came on thirteen days after probable exposure for four hours to fumes from dynamite blasting.[x] This patient had nausea and headache the day following exposure, but no illness at the time of exposure, nor any period of unconsciousness. In another case, optic neuritis with contraction of visual fields and paracentral scotomas was presumed to be due to chronic carbon monoxide poisoning in a young child, on the grounds that he and other members of his household had suffered hallucinations which were attributed to fumes escaping from a coal furnace.[zh] In a third doubtful case, a bilateral optic atrophy was attributed to fumes from a gasoline blowtorch, although the patient also had abnormal peripheral tendon reflexes and increased cells and protein in the spinal fluid, but had had no period of unconsciousness.[zh]

Examination of the optic nerves in mice by electron microscopy has shown the myelin sheaths to be scarcely affected by carbon monoxide poisoning, but some degenerative changes have been found in astrocytes.[z] Changes in the ERG of cats have suggested a direct toxic effect of carbon monoxide on the retina.[zl]

Electrical signals from the visual cortex in rats and cats evoked by flashes of light have been utilized as a means for studying the influence of carbon monoxide on function of the visual pathways and central nervous system.[h,zj] In cats the cortical potentials were reduced when potentials at lower levels were still normal. Histologically degeneration was found mainly in the optic radiation fibers.[s] Visually evoked EEG responses are also affected in man.[ze,r]

Local external effects of carbon monoxide gas on the eyes are essentially nil. One case of very severe uveitis and dermatitis resembling herpes zoster purportedly was a direct toxic effect of the gas, but this is extremely unlikely.[zc] Experimental injection of a large bubble of carbon monoxide into the anterior chamber of the eyes of rabbits has caused no injury or inflammatory reaction, and the bubble was absorbed within two days without aftereffect.[81]

In carbon monoxide poisoning, no special treatment is indicated for eye involvement other than discontinuance of exposure, and treatment that is directed at the systemic poisoning. Generally this treatment consists of administration of 100% oxygen. In special cases with neurologic sequelae, such as described by Duncan and Gumpert, dopamine infusion may be indicated.[g]

a. Abelsdorff G: Transitory blindness with eye muscle paresis after carbon monoxide poisoning. *DTSCH MED WOCHENSCHR* 46:210, 1920. (German)

b. Abt I, Witt DB: Cortical blindness and mental deterioration in a child due to carbon monoxide. *MED CLIN N AM* 5:1645, 1922.

c. Benson DF, Greenberg JP: Visual-form agnosia. *ARCH NEUROL* 20:82–89, 1969.

d. Bilchik RC, Muller-Bergh HA, Freshman ME: Ischemic retinopathy due to carbon monoxide poisoning. *ARCH OPHTHALMOL* 86:142–144, 1971.

e. Caussade G: 2 cases of severe carbon monoxide poisoning. *BULL SOC MED HOP PARIS* 50:503–507, 1934. (French)

f. Dempsey LC, O'Donnell JJ, Hoff JT: Carbon monoxide retinopathy. *AM J OPHTHALMOL* 82:692–693, 1976.

g. Duncan JS, Gumpert J: A case of blindness following carbon monoxide poisoning, treated with dopamine. *J NEUROL NEUROSURG PYSCHIATRY* 46:459–460, 1983.

h. Dyer RS: Effects of prenatal and postnatal exposure to carbon monoxide on visually evoked responses in rats. Pages 17–34 in Merigan and Weiss (1980).[358]

i. Fejer J: A case of bilateral blindness ending in recovery after breathing wood charcoal gas. *WIEN KLIN WOCHENSCHR* 87:216–217, 1924. (German)

j. Fink AI: Carbon monoxide asphyxia with visual sequelae. *AM J OPHTHALMOL* 34:1024–1027, 1951.

k. Francois J: Homonymous hemianopia in acute carbon monoxide poisoning. *OPHTHALMOLOGICA* 103:143–149, 1942. (French)

l. Friedenwald H: Hemiopia following poisoning by illuminating gas, with report of a case. *ARCH OPHTHALMOL* 29:294–296, 1900.

m. Garland H, Pearce J: Neurological complications of carbon monoxide poisoning. *QUART J MED* 36:445–455, 1967.

n. Grace TW, Platt FW: Subacute carbon monoxide poisoning. *J AM MED ASSOC* 246:1698–1700, 1981.

o. Grimsdale H: A case of gas-poisoning with unusual ophthalmological complications. *BR J OPHTHALMOL* 18:443–446, 1934.

p. Halperin MH, McFarland RA, et al: The time course of the effects of carbon monoxide on visual thresholds. *J PHYSIOL* 146:583–593, 1959.

q. Helminen T: Amaurosis in CO poisoning. *ACTA OPHTHALMOL* 25:328–329, 1947.

r. Hosko MJ: Effect of carbon monoxide on the visual evoked response in man, and the spontaneous electro-encephalogram. *ARCH ENVIRON HEALTH* 21:174–180, 1970.

s. Ikeda T: Experimental carbon monoxide poisoning: its electrophysiological effects on the visual pathway in cats. *FOLIA PSYCHIATR NEUROL* 23:135–142, 1969. (Chem Abstr 72:41126, 1970.)

t. Ingenito AH, Durlacher L: Effects of carbon monoxide on the b-wave of the cat electroretinogram. *J PHARMACOL EXP THER* 211:638–646, 1979.

u. Kelley JS, Sophocleus GJ: Retinal hemorrhages in subacute carbon monoxide poisoning. *J AM MED ASSOC* 239:1515–1517, 1978.

v. Kozlowski B: A case of disturbance of vision induced by combustion gas. *KLIN OCZNA* 16:176–182, 1938.

w. Levy-Valensi LC, Rochard A: A case of amaurosis from carbon monoxide poisoning; juxtapapillary hemorrhages. *BULL SOC MED HOP PARIS* 40:349–351; 470–472, 1924. (French)

x. Lindemann K: Report of a case of blindness from breathing products of combustion from dynamite blasting in an excavation operation. *Z AUGENHEILKD* 61:72–79, 1927. (German)

y. Murray WR: Amblyopia caused by inhalation of carbon monoxide gas. *MINNESOTA MED* 9:561–564, 1926.

z. Ohara M: The electron microscopic studies on the optic nerves of mice poisoned with carbon monoxide gas or potassium cyanide solution. *FOLIA OPHTHALMOL JPN* 19:99–123, 1968.

za. Rathery F, Gournay J: Amaurosis in a person poisoned probably by carbon monoxide. *BULL SOC MED PARIS* 40: 359–360, 1924. (French)

zb. Reynolds NC, Shapiro I: Retrobulbar neuritis with neuroretinal edema as a delayed manifestation of carbon monoxide poisoning. *MIL MED* 144:472–473, 1979.

zc. Scheuermann: Rare case of burning of the eye by carbon monoxide gas. *KLIN MONATSBL AUGENHEILKD* 88:242–243, 1932. (German)

zd. Stengel E: Peculiar visual disturbance after illuminating gas poisoning. *ZENTRALBL NEUR* 122:597–605, 1929. (German)

ze. Stewart RD, et al: Experimental human exposure to carbon monoxide. *ARCH ENVIRON HEALTH* 21:154–164, 1970.

zf. Trese MT, Krohel GB, Hepler RS: Ocular effects of chronic carbon monoxide exposure. *ANNALS OPHTHALMOL* 12:536–538, 1980.

zg. Wechsler I: Partial cortical blindness with preservation of color vision. *ARCH OPHTHALMOL* 9:957–965, 1933.

zh. Wilmer WH: Effects of carbon monoxide on the eye. *AM J OPHTHALMOL* 4:73–90, 1921.

zi. Woillez M, Blervacque A, Bisiaux-Aufort: Ophthalmologic changes in the course of carbon monoxide gassings. *BULL SOC OPHTALMOL FRANC* 64:575–580, 1964. (French)

zj. Xintaras C, Johnson BL: Application of the evoked response technique in air pollution toxicology. *TOXICOL APPL PHARMACOL* 8:77–87, 1966.

zk. Ferguson LS, Burke MJ, Choromokos EA: Carbon monoxide retinopathy. *ARCH OPHTHALMOL* 103:66–67, 1985.

Carbon tetrachloride is a volatile solvent of characteristic unpleasant odor. The vapor is slightly irritating to the eyes. The vapor or liquid may cause serious and even fatal poisoning. It has been repeatedly stated that carbon tetrachloride may affect vision by causing optic neuritis and optic atrophy, and that constriction of the visual fields is an early sign of poisoning. The evidence on which these statements are based deserves critical examination.

Attention was first called to visual effects by Wirtschafter in 1933 when three out of a group of five dry cleaners who were ill from absorbing carbon tetrachloride complained of blurred vision or spots before the eyes. The reported examinations of these patients were rather incomplete. Ophthalmoscopic examinations were essentially negative. No measurements of visual acuity were reported. Principal attention was given to perimetry and stereocampimetry using a small (1.5°) test object. All five patients were said to have had bilateral peripheral constriction of the color fields, but no central scotoma. No quantitative data were provided. All returned to normal in five weeks after cessation of exposure.[j]

A more-or-less supporting study by Smyth (1936) was carried out under factory conditions with a portable perimeter, and ten out of ninety-three men working in the presence of 40 to 117 ppm vapor in air were reported to have a restriction of field of 30° or more, toward the bottom and outer edge, with no apparent relationship between the degree of exposure and the degree of visual field abnormality.[h] Subsequently, Stewart and Witts (1944) performed a detailed examination of factory workers exposed chronically to dangerous concentrations of carbon tetrachloride and found no significant evidence of toxic amblyopia or restriction of visual field.[i]

Moeller (1973) reported a detailed eye and vision examination on 82 unexposed people and 62 workers exposed chronically to 40–60 mg/cubic meter of air for 1 to 3 hours a day, along with gross skin contact, and could not find the high percentage of pathologic fields that had been reported by Smyth, but did find occasional abnormality of the outer limits of visual fields to colored or white test objects, and could not rule out the possibility of some effect on vision from chronic exposure.[f]

In evaluating the reports from the 1930's one must be aware of the skill, experience, and time required to obtain reliable measurements of visual fields. Considering the conditions under which the constrictions reported by Smyth were measured, there must be some doubt concerning their validity. In fact, Smyth and co-workers were careful to indicate that their evaluations of visual fields were only tentative, subject to later correction.[h]

Reduction of central visual acuity following inhalation of carbon tetrachloride has been suggested by Gocher who reported a disturbance of vision lasting ten days in one case, and permanent reduction of vision in another case, but reported no details of ocular examination.[b] Similarly, Gray reported one case of a man who had temporary blurring of vision after chronic exposure to carbon tetrachloride.[c] Henggeler had recorded temporary impairment of vision along with complete deafness in a man apparently severely poisoned with carbon tetrachloride.[d] Smith described three cases in which people who had been exposed to carbon tetrachloride had disturbances of vision.[g] In none of Smith's cases was there evidence of liver or kidney damage, but one patient did suffer from headaches, weakness, nausea, etc. Two of the patients were diagnosed as having bilateral optic neuritis with permanent impairment of vision; the third was diagnosed as having retrobulbar neuritis, and this one recovered completely.

Teleky in his book on toxicology reported having seen a man who had worked exposed to carbon tetrachloride vapors for five months, noticing impairment of vision, first in one eye then the other. At that time an ophthalmologist was said to have found irregular constriction of the visual fields and optic atrophy, which subsequently did not improve.[239]

Lyle and Zavon have described a man who ultimately had vision correctable to 20/25 and 20/35 two years after his vision had been reduced to counting fingers at a few feet because of central scotomas, accompanied by paresis of the sixth nerves and nystagmus of the abducted eye. Suspicion of a toxic cause was based on a history of having been exposed two times per year during twenty-three years in fumigating with vapors consisting mainly of carbon tetrachloride (concentration in the air not greater than 2.3 ppm), plus smaller concentrations of ethylene dichloride and ethylene dibromide (not greater than 0.35 ppm).[e]

Carbon tetrachloride also was present in a mixture of solvents which caused severe intoxication and retrobulbar neuritis in a case reported by Franceschetti and Rickli.[a]

From the available clinical evidence, carbon tetrachloride does appear strongly suspect of causing retrobulbar neuritis, optic neuritis, and optic atrophy, but constriction of visual fields as an early sign of poisoning is not securely established.

Experimentally no convincing demonstration of injury to retina or optic nerve has been made.

a. Franceschetti A, Rickli JH: Retrobulbar neuritis after acute poisoning by chlorinated hydrocarbons. *OPHTHALMOLOGICA* 123:255–260, 1952.
b. Gocher TEP: Carbon tetrachloride poisoning. *NORTHWEST MED* 43:228, 1944.
c. Gray I: Carbon tetrachloride poisoning; report of 7 cases with 2 deaths. *NEW YORK J MED* 47:2311–2315, 1947.
d. Henggeler A: A serious case of poisoning (carbon tetrachloride poisoning.) *SCHWEIZ MED WOCHENSCHR* 1:223–224, 1931.
e. Lyle DJ, Zavon MR: Blindness in a fur worker. *OCCUP MED* 3:478–479, 1961.
f. Moeller W: Chronic carbon tetrachloride poisoning from the ophthalmological point of view. *Z GESAMTE HYG* 19:127–133, 1973. (German)
g. Smith AR: Optic atrophy following inhalation of carbon tetrachloride. *ARCH IND HYG* 1:348–351, 1950.
h. Smyth HF, Smyth HF Jr, Carpenter CP: The chronic toxicity of carbon tetrachloride; animal exposures and field studies. *J IND HYG* 18:277–297, 1936.
i. Stewart A, Witts LJ: Chronic carbon tetrachloride intoxication. *BR J IND MED* 1:11–19, 1944.
j. Wirtschafter ZT: Toxic amblyopia and accompanying physiological disturbances in carbon tetrachloride intoxication. *AM J PUBLIC HEALTH* 23:1035–1038, 1933.

Carbromal (Adaline), a sedative and hypnotic drug, has caused disturbances of vision, thought to be due to retrobulbar neuritis, in several cases. Sattler in 1923 described a patient who had reversible reduction of vision with central scotoma and temporal pallor of the optic nerveheads after year long daily use of carbromal.[d] Omoto in 1933 reported a case of retrobulbar neuritis with hyperemia of the optic nervehead from chronic poisoning, with improvement after the drug was stopped.[c] Stohr in 1951, describing three cases of chronic addiction and overdosage, noted that one patient complained of worsening of vision, which was associated with central scotomas and temporal pallor of the optic nerveheads, accompanied by ptosis and sluggish pupillary reactions to light. The patient improved greatly after carbromal was discontinued.[e] Copas and associates, reporting on five cases of chronic intoxication, made vague mention of temporal restriction of the visual field in one patient, irregular sluggish pupils in another, and suspicion of blurring of the optic disc and retrobulbar neuritis in a third, but gave little precise ophthalmologic information.[a] Berndt and Piper described two middle-aged women who had taken carbromal-containing sleeping medication and alcohol for about two years, and during the last months had noted decreasing visual acuity. Both had central scotomas and retinal edema, diffuse in one, and limited to the macula in the other. After discontinuing the medication, one gradually recovered, but the other already had some optic atrophy, and a follow-up was not given. Manthey and Heuer each very briefly described a case with bilateral central scotomas and pallor of the nerve heads, with partial recovery of vision when carbromal was discontinued.[g,h]

Crawford in 1959 described a patient in whom some effect on the lens was suspected but not proved.[b]

a. Copas DE, Kay WW, Longman VH: Carbromal intoxication. *LANCET* 1:703–705, 1959.
b. Crawford R: Toxic cataract. *BR MED J* 2:1231–1232, 1959.

c. Omoto K: On axial neuritis from Adalin poisoning. *ACTA SOC OPHTHALMOL JPN* 37:1634–1639, 1933. (Zentralbl Ges Ophthalmol 30:669, 1934.)

d. Sattler CH: Bromural and Adalin poisoning of the eyes. *KLIN MONATSBL AUGEN-HEILKD* 70:149, 1923. (German)

e. Stohr G: Adalin injuries. *ARZTL WOCHENSCHR* 6:1097–1098, 1951. (German)

f. Berndt K, Piper HF: Eye changes from intoxication with bromcarbamide containing sleeping medications. *KLIN MONATSBL AUGENHEILKD* 174:123–126, 1979. (German)

g. Manthey KF: Eye changes after chronic abuse of bromide-containing sleeping medication. *KLIN MONATSBL AUGENHEILKD* 172:400, 1978. (German)

h. Heuer H: Eye involvement in bromine intoxication. *KLIN MONATSBL AUGENHEILKD* 172:400, 1978. (German)

Carbutamide (aminophenurobutane), a sulfanilamide oral hypoglycemic drug used in diabetes, has been shown to be toxic to the eyes of rats when chronically administered at dosages five to forty times those employed in treatment of human beings. It has caused opacification of the lens and cornea, vascularization of the cornea, and posterior synechias, usually in eight to twenty-four months.[a] The same types of changes have been induced by *tolbutamide* and *chlorpropamide,* but not by *insulin.* In dogs, similar treatment has not affected the eyes.[a]

a. Wright HN: Corneal and lenticular opacities in eyes of rats following long-term administration of sulfonylurea derivatives. *DIABETES* 12:550–554, 1963.

Cardiac glycosides (including *acetyldigitoxin, digitalis, digitoxin, digoxin, ouabain* [*G-strophanthin*], and *strophanthus*) probably all have the same types of toxic effects on the eyes and on vision, though administered in various ways. Observations on visual disturbances in human beings have been reported from each of these drugs except *ouabain.* This last drug has been extensively studied in the laboratory for its various toxic effects on animal eyes, but seems to have been relatively little used clinically.

While most clinical descriptions of visual disturbances from excessive dosage of cardiac glycosides continue to feature the disturbances of color vision, dazzling or glare phenomena, which are reversible and provide little clue to the anatomic site of the toxic action, a number of instances of induction of central scotomas with reduction of visual acuity have been reported, and evidence has been increasing to point to the receptor cells of the retina as the principal anatomic site for the toxic influences of cardiac glycosides on vision.

Specific details on each of the drugs are given separately elsewhere under the individual names of the drugs, most extensively under *Digitalis* and *Digitoxin.*

Several of the cardiac glycosides listed above are toxic to the cornea on direct contact. (In this connection, see also *Gitalin* and *Squill.*) Several have been shown to reduce intraocular pressure by interfering with formation of aqueous humor, presumably by inhibition of the enzyme NaK–ATPase. This has been demonstrated more effectively in animals than in human beings, in whom toxicity limits the dosage. (In this connection, see also *Lanatoside C.*)

Carmustine (BCNU; BiCNU), an antineoplastic, has caused vasculitis and neuro-retinitis when given systemically. Three out of four dogs given carmustine by intracarotid injection developed progressive clouding of the ipsilateral cornea, and apparent blindness.[a] Histology showed edema of both cornea and retina. A man given carmustine in combination with procarbazine and cyclophosphamide developed acute bilateral neuroretinitis eight days later.[e] He had no light perception, widely dilated pupils, normal ERG, but extinguished visual evoked cortical response. His discs showed temporal swelling extending into the retina. Disc edema and hemorrhages in the fundus periphery resolved, but there was only slight improvement of vision. Another patient had unilateral neuroretinitis after carmustine in association with dacarbazine, fluorouracil, and vincristine.[d] Shingleton and associates have reported on 50 patients treated intravenously with carmustine, of whom two developed retinal changes after 4 weeks consisting of infarcts of the retinal nerve-fiber layer, asymptomatic in one patient, reducing vision to counting fingers in one eye of the other patient.[f] Shingleton also reported on 10 patients treated with intracarotid carmustine for supratentorial brain tumors, all of whom had severe pain in the eye on the same side during the injection, and in 2 to 14 weeks 7 out of the 10 patients had retinal arterial narrowing, nerve fiber infarcts and intraretinal hemorrhages from vasculitis and papillitis.[f] Vision decreased to no light perception in the affected eye in 3 patients, and only one of the patients maintained normal central vision.

In rabbits, injections of carmustine into and around the globe have been evaluated for toxicity to the eye. As much as 0.25 mg could be injected into the anterior chamber, or 0.5 mg into the vitreous body without significant damage.[b] For vitrectomy perfusion a concentration of 4 μg/ml produced no change in histology or ERG.[277] Subtenon and retrobulbar injection of 1.5–2 mg per day for 10 days caused corneal stromal infiltration, edema, and vascularization.[b] Also, a slow-release episcleral implantation device caused corneal clouding and conjunctival edema.[c]

a. De Wys WD, Fowler EH: Report of vasculitis and blindness after intracarotic injection of 1,3-bis(2-chloroethyl)-1-nitrosourea in dogs. *CANCER CHEMOTHER REP* 57:33–40, 1973.

b. Liu HS, Perry HD, Refojo MF: Tolerance of normal rabbit eyes to the antineoplastic carmustine. *OPHTHALMOLOGICA* 181:41–46, 1980.

c. Liu LHS, Refojo MF, et al: Sustained release of carmustine (BCNU) for treatment of experimental intraocular malignancy. *BR J OPHTHALMOL* 67:479–484, 1983.

d. Louie AC, Turrisi AT, et al: Visual abnormalities following nitrosourea treatment. *MED PEDIATR ONCOL* 5:245–247, 1978.

e. McLennan R, Taylor HR: Optic neuroretinitis in association with BCNU and procarbazine therapy. *MED PEDIATR ONCOL* 4:43–48, 1978.

f. Shingleton BJ, Bienfang DC, et al: Ocular toxicity associated with high-dose carmustine. *ARCH OPHTHALMOL* 100:1766–1772, 1982.

Carrageenan is a water-soluble colloid extracted from Irish moss (*Chondrus crispus*). It is said to stimulate production of collagen in wounds. Injection of a solution of carrageenan into the corneal stroma of guinea pigs has produced a granulomatous reaction.[a,b,d] In one study the day after injection the entire cornea became clouded, and in twelve to sixteen days became extensively vascularized, but gradually cleared and by forty days there were only faint haze and persistent blood vessels.[a,b] Histologically, the prominent features were invasion of the cornea by inflammatory cells which removed the carrageenan, and thickening of the cornea from deposition of apparently new collagen, which gradually atrophied, leaving the cornea of approximately normal dimensions and architecture. A study of the biochemical changes indicated mucopolysaccharide accumulation, but gave no evidence for synthesis of new collagen.[d]

Application of carrageenan solution to the eyes of rabbits caused irritation and an acute rise of intraocular pressure lasting less than an hour.[c] In the anterior chamber of rabbits an inflammation is induced, which involves production of prostaglandins, and a strong cellular reaction in the aqueous humor.[e]

a. Burns RP, Beighle R: Experimental carrageenin granuloma of the cornea. *ARCH OPHTHALMOL* 64:712–723, 1960.
b. Burns RP, Beighle R: Effects of triethylenethiophosphoramide on the carrageenin granuloma of the guinea pig cornea. *INVEST OPHTHALMOL* 1:666–671, 1962.
c. Altieri G: Experimental ocular hypertension induced by topical application of carrageenan and formalin. *RASS ITAL OTTALMOL* 37:196–200, 1969. (Italian)
d. Praus R, Obengerger J: Biochemical changes in guinea pig cornea following carrageenan injection. *EXP EYE RES* 2:53–64, 1963.
e. Szary A: Prostaglandins in carrageenan-induced iridocyclitis. *ARCH IMMUNOL THER EXP* 27:373–375, 1979.

Cashew nut shell oil is an irritating and sensitizing substance which has been known to cause edema of the lids and conjunctivitis as part of a widespread dermatitis,[a] but it is not selectively toxic to the eye.

a. Downing JG, Gurney SW: Dermatitis from cashew nut oil. *J IND HYG TOXIC* 22:169–174, 1940.

Cassava, a tropical plant, has been suspected of having caused slow decrease in visual acuity with constriction of visual fields, optic atrophy, deafness, ataxia, weakness of the legs, and posterior column sensory loss, so-called tropical ataxic neuropathy, in numerous middle-aged natives in Nigeria on a continuous diet mainly of cassava derivatives.[a–e] Less often the findings have suggested retrobulbar neuritis and there have been central scotomas.[e] These neuropathies have been attributed to cyanide released by hydrolysis from a cassava glycoside, *linamarin*. Studies on patients showed elevated plasma cyanide and thiocyanate as evidence of cyanide intake. However, the relationship of cyanide to the visual loss and the rest of the syndrome is still unproved.

a. Editorial: Tropical ataxic neuropathy. *BR MED J* 3: 632–633, 1968.
b. Osuntokun BO: Ataxic neuropathy in Nigeria. *BRAIN* 91:215–248, 1968.
c. Osuntokun BO, Durowoju JE, et al: Plasma amino acids in the Nigerian nutritional ataxic neuropathy. *BR MED J* 3:647–649, 1968.
d. Tuboku-Metzger AF: Diet and neuropathy. *BR MED J* 2:239, 1969.
e. Osuntokun BO, Osuntokun MB: Tropoical amblyopia in Nigerians. *AM J OPHTHALMOL* 72:708–716, 1971.

Castor beans (castor oil seeds; ricinus seeds, from *Ricinus communis*) are approximately 18 × 12 × 6 mm, oval, with a mottled, shiny brown capsule, and hard homogeneous yellow contents.[e] *Castor oil,* prepared by cold-pressing the seeds is bland and innocuous when applied to the eye.[27] However, both the original seed and the residue after pressing contain a highly toxic substance, *ricin,* which is not present in the oil. Dust originating from the dried pressed residue is strongly irritating to the eyes, causing conjunctivitis, lacrimation, and edema of the lids, accompanied by irritation of the nose and respiratory passages.[c,252] Practically all workers exposed develop these symptoms; this suggests a direct irritative effect, probably from *ricin,* but some individuals develop urticaria and asthma, suggesting that sensitization is also a factor.[129,252] During two years at least 112 men handling castor bean pomace developed these symptoms at seaports on the east coast of the United States.[b]

Direct application of particles of the seeds to the conjunctiva causes a localized conjunctival reaction with the formation of a pseudomembrane and accumulation of many polymorphonuclear leukocytes. When the foreign material is removed, healing takes place in five to six days, but repeated application may lead to local symblepharon.[e] Castor beans have been employed in self-infliction of conjunctivitis.[e,46]

The beans have been used ornamentally in necklaces. When accidentally crumbled in handling and inadvertently carried to the eye on the fingers, they have induced an acute reaction of sneezing, intense itching of the face, and great swelling of the lids.[d]

Atrophy of both optic nerves with great reduction of visual acuity has been reported in one patient after ingestion of a large number of seeds.[a,129] Severe gastrointestinal symptoms appeared promptly, and two days later pain occurred in one orbit. This was followed in two weeks by reduced visual acuity and ultimately optic atrophy with constriction of the visual fields. Six other persons who ingested the seeds did not have loss of vision. (See also *Ricin.*)

a. Belousova RV, Rafalovich SN: Optic atrophy after intoxication caused by seeds of castor plant. *VESTN OFTALMOL* (3):40–41, 1949.
b. Copper WC, Perone VB, et al: Occupational hazards from castor bean pomace: tests for toxicity. *AM IND HYG ASSOC J* 25:431–438, 1964.
c. Havel J: Davage to the eye by ricinus. *CESK OFTALMOL* 9:563, 1953. (Reference from Jaensch, P.A.)[129]
d. Lockey SD Jr, Dunkelberger L: Anaphylaxis from an Indian necklace. *J AM MED ASSOC* 206:2900–2901, 1968.
e. Somerset EJ: Self-inflicted conjunctivitis. *BR J OPHTHALMOL* 29:196–204, 1945.

Catechol (pyrocatechol; 1,2-dihydroxybenzene), a phenolic solid, is caustic and has caused burns of the eye which were slow in healing in two out of six cases.[165] Aqueous solutions up to 0.05 M tested by injection into rabbit corneas were not injurious, however.[123]

Caterpillar hairs, from the worm-like caterpillar larvae of butterflies and moths, have been known for centuries for their irritative effect on the eyes and skin. Lewin and Guillery in 1913 presented twenty-five pages of discussion and description of the effects upon the eye.[153] Numerous additional articles since that time were well reviewed by Gundersen et al in 1950,[1] by Duke Elder in 1954[46] and by Jaensch in

1958.[129] Korner (1971) listed 53 articles in the German literature.[o] Additional cases of caterpillar hair keratitis and uveitis continue to be reported.[a-w] Most reports are concerned with hairs in the conjunctiva and cornea. It has often been supposed that ocular lesions produced by the hairs are attributable not only to a mechanical effect but to some toxic substance in the hairs, yet its nature has not been demonstrated.

The hairs are sharp and sometimes barbed, penetrating conjunctiva and cornea, sometimes entering and wandering throughout the eye. In reaction to the hairs, keratoconjunctivitis and severe iridocyclitis may result. Nodular reactions about the hairs occur wherever they come to rest. This has been given the descriptive name *ophthalmia nodosa*. The microscopic appearance of the nodules, consisting of infiltration with inflammatory cells and giant cells and local necrosis, has been interpreted as probably being due to a chemical irritant, or it could be the effect of products of degeneration of the hair itself.

Migration of the caterpillar hairs tends to be in a direction opposite to what might be expected from the position of the barbs. An explanation has been proposed that some toxic substance may leak from the broken end, causing accumulation of inflammatory cells to form a nodule only at that end, and this accumulation of cells may push the hair forward.[b-d] One report is somewhat unusual in observing that the hairs of the processionary caterpillar, *Taumatopoea pityocampa*, do not migrate after entering the cornea, and that they are eventually completely absorbed and do not require surgical removal.[j] To the other extreme, chronic uveitis developed after caterpillar hairs of presumably some other variety penetrated into one eye of a patient at age three years and was still active at age twenty-four years, only partially improved after excision of portions of conjunctiva and iris to remove some of the hairs.[p]

Among the more recently noteworthy observations, Cadera and colleagues (1984) described a patient who had acute reaction to hairs in cornea and conjunctiva promptly after contact, and 4 months later complained of "floaters". At that time many subretinal and intravitreal hairs were found.[b] Subsequently severe vitritis developed with cystoid macular edema, but eventually subsided under local corticosteroid treatment, and normal vision was retained. A case of endophthalmitis from caterpillar setae was presented by Steele and colleagues (1984) in which there was much reaction to hairs in the cornea, iris, and anterior and posterior vitreous. A number of hairs were removed surgically from the anterior chamber and iris, and were examined by electron microscopy. A patch of chorioretinitis developed, but eventually under corticosteroid treatment the eye became quiet and normal visual acuity was retained. In both Cadera's and Steel's cases some hairs remained visible in the vitreous body even after inflammation subsided, apparently having become relatively inert, maybe through encapsulation.

Experimentally in rabbits, Haluska and colleagues (1983) produced inflammatory nodules resembling those of ophthalmia nodosa in human beings by implanting hairs of gypsy moth caterpillars in the cornea, but found that if the hairs were simply placed in the conjunctival cul-de-sac they produced no reaction.[m]

Caldera has provided a clinical classification of the various degrees of involvement of human eyes and advice on corresponding treatments, ranging from surface

irrigation for superficial hairs, to excision of accessible nodules, and even consideration of vitrectomy in the worst sort of case, along with corticosteroids for inflammation.[f]

a. Angebault JY, Sellier P, Mathieu M: Ocular complications from hairs of pine-tree processionary caterpillar (*Thaumetopoea pithyocampa*). *BULL SOC OPHTALMOL FRANCE* 74:373–380, 1974. (French)

b. Ascher KW: On the mechanism of wandering of caterpillar hairs in human eyes. *KLIN MONATSBL AUGENHEILKD* 143:262–264, 1964. (German)

c. Ascher KW: Mechanism of locomation observed on caterpillar hairs. *AM J OPHTHAL-MOL* 66:354–355, 1968.

d. Ascher KW: Mechanism of locomotion observed on caterpillar hairs. *BR J OPHTHAL-MOL* 52:210, 1968.

e. Bishop JW, Morton MR: Caterpillar-hair kerato-conjunctivitis. *AM J OPHTHALMOL* 64:778–779, 1967.

f. Cadera W, Pachtman MA, et al: Ocular lesions caused by caterpillar hairs (ophthalmia nodosa). *CAN J OPHTHALMOL* 19:40–44, 1984.

g. Colotto A, Santandrea R: On ocular lesions from processionary caterpillar. *ANN OTTALMOL CLIN OCUL* 105:963–968, 1979. (Italian)

h. Daman F: Caterpillar hair uveitis from the hairs of Bombyx rubi. *KLIN MONATSBL AUGENHEILKD* 153: 643–648, 1968. (German)

i. Dean RC: Ophthalmia nodosa. *ANN OPHTHALMOL* 14:1177–1178, 1982.

j. Detti S: On four cases of keratitis from caterpillars with special attention to the behavior of hairs in the cornea. *BOLL OCULIST* 46:512–529, 1967. (Italian)

k. Fau R, Andre P: Ocular lesions from caterpillar hairs. *BULL SOC OPHTALMOL FRANCE* 72:963, 1972. (French)

l. Gundersen T, Heath P, Garron L: Ophthalmia nodosa. *TRANS AM OPHTHALMOL SOC* 48:151–169, 1950.

m. Haluska FG, Puliafito CA, et al: Experimental gypsy moth (*Lymantria dispar*) ophthalmia nodosa. *ARCH OPHTHALMOL* 101:799–801, 1983.

n. Kolb H: On treatment of caterpillar hair uveitis. *KLIN MONATSBL AUGENHEILKD* 157:698–700, 1970. (German)

o. Korner H: On eye injuries from caterpillar hairs. *OPHTHALMOLOGICA* 162, 308–317, 1971. (German)

p. Kutschera E: Ophthalmia nodosa. *KLIN MONATSBL AUGENHEILKD* 153:68–70, 1968. (German)

q. Lerchavanakul A, Pearce WG, Nigam S: Ophthalmia nodosa. *CAN J OPHTHALMOL* 10:86–89, 1975.

r. Reiser KA: On caterpillar hair "wandering" in the choroid of human beings. *KLIN MONATSBL AUGENHEILKD* 141:907–912, 1962. (German)

s. Steele C, Lucas DR, Ridgway AEA: Endophthalmitis due to caterpillar setae: surgical removal and electron microscopic appearances of the setae. *BR J OPHTHALMOL* 68:284–288, 1984.

t. Velicky J: Caterpillar injury of the eye. *CESK OFTALMOL* 21:413–416, 1965. (Zentralbl Ges Ophthalmol 97:580, 1967.)

u. Watson PG, Sevel D: Ophthalmia nodosa. *BR J OPHTHALMOL* 50:209–217, 1966.

Catha edulis (kat or qat leaves, native to southern Arabia and Ethiopia) has been
employed for centuries as a mild stimulant.[171] Addiction to chewing Catha edulis
has been held responsible for disturbance of vision in a father and son.[a] The son
complained of misty vision for more than two years, and was found to have an

appearance of congestion and edema of his optic discs; however, no mention of elevation nor measurements of vision or visual fields were reported. The maculas were said to be normal and there were no hemorrhages. During two weeks in which Catha edulis was not available, the appearance of the discs gradually improved and the vision became less misty, but again no measurements were reported. The father also was said to have poor vision and was found to have discs of the same appearance as the son's. If this actually was an effect of Catha edulis, it must have been an extremely rare one.

There appears to be no danger of elevation of intraocular pressure from chewing Catha edulis. A study by Vedy and associates in 1968 showed that slow chewing of the leaves and young shoots caused a reduction of intraocular pressure in both normal and glaucomatous patients in two or three hours.[b]

   a. Baird DA: A case of optic neuritis in qat addiction. *E AFRICAN MED J* 29:325–326, 1952.
   b. Vedy J, Fretillere Y, et al: Clinical study of the effects on tonometric measurements from consumption of cath among the Somalis. *BULL SOC OPHTALMOL FRANCE* 68:386–389, 1968. (French)

Cefazolin sodium, an antibacterial, has been tested in rabbit eyes; 25 mg subconjunctivally or 2.25 mg injected into the vitreous humor appeared to be non-toxic by ophthalmoscopy, ERG, and histology.[a,b] Topically, a 5% solution had little effect on corneal epithelial healing.[382]

   a. Abel R, Boyle G, et al: Intraocular penetration of cefazolin sodium in rabbits. *AM J OPHTHALMOL* 78:779–787, 1974.
   b. Fisher JP, Civiletto SE, Forster RK: Toxicity, efficacy, and clearance of intravitreally injected cefazolin. *ARCH OPHTHALMOL* 100:650–652, 1982.

Ceftriaxone sodium (Rocephin), an antibacterial, has been tested for retinotoxicity in rabbits after intravitreal injection.[a] A 50 mg dose caused temporary clouding of cornea and lens, retinal edema, and disruption of retinal layers, but by 2 weeks the histology was normal. Doses of 7.5 to 20 mg temporarily reduced the amplitude of the ERG b-wave, but doses up to 5 mg did not.

   a. Shockley RK, Jay WM, et al: Intravitreal ceftriaxone in a rabbit model. *ARCH OPHTHALMOL* 102:1236–1238, 1984.

Cellulose sponge particles have been observed and photographed adherent to the iris, in the anterior chamber of patients, after intraocular surgery in which cellulose surgical sponges were used.[a] They caused no trouble. An analogous problem involving cellulose and other fibers from various sources is described elsewhere under the heading *Lint.*

   a. Marback RL: Cellulose sponge as a foreign body in the anterior chamber following cataract surgery. *REV BRAS OFTALMOL* 30:425–429, 1971.

Cement, Portland, is a fine, gray powder used to make *concrete.* Either dry or wet it is sufficiently alkaline to injure the cornea. A splash in the eye causes smarting and burning sensation, and induces corneal edema. The victim may immediately see colored rings or haloes about lights.[81] However, Portland cement and concrete are not as dangerous as *mortar,* which contains a greater amount of free calcium hydroxide (lime) and is more strongly alkaline. Splashes of mortar cause "lime burns" which may be very severe if irrigation is not performed promptly. After concrete or mortar have set or hardened, they slowly become less alkaline and less apt to cause chemical injury of the eye.

Cephaloridine (Cefaloridine, Loridine, Kefloridin, Ceporine) a broad spectrum antibacterial, is of special interest because of its toxicity to the retina. Early tests in which it was administered to dogs for twelve weeks produced no ophthalmoscopically detectable disturbance in the eyes.[a] However, in 1975 effects on the ERG of rabbit retina *in vitro* were found,[e] and in tests in rabbits it was shown that, while intravitreal injections of 0.25 mg or less caused no damage, 5 mg produced small retinal hemorrhages, and 10 mg caused clumping of the outer segments of the photoreceptors, destruction of retinal pigment epithelium, and extinction of the electroretinogram.[d] Intravitreal injection of 25 mg caused complete destruction of the outer segments of the photoreceptors and phagocytosis by cells from the retinal pigment epithelium; these changes proved irreversible.[h] The tests were repeated and the findings were corroborated in 1980, with additional attention to the ophthalmoscopic appearance of the fundi; which by the second day showed numerous specks of pigment scattered about over the whole fundus, with larger clumps of pigment in the periphery against a background of extensive atrophy of the pigment epithelium.[g] Despite this well-defined and severe toxic action from intravitreal cephaloridine, no retinotoxic effect was detected when this substance was injected intravenously, subconjunctivally or into the anterior chamber in rabbits in very large doses.[d,g]

In human beings the first suggestion of retinotoxic action appeared in 1967.[b] Treatment with cephaloridine in a girl with septicemia was associated with acute renal failure and blindness, with papilledema and pigmentation in the periphery of the fundi. The retinal vessels were said to be normal. After treatment by peritoneal dialysis there was partial recovery of vision in the course of three months. Toxic action from the antibiotic was suspected.[b] The patient had also received cloxacillin and fusidic acid, but neither of these was known to have this sort of toxicity.[c] Subsequently, cephaloridine was very widely used clinically, apparently without further ocular complication until 1979, when an impressive report described severe pigmentary retinopathy and loss of vision in one eye each of four patients after injection subconjunctivally or intracamerally or both.[f,g] In each patient only one eye required antibacterial treatment; the contralateral eyes did not require treatment, and remained normal. The affected eyes rapidly developed complete retinal degeneration with pigmentary retinopathy, extinction of the ERG, and complete permanent loss of vision, except in one eye which retained a 10° central field. The ophthalmoscopic appearance has been well demonstrated with fundus photographs, and consists of unilateral migration of retinal pigment from the retinal pigment epithelium to form scattered black specks, gathered into larger plaques peripherally or at the macula.[g] Retinal vessels and optic discs remained normal. The changes in the human eyes appeared to be the same as those produced experimentally in rabbits.[g]

Yet to be explained is why these four patients developed toxic retinopathy from subconjunctival or intracameral injection, when it has seemed impossible to induce by this route in rabbits, and when many other patients have received similar treatment without complications.

a. Atkinson RM, Caisey JD, et al: Subacute toxicity of cephaloridine to various species. *TOXICOL APPL PHARMACOL* 8:407–428, 1966.
b. Ballingall DLK, Turpie AGG: Cephaloridine toxicity. *LANCET* 2:835–836, 1967.
c. Crosbie RB: Cephaloridine toxicity. *LANCET* 1:422, 1968.
d. Graham RO, Peyman GA, Fishman G: Intravitreal injection of cephaloridine in the treatment of endophthalmitis. *ARCH OPHTHALMOL* 93:56–61, 1975.
e. Honda Y, Nagata M: A neurological side effect of cephaloridine: enhancement of the electroretinogram. *OPHTHALMIC RES* 7:395–400, 1975.
f. Turut P, Florin P, Malthieu D: Pigmentary pseudo-retinitis from Ceporine; 4 observations. *BULL SOC OPHTALMOL FRANCE* 79:1095–1098, 1979. (French)
g. Turut P, Malthieu D: Ocular toxicity of cephaloridine; clinical and experimental study. *J FR OPHTALMOL* 3:401–408, 1980. (French)
h. Vlchek JK, Peyman GA: Cephaloridine-induced retinopathy by intravitreal injection; an ultrastructural study. *ANN OPHTHALMOL* 7:903–914, 1975.

Cephalothin sodium (Cefalotin, Keflin), an antibacterial, has been tested by intravitreal injection in rabbits, showing that 8 mg and 4 mg could produce "mild focal disorganization of the retinal nuclear layers," but 2 mg produced no abnormality.[a] The condition of the retinal pigment epithelium was not stated. This is of some interest, because there is notable chemical similarity to *cephaloridine,* which has clearly defined retinotoxic effects, involving particularly the retinal pigment epithelium and outer segments of the photoreceptors.

Injected into the anterior chamber, cephalothin is toxic to rabbit endothelium.[270]

a. Rutgard JJ, Berkowitz RA, Peyman GA: Intravitreal cephalothin in experimental staphylococcal endophthalmitis. *ANN OPHTHALMOL* 10:293–298, 1978.

Cerium salts tested on rabbit eyes appear to have local toxic effect on the cornea similar to that of salts of lanthanum and other members of the lanthanide series. Application of 0.1 M solution of cerous chloride at pH 6 to a rabbit's eye after removal of the corneal epithelium to permit penetration into the stroma caused immediate slight bluish turbidity, progressing in the course of three weeks to complete corneal opacification.[81]

Cesium salts; caesium salts, are not known to have toxic effect on the eyes. Cesium administered systemically to animals has, however, been found to accumulate in the retina.[a] A solution of cesium chloride (0.1 M, pH 5) tested by application for ten minutes to a rabbit's eye after mechanical removal of the epithelium caused no appreciable injury.[81]

a. Scott GH, Canaga BL: Cesium in the mammalian retina. *PROC SOC EXP BIOL MED* 40:275, 1939.

Cetrimonium bromide (hexadecyltrimethylammonium bromide, Cetrimide), a cationic surfacant and antiseptic, appears to be potentially dangerous to the eyes if excessive concentrations are used, according to tests on rabbit eyes,[a] and according to experience with a commercial preparation, Savlon, which contains 15%. Severe injury of rabbit eyes and one human eye by this preparation are described under *Savlon.*

  a. Dewey WL, Malone MH, et al: *TOXICOL APPL PHARMACOL* 12:115–121, 1968.

Cetylpyridinium chloride, a topical anti-infective and pharmaceutical preservative, has lytic action on epithelial cells of the lens and of the cornea, increasing permeability by destroying cell membranes.[a,b,320] The endothelial cells of the cornea are likewise prone to injury by this substance, with potentially serious consequences to the whole cornea.[321] The effects are concentration-related, and, as with benzalkonium, it is possible to select concentrations which increase penetration of drugs into the eye without clinically evident injury.

  a. Cotlier E, Sanders D, Wyhinny G: Effects of cetylpyridinium chloride on the membranes of the lens fibers and on lens permeability, hydration and ^{22}Na and ^{86}Rb transport. *OPHTHALMIC RES* 6:107–130, 1974.
  b. Green K: Electrophysiological and anatomical effects of cetypyridinium chloride on the rabbit cornea. *ACTA OPHTHALMOL* 54:145–159, 1976.

Chelidonium majus, a plant of the papaveracia family, has a yellow-red sap or latex which has been employed in treatment of warts. In contact with the eye it is very irritating,[253] and in one case caused severe keratoconjunctivitis with iritis and hypopyon.[a] However, in this case recovery was complete in two to three weeks.

  a. Hilbert R: Iritis from the action of the latex of Chelidonium majus. *ZENTRALBL PRAKT AUGENHEILKD* 47:142–144, 1916. (German)

Chenopodium oil (American wormseed), an anthelmintic, is said very rarely to have caused temporary impairment of vision.[c,70,153] In one case, after *Chenopodium hybridum* was ingested, there was faintness, temporary dimness of vision and mydriasis.[153] In another instance a girl had headache, vomiting, unconsciousness, and convulsions after taking oil of chenopodium for worms. While recovering, she was given *santonin.* She then developed increased intracranial pressure and papilledema with impairment of vision. She ultimately recovered 0.5 vision in one eye, but only light perception in the other, because of optic atrophy.[a] It was thought that the patient observed some decrease in vision before the santonin was given, but it could not be established for certain that chenopodium was responsible. (Compare *Santonin.*)

  a. Biesin A: Risk of poisoning and idiosyncracy in administering chenopodium oil. *MUNCH MED WOCHENSCHR* 76:661–664, 1929. (German)
  c. Desoille H: The antihelminics, sensory poisons. *REV OTOL* 15:170–173, 1937. (French)

Chloral hydrate a sedative and hypnotic, generally produces miosis, but in dangerous overdosage there may be mydriasis. Moderate doses are said to affect eye movements, particularly interfering with convergence, and sometimes causing ptosis.

These effects are transitory. Chloral hydrate not uncommonly causes dermatitis and may cause swelling of the lids, hyperemia and edema of the conjunctivae, plus a sensation of irritation and tearing.[153,214,246]

There is uncertainty whether chloral hydrate has injurious action on the optic nerve or retina; Uhthoff thought it did not.[247] deSchweinitz noted cases of temporary amaurosis following daily ingestion of larger than normal doses for several months, but was not sure whether the drug was responsible.[41] Similarly, Lewin and Guillery mentioned cases of transient diminution of vision or amaurosis and were uncertain whether they were of central or peripheral origin.[153] No cases have been reported in recent times.

Chlorambucil (Leukeran), an antineoplastic, has been carefully examined for teratogenic involvement of the eye. Administration during pregnancy has been shown to be injurious to the developing retina in mice, rats, monkeys, and one human embryo,[a] and to the optic nerves and lenses in mice.[b]

Chlorambucil caused keratitis epithelialis in association with exfoliative dermatitis in one patient under treatment for lymphosarcoma. One child developed reversible pseudotumor cerebri with papilledema, but no change in vision while being treated for nephritis with this drug.[c]

   a. Rugh R, Skaredoff L: Radiation and radiomimetic chlorambucil and the fetal retina. *ARCH OPHTHALMOL* 74:382–393, 1965.
   b. Clavert A, Gabriel Robez O: Eye defects induced by chlorambucil in the mouse. *C R SEANCES SOC BIOL* 168:1115–1118, 1974.
   c. Saraux H, Laplane R, Begue H: Spontaneous reversible papilledema in the course of a treatment with chlorambucil. *BULL SOC BELGE OPHTALMOL* 160:567–569, 1972.

Chloramphenicol (Chloroptic, Chloromycetin, Chloromyxin, Econochlor, Ophthocort), antibacterial and antirickettsial, has been used systemically and topically on the eye. When first introduced, it tended to be used rather indiscriminately, but since it has become well recognized that chloramphenicol can cause depression of the bone marrow and fatal aplastic anemia, its use has become limited to specific indications.

Optic neuritis and optic atrophy with impairment of central vision from orally administered chloramphenicol have occurred in a long series of cases during the past 30 years, mostly in children with cystic fibrosis. In 1969, Kittel and Cornelius surveyed the literature (19 references), and presented two new cases. They noted that at least forty cases had been reported associating chloramphenicol treatment and optic nerve injury. (By the time of their survey at least 21 articles had been published giving case reports of optic neuropathy. References to case reports since the 1969 survey are given in the bibliography of the present synopsis.) In the 1969 survey it was noted that optic nerve injuries had been observed predominantly in children, accounting for thirty-three out of forty cases. Regularly both nerves of every patient were affected, usually at approximately the same time and fairly symmetrically. Most often the findings indicated optic neuritis, infrequently a retrobulbar neuritis. The signs that Kittel and Cornelius were impressed with in reported cases and in their own, included hyperemic papillas with indistinct margins, peripapillary edema, a little elevation of the papillas, increased tortuosity, and congestion of the retinal veins, and hemorrhages on and around the optic nerveheads. The visual disturbances consisted principally of central scotoma and paracentral scotoma, with concentric constriction of the visual fields less common. In most instances vision improved when chloramphenicol was discontinued, but atrophy with persistent severe visual loss had been reported in several patients, all children. Kittel and Cornelius observed that the injuries of the optic nerve and peripheral nerves had been associated in nearly all cases with administration of chloramphenicol at high dosage for a long time. Many of the patients had had pancreatic fibrosis and severe lung disease (Beyrer; Harley), but some patients, including their own two patients, had not had these diseases when they developed optic nerve damage from chloramphenicol. Kittel and Cornelius called attention to the potential value of the warning signs of paresthesias (tingling or burning), numbness, and cramps in the extremities, which in some cases developed before the optic nerve injuries. Polyneuritis was not present in all cases. Since that study, many additional cases have been reported, but the clinical picture has essentially remained the same (Bayer; Charache; Cogan; Harley; Inoue; Mayer; Murayama; Nakamura; Nielsen; Schmiedel; Tamura). In general, the incidence has been related to dosage and duration of treatment. Optic neuritis has been rare unless the total dose of chloramphenicol has exceeded 100 g and the duration of administration has been longer than six weeks. In most cases, much greater total dosage and much longer administration have been involved.

Atypical cases of optic neuropathy have been reported by Begg (1968), Cocke (1967), Lamba (1968), and Rothkoff (1979). The last was a case of acute monocular optic atrophy from irrigating the lacrimal duct with a 20% solution of chloramphenicol, quite different from all the other cases of optic neuropathy.

(With respect to chloramphenicol optic neuropathy, also see INDEX for *Thiamphenicol,* a closely related drug.)

In several cases of typical chloramphenicol optic neuropathy postmortem histology has been reported and characteristically has shown loss of retinal ganglion cells, particularly from the macular and perimacular regions, with atrophy of corresponding areas of the optic nerves, extending to the chiasm in long-standing cases (Cogan; Harley; Lietman). Although morphologic abnormality has been evident only in the ganglion cell and nerve fiber layer of the retina, there have been suggestions of functional disturbance of the photoreceptor layer on the basis of abnormality of the ERG to testing with red light (Godel), the presence of dyschromatopsia in some cases, and an abnormality of color vision induced experimentally with chloramphenicol in people with normal vision.[339] Histology of a biopsy of the sural nerve in a case of polyneuritis associated with chloramphenicol optic neuropathy has shown atrophy of Schwann cells and myelin sheaths (Murayama).

Animal experiments concerning effects of systemically administered chloramphenicol on the retina and optic nerves have been carried out in cats by Meier-Ruge and Werthemann.[167] They administered 70 to 180 mg/kg per day and found, even at the highest doses after thirty-five weeks of treatment, no abnormalities in the fundi recognizable ophthalmoscopically or by ordinary histology, but histochemically they found a diffuse reduction in the activity of lactic dehydrogenase. *In vitro* they found no inhibitory effect on succinic acid dehydrogenase, lactic acid dehydrogenase, glutamate dehydrogenase, or alcohol dehydrogenase. The sulfhydryl groups of the retina were not affected according to histochemical observations.[167] Saleh and Hussein have, however, reported that in rabbits large oral doses (150–200 mg/kg/day for 21–45 days) did cause degeneration in the retina and optic nerves (Saleh).

Intravitreal injection of chloramphenicol succinate, which is said to release free drug rapidly in the eye, in a dose of 5 to 10 mg in rabbits has caused the ERG to become flat, and all layers of the retina to be destroyed, though the optic nerves still looked normal after a month (Koziol). If the rabbits' lens and vitreous humor were first removed, the retina appeared to become more vulnerable, suffering widespread damage of all layers when a concentration of 0.05 mg/ml was used as irrigating fluid.[380] However, 0.02 mg/ml was tolerated.

Local toxicity of chloramphenicol to the eye has otherwise been no clinical problem. Chloramphenicol eye drops are generally well tolerated, with no irritation, and only occasional allergy. Examined microscopically, the cornea has shown very slight disturbance, or none.[120,285,354] However, healing of corneal epithelium in rabbits is said in one report to be retarded by 0.5% solution, but another report says not by 0.4% solution.[368] Rare instances of depigmentation of the skin of the lids are known from topical chloramphenicol (Chalfin; Kikuchi).

Aplastic anemia was attributed to use of eyedrops in a case reported by Rosenthal and Blackman (1965) in which a man developed hypoplasia of the bone marrow after using chloramphenicol eyedrops several times a day for several years (Rosenthal). In this case the grounds for holding chloramphenicol responsible were strengthened by a family history of blood dyscrasia from this drug.

A small number of additional cases have been reported, one by Carpenter (1975) and one by Fraunfelder (1982) attributed to eye drops, and one by Abrams (1980) attributed to chloramphenicol ophthalmic ointment, but in each of these cases it has been impossible to eliminate the possibility of coincidence, and considerable discussion has ensued on how much weight to give to these cases in estimating the risks of topical treatment (Fraunfelder; Davidoff; Dutro; Flach). To eliminate the probable risks, chloramphenicol has very widely been replaced by other drugs.

Abrams SM, Degnan TJ, Vinciguerra V: Marrow aplasia following topical application of chloramphenicol eye ointment. *ARCH INTERN MED* 140:567–577, 1980.

Begg IS, Small M, White AM: Propionate and acetate excretion in chloramphenicol toxicity. *LANCET* 2:686–687, 1968.

Beyrer CR: Chloramphenicol-induced acute bilateral optic neuritis in cystic fibrosis. *J PEDIATR OPHTHALMOL* 15:290–292, 1978.

Carpenter G: Chloramphenicol eye-drops and marrow aplasia. *LANCET* 2:326–327, 1975.

Chalfin J, Putterman AM: Eyelid skin depigmentation. *OPHTHALMIC SURG* 11:194–196, 1980.

Charache S, Finkelstein D, et al: Pherpheral and optic neuritis in a patient with hemoglobin sc disease during treatment of Salmonella osteomyelitis with chloramphenicol. *JOHNS HOPKINS MED J* 140:121–124, 1977.

Cocke JG Jr: Chloramphenicol optic neuritis. *AM J DIS CHILD* 114:424–426, 1967.

Cogan DG, Truman JT, Smith TR: Optic neuropathy, chloramphenicol and infantile genetic agranulocytosis. *INVEST OPHTHALMOL* 12:534–537, 1973.

Davidoff E: Aplastic anemia and chloramphenicol. *AM J OPHTHALMOL* 94:268–269, 1982.

Dutro MP: Chloramphenicol and aplastic anemia. *AM J OPHTHALMOL* 92:870, 1981.

Flach AJ: Chloramphenicol and aplastic anemia. *AM J OPHTHALMOL* 93:664–666, 1982.

Flach AJ: Fatal aplastic anemia following topical administration of ophthalmic chloramphenicol. *AM J OPHTHALMOL* 94:420–422, 1982.

Fraunfelder FT, Bagby GC, Kelly DJ: Fatal aplastic anemia following topical administration of ophthalmic chloramphenicol. *AM J OPHTHALMOL* 93:356–360, 1982.

Godel V, Nemet P, Lazar M: Chloramphenicol optic neuropathy. *ARCH OPHTHALMOL* 98:1417–1421, 1980.

Harley RD, Huang NN, et al: Optic neuritis and optic atrophy following chloramphenicol and cystic fibrosis patients. *TRANS AM OPHTHALMOL SOC* 74:1011–1031, 1970.

Inoue K, Mannen T, et al: Chloramphenicol opticoneuropathy. *CLIN NEUROL (Tokyo)* 13:128–135, 1973.

Kikuchi I, et al: A case of depigmentation following the use of eye drops and steroid ointment. *KUMAMOTO MED J* 28:145–150, 1975.

Kittell V, Cornelius C: Optic nerve injury by chloramphenicol. *KLIN MONATSBL AUGENHEILKD* 155:83–87, 1969. (German)

Koziol J, Peyman G: Intraocular chloramphenicol and bacterial endophthalmitis. *CAN J OPHTHALMOL* 9:316–321, 1974.

Lamba PA, Sood NN, Moorthy SS: Retinopathy due to chloramphenicol. *SCOT MED J* 13:166–169, 1968.

Lietman PS, diSant'Agnese P, Wong V: *J AM MED ASSOC* 189:924–927, 1964.

Mayer U: Changes in the optic nerve and retina from systemic administration of chloramphenicol. *KLIN PADIATR* 186:447–451, 1974. (German)

Murayama E, Miyakawa T, et al: Retrobulbar optic neuritis and polyneuritis due to prolonged chloramphenicol theraphy. *CLIN NEUROL (Tokyo)* 13:213–220, 1973.

Nakamura Y, et al: Myelo-optico-neuropathy probably due to chloramphenicol, an autopsy case. *CLIN NEUROL (Tokyo)* 16:1–7, 1976.

Nielsen EL: Optic neuritis as a complication to treatment of cystic fibrosis with chloramphenicol. *UGESKR LAEGER* 134:2328–2329, 1972.

Rosenthal RL, Blackman A: Bone-marrow hypoplasia following use of chloramphenicol eyedrops. *J AM MED ASSOC* 191:136–137, 1965.

Rothkoff L, Biedner B, et al: Optic atrophy after irrigation of the lacrimal ducts with chloramphenicol. *ANN OPHTHALMOL* 11:105–106, 1979.

Saleh AL, Hussein ZH: Ocular toxicity of chloramphenicol, an experimental approach. *J DRUG RES* 3:141–152, 1971.

Schmiedel E: Optic atrophy after a long term therapy with chloramphenicol. *PADIATR GRENZGEB* 15:109–112, 1976. (German)

Tamura K, et al: Optic and peripheral neuritis following chloramphenicol therapy. *J JPN SOC INTERN MED* 62:1678–1684, 1973.

Chlorcyclizine hydrochloride, an antihistaminic, has been shown experimentally to induce lipidosis of the retinal pigment epithelium and the sensory retina in rats when fed in high dosage for several weeks.[304]

Chlordane is a widely employed insecticide which in rare instances has caused severe but nonfatal poisoning in human beings. A girl developed diplopia, blurring of vision, and twitching of the extremities two to three hours after accidentally swallowing a teaspoonful of a 24% solution of chlordane plus 16% of related compounds in a mixture of pine oil, polyethylene glycol, and petroleum distillate. Despite nausea, vomiting, and generalized convulsion, recovery was complete in five days.[a] Experimental studies have shown that a compound used in the manufacture of chlordane, *hexachlorocyclopentadiene,* can cause behavior in mice suggesting blindness, but no such effect was demonstrable with commercial chlordane which is free of the hexachloro compound.[b]

  a. Dadey JL, Kammer AA: Chlordane intoxication: report of a case. *J AM MED ASSOC* 153:723–725, 1953.
  b. Ingle L: The toxicity of chlordane vapors. *SCIENCE* 118:213, 1953.

Chlordecone (Kepone), a chlorinated hydrocarbon insecticide related to mirex, caused an epidemic of poisonings in 1975 in one manufacturing plant in Virginia due to uncontrolled gross exposure of workers. Characteristic neuro-psychiatric disturbances were foremost tremor and fluttering eye movements (opsoclonus), also pseudotumor cerebri, stuttering, easy startling, anxiety, confusion and poor memory. The eye signs and symptoms, described in a synopsis by Taylor, Selhorst and Calabresi (1980), were present in 15 out of 23 poisoned workers.[a] Those affected complained of brief periods of blurring of vision due to series of quick eye movements or saccades, characterized as opsoclonus. These movements were both conjugate and dysconjugate. They usually occurred spontaneously, but could be induced by shifting gaze from one object to another, or in one patient by touching the lids. These disturbances of eye movements have been studied and described in detail by Taylor et al.[a] They noted that during recovery from poisoning opsoclonus subsided to a slight post-saccadic tremor of the eyes during 3 to 6 months.

Three out of 23 chlordecone-poisoned workers had papilledema associated with elevated cerebrospinal fluid pressure.

  a. Taylor JR, Selhorst JB, Calabrese VP: Chlordecone. Pages 404–421 in Spencer and Schaumburg (1980).[378]

Chlordiazepoxide (Librium), a tranquilizer drug, has been examined for influences on the eyes, particularly in relation to automobile driving.[b,c] Oral dosage from 20 to 75 mg per day has been shown principally to tend to induce exophoria, sometimes to impair depth perception, and to reduce saccadic velocity.[g,h] What significance this may have with respect to automobile driving has not been clearly demonstrated.[h,86] A single oral dose of 10 mg did not alter visual fields, oculomotor balance, or color vision.[f]

There has been no indication of toxicity to the retina or other parts of the visual system. Testing of the effect of chlordiazepoxide on the electroretinogram of isolated rabbit retina has shown it to be essentially nontoxic to this preparation.[119]

In normal and glaucomatous patients ordinary doses of chlordiazepoxide appear to have had no significant adverse influence on ocular pressure. Slight or brief reduction of pressure has occasionally been claimed, but long-term studies have shown no significant sustained reduction of ocular pressure in glaucoma by this drug.[a,d,e]

a. Fukuchi S: Balance treatment in ophthalmology. *J CLIN OPHTHALMOL* 18:195–204, 1964.
b. Miller JG: Objective measurements of the effects of drugs on driver behavior. *J AM MED ASSOC* 179:940–943, 1962.
c. Murray N: Covert effects of chlordiazepoxide therapy. *J NEUROPSYCHIATR* 3:168–170, 1962.
d. Petrosillo O, Beccaria F: Tonography and tranquillizers. *ARCH OTTALMOL* 67:135–152, 1963.
e. Roberts W: The use of psychotropic drugs in glaucoma. *DIS NERV SYST* 29 Suppl:40–43, 1968.
f. Austen DP, Gilmartin BA, Turner P: The effect of chlordiazepoxide on visual field, extraocular balance, colour matching ability and hand eye coordination in man. *BR J PHYSIOL OPT* 26:161–165, 1971.
g. Gentles W, Thomas EL: Effect of benzodiazepines upon saccadic eye movements in man. *CLIN PHARMACOL THER* 12:563, 1971.
h. Schroeder SR, Ewing JA, Allen JA: Combined effects of alcohol with methapyrilene and chlordiazepoxide on driver eye movements and errors. *J SAF RES* 6:89–93, 1974.

Chlorhexidine hydrochloride or **gluconate** is an antimicrobial that has been of interest particularly inconnection with contact lenses. Chlorhexidine has been involved in one serious accident to a human eye when a solution containing 1.5%, in addition to cetrimonium 15%, entered the anterior chamber at surgery. For further details, see INDEX for *Savlon*. Testing in rabbits has shown that 0.005% solution can be injected into the anterior chambers without causing gross injury,[a] but that irrigation of the endothelium with 0.002% causes injury discernable by scanning electron microscopy, and causes swelling of the cornea.[g]

External application to the eye has given varied results, one study indicating that rabbits tolerate 0.005% to 0.05%,[b] and another that even repeated external application of 2% solution caused no gross injury and produced no disturbance of the endothelium visible by light microscopy in flat preparations,[f] yet 0.05% to 0.1% caused swelling,[g] and scanning electron microscopy showed changes in the epithelium at concentrations of 0.001% to 0.01%,[c] with reduced drying time of the tear film at 0.01%.[305] Bathing the cornea with 0.1% caused loss of the top cell layer of corneal epithelium.[300] The criteria for diagnosing injury have been quite varied. When chronically tested in conjunction with contact lenses, it appears that even concentrations of 0.002% to 0.005% may present problems of irritation.[b,d]

In guinea pigs external application of 0.004% to 0.01% produced reversible superficial punctate keratopathy; 5% was severely irritating, causing persistent clouding of the cornea.[h]

Hibiclens, a presurgical skin antiseptic containing 4% chlorhexidine gluconate, on a rabbit eye caused edema and loss of corneal epithelial cells, but return to normal in a week.[350]

a. Crompton DO, Anderson KF: Chlorocresol in eyedrops. *LANCET* 2:1279, 1963.
b. Browne RK, Anderson II BW, et al: Ophthalmic response to chlorhexidine digluconate in rabbits. *TOXICOL APPL PHARMACOL* 32:621–627, 1975.

c. Burstein NL: Preservative cytotoxic threshold for benzalkonium chloride and chlor-hexidine digluconate in cat and rabbit corneas. *INVEST OPHTHALMOL VIS SCI* 19:308–313, 1980.

d. Davies M: Rabbit eye irritation from bactericides in soft lens soaking solutions. *J PHARM PHARMACOL* 25:134P, 1973.

e. D'Haenens J: Chlorhexidine conjunctivitis. *BULL SOC BELGE OPHTALMOL* 186:65–68, 1979.

f. Gasset AR, Ishi Y: Cytotoxicity of chlorhexidine. *CAN J OPHTHALMOL* 10:98–100, 1975.

g. Green K, Livingston V, et al: Chlorhexidine effects on corneal epithelium and endothelium. *ARCH OPHTHALMOL* 98:1273–1278, 1980.

h. Pagot R, Lautier F, Brini A: Toxic action of a solution of chlorhexidine at various concentrations on the guinea pig cornea. *BULL SOC OPHTAL FRANCE* 80:631–634, 1980.

i. Takahashi N: Cytotoxicity of chlorhexidine (Hibitane) to cultured conjunctival epithelia. *FOLIA OPHTHALMOL JPN* 30:1851–1855, 1979. (English summary)

Chlorine is a poisonous gas, having suffocating odor. Presumably severe damage to the eye would result from contact with compressed liquefied gas or high concentrations of the gas, but eye accidents of this sort seem not to have been reported. Because of severe and lethal damaging action of chlorine on the respiratory tract, it is unlikely that conditions seriously injurious to the eye would be survived. Exposure to concentrations as low as 3 to 6 ppm in air causes sensation of stinging and burning of the eyes of some individuals, with associated blepharospasm, redness, and watering, but on continued exposure sensitivity may decrease and signs and symptoms diminish.[33, 188]

In swimming pools, chlorine may be added as elemental gaseous or liquid chlorine from a tank, or in the form of the hypochlorites of calcium, sodium, or lithium to kill harmful bacteria and algae. Complex relationships between the concentration of chlorine, the pH, and the concentration of ammonia or urea in the water determine the effectiveness in killing bacteria and the irritancy to the eyes of swimmers. It is said that part of the chlorine in the water reacts with the nitrogenous compounds to form chloramines and nitrogen trichloride, and that these compounds are particularly irritating to the eye. By maintaining the pH sufficiently high, the irritating products of reaction of chlorine with water and with nitrogenous compounds tend to be eliminated and irritation of the eyes avoided, while permitting use of sufficient concentrations of chlorine to effect proper killing of bacteria and algae. (See INDEX for *Swimming pool water.*)

Chlorine dissolved in water and injected into the anterior chambers of rabbits is very damaging, causing severe inflammation, corneal opacity, iris atrophy and injury of the lens.[153, 253]

Chlorine dioxide is a reddish yellow, poisonous gas which is very irritating to the respiratory tract. Industrially men exposed to low concentrations of the gas in air have been noted occasionally to suffer from irritation of the eyes and to see haloes about lights, but these effects have been minor compared to respiratory irritation.[a] The corneas of workers seeing haloes have not been examined to determine whether epithelial edema is present and responsible for this symptom.

a. Gloemme J, Lundgren K: Health hazards from chlorine dioxide. *ARCH INDUSTR HEALTH* 16:169–176, 1957.

Chlorine monofluoride (chlorine fluoride) is an extremely reactive gas which is very corrosive and irritating to the skin, eyes, and respiratory tract.[171]

Chlorine trifluoride is an extremely reactive, corrosive and irritating gas which experimentally has been observed to cause a severe reaction in the lungs and in all exposed mucous membranes.[171] It is highly irritating to the skin and eyes, and has caused severe corneal ulcers in dogs.[a]

a. Horn HJ, Weir RJ: Inhalation toxicology of chlorine trifluoride. *ARCH IND HEALTH* 12:512–521, 1955.

Chloroacetaldehyde 2,4-dinitrophenylhydrazone, a fungicide, has been tested in chickens by feeding in high doses for sixty days, looking for development of cataracts because of a chemical relationship to the known cataractogenic compound *2,4-dinitrophenol,* but it produced no cataracts.

a. Ambrose AM, Borzelleca JF, et al: Toxicologic studies on monochloroacetaldehyde 2,4-dinitrophenylhydrazone, a foliar fungicide. *TOXIC APPL PHARMACOL* 8:472–481, 1966.

Chloroacetone (monochloracetone) is a liquid which gives off heavy vapors that are very irritating to the eyes. It causes much lacrimation at concentrations of 5 to 8 ppm in air, and at higher concentrations causes a clouding of the cornea which has not been described in detail. A concentration of 26 ppm in air is intolerable for more than a minute because of severe irritation of all mucous membranes.[56,61]

Chloroacetophenone (CN; α-chloroacetophenone; phenylchloromethylketone) is a crystalline solid, melting at 59°C, with rather low vapor pressure at room temperature. When CN is heated and dispersed in air by explosion of a tear gas shell or combustion in a cannister, or when dissolved in a solvent and sprayed, as in Chemical Mace, it is extremely irritating to the eyes and skin. Employed as a tear gas, CN disables its victims by causing strong smarting of the eyes, copious tearing and blepharospasm. These effects are usually gone within an hour after exposure is ended, with no residual injury. However, in numerous instances, when eyes have been grossly contaminated with CN from tear gas pistols at short range, permanent corneal opacification and scarring have resulted. Less severe injuries have been produced by sprays of CN in pressurized solvent at close range. (For more clinical information, see INDEX for *Tear gas weapons.*)

Experimental comparisons of the irritant lacrimogenic effects of CN vapor in human beings, rabbits, dogs, rats, mice, and guinea pigs, and comparison with other irritant substances, have been reported by several investigators.[a,g,46,61,204,205] Experimental exposure of dogs and rabbits to high concentrations of vapor has caused permanent opacification and ulceration of the corneas.[46,61]

For experimental studies on the toxic action of CN on the cornea in rabbits, the following procedures is convenient for producing standard lesions.[81] Impregnated discs of filter paper 6 mm in diameter are prepared by dipping in a 10% solution of CN in ether, and allowing the ether to evaporate. When a disc prepared in this way is applied to the vertex of the cornea for two minutes it produces a permanent gray central opacity. A similar procedure has been used by Macrae et al, employing a 9 × 9 mm square of filter paper impregnated with various amounts of CN in 1,1,1-trichloroethane.[e] This is applied to the rabbit eyes for ten minutes, and kept moistened during that time by small additions of solvent minute by minute. A different procedure for studying corneal injuries has been employed by Bleckmann and Sommer, applying 4 µl of a solution of CN in 1,1,1-trichloroethane to the cornea with a micropipette.[b] The severity of injury is dose-related. Pfannkuch and Bleckmann have described the histology in detail, noting at 21 days after exposure a granulation reaction, necrosis, and ulceration of the cornea.[f] When the solution is placed at the limbus the reaction is worse than when applied to the center of the cornea.

The same exposure methods could be used if one were searching for an effective antidote to the injurious action of CN. At present there is none, and the best available treatment probably is immediate irrigation with water.

CN action on the eye very likely has two parts, one a lacrimogenic, reversible and essentially noninjurious stimulatory effect on corneal nerve endings at low concentrations, the other an injurious, denaturing, difficultly-reversible reaction probably with other components of cornea and conjunctiva occurring at high concentrations. It is this type of reaction for which an antidote would be important.

An indication that sensory stimulation and tissue injury represent separate reactions is given by observations by Jancso and associates in 1968 that toxic effects of CN on the eye, measured by hyperemia of the conjunctiva and increased permeability of vessels of conjunctiva and lids, are not blocked by local anesthesia.[d]

Ballantyne has shown that exposure of rabbit eyes to CN can cause a transient doubling of intraocular pressure, but it is not known how this relates to the human eye.[a,276]

Seeking a biochemical explanation for lacrimatory stimulation of corneal nerves, and an explanation for the rapid reversibility of the lacrimogenic effect, Castro in 1968 studied the reaction of CN with cholinesterase *in vitro*.[c] Castro provided evidence that chloroacetophenone can inhibit cholinesterase by reacting rapidly with a non-sulfhydryl group, and showed that this reaction is readily reversible, whereas alkylating reaction with sulfhydryl groups generally produces very stable bonds. No evidence has been obtained that cholinesterase itself is involved in lacrimogenic stimulation of the cornea, but this provides an example of types of reactions which could be involved. The injurious reaction presumably involves formation of relatively stable bonds with tissue components. (For additional information, see INDEX for *Lacrimatory action,* and for more clinical observations see *Tear gas weapons.*)

a. Ballantyne B, et al: The comparative ophthalmic toxicology of 1-chloroacetophenone (CN) and dibenz(b.f)-1:4-oxazepine (CR). *ARCH TOXICOL (BERL)* 34:183–201, 1975.

b. Bleckmann H, Sommer C: Corneal damage by chloroacetophenone. *GRAEFES ARCH OPHTHALMOL* 216:61–67, 1981. (German)

c. Castro JA: Effects of alkylating agents on human plasma cholinesterase. *BIOCHEM PHARMACOL* 17:295–303, 1968.

d. Jancso N, Jancso-Gabor A, Szolcsanyi J: The role of sensory nerve endings in neurogenic inflammation induced in human skin and in the eye and paw of the rat. *BR J PHARMACOL* 33:32–41, 1968.

e. Macrae WG, Willinsky MD, Basu PK: Corneal injury produced by aerosol irritant projectors. *CAN J OPHTHALMOL* 5:3–11, 1970.

f. Pfannkuch F, Bleckmann H: Morphologic findings in the rabbit cornea after tear gas burn. *GRAEFES ARCH OPHTHALMOL* 218:177–184, 1982. (German)

g. Thatcher DB, Blaug SM, et al: Ocular effects of chemical Mace in the rabbit. *CLIN MED* 78:11–13, 1971.

1-Chloro-amitriptyline, an experimental drug, when administered to albino rats for several weeks caused abnormally large accumulation of phospholipid inclusions in retinal ganglion cells and pigment epithelium.[348] (For comparable effects from other compounds, see INDEX for *Lipidosis*.)

o-Chlorobenzylidene malononitrile (o-chlorobenzalmalonitrile, CS), a riot control agent, when dispersed in the air is a powerful sternutator and lacrimator. Although loosely spoken of as a tear gas, this agent is not a gas, but a crystalline powder that is dispersed as a cloud of finely divided particles by means of blowers, explosives, aerosol sprays, or by burning a mixture of the powder and some fuel.[a] It is said that though this agent immediately causes extremely disabling irritation of eyes and respiratory passages when used as a riot control agent, it has not been held responsible for human deaths, and it is calculated that a lethal amount for a man would be some 2,600 as great as required to cause temporary disabling.[a]

Human volunteers in a test exposure chamber have found concentrations greater than 10 mg/cu m of air to be extremely irritating, intolerable for more than thirty seconds owing to burning and pain in the eyes and in the chest, but irritation of the eyes spontaneously disappeared within an hour after removal to fresh air, and the respiratory effects disappeared within a few minutes.[h] The size of particles of the agent in air influenced the amount of irritation produced. Human volunteers experienced greater ocular and respiratory irritation from 0.9μ than from 60μ particles. However, with the larger particles the ocular irritation predominated and required a longer recovery time than with the smaller particles.[g]

Although human volunteers exposed to concentrations higher than 5 mg/cu m have found irritation of the eyes so intense that they could not keep their eyes open for even a few seconds, their visual acuity was found to be normal within a few minutes after exposure was terminated.[j]

Series of tests and dose-response studies of CS on rabbit, rat, guinea pig and human eyes have been made, with the material variously in the form of an aerosol, solid, or in different solvents, and comparisons have been made with CN (chloroacetophenone).[c–f,k,l] In essence these tests have shown the human eye to be many times more sensitive than rabbit or guinea pig to the irritating effect of CS (based on lowest concentration causing blepharospasm). The irritating effect of CS has been shown to be several times greater than that of CN, yet CS is significantly less injurious to the eyes. CS, even with extreme exposures, has mainly caused superficial reversible injuries. When CS is applied in a solvent, its effect on the cornea is very much influenced by the nature of the solvent, less injury resulting from solutions in trichloroethane or tri(2-ethylhexyl)phosphate than in methylene dichloride, corn oil, or polyethylene glycol 300. Hydrolysis products of CS, o-chlorobenzaldehyde and malononitrile, are much less irritating than CS itself.[c] A small transitory rise of intraocular pressure is produced in rabbits by CS.[276]

(Also see INDEX for *Tear gas weapons.*)

a. Anonymous: Characteristics of riot-control agent CS. *ORDNANCE* 52:286, 1968.
b. Ayers KM: Experimental injuries of the eye caused by a tear gas pen gun loaded with ortho-chlorobenzalmalononitrile. *J FORENSIC SCI* 17:547–554, 1972.
c. Ballantyne B, Gazzard MF, et al: Ophthalmic toxicology of o-chlorobenzylidene malononitrile (CS). *ARCH TOXICOL* 32:149–168, 1974.
d. Ballantyne B, Swanston DW: The irritant potential of dilute solutions of ortho chlorobenzylidene malononitrile (CS) on the eye and tongue. *ACTA PHARMACOL TOXICOL* 32:266–277, 1973.
e. Gaskins JR, Hehir RM, et al: Acute effects of chloroacetophenone and o-chloro-benzylidenemalonitrile in rats and rabbits. *TOXICOL APPL PHARMACOL* 17:295, 1970.
f. Gaskins JR, Hehir RM, et al: Lacrimating agents CS and CN in rats and rabbits. *ARCH ENVIRON HEALTH* 24:449–454, 1972.
g. Owens EJ, Punte CL: Human respiratory and ocular irritation studies utilizing o-chlorobenzylidenemalonitrile aerosols. *AM IND HYG ASSOC J* 24:262–264, 1963.
h. Punte CL, Owens EJ, Gutentag PJ: Controlled human exposures to (ortho-) Chloro-benzylidene malononitrile. *ARCH ENVIRON HEALTH* 6:366, 1963.
j. Rengstorff RH: The effects of the riot control agent CS on visual acuity. *MIL MED* 134:219–221, 1969.
k. Rengstorff RH, et al: CS(o-chlorobenzylidene malononitrile) in water. *MIL MED* 136:146–148, 149–151, 1971.
l. Rengstorff RH, Mershon MM: CS in trioctyl phosphate: effects on human eyes. *MIL MED* 136:152–153, 1971.

Chlorobromomethane (CB, methylene chlorobromide, chloromethyl bromide) under pressure is a liquid, but at atmospheric pressures and temperatures is a heavy vapor. This compound has been employed as a fire extinguisher, usually in a metal cylinder with dichlorodifluoromethane (Freon) added to increase the pressure.

The cornea was injured in one instance in which a fire extinguisher of this kind was discharged close to a person's face.[81] The victim felt the spray of liquid and vapor hit his face and eyes, causing immediate severe burning sensation in the eyes. Soon thereafter a partial loss of corneal epithelium was observed, but the deeper layers of the cornea remained clear. The conjunctivae and lids were hyperemic and edematous. Discomfort and photophobia gradually subsided in the course of three days, and the eyes returned to normal as the corneal epithelium healed. There was no direct injury of the skin and no irritation of the respiratory passages.

Experimental exposure of rabbit eyes to a spray of liquid from a fire extinguisher containing a mixture of 75% chlorobromomethane plus 25% dichlorodifluoromethane caused transient corneal epithelial injury and conjunctival edema similar to that seen in the patient.[81]

1-Chloro-3-bromopropene-1 (CBP) at a concentration of 3 ppm in air causes ocular pain and blepharospasm in human beings exposed for several minutes. This discomfort forces the subject to discontinue exposure before injury can occur. Tests of the liquid on rabbit corneas have shown that it is capable of causing injury as severe as that caused by ammonium hydroxide.[a]

    a. Hine CH, Anderson HH, et al: Toxicology and safe handling of CBP-55 (technical 1-chloro-3-bromopropene-1). *ARCH IND HYG OCCUP MED* 7:118–136, 1953.

Chlorobutanol (Chlorbutol, Chloretone) is a colorless, crystalline substance, having odor and taste like camphor, formerly used internally as a sedative and hypnotic.[171] Chlorobutanol has been widely employed as a preservative in eyedrops, usually in 0.5% concentration, without producing clinically significant ocular disturbance.[314] However, certain precautions in use of chlorobutanol in eyedrops are necessary. Hydrolysis destroys chlorobutanol in alkaline solution. It is usually employed in solution at pH 5 or lower, which is stable for at least many months. However, if unbuffered solutions are autoclaved, or allowed to stand at room temperature for several years, the pH may drop to as low as pH 2.4. Furthermore, although fresh solutions containing 0.5% chlorobutanol are quite satisfactory and innocuous for the brief applications involved in the ordinary use of eyedrops, they appear to be unsuited for prolonged bathing of the outer surface of the cornea.

When solutions containing 1.4% sodium chloride and 0.4% chlorobutanol have been employed in gonioscopy under the contact lens and this has been left on the eye for several minutes, in several patients an uncomfortable keratitis epithelialis has resulted, with fogging of vision, haloes around lights, and foreign-body type of discomfort beginning within the hour and becoming worse for several hours after the exposure.[81] Fortunately, in all such instances the eyes have recovered spontaneously and completely in a day to two.

Experiments on rabbits have established that after application of a drop of a standard local anesthetic such as 0.5% tetracaine or proparacaine hydrochloride, bathing the eyes continuously for twenty minutes with aqueous solutions containing 1.4% sodium chloride and 0.4% chlorobutanol produces definite keratitis epithelialis, which can be seen without magnification as a slight superficial haze in the cornea. The corneal epithelium becomes diffusely stainable with fluorescein, and under magnification has a ground-glass appearance. Freshly prepared solution at pH 5.5 has caused visible keratitis epithelialis after five to ten minutes of bathing. A solution which had been autoclaved, and had pH 2.7, induced grossly evident disturbance of the corneal epithelium within three to five minutes. Control experiments in which rabbit eyes were anesthetized in the same way and were bathed for twenty minutes with a simple 1.4% solution of sodium chloride in water caused no disturbance of the cornea detectable grossly, under magnification, or by staining with fluorescein.

Experiments on excised animal corneas have shown that chlorobutanol inhibits oxygen uptake,[108] interferes with the temperature reversal effect,[383] and reduces epithelial cohesion[285] and adhesion of epithelium to the corneal stroma.[107]

How much damage solutions containing chlorobutanol would produce if accidentally introduced into the anterior chamber has not been adequately evaluated. (Compare the damaging effects of other preservatives in the anterior chamber, e.g., *Benzyl alcohol* and *Chlorocresol.*)

Chlorocresol (p-chlorometacresol) was formerly utilized as a preservative and antifungal agent in eyedrops, but since it has been shown that a 0.05% solution in saline injected into the anterior chamber of a rabbit's eye causes the cornea to become opaque, this use is no longer authorized in Great Britain.[a,b,248] (Compare the injurious effect of the preservative *Benzyl alcohol* in the anterior chamber.)

    a. Cromopton DO, Anderson KF: Chlorocresol in eyedrops. *LANCET* 2:1279, 1963.
    b. Notes and News: Deletion of chlorocresol from formulae of eyedrops. *LANCET* 2:1287, 1963.

2-Chloroethanol (ethylene chlorohydrin) is a poisonous liquid which may be absorbed through the skin, the gastrointestinal tract, or by inhalation. The vapor is not sufficiently irritating to eyes and respiratory mucous membranes to prevent serious systemic poisoning.[b] In cats, poisoning is attended by temporary sluggish reaction of the pupil to light, and by nystagmus.[61] Men surviving exposure to toxic concentrations have had burning sensation in the eyes and nose, and numbness of the hands and fingers. Serious and sometimes fatal poisoning involves the nervous, hepatic, renal, and vascular systems, but no permanent ocular disturbances have been reported in survivors.[a]

Application of the undiluted liquid to eyes of rabbits caused transient clouding of the cornea, but 24 hours later the cornea appeared normal, despite some iritis and increasing conjunctival hyperemia and edema that took a week to subside.[e] Human corneal burns from a splash have been known to recover promptly, usually in forty-eight hours.[61,165] The highest non-damaging concentrations of aqueous solutions applied to eyes of rabbits were 1 to 2% as a drop every 10 minutes for 6 hours, or 10% as a drop 5 times a day for 21 days, or 10% as a single drop.[c,e,f] Aqueous solutions injected into the anterior chamber of rabbit eyes daily for 5 days at concentrations from 1% to 20% produced iritis, and corneal opacification at the high concentration.[c,d] At 10% and 20% concentration there was also cataract and rupture of the lens.[c,d] Maximum non-toxic intraocular concentration appears to be 0.5%. This is of special interest because when *ethylene oxide* is used for gas sterilization 2-chloroethanol is sometimes formed as a reaction product, and may gain access to the anterior chamber in contaminated solutions or plastic devices.

    a. Bush AF, Abrams HK, Brown HB: Fatality and illness caused by ethylene chlorohydrin in an agricultural occupation. *J IND HYG* 31:352, 1949.
    b. Goldblatt MW, Chiesman WE: Toxic effects of ethylene chlorohydrin. I. Clinical. *BR J IND MED* 1:207–223, 1944.
    c. McDonald TO, Roberts MD, Borgmann AR: Ocular toxicity of ethylene chlorohydrin and ethylene glycol in rabbit eyes. *TOXICOL APPL PHARMACOL* 21:143–150, 1972.

d. Alfieri G, Alfieri-Rolla G: On the ocular toxicity of ethylene chlorohydrin. *ARCH RASS ITAL OTTALMOL* 3:169–182, 1973. (Italian)

e. Guess WL: Tissue reactions to 2-chloroethanol in rabbits. *TOXICOL APPL PHARMACOL* 16:382–390, 1970.

f. McDonald TO, Kasten K, et al: Acute ocular toxicity for normal and irritated rabbit eyes and subacute ocular toxicity for ethylene oxide, ethylene chlorohydrin and ethylene glycol. *BULL PARENTER DRUG ASSOC* 31:25–32, 1977.

2-Chloroethyl isocyanate caused severe irritation of the rabbit eye when as little as 5 microliters was applied, and corneal clouding took 14 or more days to clear.[a]

a. Hofmann A, Neufelder M: Animal experimental investigation for evaluation of the industrial toxicology of 2-chloroethylisocyanate. *ARCH TOXICOL* 29:73, 1972. (German)

Chloroform has been used as a solvent and inhalation anesthetic.[171] Splash of liquid chloroform in the eyes causes immediate burning pain, tearing, and reddening of the conjunctiva. The corneal epithelium is usually injured and may be partially lost. However, regeneration is prompt, and as a rule the eye returns to normal in one to three days.[a, b, 46, 153, 253] Splash of a mixture of chloroform and methyl alcohol in the eye in one laboratory worker similarly caused no serious permanent injury.[81]

Intravitreal injection of a mixture of chloroform and methyl alcohol (2:1) in rats damaged the endothelial cells of the retinal vessels and rendered the vessels permeable to colloidal carbon.[c]

a. Duprat P, Delsaut L, Gradiski D: Irritant power of the principal aliphatic chlorinated solvents on rabbit skin and ocular mucosa. *EUR J TOXICOL ENVIRON HYG* 9:171–177, 1976. (French)

b. Torkelson TR, Oyen F, Rowe VK: The toxicity of chloroform as determined by single and repeated exposure of laboratory animals. *J AM IND HYG ASSOC* 37:697–705, 1976.

c. Cunha-Vaz JG: Studies on the permeability of the blood-retinal barrier. *BR J OPHTHALMOL* 50:454–462, 1966.

Chloroformic acid esters, as follows, have irritant lacrimogenic vapors:

Chloroformic acid ethyl ester (ethyl chloroformate, ethyl chlorocarbonate).[73]
Chloroformic acid methyl ester (methyl chloroformate, methyl chlorocarbonate).[171]
Chloroformic acid monochloromethyl ester (chloromethyl chloroformate, Palite), employed as a war gas.[46, 155]
Chloroformic acid trichloromethyl ester.[155]
Chloroformic acid propyl ester (propyl chloroformate, propyl chlorocarbonate).[171]

p-Chloromercuribenzene sulfonate has been reported to react primarily with the sulfhydryl groups of surface membranes. It has been used as a selective sulfhydryl reagent in study of biochemistry of the lens, where it was found to interfere with cation transport, without necessarily affecting glutathione content, and without entering lens fibers.[b] In the anterior chamber of enucleated eyes, both p-chloromercuribenzene sulfonate and p-chloromercuribenzoate caused decrease in facility of aqueous outflow (measured by quantitative aqueous perfusion), associated with swelling of cells of the trabecular meshwork found histologically.

a. Freddo TF, Patterson MM, et al: Influence of mercurial sulfhydryl agents on aqueous outflow pathways in enucleated eyes. *INVEST OPHTHALMOL VIS SCI* 25:278–285, 1984.

b. Fukui HN, Epstein DL: Effect of p-chloromercuribenzene sulfonate on lens cation transport. *OPHTHALMIC RES* 10:41–46, 1978.

p-Chloromercuribenzoate (PCMB) has been tested for possible toxic effect on the retina after administration systemically to rabbits. Some investigators have found no alteration of the ERG and no injury,[179,231] but Setogawa has reported an early depression of the ERG.[a] *In vitro* this compound is very toxic to the retina, causing histologic and metabolic disturbances of retinas of both rabbits and rats at a concentration of 0.05 mM.[157] Because of this disparity between slight toxic effect on the retina from systemic administration and high toxicity *in vitro,* Tieri and associates sought to break down the blood-retina barrier to allow greater penetration from the circulation to the retina in rabbits. They did this by injecting sodium chloride solution or glycerol into the vitreous humor close to the retina, and then gave PCMB intravenously. This was successful in inducing intense edema of the retina, which gradually absorbed, leaving areas of chorioretinal atrophy and pigment clumping.[b]

For effects on aqueous outflow, see *p-Chloromercuribenzene sulfonate.*

a. Setogawa T: ERG of experimental pigmentary degeneration of the retina. *YONAGO ACTA MED* 11:262–269, 1967. (ZENTRALBL GES OPHTHALMOL 101:152, 1969.)

b. Tieri O, Benusiglio M, et al: Clearly harmful action of sodium p-chloromercuribenzoate on the retina. *BOLL SOC ITAL BIOL SPER* 43:1119–1121, 1967. (Italian)

p-Chlorophenylalanine (parachlorophenylalanine), a phenylalanine antimetabolite, has been found to produce cataracts when injected subcutaneously or fed to very young rats. These cataracts have persisted after the injections were discontinued.[a,b,d-f] Feeding phenylalanine has a partially protective effect.[a,f] In some rats the cataracts were found to develop several months after administration of p-chlorophenylalanine was stopped.[f] Radioactive carbon-labeled compound was found to accumulate markedly in lenses of rats and rabbits.[e] Cataractous lenses were found to be deficient in most amino acids, leading to a suggestion that the cataract might be due to interference with entry of amino acids into the lens or to the aqueous humor from the ciliary body.[e,f] Some species peculiarity was suggested by a finding that monkeys given p-chlorophenylalanine daily for a year developed no abnormalities in their eyes.[a]

The optic nerves of newborn rats given p-chlorophenylalanine plus phenylalanine daily showed increased neurological activity at 20 days of life, but much later, after treatment was stopped, showed continuing gliosis, focal abnormal myelination, and axonal degeneration.[c] This was of particular interest because of possible relationship to the abnormality of myelination in the central nervous system known to occur in human congenital phenylketonuria.

a. Gralla EJ, Rubin L: Ocular studies with parachlorophenylalanine in rats and monkeys. *ARCH OPHTHALMOL* 83:734–740, 1970.

b. Watt DD, Martin PR: Phenylalanine antimetabolite effect on development. *LIFE SCI* 8:1211–1222, 1969.

c. Avins L, Guroff G, Kuwabara T: Ultrastructural changes in rat optic nerve associated with hyperphenylalaninemia induced by parachlorophenylalanine and phenylalanine. *J NEUROPATHOL EXP NEUROL* 34:178–188, 1975.

d. Brown WJ, Schalock RL, Gunter RG: The effect of parachlorophenylalanine on lens ultrastructure. *EXP EYE RES* 17:231–244, 1973.

e. Mollmann H, Knoch H, et al: A study of the pathogenesis of cataracts from p-chlorophenylalanine administration. *KLIN MONATSBL AUGENHEILKD* 158:681–684, 1971. (German)

f. Rowe VD, Zigler S, et al: Some characteristics of the p-chlorophenylalanine-induced cataract. *EXP EYE RES* 17:245–250, 1973.

Chloropicrin (trichloronitromethane) is a liquid, having extremely irritating vapors. It has been used both as a war gas and as a fumigant. At a concentration of 1 ppm in air it causes lacrimation and smarting pain in the eyes.[56] It is also severely irritating to the respiratory passages and has toxicity comparable to that of chlorine.

Chloropropionic acid esters have been described by Lohs as having vapors with irritating lacrimogenic effect on the eyes and intense effect on the skin Toxicity is greatest when the chlorine is in the beta position, considerably less when in the alpha position.[155]

Chloroquine diphosphate (Aralen, Resochin), *Chloroquine sulfate* (Nivaquine) and *Hydroxychloroquine sulfate* (Plaquenil) are quinoline derivatives used as anti-malarials and in treating rheumatoid arthritis and lupus erythematosis. Chronic administration of chloroquine can produce deposits in the cornea that are visible biomicroscopically, but of no consequence, and a retinopathy that can seriously affect vision if certain dosage limits are exceeded. More than two hundred reports on these and other toxic effects of chloroquine on the eye have been published since 1960, and these effects have become widely known. Several comprehensive reviews and bibliographies have been published concerning effects of chloroquine on the eye. The present synopsis is intended to outline the principal features of more recent developments and to provide a selected bibliography of what has seemed to be the most significant publications.

This synopsis is to be presented in the following order: *(a) reviews of chloroquine toxicity, (b) early symptoms from chloroquine, (c) corneal deposits from chloroquine, (d) retinopathy from chloroquine and methods utilized in attempting early detection, (e) extraordinary or bizarre ocular toxicity attributed to chloroquine,* and *(f) experimental studies on chloroquine effects on the eye.*

Toxic effects of drugs related to chloroquine are described under *Amodia-quin, Hydroxychloroquine,* and *Quinoline derivatives.* (See the INDEX for page numbers.)

(a) Reviews of the toxic effects of chloroquine on the eye that have provided extensive bibliographies on the subject have been published by Bernstein; Boke; Bregeat; Francois; Henkind; Meier-Ruge[356,357]; Nylander; Voipio; and one particularly comprehensive edited by Michiels.[356]

(b) Early visual complaints which have occurred in patients receiving 500 to 700 mg chloroquine diphosphate per day, which is two or three times the ordinary dosage, have consisted mainly of blur when reading and occasionally diplopia. The early complaint of blur has been thought to be due to transient increase in presbyopia in older people. These early complaints have regularly been reversible, according to Percival.

(c) Corneal deposits from chronic oral use of chloroquine have been known to do no harm and disappear gradually if the medication is discontinued or the dosage reduced. They are not considered a contraindication to continued use of the drug. Development of deposits in the cornea has no known relationship to occurrence of retinopathy. Usually the deposits in the corneas have produced no symptoms. Exceptionally, they have slightly reduced visual acuity. The deposits consist of myriads of fine white or yellowish dots in the epithelium, distributed particularly in the palpebral fissure, and often arranged in patterns of curved lines forming a fan or vortex. They do not disturb the surface of the epithelium. The deposits are said not to fluoresce in the cornea of patients when tested by clinical methods,[e] but in histological preparations under the microscope where they are seen as very fine particles within cells outside of the nucleus they are said to fluoresce strongly.[zv] Electron microscopy has shown these cytoplasmic inclusions to be of the same nature as those in Fabry's disease, or as produced by amiodarone and other cationic amphiphilic molecules. Chloroquine keratopathy has been categorized as a drug-induced phospholipidosis, which involves not only the cornea but also cells of a number of other organs of the body (Pulhorn; Seiber). The mechanism of formation of lysosomal inclusions in this condition has been especially well described by Seiler and associates in 1977.

The corneal deposits have also developed in people exposed to chloroquine dust (Eriksen).

(d) Retinopathy from chloroquine in human eyes from long time administration consists first of perifoveal change in granularity of the retinal pigment layer. An abnormal, finely granular appearance is recognizable ophthalmoscopically, best with the spot of light from the ophthalmoscope directed slightly to the side of the area being looked at, to show up the granular character of the pigment against a pink glow of choroidal background. At about the same time, subtle changes in paracentral retinal function are demonstrable, while central visual acuity may still be entirely normal. Later, a bull's-eye pattern of thinning and clumping of retinal pigment in the macular area around the fovea becomes more obvious. This is usually associated with an annular scotoma within 2° or 3° from fixation. The rods and cones are destroyed in this area, but the cones tend to survive longer at the fovea. Central vision is lost if damage is allowed to progress. Changes in peripheral visual fields and peripheral pigmentation are generally considered to be of later development. Also narrowing of retinal arteries is generally considered to be a secondary late effect, appearing in some cases, and not an early or primary effect. Pallor of the optic disc has often been mentioned as part of the late phase, and this appears to correspond to electron microscopic evidence of death of some of the

retinal ganglion cells and their optic nerve fibers. However, conspicuous whitening of the optic disc has not been characteristic.

The most insidious aspect of the chloroquine retinopathy is the fact that it can seriously injure the retina around the fovea with the patient unaware until it is too late, because his central visual acuity in a small central area may remain good while severe damage is being done to the surrounding area. When eventually this process involves the central area, central vision is irreversibly lost. Patients occasionally have clues to loss of paracentral vision from difficulty in keeping their place in reading a line of print, or in tripping over objects they fail to see, or in having difficulties in automobile driving through failing to be aware of objects very slightly out of the line of direct vision.

When retinopathy is recognized early and chloroquine is discontinued, in most cases the vision that has been lost is not recovered, but in a small proportion of cases there has been significant recovery. In a particularly unfortunate small proportion, loss of vision has been progressive despite discontinuing the medication. In several instances chloroquine retinopathy is reported to have appeared and developed years after chloroquine was no longer being taken (Burns; Nasu; Ogawa; Sassani).

The dosage of chloroquine appears to be the most fundamentally important factor determining the risk of development of retinopathy. In general it appears that serious retinopathy in nearly all instances has been caused by taking more than 250 mg of chloroquine phosphate or 200 mg of chloroquine sulfate per day to a total amount greater than 100 g of chloroquine base (Marks). By not exceeding this daily dosage it has been found possible for patients to take chloroquine for as long as nine years without developing clinically evident retinopathy. In most cases in which dosage slightly greater than 250 mg chloroquine phosphate per day has been administered, the onset of definite retinopathy has taken one to three years. According to Nylander,[zs] most patients who have developed retinopathy have received nearly a total of 300 g during three or more years.

According to Carr and associates,[r] all patients who receive more than the standard supposedly safe daily doses of chloroquine phosphate (250 mg) or of hydroxychloroquine sulfate (200 mg), if given the drugs at high enough levels for a long enough time, develop abnormalities of the retina, indicating that the retinopathy is a general toxic effect and not an idiosyncratic reaction.

In prophylaxis of malaria a considerably lower dose is prescribed than in treatment of collagen diseases, usually 300 mg once a week, and this was thought not to endanger the retina, and it presumably would be safe for 6 or 7 years. Unfortunately, there have been a number of instances of serious and unnecessary overdosage in prophylaxis of malaria, with severe retinopathy resulting.[ax] Several children have become nearly blind from this cause by age 7 or 8 years (Cordier).

The problems and methods of early detection of chloroquine retinopathy before serious and irreversible damage may be done have been reviewed by Crews.

Central visual field testing with red test objects, particularly testing the paracentral area 4° to 9° from fixation with a 7.5 mm red test object at 1 meter, has been shown by Percival to be one of the practical and effective means for early detection. Static perimetry and measurements of critical flicher fusion frequency have been recommended also on the basis of clinical trials (Hart; Alkhamis).

Color vision is known to become defective in association with chloroquine retinopathy, but apart from use of red test objects for central visual field testing, color vision tests have not been demonstrated to be a sufficiently sensitive or early indicator of beginning chloroquine retinal toxicity to be relied upon by themselves, according to a comprehensive study by Grutzner.[95] Others have concluded that color vision evaluation with the Farnsworth 100-hue test is helpful if repeated periodically and used in conjunction with visual field testing and electroretinography (Bec; Francois).

Electrodiagnostic measures, particularly electroretinography and electro-oculography, have received much attention in efforts to devise means for early detection of toxic effects of chloroquine on the retina before irreversible damage to vision occurs. Opinions on the practical value of these methods have varied widely. Some observers have felt that these methods were more sensitive than ophthalmoscopy and than functional visual tests (Babel; Francois), while others (Aklakha; Elenius), have pointed out cases in which retinopathy occurred without definite abnormality in ERG or EOG. Although a consensus is yet to be reached concerning the value of these methods, it appears that for fair evaluation these tests must be performed before treatment with chloroquine is started and periodically thereafter. The predominant tendency seems to be to regard the ERG and the EOG as adjuncts to ophthalmoscopy and evaluation of the visual field in early detection of retinopathy, but not to rely on them as the prime indicators of imminent retinopathy (Aklakha; Henkind; Kolb; Percival).

ERG induced by ultraviolet illumination of the eyes has been shown by Alfieri and Sole to be a means for demonstrating the presence of fluorescent materials such as chloroquine deposits in the retinal pigment epithelium in patients. Ultraviolet produces no ERG in normal people.

Fluorescein fundus angiography has been shown by Kearns and Hollenhorst to be a means for demonstrating dramatically the macula retinopathy of chloroquine, based on the fact that alterations of pigment in the pigment epithelium allow the choroidal fluorescence to show through in a characteristic manner. A comprehensive clinical study by Oosterhuis substantiated that migration and loss of perifoveal pigment increased the visibility of choroidal fluorescence, usually in a bull's eye pattern. However, these authors thought the procedure would not be useful for early detection of chloroquine retinopathy, because the pattern had a characteristic appearance only when retinopathy was fully developed.

Post mortem examination in patients with chloroquine retinopathy has shown destruction of rods and cones, with evidence of pigment migration from the retinal pigment epithelium to accumulate in cells in the nuclear and plexiform layers of the retina. The perifoveal region was particularly affected, with foveal cones appearing slightly more resistant to destruction (Bernstein; Wetterholm). Electron microscopy by Ramsey and Fine revealed that the retinal ganglion cells contained membranous cytoplasmic bodies resembling those of drug-induced phospholipidoses, and these were present also in the inner nuclear layer and inner segments of the photoreceptor cells.[at] Retinal lipidosis has also been induced in experimental animals (Drenckhahn).[304]

Efforts at treatment have so far had no clearly demonstrable beneficial effect on the retinopathy. Whether attempts to hasten release of chloroquine from deposits in body tissues may be advantageous or disadvantageous remains to be shown.

(e) Extraordinary or bizarre ocular effects that have been attributed to chloroquine include the following. Two children poisoned by overdosage during several days developed photophobia, with seeming reduction of visual acuity, but recovered when the medication was discontinued (Markowitz, Zabel). One child had light spots in the region of the macula which persisted and increased in number in subsequent months. Bilateral macula degeneration occurred in a man who took 625 mg per day for ten days (Paul). Isolated cases of unilateral optic neuritis with retinal exudates and hemorrhages (Agarwal), bilateral papilledema (Huismans), detachment of the retina (Begue), and anterior uveitis (Lazar), have been ascribed to chloroquine, but a relationship seems doubtful. In one noteworthy case the diagnosis of retinopathy was delayed because changes began in the periphery of the fundi, rather than in the macula region, and went undiscovered until fairly advanced (Lowes).

Congenital pigmentary retinopathy possibly due to chloroquine (Nivaquine) taken daily by the mother throughout pregnancy has been reported by Paufique.

Lens involvement seems rarely to have been related to medical use of chloroquine, although snowflake opacities in the anterior cortex were mentioned in two of the first cases of retinopathy described by Hobbs. Paufique and associates have described development of cataract in one patient on chloroquine. Experimentally in rats, opacities in the lens have been noted as part of a general phospholipidosis (Drenckhahn)[303].

(f) Animal experiments have shown that corneal lesions can be produced in rats by repeated parenteral injections or by subconjunctival administration, but with differences from those occurring in patients (Francois). In experimental animals retinopathy recognizable ophthalmoscopically or histologically has been produced by repeated administration in rats, cats, and rabbits (Babel; Francois; Hodgkinson; Ivanina; Meier-Ruge). Striking swelling of the retinal pigment epithelium has been described in rabbits and cats.[169] Histologically the retinal pigment epithelium appeared to most observers to be damaged first, then the rods and cones. Eventually, the visual cells, all layers of the retina, and the choroid became atrophic. Reinert and Rutty and others (Abraham; Gregory; Hodgkinson) reported evidence that the primary lesion was in retinal ganglion cells, and Gleiser and associates have reported retinal ganglion cell degeneration in swine without disturbance of rods, cones, or retinal pigment epithelium. Solze and McConnell found first ultrastructural changes in rats in the inner segments of receptor cells. Extensive reviews of experimental work have been published by Rubin (1968) and Meier-Ruge (1965, 1977[357]). In interpretation of ultrastructural changes shown by electron microscopy it has been difficult to assess the relationship between the formation of lysosomal inclusion or membranous cytoplasmic bodies of drug-induced phospholipidosis and actual damage to the cells involved. Inclusion bodies have been found especially in retinal ganglion cells (Ivanina; Klinghardt; Drenckhahn[304]). Perasalo and associates have reviewed particularly the controversies that have existed in interpretation of

ultrastructural changes induced in retinal pigment epithelium of animals by chloroquine, and their own experiments on lysosomal activity in albino rats.

ERG changes have been observed in chronically poisoned rats and in acutely poisoned rabbits without morphologic alterations in the retina, presumably representing functional disturbances of the pigment epithelium (Junemann; McConnell). Babel and Englert have, however, detected scattered histologic abnormalities by electron microscopy in rabbit retinas before changes in the ERG were demonstrable. ERG changes have been reported by Shearer and Cooper to appear at different rates and in different ways in rabbits, monkeys, and cats. They concluded that abnormality of the ERG was a sign of toxic effect on the retina that generally appeared before abnormalities were visible ophthalmoscopically. Berson has shown ERG changes from intravitreal injection in cats.

In monkeys the first studies on chloroquine ocular toxicity were reported in 1978 by Rosenthal and associates, presenting the results of administering the drug intramuscularly 5 times a week for as long as $4\frac{1}{2}$ years, at a dosage greater than that known to produce retinopathy in human beings. They found normal ophthalmoscopic appearance, fluorescein angiography, and ERG responses, but dramatic histologic changes. They believed what they had produced corresponded to an early phase in development of retinopathy in human beings. Early in the experiment they found morphologic changes in retinal ganglion cells and photoreceptors, with progression in later years in patchy degeneration of these cells, and lastly deterioration of pigment epithelium and choroid.

Chloroquine has been shown repeatedly to have a high affinity for melanin granules of the uveal tract, where a considerable concentration accumulates when chloroquine is given systemically, and remains stored for a very long time even after administration of the drug is discontinued (Bernstein; Lawwill; Potts; Ullberg). Accumulation in the pigment of the retinal pigment epithelium has seemed to many investigators probably to be an important factor in production of retinopathy (Meier-Ruge[357]). However, others disagree and point out that many other drugs and chemicals are stored by uveal melanin granules and do not produce retinopathy (Kuhn). A protective effect from melanin has even been suggested (Ivanina).

A comprehensive survey by Rubin of possible mechanisms involved at the molecular biochemical level in toxicity of chloroquine to the eye indicated that no special role had been demonstrated for the binding of chloroquine by melanin in the production of retinopathy. Rubin listed numerous biochemical actions of chloroquine other than binding to melanin, such as interference with formation of proteins, inhibition of a variety of enzymes, reaction with nucleic acids, and other effects, which may have a more important role in the toxicity of chloroquine than the binding to melanin. Evidence pro and con interference with retinal protein synthesis by chloroquine has been presented (Gonasun; Karlsson).

At this time, despite all the clinical and experimental data that have been collected, the fundamental mechanism for chloroquine retinopathy remains to be resolved.

Abraham R, Hendy RJ: Irreversible lysosomal damage induced by chloroquine in the retinae of pigmented and albino rats. *EXP MOL PATHOL* 12:185–200, 1970.

Agarwal RC: An unusual finding in a patient undergoing chloroquine therapy. *ORIENT ARCH OPHTHALMOL* 3:215–216, 1965.

Aklakha D, Crews SJ, et al: Electrodiagnosis in drug-induced disorders of the eye. *TRANS OPHTHALMOL SOC UK* 87:267–284, 1967.

Alfieri R, Sole P: On very short wavelength electroretinography. *OPHTHALMOLOGIC ADDIT AD* 158:661–668, 1969.

Al Khamis AR, Easterbrook M: Critical flicker fusion frequency in early chloroquine retinopathy. *CAN J OPHTHALMOL* 18:217–219, 1983.

Applemans M, Lebas, et al: Ocular changes in the course of treatment with synthetic antimalarials. *BULL SOC BELGE OPHTALMOL* 127–129:260–272, 1961.

Babel J, Englert U: Experimental study of retinopathy from chloroquine. *BULL SOC FRANC OPHTALMOL* 82:491–505, 1969. (French)

Babel J, Meyer E: Incidence and prevention of retinal lesions due to chloroquine. *SCHWEIZ MED WOCHENSCHR* 95:1125–1130, 1965.

Bec P, Belleville D, et al: Value of exploring chromatic sensitivity with Farnsworth 100 hue in detection of maculopathy from synthetic anti-malarials. *ANN OCULIST (Paris)* 210:291–296, 1977. (French)

Begue H, Negre L: Retinal detachment and synthetic antimalarials. *BULL SOC FRANC OPHTALMOL* 79:464–477, 1966. (French)

Bernstein HN: Chloroquine ocular toxicity. *SURVEY OPHTHALMOL* 12:415–447, 1967.

Bernstein HN, Ginsberg J: The pathology of chloroquine retinopathy. *ARCH OPHTHALMOL* 71:238–245, 1964.

Bernstein H, Zvaifler N, et al: The ocular deposition of chloroquine. *INVEST OPHTHALMOL* 2:384–391, 1963.

Berson EL: Acute toxic effects of chloroquine on the cat retina. *INVEST OPHTHALMOL* 9:618–628, 1970; 10:237–246, 1971.

Boke W, Baumer A, et al: On the question of chloroquine injury of the eye. *KLIN MONATSBL AUGENHEILKD* 151:617–633, 1967. (German)

Bregeat P, Grupper C, et al: Ocular complications of synthetic antimalarials. *ARCH OPHTALMOL (Paris)* 25:417–444, 1965. (French)

Burns RP: Delayed onset of chloroquine retinopathy. *N ENGL J MED* 275:693–696, 1966.

Carr RE, Henkind P, et al: Ocular toxicity of antimalarial drugs. *AM J OPHTHALMOL* 66:738–744, 1968.

Cordier C, Raspiller A, Lepori JC: Childhood form of chloroquine retinopathy. *BULL SOC OPHTALMOL FRANCE* 81:647–650, 1981. (French)

Crews SJ: Some aspects of retinal drug toxicity. *OPHTHALMOLOGICA* 158:232–244, 1969.

Elenius V, Mantyjarvi M: A case of chloroquine retinopathy examined by electro oculography. *ACTA OPHTHALMOL* 45:114–118, 1967.

Eriksen LS: Chloroquine keratopathy in chloroquine workers after topical dust exponation. *ACTA OPHTHALMOL* 57:823–825, 1979.

Francois J, DeBecker L: Ocular manifestations of chloroquine poisoning. *ANN OCULIST (Paris)* 198:513–544, 1965. (French)

Francois J, Maudgal MC: Experimental chloroquine keratopathy. *AM J OPHTHALMOL* 60:459–466, 1965.

Francois J, Maudgal MC: Experimentally induced chloroquine retinopathy in rabbits. *AM J OPHTHALMOL* 64:886–893, 1967.

Francois J, de Rouck A, et al: Chloroquine retinopathy. *OPHTHALMOLOGICA* 165:81–99, 1972.

Francois P, Constantinides G, et al: Signs of retinal disturbances requiring discontinuance of synthetic antimalarials. *BULL SOC FR OPHTALMOL* 86:158–163, 1973. (French)

Gleiser CA, Dukes TW, et al: Ocular changes in swine associated with chloroquine toxicity. *AM J OPHTHALMOL* 67:399–405, 1969.

Gonasun LM, Potts AM: In vitro inhibition of protien synthesis in the retinal pigment epithelium by chloroquine. *INVEST OPHTHALMOL* 13:107–115, 1974.

Gregory MH, Rutty DA, Wood DR: Differences in the retinotoxic action of chloroquine and phenothiazine derivatives. *J PATHOL* 102:139–150, 1970.

Hart Jr WM, Burde RM, et al: Static perimetry in chloroquine retinopathy. *ARCH OPHTHALMOL* 102:377–380, 1984.

Henkind P, Arden K, Kolb H: Screening test for chloroquine retinopathy. *LANCET* 2:40–41, 1964.

Henkind P, Carr RE, Siegel IM: Early chloroquine retinopathy: Clinical and functional findings. *ARCH OPHTHALMOL* 71:157–165, 1964.

Henkind P, Rothfield NF: Ocular abnormalities in patients treated with synthetic antimalarial drugs. *N ENGL J MED* 269:433–439, 1963.

Hobbs HE, Sorsby A, Freedman A: Retinopathy following chloroquine therapy. *LANCET* 2:478–480, 1959.

Hodgkinson BJ, Kolb H: A preliminary study of the effect of chloroquine on the rat retina. *ARCH OPHTHALMOL* 84:509–515, 1970.

Huismans H: Bilateral (toxic?) papilledema in chloroquine treatment for primary chronic polyarthritis. *KLIN MONATSBL AUGENHEILKD* 181:36–37, 1982. (German)

Ivanina TA, Zueva MB, et al: Ultrastructural alterations in rat and cat retina and pigment epithelium induced by chloroquine. *GRAEFES ARCH OPHTHALMOL* 220:32–38, 1983.

Junemann G, Schulze J: Electroretinographic studies on the development of quinine and chloroquine retinopathy. *KLIN MONATSBL AUGENHEILKD* 152:562–566, 1968. (German)

Karlsson JO, Stella-Giuffrida AM, et al: Action of chloroquine on in vivo RNA and protein biosynthesis in the retina and the optic pathway of the rabbit. *J NEUROL SCI* 30:237–245, 1976.

Kearns TP, Hollenhorst RW: Chloroquine retinopathy: Evaluation by fluorescein fundus angiography. *TRANS AM OPHTHALMOL SOC* 64:217–231, 1966; and *ARCH OPHTHALMOL* 76:378–384, 1966.

Klinghardt GW, Fredman P, Svennerholm L: Chloroquine intoxication induces ganglioside storage in nervous tissue. *J NEUROCHEM* 37:897–908, 1981.

Kolb H: Electro-oculogram findings in patients treated with antimalarial drugs. *BR J OPHTHALMOL* 49:537–590, 1965.

Kuhn H, Keller P, et al: Lack of correlation between melanin affinity and retinopathy in mice and cats treated with chloroquine and flunitrazepam. *GRAEFE S ARCH KLIN EXP OPHTHALMOL* 216:177–190, 1981.

Lawill T, Appleton B, Altstatt L: Chloroquine accumulation in human eyes. *AM J OPHTHALMOL* 65:530–532, 1968.

Lazar M, Regenbogen L, Stein R: Anterior uveitis due to chloroquine. *OPHTHALMOLOGICA* 146:411–414, 1963.

Lowes M: Peripheral visual field restriction in chloroquine retinopathy. *ACTA OPHTHALMOL* 54:819–826, 1976.

Markowitz HA, McGinley JM: Chloroquine poisoning in a child. *J AM MED ASSOC* 189:950–951, 1964.

Marks JS: Chloroquine retinopathy: Is there a safe daily dose? *ANN RHEUM DIS* 41:52–58, 1982.

McConnell DG, Wachtel L, Havener WH: Observations on experimental chloroquine retinopathy. *ARCH OPHTHALMOL* 71:552–553, 1964.

Meier-Ruge W: Experimental investigation of the morphogenesis of chloroquine retinopathy. *ARCH OPHTHALMOL* 73:540–543, 1965.

Meier-Ruge W: Morphology of experimental chloroquine retinopathy in rabbits. *OPHTHALMOLOGICA* 150:127–137, 1965. (German)

Nasu K: Studies on drug-induced retinal degeneration. *ACTA SOC OPHTHALMOL JPN* 81:883, 1977.

Nylander U: Ocular damage in chloroquine therapy. *ACTA OPHTHALMOL (Suppl)* 92:5–71, 1967.

Ogawa S, Kurumatani N, et al: Progression of retinopathy long after cessation of chloroquine therapy. *LANCET* 1:1408, 1979.

Oosterhuis JA, Boen-Tan TN: Fluorescein fundus angiography in chloroquine retinopathy. *OPHTHALMOLOGICA ADDIT AD* 158:615–630, 1969.

Pau H: Chloroquine deposits in the cornea. *BER DTSCH OPHTHALMOL GESELLSCH* 62:285–294, 1959.

Paufique L, Magnard P: Retinal degeneration in two infants as a consequence of prophylactic antimalarial treatment of the mother during pregnancy. *BULL SOC OPHTALMOL FRANCE* 69:466–467, 1969. (French)

Paul SD: Chloroquine retinopathy. *ORIENT ARCH OPHTHALMOL* 4:244–247, 1966.

Perasalo R, Rechardt L, Palkama A: Chloroquine-induced ultrastructural changes in the pigment epithelium of the albino rat. *ACTA OPHTHALMOL SUPPL* 123:94–98; 99–102, 1974.

Percival SPB, Behrman J: Ophthalmological safety of chloroquine. *BR J OPHTHALMOL* 53:101–109, 1969.

Potts AM: Further studies concerning the accumulation of polycyclic compounds on uveal melanin. *INVEST OPHTHALMOL* 3:399–404, 1964.

Pulhorn G, Thiel HJ: The ultrastructural appearance of chloroquine keratopathy. *GRAEFE S ARCH KLIN EXP OPHTHALMOL* 201:89–99, 1976. (German)

Ramsey MS, Fine BS: Chloroquine toxicity in the human eye. *AM J OPHTHALMOL* 73:229–235, 1972.

Reinert H, Rutty DA: Mechanisms of chloroquine and phenothiazine retinopathies. *TOXICOL APPL PHARMACOL* 14:635–636, 1969.

Rosenthal AR, Kolb H, et al: Chloroquine retinopathy in the rhesus monkey. *INVEST OPHTHALMOL VIS SCI* 17:1158–1175, 1978.

Rubin M: The antimalarials and the tranquilizers. *DIS NERV SYST* 29 (Suppl):67–76, 1968.

Sassani JW, Brucker AJ, et al: Progressive chloroquine retinopathy. *ANN OPHTHALMOL* 15:19–22, 1983.

Seiler KU, Thiel HJ, Wassermann O: Chloroquine keratopathy as an example of drug-induced phospholipidosis. *KLIN MONATSBL AUGENHEILKD* 170:64–73, 1977. (German)

Shearer ACI, Cooper BE: The assessment of retinal function by electrophysiological techniques. In Pigott, P.V. (Ed.): *Evaluation of Drug Effects on the Eye.* London, F.J. Parsons, 1968.

Sole P, Alfieri R, Rouher F: New method of supervising patients under treatment with synthetic antimalarials: fluorescence electroretinography. *BULL SOC OPHTALMOL FRANCE* 69:316–325, 1969. (French)

Solze DA, McConnell DG: Ultrastructural changes in the rat photoreceptor inner segment during experimental chloroquine retinopathy. *OPHTHALMOL RES* 1:140–148, 1970.

Trojan HJ: Eye injury from long-term prophylaxis of malaria with chloroquine. *KLIN MONATSBL AUGENHEILKD* 180:232–236, 1982.

Ullberg S, Lindquist NG, Sjostrand SE: Accumulation of chorioretinotoxic drugs in the foetal eye. *NATURE* 227:1257–1258, 1970.

Voipio H: Incidence of chloroquine retinopathy. *ACTA OPHTHALMOL* 44:349–354, 1966.

Wetterholm DH, Winter FC: Histopathology of chloroquine retinal toxicity. *ARCH OPHTHALMOL* 71:82–87, 1964.

Zabel R: Vision disorders and depigmentation of hair of the head following an overdose of chloroquine diphosphate. *AESTHET MED* (Berlin) 17:107–110, 1968. (German)

Chlorosilanes are highly corrosive and hazardous. Tests by application of a drop to rabbit eyes have been made on tetrachlorosilane, dichlorodimethyl silane, dichlorodiethylsilane, methyl trichlorosilane, and ethyl trichlorosilane.[211] All the chlorosilanes were found to cause severe damage of the cornea and lids. More severe damage was caused by the alkychlorosilanes than by tetrachlorosilane (silicone tetrachloride). The principal danger is from splash contamination. No specific antidote is available, but first aid treatment consists of copious irrigation with water, and subsequent treatment is as for chemical burns in general.

Chlorosulfonic acid is an extremely caustic liquid which gives off fumes very irritating to the eyes and respiratory passages.[51] When dropped into water, it decomposes with explosive violence.[171] One patient accidentally dropped some into water and the resulting explosion sprayed his face, immediately veiling his vision and hampering respiration, but he was able to wash his eyes with water from a hose within a few seconds. Burns of the cornea and conjunctiva were restricted to the palpebral fissure. Burns of the lids were more severe. However, within two weeks the lids were healing well and the corneas had only tiny areas of unhealed epithelium with slight edema and occasional stroma vessels near the limbus inferiorly. Vision was returning to normal.[81] In this case the eyes presumably were saved by very speedy irrigation with water after the accident.

Chlorosulfonic acid ethyl ester and **Chlorosulfonic acid methyl ester** have been discussed by Lohs and described as lacrimators.[155]

Chlorothiazide (Diuril), a diuretic and antihypertensive, caused yellow vision in a woman receiving 0.5 gm per day for two-week periods each month for premenstrual edema.[a] She experienced episodes of seeing yellow spots against white backgrounds. These disappeared when chlorothiazide was discontinued, and returned when it was taken again several days later. This cycle was twice repeated. Vision and eyes were otherwise normal and the patient was not taking digitalis.

Acute one-sided oculomotor palsy with retrobulbar pain developed in a man who had glucose intolerance from use of chlorothiazide, with recovery when the drug was discontinued.[c]

Chlorothiazide also is reported to have induced acute myopia lasting a day or two, apparently similar to that induced by many other drugs, including acetazolamide and hydrochlorothiazide.[b] (See INDEX for *Myopia, acute transient.*)

A unique instance of coma and cortical blindness has been attributed to severe reactions to chlorothiazide in a boy who had been very ill from infancy with nephrogenic diabetes insipidus and was very retarded physically and mentally.[c]

In glaucoma no adverse nor beneficial effect has been established for chlorothiazide.

a. Post J: Yellow vision in a patient after taking chlorothiazide. *N ENGL J MED* 263:398–399, 1960.
b. Hermann MP: Spasmodic myopia in the course of diuretic treatment. *BULL SOC OPHTALMOL FRANCE* 63:719–723, 1963.
c. Miller NR, Moses H: Transient oculomotor nerve palsy associated with thiazide-induced glucose intolerance. *J AM MED ASSOC* 240:1887–1888, 1978.

Chlorpheniramine (Chlor-trimeton, Teldrin), an antihistaminic, appears rarely to affect the eyes when taken orally in ordinary dosage. In normal volunteers 8 to 12 mg chlorpheniramine maleate taken by mouth had no significant effect on pupils or accommodation.[81] One patient developed left-sided blepharospasm and dyskinesia of the left side of the face, which improved after chlorpheniramine was discontinued.[a]

a. Davis WA II: Dyskinesia associated with chronic antihistamine use. *N ENGL J MED* 294:113, 1976.

Chlorphentermine hydrochloride (Lucofen, Pre-State) is used as an appetite depressant, but it does not alter the flicker fusion frequency in normal patients in the manner of drugs having considerable central stimulatory effect.[219] It is said to produce slight mydriasis when given systemically and on this basis there has been apprehension about its use in glaucoma, but there have been no reports of precipitation or aggravation of angle-closure glaucoma, and it seems extremely unlikely that the drug would have adverse action in chronic open-angle glaucoma.[83] Although no disturbance of vision or changes in the lens have been noted in patients taking chlorphentermine, it is intriguing that in rats this drug, like several other amphiphilic cationic drugs and chemicals, causes striking accumulation of phospholipids in the retinal pigment epithelium, and also accumulation of inclusions in the epithelial cells of rat lenses, upsetting lipid metabolism and leading to subcapsular lens opacities[303, 348].

Chlorpromazine (Thorazine, Largactil, Megaphen), the first widely used psychotropic phenothiazine derivative, has been utilized mainly in treatment of schizophrenia. There are many reports of eye examinations in large series of patients chronically treated with chlorpromazine. Except for an unsettled question of possible rare retinopathy, there have been no fundamental differences among the findings reported in these numerous surveys. Several reviews of clinical findings have been published (Baron; Boet; DeLong; Francesconi; Kalberer; Mathalone; Mason[353]). All have agreed that when the total dosage of chlorpromazine has been large enough, characteristic deposits appear first in the lenses, then the corneas, and relatively rarely in the conjunctiva (Gerhard).

In the lenses, fine dust-like granular material becomes visible by slit-lamp biomicroscopy in the pupillary area beneath the anterior capsule. The granules vary from whitish to yellowish brown. Early, they are distributed in a small disc in the pupil but later develop a stellate pattern and appear deeper in the anterior cortex (Baron; Calluaud; Cuendet; Deluise; Elder; Gerhard; Klima). The deposits in some cases eventually become heavy enough to be observable by close inspection with a focused light without a microscope, but they very rarely interfere with vision. The fine, granular deposits in the lens can also be conveniently detected with a direct ophthalmoscope with +6D lens, with the examiner focusing his attention on the pupil rather than on the fundus. Years of accumulated evidence indicate that these granular deposits do not lead to formation of ordinary cataracts (Gerhard; Hesse). They might reasonably be called pseudo-cataracts (Gerhard). Naturally some patients taking chlorpromazine do develop real cataracts (Pouget; Setogawa), but there has been no evidence of an incidence any greater than in patients not taking the drug.

In rat lenses, in vitro, thymidine uptake by epithelial cells has increased when exposed to chlorpromazine and light (Jose), but what this might relate to clinically is obscure. The same may be said of an observation that, in vitro, interference with respiratory metabolism of the lens epithelium has been shown (Howard).

In the corneas, which are affected usually less often and later than the lenses, and as a rule only when the lens has already been affected, very fine granules appear at the posterior surface, apparently within the deepest layers of the stroma next to Descemet's membrane and endothelium (Elder; Gerhard). The granules are yellowish dots similar to those seen beneath the anterior lens capsule. They tend to occur principally in the palpebral fissure. They have not been injurious to the cornea and rarely have interfered with vision. In one patient Pouget reported enough granular material in cornea and lens to reduce visual acuity, but there was no cataract and no retinopathy (Pouget). (Subsequently, this report has been misquoted in the literature as having reported formation of cataract.)

In the cornea, in addition to the fine granular deposits deep in the stroma, less often fine pigmented streaks or swirling lines have been described in the corneal epithelium in the palpebral fissure. These epithelial changes have been noted in patients who have received the largest doses of chlorpromazine (DeLong; Johnson). They closely resemble the changes produced by chloroquine and amiodarone (Sizaret), and cause no harm (Prien).

The fine, granular deposits in lens, cornea, and conjunctiva have been supposed to be similar to deposits in the skin that have caused a grossly noticeable discoloration of the skin in some patients. The deposits in lens and corneal stroma seem to remain indefinitely after administration of chlorpromazine has been discontinued. However, the epithelial keratopathy behaves quite differently, and can disappear or diminish markedly after the drug is stopped (Prien).

The predominance of changes in the palpebral fissure and the association in some patients with photosensitization of the skin by chlorpromazine has suggested that exposure to light may be a factor in producing the deposits. In one patient who had drooping of one upper lid shading the eye the density of the anterior segment deposits was less on that side than on the other side with normal lids, suggesting that difference in exposure to light might have been a factor (Deluise). However, more evidence is needed. Lens opacities in guinea pigs resembling the granular deposits seen in patients have been reported by Howard and associates after administration of chlorpromazine daily for four to twelve months and exposure to ultraviolet, but in the same animals no changes appeared in cornea, conjunctiva, or retina. An attempt to produce deposits in corneas of rabbits by combining chronic administration of chlorpromazine and ultraviolet radiation has failed (Baum). Granular deposits have been produced in the corneas of dogs, in the cytoplasm of the stromal cells, (Rubin; Tousimis) but not in the lenses of dogs, by chronic administration of the drug, independent of amount of ultraviolet radiation (Baron[278]). In bovine corneas, in vitro, chlorpromazine has been shown to have an inhibitory influence on synthesis of glycosaminoglycans, independent of illumination (Cremer-Bartels). Rabbit corneas, in vitro, have shown increase in swelling rate and greater morphologic abnormalities when they were exposed to ultraviolet in addition to chlorpromazine, but to obtain these indications of injury a concentration a thousand times greater than encountered in patients was used, and it is questionable whether the findings are relevant to clinical conditions (Hull).

Because the location of most of the deposits that are seen clinically within the lens and the cornea border on the anterior chamber, it has seemed that the material gets there by way of the aqueous humor. There are good reasons to conclude that melanin and the iris are not involved in this process (Cuendet; Elder; Gerhard; Sizaret; Verrey).

Lens opacities of different type in mice, appearing within minutes after systemic administration of chlorpromazine and subsequently spontaneously reversible, have been described by several experimenters (Smith), the same as produced by numerous other drugs that reduce blinking or cause hypothermia, with no known relationship to opacities in human beings.

Rare instances of reduced visual acuity have been mentioned in association with chlorpromazine pigmentation of lens and cornea, for example one case by McClanahan, one by Wetterholm, on by Nouri, possibly several by Siddall, but in these cases the relationship to the medication or to the pigmentation has not been clearly demonstrated, and in some there have been questions of retinal abnormality. In Pouget's case there was clear relationship to medication and pigmentation, and no retinopathy.

The intraocular pressure has not been elevated by chlorpromazine. Occasional cases of glaucoma have been found among mental patients under treatment with chlorpromazine, but there has been no indication that glaucoma occurs in higher incidence than in untreated people. There have been reliable observations of temporary reduction of intraocular pressure in glaucomatous patients by chlorpromazine. There is no risk of inducing glaucoma from pupillary effect, since chlorpromazine causes slight but measureable miosis (Carlson[26]).

Pigmentary retinopathy in association with chlorpromazine medication has been looked for and has not been found in large series of patients (Cairns; Deluise; Elder; Forrest; Gerhard; Kalberer; Mathalone; McClanhan; Santamarina; Zinn and

Marmor[389]), but a small number of cases have been reported in which pigmentary disturbances in the fundi have been observed and suspected to be related to the medication. One great problem has been that many of the patients who have been under long-term treatment with chlorpromazine have also been treated with other phenothiazine psychotropic drugs (Boet; Henkes; Petrohelos; Zelickson), and some drugs, particularly thioridazine, are definitely established to produce pigmentary retinopathy when certain dose levels are exceeded. Furthermore, pigmentary disturbances in the fundi occur occasionally in people receiving no medications. With chlorpromazine alone the number of cases of pigmentary retinopathy reported has been so small that it has not been possible to prove that chlorpromazine itself has been responsible.

Retinal pigment disturbances in patients taking chlorpromazine have been mentioned in a small number of reports. Henkes reported that fifteen patients had fine pigment deep in the macula, but the patients had been taking promazine or perazine as well as chlorpromazine (Henkes). Nouri mentioned one patient who had pigmentary disturbance of both maculas and much reduced visual acuity among 225 patients surveyed without retinal disturbance; whether the medication was responsible was quite uncertain (Nouri). Petrohelos noted abnormal retinal pigmentation in six out of three hundred patients receiving chlorpromazine and other phenothiazine derivatives, but could not be sure that the pigmentation was different from that which occurs without medication in some patients.[r] Siddall in publications from 1965 to 1968 has mentioned four cases of granular pigmentary retinopathy which later became retinal depigmentation, with apparent attenuation of retinal vessels, also with reduced visual acuity and constricted visual fields in two of these cases, thought to have been caused by chlorpromazine (Siddall). Zelickson described in three cases a variety of pigment disturbances, either clumps of pigment in the periphery or at the posterior pole and depigmented spots at the posterior pole, but in addition to chlorpromazine one patient was receiving triflupromazine and another was receiving trifluoperazine; whether the medications actually were responsible was unproven (Zelickson). Klima described greyish-white dots in the macular region, but others have not reported seeing these (Klima).

Optic atrophy in one patient taking chlorpromazine has been described by Rab, but this case seems to remain unique.

To put the changes in lens and cornea and the possible changes in the retina in perspective, it seems important to reiterate that patients under long-term treatment with chlorpromazine rarely have disturbance of their vision (Gerhard).

Experimentally, the most intriguing finding in relation to possible effects on the retina has been the demonstration by Potts that chlorpromazine is avidly taken up and concentrated by pigment granules of the uvea, amply substantiated by other investigators (Cassano; Green; Lindquist; Mason[353]; Meier-Ruge[166]; Potts[201-203]). However, the significance of this affinity to the melanin granules of the uvea in relation to retinal function is still unclear, particularly in view of the fact that a number of other drugs similarly are taken up by the uveal melanin but have not been demonstrated to affect retinal function or morphology.

The electroretinogram in cats, sheep, rabbits (both albino and pigmented), dogs, and albino rats has shown a decrease in amplitude, particularly the amplitude of the b-wave, under the influence of chlorpromazine (Bornschein; Calissendorff; Jagadeesh; Legros). However, in patients taking the drug the electroretinogram only occasionally becomes abnormal, and seems to have no established clinical significance (Gerhard; Henkes). Similarly, the electro-oculogram is reported only occasionally to be abnormal in patients, with no recognized special significance (Gerhard; Mathalone). Visually evoked occipital potentials seem to have received relatively little attention in these patients, but instances of delay have been reported (Muller).

Histologic studies of the effect of chlorpromazine on the retina in experimental animals have given results that varied with species. In a minority of tested dogs, after 4 months of medication there were slight abnormalities consisting of intraretinal cystic formation suggestively associated with a suspected change in appearance of the fundi and slight decrease in amplitude of the ERG, but not really definitive (Legros). In albino and pigmented rats no histologic lesion was recognized, although in the albino rats the ERG amplitude was reduced (Legros).

In cats, dosage many times larger than human dosage produced abnormalities of the visual cells (Gregory).

Metabolites of chlorpromazine have been of interest with regard to deposits in the lens and cornea mentioned earlier, which some have speculated might come from drug metabolites. Acute tests by injection into the anterior chamber of rabbits have shown the cornea to be severely injured by *2,3-dihydroxypromazine* and *7,8-dihydroxychlorpromazine*, less severely by *7-hydroxychlorpromazine* and *8-hydroxychlorpromazine*, while no significant change in corneal transparency were produced by chlorpromazine itself, *chlorpromazine sulfoxide, 7-methoxychlorpromazine, promazine, 2-hydroxypromazine*, or *3-hydroxypromazine* (Adams). The acute changes produced by some of the hydroxy-derivatives are quite different from the slowly developing chronic changes in the cornea observed clinically from chlorpromazine.

As a final, miscellaneous item, a Thorazine spansule placed in the conjunctival sac by a psychotic patient caused very severe injury to the eye; the component responsible was not identified (Eichenbaum).

Adams HR, Manian AA, et al: Effects of promazine and chlorpromazine metabolites on the cornea. *ADV BIOCHEM PSYCHOPHARMACOL* 9:281–293, 1974.

Baron JB, Morel P, et al: Ocular side effects of prolonged treatment with chlorpromazine associated or not with skin complications. *AGRESSOLOGIE* 9:293–304, 1968.

Baron JB, Morel P, Rivoalan Y: Long term evolution of the lens opacities induced by chlorpromazine prolonged therapy. *AGRESSOLOGIE* 12:57–60, 1971.

Baum JL; The effect of chloroquine, chlorpromazine and ultraviolet radiation on the corneas of pigmented rabbits. *ACTA OPHTHALMOL* 50:18–25, 1972.

Boet DJ; Toxic effects of phenothiazines on the eye. *DOC OPHTHALMOL* 28:1–69, 1970.

Bornschein H, Heiss WD, et al: The action of chlorpromazine on the retinal system. *WIEN Z NERVENHEILKD* 25:137–142, 1967. (German)

Cairns RJ, Capoore H, Gregory I: Oculocutaneous changes after years on high doses of chlorpromazine. *LANCET* 1:239–241, 1965.

Calissendorff B: Melanotropic drugs and retinal functions. *ACTA OPHTHALMOL* 54:118–128, 1976.

Calluaud JL, DiBattista JC, et al: Ocular pigmentation and phenothiazine derivatives. *BULL SOC OPHTHALMOL FRANCE* 77:661–664, 1977.

Cassano GB, Sjostrand SE, et al: Eye distribution of (^{35}S) chlorpromazine. *EXP EYE RES* 7:196–199, 1968.

Cremer-Bartels G, Hollwich F: The combination of light and phenothiazine effect on the incorporation of ^{14}C-glucosamine in glycosaminoglycans in bovine cornea in vitro. *KLIN MONATSBL AUGENHEILKD* 164:134–137, 1974. (German)

Cuendet JF, Verry F, et al: Ocular disturbances in the course of treatment with neuroleptics and thymoleptics. *BULL SOC BELGE OPHTALMOL* 160:601–606, 1972. (French)

DeLong SL: Incidence and significance of chlorpromazine-induced eye changes. *DIS NERV SYST* 29 Suppl:19–22, 1968.

Deluise VP, Flynn JT: Asymmetric anterior segment changes induced by chlorpromazine. *ANN OPHTHALMOL* 13:953–955, 1981.

Dewar AJ, Yates CM, et al: The effects of chronic chlorpromazine administration on the albino rat retina. *TOXICOL APPL PHARMACOL* 43:501–506, 1978.

Edler K, Gottfries CG, et al: Eye changes in connection with neuroleptic treatment. *ACTA PSYCHIATR SCAND* 47:377–385, 1971.

Eichenbaum JW, D'Amico RA: Corneal injury by a Thorazine spansule. *ANN OPHTHALMOL* 13:199–200, 1981.

Forrest FM, Snow HL: Prognosis of eye complications caused by phenothiazines. *DIS NERV SYST* 29 Suppl:26–28, 1968.

Francesconi G, DiTizio A, Cameo D: Disturbances of the eyes and skin in patients subjected to long-term treatment with neuroleptic drugs. *ANN OTTAL* 94:835–852, 1968. (Italian).

Gerhard JP, Franck H, et al: Ophthalmologic side effects of treatment with phenothiazines. *REV OTO–NEURO–OPHTHALMOL* 47:71–77, 1975. (French)

Green H, Ellison T: Uptake and distribution of chlorpromazine in animal eyes. *EXP EYE RES* 5:191–197, 1966.

Gregory MH, Rutty DA, Wood RD: Differences in the retinotoxic action of chloroquine and phenothiazine derivatives. *J PATHOL* 102:139–150, 1970.

Henkes HE: Fenothiazine-retinopathy. *NED TIJDSCHR GENEESKD* 110:789–790, 1966. (*ZENTRALBL GES OPHTHALMOL* 97:105, 1966).

Hessee RJ; Anterior lens opacities in prolonged phenothiazine therapy. *ANN OPHTHALMOL* 11:1212, 1979.

Howard RO, McDonald CJ, et al: Experimental chlorpromazine cataracts. *INVEST OPHTHALMOL* 8:413–421, 1969.

Hull DS, Csukas S, Green K: Chlorpromazine-induced corneal endothelial phototoxicity. *INVEST OPHTHALMOL VIS SCI* 22:502–508, 1982.

Jagadeesh JM, Lee HC, Salazar-Bookaman M: Influence of chlorpromazine on the rabbit electroretinogram. *INVEST OPHTHALMOL VIS SCI* 19:1449–1456, 1980.

Johnson AW, Buffaloe WJ: Chlorpromazine epithelial keratopathy. *ARCH OPHTHALMOL* 76:664–667, 1966.

Johnson AW, Buffaloe WJ: Chlorpromazine corneal toxicity. *SOUTH MED J* 61:993–994, 1969.

Jose JG, Yielding KL: Photosensitive cataractogens, chlorpromazine and methoxy-psoralen, cause DNA repair synthesis in lens epithelial cells. *INVEST OPHTHALMOL VIS SCI* 17:687–691, 1978.

Kalberer M, Atar Z, Bider E: On eye changes in long-term treatment with Largactil. *OPHTHALMOLOGICA* 161:118–124, 1970. (German)

Klima M, Klimova A: Ocular complications in long-term chlorpromazine treatment. *CESK OFTALMOL* 33:349–352, 1977. (English summary)

Legros J, Rossner I, Berger C: Ocular effects of chlorpromazine and oxypertine on beagle dogs. *BR J OPHTHALMOL* 55:407–415, 1971.

Legros J, Rossner I, Berger C: Retinal toxicity of chlorpromazine in the rat. *TOXICOL APPL PHARMACOL* 26:459–465, 1973.

Lindquist NG, Ullberg S: Autoradiography of sulfur-35-labeled chlorpromazine. *ADV BIOCHEM PSYCHOPHARMACOL* 9:413–423, 1974.

McClanahan WS, Harris JE, et al: Ocular manifestations of chronic phenothiazine derivative administration. *ARCH OPHTHALMOL* 75:319–325, 1966.

Mathalone MBR: Eye and skin changes in psychiatric patients treated with chlorpromazine. *BR J OPHTHALMOL* 51:86–93, 1967.

Mathalone MBR: Ocular effects of phenothiazine derivatives and reversibility. *DIS NERV SYST* 29 (Suppl):29–35, 1968.

Muller W: The cortical response in long-term therapy with high doses of Propaphenin/ Prothazin. *GRAEFES ARCH OPHTHALMOL* 172:164–169, 1967. (German)

Nouri A, Cuendet JF: Ocular side effects in the course of prolonged treatment with neuroleptics. *SCHWEIZ MED WOCHENSCHR* 98:1708–1711, 1968. (French)

Petrohelos MA, Tricoulis D: Ocular complications of chlorpromazine therapy. *OPHTHALMOLOGICA* 159:31–38, 1969.

Pouget R, Blayvac B: Corneal and lens deposits due to treatment by phenothiazine type neuroleptics. *ANN MED PSYCHOL* 1:403–407, 1976. (French)

Pouliquen Y, Graf B, et al: Ultrastructural study of a corneal overload in the course of treatment with chlorpromazine. *ARCH OPHTALMOL (Paris)* 30:769–782, 1970. (French)

Prien RF, DeLong SL, et al: Ocular changes occuring with prolonged high dose chlorpromazine therapy. *ARCH GEN PSYCHIATR* 23:464–468, 1970

Rab SM, Alam MN, Sadequzaman MD: Optic atrophy during chlorpromazine therapy. *BR J OPHTHALMOL* 53:208–209, 1969.

Rubin LF, Murchison TE, Barron CN: Chlorpromazine and the eye of the dog. Chronic study. *EXP MOL PATHOL* 13:111–117, 1970.

Santamarina JM: Ocular changes during prolonged treatment with neuroleptic agents. *ARCH SOC ESP OFTALMOL* 33:193–206, 1973. (English summary)

Setogawa T, Tamai A, Matsuura H: Lens changes induced by long term psychotropic agents. *JPN J CLIN OPHTHALMOL* 29:1009–1013, 1975. (English abstract)

Siddall JR: Ocular toxic changes associated with chlorpromazine and thioridazine. *CAN J OPHTHALMOL* 1:190–198, 1966.

Sidall JR: Ocular complications related to phenothiazines. *DIST NERV SYST* 29 Supp:10–13, 1968.

Sizaret P, Rosazza C, Brassart B: Ultrastructural study of ocular pigmentation due to phenothiazines. *REV OTO-NEURO-OPHTALMOL* 47:247–251, 1975. (French)

Smith AA, Gavitt JA, Karmin M: Lenticular opacities induced in mice by chlorpromazine. *ARCH OPHTHALMOL* 75:99–101, 1966.

Tousimis AJ, Barron CN: Chlorpromazine and the eye of the dog. Electron microscopic study. *EXP MOL PATHOL* 13:89–110, 1970.

Verrey F, Cuendet JF, Nouri A: Study of the aqueous humor in prolonged therapies with neuroleptic agents. *OPHTHALMOLOGICA* 165:200–202, 1972.

Wetterholm DH, Snow HL, Winter FC: A clinical study of pigmentary change in cornea and lens in chronic chlorpromazine therapy. *ARCH OPHTHALMOL* 74:55–56, 1965.

Zelickson AS, Zeller HC: A new and unusual reaction to chlorpromazine. *J AM MED ASSOC* 188:394–396, 1964.

Chlorpropamide (Diabinese), an antidiabetic, has in rare instances been suspected of causing central scotomas and reactions involving conjunctiva and cornea. Centrocecal scotomas were reported in a diabetic patient who had been taking this drug for six months and reported not seeing clearly for an hour after taking each dose for the last six weeks.[c] Vision of 20/200 and 20/70 with centrocecal scotomas and bitemporal pallor of the discs were found. After the drug was stopped and multiple vitamin treatment started, the vision recovered to 20/40 and 20/30-2. Also, a man who was given 0.25 g of chlorpropamide per day for two days complained of blurring of vision and could only count fingers at two feet with each eye.[b] Examination of the eyes was normal except for 3° central scotoma in each eye. After the drug was stopped and ACTH and B vitamins were given, the vision became essentially normal.

Exudative conjunctivitis and stomatitis with scarring of the palpebral conjunctiva and pannus simulating trachoma, or erythema multiforme exudativum is reported to have developed in one man a few weeks after starting treatment with chlorpropamide for diabetes.[a]

The cornea and lens of rats have become opacified and vascularized, and posterior synechias have developed when chlorpropamide has been administered for eight to twenty-four months at dosages five to forty times greater than those employed in human patients. None of these changes has developed in dogs.[d]

a. Crews SJ: Toxic effects on the eye and visual apparatus resulting from the systemic absorption of recently introduced chemical agents. *TRANS OPHTHALMOL SOC UK* 82:387–406, 1963.

b. George CW: Central scotomata due to chlorpropamide. *ARCH OPHTHALMOL* 69:733, 1963.

c. Givner I: Centrocecal scotomas due to chlorpropamide. *ARCH OPHTHALMOL* 66:64, 1961.

d. Wright HN: Corneal and lenticular opacities in eyes of rats following long-term administration of sulfonyl-urea derivatives. *DIABETES* 12:550–554, 1963.

Chlorthalidone (Chlortalidone, Hygroton), a diuretic and antihypertensive drug, has been tested in normal and glaucomatous patients in doses from 200 to 500 mg per day, and found to have no tendency to raise ocular pressure;[a,e] rather it was found to reduce pressure slightly, particularly in glaucomatous eyes.[192]

Acute transient myopia, apparently like that induced occasionally by acetazolamide and many other drugs, has been reported from chlorthalidone.[b,d,f–j] Typically the myopia has appeared within one to three days of starting the drug, and young pregnant women appear to be particularly prone to this side effect. Characteristically the ocular pressure and anterior chambers have remained normal, and the acute myopia has not been relieved by applying cycloplegic drugs. In one patient transient retinal edema has been reported.[b] Study of another patient with acute transient myopia from chlorthalidone, making use of 12 MHz ultrasound, showed that during the transitory myopia the crystalline lens was abnormally thick and the anterior chamber was slightly shallowed, but the distance from lens to posterior scleral wall was not altered.[f] The myopia has always been promptly and completely reversible when the drug is stopped.

a. Bucci MG, Stirpe M: Clinical investigation into the hyptonizing effect of Hygroton. *BOLL OCULIST* 42:241–254, 1963. (Italian)

b. Ericson LA: Hygroton-induced myopia and retinal edema. *ACTA OPHTHALMOL* 41:538–543, 1963.

c. Gastaldi GM: Observations on transitory myopia after administration of diuretics. *RASS ITAL OTTAL* 34:178–185, 1965–1966. (Italian)

d. Hermann MP: Spasmodic myopia in the course of diuretic treatment. *BULL SOC OPHTALMOL FRANCE* 63:719–723, 1963. (French)

e. LeFranc J, Garnier JP, Catros A: Use of a non-mercurial diuretic derived from iso-indoline in the treatment of elevated intraocular pressure. *BULL SOC OPHTALMOL FRANCE* 66:152–153, 1966. (French)

f. Pallin O, Ericsson R: Ultrasound studies in a case of Hygroton-induced myopia. *ACTA OPHTHALMOL* 43:692–696, 1965.

g. Robinson M, D'Alena P: Hygroton-induced myopia. *CALIF MED* 110:134–135, 1969.

h. Zehetbauer G: Transitory myopia after taking Hygroton. *KLIN MONATSBL AUGEN-HEILKD* 154:204–206, 1969. (German)

i. Weinstock FJ: Transient severe myopia. *J AM MED ASSOC* 217:1245–1246, 1971.

j. Stennis SD: Drug-induced myopia. *AM J OPTOM PHYSIOL OPT* 53:422–423, 1976.

Cholera toxin sounds as though it might be of interest for toxic effects on the eye, but in fact it has rather been of pharmacologic interest for its property of activating adenylate cyclase, leading to increase in cyclic AMP, with stimulation of corneal wound healing, and reduction of intraocular pressure in rabbits.[a,b]

a. Jumblatt MM, Fogle JA, Neufeld AH: Cholera toxin stimulates adenosine 3'5'-monophosphate synthesis and epithelial wound closure in the cornea. *INVEST OPHTHALMOL VIS SCI* 19:1321–1327, 1980.

b. Bartels SP, Roth HO, Neufeld AH: Effects of intravitreal cholera toxin on adenosine 3'5'-monophosphate, intraocular pressure, and outflow facility in rabbits. *INVEST OPHTHALMOL VIS SCI* 20:411–414, 1981.

Cholesterol fed to rabbits for several weeks has caused xanthomatous infiltration of the cornea, iris, ciliary processes, vitreous humor, and the choroid, eventually with complete opacification of the cornea and detachment of the retina. Systemic vascular xanthomatosis has also developed under these conditions.[a,b,f,g] Asteroid hyalopathy has been produced experimentally.[d]

Intracarotid injection of cholesterol crystals in dogs and monkeys has produced retinal emboli like those seen in patients with carotid atherosclerotic disease,[c] and in rabbits this has produced uveitic reactions.[e]

a. Cogan DG, Kuwabara T: Ocular changes in experimental hypercholesteremia. *ARCH OPHTHALMOL* 61:219–225, 1959.

b. Francois J, Neetens A: The ocular manifestations of experimental hypercholesteraemia in rabbits. *OPHTHALMOLOGICA* 148:57–79, 1964.

c. Hollenhorst RW, Lensink ER, Whisnant JP: Experimental embolization of the retinal arterioles. *TRANS AM OPHTHALMOL SOC* 60:316–334, 1962.

d. Lamba PA, Shukla KN: Experimental asteroid hyalopathy. *BR J OPHTHALMOL* 55:279–283, 1971.

e. Nakamura K: Experimental study on the uveitis induced by injection of cholesterin crystal into the common carotid artery. *ACTA SOC OPHTHALMOL JPN* 74:1087, 1970. (English summary)

   f. Rodger FC: A study of the ultrastructure and cytochemistry of lipid accumulation and clearance in cholesterol-fed rabbit cornea. *EXP EYE RES* 12:88–93, 1971.

   g. Vass Z, Tapaszto I, Polgar J: The effect of long-term feeding of cholesterol on the lipid content of rabbit cornea. *GRAEFES ARCH OPHTHALMOL* 178:306–312, 1969.

Cholestyramine (Questran), an ion-exchange resin for bile salts, has affected vision indirectly in two elderly women who were being treated for biliary cirrhosis. By interfering with vitamin A absorption it led to decrease in visual acuity, constriction of visual fields with nightblindness, and disturbance of color vision. The patients showed improvement when the medication was discontinued and vitamin A was given.

   a. Saraux H, Offret H, Levy VG: Severe amblyopia from avitaminosis A, induced by prolonged treatment with cholestyramine. *BULL SOC OPHTALMOL FRANCE* 80:367–368, 1980.

Chondroitin sulfate, a natural tissue component, forms viscous solutions that have been investigated for use in the anterior chamber during intraocular surgery, and on the surface of the eye as a mucomimetic. In experimental animals, injection of 20% solution into the anterior chamber protected the corneal endothelium from mechanical trauma, but caused a rise of intraocular pressure to 55 mm Hg if not washed out (MacRae[349]). In human eyes, use in the anterior chamber during surgery was without toxic effect in the first several hundred patients.[a]

   a. Carty JB: Chondroitin sulphate in anterior segment surgery. *TRANS OPHTHALMOL SOC UK* 103:263–264, 1983.

Chromic acid (chromic oxide, chromium trioxide) is a brown solid which dissolves readily in water to form a strongly acidic, caustic solution. Contact causes severe injury characterized by infiltration, vascularization, and opacification of the cornea.[b,81] Chronic exposure to fine droplets in the air from electroplating baths or transfer to the eyes on the fingers causes chronic conjunctival inflammation and in rare instances a brown band in the superficial layers of the cornea.[253] In rabbit eyes, the discoloration was not reproducible by application of 1% chromic acid repeatedly, but was induced by applying 5% potassium dichromate solution and exposing the eye to sunlight.[a]

   a. Koll C: A case of brown coloration of the cornea. *Z AUGENHEILKD* 13:220–225, 1905. (German)

   b. Pollet-Delille F: Characteristics of burns of the eye by chromic acid. *BULL SOC FRANCE OPHTALMOL* 52:221, 1939. (French)

Chromium metal tested by implantation in rabbit eyes was well tolerated while under observation for one year.[340]

Chromomycin A$_3$, an antineoplastic antibiotic inhibitor of synthesis of RNA, has been found when injected into the vitreous humor in rabbits to extinguish the ERG, to destroy the outer segments of the visual cells, and to fragment the nuclei in the ganglion cell and nuclear layers of the retina.

  a. Yamamoto K, Tokunga S, et al: Experimental degeneration of the retina. I. Mitomycin C and Chromomycin A_3. *FOLIA OPHTHALMOL JPN* 18:52–60, 1967.

Chrysarobin, a mixture of substances obtained from Goa powder, has been employed in treatment of psoriasis, but is notoriously irritating to the eyes and all mucous membranes,[253] causing conjunctival inflammation with discharge. *Chrysophanic acid* is said to be responsible for some of the ocular inflammation induced by chrysarobin, of which it is a constituent.[46] Occasionally the corneal epithelium has been injured, manifested by punctate defects in the epithelium and foreign-body type of discomfort.[a] This toxic effect is demonstrable in animal eyes.[53]

It has been reported that following application of a solution of chrysarobin in chloroform to the skin some distance from the eyes there appeared in both eyes in twelve to twenty-four hours a very uncomfortable keratoconjunctivitis.[153] In general, after either direct or indirect irritation of the eyes, symptoms have diminished in two to four days. In exceptional instances, superficial corneal opacities have persisted for weeks.[153]

  a. Igersheimer J: On injury of the eyes by chrysarobin. *KLIN MONATSBL AUGENHEILKD* 50:518–527, 1912. (German)

Chymotrypsin (Quimar, Chymar, Quimotrase, Zolyse), a proteolytic enzyme, has been widely used in ophthalmology as an aid to surgical extraction of cataracts since it was introduced by Barraquer in 1958 to weaken the zonules and facilitate removal of the lens. Many articles have been published, and reviewed (Hofmann), concerning series of patients operated upon with and without the enzyme. Possibly related to differences in technique, some observers have reported increased incidence of postoperative glaucoma, adhesion of iris to vitreous and pupillary block, weakness of the wound unless extra sutures are used, greater incidence of postoperative corneal edema, and a variety of minor complications, but many other observers have found no greater incidence of complication when the enzyme is used, or even a reduction of complications because of the greater ease with which the cataract can be extracted when the enzyme is employed. Glaucoma, as a complication of use of chymotrypsin in cataract extractions in patients, has occurred usually within two to five days after operation, and usually the intraocular pressure has returned to normal within a week. Kirsch has been foremost in calling attention to this early postoperative complication, reporting an elevation of pressure in about 70 per cent of patients after use of 2 cc of enzyme solution, and in about 55 per cent after use of 0.25 cc of solution. In most instances the elevation of tension was slight, but in one series a pressure as high as 60 mm Hg was reported. Both Kirsch and Galin found evidence of obstruction to aqueous outflow by tonographic measurements in association with the postoperative glaucoma while the angle remained open and clinically apparently normal. Besides Kirsch, Bloomfield, Galin, Papolczy, Lantz, and Menezo have reported significantly higher incidence of elevated tensions early postoperatively in patients in whom the enzyme has been used, while others have found the incidence low and not a sufficient problem to be of concern, particularly if minimum volumes and times of application are observed, as described by Barraquer, Bedrossian and Gombos.

There has been no evidence in human beings of persistent alteration of intraocular pressure or alteration of facility of aqueous outflow measured tonographically, or alterations in the angle of the anterior chamber visible gonioscopically, according to Jocson and Leydhecker.

Experimental attempts to induce glaucoma acutely in animal eyes by injection of α-chymotrypsin into the anterior chamber have been unsuccessful; but glaucoma has been produced when the enzyme has been injected into the posterior chamber in contact with zonules and vitreous humor in monkeys and rabbits (Araki; Best; Blumenthal; Dymitrouska; Gotok; Hamasaki; Kalvin; Lessell; Sears; Skrzypzak; Vareilles; Wind). It has been established that it is necessary for the enzyme to come in contact with some structures bordering the posterior chamber (Kalvin), and that it is not prevented by previous removal of the lens or performance of iridectomy (Lessell). An attractive elucidation of the mechanism has been advanced by Anderson, who discovered that the lens zonules in the monkey eye under the action of the enzyme gather into microscopic balls having a characteristic appearance readily identifiable by scanning electron microscopy, and that these balls disseminate from the zonules and accumulate in the corneoscleral trabecular meshwork of the monkey eye in a situation where they could obstruct aqueous outflow. Strong evidence that these products of lysis of the zonules are the actual obstructions to the outflow of aqueous has been presented by Chee and Hamasaki, who found in owl monkeys that a rise of pressure was induced by the enzyme only when lens zonules were present, regardless of whether the eye was phakic or aphakic. Furthermore, they showed that fluid transferred from the anterior chamber of a monkey with enzyme-induced pressure elevation to the anterior chamber of another animal could evoke a pressure rise, and that this could be prevented by passing the fluid through a Millipore filter, suggesting that particles were responsible for blocking the outflow of aqueous humor. However, observations on humans have been discordant.

In human eyes, Worthen obtained evidence that alpha-chymotrypsin breaks down the zonules, and that occasionally the products are detectible in the trabecular meshwork, but found in eyes perfused with the enzyme postmortem via the posterior chamber that the facility of aqueous outflow remained normal. In eyes of patients after cataract extraction with the aid of the enzyme, Leydhecker and Meyerratken found no histologic lesion attributable to the enzyme, while Landolt and Fanta have described some abnormalities which might be attributable to the enzyme, or might represent some unrelated reaction to surgery, but did not provide a conclusive explanation for the occasional instances of early transient postoperative glaucoma. Leydhecker examined the angles of cattle and pig eyes exposed to alpha-chymotrypsin and found no changes induced in them by action of the enzyme.

In rabbits, as in monkeys, little change in intraocular pressure has been induced by alpha-chymotrypsin in the anterior chamber (Wind), but by injecting or irrigating into the posterior chamber several investigators have induced pressures in the neighborhood of 40 mm Hg lasting for many months (Best; Blumenthal; Dymitrouska; Gotok; Sears; Vareilles). Initially there is a considerable inflammatory reaction involving ciliary body, iris, and cornea, with dislocation of the lens backward, and formation of some peripheral anterior synechias. Sears has concluded that the extent of synechias is insufficient to account for the degree of obstruction of aqueous outflow and rise of pressure and has observed abnormality of the architecture of the trabecular meshwork itself, which may be secondary to severe changes in the adjacent ciliary body. Involvement of a prostaglandin mechanism is suggested by a demonstration by Sears that most of the reaction and elevation of pressure could be prevented by giving indomethacin. Chymotrypsin glaucoma in the rabbit appears to differ in important respects from the transient glaucoma observed in human patients.

The cornea in patients who have had cataract extractions with alpha-chymotrypsin has received considerable attention, with some authors concluding that the incidence of striate keratopathy is increased, but with many observers feeling that the effect of the enzyme is clinically negligible compared to the effect of operation itself. Cases which have been quite extraordinary include three mentioned by Hogan in which "total opacification of the cornea following use of chymotrypsin" was noted, and one case recorded by Ray in which accidentally an enzyme solution two hundred times the usual concentration was introduced into a patient's eye for cataract extraction and produced "a deep milky opacity of the central cornea", which cleared completely in fourteen days.

The rabbit cornea appears to differ significantly from the human cornea in its reaction to alpha-chymotrypsin. It has been noted repeatedly that introduction of alpha-chymotrypsin solution into the corneal stroma either by injection or through a wound of the endothelium leads to severe swelling reaction of the cornea, much more than is seen in human beings, and in some instances leading to perforation of the cornea (Bedrossian; Hofmann; Honegger; Huckel; Radnot). Reviews and experiments by Honegger and Skrzypczak indicate that the normal endothelium of the rabbit's cornea protects it from gross injury by the enzyme in the anterior chamber, but permits microscopic alterations. Exposure of rabbit corneas to alpha-chymotrypsin on the anterior surface with the epithelium injured also has been shown to cause swelling and destruction of the cornea (Ing). The cat cornea appears to be more like the human cornea in its resistance to chymotrypsin injected into the anterior chamber (Olson[366]).

The retina has been observed to be injured in animal eyes in which alpha-chymotrypsin has been injected into the vitreous or close to the retina, producing damage evident histologically, and altering the ERG (Hamasaki; Maumenee; O'Malley; Radnot). In rabbits, Vareilles has observed destruction of all layers of the retina when the enzyme was injected into the vitreous humor. Retinal detachment reported in one patient by Lugossy after cataract extraction with the enzyme evoked a great deal of discussion when presented at a meeting, with the consensus that the retinal detachment was coincidental and unrelated to use of the enzyme. A study by Sachsenweger in 1968 concluded that the use of alpha-chymotrypsin caused neither an increase nor a decrease in incidence of retinal detachment. The enzyme has been shown by Munich to have a proteolytic effect on vitreous humor from human eyes *in vitro*, but apparently it is not enough to be of clinical significance.

Anderson DR: Experimental alpha chymotrypsin glaucoma studied by scanning electron microscopy. *AM J OPHTHALMOL* 71:470–476, 1971; *ibid* 71:619–625, 1971.

Araki M: Observations on the corrosion casts of the capillaries of the iris and the ciliary body in the enzyme-induced glaucoma. *ACTA SOC OPHTHALMOL JPN* 80:952, 1976. (English summary)

Barraquer J, Rutllan J: Enzymatic zonulolysis and postoperative ocular hypertension. *AM J OPHTHALMOL* 63:159, 1967.

Bedrossian R: Letter to the Editor. *ARCH OPHTHALMOL* 74:882–883, 1965.

Bedrossian RH, Lalli RA: Clinical application of new laboratory data on alpha chymotrypsin. *ARCH OPHTHALMOL* 67:616–621, 1962.

Best M, Rabinovitz AZ, Masket S: Experimental alphachymotrypsin glaucoma. *ANN OPHTHALMOL* 7:803–810, 1975.

Bloomfield S: Failure to prevent enzyme glaucoma. *AM J OPHTHALMOL* 65:405–406, 1968.

Blumenthal M, Yankelev S, Dikstein S: Method for antiglaucoma drug screening on rabbits. *OPHTHALMIC RES* 8:259–261, 1976.

Chee P, Hamasaki DI: The basis for chymotrypsin-induced glaucoma. *ARCH OPHTHALMOL* 85:103–106, 1971.

Dymitrouska M, Maciejewska J: Experimental glaucoma. *KLIN OCZNA* 42:477–481, 1972. (English summary)

Fanta H: Changes in histologic morphology after enzymatic zonulolysis. *KLIN MONATSBL AUGENHEILKD* 142:1011–1020, 1963. (German)

Galin MA, Barasch KR, Harris LS: Enzymatic zonulolysis and intraocular pressure. *AM J OPHTHALMOL* 61:690–691, 1966.

Gombos GM, Oliver M: Cataract extraction with enzymatic zonulolysis in glaucomatous eyes. *AM J OPHTHALMOL* 64:68–70, 1967.

Gotok I: A study on experimental α-chymotrypsin glaucoma. *ACTA SOC OPHTHALMOL JPN* 74:1277, 1970. (English summary)

Hamasaki DI, Ellerman N: Abolition of the electroretinogram. *ARCH OPHTHALMOL* 73:843–850, 1965.

Hofmann H: *Cataract Operation by Enzymatic Zonulolysis.* Translated from the German by D. Shukri. New York, Grune, Toronto, Reyerson, 1965.

Hofmann H, Propst A: Experimental investigations of injury of the cornea by α-chymotrypsin and trypsin. *GRAEFES ARCH OPHTHALMOL* 162:255–268, 1960. (German)

Hogan MJ: Alpha Yes? or Alpha No? (Editorial). *ARCH OPHTHALMOL* 76:3, 1966.

Honegger H: Experimental investigations of injury of the cornea by α-chymotrypsin. *KLIN MONATSBL AUGENHEILKD* 143:75–90, 1963. (German)

Huckel H: On the influence of alpha-chymotrypsin on the healing of endothelial wounds. *GRAEFES ARCH OPHTHALMOL* 166:335–344, 1963. (German)

Ing MR, Deiter P, Wong AS: Chymotrypsin for experimental herpes simplex keratitis. *ARCH OPHTHALMOL* 71:554–555, 1964.

Jocson VL: Tonography and gonioscopy before and after cataract extraction with alpha chymotrypsin. *AM J OPHTHALMOL* 60:318–322, 1965.

Kalvin NH, Hamasaki DI, Gass JDM: Experimental glaucoma in monkeys. *ARCH OPHTHALMOL* 56:82–93, 94–103, 1966.

Kirsch RE: Glaucoma following cataract extraction associated with use of alpha-chymotrypsin. *ARCH OPHTHALMOL* 72:612–620, 1964.

Kirsch RE: Further studies on glaucoma following cataract extraction associated with the use of alpha-chymotrypsin. *TRANS AM ACAD OPHTHALMOL OTOL* 69:1011–1023, 1965.

Kirsch RE: Dose relationship of alpha-chymotrypsin in production of glaucoma after cataract extraction. *ARCH OPHTHALMOL* 75:774–775, 1966.

Landolt E, Heinzen H: Pathologic-anatomic findings in two eyes operated for cataract with alpha-chymotrypsin. *OPHTHALMOLOGICA* 139:313–322, 1960. (German)

Lantz JM, Quigley JH: Intraocular pressure after cataract extraction. *CAN J OPHTHALMOL* 8:339–343, 1973.

Lessell S, Kuwabara T: Experimental α-chymotrypsin glaucoma. *ARCH OPHTHALMOL* 81:853–864, 1969.

Leydhecker W: Is there injury to the eye from cataract operation with alpha-chymotrypsin? *KLIN MONATSBL AUGENHEILKD* 138:381–387, 1960. (German)

Leydhecker W, Dardenne U: Histologic studies of the trabecular system after brief action of alpha-chymotrypsin. *KLIN MONATSBL AUGENHEILKD* 142:554–559, 1963. (German)

Lugossy G: Retinal complications of enzymatic zonulolysis. *BULL SOC FRANC OPHTALMOL* 77:238–251, 1964. (French)

Maumenee AE: Effects of alpha-chymotrypsin on the retina. *TRANS AM ACAD OPHTHALMOL OTOL* 64:33–36, 1960.

Menezo JL, Marco M, Mascarell EV: Statistical study of enzymatic hypertension. *J FR OPHTALMOL* 1:289–296, 1978. (French)

Meyerratken E: Comparative gonioscopic examinations before and after cataract extraction without and with enzymatic zonulolysis. *KLIN MONATSBL AUGENHEILKD* 140:788, 1962. (German)

Munich W: Experimental studies on the influence of alpha-chymotrypsin on human vitreous body. *GRAEFES ARCH OPHTHALMOL* 163:88–98, 1961. (German)

Munich W: Experimental studies on the influence of alpha-chymotrypsin on the uptake of S^{35} sulfate in corneal tissue. *GRAEFES ARCH OPHTHALMOL* 164:145–150, 1961.

O'Malley C, Moskovitz M, Straatsma BR: Alpha-Chymotrypsin. *ARCH OPHTHALMOL* 66:539, 1961.

Papolczy F: Evaluation of enzymatic zonulolysis. *KLIN MONATSBL AUGENHEILKD* 147:805–817, 1965. (German)

Radnot M, Pajor R: The effect of alpha-chymotrypsin on the retina. *KLIN MONATSBL AUGENHEILKD* 136:370–376, 1960. (German)

Ray PK: Use of 200 times the recommended dose of alpha-chymotrypsin without complications. *BR J OPHTHALMOL* 48:230–231, 1964.

Sachsenweger R: The incidence of retinal detachment after cataract operations with enzymatic zonulolysis. *KLIN MONATSBL AUGENHEILKD* 153:530–533, 1968. (German)

Sears D, Sears M: Blood-aqueous barrier and alpha-chymotrypsin glaucoma in rabbits. *AM J OPHTHALMOL* 77:378–383, 1974.

Skrzypczak KE: Effect of alpha-chymotrypsin on endothelial lining of anterior chamber of eye. *ARCH IMMUNOL THER EXP* 11:671–682, 1963.

Vareilles P, Durand G, et al: The experimental glaucoma model with alpha-chymotrypsin in the rabbit. *J FR OPHTHALMOL* 2:561–568, 1979. (French)

Wind CA, Gassett AR: The effect of alpha-chymotrypsin on intraocular pressure and corneal wound healing. *ANN OPHTHALMOL* 4:32–39, 1972.

Worthen DM: Scanning electron microscopy after alpha chymotrypsin perfusion in man. *AM J OPHTHALMOL* 73:637–642, 1972.

Zimmerman LE, de Venecia G, Hamasaki DI: Pathology of the optic nerve in experiments acute glaucoma. *INVEST OPHTHALMOL* 6:109–125, 1967.

Cimetidine (Tagamet), antagonist to H_2 receptors, was reported in one patient with chronic glaucoma to have been associated with ocular pain and blurred vision, with intraocular pressure up to 24 mm Hg, with relief when the drug was stopped. A year later a trial of *ranitidine* was associated with similar symptoms.[a] It is noteworthy that glaucomatous patients rarely experience pain at such modest pressure, and it is open to question whether variation in pressure in this case was induced or coincidental. Investigation by administering cimetidine (2 mg/kg during an hour) to 4 normal people and to 4 patients with medically controlled glaucoma induced no change in intraocular pressure, although this dose was enough to abolish basal gastric acid secretion.[b,c]

Oculomotor paresis is reported in one case to have occurred, and recurred, when both cimetidine and sulpiride were taken, but not when either was taken separately. Visual hallucinations have been reported.[312]

a. Dobrilla G, Felder M, et al: Exacerbation of glaucoma associated with both cimetidine and ranitidine. (Letter) *LANCET* 1:1078, 1982.
b. Feldman F, Cohen MM: Effect of histamine −2 receptor blockade by cimetidine on intraocular pressure in humans. *AM J OPHTHALMOL* 93:351–355, 1982.
c. Cohen MM, Feldman F, et al: Effect of cimetidine on intraocular pressure in patients with glaucoma. *CAN J OPHTHALMOL* 19:212–214, 1984.
d. Malbrel PH, Woillez M: A case of iatrogenic oculomotor paresis. *BULL SOC OPHTAL-MOL FRANCE* 82:1285–1287, 1982. (French)

Cinchona derivatives consist of about thirty-five alkaloids obtained from the dried bark of cinchona.[171] In addition to *quinine,* of principal interest with regard to the eye are *cinchonidine* and its stereoisomer, *cinchonine.* Derivatives that are noteworthy for ocular toxicity include *apoquinine (apocupreine), ethylapoquinine (ethylapocupreine), ethylhydrocupreine (Optochin), hydroxyethyl apocupreine* and *isoamylhydrocupreine,* usually known as *Eucupine.* Synthetic 8-aminoquinoline derivatives, which are chemically related to the above listed cinchona derivatives, and which have also had toxic visual effects, are *Pamaquine* and *Plasmocid.*

All of these compounds have been of medical interest, primarily as antibiotic chemotherapeutic agents, mostly as antimalarial agents. The derivatives of apoquine or apocupreine, in particular Optochin, were formerly of interest mainly because of antipneumococcal activity, and were employed systemically in treatment of pneumonia and topically in the eye for pneumococcal ulcers.

Concerning the toxic effects of the cinchona derivatives on the eye, a large literature exists on effects of *quinine, Optochin,* and *Eucupine.* (These are described elsewhere under their individual headings.) Relatively little information is available on the others. *Cinchonidine* was reputed in 1899 to resemble *quinine* in causing disturbances of hearing and impairment of vision of long duration, but there appear to be no more recent observations.[153] *Cinchonin* was reported, also at the turn of the century, to cause damage to the retina of dogs similar to that caused by *quinine,* and in human beings it was found that a dose of *cinchonine sulfate* which would produce weakness, tremor, and irregular heart action would regularly induce nearly complete paralysis of accommodation, lasting eight to twelve hours.[153,214]

Apoquinine and *ethylapoquinine* are reported to have caused visual changes the same as those of *quinine* in a woman treated with these drugs for pneumonia.[255] *Ethylhydrocupreine (Optoquin), ethylapocupreine,* and *isopropylapocupreine* injected subcutaneously in large doses in dogs have damaged the retinal ganglion cells.[a]

a. Dawson WT, Perman HH, et al: An experimental study of the variations in the production of visual disturbance by certain new cinchona derivatives. *AM J MED SCI* 193:543, 1937.

Cisplatin (cis-platinum II; cis-diamminedichloroplatinum; Platinol), an antineoplatic, has caused papilledema and headache without disturbance of vision in one patient, and retrobulbar neuritis with great reduction of vision, but normal optic disc, in another patient.[b] The patient with papilledema had also received doxorubicin, but this has not been known to cause papilledema. In this patient the cerebrospinal fluid pressure decreased and the papilledema resolved soon after systemic corticosteroid was given. Papilledema was also observed in a young child treated with cisplatin and *doxorubicin.*[c] The papilledema was diagnosed ophthalmoscopically and was confirmed histologically postmortem, but there was no evidence of elevated intracranial pressure. Cisplatin has been shown in rats to produce axonal lesions in the optic nerves and spinal cord.[a]

Intravitreal injection in rabbit eyes has shown that as much as 0.1 μg can be injected without toxic effect (Peyman[369]).

a. Clark AW, Parhad IM, et al: Neurotoxicity of cisplatinum. *NEUROLOGY* 30:429, 1980.
b. Ostrow S, Hahn D, et al: Ophthalmologic toxicity after cisdichlorodiammineplatinum (II) therapy. *CANCER TREATMENT REPORTS* 62:1591–1594, 1978.
c. Walsh TJ, Clark AW, et al: Neurotoxic effects of cisplatin therapy. *ARCH NEUROL* 39:719–720, 1982.

Citraconic acid (methyl maleic acid) tested by application of two drops of 11% solution in water to a rabbit's eye caused only slight transient injury.[81] However, *citraconic acid anhydride* tested full strength by drop application to rabbit eyes caused severe injury like that caused by acetic anhydride.[222]

Citral once was alleged to cause increase in intraocular pressure in monkeys,[149] but this has not been confirmed,[a] nor has an influence on intraocular pressure been found in rabbits.[b]

a. Rodger FC, Grover AD, Saiduzzafar MS: The effect of citral on intraocular dynamics in monkeys. *ARCH OPHTHALMOL* 63:77–82, 1960.
b. Rodger FC, Saiduzzafar MS, Grover AD: The effect of citral and vitamine A on the intraocular dynamics of rabbits. *AM J OPHTHALMOL* 50:309–313, 1960.

Citric acid tested on rabbit eyes as a single drop of 2% to 5% solution in water caused little or no injury.[27,81] However, irrigation for thirty minutes with 0.5% to 2% solutions causes severe injury; the 0.5% solution causes permanent cloudiness of the cornea, and the 2% solution causes severe dense opacification. The same kind of irrigation applied to eyes which had been burned with sodium hydroxide gave much worse ultimate results than did the control eyes irrigated with sodium chloride solution.[27] In one patient a splash of a large quantity of saturated solution of citric acid in the eyes caused severe conjunctival reaction and ulceration of the cornea, resulting in extensive adherent leukoma.[249]

Sodium citrate, unlike citric acid, is very well tolerated by the eye. Sodium citrate 10% eyedrops have been used beneficially in treatment of chemical burns. (See Chapter III, *Treatment of Chemical Burns of the Eye.*)

Clindamycin (Cleocin) hydrochloride or phosphate, an antibacterial, has been evaluated for injection into or around the eye. In rabbits it was found that 1 mg could be safely injected into the vitreous body,[a] but for use in an irrigating solution during vitrectomy it was necessary to limit the concentration to 10 μg/ml to avoid damage to the retina.[361,380] When 20 μg/ml was used, it caused histologic abnormality of the retina, and 50 μg/ml extinguished the ERG and damaged all layers of the retina.[380] Subconjunctival injection of 150 mg in rabbits injured the corneal epithelium, and caused severe inflammation and corneal edema.[b] In experimental treatment of six patients with serious ocular toxoplasmosis, two patients were given retrobulbar injections of 75 and 150 mg, causing papillitis, which recovered in the first, but resulted in optic atrophy with impairment of vision in the other.[c] Subtenons injections of 75 mg in some of the other patients was irritating temporarily. Subtenons injection of 450 mg in divided doses in one patient produced temporary restrictive tenonitis and diplopia.[c]

   a. Paque J, Peyman G: Intravitreal clindamycin phosphate in the treatment of vitreous infection. *OPHTHALMIC SURG* 5:34, 1974.
   b. Tabbara KH, O'Connor R: Ocular tissue absorption of clindamycin phosphate. *ARCH OPHTHALMOL* 93:1180–1185, 1975.
   c. Tate GW Jr, Martin RG: Clindamycin in the treatment of human ocular toxoplasmosis. *CAN J OPHTHALMOL* 12:188–195, 1977.

Clioquinol (Iodochlorhydroxyquin, Chinoform, Entero-Vioform, Vioform, Mexoform), an anti-amebic, formerly widely used in treating diarrhea, is selectively toxic to axons of the optic nerves and tracts of the spinal chord. The neurotoxic properties of clioquinol were discovered only after the drug had been used by many people for many years without obvious difficulty[m]. Some of the earliest suspicions of toxicity affecting vision were in relation to children who were being treated for acrodermatitis enteropathica for long periods with large doses when their vision was found to be much impaired, and optic atrophy was diagnosed[c,d,k,l,r,y]. Some children had difficulty in walking as well as poor vision[a]. An investigating committee reported in 1974 knowledge of more than a dozen children with optic neuropathy from clioquinol[294]. Less than half had symptoms of peripheral neuropathy.

   In adults a rare case of decreasing vision had been recorded in association with clioquinol in 1968[d], and by 1971 serious concern over possible neurotoxicity of clioquinol had developed as a result of an epidemic affecting thousands of people in Japan who suffered subacute myelo-optico-neuropathy ("S.M.O.N."). Typically, those affected had abdominal discomfort or pain, numb feet and discomfort in the legs, spastic difficulty in walking, and about a quarter had impaired vision, about 5%

developing optic atrophy[u]. Autopsies showed the loss of vision to be explained by degeneration of optic nerve axons, most severe adjacent to the geniculate nucleus, but extending also to the retina with degeneration and disappearance of retinal ganglion cells[q,w]. There is a large literature on controversy that followed over whether or not clioquinol was responsible.

Early attempts to reproduce the condition in animals gave varied results, but more recent testing has shown that the same disabilities and the same neuropathology as found in patients can be reproduced in dogs and cats[p,t,u,x,z]. In dogs, clioquinol caused decrease of visual acuity, with vacuolation and loss of axons in the optic tract[x]. There seems to be agreement that peripheral nerves are not primarily affected, but that long tracts in the spinal cord show degeneration, and that the relatively short axons of the optic nerves are especially vulnerable. The seemingly unique distribution has been termed "central distal axonopathy[t]." Demyelination follows axon degeneration[x].

Apart from the experience in Japan, there have been many similar cases of the typical syndrome scattered in various parts of the world affecting adults, with convincing histories relating clioquinol to disturbances of vision, with varying degrees of spinal chord involvement[b,e-j,n,v]. Visual disturbances have ranged from impairment of discrimination of colors to blindness from optic atrophy, with moderate involvement in the form of central scotomas with symmetrically reduced visual acuity. Clinical ophthalmoscopic abnormality appears to be limited to pallor of the disc in eyes with optic atrophy. In a number of cases there has been improvement of vision during several months after administration of clioquinol was discontinued. No treatment has been effective other than stopping administration of clioquinol.

It is noteworthy that since the early 1970's the number of cases of clioquinol neurotoxicity has decreased markedly both in children and adults. In children this is explained by discovery that administration of zinc sulfate is far more effective than clioquinol in treatment of childhood acrodermatitis enteropathica. In adults the decrease is explained by limitation of the use of clioquinol for diarrhea, because of awareness of potential toxicity.

(The following bibliography represents a small portion of what has been published on *clioquinol neurotoxicity,* omitting a number of case reports that do not provide new or different information, and omitting earlier publications of authors who have a series of publications on the subject.)

a. Aron JJ, Bebuisson DA, Gidi M: Optic neuritis from derivatives of clioquinol in the child. *BULL SOC OPHTALMOL FRANCE* 77:409–411, 1977. (French)

b. Bawmgartner G, Gawel MJ, et al: Neurotoxicity of halogenated hydroxyquinolines. *J NEUROL NEUROSURG PSYCHIATRY* 42:1073–1983, 1979.

c. Berggren L, Hansson O: Treating acrodermatitis enteropathica. *LANCET* 1:52, 1966.

d. Berggren L, Hansson O: Absorption of intestinal antiseptics derived from 8-hydroxyquinolines. *CLIN PHARMACOL THER* 91:67–70, 1968.

e. Biard L, Decroix G, et al: A new case of toxic neuro-opticomyelitis from a quinoline. *BULL SOC OPHTALMOL FRANCE* 73:1173–1177, 1974. (French)

f. Billson FH, Reich J, Hopkins IJ: Visual failure in a patient with ulcerative colitis treated by clioquinol. *LANCET* 1:1015–1016, 1972.

g. Boergen KP: Optic nerve damage through antidiarrheal preparations containing 8-quinolol. *KLIN MONATSBL AUGENHEILKD* 163:217–219, 1973. (German)

h. Cambier J, Masson M, et al: Sensory neuropathy and optic neuritis after prolonged intake of clioquinol. *NEUV PRESS MED* 1:1991–1992, 1972. (French)

i. Danis P: Optic neuritis and clioquinol. *BULL SOC BELGE OPHTALMOL* 159:671–675, 1971. (French)

j. Derakhshan I, Forough M: Progressive visual loss after years on clioquinol. *LANCET* 1:715, 1978.

k. Etheridge Jr JE, Stewart GE: Treating acrodermatitis enteropathica. *LANCET* 1:261, 1966.

l. Garcia Perez A, Castro C, et al: A case of optic atrophy possibly induced by quinoline in acrodermatitis enteropathica. *BR J DERMATOL* 90:453–455, 1974.

m. Gholz LM, Arons WL: Prophylaxis and therapy of amebiasis and shigellosis with iodochlorhydroxyquin. *AM J TROP MED* 13:396–401, 1964.

n. Heilig P, Thaler A: Subacute myelo-optico-neuropathy (S.M.O.N.). *KLIN MONATSBL AUGENHEILKD* 164:386–388, 1974. (German)

o. Kaeser HE, Wuthrich R: On the question of the neurotoxicity of hydroxyquinolines. *DTSCH MED WOCHENSCHR* 95:1685, 1970.

p. Krinke G, Schaumburg HH, et al: Clioquinol and 2,5-hexanedione induce different types of distal axonopathy in the dog. *ACTA NEUROPATHOL* 47:213–221, 1979.

q. Okuda K, Matsuo H, Ueno H: Ocular disorders in S.M.O.N., especially neuroretinal lesions. *ACTA SOC OPHTHALMOL JPN* 75:1937, 1971.

r. Reich JA, Billson FA: Toxic optic neuritis; clioquinol ingestion in a child. *MED J AUST* 2:593–595, 1973.

s. Schaumburg HH, Spencer PS, et al: The CNS distal axonopathy in dogs intoxicated with clioquinol. *J NEUROPATHOL EXP NEUROL* 37:686a, 1978.

t. Schaumburg HH, Spencer PS: Toxic models of certain disorders of the nervous system. *NEUROTOXICOLOGY* 1:209, 1979.

u. Schaumburg HH, Spencer PS: Clioquinol. Chapter 27 in Spencer and Schaumburg (1980).[378]

v. Selby G: Subacute myelo-optic neuropathy in Australia. *LANCET* 1:123–125, 1972.

w. Shiraki H: The neuropathy, S.M.O.N., in humans. *JPN J MED SCI BIOL* 28 Suppl:101–164, 1975.

x. Tateishi J, Kuroda S, et al: Experimental myelo optic neuropathy induced by clioquinol. *ACTA NEUROPATHOL* 24:304–320, 1973.

y. van Balen ATM: Toxic damage to the optic nerve caused by iodochlorhydroxyquinoline (Enterovioform). *OPHTHALMOLOGICA* 163:8–9, 1971.

z. Worden AN, Heywood R, et al: Clioquinol toxicity in the dog. *TOXICOLOGY* 9:227–238, 1978.

Clofazimine (Lamprene), an antibacterial and anti-psoriatic, causes reddish-brown discoloration of the skin, discoloration of the conjunctiva, and fine brownish lines composed of very fine granules in the superficial layers of the cornea.[a,b] Except for the brownish color, the fine material in the cornea resembles in several respects the material seen in the corneas of patients receiving chloroquine or amiodarone. It has the same tendency to develop in lines which may have a cats-whiskers distribution. It causes no symptoms, does not interfere with vision, and slowly disappears when the medication is discontinued. In two cases described in detail the appearance was well developed after 100 to 400 mg of clofazimine daily for two months, and disappeared within 6 to 12 months after medication was stopped.[b]

A finely granular appearance or "speckled pigmentation" in the maculas has been attributed to the drug in 3 patients out of 45 examined under treatment,[a,b] but no decrease in vision was reported in those cases.[a,b] There was no change in appearance of the retinal pigment after 4 to 6 months without medication. (Also see INDEX for *Lipidosis.*)

a. Ohman L, Wahlberg I: Ocular side-effects of clofazimine (Letter). *LANCET* 2:933–934, 1975.
b. Walinder PE, Gip L, Stempa M: Corneal changes in patients treated with clofazimine. *BR J OPHTHALMOL* 60:526–528, 1976.

Clofenamide (Monochlorphenamide, Aquedux), a diuretic, has caused acute transitory myopia like that induced by many other diuretics.[a,b] (See INDEX for page number of *Myopia, acute transient.*) The onset has been soon after starting the medication, and return to normal has been spontaneous in two or three days after medication was stopped.

a. Hermann MP: Spasmodic myopia in the course of diuretic treatment. *BULL SOC OPHTALMOL FRANCE* 63:719–723, 1963. (French)
b. Voisin J, Lombard G: Transitory myopia, a possible complication of use of the new diuretics. *BULL SOC OPHTALMOL FRANCE* 63:495–497, 1963. (French)

Clomacran phosphate (Devryl, Olaxin), an antipsychotic, has been reported to produce deposits in the lenses of patients like those produced by chlorpromazine.[a] They are reversible.

a. Lampe WT: Adverse effects with clomacran. *J CLIN PHARMACOL* 10:171–174, 1970.

Clomiphene citrate (Clomifene, Clomid), a gonad-stimulating principle, has several times been mentioned as producing blurring of vision without description of the cause,[a-c] but there were no opacities of the lenses. A review of the literature concerning visual complaints in patients taking clomiphene indicated an incidence generally around 5 or 10 percent, severe enough in a much smaller proportion to require stopping treatment.[e] In a study of fifty-eight patients taking clomiphene citrate, four developed visual symptoms of phosphenes, consisting of episodes of flashing lights, or complaint of blurred vision, and two of these patients were found to have reduced visual acuity with central scotomas.[e] In one of these patients the scotomas disappeared while the drug was still being administered. In the other patient the scotomas disappeared when the drug was stopped and reappeared when it was readministered.[e] One good observer noted that the so-called flashing lights had a pulsatile, rather than a streaking, character, and they were most evident in artificial illumination at night, rather than in the dark.[i] A patient seen by Carroll five months after a suspected unilaterial retrobulbar neuritis from clomiphene had regained 20/30 vision in the affected eye, but was unable to identify red color with that eye; color vision was normal in the other eye.[f]

Clomiphene taken during pregnancy has been associated with congenital retinal aplasia in one otherwise normal infant, with poor visual acuity, worse in bright light than dim light, fine pigmentary stippling in the fundi, especially in the periphery, and markedly subnormal electroretinograms.

In rats given clomiphene grossly visible lens opacities have been reported, corresponding to "degeneration of the subcapsular protein fibers" histologically.[d] Congenital cataracts have also been produced in rats.

In dogs no opacities were observable ophthalmoscopically in the media, but by slit-lamp very minute opacities of questionable significance were seen in a small proportion of the eyes. In one dog "bilateral retinitis" believed to be due to incidental infection rather than the test drug was discovered histologically.[d] The ocular pressure in dogs was unaltered.

(For effects of related drugs, see INDEX for *Chlorotrianisene, Tamoxifen,* and *Triparanol.*)

a. Editorial: Clomiphene. *CAN MED ASSOC J* 98:653, 1968.
b. Today's Drugs: Clomiphene citrate. *BR MED J* 1:363–364, 1968.
c. A drug to induce ovulation. *MED LETT* 8:47–49, 1966.
d. Newberne JW, Kuhn WL, Elsea JR: Toxicologic studies on clomiphene. *TOXICOL APPL PHARMACOL* 9:44–56, 1966.
e. Roch LM II, Gordon DL, et al: Visual changes associated with clomiphene citrate therapy. *ARCH OPHTHALMOL* 77:14–17, 1967.
f. Carroll FD: Personal communication, 1972.
g. Eneroth G, Forsberg V, Grant CA: Hydramnios and congenital cataracts induced in rats by clomiphene. *PROC EUR SOC STUDY DRUG TOXICITY* 12:299–306, 1971.
h. Laing IA, Steer CR, et al: Clomiphene and congenital retinopathy (Letter). *LANCET* 2:1107–1108, 1981.
i. Scott AW: Personal communication, 1981.

Clomipramine, an antidepressant, when fed to rats produces cytoplasmic inclusions in retinal pigment epithelium and retinal ganglion cells characteristic of lipidosis or phospholipidosis (Lullmann-Rauch[348]).

Clonidine hydrochloride (Catapres, Dixarit), a systemic and ocular antihypertensive, which has been used in treatment of glaucoma, was found in chronic toxicity tests in rats to cause an increased incidence of light-induced retinal degeneration.[c,d] This was explicable by the fact that the drug caused mydriasis in rats, and thereby allowed greater exposure of the retina to light. In rats, clonidine also produces a species specific keratoconjunctivitis sicca.[d]

A clinical study limited to 19 clonidine-treated patients utilizing a comprehensive battery of retinal function tests, showed, except for some lower EOG values of uncertain significance, there were no more abnormalities in these patients than in a matched group of patients treated with other antihypertensive agents.[b] A large number of eye examinations during clinical testing of the drug have given no evidence of retinopathy.[a]

a. Kosman ME: Evaluation of clonidine hydrochloride (Catapres). *J AM MED ASSOC* 233:174–176, 1975.
b. Turacli ME: The clonidine side effect in the human eye. *ANN OPHTHALMOL* 6:699–710, 1974.

c. Weisse I, Stoetzer H, et al: Effects of clonidine on the pupil diameter and the retina in rats, assessed in relation to the intensity of light. *ARZNEIM-FORSCH* 21:821–825, 1971.
d. Weisse I, Hoefke W, et al: Ophthalmological and pharmacological studies after administration of clonidine in rats. *ARCH TOXICOL* 41:89–98, 1978.

Clove oil injected into the cornea in rabbits causes necrosis within the cornea, with infiltration by inflammatory cells and with fibrin and gross hypopyon in the anterior chamber. This provides a reproducible model which has been the basis of a test method for evaluating antiinflammatory agents.[a,b] Clove oil splashed in the eyes of a patient caused severe pain, blepharospasm, lacrimation, and conjunctival edema with loss of corneal epithelium. Recovery was complete, except for slight residual superficial opacity in one eye.[c]

a. Chusid MJ, Starkey DD: Polymorphonuclear leukocyte kinetics in experimentally induced keratitis. *ARCH OPHTHALMOL* 103:270–274, 1985.
b. Leibowitz HM, Lass JH, Kupferman A: Quantitation of inflammation in the cornea. *ARCH OPHTHALMOL* 92:427–430, 1974.
c. Libby GF: Ocular injury from oil of cloves. *OPHTHALMIC REC* 21:189, 1912.

Coal tar is a high-boiling, crude mixture obtained by the destructive distillation or coking of coal. The most extensive survey and bibliography on injuries of the eye from coal tar from 1893 to 1927 has been given by D'Asaro Biondo.[123] The same author has presented the most extensive testing on rabbit eyes of crude coal tar, various crude fractions and oils, and of purified constituents from coal tar. Coal tar and its various crude fractions appear principally to cause reddening and squamous eczema of the lid margins, with only small erosions of the corneal epithelium and superficial changes in the stroma which disappear in a month following exposure.[123] (For descriptions of effects of related substances, see *Tar*, page number in INDEX.)

Cobalt and **Cobalt compounds** have been found to induce a variety of toxic effects in the eyes of experimental animals, but reports of injury to human eyes have been rare.

Cobalt metal introduced in to rabbit eyes has caused a severe reaction, with abscess involving lens, ciliary body, vitreous humor and retina.[340]

Cobalt chloride is seriously toxic to the cornea in rabbits when brought into direct contact with the corneal stroma after removal of the epithelium, causing dense opacity and vascularization.[81,90]
Systemic poisoning of rats and rabbits with cobalt chloride has induced vacuoles and slight clouding in the lenses, edema of the retina, and degenerative changes in the choroid, retina, and optic nerve.[a] Partial protection has been afforded by simultaneous administration of cysteine[a] or calcium edetate.[b]
In human beings, accounts of eye disturbance from systemic cobalt tend to be rather bizarre and difficult to evaluate. It is noteworthy that in epidemics of cardiomyopathy believed to be attributable to addition of cobalt to beer, no mention has been made of disturbance of the eyes. (See *Beer*, page number in INDEX.)

However, optic atrophy has been reported in a case in which a patient was treated with cobalt chloride for pancytopenia.[e] Allergy to cobalt in fragments of metal in a war injury was held to be responsible for unilateral exophthalmos and paresis of eye muscles on the basis of skin tests and observation that the condition became worse on an occasion when a cobalt-containing medication was administered for anemia.[f]

A cobalt compound, thought to be cobaltous aluminate pigment, used as a light-blue skin tatto, is believed to have caused both local granulomatous reactions and uveitis in three patients. The uveitis appeared to become worse each time there was a flareup of the reaction at the tattoo site. Skin testing with cobalt chloride gave evidence of delayed sensitivity reaction in two of the patients. The uveitis was relieved by excision of the tattoo material in two out of three patients. (See *Tattooing*.)

Chronic exposure of animal eyes to dusts of minerals containing both cobalt and arsenic has also caused corneal injury. *Smaltite* ($CoAs_2$) caused serious reaction, and *cobaltite* (CoSAs) caused slight reaction.[188]

A slight teratogenic effect (incidence 2.7 to 2.8%) involving gross abnormalities of the eyes and lower extremities is reported from injecting cobaltous chloride into the yolk sac of hen's eggs on day four of incubation.[d]

a. Alagna G, D'Aquino S: Disturbance of the eye from cobalt chloride. *ARCH OTTALMOL* 60:5–29, 1956. (Italian)

b. DiMartino C: On the beneficial effect of calcium disodium ethylenediaminetetraacetate on ocular disturbances from $CoCl_2$. *ARCH OTTALMOL* 62:414–423, 1958.

d. Kury G, Crosby RJ: Studies on the development of chicken embryos exposed to cobaltous chloride. *TOXICOL APPL PHARMACOL* 13:199–206, 1968.

e. Licht A, Oliver M, Rachmilewitz EA: Optic atrophy following treatment with cobalt chloride in a patient with pancytopenia and hypercellular narrow. *ISR J MED SCI* 8:61–66, 1972.

f. Nover A, Heinrich I: Cobalt-allergy as cause of lid edema, exophthalmos and paresis of eye muscles. *KLIN MONATSBL AUGENHEILKD* 158:546–550, 1971.

Cocaine a local anesthetic and sympathomimetic, causes transient irregularity of the corneal epithelium, pupillary dilation with the attendant hazard of precipitating acute glaucoma in individuals having abnormally shallow anterior chambers, and in overdosage may cause death.[a] Many cases of acute glaucoma were reported around 1900 from cocaine eyedrops, presumably representing angle-closure glaucoma secondary to mydriasis.

The endothelium of the cornea in rabbits is found not to be injured by applying 4% cocaine to the outer surface of the eye for fifteen minutes and then reapplying it frequently during five days.[120] However, the epithelium and stroma of the cornea can be injured by repeated application of cocaine, as by other local anesthetics, and in one bizarre case corneal ulceration and scarring have been reported in an addict who used the conjunctival sac as the route for self-administration.[c]

In rabbits a single application of 10% cocaine hydrochloride and rubbing of the cornea with an applicator stick easily removes the corneal epithelium without permanent damage to the stroma.[330]

Systemically, cocaine has no selective ocular toxic action, but there have been instances of transient blackouts of vision with the onset of unconsciousness in systemic poisoning.[41] In association with pupillary dilation, the lids become elevated and the eyes appear staring, owing to the contraction of sympathetically innervated smooth muscle attached to the lid. Systemically administered cocaine has been found to have no influence on ocular pressure or on facility of aqueous outflow in rabbits.[b]

a. Meyers EF: Cocaine toxicity during dacryocystorhinostomy. *ARCH OPHTHALMOL* 98:842–843, 1980.
b. Paterson CA: The effect of sympathetic nerve stimulation on the aqueous humor dynamics of the cocaine pretreated rabbit. *EXP EYE RES* 5:37–44, 1966.
c. Ravin JG, Ravin LC: Blindness due to illicit use of topical cocaine. *ANN OPHTHALMOL* 11:863–864, 1979.

Coconut shell fragments deep in the cornea have been reported in a single case to have produced protracted inflammation of a patient's eye, with leukoma, iritis, and at times hypopyon, all relieved when the particles were removed surgically.[a] Foreign bodies of vegetable origin commonly tend to produce this kind of reaction.

a. Steahly LP, Almquist HT: Corneal foreign bodies of coconut origin. *ANN OPHTHAL-MOL* 9:1017–1021, 1977.

Colchicine is a drug extracted from *Colchicum atumnale,* employed in the treatment of gout, and in research on mitosis and intracellular transport. Only one case of eye involvement associated with systemic poisoning in a human being seems to have been reported, and this was a fatal poisoning, accompanied by keratitis, hypopyon, cataract, pupillary membrane, and disturbance of eye movements.[153] A decidedly minor disturbance has been reported in two children who were receiving colchicine when they had strabismus surgery, and developed dellen which healed only when colchicine was discontinued.[i]

In rabbits, colchicine given intravenously has been observed by DeOcampo to cause degenerative changes in the ciliary body observable histologically, but not to alter the intraocular pressure at doses which produce no clinical signs of disturbance of the eye.[b] When the drug was applied to the eye, or injected into the eye, it did reduce intraocular pressure,[h] and this was shown to be due to increase in facility of aqueous outflow.[m] The effect was maximal in 24 hours, and gone in 4 days, despite continued administration. It has been suspected that action of colchicine on intracellular microtubules somewhere in the aqueous outflow system is responsible for this phenomenon.[h,m]

Toxic effects on the cornea in experimental animals have been observed to follow local application, ranging from almost no disturbance from 0.05% solution to a serious reaction from 1% solution.[g,m,46,53,63] In human eyes application of one drop of 1% solution has caused clouding of the corneal stroma, reducing vision to 1/50, but the cornea cleared in the course of a few weeks. In rabbit eyes the same solution caused cellular infiltration of the cornea and vascularization, with considerable opacification. Cortisone was beneficial in preventing this toxic effect.[63] In cultured rabbit corneas having an epithelial defect, colchicine has been seen to inhibit migration of cells surrounding the defect,[q] while in similar corneas from rats, colchicine only slowed the migration.[i]

Several studies on the epithelium of the cornea have shown colchicine to arrest mitosis in metaphase without influencing the entrance of the cells into mitosis.[a,d,e]

Effects on the retina from colchicine have been studied after intravitreal injection in animals. In rabbits injection of 2.5μg into the vitreous body had only slight effect on protein synthesis in the retina, but almost completely blocked fast transport in the axons of retinal ganglion cells.[f,o] In rats, 1μg not only blocked axonal transport but also caused nearly complete, temporary disappearance of outer segments of photoreceptors, and signs of increased metabolic activity of the retinal pigment epithelium.[k,l,n] Injection of 10 μg caused vitreous opacities, lens opacities, and reduced intraocular pressure.[l] In cats, intravitreal injection of 20 μg caused temporary blindness associated with changes in the retinal pigment epithelium, marked changes in the photoreceptors, and blocking of axoplasmic flow.[p] In monkeys, optic atrophy was evident 4 weeks after intravitreal injection of 10 μg, and there were extensive changes in the retina.[r]

Teratogenic action causing malformations of the eye have been reported from colchicine given systemically to hamsters. This has been explained by histologic finding of arrest of mitosis in metaphase in the fetus three hours after a single dose given to the mother.[c]

a. Buschke W, Friedenwald JS, Fleischmann W: Studies on the miotic activity of the corneal epithelium. *JOHNS HOPKINS HOSP BULL* 73:143–168, 1943.

b. DeOcampo G: Inhibition of reaction to freezing injury of the ciliary body by colchicine. *J PHILIPP MED ASSOC* 42:573–598, 1966.

c. Ferme VH: Effect of transplacental miotic inhibitors on the fetal hamster eye. *ANAT REC* 148:129–137, 1964.

d. Fleischmann W, Goldin A, et al: Studies of colchicine derivatives: toxicity and antimiotic effect. *FED PROC* 8:47, 1949.

e. Friedenwald JS, Busche WJ, Moses SG: Comparison of effects of mustard, ultraviolet and x-radiation, and colchicine on cornea. *JOHNS HOPKINS HOSP BULL* 82:312–325, 1948.

f. Karlsson JO, Sjostrand J: Effect of colchicine on the axonal transport of protein in the optic nerve and tract of the rabbit. *BRAIN RES* 13:617–619, 1969.

g. Akinosho EA, Basu PK: The control of corneal graft reaction by topical application of antimitotic agents. *CAN J OPHTHALMOL* 6:109–114, 1971.

h. Bhatteracherjee P, Eakins KE: The intraocular pressure lowering effect of colchicine. *EXP EYE RES* 27:649–653, 1978.

i. Biedner BZ, Rothkoff L, et al: Colchicine suppression of corneal healing after strabismus surgery. *BR J OPHTHALMOL* 61:496–497, 1977.

j. Gipson IK, et al: Effects of cytochalasins and colchicine on migration of corneal epithelium. *INVEST OPHTHALMOL VIS SCI* 22:633–642, 643–650, 1982.

k. Hanson H–A: A histochemical study of retinal changes induced by treatment with colchicine. *EXP EYE RES* 12:198–205, 1971.

l. Hanson H–A, Sjostrand J: Ultrastructural changes induced in the rat retina by treatment with colchicine. *DOC OPHTHALMOL* 31:29–63, 1972.

m. Ritch R, Mulberg A, et al: The effect of colchicine on aqueous humor dynamics. *EXP EYE RES* 32:143–150, 1981.

n. Sjostrand J, Hannson H–A: Effect of colchicine on the transport of axonal protein in the retinal ganglion cells of the rat. *EXP EYE RES* 12:261–269, 1971.

o. Sjostrand J, Karlsson J–O: Axonal transport in the retinal ganglion cells of the rabbit under different experimental conditions. *ACTA OPHTHALMOL* Suppl 123:31–40, 1974.

p. Vaccarezza OL, Pasqualini E, Pecci Saavedra J: Retinal alterations induced by intravitreous colchicine. *VIRCHOWS ARCH ABT B CELL PATHOL* 12:159–167, 1973.

q. Weimar V, Fellman M: Connective tissue cell mobilization and migration following wounding. *EXP EYE RES* 9:12–21, 1970.

r. Davidson C, Green WR, Wong VG: Retinal atrophy induced by intravitreous colchicine. *INVEST OPHTHALMOL VIS SCI* 24:301–311, 1983.

Collagen derivatives from animal skin in the form of a viscous solution or a gel produced by ultraviolet irradiation have been tested as substitute for vitreous humor, with potential use in treatment of retinal detachment in mind, but in normal monkeys the solutions produced vitreous opacities, and the gel lacked the desired rigidity.[a] Inflammation was not excessive in normal eyes, but more severe in eyes subjected to scleral diathermy or cryotreatment.[b]

Collagen itself in rabbit eyes caused moderate reaction.[c]

a. Pruett RC, Calabria GA, Schepens CL: Collagen vitreous substitute. *ARCH OPHTHALMOL* 88:540–543, 1972.

b. Constable IJ, Swann DS: Biological vitreous substitutes. *ARCH OPHTHALMOL* 88:544–548, 1972.

c. Pfeiffer RL, Safrit HD, et al: Intraocular response to cotton, collagen, and cellulose in the rabbit. *OPHTHALMIC SURG* 14:582–587, 1983.

Collagenase enzyme in purified form from bacteria has been investigated as an aid to vitrectomy in removing scar tissue strands in the vitreous body in rabbits, and has been found to be adequately tolerated by the retina and lens.[a]

a. Moorhead LC, Chu HH, Garcia CA: Enzyme-assisted vitrectomy with bacterial collagenase. *ARCH OPHTHALMOL* 101:265–274, 1983.

Concanavalin A is a protein from jack beans that has been shown to bind to the plasma membrane of the outer segments of photoreceptors and retinal pigment epithelium in rats and frogs. When injected into the vitreous body in rats it has caused a temporary increase in large phagosomes in the retinal pigment epithelium, which could be explained by an increase in phagocytosis of rod outer segments, or a decrease in the rate of their degradation in the retinal pigment epithelium.[a] This is primarily of interest as an investigative tool. Incidentally, and thought unrelated, the injection causes bleeding into the vitreous body, but not into the retina. The retina and optic nerves appear to be uninjured.

a. Pedersen OO, Karlsen RL: Effects of the plant lectin concanavalin A on the retinal pigment epithelium. *ACTA OPHTHALMOL* 59:901–908, 1981.

Contact lenses have caused conjunctival and corneal disturbances attributed to substances accumulated on their surfaces, to physical effects, or to the solutions used with them. More relevant to a toxicologic inquiry is the question whether wearing contact lenses is advantageous or disadvantageous to people exposed to irritant atmospheres or splashes of dangerous chemicals, and especially when also wearing standard safety goggles or face shield. A survey of opinions obtained by Kandel in 1980 indicated that most respondents thought that contact lenses were disadvantageous, but these opinions seemed to be based on hypothetical reasoning, whereas the opinions of a minority who had actual case experience or had performed experimental tests were that contact lenses were advantageous and partially protective. Tests in rabbits of splashes of acetic acid, n-butylamine and acetone by Guthrie and Seitz in 1975 were specifically noted as showing some protection.

In 1982, Nilsson and Andersson investigated the behavior of soft contact lenses in the presence of trichloroethylene and xylene vapors, finding that these vapors were absorbed and concentrated by the lenses, but were released so slowly to a simulated tear film that for a considerable period the eye itself would be exposed to a lower concentration than by direct exposure. The same investigators, in experiments on rabbits, applied a drop of solution of sodium hydroxide or of hydrochloric acid to both eyes, with a soft contact lens on one, then removed the lens after one or two minutes (no irrigation mentioned). With sodium hydroxide the eye with the lens was no better or worse than the control eye. With hydrochloric acid, the eye with the lens was slightly less injured than the control eye, indicating partially protective effect.

Guthrie JW, Seitz GF: An investigation of the chemical contact lens problem. *J OCCUP MED* 17:163, 1975.

Kandel M: Summary on contact lenses. *CHEM ENGIN NEWS* 58:2 and 65, 1980.

Nilsson SG, Andersson L: The use of contact lenses in environments with organic solvents, acids or alkalis. *ACTA OPHTHALMOL* 60:599–608, 1982.

Contraceptive hormones (oral contraceptives, ovulation inhibitors, "the pill"), composed of various proportions of estrogens and progestins, came into widespread use in the 1960's as birth control agents.

The resume of reported adverse neuro-ophthalmic and ophthalmic effects to be given here is arranged to present first the clinical and then the experimental animal studies. Under the clinical heading will be a listing of other reviews, controlled surveys of series of patients, and then specific reported clinical side effects. A selected bibliography of more than 90 references is given at the end of this report on contraceptive hormones; still others are to be found in some of the review articles listed. Practically all the clinical information to be discussed concerns women of child-bearing age.

By 1970 the oral contraceptives had been shown to have significantly fewer adverse side effects than pregnancy itself, but retrospective statistical studies, especially in Great Britain, indicated that women who were taking these agents, especially those taking preparations having higher estrogen content, had significantly higher incidence of thromboembolic phenomena, particularly pulmonary embolism, than nonpregnant unmedicated women. Whether taking oral contraceptives of the progestin-estrogen type produced a higher incidence of ocular and ophthalmoneurologic diseases than would occur spontaneously in unmedicated women or in pregnant women was not answered conclusively, though much attention had been given to the question.

Walsh and Hoyt in 1969 gave a comprehensive discussion of the evolution and status of studies on the question of association of ophthalmic and neurologic diseases with the progestin-estrogen oral contraceptives.[256] Reviews with numerous references have been published by Walsh (1965), Lieberman (1968), Mayo (1968), Salmon (1968), Chizek (1969), Levinson (1969), Nicholson (1969), McQueen (1971), Corcelle (1972, 1973), Bonnet (1976), and Petursson (1981).

There have been numerous case reports of neuro-ophthalmic and ophthalmic diseases in patients taking oral contraceptives, but most of the same diseases occur sporadically also in the absence of oral contraceptives, and it will take many observations and much analysis of statistics to determine whether the contraceptive hormones have actually been responsible for the disturbances reported. The main considerations that have often molded clinical opinion into blaming these agents have been case reports in which ophthalmic disease has appeared in formerly normal women soon after medication was started, and case reports in which the ophthalmic disease disappeared or greatly improved after contraceptive hormones were discontinued. However, in some cases, ophthalmic disease appeared only after months or years of medication.

Ophthalmologic surveys of large groups of patients taking oral contraceptives have been carried out as a first necessary step in an attempt to determine whether ophthalmic disease is present in greater incidence than in unmedicated women. Faust (1966), studying 212 patients on oral contraceptives, found no greater incidence of disease than in the general population. Connell (1969), examining 611 patients prior to medication and 305 after use of oral contraceptives for one to three years, found no significant difference in incidence of eye abnormalities in association with the treatment. Corcelle (1972, 1973) and Davidson (1971) evaluating incidence reports found no direct evidence to prove the oral contraceptives responsible. Gossele (1971) found no difference in Goldmann perimetry or dark adaptation measurements with and without medication. McQueen (1971) reviewed these and other studies of a series of patients indicating no significant increase in eye disease in association with oral contraception. Tiburtius (1973) compared visual fields, dark adaptation, and intraocular pressures in women taking the pill intermittently and found no significant differences during periods with or without. On the contrary, Verbeck (1973) in a survey of 60 women taking the pill reported abnormalities of retina and optic nerves in 10, which seemed remarkable, but without a comparable control series evaluated by the same criteria it is difficult to assess the significance. More frequent abnormalities of color vision have been detected by Neubauer (1973), Marre (1974), and Lakowski (1977) in women taking contraceptive hormones than in those not taking them, and there appears to be an increase in incidence with time.

Despite the several surveys that have failed to prove an association statistically, there have been such strong clinical impressions and so many individually impressive case reports that it seems necessary to keep an open mind to the likelihood that contraceptive hormones have an important role in a small proportion of cases.

The abnormal conditions that have been reported in patients taking oral contraceptives have fallen mainly into two groups: (a) those affecting the CNS primarily and affecting the eyes secondarily, and (b) those involving primarily the optic nerve and retina. In both categories the strongest suspicions have been focused on vascular abnormalities because of the general agreement that thromboembolic phenomena in general may be greater when oral contraceptives are taken, though not as great as in pregnancy.

Walsh (1965) in a classical assembly of sixty-nine cases from all available sources, found these included four cases of pseudotumor cerebri, seventeen cases of stroke syndrome, and ten cases of migraine. Since then, additional cases of pseudotumor cerebri have been reported by Arbenz (1965), Huismans (1974), Janzik (1973), Saracco (1971), and Van Dyk (1969).

Additional cases of cerebrovascular thrombosis, both venous, and arterial have been reported by Atkinson (1970), Beeckman (1975), Mayer (1979), Reisner (1973), and Zanin (1977). According to Beeckman (1975) the greatest number of cases were internal carotid artery and collaterals thrombosis; second were vertebro-basilar obstructions.

Homonymous hemianopia or quadrant-anopia, as signs of cerebrovascular accidents, have been reported in individual cases by Behrman (1967), Salmon (1968), Eichholtz (1975), and Vola (1976).

Onset of migraine, or conspicuous worsening of migraine, or other types of headache, in association with taking contraceptive hormones have been mentioned in numerous reports since called to attention by Walsh,[256] and studied by Carroll (1973). Many patients have been described as having to discontinue the treatment because of headache, and to be much relieved after discontinuing.

Involvement of the optic nerves has been attributed to contraceptive hormones in a number of cases, without sufficient numbers or comparisons in untreated women to be sure of the association.

Bilateral optic neuritis has been reported in individual cases by Hollwich (1969) and Hopping (1969) in five cases by McGrand (1969), as well as by Payeur (1970), Verbeck (1973), and Huismans (1982). Retrobulbar neuritis in two cases was reported by Caffi (1968), and in other cases by Smith (1970) and Follman (1973).

Disturbances of retinal blood vessels have been by far the most common ocular abnormality reported in patients taking oral contraceptives, though there is little to indicate that the incidence is significantly greater than in unmedicated patients. Occlusions of central branch retinal arteries or veins have been reported by Caffi (1968), Hollwich (1969), Hopping (1969), McGrand (1969), Neubauer (1969), Paufique (1968), Thiel (1969), Beeckman (1975), Blade (1971), Boissini (1971), Delpech (1971), Fanta (1973), Fulmek (1974), Gervais (1977), Gombos (1975), Huismans (1976), Jamotton (1972), Jampol (1976), Leff (1976), Mayer (1979), Perry (1977), Stowe (1978), Varga (1973, 1976), and Verbeck (1973). Histopathology was reported by Stowe (1978). In a large majority of these cases vascular occlusions have been uniocular. In some of the reports, retinal vein occlusions appeared imminent, rather than complete.

Retinal edema has been described by Flynn (1966) and Goren (1967), and retinal hemorrhages by Svarc (1977), Verbeck (1974), and Zirm (1974).

Maculopathy attributed to contraceptive hormones has been reported by McGrand (1969), Huismans (1974), Rush (1977), Svarc (1977), Verbeck (1974), and Zirm (1974). Pigmentary degeneration of the maculas but normal ERG has been reported by Paufique (1969) with the particularly interesting observations that when the contraceptive hormones were discontinued, the vision returned to normal in the course of a few months on two occasions, and that achromatopsia and central scotoma reappeared when the medication was resumed. Bilateral macular hemorrhages have been reported by Paton (1969) in a young woman who had severe megaloblastic anemia with very low serum folate, possibly due to oral contraceptives, and she recovered well when folic acid was administered.

Apart from the reports of disturbances of the CNS and retinal vascular disease, or optic neuritis, there have been several articles expressing opinions concerning the possible induction of lens opacities or cataracts in women taking contraceptive hormones, by Godde-Jolly (1972), Morizot-Leite (1978), Offret (1974), Trux (1975), and Varga (1973, 1976). However, evidence is lacking to establish whether the incidence is significantly greater than in women not taking the hormones. Most of the opacities have been described as posterior cortical and often dust-like. In some reports there has been no indication whether the opacities were actually sufficient to interfere with vision.

There has been considerable interest in possible influences of contraceptive hormones on tear production and on the cornea that might influence wearing of contact lenses. Various beliefs or impressions concerning alterations of curvature or tendency to edema that might be produced by the hormones have been expressed by Caran (1966), Koetting (1966), Malbrel (1968), Peter (1967), Reuben (1966), and Sarwar (1966). However, Reilingh (1978) in a controlled evaluation found no difference in tolerance to contact lenses among 199 women on the pill, 242 not on the pill, and 76 men, and noted that also Connell, Davidson, Fausst, and Ruben had found no relationship in series of patients. Similarly, although Verbeck (1973) had reported frequent subnormal tear production, no evidence for this was found in controlled series by Ruprecht (1976) and Frankel (1978).

The intraocular pressure has been no problem under the influence of the pill. In fact, several authors have reported a modest reduction, and it has been used with some small benefit in treatment of open-angle glaucoma, as noted by Corcelle (1972, 1973). A series of comparative observations in non-glaucomatous women by Tiburtius (1973) showed no significant difference in pressure on or off the pill. In one exceptional case report by Mortada (1975), unilateral proptosis and open-angle glaucoma limited to the same eye disappeared after the hormones were stopped, but it now appears quite probable that this was an instance of dural shunt with glaucoma due to elevation of episcleral venous pressure, a condition that occurs in the absence of hormonal treatment and typically spontaneously gets better.

In experimental animals little has been established so far relative to ophthalmic complications of oral contraceptives. In owl monkeys Kulvin (1965) observed dilation of retinal veins after daily administration of oral contraceptive hormones, but no papilledema or hemorrhages. In monkeys Lee (1969) observed small dots of opacity in the anterior cortex of the lenses at dosages twenty-five to forty times the human dosage, also transient dilation of retinal veins in two out of forty-seven rabbits, and papilledema and optic atrophy in one rabbit out of forty-seven. Several months after norethynodrel had been given and then stopped, two out of twelve rabbits were found to develop retinal vein occlusions. In rats Ray (1969) found cataracts in females after fifteen to eighteen months medication at low dosage, but no abnormality of the lenses in four months at very high dosage.

In rabbit lenses maintained in tissue culture, Lambert (1968) found that a series of progestins and estrogens added to the medium caused increase in permeability to cations and loss of clarity of the lenses associated with alteration of cation content and increase in water content, but these hormones did not affect active cation transport by the lenses.

More recently, Drill (1975) administered commercial contraceptive hormone preparations to dogs and rhesus monkeys in dosages 25 to 50 times the human dose for 5 years, and found no significant differences between the eyes of medicated and unmedicated control animals. However, Kraeer (1981) in a 22 month study with monkeys found that while no ocular lesions developed when safflower oil was fed with the hormones, there was a difference when butter was fed with the hormones, leading to perivascular and sub-intimal abnormalities of the central retinal vessels, and thickening of the stroma of the cornea.

Arbenz JP: Cerebral pseudotumor from oral contraceptives. *SCHWEIZ MED WOCHENSCHR* 95:1654, 1965.

Atkinson EA, Fairburn B, Heathfield KWG: Intracranial venous thrombosis as complication of oral contraception. *LANCET* 1:914–918, 1970.

Beeckman G, Brihaye-Van Geertruyden M, et al: Neuro-ophthalmologic vascular disturbances from contraceptive hormones. *BULL SOC BELGE OPHTALMOL* 171:754–767, 1975. (French)

Behrman S: Homonymous hemianopia after oral contraceptives. *BR MED J* 683, 1967.

Blade J, Darleguy P, Chanteau Y: Early onset of thrombosis of the central retinal artery and oral contraceptives. *BULL SOC OPHTALMOL FRANCE* 71:48–49, 1971. (French)

Boisson J–P: The pill and ophthalmic artery pressure. *BULL SOC OPHTALMOL FRANCE* 71:872–874, 1971. (French)

Bonnet M: The visual apparatus and oral contraceptives. *ANN OCULIST* 209:213–220, 1976. (French)

Caffi M: Oral contraceptives and ocular complications. *ANN OTTALMOL CLIN OCUL* 94:149–154, 1968. (Italian)

Caran GA: Contact lenses and oral contraceptives. *BR MED J* 5493:980, 1966.

Carroll JD, Grant ECG: The effect of oral contraceptives on blood vessels and migraine. *KLIN MONATSBL AUGENHEILKD* 163:212–215, 1973. (German)

Chizek DJ, Franceschetti AT: Oral contraceptives: their side effects and ophthalmological manifestations. *SURV OPHTHALMOL* 14:90–105, 1969.

Cogan DG: Do oral contraceptives have neuro-ophthalmic complications? (Editorial) *ARCH OPHTHALMOL* 73:461–462, 1965.

Connell EB, Kelman CD: Ophthalmologic findings with oral contraceptives. *OBSTET GYNECOL* 31:456–460, 1968.

Connell EG, Kelman CD: Eye examinations in patients taking oral contraceptives. *FERTIL STERIL* 20:67–74, 1969.

Corcelle L: Eye and pill. *KLIN MONATSBL AUGENHEILKD* 160:235–239, 1972; 163:204–211, 1973. (German)

Davidson SI: Reported adverse effects of oral contraceptives on the eye. *TRANS OPHTHALMOL SOC UK* 91:561–574, 1971.

Delpech J, Amalric P, Cuq G: Retinal arterial thrombosis and oral estrogen-progestins. *BULL SOC OPHTALMOL FRANCE* 71:306–309, 1971. (French)

Drill VA, Rao KS, et al: Ocular effects of oral contraceptives. I. Studies in the dog. *FERTIL STERIL* 26:908–913, 1975.

Drill VA, Martin DP, et al: Ocular effects of oral contraceptives. II. Studies in the rhesus monkey. *FERTIL STERIL* 26:914–918, 1975.

Eichholtz W: A collection of homonymous visual field defects with vascular basis in young women. *MUNCH MED WOCHENSCHR* 117:571–574, 1975. (German)

Fanta H: Changes in vessels in the ocular fundus caused by contraceptives. *KLIN MONATSBL AUGENHEILKD* 163:13–17, 1973. (German)

Faust JM, Tyler ET: Ophthalmologic findings in patients using oral contraception. *FERTIL STERIL* 17:1–6, 1966.

Flynn MA, Esterly DB: Ocular manifestations after Enovid. *AM J OPHTHALMOL* 61:907–910, 1966.

Follmann P, Mucsi G, Varga M: Functional disturbances of the optic nerve associated with use of contraceptives. *KLIN MONATSBL AUGENHEILKD* 162:643–648, 1973.

Frankel SH, Ellis PP: Effect of oral contraceptives on tear production. *ANN OPHTHALMOL* 10:1585–1588, 1978.

Fulmek R: Branch occlusion of central retinal artery after long-term prophylaxis with antiovulation medications. *KLIN MONATSBL AUGENHEILKD* 164:371–377, 1974. (German)

Gervais C, LeRebeller MJ, Fontanges F: Bilateral widespread retinal periphlebitis in a young woman under contraceptive treatment. *BULL SOC OPHTALMOL FRANCE* 77:191–192, 1977. (French)

Giovanni A, Consolani A: Contraceptive-induced unilateral retinopathy. *OPHTHALMOLOGICA* 179:302–305, 1979.

Godde-Jolly D, Ruellan YM, et al: Three observations of cataract that appeared in women taking the same oral contraceptive. *BULL SOC OPHTALMOL FRANCE* 72:441–442, 1972. (French)

Gombos GM, Moreno DH, Bedrossian PB: Retinal vascular occlusion induced by oral contraceptives. *ANN OPHTHALMOL* 7:215–217, 1975.

Goren SB: Retinal edema secondary to oral contraceptives. *AM J OPHTHALMOL* 63:447–453, 1967.

Gossele I, Tiburtius H: Visual field and dark adaptation after giving contraceptives. *KLIN MONATSBL AUGENHEILKD* 158:856–861, 1971. (German)

Hollwich F, Verbeck B: Side effects of antiovulation medications on the eye. *DTSCH MED WOCHENSCHR* 35:1761–1765, 1969. (German)

Hollwich F, Junemann G, Verbeck B: On side effects of anti-ovulation medications on the retinal venous system and the optic nerve. *KLIN MONATSBL AUGENHEILKD* 154:830–837, 1969. (German)

Hopping W, Wessing A: Bilateral optic neuritis and occlusion of the superior macular arteriole in a 24-year-old woman. *KLIN MONATSBL AUGENHEILKD* 154:847–850, 1969. (German)

Huismans H: (Complications of contraceptive hormones.) *KLIN MONATSBL AUGENHEILKD* 165:344–347, 1974; 169:505–507, 1976; 171:781–786, 1977; 180:173–175, 1982.

Jamotton L, Michiels J: Retinal arterial accidents with anovulatory medications. *BULL SOC BELGE OPHTALMOL* 161:669–682, 1972. (French)

Jampol LM, Isenberg SJ, Goldberg MF: Occlusive retinal arteriolitis with neovascularization. *AM J OPHTHALMOL* 81:583–589, 1976.

Janzik HH: Benign increase in intracranial pressure during oral contraception. *DTSCH MED WOCHENSCHR* 98:2028–2029, 1973.

Koetting RA: Influence of oral contraceptives on contact lens wearing. *J OPTOM* 43:2368–2374, 1966.

Kulvin SM, Harner RE, Smith JL: Acute norethynodrel toxicity in the primate. *INVEST OPHTHALMOL* 4:957, 1965.

Lakowski R, Morton A: The effect of oral contraceptives on colour vision in diabetic women. *CAN J OPHTHALMOL* 12:89–97, 1977.

Lambert BW: The effects of progestins and estrogens on the permeability of the lens. *ARCH OPHTHALMOL* 80:230–234, 1968.

Lee P, Donovan RH, Mukai N: Effects of norethynodrel with mestranol on the rabbit eye. *ARCH OPHTHALMOL* 81:89–98, 1969.

Lee PF, Schepens CL, Donovan RH: Norethynodrel with mestranol and the rabbit eye. *INVEST OPHTHALMOL* 7:119, 1968.

Leff SP: Side effect of oral contraceptives. Occlusion of branch artery of the retina. *BULL SINAI HOSP DETROIT* 24:227–229, 1976.

Levinson JM: The birth control pill and its ophthalmologic side effects. *DELAWARE MED J* 41:118–120, 1969.

Lieberman TW: Ocular effects of prolonged systemic drug administration. *DIS NERV SYST* 29:44–50, 1968.

Malbrel PH, Woillez M, Dhedin G: The influence of the pill on the wearing of contact lenses. *BULL SOC OPHTALMOL FRANCE* 68:1035–1039, 1968. (French)

Marre M, Neubauer O, Nemetz U: Colour vision and the "pill". *MOD PROBL OPHTHALMOL* 13:345–348, 1974.

Mayer H: A contribution concerning serious eye disturbances by ovulation inhibitors. *KLIN MONATSBL AUGENHEILKD* 175:677–680, 1979. (German)

Mayo CM, et al: Neurologic complications of oral contraceptives. *ILLINOIS MED J* 133:619–621, 1968.

McGrand JC, Cory CC: Ophthalmic disease and the pill. *BR MED J* 187, 1969.

McQueen EG: Hormonal steroid contraceptives. *DRUGS* 2:20–44, 1971.

Mortada A: Oral contraceptive and unilateral proptosis with glaucoma simplex. *BULL SOC OPHTHALMOL EGYPT* 68:485–488, 1975.

Morizot-Leite LA, Chagas RJV: Cataract induced by oral contraceptives. *REV BRAS OFTALMOL* 37:161–165, 1978. (Portuguese)

Neubauer H: Disturbances of retinal blood circulation under ovulation inhibitors. *KLIN MONATSBL AUGENHEILKD* 154:838–845, 1969. (German)

Neubauer O: Color disturbances during long-term use of ovulation inhibitors. *KLIN MONATSBL AUGENHEILKD* 162:803–806, 1973. (German)

Nicholson DH, Walsh FB: Oral contraceptives and neuroophthalmologic disorders. *J REPROD MED* 3:73–79, 1969.

Offret G, Haut J: Contraceptive pills and cataract. *BULL SOC OPHTALMOL FRANCE* 74:1119–1123, 1974. (French)

O'Steen WK, Kraeer SL, St.Clair RW: Influence of fatty acids on the eyes of a non-human primate. *EXP MOL PATHOL* 34:43–51, 1981.

Paton A: Oral contraceptives and folate deficiency. *LANCET* 1:418, 1969.

Paufique L, Lequin M: Retinal arterial thrombosis and oral contraceptives. *BULL SOC OPHTALMOL FRANCE* 68:512–515, 1968. (French)

Paufique L, Magnard P: Manifestations of macular disturbances while using the pill. *BULL SOC OPHTALMOL FRANCE* 69:467–468, 1969. (French)

Payeur G, Bronner A: Ocular problems and contraceptives. *BULL SOC OPHTALMOL* 70:699–703, 1970. (French)

Perry HD, Mallen FJ: Cilioretinal artery occlusion associated with oral contraceptives. *AM J OPHTHALMOL* 84:56–58, 1977.

Peter PA, Parsons CP: Observations of some contact lens wearers using oral contraceptives. *J CONTACT LENS SOC* 1:9–14, 1967.

Petursson GJ, Fraunfelder FT, Meyer SM: Oral contraceptives. *OPHTHALMOLOGY* 88:368–371, 1981.

Ray JA, Schut AL: Cataracts and other lesions in rats receiving a synthetic progestin-estrogen. *TOXICOL APPL PHARMACOL* 14:634, 1969.

Reilingh AD, Reiners H, Van Bijsterveld OP: Contact lens tolerance and oral contraceptives. *ANN OPHTHALMOL* 10:947–952, 1978.

Reisner H: Cerebral disturbances in connection with use of oral contraceptives. *KLIN MONATSBL AUGENHEILKD* 163:6–12, 1973. (German)

Reuben M: Contact lenses and oral contraceptives. *BR MED J* 5497:1235, 1966.

Ruprecht KW, Loch EG, Giere W: Sandy feeling in the eyes and contraceptive hormones. *KLIN MONATSBL AUGENHEILKD* 168:198–204, 1976.

Rush JA: Acute macular neuroretinopathy. *AM J OPHTHALMOL* 83:490–494, 1977.

Salmon ML, Winkelman JZ, Gay AJ: Neuroophthalmic sequelae in users of oral contraceptives. *J AM MED ASSOC* 206:85–91, 1968.

Saracco JB, et al: Hemorrhagic papilledema associated with oral contraceptives. *BULL SOC OPHTALMOL FRANCE* 71:43–48, 1971. (French)

Sarwar M: Contact lenses and oral contraceptives. *BR MED J* 5497, 1235, 1966.

Smith MS, Krieger A: Visual loss associated with oral contraceptives. *AM J OPHTHALMOL* 69:874–876, 1970.

Stowe GC III, Zakov ZN, Albert DM: Central retinal vascular occlusion associated with oral contraceptives. *AM J OPHTHALMOL* 86:798–801, 1978.

Svarc ED, Werner D: Isolated retinal hemorrhages associated with oral contraceptives. *AM J OPHTHALMOL* 84:50–55, 1977.

Thiel H–L: Observations on the effect of ovulation inhibitors on the eye. *KLIN MONATSBL AUGENHEILKD* 154:845–847, 1969. (German)

Tiburtius HF: Investigations of the influence of contraceptives on the visual field, dark adaptation and the intraocular pressure. *KLIN MONATSBL AUGENHEILKD* 163:215–216, 1973. (German)

Trux E, Varga M, Follman P: Ocular complications in the course of oral contraceptive treatment. *BULL MEM SOC FR OPHTALM* 87:310–312, 1975. (French)

Varga M: Ophthalmologic complications after oral contraception. *KLIN MONATSBL AUGENHEILKD* 162:621–629, 1973. (German)

Varga M: Recent experiences on the ophthalmologic complications of oral contraceptives. *ANN OPHTHALMOL* 8:925–934, 1976.

Verbeck B: Eye findings and metabolic conditions associated with taking ovulation inhibitors. *KLIN MONATSBL AUGENHEILKD* 162:612–621, 1973. (German)

Verbeck B, Schiffer HP: Does long-term medication with ovulation inhibitors cause premature arteriosclerotic fundus changes? *KLIN MONATSBL AUGENHEILKD* 165:296–304, 1974. (German)

Vola JL, Boudouresques J, et al: Hemianopsia and oral contraceptives. *BULL SOC OPHTALMOL FRANCE* 76:489–491, 1976.

Walsh FB, Clark DB, et al: Oral contraceptives and neuro-ophthalmologic interest. *ARCH OPHTHALMOL* 74:628–640, 1965.

Zanin A, Bourgeois R, et al: Bilateral aseptic thrombosis of the cavernous sinuses. *BULL SOC BELGE OPHTALMOL* 176:7–18, 1977. (French)

Zirm M, Schmut O, Bartl G: Lipoprotein elevation and possible simultaneous retinal disturbance by an oral contraceptive. *KLIN MONATSBL AUGENHEILKD* 165:470–474, 1974.

Copper compounds. External contact effects are described for *copper acetoarsenite, copper chloride, copper cyanide, copper sulfate,* and *verdigris* (copper carbonate and oxide) as follows:

Copper acetoarsenite (Paris green, Schweinfurth green) in farmers exposed to the dust has caused dry scaly dermatitis with brown pigmentation and irritation of the eyes and upper respiratory tract.

Copper chloride applied in 0.08 to 0.16 M solution to the corneas of rabbits after the removal of the epithelium, or injected into the stroma, causes severe reaction with permanent opacification.[81,123]

Copper cyanide plating bath employed in electroplating of copper can cause severe burns of the human eye, owing principally to the strong alkalinity of the solution. The type of corneal damage appears to be the same as in alkali burns such as produced by sodium hydroxide.[81]

Copper sulfate formerly was widely employed in treatment of trachoma by repeated topical application of the solid material to the diseased conjunctiva. This resulted in temporary inflammation and purulent reaction, and eventually induced discoloration of the cornea, beginning as a reddish brown or greenish ring distributed like arcus senilis, in advanced cases covering the whole cornea, but causing slight or no interference with vision.[a] The deposit resembled that seen in ocular chalcosis from intraocular metallic copper, appearing most dense in the region of Descemet's membrane.[b] The same uncomplicated discoloration of the cornea has been produced by use of eyedrops containing copper sulfate for many years.[c] If a particle of copper sulfate was left accidentally in the conjunctival sac, it could cause local inflammation and necrosis, corneal opacity, and symblepharon.[153] Experimentally in rabbit eyes the severity of reaction to locally applied copper sulfate varies with concentration, duration and exposure, and condition of the corneal epithelium.[123,377] Rabbit corneas have been noted to become more densely opacified than ox corneas.[153]

Verdigris, formed by atmospheric corrosion of the surface of metallic copper and presumably composed of copper carbonates and oxides, causes immediate irritation and conjunctival inflammation when accidentally dropped or dusted on the eyes of patients, but the reaction subsides without permanent damage soon after the eye is cleaned by irrigation.[81,153]

a. Stephenson S: Corneal opacity from the use of copper sulphate. *OPHTHALMOL REV* Feb. 1903, p. 54.
b. vonSallmann L: On atypical chalcosis of the cornea from incorrect use of the copper stick. *Z AUGENHEILKD* 62:180–182, 1927. (German)
c. Sundmacher R, Alpers K: Corneal chalcosis from misuse of copper sulfate eye drops. *KLIN MONATSBL AUGENHEILKD* 182:325–327, 1983. (German)

Copper metal foreign bodies, and foreign bodies of copper alloys such as *brass* and *bronze,* have had such serious toxic effects within the eye, and have presented such problems in clinical management that hundreds of articles have been written on the subject. Notable reviews have been published by Fontana (1938); Jess (1924); Neubauer (1979); Pau (1969)[189] and Rosenthal (1974, 1975, 1977). The proceedings of a symposium on intraocular foreign bodies and resultant ocular metalloses sponsored by the German Ophthalmological Society in 1977 are particularly noteworthy.[364] (The term *metallosis* signifies impregnation of eye tissues with a foreign metal; *chalcosis* signifies impregnation with copper, which may be exogenous as from a foreign body, or endogenous as in Wilson's disease; the endogenous form will be described in a subsequent separate section entitled "Copper, systemic".)

Intraocular foreign bodies of copper, or its alloys, have been notorious for destructive effect on the eye for over a century. The fact that they are non-magnetic generally makes them more difficult to remove than iron or steel, and no effective medical treatment has been devised for those that cannot be removed surgically. Copper intraocular foreign bodies are less common than those of iron, and their source is different. Copper and its alloys are usually driven into the eye by an explosion, most characteristically by explosion of brass cartridges, blasting caps, or war-time mines. The seriousness of injury depends primarily on the size and location of the foreign body within the eye, and the amount of hemorrhage and physical injury to eye tissues. In most animal experiments in which copper has been inserted into the eye, physical trauma has been minimized. Accordingly, conditions induced for study in animal eyes have not been as serious as some encountered clinically (Neubauer 1974, 1975; Walzer 1977).

In the worst cases seen clinically the copper particle penetrates the vitreous body to the retina. This is accompanied by hemorrhage, and rapid formation of an abscess, soon followed by some degree of encapsulation by connective tissue. The vitreous body characteristically is disorganized and destroyed. Total retinal detachment and phthisis bulbi follow. In these circumstances there is no time for copper to migrate forward and cause the discoloration of lens, cornea, and iris as is seen in chronic chalcosis associated with less serious injuries. Encapsulation of the foreign body may prolong the process in some cases, but copper has a tendency eventually to escape its encapsulation and to continue to do damage.

Clinical experience and experiments in animals have shown that, when a copper foreign body is in the vitreous body, it causes less disturbance the further it is from the retina, and the smaller it is. (Brunette 1980; Neubauer 1979; Rosenthal 1974). Small fragments of copper or brass in the anterior vitreous just behind the lens in a number of cases have been observed for years, gradually dissolving and disseminating copper to lens, cornea and iris, where copper has a predilection for the basement membranes, (Rao 1976; Rosenthal 1975). In the lens, most characteristically greenish-brown discoloration of the anterior capsule in the form of a sunflower is visible by slit-lamp microscope, sometimes accompanied by posterior subcapsular opacities (Hanna 1973; Jess 1922; Rosenthal 1979; Seland 1976; Michiels 1978.[360]) In the cornea, Descemet's membrane may show brownish discoloration peripherally similar to the Kayser-Fleischer ring of Wilson's disease (Jess 1924), and the iris may appear of a different, greenish, color than in the other eye. (Chalcosis in rabbits, unlike that in human beings, is said not to lead to discoloration of lens and cornea (Rosenthal 1975), but sunflower pseudocataract has been reported in rare instances (Palimeris 1977). Some of the interactions of copper and lens have been investigated in culture (Awasthi 1975; Coulter 1978).

A number of cases of long survival of vision with sequestered or anteriorly located copper foreign bodies have been described (Beckerman 1972; Rosenthal 1979). Copper alloys, such as brass, tend to produce the same effects as copper, but a little more slowly (Shereshevska 1960; Welge-Lussen 1977).

There has been some discussion of maculopathy that may be produced by copper, and be reversed by removal of the foreign body, but so far there is little documentation (Delaney 1975; Rosenthal 1979).

The reason for the less severe reaction when the foreign body is at a distance from the retina has been proposed to be on the grounds that near the retina and its blood vessels there is greater oxygen tension than at a distance, which causes metallic copper to oxidize to toxic copper compounds more rapidly close to or in contact with the retina than at a distance. Furthermore, the abscess formation that is characteristic of copper undergoing oxidation close to the retina and choroid can be attributed to attraction of polymorphonuclear leukocytes from these nearby vascular tissues, which become heavily infiltrated. Liquefaction and disorganization of the vitreous body has been explained on the basis of copper catalysis of oxidation of ascorbic acid, leading to depolymerization of the hyaluronic acid of the vitreous humor (Neubauer 1979; Pirie 1956; Ruessmann 1977). Changes in protein and hexosamine content have also been related to decrease in viscosity of the vitreous humor (Gundorova 1966).

Increased content of amino acids in the vitreous humor has been consistent with proteolysis of the vitreous body, but decreased concentration in the aqueous humor has suggested suppression of secretion of amino acids by the ciliary body under the influence of copper (Welge-Luessen 1969, 1977).

Based on the hypothesis that retinal and choroidal circulations near a copper foreign body provide an environment of high oxygen and abundant cells for the dissolution of the foreign body, photocoagulation or diathermocoagulation around fragments in the retina and choroid had been proposed as a method for suppressing the reaction (Gundorova 1973; Reussmann 1977).

The electroretinogram has been of much interest for detection of injury to the retina by intraocular copper. Clinical studies by Gorgone (1966) and Knave (1969)[136] have given evidence of the value of the ERG as a guide to treatment. They concluded that once the ERG started to become abnormal there was serious danger to vision, unless the foreign body was removed. Subsequent clinical studies have provided additional evidence of clinical usefullness of initial and sequential ERGs in cases in which the clinical conditions suggest that a fragment of copper may be tolerated by the eye (Jayle 1970; Kozousek 1974; Leuenberger 1977; Schmidt 1977). However, a sudden flattening of the ERG may signal retinal detachment rather than copper poisoning of the retina (Jayle 1970). In cases of fulminating inflammatory reaction to intraocular copper, it has been said that if the foreign body is removed within 10 days, a somewhat abnormal ERG may eventually return to normal (Neubauer 1975). The ERG in rabbits has been studied after implantation of copper in various positions in the vitreous body, using particles of various sizes, and studying the effects on the ERG (Brunette 1980; Moschos 1977; Palimeris 1977; Rosenthal 1974; Schmidt 1977; Sickel 1977). Interesting observations have been made. If several copper particles were introduced, the ERG might become extinguished within hours, before an inflammatory reaction was observed (Brunette 1980). Small particles in the vitreous body well away from the retina might not affect the ERG, and if near the retina, but encapsulated, might take months to extinguish the ERG (Brunette 1980; Palimeris 1977). In most experiments in rabbits, changes in the ERG became evident in a week or less; if the copper fragment was large, there was parallel reduction of a- and b-waves, but if the particle was small the b-wave decreased while the a-wave was unaffected or became greater (Moschos 1977; Palimeris 1977). Reduction of the ERG response has also been studied in rats (Schmidt 1977), and in frog retina *in vitro* (Sickel 1977).

Several methods have been developed to identify and to measure copper in the eye. These methods have been used to help in diagnosis and choice of time to operate, and to help in study of the mechanisms of toxic action of copper in the eye. For diagnostic purposes, these methods have been utilized especially in cases in which a non-magnetic foreign body has been shown to be in the eye by x-ray or by ultrasonography, but it is hidden from view by blood or other opaque media, and its composition is not known. For experimental investigative purposes, these methods have been utilized in studies of the rate of dissolution, and the patterns of dissemination of copper in the eye.

Chemical assay (Gerhard 1964, 1974), and atomic absorption spectrophotometry (Chechan 1968; Rosenthal 1974) have been used for analysis of aqueous humor obtained from patients by paracentesis, and for analysis of aqueous and vitreous humors from rabbits (Runyan 1979, Yassur 1979). X-ray fluorescence spectrometry has been utilized as a noninvasive procedure for identification and measurement of copper in the anterior chamber, cornea and sclera in patients (Belkin 1979) and in the vitreous body and retina in rabbits (Belkin 1976; Gorodetsky 1977; Loewinger 1976; Zeimer 1978). Electron probe x-ray analysis has been employed to determine the composition of an extracted foreign body (Chisholm 1977). In excised eyes, copper foreign bodies have been analyzed by atomic absorption spectrophotometry and x-ray diffraction (Rao 1976). Paramagnetic resonance spectroscopy has been employed to demonstrate the distribution of cupric ions in tissues of an enucleated eye (Shiga 1967). The specificity of histochemical staining procedures for copper deposits in the eye have been significantly improved and usefully applied (Rao 1976; Rosenthal 1975).

Comparing the measurement of copper in the aqueous humor and examination of the ERG as guides to clinical management, it has been pointed out that finding excessive copper in the aqueous humor indicates the foreign body is dissolving and warns of potential harm, whereas abnormality of the ERG signals that harm is actually occurring or has already occurred. It has been pointed out that elevated copper concentration is helpful in identifying a non-magnetic intraocular foreign body as copper or copper alloy, but that the concentration may not correlate with the amount of damage done (Leuenberger 1977; Zeimer 1978). However, normal copper concentration has been found to correlate with a quiescent foreign body which may be tolerated for a long time (Belkin 1979). A note of caution in interpretation of copper concentration in the aqueous humor has come from a study that showed that experimentally a piece of iron put into the vitreous body caused as much rise in aqueous and vitreous copper as did a copper particle (Yassur 1975). Also, caution is indicated by an observation that breaking down the blood-aqueous barrier causes increase in aqueous copper concentration, in rabbits at least (Rosenthal 1977). Another cautionary note comes from a clinical case in which treatment with penicillamine reduced the copper concentration in the aqueous humor and cornea, but did not prevent progression of severe damage in the posterior segment where the foreign body was located (Gerhard 1974).

The intraocular pressure in eyes with copper foreign bodies is most often not mentioned, but experienced observers have pointed out that when there is a strong ocular reaction to copper in human or rabbit eyes, the pressure characteristically is low (Neubauer 1974, 1979; Ruessman 1974, 1977). This may be due to reduction of aqueous formation. However, in rabbits some enzyme activities in the ciliary epithelium were found to be increased, rather than decreased (Ruessmann 1974). Ciliary carbonic anhydrase activity was reduced by about a third (Ruessmann 1977), but not enough to account for ocular hypotony.

In rare instances open-angle glaucoma has developed in eyes with disseminated chalcosis from copper foreign bodies, but not in endogenous chalcosis of Wilson's disease (Hanna 1973; Jess 1924, 1924; Pischel 1925; Sedan 1961; Teichmann 1978). Little has been known about the mechanism of induction of the glaucoma. A case reported by Sedan is an example. The patient had an intraocular copper foreign body for ten years with characteristic discoloration of the lens, and after the first several years developed glaucoma with pressures up to 55 mm Hg, responding partially to treatment with pilocarpine. Sedan, though providing a large bibliography on chalcosis, gave no information on the basis for the glaucoma. However, Stankovic, in discussing Sedan's case, reported a case of his own which was more informative. In this case, in which the glaucoma was associated with chalcosis of the lens and retina, Stankovic established that it was of open-angle type. It had been so severe and caused so much pain that iridencleisis was necessary. In the surgical coloboma the ciliary processes could be seen to be covered by a green dust, especially on their basal portions, presumably some sort of copper-containing material. Also the zonules had slight green discoloration. The corneoscleral trabecular meshwork was covered by ordinary brown pigment, but it was uncertain whether this pigmentation played a role in producing the open-angle glaucoma, or whether this pigment had been disseminated by the surgery.

Findings in another patient, who was shown to me by Warren Haley, have been additionally instructive. The patient had multiple fine intravitreal foreign bodies of brass from rupture of a rifle cartridge in 1960. These particles were too numerous and fine to remove. Within the next year characteristic discoloration appeared in the anterior lens capsule, but eight years later the vision was still 20/25. The anterior segment had never shown clinical evidences of inflammation, but eight years after the injury the intraocular pressure became elevated to 36 mm Hg. At that time there was a moderate amount of vitreous opacities, but the optic nervehead could be seen and appeared normal. There was slight yellow-green discoloration of the anterior lens capsule, and similar bilious sort of discoloration was strikingly present in the posterior layers of the cornea. This discoloration of the cornea was particularly striking during gonioscopic examination, and could be seen to change abruptly at Schwalbe's line, with corneoscleral trabecular meshwork and the scleral background distinctly less colored than the cornea. The angle of the anterior chamber was wide open all around. The trabecular meshwork had a distinct jaundiced sort of discoloration, mostly in the filtration area, and this area appeared to lack the fine, glittering surface characteristics of the normal contralateral eye. One tiny foreign body was visible in the angle of the anterior chamber, blackened, but with areas of slight metallic glistening. The contralateral eye, which was uninjured, was entirely normal, with normal intraocular pressure and no discoloration. In this case there appeared to be a very clear relationship between intraocular copper and the development of open-angle glaucoma, which appeared almost surely attributable to the action of copper on the trabecular meshwork, rather than due to inflammatory, mechanical, or synechial changes in the angle, since these were absent.

Copper or its alloys as foreign bodies in the cornea, conjunctiva or sclera provokes a purulent inflammatory reaction (Thiel 1977), which may lead to expulsion of the particle, but sometimes a particle in the cornea is tolerated (Verin 1973).

If the foreign body is in the anterior chamber, a purulent and fibrinous iritis soon appears, especially immediately around the foreign body, and soon completely covering it. In the angle of the anterior chamber copper may induce iritis and purulent infiltration of the adjacent cornea, which may go on to perforation and extrusion of the particle. When completely embedded in the lens, the foreign body causes the least inflammatory reaction. The gonioscopic appearance of copper and brass foreign bodies in the anterior chamber angle have been described by Thorpe.[243]

Embedded in iris or ciliary body, copper is poorly tolerated (Verin 1973).

Treatment of intraocular foreign bodies of copper and brass has generally been surgical when the particle has been sufficiently accessible so that its removal would not involve excessive physical damage to the eye, and results indicate that surgical removal often is successful and that it is particularly advantageous when done early before chalcosis develops.

Medical treatments for copper and brass foreign bodies in the eye were reviewed by Neubauer (1968).

The following agents have been tried experimentally in animals or clinically. Systemic *penicillamine* has been used by Delbecque (1966); Segal (1977), and Soyeux (1980); *sodium thiosulfate* topically and systemically by Muller (1937) and Habig (1951); *dimercaprol* parenterally, topically and intracamerally by Newell (1949), Rouher (1958), and Segal (1977); *hydrogen sulfide* intravitreally by Krwawicz (1966); *calcium and sodium edetate* orally by Mine (1958); and *electrolytic plating* by Krwawicz (1958). Unfortunately, none of these has been very successful.

Awasthi YC, Miller SP, et al: The effect of copper on human and bovine lens and on human cultured lens epithelium enzymes. *EXP EYE RES* 21:251–257, 1975.

Becherman BL: Intraocular foreign body extraction in early chalcosis. *ARCH OPHTHALMOL* 87:444–446, 1972.

Belkin M, Loewinger E, et al: A non-invasive method for detection and analysis of metals in the eye. *INVEST OPHTHALMOL* 15:770–773, 1976.

Belkin M, Zeimer R, et al: Management of nonmagnetic intraocular foreign bodies. *ARCH OPHTHALMOL* 97:106–108, 1979.

Brunette JR, Wagdi S, Lafond G: Electroretinographic alterations in retinal metallosis. *CAN J OPHTHALMOL* 15:176–178, 1980.

Chechan C, Francois P, Hache J–C: Application of atomic absorption spectrometry in assaying metals in the aqueous humor. *BULL SOC OPHTALMOL FRANCE* 68:113–120, 1968. (French)

Chisholm IA, Lalonde JMA, Ghadially FN: Electron probe x-ray analysis of an intraocular foreign body. *CAN J OPHTHALMOL* 12:315–317, 1977.

Coulter JB II, Oliver SS, et al: Toxic effects of copper on cultured rat lenses. *EXP EYE RES* 26:547–554, 1978.

Delaney WV Jr: Presumed ocular chalcosis and a reversible maculopathy. *ANN OPHTHALMOL* 7:378–830, 1975.

Delbecque P, Sourdille J, Delthil S: Treatment of traumatic ocular chalcosis with penicillamine. *BULL MEM SOC FR OPHTALMOL* 79:275–282, 1966. (French)

Fontana G: Behavior of ocular tissues in the presence of intraocular metal splinters. *RASS ITAL OTTALMOL* 7:695–720, 1938. (Italian)

Gerhard JP, Calme P: The measurement of copper in human aqueous humor and its pathologic variations. *BULL SOC OPHTALMOL FRANCE* 64:929–935, 1964. (French)

Gerhard JP, Flament J, et al: Chemical study in a case of chalcosis. *BULL SOC OPHTALMOL FRANCE* 74:699–703, 1974. (French)

Gorodetsky R, Weinreb A, et al: Noninvasive copper measurement in chalcosis. *ARCH OPHTHALMOL* 95:1059–1064, 1977.

Gorgone G: Clinical importance of the ERG in siderosis and chalcosis. *BOLL OCULIST* 45:638–649, 1966.

Gundorova RA: Clinical and biochemical changes involving the vitreous body in the presence of iron and copper foreign bodies. *VESTN OFTALMOL* 79(5):21–26, 1966. (English summary)

Gundorova RA, Malaev AA: A method of neutralizing chemical activity of metallic foreign bodies. *VESTN OFTALMOL* (4):37–38, 1973. (English summary)

Habig JM, Lumen A, Snacken J: Trial of chemical treatment for intraocular copper. *ANN OCULIST (PARIS)* 184:944, 1951. (French)

Haley W: Personal communication, 1968.

Hanna C, Fraunfelder FT: Lens capsule change after intraocular copper. *ANN OPHTHALMOL* 5:9–22, 1973.

Jayle GE, Tassy AF: Electroretinography in the case of intraocular metallic foreign bodies. *ARCH OPHTALMOL (PARIS)* 30:633–638, 1970. (French)

Jess A: The histologic appearance of copper discoloration of the lens. *KLIN MONATSBL AUGENHEILKD* 68:433–443, 1922. (German)

Jess A: The histologic appearance of copper in the cornea. *BER DTSCH OPHTHALMOL GESELLSCH* 251–253, 1924. (German)

Jess A: Glaucoma from copper impregnation of the eye. *KLIN MONATSBL AUGENHEILKD* 72:128–133, 1924. (German)

Kozousek V: Electroretin metalloses.ography and electroculography in *VIE MED CAN FR* 3:1185–1189, 1974. (French)

Krwawicz T, Zagorski K: Experimental electro-chemical removal of copper splinters from the isolated vitreous. *BR J OPHTHALMOL* 42:494–500, 1958.

Krwawicz T, Zagorski K, Szwarc B: Experimental investigations on the possibility of stopping the chemical activity of copper splinter in the vitreous body. *KLIN OCZNA* 36:1–5, 1966. (English summary)

Leuenberger PM: Ultrastructure of the retina, ERG, and aqueous humor studies in metalloses. pp. 141–149 in Neubauer (1977.[364d (German)]

Loewinger E, Weinreb A, Zeimer R: A noninvasive method for detection and analysis of metals in the eye. *INVEST OPHTHALMOL* 15:770–773, 1976.

Mine H: Experimental studies on chalcosis bulbi. *ACTA SOC OPHTHALMOL JPN* 62:470–478, 1958. (English summary)

Moschos M, Panagakis E, et al: Alterations of the ERG in experimental metalloses. *ARCH OPHTALMOL (Paris)* 37:285–293, 1977. (French)

Muller HK: On copper impregnation of the eye and its treatment. *SCHWEIZ MED WOCHENSCHR* II:790–791, 1937.

Neubauer H, Bos W: Chalcosis of the vitreous body. *BER DTSCH OPHTHALMOL GESELLSCH* 68:98–102, 1968. (German)

Newell F, Cooper JAD, Farmer CJ: Effect of BAL (2,3-dimercaptopropanol) on intraocular copper. *AM J OPHTHALMOL* 32:161–167, 1949.

Palimeris G, Moschos M, et al: ERG findings in clinical and experimental metallosis. pp. 127–135 in Neubauer (1977).[364]

Pirie A, Van Heyningen R: The Biochemistry of the Eye. Blackwell, Oxford (1956).

Pischel K: Copper in the lens. Glaucoma. *AM J OPHTHALMOL* 8:579, 1925.

Rao NA, Tso MOM, Rosenthal AR: Chalcosis in the human eye. *ARCH OPHTHALMOL* 94:1379–1384, 1976.

Rosenthal AR, Hopkins JL, Appleton B: Studies on intraocular copper foreign bodies. *ARCH OPHTHALMOL* 92:431–436, 1974.

Rosenthal AR, Appleton B, Hopkins JL: Intraocular copper foreign bodies. *AM J OPHTHALMOL* 78:671–678, 1974.

Rosenthal AR, Appleton B: Histochemical localization of intraocular copper foreign bodies. *AM J OPHTHALMOL* 79:613–625, 1975.

Rosenthal AR: Experimental aspects of implantation of copper in the vitreous of the rabbit eye. pp. 54–61 in Neubauer (1977).[364]

Rosenthal AR, Marmor MF, et al: Chalcosis—a study of natural history. *OPHTHAL-MOLOGY* 86:1956–1972, 1979.

Rouher MF: Chalcosis of the lens—effects of BAL. *BULL SOC OPTALMOL FRANCE* 19–20, 1958. (French)

Reussmann W: Intraocular pressure, aqueous humor copper and enzymes of the ciliary epithelium in experimental chalcosis. *GRAEFES ARCH OPHTHALMOL* 189:179–189, 1974. (German)

Ruessmann W, Angele W: Intraocular pressure and ciliary process carbonic anhydrase activity in acute experimental chalcosis. *TRANS OPHTHALMOL SOC UK* 97:709–714, 1977.

Ruessmann W: Biochemistry of metalloses. pp. 45–53 in Neubauer (1977).[364] (German)

Runyan TE, Levri EA: Vitreous analysis in eyes containing copper and iron intraocular foreign bodies. *AM J OPHTHALMOL* 69:1053–1057, 1970.

Schmidt JGH: Experimental animal studies on the effect of intraocular foreign bodies on ERG. pp. 136–139 in Neubauer (1977).[364] (German)

Schmidt JGH: Metallosis of the retina—pathophysiology and clinical findings. pp. 670–676 in Neubauer (1977).[364] (German)

Sedan J: On the development of chalcosis of the lens. *BULL MEM SOC FR OPHTALMOL* 74:169–173, 1961. (French)

Segal N: The effect of some chelating agents in prevention of exogenous siderosis and chalcosis. pp. 97–104 in Neubauer (1977).[364] (French)

Seland JH: The nature of capsular inclusions in lenticular chalcosis. *ACTA OPHTHALMOL* 54:99–108, 1976.

Sherreshevska SF: Intraocular bronze fragments and chalcosis. *VESTN OFTALMOL* 73(2):3–7, 1960.

Shiga S: Intraocular localization of copper by paramagnetic resonance spectroscopy. *AM J OPHTHALMOL* 63:133–134, 1967.

Sickel W: Experimental electroretinography in metalloses. pp. 111–118 in Neubauer (1977).[364d (French)]

Soyeux A: Treatment of copper intraocular foreign bodies with D-penicillamine. *BULL SOC OPHTHALMOL FRANCE* 80:727–729, 1980. (French)

Teichmann KD, Puelhorn G: Glaucoma associated with chalcosis. *KLIN MONATSBL AUGENHEILKD* 173:295–298, 1978. (German)

Thiel HJ, Puelhorn G: Clinical and morphological aspects of corneal damage after metal implantation. pp. 16-in Neubauer (1977).[364d] (German)

Verin P, Vildy A: Discouraging prognosis for intraocular foreign bodies of copper from war injuries. *BULL SOC OPHTALMOL FRANCE* 73:1051–1058, 1973.

Walzer P, Heimann K: Morphology of intraocular tissue changes after foreign body injuries. pp. 31–36 in Neubauer (1977).[364d (German)]

Welge-Luessen L, Oppermann W: Changes in the amino-acid spectrum in the rabbit eye from metallic copper. *BER DTSCH OPHTHALMOL GESELLSCH* 69:465–469, 1969. (German)

Welge-Luessen L, Meissner T: Intraocular brass splinters and their effect on the amino acid spectrum. pp. 78–88 in Neubauer (1977).[364d] (German)

Yassur Y, Zauberman H, Zidon M: Identification of copper ions in aqueous and vitreous of eyes containing copper and iron foreign bodies. *BR J OPHTHALMOL* 59:590–592, 1975.

Zeimer R, Gorodetsky R, et al: Experimental chalcosis. *ARCH OPHTHALMOL* 96:115–119, 1978.

Copper, systemic. In Wilson's hepatolenticular degeneration numerous patients have been described with typical Kayser-Fleischer ring consisting of discoloration of the peripheral portions of the corneas by copper as a result of abnormal copper metabolism, and several cases have been described in which the discoloration became less or disappeared during several years of systemic treatment with D-penicillamine,[h] or after liver transplantation.[n] Sunflower-type discoloration of the most anterior layers of the lens has also been described.[a] Other causes of discoloration of the cornea from deposition of copper like that in Wilson's disease have been recognized in a few patients who did not have Wilson's disease but who had hypercupremia. These conditions have included multiple myeloma,[c,j] cirrhosis of the liver,[d] and monoclonal gammopathy with carcinoma of the lung.[l] In these conditions, for unknown reasons, the discoloration of Descemet's membrane may tend to involve the more axial portions of Descemet's membrane. In rare instances the central deposit has been considered to be dense enough to reduce visual acuity.[l] Otherwise, these discolorations of cornea and lens by copper in Wilson's disease or the other systemic diseases have had no significant injurious effect on the eye. The discoloration does not extend to the trabecular meshwork, and there is no known tendency to glaucoma.

Several methods of analysis have proved beyond question that there is an abnormal amount of copper in cornea and lens, and histological studies have pin-pointed its location,[g,i,p] but it remains to be determined in what chemical combination the copper is present.

There has been controversy over whether systemic copper metabolism is abnormal in retinitis pigmentosa and other pigmentary retinopathies. Some have said so,[e,m] and some have said not.[b,k] Others have suggested a possible association,[o] or possible differences on a racial basis,[m] but there has been no suggestion that there is enough abnormality to require copper-binding medication.[m] Thers has been one report of experiments in albino rabbits in which copper sulfate was injected intraperitoneally, and later photoreceptor degeneration and pigment epithelial changes were found.[f]

a. Cairns JE, Williams HP, Walshe JM: "Sunflower cataract" in Wilson's disease. *BR MED J* 3:95, 1969.

b. Ehlers N, Buelow N: Clinical copper metabolism parameters in patients with retinitis pigmentosa and other tapeto-retinal degenerations. *BR J OPHTHALMOL* 61:595–596, 1977.

c. Ellis PP: Ocular deposition of copper in hypercupremia. *AM J OPHTHALMOL* 68:423–427, 1969.

d. Fleming CR, Dickson ER, et al: Pigmented corneal rings in nonWilsonian liver disease. *ANN INTERN MED* 86:285–288, 1977.

e. Gahlot DK, Khosla PK, et al: Copper metabolism in retinitis pigmentosa. *BR J OPHTHALMOL* 60:770–774, 1976.

f. Gahlot DK, Khosla PK, et al: Effect of copper on rabbit retina. *EXP OPHTHALMOL* 2:76–78, 1976.

g. Harry J, Tripathi R: The Kayser-Fleischer ring. *TRANS OPHTHALMOL SOC UK* 90:191–193, 1970.

h. Hiti H, Harpf H, et al: Regression of a Kayser-Fleischer ring in a case of Wilson's disease on penicillamine therapy. *KLIN MONATSBL AUGENHEILKD* 176:235–238, 1980. (German)

i. Kanai A, Yamaguchi T, et al: Histopathological study of Wilson's disease. *FOLIA OPHTHALMOL JPN* 25:237–248, 1979. (English summary)

j. Lewis RA, Falls HF, Troyer DO: Ocular manifestations of hypercupremia associated with multiple myeloma. *ARCH OPHTHALMOL* 93:1050–1053, 1975.

k. Marmor MF, Nelson JW, Levin AS: Copper metabolism in American retinitis pigmentosa patients. *BR J OPHTHALMOL* 62:168–171, 1978.

l. Martin NF, Kincaid MC, et al: Ocular copper deposition associated with pulmonary carcinoma, IgG monoclonal gammopathy and hypercupremia. *OPHTHALMOLOGY* 90:110–116, 1983.

m. Rao SS, Satapathy M, Sitaramayya A: Copper metabolism in retinitis pigmentosa patients. *BR J OPHTHALMOL* 65:127–130, 1981.

n. Schoenberger M, Ellis PP: Disappearance of Kayser-Fleischer rings after liver transplantation. *ARCH OPHTHALMOL* 97:1914–1915, 1979.

o. Silverstone B, Berson D, et al: Copper metabolism changes in pigmentary retinopathies and high myopia. *METAB PEDIATR OPHTHALMOL* 5:49–53, 1981.

p. Tso MOM, Fine BS, Thorpe HE: Kayser-Fleischer ring and associated cataract in Wilson's disease. *AM J OPHTHALMOL* 79:479–488, 1975.

Cortex granati (pomegranate bark), and its active principle *pelletierine tannate,* formerly were used in treatment of tapeworms, and were known to cause decrease in visual acuity similar to that from *filix mas.*[153,214] Observations were sometimes complicated by a practice of giving *filix mas* along with cortex granati. In the past half-century visual disturbance from this cause has become practically unknown. (See also *Aspidium.*)

Corticosteroids, (glucocorticoids) have been involved in many ocular complications. Hundreds of relevant publications have been published since 1960. It would take too much space to provide all the references. What will be presented here is a general summary with representative more recent references. The following corticosteroid complications or side effects involving the eyes will be summarized:

(a)	Cataract	(b)	Glaucoma
(c)	Induced Uveitis	(d)	Cornea and Sclera
(e)	Intraocular injections	(f)	Retina
(g)	Embolism	(h)	Pseudotumor Cerebri
(i)	Eyelids	(j)	Exophthalmos
(k)	Pupil	(l)	Teratogenesis
(m)	Systemic effects		

The effects of local and systemic corticosteroids in patients and the results of investigations in experimental animals will be included under each of these headings.

(a) Cataract. As a complication of both local and systemic long-term corticosteroid treatment cataract has become well recognized. Fortunately, the great majority of cataracts reported have consisted of a posterior subcapsular opacity and vacuolation that could be recognized by slit-lamp examination, but too delicate to interfere appreciably with vision or to be recognized with the ophthalmoscope. These could be arrested upon stopping treatment, and some regressed. However, a small proportion have progressed to interfere with vision and require operation. Corticosteroid lens opacities have in many instances developed in children under long-term treatment, as well as in young adults. Myopia from change in lenticular refraction has been noted (Koch).

Cataracts from corticosteroid eye drops or ointment have usually appeared after many months or years of daily application for chronic conditions, such as vernal conjunctivitis, or after keratoplasty (Bietti; Charleux; Donshik; Espildora; Gasset; Saracco; Wood; Yablonski). When chronic corticosteroid treatment has been limited to one eye, the lens opacity has been limited to the treated eye (Cronin; Donshik; Valerio).

Corticosteroid glaucoma has developed in some eyes in company with corticosteroid cataract.

Systemic long-term corticosteroid treatment has produced many posterior subcapsular lens opacities among patients under treatment for arthritis, asthma, eczema, and particularly after renal transplantation, and in children with nephrosis. Several series of cases of these conditions have been published with a high incidence of cataracts (Adhikary; Astle; Bachmann; Berkowitz; Forman; Hilton; Hovland; Kern; Kobayashi; Koch; Kollarits; Loredo; Loreto; Molnar; Ohguchi; Pfefferman; Porter;

Rintelen; Rodrigues-Alves; Sevel; Shiono; Skalka; Williamson). Most authors have concluded that incidence of cataract is related mainly to total dose, and that generally daily dosage over 15 mg prednisone and at least a year of medication is involved. However, there have been reports of detectible posterior subcapsular changes in considerably less than a year (Loredo). Differences in individual susceptibility appear important.

In experimental animals, efforts to induce cataracts with corticosteroids have met with little success, though Tamada has reported producing posterior subcapsular opacities in rabbits after 6 months of subconjunctival injections. Others have reported small or no changes in transparency (Bocci; Tarkkanen; Wood). Koch, and others earlier, reported in rats a slight acceleration of induction of cataracts from galactose poisoning when corticosteroids were administered. The lens epithelium has been shown to have a specific receptor with high affinity for dexamethasone, providing for at least the first step in an unelucidated mechanism for disturbance of the lens epithelium (Southren; Van Venrooif). Studies of animal lenses in vivo and in culture have shown a variety of changes in composition and metabolism under the influence of corticosteroids, but without much progress toward explaining the cataractogenesis in human beings (Mayman).

(b) Glaucoma.

(b) Glaucoma. Elevation of intraocular pressure from repeated application of corticosteroids to the eyes of human beings has been extensively documented. Corticosteroid glaucoma has been known at all ages, including a considerable number of children and very young adults. The degree of elevation of pressure has not been consistently related to the duration of exposure, though the highest pressures generally have developed after several months or years. Typically, corticosteroid glaucoma has been poorly responsive to standard antiglaucoma medical treatment. In most cases when the application of corticosteroids has been discontinued the intraocular pressure has subsided. The time required for return of pressure to normal has not necessarily been related to the length of exposure, the height of the intraocular pressure, or the degree of impairment of facility of outflow. In one series of cases the time required for recovery ranged from one week to four and one-half months after corticosteroids were discontinued.[31]

The mechanism by which locally applied corticosteroids cause glaucoma is yet to be established. There has been some evidence of a small increase in aqueous formation (Kim; Linner), though Rice has not confirmed this. The predominant effect reported by many authors appears to be a reduction of facility of aqueous outflow, which is usually reversible. Preliminary reports of relief of glaucoma by trabeculotomy have suggested that the glaucoma may be due to changes in the corneoscleral trabecular meshwork, possibly an abnormal accumulation of mucopolysaccharides.

The damage done to the optic nerve and the vision by corticosteroid glaucoma depends on the height of the intraocular pressure, the duration of the glaucoma, and the vulnerability of the individual eye. In some cases the damage has been so great that the eye has become essentially blind.

In many unfortunate cases corticosteroid drops or ointment have been used for many months or years in treatment of vernal conjunctivitis and other chronic conditions in young people without attention to the intraocular pressure, and with serious results. Especially instructive reports have been published by Bietti; Charleux; Espildora; Roberts; Saracco. Bietti reported on 69 patients with corticosteroid glaucoma in young people, mostly 11 to 30 years of age, diagnosed usually after a year of topical applications, when two thirds already had posterior subcapsular lens opacities. Bietti considered that a third of the eyes had glaucoma of such severity and lack of responsiveness to discontinuing corticosteroids and giving medical anti-glaucoma treatment that he performed goniotrabeculotomy in four-fifths of the circumference, reporting success in 98%. Charleux described similar results in two cases. Espildora studied 44 eyes of 22 mostly young patients with intraocular pressure mostly in the range 37 to 47 mm Hg from topical corticosteroids, and noted an apparent relationship between the length of exposure and the tendency for the pressure to return to normal after corticosteroids were discontinued. All exposed for only 2 to 8 weeks returned spontaneously to normal, while of those exposed for 2 to 12 months only 50% did so. After exposure for 1 to 4 years most eyes with elevated pressure, and all with damage to optic discs and visual fields, showed a relatively small drop of pressure and poor responsiveness to medical treatment for glaucoma. Espildora reported success with trabeculotomy similar to Bietti. Both Bietti and Espildora called attention to the fact that the pressure commonly differed in the two eyes of a patient although they were thought to have applied corticosteroids equally to both. Some patients in 6 months or less can suffer severe damage to the discs and loss of visual field from corticosteroid glaucoma with high pressure, as in single cases reported by Roberts and Saracco.

Corticosteroid ointments applied to the skin of the eyelids can spread to the conjunctival sac (Norn), and when applied repeatedly can cause glaucoma in corticosteroid responders. Severe cases of glaucoma with high intraocular pressures induced in this way have been reported (Cubey; Vie; and Zugerman).

Sub-Tenon's capsule injections of repository corticosteroids (especially triamcinolone acetate or acetonide, and methylprednisolone acetate) pose a special threat, since this treatment can raise intraocular pressure to dangerous levels in susceptible individuals, even if they do not suffer a rise from corticosteroid eyedrops, and surgical excision of the material from ocular tissues may be necessary. This is documented in series of cases reported by Herschler and by Kalina.

Investigational testing of corticosteroid eyedrops in patients by many investigators, especially by Becker and Armaly, has furnished a great deal of information concerning genetic relationships of responsiveness of intraocular pressure to corticosteroids, and also concerning the genetics of various types of glaucoma. About one-third of the human adult population has been shown to respond with definite rise of intraocular pressure when tested with repeated application of corticosteroid eyedrops. A smaller fraction have dangerous elevation. Most, but not all, patients who have primary open-angle glaucoma, and many of their relatives, have a significant rise of pressure.

In patients who have uveitis and are treated with topical corticosteroids, the effect on intraocular pressure is peculiarly varied. If there is glaucoma with elevated pressure secondary to the uveitis, treatment with corticosteroids may relieve both the inflammatory process and the glaucoma. If there is obstructed aqueous outflow due to uveitis, but no elevation of pressure because aqueous formation has been reduced by the uveitis, treatment with corticosteroids may cause a rise of intraocular pressure, if the treatment brings about improvement in formation of aqueous humor before it relieves the inflammatory obstruction to aqueous outflow. Furthermore, a certain proportion of uveitic patients presumably would have elevation of intraocular pressure in response to repeated application of corticosteroids from genetically determined corticosteroid interference with aqueous outflow whether uveitis was present or not.

Investigational testing in animals for induction of glaucoma by local administration of corticosteroids was initially unsuccessful in many attempts in both rabbits and monkeys, but Wood and Lorenzetti succeeded in causing the intraocular pressure to rise several mm Hg by application of very large amounts of corticosteroids repeatedly to the eyes, enough to cause systemic toxic effects. This response has been confirmed by Bonomi; de Juan; Dueker; Levene; Ticho; and Virno, utilizing eyedrops or subconjunctival injections. Generally the pressure has been noted to be raised in 3 weeks, but to begin to fall after 4 weeks, even if the medication is continued. Oppelt reported flow measurements with radioactive inulin showed in cats a slight decrease of aqueous formation but a greater reduction of facility of outflow. Histologic changes of uncertain significance have been described in the anterior chamber angles of rabbits by de Juan; Fossarello; Francois; and Pantlieva.

Dueker found by scanning electron microscopy that as the intraocular pressure in rabbits rose 10 mm Hg during 5 weeks of topical treatment with dexamethasone spaces developed between the cells lining the pectinate ligaments, baring the underlying collagen. The large spaces normally found between pectinate ligaments were gradually occluded by a layer of cells which appeared to arise from the anterior surface of the iris and move anteriorly along the ligaments and fibrous elements in the spaces.

Systemic administration of corticosteroids to human beings has induced intraocular pressure elevation or aggravated chronic open-angle glaucoma in a number of cases, but much less often than when corticosteroids have been administered topically. An idea of the incidence of this side effect can be obtained from the several publications already mentioned in which series of patients were examined for cataracts while receiving long-term systemic corticosteroids for arthritis, asthma, nephrosis, or after renal transplantation. Adhikary noted among 62 patients only 6 had pressures of 24 to 33 mm Hg, with no damage to discs or fields, after treatment that produced posterior subcapsular opacities in 36. Of Astle's 312 patients, 14 had pressures of 21 to 30 mm Hg detected on average after 7 months of oral corticosteroid in dosage that produced cataracts in 52. Lee found one pressure of 26 mm Hg among 13 patients under systemic corticosteroid treatment for severe asthma for two or more years. In Loreto's series of children 33% of whom developed cataracts, a sample of 18 had average pressure of 18 mm Hg. Among Pfefferman's 78 patients, only one had pressures of 25 mm Hg, while 41 had cataracts. However, among Porter's 39 patients (23% with corticosteroid cataracts), while one patient had pressures of 25 mm Hg, another had 38 and 40 mm Hg with arcuate scotoma; these pressures dropped to 26 and 30 mm Hg in two weeks after the dosage of corticosteroid was reduced. It appears that severe rises of intraocular pressure from systemic corticosteroid treatment are rare compared to induced lens opacities. Individual instances have been reported by Nagai and by Wilson. Nagai described a 16 year old boy who became Cushingoid and developed cataracts during 3 years of treatment, then was discovered to have pressures of 63 and 78, with severe glaucomatous damage of discs and fields. The provocative role of the corticosteroid was confirmed by observing that after this medication was discontinued the pressures became normal in 3 weeks, and remained normal without antiglaucoma treatment.

In a synopsis of complications of corticosteroid therapy Francois made an interesting comment saying that it seemed curious that the glaucoma produced by intensive systemic treatment may be acute, with pain, ciliary injection, corneal edema, and pressure above 50 mm Hg, yet it was an open-angle type of glaucoma. There appears to be very little documentation in the literature on this type of glaucoma.

It has been the clinical experience of Chandler that systemic corticosteroid treatment can definitely make medical control of primary open-angle glaucoma more difficult.[291] Also it has been Chandler's experience that in people who are given both systemic and topical ophthalmic corticosteroids the tendency to raise the intraocular pressure is appreciably greater than when corticosteroids are given by a single route.

Angle-closure glaucoma in patients who were under treatment with systemic corticosteroids has been reported in very rare instances, but there is little to indicate more than coincidence.

In animals repeated attempts to induce glaucoma by *systemic administration* of corticosteroids has so far been essentially unsuccessful.

(c) Induced Uveitis. Corticosteroids are regularly beneficially employed in treatment of uveitis, but an occasional peculiar induction of uveitis by corticosteroid eye drops in apparently normal eyes was discovered during provocative testing of patients for elevation of intraocular pressure in response to the drops (Kass; Krupin; Martins; Shin). Characteristically, after dexamethasone drops had been administered four times a day for several weeks and then were discontinued, after a few days the eyes became red, painful, blurred, and photophobic with a few cells and moderate flare in the aqueous humor, and a drop in the intraocular pressure. Under cycloplegic treatment the eyes recovered in 3 to 10 days. This uveitis occurred in black patients in 14 out of 16 instances, affecting 5.4% of the black patients tested, compared to 0.5% of white patients. It did not relate to the nature of pressure response, but 14 out of 17 who had the uveitis had a positive FTA–ABS test.

(d) Cornea and Sclera. Clinically, there has been awareness that topical corticosteroids can have adverse effects on herpes simplex virus and fungus infections of the cornea, and that high dosage of systemic corticosteroids occasionally cause ulceration or perforation of the cornea or sclera (Cornand; Loffredo). Also, the incidence of unwanted filtering blebs from improper wound healing after cataract extraction has appeared to be increased from 1.6% to 8.7% by topical corticosteroid (Kirk).

In treatment of superficial inflammations there has been a somewhat controversial tendency to use topical preparations containing both a corticosteroid and an antimicrobial, even in conditions clearly calling for only one or the other, and there has been some apprehension that the risk of adverse reactions might be increased by the seemingly superfluous corticosteroid or antimicrobial. However, a survey by Bettman has not disclosed any greater incidence from the use of the combinations.

Corneal wound healing under the influence of corticosteroids has received a great deal of attention and investigation. Much thought has been given to weighing the potential clinical advantages and disadvantages in corticosteroid treatment of eyes that have been operated upon, burned by chemicals, or otherwise injured, in which suppression of inflammation and vascularization of the cornea would presumably be beneficial, if not outweighed by undesirable effects of the treatment on the cornea and on the course of healing. The considerations have been reviewed by Dohlman.

More quantitative information on the effects of corticosteroids in these conditions appears to have been obtained through animal and laboratory investigations than from clinical studies. Investigations of more than a decade ago will not be reviewed here, but in more recent years reports by Petroutsos and by Srinivasan have confirmed that the more potent anti-inflammatory topical corticosteroids retard healing of the rabbit corneal epithelium when the cornea has been mechanically denuded, but that this may be evident only when the cornea has been widely or completely denuded. In a report by Phillips it is confirmed that corticosteroid eyedrops suppress development of strength in corneal stromal wounds in rabbits, and reduce the amount of collagen formed. However, in the same report it is shown that when the eyedrops were applied immediately after injury the treatment beneficially reduced ulceration, and suppressed inflammation and corneal vascularization. This provides an argument for not delaying corticosteroid treatment of injured corneas, though it has also been held that withholding the treatment until the stroma had become covered by epithelium should avoid aggravation of the melting effect of collagenase. Scanning electron microscopy by Takashima and by Maudgal have shown that corticosteroids damage the microvilli of the corneal epithelium of rabbits, but the clinical import is unclear.

(e) Intraocular Injection of Corticosteroid.

In treatment of keratitis and uveitis Francois has reported injecting various corticosteroid suspensions into the anterior chamber several hundred times, and that they were well tolerated. Although crystals could be seen in the anterior chamber for several days, no glaucoma was observed. In rabbits, intravitreal injections of dexamethasone by Graham, methylprednisolone acetate by Moschini, and triamcinolone acetonide by McCuen and by Tano were without serious adverse effect. Clinically, there have been accidental injections of corticosteroid suspensions into the vitreous body when the injection needle penetrated the eye instead of remaining between Tenon's capsule and sclera as intended, or in one instance when Dermojet injection, which was intended for the skin of the upper lid, penetrated both lid and sclera (Perry). In two cases reported by Giles, 2 cases by Schlaegel, and individual cases by McLean and by Perry, methylprednisolone acetate (Depo-Medrol) or triamcinolone acetonide injected into the vitreous body caused immediate pain and loss of vision, apparently partly from immediate but transient high intraocular pressure and partly by clouding of the media by the injected white material. However, within weeks to months these patients regained their vision, suggesting, as did the report of Francois and the rabbit experiments, that intraocular corticosteroid suspension is not dangerously toxic.

Different results were reported by Moschini and by Schlaegel. In five cases with accidental intravitreal injections of methylprednisolone acetate, or triamcinolone diacetate or acetonide, the early course was similar, but after some weeks four of them developed retinal detachments from vitreoretinal traction bands, and the fifth developed preretinal fibrosis and retinal degeneration in an eye that prior to the accident had required much treatment for retinochoroiditis. These cases leave open a question whether corticosteroid suspensions for extraocular repository injection are toxic within the eye, or whether the retinal complications were the result of physical injury when the globes were penetrated. Interestingly, Zinn so strongly assumed dangerous toxic properties that in still another case he performed extensive intraocular surgery as an emergency procedure within hours after an accident of this type.

(f) Retina. Apart from the question raised in the paragraph on *Intraocular Injection of Corticosteroid* as to whether retinal detachments were attributable to toxicity or to physical injury, there has been a question whether corticosteroids might aggravate development of diabetic retinopathy, but this has been answered in the negative by Toussaint and by Krupin. Maculopathy as a rare possible adverse effect of systemic corticosteroids has been recorded in two cases, appearing in one as "striate and circular pigmental fissures," and in the other as exudates and edema (Pau; Williamson). An effect of systemic corticosteroid on retinal function has been more directly shown by Zimmerman based on a significant increase of E.R.G. and V.E.R. potentials in 6 eyes of normal people after 3 weeks of medication, returning toward normal during 4 weeks off medication.

In young rabbits retinopathy has been reported by Aihara after repeated systemic administration of dexamethasone, consisting of fanshaped neovascularization and tortuous vessels, but no fluorescein leakage.

(g) Embolism from Injections about the Head. Since 1970 there have been at least eleven publications describing embolic occlusion of blood vessels of the eye, mostly of retinal arteries, from injections of corticosteroid suspensions about the head or neck (e.g. in the scalp, nose, tonsil bed, orbit) as reviewed by Evans. The adverse effects were from physical embolization rather than toxic action. They will not be discussed further here.

(h) Pseudotumor Cerebri. Intracranial hypertension from systemic corticosteroids has been reported many times. Van Dyk gave a succinct synopsis of the characteristics, pointing out that it tended to occur in the young age range of 2 to 19 years, after corticosteroid administration for 3 months to 7 years. It is usually precipitated by a change in dose or type of steroid. The patients have headache and low-grade papilledema, 33% have 6th nerve palsy, sometimes with diplopia. Effective treatment usually has consisted of temporarily increasing the corticosteroid and then reducing it more slowly. Walker has provided a survey of 28 cases. In an unusual case reported by Hosking a child developed pseudotumor cerebri from

absorption of corticosteroid from the skin during 3 years of treatment of eczema with an ointment.

(i) Eyelid Effects of Topical Corticosteroids. Slight, reversible ptosis or drooping of the upper lid from use of corticosteroid eye drops has been noted by Miller and by Newsome. Atrophy and telangiectasia of the skin of the eyelids from prolonged application of hydrocortisone cream has been described by Guin. The same effect on the skin of the eyelids is seen from prolonged use of corticosteroid eye drops, presumably owing to overflow from the conjunctival sac. (Spread in the other direction from the skin of the eyelids to the conjunctival sac, with production of glaucoma, is documented in the section on *Glaucoma*.)

(j) Exophthalmos. This was reported by Slansky as a reversible complication of long-term systemic corticosteroid therapy, calling attention also to the fact that exophthalmos has been recognized in 6 to 8 percent of patients with Cushing's disease from elevated endogenous corticosteroid production.

(k) Pupil. A slight enlargement of the pupil in human beings has been noted when corticosteroids have been applied repeatedly for several days to one eye and the size of the pupil has been compared with that of the contralateral untreated eye (Miller; Newsome).

(l) **Teratogenesis.** Corticosteroids applied to the eyes of pregnant mice are reported by Ballard to have caused an increased incidence of cleft palates in the fetuses. Bilateral congenital nuclear cataracts have been reported in an otherwise normal child whose mother had received systemic corticosteroids throughout much of her pregnancy (Kraus).

(m) Systemic Poisoning from Ophthalmic Corticosteroids. Eye drops and ointment containing corticosteroids can depress plasma cortisol levels, and injections of dexamethasone phosphate about the eye can depress cortisol synthesis considerably (Meredig). Death of an 11-month-old girl from complications of Cushing's syndrome followed 3 months of treatment with corticosteroid eyedrops and sub-Tenon's capsule injections (Romano).

Adhikary HP, Sells RA, Basu PK: Ocular complications of systemic steroid after renal transplantation. *BR J OPHTHALMOL* 66:290–291, 1982.

Aihara Y: A study by fluorescein angiography on steroid-induced retinopathy in rabbit. *JPN J OPHTHALMOL* 24:196–204, 1980.

Armaly MF: Factors affecting the dose-response relationship in steroid-induced ocular hypertension. Pp 88–105 in *Symp. Ocul. Anti-Inflamm. Ther.* Edited by HE Kaufman. Thomas: Springfield, IL, 1970.

Astle JN, Ellis PP: Ocular complications in renal transplant patients. *ANN OPHTHAL-MOL* 6:1269–1274, 1974.

Bachmann HJ, Schildberg P, et al: Cortisone cataract in children with nephrotic syndrome. *EUR J PEDIATR* 124:277–283, 1977.

Ballard PD, Hearney EF, et al: Comparative teratogenicity of selected glucocorticoids applied ocularly in mice. *TERATOLOGY* 16:175–180, 1977.

Becker B: The genetic problem of chronic simple glaucoma. *ANN OPHTHALMOL* 3:351–354, 1971.

Berkowitz JS, et al: Ocular complications in renal transplant recipients. *AM J MED* 55:492–495, 1973.

Bettman JW, Aronson SB, et al: The incidence of adverse reactions from steroid/antinfective combinations. *SURV OPHTHALMOL* 20:281–290, 1976.

Bietti GB, Quaranta CA, et al: Contribution to the clinical picture of cortisone glaucoma and to its treatment. *BULL SOC FR OPHTALMOL* 86:167–173, 1973. (French)

Bocci N, Fiore C: Effect of cortisone acetate, administered topically, on the lens of rabbits. *BOLL OCULIST* 54:141–145, 1975. (Italian)

Bonomi L, Perfetti S, et al: Experimental corticosteroid ocular hypertension in the rabbit. *GRAEFES ARCH OPHTHALMOL* 209:73–82, 1978.

Charleux J, Montibert J, et al: Ocular complications after long-term treatment with topical corticosteroids. *BULL SOC OPHTALMOL FRANCE* 72:479–482, 1972. (French)

Cornand G, Cozette P, Landes J: Corneal perforation in the course of a prolonged cortico-therapy for rheumatoid polyarthritis. *BULL SOC OPHTALMOL FRANCE* 75:253–256, 1975. (French)

Cronin TP: Cataract with topical use of corticosteroid and idoxuridine. *ARCH OPHTHALMOL* 72:198–199, 1964.

Cubey RB: Glaucoma following the application of corticosteroid to the skin of the eyelids. *BR J DERMATOL* 95:207–208, 1976.

de Juan E Jr, Maumenee AE: Steroid glaucoma. *INVEST OPHTHALMOL VIS SCI* 22(Suppl):Abst 23, 1982.

Dohlman CH: Corticosteroids in corneal surgery. In Schwartz, B. (Ed.): *Corticosteroids and the Eye.* Boston, Little; and *INT OPHTHALMOL CLIN* 6:845–868, 1966.

Donshik PC, Cavanagh HD, et al: Posterior subcapsular cataracts induced by topical corticosteroids following keratoplasty for keratoconus. *ANN OPHTHALMOL* 13:29–32, 1981.

Dueker DK, de Tineo AB, Grant WM: Scanning electron microscopy of steroid-induced glaucoma in rabbits. *INVEST OPHTHALMOL VIS SCI* 22(Suppl):Abst 22, 1982.

Espildora CJ, Vicuna CP, Diaz BE: Cortisone glaucoma; concerning 44 eyes. *J FR OPHTALMOL* 4:503–508, 1981. (French)

Evans DE, Zahorchak JA, Kennerdell JS: Visual loss as a result of primary optic nerve neuropathy after intranasal corticosteroid injection. *AM J OPHTHALMOL* 90:641–644, 1980.

Forman AR, Loreto JA, Tina LU: Reversibility of corticosteroid-associated cataracts in children with the nephrotic syndrome. *AM J OPHTHALMOL* 84:75–78, 1977.

Fossarello M, Carta S, et al: Quantitative ultrastructural study of the anterior chamber angle of the rabbit with corticosteroid-induced ocular hypertension. *OPHTHALMIC RES* 14:40–45, 1982.

Francois J: Secondary effects and ophthalmologic complications of cortisone therapy. *BULL SOC BELGE OPHTALMOL* 186:47–55, 1979. (French)

Francois J, Victoria-Troncoso V, et al: Appearance of the sclerocorneal trabeculum after cortisone treatment and perfusion of the anterior chamber with hyaluronidase. *KLIN MONATSBL AUGENHEILKD* 180:68–69, 1982. (German)

Francois P, Constantinides G, et al: Intracameral injections of corticosteroids. *BULL SOC FR OPHTALMOL* 84:331–340, 1971. (French)

Gasset AR, Lorenzetti DWC, et al: Quantitative corticosteroid effect on corneal wound healing. *ARCH OPHTHALMOL* 81:589–591, 1969.

Gasset AR, Bellows RT: Posterior subcapsular cataracts after topical corticosteroid therapy. *ANN OPHTHALMOL* 6:1263–1265, 1974.

Giles CL: Bulbar perforation during periocular injection of corticosteroids. *AM J OPHTHALMOL* 77:438–441, 1974.

Graham RO, Peyman GA: Intravitreal injection of dexamethasone. *ARCH OPHTHALMOL* 92:149–156, 1974.

Guin JD: Complications of topical hydrocortisone. *J AM ACAD DERMATOL* 4:417–422, 1981.

Herschler J: Intractable intraocular hypertension induced by repository triamcinolone acetonide. *AM J OPHTHALMOL* 74:501–504, 1972.

Herschler J: Increased intraocular pressure induced by repository corticosteroids. *AM J OPHTHALMOL* 82:90–93, 1976.

Hilton AF, Harrison JD, et al: Ocular complications in haemodialysis and renal transplant patients. *AUST J OPHTHALMOL* 10:247–253, 1982.

Hosking GP, Elliston H: Benign intracranial hypertension in a child with eczema treated with topical steroids. *BR MED J* 1:550–551, 1978.

Hovland K, Ellis PP: Ocular changes in renal transplant patients. *AM J OPHTHALMOL* 63:283–289, 1967.

Lee PF: The influence of systemic steroid therapy on the intraocular pressure. *AM J OPHTHALMOL* 46:328–331, 1958.

Levene R, Rothberger M, Rosenberg S: Corticosteroid glaucoma in the rabbit. *AM J OPHTHALMOL* 78:505–510, 1974.

Linner E: Adrenocortical hormones and glaucoma. *ACTA OPHTHALMOL* 44:299–305, 1966.

Loffredo A, Sammartino A, et al: Prolapse of the iris from spontaneous perforation of the cornea and pathologic rib fracture after cortisone treatment for rheumatoid arthritis. *J FR OPHTALMOL* 1:439–442, 1978. (French)

Loredo A, et al: Cataracts after short-term corticosteroid treatment. *N ENGL J MED* 286:160, 1972.

Lorenzetti OJ: Steroid-induced elevated intraocular pressure in rabbits. *TOXICOL APPL PHARMACOL* 12:304–305, 1968.

Loreto JA, Limaye SR, et al: Steroid associated cataracts in nephrotic syndrome. *J PEDIATR OPHTHALMOL* 11:112–115, 1974.

Kalina RE: Increased intraocular pressure following subconjunctival corticosteroid administration. *ARCH OPHTHALMOL* 81:788–790, 1969.

Kass MA, Gieser DK, et al: Corticosteroid-induced iridocyclitis. *AM J OPHTHALMOL* 93:368–369, 1982.

Kern R, Zaruba K, Scheitlin W: Ocular side-effects of long-term immunosuppressive therapy in recipients of cadaver kidney transplants. *OPHTHALMIC RES* 1:21–30, 1970.

Kimura R, Honda M: Effect of orally administered hydrocortisone on the rate of aqueous flow in man. *ACTA OPHTHALMOL* 60:584–589, 1982.

Kirk HQ: Corticosteroids as a cause of filtering blebs after cataract extraction. *AM J OPHTHALMOL* 77:442, 1974.

Kobayashi Y, et al: Posterior subcapsular cataract in nephrotic children receiving steroid therapy. *AM J DIS CHILD* 128:671–673, 1974.

Koch HR, Weikenmeier P, Siedek M: Corticosteroid cataract after kidney transplantation. *GRAEFES ARCH OPHTHALMOL* 194:39–53, 1975. (German)

Koch HR, Heinz E, Wendt H: Investigations on the influence of different corticosteroids on the development of galactose cataracts in rats. *GRAEFES ARCH OPHTHALMOL* 198:105–112, 1976.

Koch HR, Siedek M: Lenticular myopia in steroid cataract. *KLIN MONATSBL AUGENHEILKD* 171:620–622, 1977. (German)

Kollarits CR, Swann ER, et al: HLA–A1 and steroid-induced cataracts in renal transplant patients. *ANN OPHTHALMOL* 14:1116–1118, 1982.

Kraus AM: Congenital cataract and maternal steroid ingestion. *J PEDIATR OPHTHALMOL* 12:107–108, 1975.

Krupin T, LeBlanc RP, et al: Uveitis in association with topically administered corticosteroid. *AM J OPHPTHALMOL* 70:883–885, 1970.

Krupin T, Schoch LH, et al: Lack of correlation between ocular hypertensive response to topical corticosteroids and progression of retinopathy in insulin-dependent diabetes mellitus. *AM J OPHTHALMOL* 96:52–56, 1983.

Martins JC, Wilensky JT, et al: Corticosteroid-induced uveitis. *AM J OPHTHALMOL* 77:433–437, 1974.

Maudgal PC, Cornelis H, Missotten L: Effects of commercial ophthalmic drugs on rabbit corneal epithelium. *GRAEFES ARCH OPHTHALMOL* 216:191–203, 1981.

Mayman CI, Miller D, Tijerina ML: In vitro production of steroid cataract in bovine lens. *ACTA OPHTHALLMOL* 57:1107–1116, 1979.

McCuen BW, Bessler M, et al: The lack of toxicity of intravitreally administered triamcinolone acetonide. *AM J OPHTHALMOL* 91:785–788, 1981.

McLean EB: Inadvertent injection of corticosteroid into the choroidal vasculature. *AM J OPHTHALMOL* 80:835–837, 1975.

Meredig WE, Jentzen F, Hartmann F: The influence of glucocorticoids applied to the eye on adrenal gland function. *KLIN MONATSBL AUGENHEILKD* 176:907–910, 1980. (German)

Miller D, Peczon JD, Whitworth CG: Corticosteroids and functions in the anterior segment of the eye. *AM J OPHTHALMOL* 59:31–34, 1965.

Molnar L, Lazar J: On corticosteroid-induced cataract. *KLIN MONATSBL AUGENHEILKD* 158:578–584, 1971. (German)

Moschini GB: Accidental introduction of repository corticosteroid into the vitreous body. *BOLL OCULIST* 48:426–432, 1969. (Italian)

Nagai T, Uchida S: A case of glaucoma induced by long-term systemic corticosteroid therapy. *FOLIA OPHTHALMOL JPN* 24:532, 1973.

Newsome DA, Wong VG, et al: "Steroid-induced" mydriasis and ptosis. *INVEST OPHTHALMOL* 10:424–429, 1971.

Norn MS: Eyelid ointment penetrating into conjunctival sac. *ACTA OPHTHALMOL* 50:206–209, 1972.

Ohguchi M, Ohno S, et al: Posterior subcapsular cataracts in children on long-term corticosteroid therapy. *JPN J OPHTHALMOL* 19:254–260, 1975.

Oppelt WW, White EO, Halpert ES: The effect of corticosteroids on aqueous humor formation rate and outflow facility. *INVEST OPHTHALMOL* 8:535–541, 1969.

Pantieleva VM, Shapkina AM: Glucocorticoids and intraocular pressure. *GRAEFES ARCH OPHTHALMOL* 199:303–310, 1976.

Pau H: Macula changes from corticosteroids. *KLIN MONATSBL AUGENHEILKD* 174:557–560, 1979. (German)

Perry HT, Cohn BT, Nauheim JS: Accidental intraocular injection with Dermojet syringe. *ARCH DERMATOL* 113:1131, 1977.

Petroutsos G, Guimaraes R, et al: Corticosteroids and corneal epithelial wound healing. *BR J OPHTHALMOL* 66:705–708, 1982.

Pfefferman R, Gombos GM, Kountz SL: Ocular complications after renal transplantation. *ANN OPHTHALMOL* 9:467–470, 1977.

Phillips K, Arffa R, et al: Effects of prednisolone and medroxyprogesterone on corneal wound healing, ulceration, and neovascularization. *ARCH OPHTHALMOL* 101:640–643, 1983.

Porter R, Crombie AL, et al: Incidence of ocular complications in patients undergoing renal transplantation. *BR MED J* 3:133–136, 1972.

Rice SW, Bourne WM, Brubaker RF: Absence of an effect of topical dexamethasone on endothelial permeability and flow of aqueous humor. *INVEST OPHTHALMOL VIS SCI* 24:1307–1311, 1983.

Rintelen F, Dobrivojevic D: On cortisone-cataract in kidney transplantation. *OPHTHAL-MOLOGICA* 161:125–131, 1970.

Roberts W: Rapid progression of cupping in glaucoma. *AM J OPHTHALMOL* 66:520, 1968.

Rodrigues-Alves CA, Sabbaga E, Chocair PR: Ophthalmological findings in renal transplant patients. *REV BRASIL OFTAL* 35:205–215, 1976.

Romano PE, Traisman HS, Green OC: Fluorinated corticosteroid toxicity in infants. *AM J OPHTHALMOL* 84:247–250, 1977.

Saracco JB, Estachy G, Llavador M: Complications of corticotherapy in the treatment of vernal conjunctivitis. *BULL SOC OPHTALMOL FRANCE* 79:185–187, 1979. (French)

Schlaegel TF Jr, Wilson FM: Accidental intraocular injection of depot corticosteroids. *TRANS AM ACAD OPHTH OTOL* 78:847–855, 1974.

Sevel D, Weinberg EG, Van Niekerk CH: Lenticular complications of long-term steroid therapy in children with asthma and eczema. *J ALLERGY CLIN IMMUNOL* 60:215–217, 1977.

Shin DH, Kass MA, et al: Positive FTA–ABS tests in subjects with corticosteroid-induced uveitis. *AM J OPHTHALMOL* 82:259–260, 1976.

Shiono H, Oonishi M, et al: Posterior subcapsular cataracts associated with long-term oral corticosteroid therapy. *CLIN PEDIATR* 16:726–728, 1977.

Skalka HW, Prchal JT: Effect of corticosteroids on cataract formation. *ARCH OPHTHAL-MOL* 98:1773–1777, 19801.

Slansky HH, Kolbert G, Gartner S: Exophthalmos induced by corticosteroids. *ARCH OPHTHALMOL* 77:579–581, 1967.

Southern AL, Gordon GG, et al: Receptors for glucocorticoids in the lens epithelium of the calf. *SCIENCE* 200:1177–1178, 1978.

Srinivasan BD, Kukarni PS: The effect of steroidal and nonsteroidal anti-inflammatory agents on corneal re-epithelialization. *INVEST OPHTHALMOL VIS SCI* 20:688–691, 1981.

Takashima R: Corticosteroid effects on the corneal surface of rabbits studied by scanning electron microscopy. *JPN J OPHTHALMOL* 19:393–400, 1975.

Tamada Y, Sase Y, et al: Steroid cataract produced by long-term local administration of steroid. *FOLIA OPHTHALMOL JPN* 29:568, 1978.

Tano Y, Chandler D, Machemer R: Treatment of intraocular proliferation with intravitreal injection of triamcinolone acetonide. *AM J OPHTHALMOL* 90:810–816, 1980.

Tarkkanen A, Esila R, Liesmaa M: Experimental cataracts following long-term administration of corticosteroids. *ACTA OPHTHALMOL* 44:665–668, 1966.

Ticho V, Lahav M, et al: Ocular changes in rabbits with corticosteroid-induced ocular hypertension. *BR J OPHTHALMOL* 63:646–650, 1979.

Toussaint D, Farnir A: Study of the retinal vessels of patients treated with cortisone. *BULL SOC BELGE OPHTALMOL* 143:568–577, 1966. (French)

Valerio M, Carones AV, DePoli A: Monolateral cataract from monolateral local cortisone therapy. *BOLL OCULIST* 44:127–133, 1965. (Italian)

Van Venrooif WJ, Groeneveld AA, et al: Cultured calf lens epithelium. *EXP EYE RES* 18:527–536, 1974.

Vie R: Glaucoma and amaurosis associated with long-term application of topical corticosteroids to the eyelids. *ACTA DERM VENEREOL* 60:541–542, 1980.

Virno M, Schirru A, et al: Aqueous humor alkalosis and marked reduction in ocular ascorbic acid content following long-term topical cortisone. *ANN OPHTHALMOL* 6:983–992, 1974.

Walker AE, Adamkiewicz JJ: Pseudotumor cerebri associated with prolonged corticosteroid therapy. *J AM MED ASSOC* 188:779–784, 1964.

Williamson J, Paterson RWW, et al: Posterior subcapsular cataracts and glaucoma associated with long-term oral corticosteroid therapy. *BR J OPHTHALMOL* 53:361–372, 1969.

Williamson J, Nuki G: Macular lesions during systemic therapy with tetracosactrin. *BR J OPHTHALMOL* 54:405–409, 1970.

Wilson DM, Martin JHS, Niall JF: Raised intraocular tension in renal transplant recipients. *MED J AUST* 1:482–484, 1973.

Wood DC, Contaxis L, et al: Response of rabbits to corticosteroids. I. *AM J OPHTHALMOL* 63:841–848, 1967.

Wood DC, Sweet D, et al: Response of rabbits to corticosteroids. II. *AM J OPHTHALMOL* 63:849–856, 1967.

Wood TO, Waltman SR, Kaufman HE: Steroid cataracts following penetrating keratoplasty. *ANN OPHTHALMOL* 3:496–498, 1971.

Yablonski ME, Burde RM, et al: Cataracts induced by topical dexamethasone in diabetes. *ARCH OPHTHALMOL* 96:474–476, 1978.

Zimmerman TJ, Dawson WW, Fitzgerald CR: Electroretinographic changes in normal eyes during administration of prednisone. *ANN OPHTHALMOL* 5:757–759, 761, 763–765, 1973.

Zinn KM: Iatrogenic intraocular injection of depot corticosteroid and its surgical removal using the pars plana approach. *OPHTHALMOLOGY* 88:13–17, 1981.

Zugerman C, Saunders D, Levit F: Glaucoma from topically applied steroids. *ARCH DERMATOL* 112:1326, 1976.

Cosyntropin (Tetracosactrin), an adrenocorticotropic hormone, when administered in excessive dosage made one man Cushingoid, and during the fourth month of treatment was associated with decrease in vision because of small exudates, hemorrhages and edema in the maculas.[a] The maculas recovered after the drug was stopped. However, cause and effect was certain.

a. Williamson J, Nuki G: Macular lesions during systemic therapy with depot tetracosactrin. *BR J OPHTHALMOL* 54:405–409, 1970.

Co-trimoxazole (Bactrim, Septrin), a mixture of trimethoprim and sulfamethoxazole, has been known to cause conjunctival hyperemia and irritation with blurring of vision, and other signs and symptoms of Stevens-Johnson syndrome.[a]

a. Kikuchi S, Okazaki T: Stevens-Johnson syndrome due to co-trimoxazole. *LANCET* 2:580, 1978.

Creosote, used for impregnating wood to protect it from rot and worms, is irritating to the skin and conjunctiva of people handling and sawing treated wood, especially on sunny days, owing to photosensitization. The most common effect has been erythema of the whole face with sensation of burning and itching. In a smaller proportion, conjunctivitis with mild hyperemia, photophobia, and discharge occurs.[b]

Contact of liquid creosote with the eye has caused painful protracted keratoconjunctivitis. This has involved loss of corneal epithelium, clouding of the cornea, miosis, and long-lasting irritability and photophobia.[153,188,253] One report concerned with creosote describes two patients, one examined two weeks and the other two months after working with this material, both complaining of haziness of vision, which was found to be associated with numerous gray spots of varied size in the corneas, plus superficial keratitis.[a] However, this is not a typical picture.

    a. Birdwood GT: Keratitis from working with Creosote. *BR MED J* 2:18, 1938.
    b. Jonas AD: Cresote burns. *J IND HYG TOXIC* 25:418–420, 1943.

Cresols (Cresylic acids) are methyl phenols, usually mixed with phenol and xylenols. They have had wide use in disinfectants, in degreasing compounds, in paintbrush cleaners, and as additives to lubricating oils.

Among the disinfectants identified in the literature as containing significant amount of cresols are Lysol and Creolin. The phenolic substances in such preparations are commonly combined with soaps to produce an emulsion on mixing with water. Systemic toxicity and contact burns of the skin and eyes resemble those of phenol.[a,153] (See INDEX for *Phenol.*)

Blindness with optic atrophy but normal ERG has been described by Walsh and Hoyt (1969) to have developed in one young woman after intrauterine injection of Lysol for abortion, which caused unconsciousness, swelling of the brain, optic nerves, and chiasm.[256]

Burns of human eyes by Lysol have been reported.[b,35,153,165,249,252] For example, a splash of 2.5% Lysol solution caused hyperemia and swelling of the conjunctiva with opacification and superficial vascularization of the cornea which cleared partially in the course of several months to give a vision of 4/60.[153]

In other cases there has been eventually more complete recovery, despite slow-healing injuries of the corneal epithelium accompanied by severe conjunctival and lid reaction and much pain.[249] Experimentally, application of 2% to 2.5% Lysol solution to rabbit, guinea pig, and monkey eyes caused only an epithelial defect which soon healed, but a 10% to 12% solution applied to rabbit eyes caused pain, redness and swelling of the conjunctiva, and corneal clouding which became denser in the course of several weeks.[c,153]

Pure cresols, without the added soaps present in disinfectants, have caused permanent opacification and vascularization when applied full strength to rabbit eyes.[35,101] However, a drop of 33% solution applied to rabbit eyes and removed by irrigation within sixty seconds caused only moderate injury, from which the corneas recovered.[101] Both the clinical course and histologic findings in cresol-burned rabbit eyes have been described in the greatest detail by D'Asaro Biondo.[35] A case with fortunate outcome, involving particularly *2-methoxy-4-methyl phenol,* has been reported by Schutte (1979).[g]

Glaucoma has been induced experimentally in rabbits and monkeys by injection of 0.5% to 1% p-cresol emulsion in physiologic saline into the anterior chamber.[d-f] In rabbits this dilute cresol caused strong cellular proliferative reaction in the angle of the anterior chamber with formation of peripheral anterior synechia and obstruction of aqueous outflow. The cornea, lens, iris, and ciliary body were not affected except that the cornea became enlarged secondary to elevated ocular pressure. In monkeys the injected cresol caused increase in cells in the trabecular meshwork, hyalinization and thickening of the trabeculae, and impregnation with acid mucopolysaccharides. In four to six weeks a fibrous tissue formed in the angle, growing into the iris and ciliary body.

a. Clinton M: Cresol. *AM PETROL INST TOXIC REV* Mar. 1948.
b. Kraupa-Runk M: On Lysol burn of the eye. *KLIN MONATSBL AUGENHEILKD* 76:698–700, 1926. (German)
c. Yamashita K: Studies of the caustic action of silver nitrate and some disinfectants on the eye. *ZENTRALBL GES OPHTHALMOL* 26:523, 1932. (German)
d. Rohen JW: Experimental studies on the trabecular meshwork in primates. *ARCH OPHTHALMOL* 69:335–349, 1963.
e. Rohen JW: Morphologic changes in eyes with experimentally raised intraocular pressure. *VERH ANAT GES* 1963, pp. 293–297. (*ZENTRALBL GES OPHTHALMOL* 91(1);40, 1964.) (German)
f. Rohen JW: Comparative morphologic studies of tissue of the anterior chamber angle of eyes of rabbits and monkeys, carried out with thin-section methods. *GRAEFES ARCH OPHTHALMOL* 169:218–237, 1966. (German)
g. Schutte E, Horster B, Schafer R: On cresol burn of the eye. *KLIN MONATSBL AUGENHEILKD* 175:539–543, 1979. (German)

Cromolyn sodium (disodium cromoglycate, Intal, Aarane, Opticrom collyrium) has been utilized by inhalation as an anti-asthmatic, and as 1% to 4% eye drops in treatment of external allergic or atopic conditions of the eyes. Numerous publications have reported benefit in treatment of vernal conjunctivitis, but no side effects, except occasional slight stinging sensation, until Ostter (1982) described two adult patients who had used the drops for many months before they began to complain of acute redness, swelling of the conjunctiva and itching when the drops were applied. Ostter studied these patients and concluded that they had become allergic to the cromolyn.[a] No significant harm was done to the eyes.

a. Ostter HB: Acute chemotic reaction to cromolyn. *ARCH OPHTHALMOL* 100:412–413, 1982; and *LANCET* 2:1287, 1982.

Crotonaldehyde vapor is so highly irritant to the eyes that people are unable to remain in the presence of dangerous concentrations; at 45 ppm the odor is extremely obnoxious and there is considerable eye discomfort.[a] Crotonaldehyde liquid causes severe injury to rabbit eyes similar to that caused by acetic anhydride.[218,222] However, in eight instances of industrial corneal injury from this substance, healing is reported to have been complete in forty-eight hours; the severity of exposure was not specified.[165]

a. Rinehart WE: The effect on rats of single exposures to crotonaldehyde vapor. *AM IND HYG ASSOC J* 28:561–566, 1967.

Crotonic acid (β-methylacrylic acid) tested by drop application to rabbit eyes was severely injurious, similar to acetic anhydride.[222]

Croton oil is a violently irritant, vesicant oil expressed from the seeds of *Croton tiglium.*[171] In contact with the eye it has caused severe keratoconjunctivitis with pain, swelling, and purulent discharge. The degree of recovery has been varied, complete in some cases, but with residual corneal opacity in others.[46,153,253] Experimentally introduced into the anterior chamber of rabbits, it causes a violent iritis and necrosis of the cornea. In the vitreous body it causes devastating endophthalmitis.[a,150]

a. Kuchle HJ: Neural disturbance and the eye. *BIBL OPHTHALMOL* 51:1–106, 1958.

Crownflower (*Calotropis gigantea*), a flower used in making the Hawaiian lei, has a milky juice which in several cases has accidentally contaminated the eyes and produced severe irritation, usually prompt burning sensation, swelling of the lids, and subsequent blurring of vision from corneal edema involving both epithelium and stroma, sometimes with loss of corneal epithelium and wrinkling of Descemet's membrane. One case has been reported in which the irritation and blurring were delayed in onset, developing in the evening and the following day after probable exposure to the juice. In all reported cases recovery has been spontaneous and complete within two to ten days. No specific treatment is known or required.[a–c,142]

a. Crawford HE: Crown flower keratoconjunctivitis. *HAWAII MED J* 17:244–245, 1958.
b. Sugiki S: Crownflower or cornflower. (Correspondence.) *ARCH OPHTHALMOL* 75:736, 1966.
c. Wong WW: Keratoconjunctivitis due to crownflower. *HAWAII MED J* 8:339–341, 1949.

Curare (Curarine, tubocurarine), muscle relaxants, systemically administered, cause weakness of convergence, diplopia, and disturbed perception of the visual world on attempted eye movement,[a,255] but application of tubocurarine to the surface of the lids has no perceptible effect on the orbicularis muscle, probably owing to poor absorption.[81]

a. Stevens JK, Emerson RC, et al: Paralysis of the awake human: visual perceptions. *VISION RES* 16:93–98, 1976.

Cyalume Lightstick is a chemiluminescent device containing two solutions which are mixed to start chemical reaction and emission of light without heat. When the reaction mixture is dropped on the eye or injected into the nasolacrimal system of monkeys and rabbits, it appears not to be significantly injurious.[a,b] However, when injected subconjunctivally or into the anterior chamber of rabbits, it has produced severe reactions with opacification and vascularization of the cornea.[b]

a. Cohen SW, Sherman M, et al: Lacrimal outflow patency demonstrated by chemiluminescence. *ARCH OPHTHALMOL* 98:126–127, 1980.
b. Vettese T, Hurwitz JJ: Toxicity of the chemiluminescent material Cyalume in anatomic assessment of the nasolacrimal system. *CAN J OPHTHALMOL* 18:131–135, 1983.

Cyanimide is a name applied both to *carbodiimide* and to *calcium cyanamide.* The latter in commercial form may contain calcium hydroxide, calcium carbonate, and carbon.[171,252] Cyanamide is severely irritating and caustic to the eye,[a,46,129,215] as well as to moist skin, in which it induces ulceration.[171,252] The dust irritates the eyes and respiratory tract.[a,171,252]

Cyanamide poisoning of human beings and rats characteristically induces parasympathetic overactivity, causing miosis, salivation, lacrimation, and twitching.[b,c] In rats undergoing severe poisoning the pupils may initially constrict, but then dilate, and the vessels of the iris and retina become congested, and papilledema is said to occur. These congestive effects in rats appear to be due to swelling of the Harderian gland, and can be blocked by atropine.[c]

    a. Abramyan RA, Grigorian SK, Antoniev AA: Cyanamide-caused burns of the eye. *VESTN OFTALMOL* (1):44–45, 1973. (English summary)

    b. Barnard RD: Cholinergic porphyrine lacrimation and paradoxical mydriasis in the rat. *PROC SOC EXP BIOL MED* 54:254–258, 1942.

    c. Mellinghoff K, Thomas D: Calcium cyanamide poisoning. *DTSCH MED WOCHENSCHR* 65:1636, 1939. (German)

Cyanate, sodium or potassium, has been used experimentally in treatment of patients with sickle cell anemia. Peripheral neuropathies have developed, with axonal degeneration of both motor and sensory nerves, but with no involvement of nerves of the eyes as yet. Cyanate carbamylates proteins, and in rabbit lenses that are maintained in culture cyanate has caused opacities and has interfered with transport of cations at concentrations less than required for antisickling treatment of red cells.[a] In two young patients being treated for sickle-cell hemoglobinopathy by prolonged oral administration of sodium cyanate under careful observation, bilateral posterior subcapsular cataracts developed, and in one of these patients the cataracts spontaneously regressed when the treatment was discontinued.[b] In Beagle dogs chronic administration has also produced posterior subcapsular cataracts, and a small proportion of the animals have developed lesions of the corneas.[c]

Cyanate in natural equilibrium with urea has been postulated to have a role in development of cataracts in patients with diarrhea and uremia in Pakistan, with some suggestive supporting chemical evidence.[d]

    a. Kinoshita JH, Merola LO: Cyanate effects on the lens in vitro. *INVEST OPHTHALMOL VISUAL SCI* 12:544–547, 1973.

    b. Nicholson DH, Harkness DR, et al: Cyanate induced cataracts in patients with sickle-cell hemoglobinopathies. *ARCH OPHTHALMOL* 94:927–930, 1976.

    c. Kern HL, Bellhorn RW, Peterson CM: Sodium cyanate induced ocular lesions in the beagle. *J PHARMACOL EXP THER* 200:10–16, 1977.

    d. Harding RJ, Rixon KC: Carbamylation of lens proteins: a possible factor in cataractogenesis in some tropical countries. *EXP EYE RES* 31:567–571, 1980.

Cyanic acid (hydrogen cyanate) has an acrid odor and is strongly lacrimatory, vesicant, and a respiratory irritant.[171] (For cyanic acid salts, see *Cyanate, sodium or potassium.*)

Cyanides have definitely affected the optic nerve and retina in experimental animals lethally or sublethally poisoned, and there have been suggestions of human beings having had similar injuries. However, in human beings, despite many known episodes of acute exposure and acute poisoning, there appears to be no really clear or conclusive evidence of acute damage of retina or optic nerves. Whether chronic poisoning by very small amounts of cyanide can affect vision in human beings is uncertain, but a theory to this effect has been of much interest in relation to tobacco smoking and in connection with Leber's hereditary optic atrophy, optic neuropathy of pernicious anemia, and optic neuropathy associated with eating cyanogenic foods such as cassava. The effects of acute poisonings will be considered first.

Cyanides such as *hydrocyanic acid, hydrogen cyanide, potassium cyanide,* and *sodium cyanide* are acutely poisonous, interfering with metabolic processes and causing rapid death. In severe poisoning the pupils characteristically are widely dilated.[153,214,247] Transient blindness of unknown mechanism has been reported in rare instances of sublethal cyanide poisoning (Blyth).[153] Ophthalmoscopic and histologic examination in a child supposedly killed by cyanide showed central retinal edema (Alagna). This patient died in convulsions several hours after eating thirty bitter seeds of apricot. In another case a man who was using cyanide to clean gold became acutely ill with headache, paresis of the arm and leg on the left side, and hemianopia on the left. Right carotid angiography and encephalography were normal. Within 4 months the paresis improved and the hemianopsia "had subsided considerably". No examination of the eyes or other information on the vision was reported (Sandberg). (The abnormalities in this case suggest CNS disturbance, rather than disturbance of retina or optic nerves.)

It is interesting that in fire fighters exposed to burning plastics, and in patients treated with nitroprusside, both involving exposure to high concentrations of cyanide, so far no ocular toxic effects have been reported.

Chronic exposure of rats to hydrogen cyanide is reported not to have damaged the optic nerves or retina (Leinfelder), but daily subcutaneous injections of potassium cyanide increasing to lethal levels has caused nystagmus and periods of blindness in monkeys, cats, dogs, and rats, with histologically demonstrable degeneration in the optic nerves, chiasm, and optic tract (Jedlowski).[194]

Lessell, in particular, has reviewed the literature on animal experiments with cyanide with respect to the eye, and he has investigated the effects of repeated near lethal or lethal injections of cyanide in rats. While finding no histological disturbance of the retina, he frequently found severe damage localized in the retrobulbar portion of the optic nerves. However, the corpus callosum was more regularly damaged than the optic nerves. Lessell found the retrobulbar portion of the optic nerves of normal rats to have a relative deficiency of capillaries, and he postulated that this anatomic peculiarity may render this zone particularly susceptible to the effects of cyanide. However, he found no evidence of cumulative toxic action on the optic nerves from repeated doses.

In rabbits, after sublethal doses of cyanide, changes in the electroretinogram have been observed.[179] Injection of sodium cyanide into the vitreous humor in rabbits to produce an estimated concentration of 0.0012 M blocked the optic nerve potential before it affected the ERG.[245] Cultured rabbit retina exposed to 0.005 M sodium cyanide, according to Lucas and Hansson, has shown unselective cellular degeneration and metabolic changes.[157,99] However, in studies by Marmor concerning the mechanisms which normally maintain retinal adhesion, and prevent detachment, cyanide caused no more inhibition of resorption of subretinal fluid or peeling of the retina than did similar concentrations of sodium chloride.

Quite apart from acute poisoning, the possibility of adverse effects on the visual system from chronic low level cyanide exposure became the subject of much interest and speculation in the 1960's. It was postulated that cyanide might have a key role in producing optic neuropathies in such diverse conditions as tobacco smoking, cassava eating, pernicious anemia, and Leber's optic atrophy. These hypotheses have been reviewed (Chisholm; Foulds; Osuntokun). Several investigators hypothesized that in tobacco smoking and in habitual eating of cassava there was chronic intake of excessive cyanide, which they thought was responsible for producing optic neuritis. In patients who smoked excessively or habitually ate cassava, the plasma thiocyanate was found to be abnormally high (Osuntokun). This was considered to be evidence for abnormally high cyanide intake, because one mechanism for detoxication of cyanide is conversion to thiocyanate (Pettigrew). Also in support of the hypothesis it was pointed out that binding of cyanide by hydroxocobalamin was another mechanism for detoxication, and that in treatment of the optic neuritis in these particular conditions greater benefit resulted from administration of hydroxocobalamin than from administration of cyanocobalamin. It was postulated that tobacco smoking and excess cyanide absorption was a significant toxic factor also in patients with pernicious anemia who developed optic neuropathy and in patients with Leber's optic atrophy. Elevated cyanocobalamin concentrations have been found in plasma of patients with these conditions (Wilson).

In Leber's hereditary optic atrophy, apart from the adverse effect of tobacco smoking postulated by some writers, there has been evidence to suggest that the disease may be due to an inherited deficiency in ability to detoxicate cyanide by converting it to thiocyanate, since in this condition plasma thiocyanate has been found low, rather than high (Osuntokun; Wilson). Improvement of the vision in this condition under treatment with hydroxocobalamin after failure of treatment with cyanocobalamin has been interpreted as support for the hypothesis that cyanide toxicity is important in the condition (Foulds). However, it is possible that the improvement was spontaneous.

While these hypotheses in which cyanide is blamed for the optic neuropathy from tobacco smoking, cassava eating, pernicious anemia and Leber's hereditary optic atrophy may be correct, there has been little clinical evidence apart from the measurements on plasma thiocyanate and the therapeutic effectiveness of hydroxocobalamin. However, there is potentially important new support in a finding by Cagianut in 1981 of an abnormally low activity of the enzyme rhodanese in the livers of two patients with Leber's disease. This enzyme normally converts cyanide to thiocyanate.

While it has been known from experiments on rats and monkeys that repeated administration of cyanide could cause lesions in the central nervous system involving particularly degeneration of myelin, and that this could be partially blocked by administering hydroxocobalamin, (Lumsden; Smith), there seems to have been no specific demonstration of optic neuropathy in animals by chronic administration of the very small doses or very low concentrations that have been supposed in the cyanide hypotheses to have caused optic neuropathy in human beings. The doses that have produced definite damage to the optic nerve or retina have approached the lethal.

If chronic absorption of very small amounts of cyanide is a factor in producing optic neuropathy as proposed in the hypotheses already mentioned, one might expect that chronic industrial exposure to cyanide would have led to comparable cases of optic neuropathy, but no such effect of chronic industrial cyanide exposure seems to have been reported. In the few patients in whom there have been definite disturbances of vision or damage to the optic nerve or retina attributable to cyanide poisoning, the poisoning has been acute and severe, lethal or near lethal.

(For additional information on these specific subjects, see also *Cassava* and *Tobacco*.)

The cornea is reported to have been injured by cyanide in a single instance in which a man was exposed to hydrocyanic acid vapors employed in fumigating. Within an hour or two the patient developed edema of the cornea, which gradually subsided to leave the appearance of a Kayser-Fleischer ring in the periphery of the cornea a month later (Amsler). No similar corneal disturbance has been produced in animal eyes by exposure to cyanides (Amsler).

Application of 10% potassium cyanide neutralized with acetic acid to the eye of a guinea pig produced no injury discernible by slit-lamp or by testing with fluorescein.[81] Cyanide is reported to have no influence on the water uptake of the cornea, nor does it cause loosening of the epithelium.[107,198] Studies of the effect of cyanide on metabolism of excised pieces of cornea have shown that respiration is readily inhibited, presumably by poisoning of cytochrome oxidase, but that spontaneous recovery of oxygen consumption can occur even after several hours if glucose is available (Robbie).

It is intriguing that hydrogen cyanide appears to be less selective than hydrogen sulfide in toxicity to the corneal epithelium, yet these substances are otherwise about equally toxic, and both probably owe their toxicity to inhibition of metal-dependent enzymes. Hydrogen sulfide has become notorious for highly selective toxicity to the corneal epithelium, but only occasionally has reference been made to an irritation of the eye, conjunctivitis, or superficial keratitis developing after chronic exposure to hydrogen cyanide gas.[33,61] (Compare *Hydrogen sulfide*.)

Secretory pumping by ciliary processes studied *in vitro* by Gerggren[10] has been shown to be inhibited by cyanide, but apparently no relationship has yet been shown or claimed between systemic cyanide *in vivo* and formation of aqueous humor.

Alagna G: Poisoning by hydrocyanic acid and the eye. *ANN OTTALMOL CLIN OCUL* 72:217–233, 1946. (Italian)

Amsler M: Hydrogen cyanide poisoning, acute segmental corneal edema, Kayser-Fleischer ring, renal diabetes. *SCHWEIZ MED WOCHENSCHR* 69:1012–1015, 1939. (French)

Blyth AW, Blyth MW: *Poisons, their effects and detection*, 5th ed. London, C. Griffin, 1920.

Cagianut B, Rhyner K, et al: Thiosulphate-sulphur transferase (rhodanese) deficiency in Leber's hereditary optic atrophy. *LANCET* 2:981–982, 1981.

Chisholm IA, Pettigrew AR: Biochemical observations in toxic optic neuropathy. *TRANS OPHTHALMOL SOC UK* 90:827–838, 1970.

Foulds WS, Cant JS, et al: Hydroxocobalamin in the treatment of Leber's hereditary optic atrophy. *LANCET* 1:896–897, 1968.

Foulds WS, Chisholm IA, et al: Cyanide induced optic neuropathy. *OPHTHAL-MOLOGICA ADDIT AD* 158:350–358, 1969.

Foulds WS, Freeman AG, et al: Cyanocobalamin: a case for withdrawal. *LANCET* 1:35, 1970.

Foulds WS, Chisholm IA, Pettigrew AR: The toxic optic neuropathies. *BR J OPHTHAL-MOL* 58:386–390, 1974.

Jedlowski P: Amblyopia experimentally induced by potassium cyanide and early lesions of optic nerve fibers. *BULL SOC ITAL BIOL SPER* L2:87–88, 1937. (Italian)

Leinfelder PJ, Robbie WA: Experimental studies in retrobulbar neuritis. *AM J OPHTHALMOL* 30:1135–1143, 1947.

Lessell S: Experimental cyanide optic neuropathy. *ARCH OPHTHALMOL* 86:194–204, 1971.

Lessell S, Kuwabara T: Fine structure of experimental cyanide optic neuropathy. *INVEST OPHTHALMOL VIS SCI* 13:748–756, 1974.

Lessell S: Capillaries of rat optic nerve: relationship of anomalies to cyanide lesions. *ARCH OPHTHALMOL* 91:308–310, 1974.

Lumsden CE: Cyanide leucoencephalopathy in rats and observations on the vascular and ferment hypotheses of demyelinating diseases. *J NEUROL NEUROSURG PSY-CHIATRY* 13:1, 1050.

Marmor MF, Abdul-Rahim AS, Cohen DS: The effect of metabolic inhibitors on retinal adhesion and subretinal fluid resorption. *INVEST OPHTHALMOL VIS SCI* 19:893–903, 1980.

Onsuntokun BO: An ataxic neuropathy in Nigeria. *BRAIN* 91 (Part II):215–248, 1968.

Pettigrew AR, Fell GS: Microdiffusion method for estimation of cyanide in whole blood and its application to the study of conversion of cyanide to thiocyanate. *CLIN CHEM* 19:466–471, 1973.

Robbie WA, Leinfelder PJ, Duane TD: Cyanide inhibition of corneal respiration. *AM J OPHTHALMOL* 30:1381–1387, 1947.

Sandberg CG: A case of chronic poisoning with potassium cyanide? *ACTA MED SCAND* 181:233–236, 1967.

Smith ADM, Duckett S: Cyanide, vitamin B_{12} experimental demyelination and tobacco amblyopia. *BR J PATH* 46:615–622, 1965.

Wilson J: Leber's hereditary optic atrophy—A possible disorder of cyanide detoxication. *EXCERPTA MED INT CONGR SERIES* 154:70, 1967.

Wilson J, Langman MJS: Relation of sub-acute combined degeneration of the cord to vitamin B_{12} deficiency. *NATURE* 5064:787–789, 1966.

Wilson J, Linnell JC, Matthews DM: Plasma-cobalamins in neuroophthalmological diseases. *LANCET* 1:259–261, 1971.

Cyanoacetic acid (malononitrile) has been reported to have caused histologic lesions in the optic nerves and tracts of two out of fifteen severely poisoned rats.[a] In rabbits no effect on the ERG has been reported from cyanoacetic acid.[179]

a. Hicks SP: Brain metabolism *in vivo*. *ARCH PATHOL* 50:545–561, 1950.

2-Cyanoacrylic acid esters from methyl to decyl polymerize to form plastic-like polymers which have been extensively tested and utilized as adhesives for tissues. Particular use has been made of these substances as adhesives applied to the cornea. There are numerous reports concerning the practical techniques of using these adhesives, but in the present synopsis, only those that contain some noteworthy information concerning toxicity to the eye will be included. Comparisons in experimental animals and in patients indicate that toxicity to tissue has been greatest with the methyl ester, and has decreased with increase in size of the alkyl group, little or no toxicity being notable in the series from isobutyl or decyl. However, the highest esters seem to have been inferior as tissue adhesives. In practice, there has been a tendency to compromise, and the intermediate esters, particularly n-butyl, isobutyl, and n-heptyl have been favored.[b,c,g,h,i,j,n]

A comprehensive review of the chemical and toxicologic properties of cyanoacrylate tissue adhesives was published in 1976.[a]

2-Cyanoacrylic acid methyl ester (methyl-2-cyanoacrylate, Krazy-Glue, Eastman 910, Borden Ad/Here) applied as an adhesive to rabbit or human eyes was originally found to produce undesirable reaction, causing haze in the cornea and inflammation, but generally without significant permanent injury.[a,c,e,i,l,m] However, highly purified material has been said to be less toxic to the cornea.[d] Clinically the purest methyl ester tested for gluing plastic lenses to the cornea after epithelium was scraped off proved unsatisfactory, inducing excessive reaction and detachment of the plastic lens.[b] However, the methyl ester has been used satisfactorily for a special purpose in patients, applied to the skin of the eyelids and to the eye lashes to glue the lids temporarily closed, and in this application it has produced no ocular inflammation.[k]

Accidentally, *cyanoacrylate glues* that are in common household use have been applied to the eye mistakenly as eyedrops, causing immediate brief smarting, and firm gluing of the lids together.[t,u,z] Fortunately, acetone is a good solvent for the polymerized glue, and can be used with a swab to unglue the lids,[t] and even to remove glue from the cornea.[y] In the common accidental dropping of the glue on the eye or similar splashing, the glue may cause transient punctate epithelial keratopathy, but as a rule it does not adhere to the cornea or conjunctiva. The use of acetone involves risk of temporary loss of corneal epithelium only if it comes in actual contact with the cornea, and, as described elsewhere under *Acetone,* the cornea can be expected to recover well.[y]

2-Cyanoacrylic acid ethyl ester is probably too toxic to use for tissue adhesive.[b,g]

2-Cyanoacrylic acid higher esters that have been tested and found to have essentially negligible toxicity to the cornea are *isobutyl,*[c,g,h] *n-butyl,*[g,i,h] *hexyl,*[c] *heptyl,*[b,g,i,n] and *octyl.*[c,g] However, even the *octyl* ester produced some inflammation when injected into guinea pig corneas,[o] and clinically an unusual granulomatous reaction has resulted from application of the *isobutyl* ester to a cornea that allowed easy access to the stroma because of the extent of pre-existing necrosis.[q]

Radioactive tracer studies with the *isobutyl* ester in rabbits have shown that the polymer degrades very slowly in the cornea, and no degradation products are detectible within the eye within 9 weeks.[w]

As an adhesive for broad conjunctival flaps, *butyl cyanoacrylate* has been reported to cause necrosis and be unsuitable.[s]

If introduced into the anterior chamber, even the higher esters produce a transient iritis in rabbits.[r]

In the posterior segment of the eye, tests of *n-butyl cyanoacrylate* (Histoacryl) have produced mild reactions in the retina and choroid, and none in the vitreous body.[p,x]

a. Bloomfield S, Barnert AH, Kanter PD: The use of Eastman 910 monomer as an adhesive in ocular surgery. *AM J OPHTHALMOL* 55:742–748, 1963.

b. Dohlman CH, Payrau P, Pouliquen Y: Application of contact lenses with the aid of adhesive materials. *ARCH OPHTALMOL (Paris)* 28:533–536, 1968. (French)

c. Girard LJ, Cobbs S, et al: Surgical adhesives and bonded contact lenses; an experimental study. *ANN OPHTHALMOL* 1:65–74, 1969.

d. Hanna C, Shibley S: Tissue reaction to intracorneal silicone rubber (Silastic RTV382) and methyl-2-cyanoacrylate. *AM J OPHTHALMOL* 60:323–328, 1965.

e. Levine AM: Sutureless ocular surgery: results of recent experiments. *EYE EAR NOSE THROAT MONTHLY* 43:55–58, 1964.

f. McGee WA, Oglesby FS, et al: The determination of a sensory response to alkyl 2-cyanoacrylate vapor in air. *AM IND HYG ASSOC J* 29:558–561, 1968.

g. Payrau P, Pouliquen Y, Lecoq J: Corneal lenses glued on with the aid of surgical adhesives. *ARCH OPHTALMOL (Paris)* 29:299–304, 1969. (French)

h. Price JA, Wadsworth JAC: Evaluation of an adhesive in cataract wound closure. *AM J OPHTHALMOL* 68:663–668, 1969.

i. Refojo MF, Dohlman CH, et al: Evaluation of adhesives for corneal surgery. *ARCH OPHTHALMOL* 80:645–656, 1968.

j. Reim M, Vogt M: Gluing of corneal wounds in rabbit experiments. *GRAEFES ARCH OPHTHALMOL* 179:53–64, 1969. (German)

k. Schimek BA, Ballou GS: Eastman 910 monomer for plastic lid procedures. *AM J OPHTHALMOL* 62:953–955, 1966.

l. Straatsma BR, Allen RA, et al: Experimental studies employing adhesive compounds in ophthalmic surgery. *TRANS AM ACAD OPHTHALMOL OTOLARYNG* 67:320–332, 1963.

m. Straatsma BR: Experimental ophthalmic surgery employing cyanoacrylate adhesives. *TRANS AM OPHTHALMOL SOC* 66:986–1021, 1968.

n. Webster RG Jr, Slansky HH, et al: The use of adhesive for the closure of corneal perforations. *ARCH OPHTHALMOL* 80:704–709, 1968.

o. Aronson SB, McMaster PRB, et al: Toxicity of the cyanoacrylates. *ARCH OPHTHALMOL* 84:342–349, 1970.

p. Faulborn J, Witschel H: Intraocular application of tissue adhesive (Histoacryl) in retinal detachment surgery. *GRAEFES ARCH OPHTHALMOL* 207:15–20, 1978.

q. Ferry AP, Barnert AH: Granulomatous keratitis resulting from use of cyanoacrylate adhesive for closure of perforated corneal ulcer. *AM J OPHTHALMOL* 72:538–541, 1971.

r. Gasset AR, Hood DI, et al: Ocular tolerance to cyanoacrylate monomer tissue adhesive anologues. *INVEST OPHTHALMOL* 9:3–11, 1970.

s. Giessmann HG, Schlote SW, et al: Use of tissue adhesives in the rabbit eye. *GRAEFES ARCH OPHTHALMOL* 184:309–313, 1972. (German)

t. Margo CE, Trobe JD: Tarsorrhaphy from accidental instillation of cyanoacrylate adhesive in the eye. *J AM MED ASSOC* 247:660–661, 1982.

u. Mindlin AM: Acetone used as a solvent in accidental tarsorrhaphy. *AM J OPHTHALMOL* 83:136–137, 1977.

v. Priluck IA, Doughman DJ, et al: Tissue adhesives. *SYMPOSIUM ON OCULAR THERAPY,* edited by JH Leopold and RP Burns, Chap. 9, pp. 137–153, John Wiley and Sons, New York, 1976.

w. Sani BP, Refojo MF: β^{14} C-Isobutyl-2-cyanoacrylate adhesive. *ARCH OPHTHALMOL* 87:216–221, 1972.

x. Spitznas M, Lossagk H, et al: Intraocular histocompatibility and adhesive strength of butyl-2-cyanoacrylate. *GRAEFES ARCH OPHTHALMOL* 187:102–110, 1973.

y. Turss U, Turss R, Refojo MF: Removal of isobutyl cyanoacrylate adhesive from the cornea with acetone. *AM J OPHTHALMOL* 70:725–728, 1970.

z. Morgan SJ, Astbury NJ: Inadvertent self administration of superglue: a consumer hazard. *BR MED J* 289:226–227, 1984.

Cyanogen (ethanedinitrile) is reported to cause irritation of eyes and nose at 16 ppm in air,[a] but apparently not sufficiently unpleasant to prevent exposure to lethal concentrations.

a. McNerney JM, Schrenk HH: The acute toxicity of cyanogen. *AM IND HYG ASSOC J* 21:121–124, 1960.

Cyanogen chloride (chlorine cyanide) has been employed as a war gas.[155] Human beings can tolerate 50 mg/cu m of air, but 100 mg/cu m causes immediate irritation of the respiratory passages and smarting of the eyes, with severe blepharospasm and lacrimation.[a] Chronic exposure causes hoarseness, conjunctivitis, and edema of the lids.[b]

a. Aldridge WN, Evans CL: The physiological effects and fate of cyanogen chloride. *Q J EXP PHYSIOL* 33:241–266, 1946.

b. Reed CI: Chronic poisoning from cyanogen chloride. *J IND HYG* 2:140–143, 1920.

Cyanuric acid (sym. triazinetriol) has been employed as a selective herbicide,[171] and also in preparation of chlorinating agents such as dichloroisocyanuric acid and trichloroisocyanuric acid. These chlorinated derivatives are employed as bleaching and sanitizing agents (e.g. in swimming pools). When the chlorocyanuric compounds release their chlorine, cyanuric acid remains. In swimming pools, it is thought that irritancy to the eye is governed by the concentrations of chlorine, chloramines, and pH of the water, and no special or additional irritant effect appears to have been attributed to the cyanuric chloro compounds or cyanuric acid. In chronic experiments on rabbit eyes not described in detail, it is reported that no irritant effect was observable in the course of a month from tests with 100 ppm of cyanuric acid, nor from monosodiumcyanurate equivalent to 6.8% cyanuric acid.[a] (Also see INDEX for *Swimming Pool Water.*)

a. Svirbely JL: New sources of available chlorine. *SWIMMING POOL AGE,* March 1960, pp. 39–42.

Cycasin (methylazoxymethanol, MAM), a neurotoxic substance from cycad leaves and seeds, is damaging to the brain and has caused abnormalities in the retinas of newborn mice, hamsters, and rats. (Also see Methylazoxymethanol, page 607.)

    a. Shimada M, Langman J: Repair of the external granular layer of the hamster cerebellium after administration of methylazoxymethanol. *TERATOLOGY* 3:119–133, 1970.

    b. Fushimi K, et al: Induction of a retinal disorder with cycasin in newborn mice and rats. *ACTA PATHOL JPN* 23:307–314, 1973.

Cyclamate sodium a sweetener, has been tested for effects on fetal eyes in rats by administering it to females in their food 20 days after mating. Histological examination at that time showed no abnormalities in the lens, vitreous body, optic nerve, or other parts of the eye.[a]

    a. Luckhaus G, Machemer L: Histological examination of perinatal eye development in the rat after ingestion of sodium cyclamate and sodium saccharin during pregnancy. *FOOD COSMET TOXICOL* 16:7–11, 1978.

Cyclandelate (Cyclomandol, Cyclospasmol, Spasmocyclon), an antispasmodic peripheral vasodilator, has been tested by administration of customary 200 mg doses by mouth to patients with open-angle glaucoma. No significant alteration of intraocular pressure was found during four to five hours, and the axial depth of the anterior chamber did not change appreciably.[193] From other studies it has been claimed that cyclandelate reduced ophthalmic blood pressure but increased flow in retinal arteries.[a] It appears that cyclandelate presents no significant threat of raising ocular pressure in open-angle glaucoma nor any threat of precipitating angle-closure glaucoma. (See also *Vasodilators.*)

    a. Hayatsu H, Suda S, Yaoeda H: Ophthalmic use of cyclandelate. *JPN J CLIN OPHTHALMOL* 20:85–91, 1966. (*ZENTRALBL GES OPHTHALMOL* 98:531, 1967.

Cyclazocine, an analgesic drug, constricts the pupils when administered systemically to normal human beings, but causes mydriasis when given to people who have become dependent on opioid drugs.[a,b]

    a. Jasinski DR, Martin WR, Hawrtzen C: The human pharmacology and abuse potential of N-allynoroxymorphone (naloxone). *J PHARMACOL EXP THER* 157:420–426, 1967.

    b. Martin WR: Opioid antagonists. *PHARMACOL REV* 19:463–506, 1967.

Cyclizine (Marazine, Marezine, Marzine), an antihistaminic used in treatment of sickness from motion and from pregnancy, was put under suspicion of having teratogenic effects by tests of very high doses in mice and rats that demonstrated induction of cataracts, microphthalmia, and anophthalmia.[g] After abnormal fetal development was reported in animals, McBride in 1963 reported that among the offspring of an estimated several thousand women who had received approximately 150 mg cyclizine per day during pregnancy, only one baby had congenital abnormalities of eyes (bilateral congenital cataracts). The mother of this baby had not been given cyclizine until the twenty-eighth week of pregnancy, and the dose she received was about one fiftieth of that reported to cause eye abnormalities in animals.[e] Other babies in the series had a variety of nonocular abnormalities, but the statistical significance in relation to cyclizine was uncertain. In 1967 Algan observed two children who at one year of age had very poor vision attributable to peripheral and central tapetoretinal degeneration which they considered might have been a result of use of cyclizine early in pregnancy.[a,b] No further change was noted in the eyes of these two children up to ages seven and nine years.

In 1965 an ad hoc committee of the U.S. Food and Drug Administration concluded that the evidence of teratogenic effects in human beings was not significant, but it made no specific mention of the eyes.[f]

Cyclizine hydrochloride administered orally in doses of 15 to 100 mg to normal young subjects had no effect on accomodation, but three patients who took 750 mg for hallucinogenic effect developed an intoxication resembling that from atropine, with dilated slowly reactive pupils and hallucinations. The reaction lasted about six hours.[d]

a. Algan B, Marchal H: Concerning drug-induced tapetoretinal degenerations. *BULL SOC OPHTALMOL FRANCE* 67:1151–1167. (French)
b. Algan B, Afarchal H: Concerning two observations of drug-induced teratogenesis: tapetoretinal degeneration produced in a brother and sister by cyclizine hydrochloride. *EXCERPTA MED INT CONG SERIES* 154:63, 1967. (French)
c. Brand JJ, Colquhoun WP, Perry WLM: Side-effects of l-hyoscine and cyclizine studied by objective tests. *AEROSPACE MED* 39:999–1002, 1969.
d. Gott PH, Cyclizine toxicity — Intentional drug abuse of a proprietary antihistamine. *N ENGL J MED* 279:596, 1968.
e. McBride W: Cyclizine and congenital abnormalities. *BR MED J* 5338:1157–1158, 1963.
f. Sadusk JF Jr, Palmisano PA: Teratogenic effect of Meclizine, cyclizine and chlorcyclizine. *J AM MED ASSOC* 194:987–989, 1965.
g. Tuchmann-Duplessis H, Mercier-Parot L: Influence of cyclizine hydrochloride on the gestation and embryonic development of the rat, mouse and rabbit. *CR ACAD SCI (Paris)* 256:3359–3362, 1963. (French)

Cyclododecatriene (cyclododeca-1,5,9-triene) on the skin of animals causes severe contact dermatitis and readily induces sensitization. On the eyes of rabbits it has caused immediate signs of irritation with mild conjunctivitis which faded within forty-eight hours. The main effect was on the lids, which became red and swollen with accompanying discharge. The lids took several days to heal. From these tests it has been anticipated that in human beings a splash in the eye would be painful and would cause uncomfortable contact dermatitis of the lids, but no permanent damage.[a] (Compare *Cycloocta-1,5-diene* and *Cyclopentadiene.*)

a. Brown VKH, Hunter CG: Experimental studies on skin hazard with cycloocta-1, 5-diene and cyclododeca-1, 5,9-triene. *BR J IND MED* 25:75–76, 1968.

1,3,5-Cycloheptatriene (Tropilidene) is reported to be a severe primary skin irritant but not a sensitizer, and its vapors are said to be lacrimatory.[a]

a. Brown VKH, Ferrigan LS, Stevenson DE: Acute toxicity and skin irritant properties of tropilidene (1,3,5-cycloheptatriene). *ANN OCCUP HYG* 10:123–126, 1967.

Cyclohexane has no notable irritant effect on human eyes, nor on rabbit eyes tested by exposure to concentration of 11 mg/cu m of air. *Methyl cyclohexane* is similarly nonirritating.[a]

    a. Treon JF, Crutchfield WE Jr, Kitzmiller KV: The physiological response of animals to cyclohexane, methylcyclohexane and certain derivatives of these compounds. *J IND HYG* 25:323–346, 1943.

Cyclohexanol (hexalin) vapor is irritating to human eyes at a concentration of 100 ppm.[183] Testing by application of a drop to rabbit eyes causes moderate injury, graded 7 on a scale of 1 to 10 after twenty-four hours.[27,228] Rabbits show ocular irritation at 270 ppm in air.[a]

Browning has remarked concerning cyclohexanol that "even without direct contact of the vapour with the eyes, it can cause lacrimation in animals when applied to the skin as a constituent of soaps." Browning also noted that it could cause lacrimation after oral administration.[21]

    a. See reference to Treon, et al under *Cyclohexane.*

Cyclohexanone is irritating to human eyes at a concentration of 75 ppm in air,[183] and to rabbits at about 300 ppm.[a] Testing by application of the liquid to rabbit eyes causes moderate temporary injury, graded 5 on a scale of 1 to 10 after twenty-four hours.[27]

In the periphery of the crystalline lenses of guinea pigs vacuoles have been described occurring extensively after repeated application of cyclohexanone to the skin, or after subcutaneous injections; no such changes were found in untreated animals.[b] After 0.5 ml was dropped on the skin of the back 3 times a week for 3 weeks, and after observation for 6 months, extensive lens changes were reported in 2 out of 12 animals, but after daily subcutaneous administration of 0.05 ml of a mixture of 50% or 5% cyclohexanone with saline according to the same schedule similar lens changes were found in only 1 out of 16 animals, and were partially spontaneously reversible. By ophthalmoscopy the vacuoles gave a lace-work or spider web appearance of the periphery of the lenses against the pink fundus reflex. (In parallel experiments with *acetone* and *dimethyl sulfoxide* a similar appearance developed, but in higher incidence.)

    a. See reference to Treon, et al under *Cyclohexane.*
    b. Rengstorff RH, Petrali JP, Sim VM: Cataracts induced in guinea pigs by acetone, cyclohexanone, and dimethyl sulfoxide. *AM J OPHTHALMOL* 49:308–319, 1972.

Cyclohexanone peroxide is employed as a catalyst in polymerization of plastics. Industrially it has caused ocular irritation, and tests on rabbit eyes by application of a 40% to 50% solution in cyclohexanone or in dimethyl phthalate have shown that cyclohexanone peroxide can cause moderately severe corneal injury with superficial opacity and associated conjunctival inflammation.[a,b] (See also *Peroxides, organic.*)

    a. Kuchle (1958)—see *Peroxides, organic*
    b. Oettel H: Health endangerment by plastics. *NAUNYN-SCHMIEDEBERG'S ARCH EXP PATH PHARMAK* 232:77–132, 1957. (German)

Cyclohexylamine is a strongly basic liquid which is very irritating to the skin, and its vapor at concentrations from 150 to 1,200 ppm in air is extremely irritating and injurious, causing the corneas of guinea pigs and mice to become opaque.[a] Presumably a splash in the eye would also be severely injurious.

a. Watrous RM, Schulz HN: Cyclohexylamine, p-chloronitrobenzene, 2-amino-pyridine. Toxic effects in industrial use. *IND MED SURG* 19:317–320, 1950.

Cycloocta-1,5-diene has essentially the same toxic properties as described elsewhere for *cyclododeca-1,5,9-triene.*

Cyclopentolate (Cyclogyl, Ciclolux, and a component of Cyclomydril) is an anticholinergic cycloplegic agent administered in eyedrops. Its effects on the eye appear to be the same as those of other anticholinergic eyedrops except for differences in duration of action, concentrations employed, and possibly in rate of penetration. As with other agents discussed under the heading *Anticholinergic drugs,* cyclopentolate dilates the pupil and paralyzes accommodation, but rarely affects intraocular pressure in normal eyes.[a,i,r] However, it can induce angle-closure glaucoma in eyes that are peculiarly predisposed anatomically because of shallow anterior chambers and abnormally narrow angles. Also in some patients who have open-angle glaucoma it causes a rise of pressure with the angle remaining open.[a,h,j,n,r,102]

In the absence of glaucoma there has been no evidence of injurious effect on the eye. Experiments in young dogs to which 1% cyclopentolate eyedrops were administered twice a day for twelve months produced no abnormality discoverable by light and electron microscopy.[v,w]

Systemic toxic reactions from cyclopentolate eyedrops have been reported several times, as they have also from other anticholinergic eyedrops, particularly those containing atropine and scopolamine. Missiroli in 1969 reviewed previous reports and described a new case in which a young woman with normal medical and neurologic history had received a drop of 1% cyclopentolate in each eye every fifteen minutes three times, and about fifteen minutes after the last drop developed vertigo. Within the next hour she became dysarthric, could not stand, and could not articulate words. This condition lasted two hours and then rapidly improved without treatment, with complete recovery within four hours of the onset. During this reaction the pulse was rapid and irregular, but the patient's temperature remained normal.[p]

There are several reports describing psychotic behavior, suggestive of schizophrenia, in some instances with hallucinations and with difficulty in talking, usually associated with loss of equilibrium and ataxia.[e,f,o,q,t,u] Children seem to be particularly subject to reactions of this sort, especially when 2% eyedrops have been used.[b,f,k,l,u] In 2 children (one epileptic, one not epileptic) grand mal seizures have been induced.[l]

Systematic questioning of patients has brought out that milder systemic reactions, such as nausea, weakness, and lightheadedness, may be induced by cyclopentolate eyedrops more frequently than has been appreciated.[c,d] The onset has usually been in 20 to 30 minutes after application of drops, and symptoms usually have spontaneously passed in an hour. However, the onset in some cases has been delayed for an hour or two, and symptoms have sometimes lasted 2 to 4 hours. Reactions involving change in mood, uncontrolled crying, and disorientation are not rare.

Even in overt cases of systemic reaction the blood pressure has generally been unaffected, though characteristically the pulse rate is elevated.

Physostigmine parenterally is a potential antidote, but the systemic reactions to cyclopentolate have generally proven to be so self-limited that there has not been a need for it.

In one instance permanent mental derangement persisted after only four drops of 0.2% cyclopentolate hydrochloride were used in an elderly patient, an eighty-two-year-old man who had previous "compensated chronic dementia." This could not be considered an instance of toxic induction of permanent psychosis in a normal person.

a. Abraham SV: The use of several new drugs as substitutes for homatropine. *AM J OPHTHALMOL* 36 (part 2):69–74, 1953.

b. Adcock EW: Cyclopentolate (Cyclogyl) toxicity in pediatric patients. *J PEDIATR* 79:127–129, 1971.

c. Awan KJ: Adverse systemic reaction of topical cyclopentolate hydrochloride. *ANN OPHTHALMOL* 8:695–698, 1976.

d. Awan KJ: Systemic toxicity of cyclopentolate hydrochloride in adults following topical instillation. *ANN OPHTHALMOL* 8:803–806, 1976.

e. Beswick JA: Psychosis from cyclopentolate. *AM J OPHTHALMOL* 53:879, 1962.

f. Binkhorst RD, et al: Psychotic reaction induced by cyclopentolate. *AM J OPHTHALMOL* 55:1243, 1963.

g. Carpenter WT Jr: Precipitous mental deterioration following cycloplegia with 0.2% cyclopentolate HCl. *ARCH OPHTHALMOL* 78:445–447, 1967.

h. Galin MA: The mydriasis provocative test. *ARCH OPHTHALMOL* 66:353–355, 1961.

i. Gordon DM, Ehrenberg MH: Cyclopentolate hydrochloride: a new mydriatic and cycloplegic agent. *AM J OPHTHALMOL* 38:831–838, 1954.

j. Harris LS, Galin MA: Cycloplegic provocative testing. *ARCH OPHTHALMOL* 81:544–547, 1969.

k. Huismans H: Intoxication-psychosis after cyclopentolate hydrochloride (Zyklolat). *KLIN MONATSBL AUGENHEILKD* 175:100–102, 1979. (German)

l. Kennerdell JS, Wucher FP: Cyclopentolate associated with two cases of grand mal seizure. *ARCH OPHTHALMOL* 87:634–635, 1972.

m. Lazenby GW, Reed JW, Grant WM: Short term tests of anticholinergic medication in open-angle glaucoma. *ARCH OPHTHALMOL* 80:443–448, 1968.

n. Lowe RF: Angle-closure, pupil dilation, and pupil-block. *BR J OPHTHALMOL* 50:385–389, 1966.

o. Mark HH: Psychotogenic properties of cyclopentolate. *J AM MED ASSOC* 186:214–215, 1963.

p. Missiroli A: Toxic effects of cyclopentolate. *BOLL OCULIST* 48:433–438, 1969. (Italian)

q. Praeger DL, Miller SN: Toxic effects of cyclopentolate (Cyclogel). *AM J OPHTHALMOL* 58:1060–1061, 1964.

r. Priestly BS, Medine MM: A new mydriatic and cycloplegic drug. *AM J OPHTHALMOL* 34:572–575, 1951.

s. Schimek RA, Lieberman WJ: The influence of Cyclogyl and Neo-Synephrine on tonographic studies of miotic control in open-angle glaucoma. *AM J OPHTHALMOL* 51:781–784, 1961.

t. Shihab ZM: Psychotic reaction in an adult after topical cyclopentolate. *OPHTHAL-MOLOGICA* 181:228–230, 1980.

u. Simcoe CW: Cyclopentolate (Cyclogyl) toxicity. *ARCH OPHTHALMOL* 67:406, 1962.

v. Watanabe C: Histological findings on ciliary body performed the long-dated administration of the cycloplegics for pseudomyopia. *ACTA SOC OPHTHALMOL JPN* 73:1494–1511, 1968.

w. Yamaji D, et al: Study on pseudomyopia. *ACTA SOC OPHTHALMOL JPN* 72:2083–2150, 1968.

Cyclophosphamide (Cytoxan, Endoxan), an alkylating antineoplastic agent used orally or intravenously, has been tested by injection into the anterior chamber of rabbit eyes, but proved excessively damaging to the cornea to allow its use in treatment of epithelial invasion of the anterior chamber.[p] However, injections into the vitreous body in rabbits in concentrations up to 10 mg/ml have been tolerated without excessive inflammation and without alteration of the ERG.[d]

Parenteral administration to rats has induced cyclitis,[j] and this is made worse by nephrectomy.[k]

Teratogenic effects involving the eyes have been extensively studied in experimental animals.[a,b,c,e,f,n,o]

In children treated with cyclophosphamide a transient blurring of vision has been reported in 5 out of 59, coming on in minutes after intravenous injection in two, and within 24 hours in the other three.[h] The duration of blurring ranged from one hour to two weeks, but vision returned to normal in all. Ophthalmological examination did not disclose the mechanism of blurring.

A systematic study of 90 patients who received large doses of cyclophosphamide, total body irradiation, and marrow transplants showed eye complications to be common, consisting of dry eye syndrome, viral and other keratitis, and severe keratoconjunctivitis associated with graft-versus-host disease leading to scarring of the corneas.[g]

Blepharoconjunctivitis, first reported in 1965[333], has occurred in several cases reported to Fraunfelder's National Registry.[313]

Optic neuroretinitis reported in one patient under treatment with cyclophosphamide was thought more likely to be attributable to carmustine and procarbazine which were also being administered.[i]

Acute necrotizing retinitis in both eyes of one patient receiving clyclophosphamide after renal transplantation has been considered most likely to have been caused by cytomegalovirus.[l]

Cataracts have been observed in occasional patients who have received cyclophosphamide after renal transplantation, but a review of the circumstances, especially the associated use of high doses of corticosteroids, has made it seem unlikely that cyclophosphamide was specifically responsible.[m]

a. Clavert A: Modifications of cyclophosphamide induced colobomic eye lenses in the rabbit. *C R SOC BIOL* 165:2004–2007, 1971. (French)

b. Clavert A: Role of the lens in the differentiation of ciliary body and iris. *BULL ASSOC ANAT* 58:263–268, 1973. (French)

c. Clavert A: Influence of anomalies of the fetal fissure on migration of the optic fibers. *ARCH OPHTALMOL* (Paris) 34:215–224, 1974. (French)

d. Ericson L, Karlberg B, Rosengran BHQ: Trials of intravitreal injections of chemotherapeutic agents in rabbits. *ACTA OPHTHALMOL* 42:721–726, 1964.

e. Foerster H, et al: Vulnerability of early postnatal differentiation processes of the retina and the teratogenic effect of cyclophosphamide. *ACTA ANAT* 93:161–170, 1975. (German)

f. Hashimoto M, Shirai S, Majima A: Eye abnormalities in mice embryos caused by cyclophosphamide. *FOLIA OPHTHALMOL JPN* 27:42, 1976. (English abstract)

g. Jack MK, Hicks JD: Ocular complications in high dose chemoradiotherapy and marrow transplantation. *ANN OPHTHALMOL* 13:709–711, 1981.

h. Kende G, Sirkin S, et al: Blurring of vision—a previously undescribed complications of cyclophosphamide therapy. *CANCER* 44:69–71, 1979.

i. Lennan RM, Taylor HR: Optic neuroretinitis in association with BCNU and procarbazine therapy. *MED PEDIATR ONCOL* 4:43–48, 1978.

j. Levine S, Sowinski R: Cyclitis produced in rats by cyclophosphamide. *INVEST OPHTHALMOL* 13:697–699, 1974.

k. Levine S, Sowinski R: Role of the kidney in development of cystitis and other toxic effects of cyclophosphamide. *INVEST UROL* 13:196–199, 1975.

l. Porter R: Acute necrotizing retinitis in a patient receiving immunosuppressive therapy. *BR J OPHTHALMOL* 56:555–558, 1972.

m. Porter R, Crombie AL: Cataracts after renal transplantation. *BR MED J* 2:766, 1972.

n. Singh S, et al: Eye anomalies induced by cyclophosphamide in rat fetuses. *ACTA ANAT* 94:490–496, 1976.

o. Stuhltrager U: Cyclophosphamide-induced developmental disturbances of the nasolacrimal ducts in the mouse. *FOLIA OPHTHALMOL* (Jena) 7:207–211, 1982. (English summary.)

p. Verry F: Epithelial invasion of the anterior chamber: anatomical confirmation by cytological examination of the aqueous humor. *OPHTHALMOLOGICA* 153:467, 1967. (French)

Cycloserine (D-4-Amino-3-isoxazolidinone, Seromycin), an antimicrobial, has several times been said to have caused ill-defined visual disturbances in addition to drowsiness and mental confusion. The allusions to vision have been vague. For instance, Isebarth and Wiedemann in a long list of side effects have merely indicated that five out of 414 patients had eye symptoms consisting of flickering or feeling of pressure,[b] and Butt merely listed one instance of flickering vision and one of conjunctivitis among twenty-seven patients under treatment.[a] The only definite information seems to be a statement of Honegger and Genee (1969) that cycloserine had no effect on accommodation.[121]

a. Butt H: A clinical experience report on combined therapy of pulmonary tuberculosis with cycloserine-pyrazinamide. *WIEN MED WOCHENSCHR* 111:57–61, 1961.

b. Isebarth R, Wiedemann O: D–Cycloserin in pulmonary tuberculosis. *TUBERKULOSEARZT* 14:144–162, 1960. (German)

Cysteine, an amino acid, has been applied as a 3% near-neutral solution to animal and human eyes in treatment of chemical burns, attempting to accelerate regeneration of epithelium and impede vascularization of the cornea. Some benefit, and no adverse effect is reported.[a, 18, 19, 20, 127] A rationale for this application has been found in demonstrations that it inhibits the collagenase of alkali burned corneas, interfering with a mechanism believed to be involved in melting of such corneas, and it is mucolytic, helping to cleanse mucous secretions from the eye.[d,e,f,g]

In the disease cystinosis an oxidized form of cysteine is deposited in the cornea and in many other tissues. In some patients a peripheral pigmentary retinopathy is seen, and rarely a maculopathy.[b] These abnormalities have not been regarded as toxic effects. However, in young rats and mice parenteral injection of cysteine hydrochloride has damaged retinal neurons in the inner nuclear layer, the retinal ganglion cells, and the brain.[j,k,l,m] Cysteine appears to damage cells other than those affected by other neurotoxic agents such as glutamate, acting selectively upon certain subpopulations of the amacrine and ganglion cells of the retina.[c,h] In excised rabbit eye tissues exposed to cysteine the c-wave of the ERG is conspicuously increased, more than by a series of related compounds.[i] These observations of effects on the retina suggest potential for further scientific neurotoxicologic investigations utilizing cysteine as a selective tool, without as yet implying that these experimental effects have clinical counterparts.

a. Imre G, Opauszki A: The effect of local cysteine treatment in the diseases of the cornea. *SZEMESZET (Budapest)* 105:205–207, 1968.

b. Hammerstein W: Retinopathy and maculopathy in cystinosis. *KLIN MONATSBL AUGENHEILKD* 169:123–126, 1976. (German)

c. Karlsen RL, Pedersen OO: A morphological study of the acute toxicity of L-cysteine on the retina of young rats. *EXP EYE RES* 34:65–69, 1982.

d. Krause U, Nevasaari K: Treatment of corneal ulcers with cysteine. *ACTA OPHTHALMOL* 50:385–389, 1972.

e. Krejci L, Brettschneider I, Praus R: Cysteine in clinical practice. *CESK OFTALMOL* 30:355–359, 1974. (Czech)

f. Mehra KS, Singh R: Cysteine in corneal ulcer. *ANN OPHTHALMOL* 7:1329–1331, 1975.

g. Moriyama H, Kishida K, Manabe R: Effects of germanium oxide-cysteine eye drops. *FOLIA OPHTHALMOL JPN* 31:908–916, 1980. (English summary)

h. Pedersen OO, Karlsen RL: The toxic effect of L cysteine on the rat retina. *INVEST OPHTHALMOL VIS SCI* 19:886–892, 1980.

i. Shibata N: Effects of L-cysteine on the rabbit ERG. *ACTA SOC OPHTHALMOL JPN* 79:1163, 1975. (English summary)

j. Olney JW, Ho OL, Rhee V: Cytotoxic effects of acidic and sulphur containing amino acids on the infant mouse central nervous system. *EXP BRAIN RES* 14:61, 1971.

k. Olney JW, Ho OL, et al: Cysteine-induced brain damage in infant and fetal rodents. *BRAIN RES* 45:309, 1972.

l. Olney JW: Brain damage and oral intake of certain amino acids. *ADV EXP MED BIOL* 69:497, 1976.

m. Olney JW, Misra CH, de Gubareff T: Cysteine-S-sulfate: brain damaging metabolite in sulfite oxidase deficiency. *J NEUROPATHOL EXP NEUROL* 34:167–177, 1975.

Cytarabine (cytosine arabinoside), an inhibitor of DNA synthesis and antiviral agent, has been tested for toxicity to the cornea in rabbits, monkeys, and human beings. A solution of 0.1% cytarabine hydrochloride applied six times a day for six to ten days was not injurious, but concentrations of 0.5% or more, caused reversible changes in the corneal epithelium.[a,b,e] Some patients with normal corneas treated in this way for seven days developed glittering opacities in the lower layers of the epithelium, usually without stainability by fluorescein. Some had pain and developed signs of iritis. The severity was related to the concentration used and the time of exposure. After the applications were discontinued, all corneas cleared gradually during three weeks.[b]

A number of patients who have been treated systemically for leukemia or lymphoma with high doses have developed similar signs and symptoms, with punctate epithelial keratitis and photophobia in up to 46% of those treated with the drug intravenously.[d,f,i] Fraunfelder's National Registry has received additional unpublished reports of this painful keratitis.[313] Topical corticosteroid treatment has been disappointing. The keratitis has usually cleared in 1 to 2 weeks without this treatment.[d]

In rabbits glittering opacities which were induced in the lower layers of the corneal epithelium by repeated application of 1% solution were preventable by simultaneous administration of deoxy-cytidine, which was shown to reverse the inhibitory effect of the cytarabine on the synthesis of DNA.[b]

Corneal wound healing in rabbits is delayed by 1% cytarabine.[c]

Single subconjunctival injections of 37.5 mg/kg in rabbits has caused a inflammatory response in the conjunctiva lasting less than 24 hours, without disturbance of other parts of the eye.[j]

Retinal dysplasia has been produced in newborn rats by subcutaneous injections of cytarabine, and this has been studied in great detail.[g,h]

Intravitreal injection in rabbits have been "non-toxic" to the retina if a concentration of 1.2 μg/ml, or a dose of 30 μg was not exceeded.[277,369]

a. Elliott GA, Schut AL: Studies with cytarabine HCl (CA) in normal eyes of man, monkey and rabbit. *AM J OPHTHALMOL* 60:1074–1082, 1965.
b. Kaufman HE, Capella JA, et al: Corneal toxicity of cytosine arabinoside. ARCH OPHTHALMOL 72:535–540, 1964.
c. Gass AR, Katzin D: Antiviral drugs and corneal wound healing. *INVEST OPHTHALMOL* 14:628–630, 1975.
d. Gressel MG, Tomsak RL: Keratitis from high dose intravenous cytarabine. *LANCET* 2:273, 1982.
e. Hara J: Experimental studies on the corneal toxicity of antiviral agents. *ACTA SOC OPHTHALMOL JPN* 75:1399–1403, 1971. (English summary)
f. Hopen G, Mondino BJ, et al: Corneal toxicity with systemic cytarabine. *AM J OPHTHALMOL* 91:500–504, 1981.
g. Percy DH, Danylchuk KD: Experimental retinal dysplasia due to cytosine arabinoside. *INVEST OPHTHALMOL VIS SCI* 16:353–364, 1977.
h. Shimada M, et al: Developmental abnormality of retina caused by postnatal administration of cytosine arabinoside. *BIOL NEONATE* 26:359–366, 1975.
i. Ritch PS, Hansen RM, Heuer DK: Ocular toxicity from high-dose cytosine arabinoside. *CANCER* 51:430–432, 1983.
j. Rootman J, Gudauskas G, Kumi C: Subconjunctival versus intravenous cytosine arabinoside. *INVEST OPHTHALMOL VIS SCI* 24:1607–1611, 1983.

Cytisine is the alkaloid present in *Cytisus laburnum* or *Laburnum anagyroides* which causes severe vomiting and collapse in children who chew the pods and seeds of this plant. Maximum pupillary dilation is characteristic.[46,153]

Cytochalasin B, a mould or fungal metabolite, has been used experimentally injected into the anterior chamber of eyes of monkeys to cause widespread structural changes in the aqueous outflow system and increase in facility of outflow.[a,b,c] This was followed by remarkably rapid recovery. (Also see *Cytochalasin D.*)

a. Johnstone M, Tanner D, et al: Concentration-dependent morphologic effects of cytochalasin B in the aqueous outflow system. *INVEST OPHTHALMOL VIS SCI* 19:835–841, 1980.
b. Kaufman PL, Bill A, Barany EH: Effect of cytochalasin B on conventional drainage of aqueous humor in the cynomolgus monkey. *EXP EYE RES* 25(Suppl):411–414, 1977; also, *INVEST OPHTHALMOL VIS SCI* 16:47–53, 1977.
c. Svedbergh B, Lutjen-Drecoll E, et al: Cytochalasin B induced structural changes in the anterior ocular segment of the cynomolgus monkey. *INVEST OPHTHALMOL VIS SCI* 17:718–734, 1978.

Cytochalasin D, a mould or fungal metabolite, added to incubated rat lenses has produced cortical cataracts with globular cortical degeneration. During the first 24 hours both the opacification and globular degeneration were reversible, possibly related to the reversibility of the effect of cytochalasin D on actin microfilaments.[b] A similar mechanism may be involved in changes in trabecular meshwork structure and increase in facility of aqueous outflow by both cytochalasin B and D.[a]

a. Kaufman PL, Erickson KA: Cytochalasin B and D dose-outflow facility response relationships in the cynomolgus monkey. *INVEST OPHTHALMOL VIS SCI* 23:646–650, 1982.
b. Mousa GY, Creighton MO, Trevithick JR: Eye lens opacity in cortical cataracts associated with actin-related globular degeneration. *EXP EYE RES* 29:379–391, 1979.

Dacarbazine (DTIC), an antineoplastic, has been tested for ocular toxicity in monkeys and rabbits by series of retrobulbar and intraocular injections. By either route, when the dosage was excessive, there was destructive chorioretinopathy and vitreous hemorrhage.[a,b]

a. Wilczek ZM: Experimental intraocular penetration of dacarbazine. *AM J OPHTHALMOL* 84:299–304, 1977.
b. Lin HS, Perry HD, et al: Tolerance of DTIC in normal rabbit eyes. *METAB OPHTHALMOL* 2:33–39, 1978.

Dactinomycin (Cosmegen), an antineoplastic, tested by intravitreal injection in rabbits is reported not to be toxic to the retina at a dose of 0.05 µg,[369] or at a concentration of 0.02 µg/ml as a vitrectomy infusion fluid after extracapsular lens extraction.[277]

Dapiprazole, an alpha-adrenergic blocking agent of potential interest in treatment of glaucoma, was found to be well tolerated topically in rabbits and monkeys, and then was tested in human volunteers. Eyedrops containing 1.0 or 1.5% caused conjunctival hyperemia lasting 2 hours, miosis, and short-lasting ptosis, but no other ocular or systemic effects. Repeated application of 0.25% during 3 weeks was satisfactorily tolerated.[a]

a. Iuglio N: Ocular effects of topical application of dapiprazole. *GLAUCOMA* 6:110–116, 1984.

Dapsone (diaminodiphenylsulfone), an antibacterial drug, has been used in treatment of leprosy since 1941, and is known sometimes to cause peripheral motor neuropathy, but the first cases of retinal damage or optic atrophy from this drug were published in 1980, from overdosage. In one case, a 20-year-old man took 600 mg daily for 10 days. Five days after stopping the medication he had counting-fingers vision, also weakness from peripheral neuropathy. In both fundi there were hemorrhages and exudates. In a month some of these cleared, but optic atrophy developed, and poor vision was permanent.

Another patient, who had been under treatment with 50 mg dapsone daily, became seriously ill after he took 7.5 g in a suicide attempt.[b] He had massive intravascular hemolysis, severe methemoglobinemia, and acute renal failure requiring peritoneal dialysis. Two weeks later visual acuity was 6/36 in each eye, associated with a yellow-white appearance and small hemorrhages in the central fundus, also localized capillary non-perfusion by angiography. In a further 3 weeks the fundus regained more normal appearance, but vision did not improve beyond 6/18 in either eye. It was suggested that retinal necrosis in the macular area had been produced by a combination of effects of severe hypoxemia and vascular occlusion by fragmented red blood cells.[b] It seemed possible that dapsone at normal dosage might sufficiently affect the blood in some patients to produce foveal capillary changes, and it was recommended that patients experiencing blurring of vision while receiving dapsone should have their macular function carefully examined, including fluorescein angiography.

Some clinical investigators have questioned whether dapsone at normal dosage is a threat to retinal blood flow, reporting normal results from careful examinations of the retinal vessels in 7 patients with normal vision, despite significant proven hemolysis and damaged red blood cells as a concomitant of chronic treatment of skin disease with dapsone.[c]

Patients under treatment with dapsone for leprosy have been known to develop posterior synechias, but this appears to be attributable to the disease, rather than to the drug.[d]

a. Homeida M, Babikr A, Daneskmend TK: Dapsone-induced optic atrophy and motor neuropathy. *BR MED J* 281:1180, 1980.
b. Kenner DJ, Holt K, et al: Permanent retinal damage following massive dapsone overdose. *BR J OPHTHALMOL* 64:741–744, 1980.
c. Leonard JN, Tucker WFG, et al: Dapsone and the retina. *LANCET* 1:453, 1982.
d. Brandt F, Adiga RB, Pradhan H: Lagophthalmos and posterior synechias during treatment of leprosy with diaminodiphenylsulfone. *KLIN MONATSBL AUGENHEILKD* 184:28–31, 1984.

Datura stramonium (*Datura arborea*, jimson weed, Jamestown weed) grows wild in all parts of the United States, as well as in Europe, Asia, Africa, and South America.

All parts of the weed contain hyoscyamine, atropine, and scopolamine. Temporary dilation of the pupils and paralysis of accommodation characteristically accompany systemic poisoning by jimson weed, which is fairly common, particularly in children who chew the leaves or swallow the seeds. The seeds are said to have little taste. The systemic effects, which are essentially like those in poisoning by atropine or stramonium, have been well described, and the appearance of the plant, its flower, seedpod, and leaves well illustrated.[c] The systemic effects generally consist of disorientation, incoordination, visual and other types of hallucination, elevated temperature and pulse rate, with reddish, dry skin and dilated, unreactive pupils. The ocular effects may also occur simply from getting seeds from the plant in the conjunctival sac without systemic poisoning and without ocular inflammation. This has occurred accidentally in farmers at harvest time.[d] Pupil and accommodation return to normal in a few days in either case. Similar dilation of the pupil has been caused by seeds of *Datura cornigera* (Angel's trumpet) and *Datura wrightii*.[e,f]

Asthmador, a preparation of dried leaves of Datura stramonium intended for use in relief of symptoms of asthma, has caused several cases of typical stramonium poisoning with hallucinations. In one extraordinary instance bilateral central scotoma has been suspected to have been caused by smoking the dried leaves of *Datura stramonium*,[225] but no comparable effect has thus far been observed in many other cases of poisoning by jimson weed, Asthmador, or the known active components of these. (Intoxications by *Asthmador* are further described elsewhere under *Stramonium*.)

a. Eichner ER, Gunsolus JM, Powers JF: "Belladonna" poisoning confused with botulism. *J AM MED ASSOC* 20:695–696, 1967.
b. Mitchell JE, Mitchell F: Jimson weed poisoning in childhood. *J PEDIATR* 47:227–230, 1955.
c. Rosen CS, Lechner M: Jimson-weed intoxication. *N ENGL J MED* 267:448–450, 1962.
d. Simmons FH: Jimson weed mydriasis in farmers. *AM J OPHTHALMOL* 44:109, 1957.
e. Wallman JDR: An odd eye. *MED J AUST* 1:153, 1963.
f. Reader AL: Mydriasis from Datura wrightii. *AM J OPHTHALMOL* 84:263–264, 1977.

DDT (dichlorodiphenyltrichloroethane) was a very widely employed insecticide which could induce poisoning in human beings, but it has not been demonstrated to have a selective toxic effect on the eyes. Pure DDT dissolved in purified kerosene was tested in a concentration of 0.01% on a human eye and caused no discomfort or irritation; it also proved non-irritating at 4% concentration on rabbit eyes.[81] Rare instances have been reported of ocular irritation following contamination of the eye by powders containing DDT,[d,e] and in one instance chronic superficial punctate keratitis was associated with fatal poisoning from long exposure to the dust,[c] but it is probable that constituents other than DDT were responsible, or that there was hypersensitivity.

Monocular transient retrobulbar neuritis was reported in three people exposed to a partially identified mixture of DDT, o- and p-dichlorobenzene, and pentachlorophenol.[a] In seven additional cases an association of DDT with retrobulbar neuritis was suspected, but without sufficient evidence definitely to incriminate it.[a]

In experimental exposure of two men to skin contact with DDT one developed many complaints including "yellow vision" for less than an hour on two occasions.[b]

Evidence to make one think that significant poisoning or disturbance of eyes or vision is unlikely from prolonged occupational exposure has been provided by a study of thirty-five men exposed for eleven to nineteen years to large amounts of DDT in its manufacture, with body fat concentrations of DDT and its isomers and metabolites ranging from 38 to 647 ppm, contrasting with the average of 8 ppm for the general population.[g] Among these men and in other employees of the manufacturing plant, no instances of clinical poisoning were recognized. Though little specific ophthalmologic information was reported, none of the thirty-five patients in the special study had eye complaints. Apparently the only significant pathology observed was moderate hypertensive retinopathy in one patient, with no suggestion that it was related to DDT.[g]

In experimental animals there is a note of visual perceptual deficit in the American bobwhite from sublethal amounts of DDT.[f] In newborn monkeys, high levels of DDT attained by prenatal administration produced no abnormality in visual-evoked potentials.[h] In mice, intraperitoneal administration caused changes in the b-wave of the ERG.[289]

a. Campbell AMG: Neurological complications associated with insecticides and fungicides. *BR MED J* 2:415–417, 1952.
b. Case RAM: Toxic effects of 2,2-bis-chlorphenyl-1,1-trichloroethane (DDT) in man. *BR MED J* 2:842–843, 1945.
c. Hertel H: Chronic DDT intoxication. *DTSCH ARCH KLIN MED* 199:256–274, 1952. (German)
d. Mackerras IM, West RFK: DDT poisoning in man. *MED J AUST* 1:400, 1946.
e. Theodorides E: Intentional or accidental unilateral conjunctivitis caused by DDT powder. *ANN OCULIST (Paris)* 182:397, 1949. (French)
f. James D, Davis KB: The effect of sublethal amounts of DDT on the discriminational ability of the bobwhite, *Colinus Virginianus (Linn)*. *AM ZOOL* 5:229, 1965.
g. Laws ER, Curley A, Biros FJ: Men with intensive occupational exposure to DDT. *ARCH ENVIRON HEALTH* 15:766–775, 1967.
h. Pearson TR, Talens GM, Woolley DE: Effects of DDT–treatment on visual-evoked potentials in immature monkeys. *FED PROC* 31:821, 1972.

Decahydronaphthalene (Decalin; perhydronaphthalene; naphthalane) tested by dropping on rabbit eyes, causes no injury. Administered systemically to rabbits and guinea pigs, it causes cataract even more readily than naphthalene.[a,b,225] No serious industrial poisonings are known.[70] (Compare *Naphthalene.*)

a. Badinand A, Paufique L, Rodier J: Experimental intoxication by 1,2,3, 4-tetra-hydronaphthalene. *ARCH MAL PROF* 8:124–130, 1947. (*CHEM ABST* 42, 7878.)
b. Basile G: The action of some products of hydrogenation of naphthalin (tetralin and decalin) on the lens and deep ocular membranes of the rabbit. *BOLL OCULIST* 18:951–957, 1939. (Abstr: *AM J OPHTHALMOL* 24:237, 1941.)

Decahydronitronaphthalene (nitrodecalin) may have a unique toxic effect on the eye. Observations are limited to a single accident in which a flask containing "Nitrodekalin", and possibly other substances not identified, broke and contaminated the hands of three people. In a few hours the three victims noted gradual clouding of vision, and by the next day their vision was so reduced that they could not see objects as large as a chair. They appeared apathetic and helpless. Their eyes had no external evidences of inflammation, but in the anterior chambers was an intense red-brown discoloration and clouding of the aqueous humor, which by slit-lamp biomicroscope appeared to be due to fine dust-like material suspended in the aqueous humor and deposited on the back surface of the corneas. The material was so thick that details of the iris could not be discerned, and the fundi could not be examined. In one patient it was almost impossible to see the pupil. The tensions were normal in all eyes. Vision was reduced to distinguishing hand movements. Nevertheless, all recovered rapidly; within six days the eyes and the vision had returned to normal. The nature of the material which had appeared on the aqueous humor was not established.[a]

a. Thies O: On effect of nitro-compounds on the human eye. *KLIN MONATSBL AUGEN-HEILKD* 111:33–34, 1946. (German)

Decamethonium bromide (Syncurine), a skeletal muscle relaxant, has been noted in patients occasionally to cause a transient rise of ocular pressure, similar to that caused by succinyl choline, not a sustained elevation.[a] The same sort of pressure rises in eyes of cats have been demonstrated to be produced by contractions of extraocular muscles, which are induced by decamethonium, or by stimulation of the third nerve.[b]

a. Maier ES: Effect of decamethonium on intraocular pressure in man. *ANESTH ANAL CUR RES* 44:753–757, 1965.
b. Macri FJ, Wanko T, Grimes P: The effect of extraocular muscle contraction on the elasticity of the eye. *ARCH OPHTHALMOL* 61:424–430, 1959.

Deferoxamine (desferioxamine, Desferal, Desferol) is a chelating agent for iron that has been used clinically both systemically and locally in the eye for ocular siderosis and for iron foreign bodies in the eye. Although deferoxamine has been found to penetrate poorly into the aqueous humor after intravenous injection in rabbits,[i] it has produced opacities in the crystalline lens in dogs, cats, and rats when given by daily subcutaneous injection for long periods at dosages so large that they produced severe gastroenteritis.[b] About half the animals in these experiments died. The clouding of the lenses started with vacuoles in the periphery, spreading toward the axis. Later, changes in the lens fibers appeared and water clefts developed, proceeding to liquefaction, and in some dogs to gradual resorption of the cortex.[a] There were no signs of inflammation, and the ciliary body showed no abnormality histologically. Deferoxamine was not detected chemically in the aqueous humor in these experiments.[b]

Ferrioxamine, the iron complex of deferoxamine, administered to dogs and rats by repeated subcutaneous injection in the same manner as employed in the production of cataracts by deferoxamine, did not cause changes in the lenses.[b]

In patients, careful ophthalmic examination after treatment for three to six months with standard oral or parenteral dosage of deferoxamine for poisoning from ingestion of iron or for treatment of ocular siderosis have shown no opacities in the cornea or lens attributable to the treatment.[c,f,h,k,n,o] However, apart from these systematic studies, mention has been made without details, that cataracts in three human beings have occurred in association with long-term deferoxamine administration.[d,f]

Rarely patients given extraordinarily large doses have had temporary disturbance of color vision and visual acuity, with abnormal ERG in two cases.[e,l] Eight patients who received daily intravenous deferoxamine for 4 to 11 days (total 12 to 96 g) had decrease in visual acuity, abnormal color vision and night blindness.[g] Six of the patients appeared to have bilateral retrobulbar neuritis, which cleared after treatment had been discontinued. Later, seven of the eight patients developed retinal pigmentary degeneration, in the macula in six. Clinical studies suggested a toxic action at the level of the retinal pigment epithelium and photoreceptors.

In treatment of rust rings of the cornea, 5% solution and 10% ointment have been applied repeatedly to the surface of the eye in patients, without evident adverse effect.[j,m] After application to the surface of the eye, deferoxamine has been shown in rabbits to penetrate very poorly into the aqueous humor. Greater penetration has been obtained by subconjunctival injection.[i,m] Injection of 28.5% solution subconjunctivally has caused slight chemosis and hyperemia, which was gone in three days. This produced no other ocular disturbance.[i] Injection of 50 mg subconjunctivally was tolerated by the eyes of monkeys, and 50 mg injected subconjunctivally in rabbits every one to three days for several months was tolerated also, but 200 mg subconjunctivally in rabbits caused reduction in the response of the pupil to light, congestion of the uvea, and exudative detachment of the choroid and retina, without affecting the ERG.[p]

Intravitreal injections of 5 mg deferoxamine in rabbits proved very toxic, causing widespread hemorrhagic necrosis, particularly affecting the rods and cones of the retina and extinguishing the ERG.[p]

a. Barnett KC, Noel PRB: The eye in general toxicity studies. In Pigott, P.V. (Ed.): *Evaluation of Drug Effects on the Eye.* London, FJ Parsone, 1968.
b. Bruckner R, Hess R, et al: Pathologic lens changes in experimental animals after prolonged administration of high doses of deferoxamine. *HELV PHYSIOL PHARMACOL ACTA* 25:62–77, 1967. (German)
c. Chavanne H, Demilliere B: Trial of a new iron chelator, deferoxamine, in a case of siderosis of the eye. *BULL SOC OPHTALMOL FRANCE* 64:810–814, 1964. (French)
d. Ciba Pharmaceutical Company: Official literature on new drugs: Deferoxamine mesylate. *CLIN PHARMACOL THER* 10:595–596, 1969.
e. Davies SC, Hungerford JL, et al: Ocular toxicity of high dose intravenous desferrioxamine. *LANCET* 2:181–184, 1983.
f. Jacobs J, Greene H, Gendel BR: Acute iron intoxication. *N ENGL J MED* 273:1124–1127, 1965.
g. Lakhanpal V, Schocket SS, Jiji R: Deferoxamine (Desferal) induced toxic retinal pigmentary degeneration and presumed optic neuropathy. *OPHTHALMOLOGY* 91:443–451, 1984.
h. McEnery JT, Greengard J: Treatment of acute iron ingestion with deferoxamine in 20 children. *J PEDIATR* 68:773–779, 1966.
i. Melchionda C, Leonardi A, Valvo A: Experimental investigation on the passage of

deferoxamine into the anterior chamber. *ANN OTTALMOL CLIN OCUL* 91:1266–1272, 1965. (Italian)

j. Morawiecki J, Jablonski J: Removing of rust from the cornea by means of pharmacological compounds. *KLIN OCZNA* 38:491–492, 1968.

k. Paufique L, Bonnet M, Didierlaurent A: Our experience with deferoxamine in treatment of siderosis of the eye. *BULL SOC OPHTALMOL FRANCE* 66:774–781, 1966. (French)

l. Simon P, Ang KS, et al: Desferrioxamine, ocular toxicity, and trace metals. *LANCET* 2:512–513, 1983.

m. Valvo A: Desferrioxamine B in ophthalmology. *AM J OPHTHALMOL* 63:98–103, 1967.

n. Valvo A, Del Duca A: Applications of a new chelating compound in ophthalmology. *ANN OTTALMOL CLIN OCUL* 91:497–512, 1965. (Italian)

o. Valvo A, Melchioda C, Leonardi A: Treatment of blood in the cornea with deferoxamine. *ANN OTTALMOL CLIN OCUL* 91:1463–2470, 1965. (Italian)

p. Wise JB: Treatment of experimental siderosis bulbi vitreous hemorrhage, and corneal bloodstaining with deferoxamine. *ARCH OPHTHALMOL* 75:698–707, 1966.

Depilatories are preparations applied to the skin for removal of hair. Most notable in the past were depilatories containing thallium salts which produced many cases of poisoning. (See *Thallium*.) More recently dipilatories have contained calcium thioglycolate. A report by Eckermann in 1966 has described three cases of severe burns and permanent corneal scarring from accidental contamination of the eye with Eva depilatory cream, which contained an excess of calcium hydroxide in addition to calcium thioglycolate. Particles of the material were found in the conjunctival sac even after the eyes were irrigated with water. The injuries of the cornea resembled severe calcium hydroxide burns.[a] Thioglycolates seem not to have been excessively injurious except at extremes of pH. (See also *Thioglycolates*.)

a. Eckermann M, Gessner L: On eye injuries from modern cosmetics. *Z ARTZTL FORTBILD* (Jena) 60:612–615, 1966. (German)

Derris (Derris root) is employed as a fish poison and insecticide and as a source of rotenone. Contact with the powder causes severe dermatitis associated with conjunctivitis and inflammation of all mucous membranes.[a]

a. Simons CP: A tropical occupational disease due to derris. *ACTA DERMATOVENER* (Stockholm) 28:601, 1948. (Abstr: *BR J IND MED* 6:265, 1949.)

Desipramine (desmethylimipramine, Norpramine, Pentrofane, Pertofran), an antidepressant drug with some anticholinergic atropine-like activity. In cats under anesthesia intravenous injection of desipramine has been found to reduce the spontaneous activity of the retinal neurones. Doses of 5 to 20 mg/kg increased the c-wave in the ERG, and doses of 20 to 35 mg/kg reduced the b-wave.[a]

a. Heiss WD, Heilig P, Hoyer J: Effect of desipramine on retinal impulse activity and electroretinogram. *EXPERIENTIA* 23:728–729, 1967.

Desoxycortone (desoxycorticosterone), an adrenocortical salt-regulating steroid, is reported to have caused a significant elevation of ocular pressure in one out of nine patients who had primary open-angle glaucoma and were given 30 mg in oil per day intramuscularly for three to six days. The tonographic facility of outflow did not decrease, but the elevation of ocular pressure persisted in the one exceptional patient while the drug was being administered.[a]

> a. Frenkel M, Krill AE: Effects of two mineralocorticoids on ocular tension. *ARCH OPHTHALMOL* 72:315–318, 1964.

Detergents, or cleansing agents fall into three convenient categories: *Inorganic detergents, Organic detergents,* and *Oil-soluble detergents,* though some commercial detergents contain a mixture of Inorganic and Organic.[322]

Inorganic detergents, used for laundering and dishwashing, are made up mainly of sodium carbonate, sodium silicates, and sodium phosphates, as mixtures in varying proportions in different commercial brands.[a,b,c] Those containing predominantly sodium silicate or metasilicate and sodium carbonate usually are more alkaline and more injurious to rabbit eyes when tested as dry powders than are detergents which are composed predominantly of phosphates. The strongly alkaline detergents can cause permanent opacification of rabbit corneas, but may not be so injurious to monkey corneas. The inorganic detergents are generally more injurious to the eye than is laundry soap. (See INDEX for *Sodium carbonate,* and for *Soap.*)

Organic detergents, used in skin-cleansers and shampoos, as well as in laundrying, dishwasing, and general cleaning, are made up of soaps and a large variety of synthetic organic surfactants (surface active agents, or wetting agents). These are described in detail elsewhere under those special headings. (See INDEX for *Soap* and for *Surfactants.*)

A typical combination-detergent, combining organic and inorganic detergents, composed of a mixture of sodium dodecylbenzene sulfonate, sodium tripolyphosphate, sodium silicate, and sodium sulfate, has been tested in great detail in rabbit and monkey eyes by W.R. Green et al in 1978, utilizing clinical and histological methods.[322] A spray-dried powder (0.1 ml) applied to the eyes caused injuries and areas of corneal opacification which tended to clear in subsequent days and weeks, better in monkeys than in rabbits.

Oil soluble detergents are used as additives to lubricating oils to hold foreign matter in suspension. No eye hazard was found in one test reported on rabbit eyes.[d]

> a. Feldman DB, Rall DP, Moore JA: Dry detergent and soap effects on the rabbit eye. *J AM MED ASSOC* 221:1055, 1972.
> b. Scharpf LG Jr, Hill ID, Kelly RE: Relative eye-injury potential of heavy-duty phosphate and nonphosphate laundry detergents. *FOOD COSMET TOXICOL* 10:829–837, 1972.
> c. Schleyer WL: Detergent hazards. *J AM MED ASSOC* 222:1310, 1972.
> d. Weisser CW, Westrick ML, Schrenk HH: Action of detergents in white mineral oil upon rabbit corneal epithelium. *ARCH INDUSTR HEALTH* 14:265–268, 1956.

Dexamphetamine (dextroamphetamine, D-amphetamine, Desoxyn, Dexedrine, Sympamin), an adrenergic or sympathomimetic CNS stimulant, has been noted in cases of systemic overdosage to make the pupils dilate but to continue to react to light.[a] In five patients with open-angle glaucoma 5 to 15 mg orally produced no significant changes in diurnal ocular pressure curves.[190]

a. Ong BH: Dextroamphetamine poisoning. *N ENGL J MED* 266:1321–1322, 1962.

Dextran (Macrodex), a polysaccharide of varied molecular weights, used as a plasma expander in emergencies, has been found in rabbits to reduce ocular pressure and at the same time to produce a flare in the aqueous humor when material of large molecular size is given intravenously, but to produce no significant effect if partially hydrolyzed to small molecular size before injection.[a] Toxic effect on the blood aqueous barrier has been suspected as the cause of reduced ocular pressure. However, when dextran has been administered in a purified form as Macrodex made isotonic with glucose, it also reduced the pressure in rabbit eyes as much as 10 mm Hg.[c]

Intravitreal injections of dextran 500 in cats is reported not to have clouded the vitreous, but dextran 2000 at low concentrations has caused clouding of the vitreous and at higher concentrations has caused phthisis bulbi.[b]

As a component for intraocular irrigating solutions for use during sugery, experiments on rabbit eyes have shown dextran and dextran-40 to be protective against effects of artificial stresses (ouabain or low calcium) on the cornea and lens.[e–g]

In monkeys adding dextran of molecular weight 200,000 to 300,000 to the blood circulation has increased the viscosity of the blood to such a degree that retinal hemorrhages have resulted.[d]

a. Barany E: The influence of gum arabic and dextran on the blood aqueous barrier and intraocular pressure. *OPHTHALMOLOGICA* 116:65–79, 1948.
b. Gombos GM, Berman ER: Chemical and clinical observations on the fate of various vitreous substitutes. *ACTA OPHTHALMOL* 45:794–806, 1967.
c. Preste E, Traverso G: The use of the dextran (Macrodex Baxter) as an ocular pressure reducing agent. *ANN OTTAL CLIN OCUL* 92:1245–1265, 1966.
d. Maurolf FA, Mensher JH: Experimental hyperviscosity retinopathy. *ANN OPHTHAL-MOL* 5:205–209, 1973.
e. Peyman GA, Stainer GA, et al: Corneal thickness after vitrectomy and infusion with dextran solution. *ANN OPHTHALMOL* 9:1241–1244, 1977.
f. Peyman GA, Sanders DR, Ligara TH: Dextran 40- containing infusion fluids and corneal swelling. *ARCH OPHTHALMOL* 97:152–155, 1979.
g. Sanders DR, Bokosky J, et al: Dextran's effect on stressed lenses. *ARCH OPHTHALMOL* 97:1948–1953, 1979.

Dextran sulfate injected into the vitreous humor of rabbits is reported to have caused severe iritis, intraocular hemorrhage, and distension of the globe.[44] In cats intravitreal injection of dextran sulfate 500 did not cloud the vitreous, but dextran sulfate 2000 caused clouding, and at high concentration caused severe vitreous opacities.[a] (See also *Dextran.*)

a. See under Dextran reference b.

Diacetin (glyceryl diacetate) tested on a human eye caused severe smarting and hyperemia of the conjunctiva, but no appreciable injury.[a]

>   a. Gomer JJ: Corneal clouding by pure acetone. *GRAEFES ARCH OPHTHALMOL* 150:622–644, 1950.

Di(acetylcyanide) tested by exposure of animals to its vapor caused irritation of the eyes, mydriasis, and cornea ulceration at concentrations which also caused respiratory distress and prostration.[a]

>   a. Treon JF, Deutra FR, Cappel J: Toxicity of di(acetyl-cyanide). *ARCH IND HYG* 4:573, 1951.

Diacetylmonoxime (DAM) has been employed experimentally to counteract the inhibition of cholinesterase induced by certain poisonous organic phosphate esters. In human volunteers intravenous injection of 15 to 20 mg/kg caused blurred vision in four out of nineteen subjects for a period of two to eight minutes, but no change in pupillary size nor nystagmus. Three individuals were tested for ability to accommodate, and accommodation was found to be unimpaired. The cause of the transient blurring of vision has not been established. No measurements of visual acuity and no examination of the fundi were reported. More common side effects have been dizziness, loss of consciousness, and diffuse tingling.[a] (Compare *Pyridine-2-aldoxime.*)

>   a. Jager BV, Stagg GN: Toxicity of diacetylmonoxime and of pyridine-2-aldoxime methiodide in man. *BULL JOHNS HOPKINS HOSP* 102:203–211, 1958.

Diacetyl peroxide has been recognized as a serious industrial hazard to the eye. Testing on rabbit eyes by application of two drops of 30% solution in dimethyl phthalate caused very severe corneal damage.[a]

>   a. Kuchle (1958); see *Peroxides, organic.*

N,N–Diallyl-2-chloroacetamide (CDAA, Randox), a herbicide, is reported to be strongly irritant on the skin, and is said to have produced "serious ocular damage" by contact of undiluted material with the eye, but no details of the injury seem to have been published.[70,171]

Diamide is a reagent utilized in biochemical investigations to oxidize cellular glutathione from GSH to GSSG. It has been shown that depletion of GSH in this way in the lens and in the cornea seriously disturbs membrane functions in these tissues, causing leakiness and abnormal fluid accumulation.[a,b]

>   a. Epstein DL, Kinoshita JH: The effect of diamide on lens glutathione and lens membrane functions. *INVEST OPHTHALMOL* 9:629–638, 1970.
>   b. Geroski DH, Edelhauser HF, O'Brien WJ: Hexose-monophosphate shunt response to diamide in the component layers of the cornea. *EXP EYE RES* 26:611–619, 1978.

4,4'-Diaminodiphenylmethane (methylenedianiline) has been found to cause blindness in cats, but not in dogs, rabbits, guinea pigs, or rats. A single near-lethal dose of 100 mg/kg produced selective atrophy of rods, cones, and nuclei in the outer granular layer.[a] It is noteworthy that *ethylenimine* has had a similar effect on the retina of cats, and that compounds not greatly dissimilar chemically, listed under *Aminophenoxyalkanes,* are also retinotoxic.

This compound has been used industrially for more than 30 years, mostly as an epoxy resin hardener, and it has caused toxic hepatitis and myocardiopathy in workers, but there appears to be no report of retinopathy in human beings.[b,c]

a. von Canstatt BS, Hofmann HT, et al: Retinal changes of the cat in poisoning by orally or percutaneously administered chemicals. *VERH DTSCH GES PATHOL* 50:429–435, 1966.

b. Brooks LJ, Neale JM, Pieroni DR: Acute myocardiopathy following tripathway exposure to methylenedianiline. *J AM MED ASSOC* 242:1527–1528, 1979.

c. McGill DB, Motto JD: An industrial outbreak of toxic hepatitis due to methylenedianiline. *N ENGL J MED* 291:278–282, 1974.

2,4-Diaminophenol dihydrochloride has been tested by irrigating a rabbit eye with 0.02 M (pH 5.3) aqueous solution for ten minutes, after removal of the corneal epithelium to facilitate penetration. This produced dark brown staining of the corneal stroma, permanent corneal opacification, and vascularization.[81] 2,4-Diaminophenol has been used as a photographic developer and for dyeing furs and hair.[171] It is oxidized readily to brown substances which behave like quinones in their toxicity and protein-staining. (See also *p-Phenylenediamine* and *Quinones.*)

Diazacholesterol, an inhibitor of desmosterol reductase, has been given to rats in a study of myotonia, and was found to produce cataracts in 6 out of 16 animals.[a] There was a large accumulation of desmosterol, and whether this or a lack of cholesterol was responsible for the cataracts was unsettled, but it was noteworthy that similar conditions are produced by *triparanol,* which produces cataracts in human beings as well as animals.

a. Peter JB, Andiman RM, et al: Myotonia induced by diazacholesterol. *EXP NEUROL* 41:735–744, 1973.

Diazepam (Valium), a tranquilizer and muscle relaxant, has been the subject of many psychophysical studies relating to visual physiology, but few reports of significant adverse or toxic effects on the eye. There has been confusion on whether diazepam is safe in the presence of glaucoma. Advertising literature has for many years included a warning against use in "acute narrow-angle glaucoma", yet there appears to be but a single case report in which this drug has been presumed to be responsible for angle-closure glaucoma, and there are good reasons for doubting such a connection.[e]

The drug has been given to large numbers of patients and to experimental animals without evidence of visual disturbance, and without change in accommodation or change in the size of the pupils.[c] The drug appears to have no significant autonomic effects on the eye. Search of English language literature by the manufacturer of Valium has disclosed no report of mydriasis except one mention of "dilated pupils" in a child.[h,n] This appeared, without comment in a table, among a variety of side effects purportedly observed by parents and "therapists" in a series of sixty-eight children, and cannot be considered an authoritative type of observation.[h]

In open-angle glaucoma, actual tests by Roberts, giving diazepam in doses of 5 to 20 mg orally per day to twenty-four glaucomatous patients who were already under standard medical treatment for open-angle glaucoma, produced no statistically significant change in ocular pressure in the course of one and one-half to two years.[m] Aqueous formation as estimated with the perilimbal suction cup method has shown no change in normal human beings given diazepam 4 mg orally per day for three days.[k] Reduction of ocular pressure by 6 mg per day has been claimed in cases of "simple glaucoma."[f] The pressure is lowered in narcoataralgesia.[j] McTigue and Urweider (1969) have reported that in ordinary intravenous use of less than 10 mg the intraocular pressure was unaffected or reduced in sixty-eight out of seventy-two patients, raised less than 4 mm Hg in three patients, and raised 11 mm Hg in one patient with open-angle glaucoma (from 15 to 26 mm Hg).[j]

There appears to be no basis for apprehension over use of diazepam in glaucoma of any sort, since the intraocular pressure is rarely adversely influenced, the pupils are not dilated, and accommodation is unaffected.[c]

In children, in preparation for procedures such as ocular fundus photography, diazepam 4 to 7.2 mg/kg intravenously has induced transient nystagmus, but then has reduced eye movements below normal and has abolished the blink reflex to touching the cornea.[a] Diplopia has also been noted prior to onset of sedation or light sleep in three normal adult volunteers who were given 10 mg rapidly intravenously.[g]

Visual flicker fusion threshold in normal human beings is reduced by diazepam, as by other tranquilizing and sedative drugs.[b]

A unique case of brown discoloration of the lenses in the pupillary areas has been described in a patient who had been taking diazepam for 3 years, but the patient had also been taking phenylephrine eyedrops 1 to 3 times a day for years.[l] The description of the brown homogeneous disc-shaped discoloration in and just beneath the lens capsule seems strongly suggestive of mercurialentis which could have come from a mercurial preservative in the eyedrops. (Whether the drops contained such a preservative was not stated.)

a. Baird HW, Pileggi AJ: Diminished corneal reflex after diazepam. *LANCET* 2:106, 1968.
b. Besser GM, Duncan C: The time course of action of single doses of diazepam, chlorpromazine and some barbiturates. *BR J PHARMACOL* 30:241–248, 1967.
c. Brunette JR, Gaudreault G, Gareau J: Influence of diazepam on the ciliary muscle. *CAN J OPHTHALMOL* 7:358–365, 1972.
d. Campan L, Couadau A, Couadau H: Ocular tonus during narcoataralgesia with diazepam. *ANN ANESTH FRANC* 10:199–204, 1969. (French)
e. Hyams SW, Keroub C: Glaucoma due to diazepam. *AM J PSYCHIATRY* 134:447–448, 1977.
f. Kabayama H, Saito H: Clinical application of Cercine to eye diseases. *JPN J CLIN OPHTHALMOL* 20:1001–1003, 1966.
g. Katz J, Finestone SC, Pappas MT: Circulatory response to tilting after intravenous diazepam in volunteers. *ANESTH ANALG CURR RES* 46:243–246, 1967.

h. Keats S, Morgese A, Nordlund T: Symposium on Diazepam. *WESTERN MED* (Spec. Suppl. 1) 4:22–25, 1963.

i. Lutz EG: Allergic conjunctivitis due to diazepam. *AM J PSYCHIATRY* 132:548, 1975.

j. McTigue JW, Urweider HA: The use of diazepam (Valium) in ophthalmic surgery. *TRANS AM ACAD OPHTHALMOL OTOL* 73:78–84, 1969.

k. Noguchi J: Studies on aqueous dynamics in glaucoma. *JPN J CLIN OPHTHALMOL* 21:215–220, 1967.

l. Pau H: Brown deposits in the lens after administration of diazepam (Valium). *KLIN MONATSBL AUGENHEILKD* 164:446–448, 1974.

m. Roberts W: The use of psychotropic drugs in glaucoma. *DIS NERV SYST* 29Suppl.:40–43, 1968.

n. Withers REE: Personal communication, Sept. 1968.

Diazomethane (azimethylene) is a highly toxic gas which has caused deaths from action on the respiratory system. It is a powerful methylating agent, and like other methylating agents (such as methyl bromide, methyl silicate, and methyl sulfate) is insidious in its poisonous actions, causing no evident reaction at the time of contact, though serious effects may develop several hours later.[170]

On the skin and respiratory mucous membranes diazomethane causes a severe, delayed inflammatory reaction. A splash of concentrated solution in the eye would probably produce serious damage, increasing in severity for several hours or days after exposure. Irritation of the eye from exposure to the gas has developed occasionally among those working with this substance, but so far no serious ocular injuries have been reported.[a, 258]

a. Stokinger HE: Diazomethane, a poisonous laboratory chemical. *OCCUP HEALTH* 13:110–111, 1953.

Diazoxide, a nondiuretic antihypertensive, when given in doses of 200 to 400 mg to thirty patients caused lacrimation in six, persistent but not disabling in four who continued taking the drug.[a] The basis for this peculiar side effect remains to be elucidated.

Extrapyramidal symptoms have developed in some patients, with oculogyric crisis in one case.

Beagle dogs given diazoxide at a dosage 10 to 40 times that used in man have developed hyperglycemia and reversible cataracts.[c, d]

a. Thomson A, Nickerson M, et al: Clinical observations on an antihypertensive chlorothiazide analogue devoid of diuretic activity. *CAN MED ASSOC J* 87:1306–1310, 1962.

b. Neary D, Thurston H, Pohl JEF: Development of extrapyramidal symptoms in hypertensive patients treated with diazoxide. *BR MED J* 3:474–475, 1973.

c. Schiavo DM, Field WE, Vymetal FJ: Cataracts in beagle dogs given diazoxide. *DIABETES* 24:1041–1049, 1975.

d. Schiavo DM: Reversible lenticular aberrations in beagle dogs given diazoxide intravenously. *VET MED SMALL ANIM CLIN* 71:190–195, 1976.

Dibenzepin, an antidepressant, has been mentioned as possibly involved in one case of glaucoma in a woman with shallow anterior chambers.[210] It was not proved to be responsible.

Dibenz[b,f][1,4]oxazepine (CR) is a riot-control agent that causes rapid transient irritation of the eyes, respiratory tract and skin.[b,e] It is more irritant to the eye in aerosol form than in solution, and severalfold more irritant than another widely used agent, o-chlorobenzylidene malononitrile (CS).[c] It causes much less inflammation and damage to the eyes of rabbits than an earlier standard tear gas compound chloroacetophenone (CN) in similar concentrations.[d] Rabbit eyes have been shown to withstand the effect of daily application of a drop of 5% solution in propylene glycol for 4 weeks without significant injury of the cornea.[g] When dissolved in 50% aqueous polyethylene glycol 300, and tested for effect on the intraocular pressure by application to the eye, in rabbits a 0.05% solution caused a 4% rise of pressure, 1% caused 20% rise, and on human eyes 0.05% caused 40% pressure rise in 5 minutes, gone in 15 minutes.[276] Methylated derivatives are less irritating to the eyes.[f]

a. Balfour DJK: Studies on the uptake and metabolism of dibenz(b,f)-1,4-oxazepine (CR) by guinea-pig cornea. *TOXICOLOGY* 9:11–20, 1978.
b. Ballantyne B, et al: The presentation and management of individuals contaminated with solutions of dibenzoxazepine (CR). *MED SCI LAW* 13:265–268, 1973.
c. Ballantyne B, Swanston DW: Irritant effects of dilute solutions of dibenzoxazepine (CR) on the eye and tongue. *ACTA PHARMACOL TOXICOL* 35:412–423, 1974.
d. Ballantyne B, Gazzard MF, et al: Comparative ophthalmic toxicology of 1-chloroacetophenone (CN) and dibenz[b,f]-1,4-oxazepine (CR). *ARCH TOXICOL* 34:183–201, 1975.
e. Ballantyne B, Gall D, Robson DC: Effects on man of drenching with dilute solutions of o-chlorobenzylidene malononitrile (CS) and dibenz(b,f)-1,4-oxazepine. *MED SCI LAW* 16:159–170, 1976.
f. Green DM, Balfour DJK: Effect of methyl substitution on the irritancy of dibenz[b,f]-1,4-oxazepine (CR). *TOXICOLOGY* 12:151–153, 1979.
g. Rengstorff RH, Petrali JP: The effect of the riot control agent dibenz(b,f)1,4 oxazepine (CR) in the rabbit eye. *TOXICOL APPL PHARMACOL* 34:45–48, 1975.

1,2-Dibromo-3-chloropropane (Nemagon), a soil fumigant fungicide, tested on animal eyes both undiluted and as a 1% solution in propylene glycol caused slight pain and signs of irritation that lasted for one to two days, but no damage to the cornea.[a]

a. Torkelson TR, Sadek SE, et al: Toxicologic investigations of 1,2-dibromo-3-chloropropane. TOXICOL APPL PHARMACOL 3:545–559, 1961.

1,2-Dibromoethane (ethylene dibromide) applied as a drop to rabbit eyes has caused only transient corneal epithelial damage.[b] However, three dogs exposed for one to one and one-half hours to the vapors of 1 to 5 cc of 1,2-dibromoethane in 1,000 liters of air developed clouding of the corneas several hours after removal from the exposure chamber. Only one of the dogs survived long enough for the subsequent course to be observed, and in this dog a purulent, presumably infectious, ulceration of one cornea complicated the situation and led to scarring in that eye.[a] Clouding of corneas in these dogs, after a latent period, may be like that induced by *1,2-dichloroethane.*

In men, the vapor is said to be irritating to the upper respiratory tract and eyes, but there appears to have been no instance of corneal opacification in human beings despite lethal poisonings. (Compare *1,2-Dichloroethane.*)

a. Merzbach L: On the pharmacology of methyl bromide and some of its relatives. *Z GES EXP MED* 63:383–392, 1928.
b. Rowe VK, Spencer HC, et al: Toxicity of ethylene dibromide determined on experimental animals. *ARCH IND HYG* 6:158, 1952.

Dibromomannitol (Myelobromol), a substance used in treatment of myelogenous leukemia, has been suspected of causing lens changes in patients.[a] In rats, it has been shown to affect both DNA synthesis and mitosis in the lens epithelium.[b] Administered chronically to rats, it has depleted the population of lens epithelial cells and caused cataract in a manner similar to busulfan.[b]

a. Podos SM, Canellos GP: Lens changes in chronic granulocytic leukemia. Possible relationship to chemotherapy. *AM J OPHTHALMOL* 68:500–504, 1969.
b. von Sallmann L, Grimes P: The cataractogenic effect of dibromomannitol in rats. *INVEST OPHTHALMOL* 9:291–299, 1970.

Dibromomethyl ether (sym) has been listed by Lohs as a potent lacrimator.[155]

Dibutyl oxalate injected subcutaneously in rabbits has produced an appearance in the eye resembling fundus albipunctatus due to accumulations of calcium oxalate in cells of the retinal pigment epithelium, similar to oxalate retinopathy in human beings with high circulating oxalate levels.[a]

a. Caine R, Albert DM, et al: Oxalate retinopathy, an experimental model of flecked retina. *INVEST OPHTHALMOL* 14:359–363, 1975.

Dibutyl phthalate (butyl phthalate) is an oily liquid employed as a plasticizer in plastics. Contact with the surface of human eyes has occurred by accidental droplet splash as well as by experimental application, and this has caused immediate severe stinging pain. The pain stimulated profuse tearing which washed the oily liquid away, and the eyes were not damaged.[81]

Only one case of ocular involvement has been reported from ingestion of dibutyl phthalate,[a] and much skepticism has been expressed about this case.[b] A chemical worker is said to have swallowed 10 g by mistake, with no symptoms until several hours later when he developed a severe transient keratitis in both eyes with loss of corneal epithelium, also a transitory toxic nephritis, characterized by presence of red and white blood cells and many oxalate crystals in the urine.[a] However, the history of ingestion was obtained with difficulty from the patient, and the question has been raised whether one could actually drink dibutyl phthalate by mistake without immediate revulsion, because its taste is so strong and bitter.

Feeding of dibutyl phthalate and other phthalate esters to animals has shown low acute toxicity,[d] with lethal doses in rats ranging from 20 to 30 g/kg after oral administration.[b,c] However, in rats dying within a few days, note has been made of edema of the eyelids and conjunctivitis.[c]

a. Cagianut B: Corneal erosion and toxic nephritis from ingestion of dibutyl phthalate. *SCHWEIZ MED WOCHENSCHR* 84:1243–1244, 1954. (German)

b. Oettel H: Health hazard from synthetic plastics? *NAUNYN-SCHMIEDEBERG'S ARCH EXP PATHOL PHARMAKOL* 232: 77–132, 1957. (German)

c. Radeva M, Dinoeva S: Toxicity of dibutylphthalate by oral application in albino rats. *KHIG ZDRAVEOPAZVANE* 9:510–516, 1966. (*Chem Abstr* 66(12):103632, 1967.)

d. Krauskopf LG: Studies on the toxicity of phthalates via ingestion. *ENVIRON HEALTH PERSPECT* 3:61–72, 1973.

Dibutyl tin dichloride is a liquid which is employed in manufacture of plastics. One instance of eye injury is reported in a worker who accidentally splashed the liquid in his face and eyes. Despite immediate washing with water, lacrimation and conjunctival hyperemia appeared within minutes and persisted for four days. At the end of a week the skin was still erythematous, but the eyes appeared normal.[a] (Also see INDEX for *Tin alkyl compounds.*)

a. Lyle WH: Lesions of the skin in process workers caused by contact with butyl tin compounds. *BR J IND MED* 15:193–196, 1958.

Dichlorisone (Diloderm, Disoderm), a dichloro analog of prednisolone, and closely related 16-α-methyldichlorosone analogs (Sch-5882, Sch-10915) have been administered orally in treatment of alopecia, but posterior subcapsular cataracts have been reported in six out of ten patients treated with these compounds for more than eighteen months.[a] This seems to be analogous to induction of posterior subcapsular opacities by the anti-inflammatory corticosteroids. (See also *Corticosteroids.*)

a. Griboff SI, Futterweit W: Effects of new 9,11-dihalogenated corticosteroids in various types of alopecia. *J MOUNT SINAI HOSP NY* 32:121–129, 1967.

Dichloroacetate, as the sodium or di-isopropylammonium salts, has been investigated as a vasodilator and hypotensive, and for treatment of lactic acidosis.[a] In rabbits an attempt was made to prevent galactose cataracts by administering this compound, but without success.[c] In dogs, chronic oral administration has produced in some animals irreversible lens opacities and superficial corneal vascularization.[d] When administered to normal human beings, it did not alter the ERG, but in patients with retinal vascular disease it is said to have increased the amplitude of the b-wave.[b] In one instance, administration for 16 weeks to a young man with familial hypercholesterolemia was associated with reversible polyneuropathy, but no abnormality of visual fields or changes in the anterior segments.

a. Editorial: Dichloroacetate. *LANCET* 2:456, 1978.

b. Cordella M, Vinciguerra E: Action of diisopropylammonium dichloroacetate on the ERG of normal subjects and of subjects affected by retinal vasculopathy. *ANN OTTALMOL CLIN OCUL* 93:443–452, 1967. (Italian)

c. Cricchi M: On the effect of diisopropylammonium dichloroacetate in the experimental cataract from galactose. *MINERVA OFTALMOL* 5:57–61, 1963.

d. Stacpoole PW, Moore GW, Kornhauser DM: Toxicity of chronic dichloroacetate. *N ENGL J MED* 300:372, 1979.

Dichloroacetylene (dichloroethyne) is a very reactive and explosive liquid of about the same volatility as ether.[d] Dichloroacetylene has long been suspected of being responsible for certain paralyses of the cranial nerves which have been reported from medical and industrial exposure to trichloroethylene under circumstances in which the trichloroethylene may have been impure or subject to decomposition, especially in a series of poisonings from trichloroethylene used in general anesthesia. (Compare *Trichloroethylene.*) So far, no proof has been presented to incriminate dichloroacetylene, but people working with this compound and with lower aliphatic alkylchloroacetylenes are said to have experienced depression and exhaustion, and occasionally to have had disturbances of peripheral nerves with weakness of the legs and disturbances of vision.[d,e]

The possible role of chloroacetylenes might also be considered in an instance reported by Flury in which serious poisoning with injury of the optic nerve, loss of smell and taste, and corneal ulceration occurred during purification of acetylene with calcium hypochlorite and other oxidizing agents.[a]

Experimentally, in 1944 Cox exposed rabbits and rats to vapors containing 0.5% to 1% dichloroacetylene in combination with trichloroethylene, with and without ether, at concentrations sufficient to induce anesthesia. The animals were anesthetized for twenty minutes, three times at five-day intervals. A week later they were killed and examined microscopically. Meningeal reaction with perivascular cuffing, glial proliferation, and foci of necrosis were found, but selective toxicity to cranial nerves was not established.[c]

In 1971 Siegel reported that prolonged exposure to an atmosphere containing 2.8 ppm of dichloroacetylene caused "blindness" in one rat.[h]

Dichloroacetylene has been the prime suspect among a large number of volatile compounds in incidents in which groups of men became ill in a hermetically sealed chamber and in a submarine where very small amounts of chlorinated hydrocarbons in the atmosphere had been exposed to thermal decomposition in a system intended to purify the atmosphere.

Saunders described how a crew of a nuclear submarine was incapacitated by dichloroacetylene which was most likely produced by breakdown of residual traces of trichloroethylene that had been used for cleaning purposes.[f] Analyses of the atmosphere showed trichloroethylene to be present and monochloroacetylene as well as dichloroacetylene. The decomposition of the trichloroethylene was believed to have taken place in an air-purifying system containing the alkalies lithium hydroxide and sodium peroxide as well as a hot catalytic burner. Saunders described the crew as developing nausea progressing to vomiting after three or four days of exposure. Also the men had itching around the eyes, headaches, sore gums, and painful jaws, but no definite trigeminal palsies or disturbances of vision. Particularly interesting, however, they developed "cold sores" after the exposure, reminiscent of several cases of facial herpes that have developed in people poisoned by trichloroethylene decomposition during general anesthesia.

Saunders also pointed out that methylchloroform, or 1,1,1-trichloroethane, another solvent which may be present in adhesives used in construction, could be decomposed by heat in the presence of a catalyst and produce vinylidine chloride and trichloroethylene, both of which can be decomposed to produce monochloroacetylene and dichloroacetylene.

An accidental poisoning of somewhat similar nature has been described by Henschler in 1970 involving the production of monochloroacetylene and dichloro-acetylene as contaminants in the atmosphere of a tank car, affecting several of the cranial nerves, particularly the trigeminal nerves, and the eye muscles of two workers.[b,g] The substances involved in this accident was an aqueous dispersion of polyvinylidenechloride, vinylidene chloride, tetrachloroethane, and trichloroethylene. While the men were cleaning residues from a tank car that had been emptied they noticed irritation of their eyes and upper respiratory tract. Several hours later they developed fatigue, headache, nausea, and vomiting, then a loss of sensation in lips and mucous membranes of the mouth. One of the men developed fifth and sixth nerve palsies affecting the eye muscles. Both men developed herpes of the lips three to five days after the poisoning. They recovered in two to six weeks, except for altered sensation in the distribution of trigeminal nerve persisting for at least four years. There was no mention of alteration of vision in these patients. Chemical investigations established the presence of several chlorinated hydrocarbons which could be decomposed to give monochloroacetylene and dichloroacetylene, and it was supposed that in the cleaning of the tank car with alkalies, the conditions were right for production of the chloroacetylenes, but their presence was not actually proven in this case.[b,g]

More recently, with improved methods of preparing, handling and measuring dichloroacetylene, Reichert has established in rabbits that exposure to this compound severely and selectively affects the sensory trigeminal nucleus, also the facial and oculomotor nerves, and less severely the motor trigeminal nucleus, giving strong support to the earlier hypotheses.[i]

a. Flury F: Modern occupational poisoning in pharmacologic-toxicologic perspective. *NAUNYN-SCHMIEDEBERG'S ARCH EXP PATH PHARMAKOL* 138:65, 1928. (German)

b. Henschler D, Broser F, Hopf HC: "Polyneuritis cranialis" from poisoning with chlorinated acetylenes, from association with vinylidene chloride-copolymers. *ARCH TOXIK* 26:62–75, 1970. (German)

c. Humphrey JH, McClelland M: Cranial nerve palsies with herpes following general anesthesia. *BR MED J* 1:315–318, 1944.

d. Ott E: Concerning dichloroacetylene. III. *CHEM BER* 75:1517–1522, 1942.

e. Ott E, Bossaller W: Concerning dichloroacetylene. VI. Lower aliphatic alkylchloroacetylenes. *CHEM BER* 76B:88–91, 1943. (*Chem Abstr* 37:5014, 1943.)

f. Saunders RA: A new hazard in closed environmental atmospheres. *ARCH ENVIRON HEALTH* 14:380–384, 1967.

g. Broser F, Henschler D, Hopf HC: Chloro-acetylene as cause of an irreversible trigeminal disturbance in two patients. *DTSCH Z NERVENHEILK* 197:163–170, 1970. (German)

h. Siegel J, Jones RA, et al: Effects on experimental animals of acute, repeated and continuous inhalation exposures to dichloroacetylene mixtures. *TOXICOL APPL PHARMACOL* 18:168–174, 1971.

i. Reichert D, Liebaldt G, Henschler D: Neurotoxic effects of dichloroacetylene. *ARCH TOXICOL* 37:23–38, 1976.

o-Dichlorobenzene is somewhat irritating to the skin and when dropped on rabbit eyes causes pain. The conjunctiva becomes hyperemic, but recovery is complete within seven days.[a] The vapors are irritating to the eyes, skin and mucous membranes,[b] but in a survey of industrial experience with this substance at concentrations up to 100 ppm in air no other ill effects were noted than eye and respiratory irritation.[51] There has been no evidence of cataractogenesis, either in human beings or experimental animals.

a. Hollingsworth RL, Rowe VK: Toxicity of o-dichlorobenzene. *ARCH IND HEALTH* 17:180–187, 1958.

b. Riedel H: Some observations on o-dichlorobenzene. *ARCH GEWERBEPATH* 10:546, 1941. (German)

p-Dichlorobenzene (paradichlorobenzene, Paracide, Di-Chloricide) is a white crystalline solid which vaporizes with strong odor at ordinary temperatures. It is a familiar household material used to protect clothing against moths. The vapor has been noted to be painful and irritating to the eyes and nose of human beings at concentrations between 50 and 160 ppm in air.[b] Solid particles cause pain when in contact with the eye, but no serious injury and no noteworthy irritation.[b]

A suspicion that p-dichlorobenzene might be cataractogenic has been based on a single report.[a] According to this report the lenses of a twenty-seven-year-old woman became completely cataractous twelve to fourteen months after an attack of hepatic enlargement, jaundice, and loss of weight which was ascribed to excessive exposure to vapors of "paradichlorobenzene" in her home; the exposure had been discontinued for one year before development of cataracts. In the same report a second woman, aged twenty-five, had monocular, immature, anterior peripheral cortical cataract with a history of jaundice and weight loss six months earlier; it was suspected that she had been poisoned by vapors from two cans of "paradichlorobenzene" which were kept in a closet in which in the previous year the patient spent considerable time sewing.

The same material administered by inhalation to rabbits and guinea pigs caused liver damage, but caused no cataract. However, a single rabbit which was fed 5 g of the material a day for four weeks, until it died, was noted after three weeks to have opacities in each lens and swelling of the cortex of one lens.[a] No information has been presented to establish the identity or purity of the substance involved in these instances of cataract attributed to p-dichlorobenzene.

In no instance have cataracts been reported in animals or human beings after exposure to p-dichlorobenzene which was assuredly pure. Thorough experimental investigations of pure p-dichlorobenzene, utilizing mice, rabbits, monkeys, guinea pigs, and ducks, with exposures to high concentration of vapor and feeding of the material dissolved in olive oil to rabbits (0.5 to 1 g/kg per day for 260 days in a year) has failed in all instances to induce cataracts.[b,c] The feeding experiments caused weakness, tremors, and death, but no abnormalities of optic nerves or retina. However, rabbits exposed repeatedly to 770 to 880 ppm in air for eight hours a day developed transient edema of the cornea, and as much as 3 to 5 diopters of edema of the optic nerveheads, edema of neighboring retina, and congestion of retinal veins, but no hemorrhages or exudates; the eyes returned to normal in seventeen days after discontinuing exposure.[c]

Workmen exposed to p-dichlorobenzene for periods varying from eight months to twenty-five years have developed no abnormalities in their lenses.[b,c] In rare instances of serious poisoning of human beings reviewed in 1955 by von Oettingen, there was no report of retinal disturbance or cataract other than that discussed above.[d]

a. Berliner ML: Cataract following the inhalation of Paradichlorobenzene vapor. *ARCH OPHTHALMOL* 22:1023–1034, 1939.
b. Hollingsworth RL, Rowe VK, et al: Toxicity of Paradichlorobenzene. *ARCH IND HEALTH* 14:138–147, 1956.
c. Pike MH: Ocular pathology due to organic compounds. *J MICHIGAN MED SOC* 43:581–584, 1944.
d. von Oettingen, WF: The Halogenated Hydrogenated Hydrocarbons, Toxicity and Potential Dangers. US Dept Health, Education, and Welfare. Public Health Serv, Pub. No. 414, US Printing Office, Washington, 1955.

Dichlorobutenes (1,4-dichlorobutene-2 and 3,4-dichlorobutene-1) have been sold with the warning that both liquid and vapor are highly dangerous to the skin, eyes, lungs, and internal organs.[a] Protracted contact with the skin causes dermatitis and blistering. High concentrations of vapor apparently have delayed toxic effect on the eyes, causing onset of irritation and lacrimation several hours after the exposure, seeming similar to dimethyl sulfate and other alkylating agents in mode of action. 1,4-Dichlorobutene-2 appears to be the more toxic compound. Surprisingly, test by drop application to rabbit eyes has been reported to cause only moderate injury, graded 5 on a scale of 10 after twenty-four hours.[225]

a. Petro-tex Chemical Corp. Manufacturer's literature, 1968.

Dichlorodifluoromethane (F-12, Freon-12) is a chemically inert and essentially nontoxic gas, widely employed in mechanical refrigerators and as a propellant in pressurized aerosol spray cans. Ordinary occupational and domestic exposure to the gas causes neither ocular nor respiratory irritation. Dogs, monkeys, and guinea pigs exposed to 20% of the gas in air for several hours a day for several days showed temporary intoxication with tremors, ataxia, and associated tendency to stare, salivate and lacrimate, but no cumulative toxic effect and no specific ocular disturbance.[d] However high concentration of the gas can kill by asphyxiation, and if F-12 is decomposed by contact with a flame or very hot filament, it yields products (including hydrogen chloride and hydrogen fluoride) that are very irritating to the eyes and to mucous membranes.[b]

Occasionally liquid or gaseous F12 sprays unexpectedly from a pressurized container or a refrigerator into a person's eyes, but no significant injuries from this source are reported. Because of the speed of reflex closure of the eyes, it seems extremely unlikely that any serious injury would result from an accidental spray of F-12 in the eyes of conscious or unanesthetized human beings. A suggestion was made many years ago that eyes exposed to F-12 be treated with olive oil,[a] but there is no need for this treatment. F-12 is so volatile that nothing is likely to remain after a few seconds except the inert lubricating oil with which it becomes mixed in refrigerators. F-12 does not persist and is not chemically corrosive or caustic. In experimental spraying of the eyes of rabbits, if the spraying is sufficiently brief, less than a second, there is no significant injury.[c,81] With enforced longer exposures the results are different.

When the lids of a rabbit's eye have been held open and a blast of a mixture of liquid F-12 and lubricating oil from a refrigerator has been applied directly to the open eye continuously for a second or two, this has caused momentary freezing of the anterior segment of the eye followed by slight epithelial edema and partial loss of epithelium, but complete recovery in three days. Spraying of rabbit eyes with pure liquified F-12 for five to ten seconds caused damage of the corneal endothelium, shedding in gray sheets from the posterior surface of the cornea, and this led to swelling of the stroma. However, there was gradual recovery so that only a small axial nebula persisted after six weeks. Exposure to the liquid spray continuously for thirty seconds caused much more severe corneal damage, the cornea ultimately becoming opaque and the globe phthisical.[79,81]

A similar type of exposure to liquid F-12 spray has been reported in two patients in whom cataract extraction was being performed. When vitreous was seen protruding from the wound, liquid F-12 was sprayed on the wound to freeze the vitreous so that the sutures could be tied with less slipping. In both cases corneal edema developed, and persisted.[c] Whether this undesirable result was caused by injury from the F-12 or by adhesion of vitreous to the cornea was not established.

In gaseous or vapor form at room temperature or body temperature, F-12 has very little toxicity to the eye inside or outside. A bubble of the gas injected into the anterior chamber of rabbit eyes has not proved damaging to the cornea.[81] Exposure of a rabbit eye to pure F-12 gas at room temperature for one and one-half minutes induced a slight irregularity of the corneal epithelium, but the eye was completely normal the next day.[81]

a. Cordes FC: Emergency treatment of chemical burns of the eye. *POST GRAD MED* 7:45, 1950.

b. Leeuwe H: The possible dangers involved in the use of Freon 12. *AEROMED ACTA* 8:103–125, 1961/2. (*Chem Abstr* 61:9943, 1964.)

c. Miller HA, Perdriel G, et al: Preliminary note on utilisation of refrigerant gas in ocular surgery. *BULL SOC OPHTALMOL FRANCE* 64:358–364, 1964. (French)

d. Sayers RR, Yant WP, et al: Toxicity of Dichlorodifluoromethane: A New Refrigerant. US Bureau of Mines, RI 3013, May, 1930.

Dichlorodinitromethane, according to Browning, causes severe irritation of the eyes, nose, and respiratory tract in man, with potentially severe injurious effect on the lungs.[21] (Compare *Chloropicrin.*)

1,2-Dichloroethane (ethylene dichloride) is a pleasant-smelling, volatile solvent. Acute illness in human beings from inhalation of the vapor and several fatalities from ingestion of the liquid have been reported between 1935 and 1951, but in none of these cases was corneal damage reported. Experimental exposure of the eyes to a high concentration of the vapor or to a drop of the liquid is known, however, to cause immediate discomfort in all species, and hyperemia of the conjunctiva and slight corneal epithelial disturbance may result, but the eyes return to normal within a day or two.[g] Twenty cases of corneal burns have been listed as caused by dichloroethane in workmen, presumably from splashes, but all recovered quickly.[165] On rabbit eyes the reaction to a drop of dichloroethane at twenty-four hours has been graded 3 on a scale of 1 to 10.[27]

Systemic intoxication with 1,2-dichloroethane causes ocular injury in a highly selective manner only in the canine species. In dogs, narcosis induced by inhalation or by subcutaneous injection of 1,2-dichloroethane is followed by striking opacification of the corneas. A similar effect has been observed in one fox, but no such effect is found in rats, mice, rabbits, guinea pigs, hogs, cats, raccoons, chickens, rhesus monkeys, or human beings.[d,e,g] The highly selective toxic effect of 1,2-dichloroethane on canine corneas was first established by DuBois and Roux in 1887,[b] and has since been several times reinvestigated and confirmed.[a,c-h] It appears that the selectivity may be explained simply by difference in amount of dichloroethane that gets into the aqueous humor from the blood circulation in different species, since it has been demonstrated that when dichloroethane is injected directly into the anterior chamber in very small amounts the endothelium is damaged in identical manner in cats and rabbits as well as in dogs.[h] Assays of dichloroethane in the aqueous humor of different species after standard systemic doses remain to be made to test this explanation.

In dogs, investigators have found fairly consistently that in ten to fifteen hours after systemic administration of 1,2-dichloroethane, either by inhalation or subcutaneous injection, both corneas begin to become blue-gray and swollen. Clouding increases to a maximum about two to three days after the intoxication, then subsides in the course of several days to several months, depending on the severity. Ultimately the corneas return to normal. Evacuation of the aqueous humor from the anterior chamber immediately after exposure is said to prevent the swelling and opacification of the cornea.[c,f] After recovery from corneal opacification from 1,2-dichloroethane it has been noted that dogs tend to become resistant to this type of injury on subsequent exposures.

Microscopic studies have shown that the corneal endothelium is injured early, and presumably the cornea becomes edematous secondarily, owing to disturbance of the normal deturgescing mechanism. Pressure with a hard object on the animal's cornea for several minutes results in an area of thinning and transparency, presumably from pressing edema fluid away. The thickening and gray opacity returns within an hour or two. The most careful study of effects on the cornea, utilizing flat preparations for light and electron microscopic examination, has shown in Norwegian elkhounds and mongrel dogs that after a near-lethal dose (0.75 ml/kg subcutaneously) the dogs began to blink frequently in about three hours, and by ten hours had a milky ring of stromal swelling in the periphery of the corneas, extending to involve the whole cornea by fifteen hours.[h] The swelling of the cornea persisted for about two days, then rapidly began to resolve; by the fifth day the corneas became completely clear. In association with these gross changes the corneal endothelium developed vacuoles progressively from periphery toward central zone. The endothelial cells became severely damaged, swollen, loosened, and finally detached from the cornea. Healing of the endothelium began within twenty-four hours with cells sliding like amoebas to cover the denuded posterior surface of Descemet's membrane. By forty-eight hours the endothelium was practically healed. No explanation has been found for the purported resistance of the cornea to repetition of injury by repeated exposures.

Direct injection of 1,2-dichloroethane into the anterior chamber of dogs, cats and rabbits, using a very small dose (about 0.0015 ml for each dog's eye) has produced severe selective damage of the corneal endothelium, just like that resulting from subcutaneous injection of near lethal doses in dogs. No inflammatory reaction has been observed at these doses, but larger doses injected into the anterior chamber have caused a severe nonspecific inflammatory reaction that is not seen after systemic administration, presumably because comparably large systemic doses are too soon lethal.

When enucleated dog eyes have been exposed to 1,2-dichloroethane by soaking in a saline solution of the solvent or by injection into the anterior chamber, in twenty-four hours there is said to be no difference in appearance from eyes soaked in saline alone.[e] This suggests that toxic action of 1,2-dichloroethane on the endothelium involves more than physical effect of a fat solvent on cell structures, presumably a more complex disturbance of biological processes.

Among compounds closely related to 1,2-dichloroethane, only *1,2-dibromoethane* and *1,2-dichloroethylene* appear to have any similar selective toxic effect on canine corneas. (See those compounds for further details.)

Disturbances of optic nerve or retina have been reported in two patients from exposure to mixtures of chlorinated hydrocarbon solvents containing a small proportion (8% to 12%) of 1,2-dichloroethane, but with no evidence to point specifically to 1,2-dichloroethane as the cause.[i,j]

a. Bullot: *SOC BELG OPHTALMOL,* 1896. (French)
b. Dubois and Roux. *CR ACAD SCI (Paris)* 104:1869, 1887. (French)
c. Dubois R: Physiologic action of chlorinated ethylene on the cornea. *CR ACAD SCI (Paris)* 107:482, 1888. (French)
d. Fravelli: *ARCH SCI MED* 16:79, 1892.
e. Heppel LA, Neal KM, et al: Toxicology of dichloroethane. I. Effect on the cornea. *ARCH OPHTHALMOL* 32:391–394, 1944.
f. Panas: *CR ACAD SCI (Paris)* 107:921, 1888. (French)
g. Steindorff K: On the effect of some chlorinated derivatives of methane, ethane and ethylene on the cornea of animal eyes. GRAEFES ARCH OPHTHALMOL 109:252–264, 1922. (German)
h. Kuwabara T, Quevedo AR, Cogan DG: An experimental study of dichloroethane poisoning. *ARCH OPHTHALMOL* 79:321–330, 1968.
i. Lyle DJ, Zavon MR: Blindness in a fur worker. *J OCCUP MED* 3:478–479, 1961.
j. Tabacchi G, Corsico R, Gallenelli R: Retrobulbar neuritis from suspected chronic intoxication by trichloroethylene. *ANN OTTALMOL CLIN OCUL* 92:787–792, 1966. (Italian)

Dichloroethyl acetate is an irritating and moderately vesicant substance. A splash in the eye causes corneal ulceration, and low vapor concentrations produce conjunctivitis and tracheitis.[258]

1,2-Dichlorethylene (acetylene dichloride, Dioform) is a volatile liquid. Some but not all dogs narcotized by inhaling the vapor have been observed to develop delicate

superficial corneal turbidity. The first observation of corneal disturbance was made
on three dogs repeatedly exposed to dichloroethylene by evaporation of 10 to 15 cc
in a chamber of 0.115 cu m volume. Haziness was observed in both corneas of one
dog after the second exposure and slight haziness of one eye of another dog after
fourteen exposures, but no ocular disturbance was found in the third dog.[b] A more
detailed study subsequently showed that the corneal haziness occurring in dogs was
attributable to many fine gray flecks in the endothelium, and that this usually
cleared in twenty-four hours, or forty-eight hours at the most.[c]

One dog narcotized with dichloroethylene vapor with the eyes protected from
direct contact was found to have no gross corneal turbidity. However, slight disturbance of the corneal endothelium and slight stromal edema were found microscopically. Apparently the endothelial changes are induced only by systemic
absorption, and not by a direct irritative or injurious action of the vapor on the
cornea. The effects of 1,2-dichloroethylene on the cornea have been much less than
those observed with 1,2-dichloroethane.

In human beings, 1,2-dichloroethylene has been employed in combination with
ether as a general anesthetic known as Dichloren in at least 2,000 cases, with no
evidence of ocular toxicity.[a] (Compare *1,2-Dichloroethane.*)

   a. Browning E: Toxicity of Industrial Organic Solvents. NEW YORK, CHEM PUB, 1938,
      p. 166.
   b. Joachimoglu G: The pharmacology of trichloroethylene. *BER KLIN WOCHENSCHR*
      58:147, 1921. (German)
   c. Steindorff K: (1922)—see reference under *1,2-Dichloroethane.*

Dichloroethyl ether (bis [2-chloroethyl] ether; β,β'-dichloroethyl ether; sym.
dichloroethylether; Chlorex), employed as a solvent and soil fumigant, its vapor is
irritating to the eyes and respiratory passages. The irritant properties are said to be
sufficient to warn against concentrations which would be poisonous by inhalation.
Irritation is objectionable but not intolerable at 260 ppm in air, and at 550 to 1,000
ppm even brief exposure produces profuse lacrimation and irritation of the nose,
also nausea, making further exposure intolerable.[a,55,188] Similar responses have
been evidenced in animals.

One instance of a burn of a human cornea, possibly from a splash, has been listed
without details.[165] Tests on rabbit eyes by application of a drop have caused mild
transient injury, graded 4 on a scale of 1 to 10 after twenty-four hours.[27,223] (It is
noteworthy that although this compound is the oxygen analog of mustard gas, it
does not possess the high alkylating type of reactivity which is characteristic of
2-chloroethyl sulfides and amines.)

   a. Clinton M: β,β'-Dichloroethyl ether (Chlorex). *AM PETROL INST TOXIC REV,* Mar
      1948.

Dichloroformoxime (dichlorformoxim, phosgenoxim) may be prepared by reduction of chloropicrin. Like chloropicrin it has been reported to be very toxic and to
attack the skin and eyes, causing severe irritation and lacrimation.[a,b,155] Both
dichloroformoxime and monochloroformoxime are said to be very effective tear

gases, and to have caused blindness.[b] Information on the nature or duration of this blindness was not available.[b]

    a. Gryzskiewicz-Trochimowsli, et al: New method for preparation of dichloroformoxime. *BULL SOC CHIM FRANCE* 597–598, 1948. (*Chem Abstr* 42:8165.)

    b. Wiedling S: The relation between the chemical composition of war gases and their physiological action. SVENSKA LAKARTIDN 51:6, 1940. (*Chem Abstr* 35:7575.)

Dichloromethyl ether (sym. chloromethyl ether, bis-chloromethyl ether, dichloro-dimethyl ether) vapor is strongly irritant to the eyes and respiratory tract.[155,171] In one accident in which a workman was sprayed with this substance mixed with aluminum chloride and methylene chloride the eyes and skin were severely irritated, leading to 2nd and 3rd degree burns, corneal opacities, and purportedly atrophy of the optic nerves.[a] Records from the same factory indicated two previous incidents of deep corneal erosion from spraying with dichloromethyl ether.[a] Exposure of rats for 3 minutes to an atmosphere saturated with the vapor caused milky corneal opaciity and narcosis. A 0.05 ml drop on a rabbits eye caused conjunctival erosion and corneal opacity.[a]

    a. Thiess AM, Hey W, Zeller H: On the toxicity of dichlorodimethyl ether. *ZENTRALBL ARB MED ARB SCHUTZ* 23:97, 1973.

2,6-Dichloro-4-nitroaniline (Allosan, Botran, Dichloran), a substance applied to the outside of vegetables and fruit to retard spoilage from mold, has been reported to produce opacities in the cornea beneath the epithelium and at the anterior sutures of the lens in dogs fed 48 mg/kg per day for fifty days.[b] The shiny spots in the cornea seen with a slit-lamp were first interpreted as lipoid deposits, but subsequently appeared to be areas of collagen degeneration.[b] In albino rats no ocular abnormality has been detected histologically after feeding of this compound for two years.[c] There has been no suggestion of toxic effect in human beings.

The opacities induced in the cornea and lens in dogs were irreversible, and according to studies reported in 1970 consisted of "discrete areas of degeneration of the anterior corneal lamellae associated with histiocytes containing lipid granules." In the lens there was edema around the anterior Y suture.[a] It was reported that these effects on cornea and lens could be produced only when the dogs were exposed to sunlight, implicating a phototoxic reaction.[a]

    a. Bernstein HN, Curtis J, et al: Phototoxic corneal and lens opacities in dogs receiving a fungicide, 2,6-dichloro-4-nitroaniline. *ARCH OPHTHALMOL* 83:336, 1970.

    b. Curtis JM, Bernstein H, et al: Corneal and lens opacities in dogs treated with 2,6-dichloro-4-nitroaniline. *TOXICOL APPL PHARMACOL* 12:305, 1968.

    c. Johnston CD, Woodard G, Cronin MT: Safety evaluation of Botran (2,6-dichloro-4-nitroaniline) in laboratory animals. *TOXICOL APPL PHARMACOL* 12:314–315, 1968.

    d. Kuwabara T: Personal communication, 1968.

1,1-Dichloro-1-nitroethane, a fumigant insecticide, has an irritant, lacrimogenic effect which gives adequate warning to prevent dangerous exposure.[181]

2,4-Dichlorophenoxyacetic acid (2,4-D), a herbicide, when administered parenterally to dogs has caused sneezing, lacrimation, and rubbing of the eyes, along with gastrointestinal disturbances.[a] In three human beings, absorption of an unspecified ester of dichlorophenoxyacetic acid through the skin caused polyneuritis, but with no disturbance of the eyes or vision.[b] *Herbatox,* a weed-killer containing both 2,4-dichlorophenoxyacetic and 2,4-dichloropropionic acids, has caused a number of cases of polyneuritis and one case of disturbance of color vision.[c]

   a. Bucher NLR: Effect of 2,4-dichlorophenoxyacetic acid on experimental animals. *PROC SOC EXP BIOL MED* 63:204–205, 1946.
   b. Goldstein NP, Jones PH, Brown JR: Peripheral neuropathy after exposure to an ester of dichlorophenoxyacetic acid. *J AM MED ASSOC* 171:1306–1309, 1959.
   c. Brandt MR: Herbatox poisoning. *UGESKRIFT LAEGER* 133:500–503, 1971. (English abstract)

2,4-Dichlorophenyl-p-nitrophenyl ether (TOK), a herbicide, when given to pregnant mice has an effect on eye development in the offspring that is not evident until sometime after birth. Opening of the eyes is delayed. The eyes may then be twice as large as normal, but, owing to failure of development of the Harderian glands in the orbits, the eyes may actually be sunken in the orbits, the palpebral fissures may be narrowed, and the condition may be misinterpreted as microphthalmia.

   Gray LE Jr, Kavlock RJ, et al: Prenatal exposure to the herbicide 2,4-dichlorophenyl-p-nitrophenyl ether destroys the rodent Harderian gland. *SCIENCE* 215:293–294, 1982.

1,2-Dichloropropane (propylene dichloride) is a volatile solvent. Applied by drop to rabbit corneas it was found moderately injurious.[b]

Human eye injury from a spray of 1,2-dichloropropane occurred when a pipeline burst and sprayed one side of the face of a workman. Smarting of the eye on that side persisted for several hours. The corneal epithelium was damaged in several small areas in the palpebral fissure, but recovery was prompt with no special treatment.

   a. Heppel LA, Neal PA, et al: Toxicology of 1,2-dichloropropane (propylene dichloride) I. Studies on effects of daily inhalations. *J IND HYG* 28:1–8, 1946.
   b. Hine CH, et al: Toxicology and safe handling of CBP-55 (Technical 1-chloro-3-bromopropene-1). *ARCH IND HYG* 7:118–136, 1953.

1,3-Dichloropropene (Telone), a soil fumigant and a component of DD mixture with 1,2-dichloropropene, is highly irritating to skin, eyes, and all mucous membranes, according to information quoted from a manufacturer.[70,171]

$\alpha\alpha$**-Dichlorotoluene** (benzal chloride) is a liquid which has a pungent odor, fumes in moist air, and reacts with water to release hydrochloric acid. The vapors are irritating to the eyes.[171]

Dichlorphenamide (diclofenamide, Daranide, Oratrol), a carbonic anhydrase inhibitor and diuretic employed to reduce intraocular pressure, has side effects similar to those of acetazolamide, causing reversible paresthesia of hands and face, anorexia and loss of weight in some patients. Excretion of citrate in the urine is reported to be suppressed by this drug, as by acetazolamide, and this presumably facilitates formation of urinary calcium stones.[a]

Acute transient myopia, like that occasionally produced by acetazolamide and many other drugs, has been reported in one young woman who had the interesting combination of aphakia plus glaucoma in one eye, but in her other eye the lens was present and that eye had no glaucoma. She had received acetazolamide for ten days without complication, but two days after acetazolamide was stopped and dichlorphenamide was given, she developed acute myopia of $-5D$ in the normal eye with the lens present, no change in the aphakic eye. The myopia was not relieved by homatropine, but gradually disappeared in five days after the dichlorphenamide was stopped.[b] Considered with observations on the same phenomenon induced by other drugs, this case suggests that change in the lens was responsible for the myopia, though it was not due to a parasympathetically induced cyclotonia. (See also *Myopia, acute transient.*)

a. Constant MA, Becker B: The effect of carbonic anhydrase inhibitors on urinary excretion of citrate by humans. *AM J OPHTHALMOL* 49:929–941, 1960.

b. Neuschuler R. Transitory myopia in the course of treatment with dichlorphenamide. *BOLL OCULIST* 43:507–513, 1964. (Italian)

2,6-Dichlorthiobenzamide (Chlorthiamide, Prefix), a herbicide, has been tested on the skin and eyes and reported nonirritant.[a]

a. Brown VKH, Chambers PK: Toxicological studies with the herbicide 2,6-dichlorthiobenzamide (Chlorthiamide "Prefix"). *ARCH TOXIK* 23:42–51, 1967. (*Excerpta Med* (Sect. 2C), 21:806, 1968.)

Dichromates (bichromates) as ammonium, sodium, or potassium salts are watersoluble crystalline substances which have a peculiar injurious effect on the cornea, causing great swelling of the corneal stroma. This type of injury has been reported in a patient who had one eye contaminated with *potassium dichromate.*[b] A soft, transparent bulging of the lower half of the cornea developed, with opacity along the upper edge of the bulge. The cornea gradually returned to normal shape, but much irregular astigmatism and anesthesia of the affected area persisted.

Experimentally this was reproduced in a rabbit eye by applying a crystal of potassium dichromate to a small area on the cornea for two minutes. This was followed in the course of the next several days by striking local thickening of the stroma, with forward bulging of the anterior surface, but only slight discoloration or turbidity. The endothelium appeared granular in the affected area, but the epithelium remained essentially normal. In the course of three weeks the cornea returned to normal except for slight granularity and grayness of the posterior surface by slit-lamp biomicroscope.[81]

Sodium dichromate tested in 0.08 M solution by injection into the corneal stroma or by application to the corneas of rabbits after removal of the epithelium has been reported to produce a rather severe reaction, graded 70 on a scale of 1 to 100.[123]

A solution of *sodium chromate* of the same concentration was found to produce injury of equal severity.[123] Crystals of sodium chromate applied for two and one-half minutes to the intact cornea caused localized endothelial injury and blue stromal edema similar to that produced by the dichromate, but of relatively slight degree, with no gross bulging of the cornea.[81]

Chromic chloride crystals applied in the same manner also failed to cause the forward bulging of essentially clear cornea caused by dichromate; instead a permanent gray vascularized opacity resulted.[81]

Crystals of reduced *chrome alum* (Koreon M and X) caused only a transient injury of the epithelium.[81]

In treatment of eyes contaminated with dichromate it has been suggested that application of vitamin C and EDTA might be beneficial, in analogy to the treatment of potassium permanganate, but this apparently has not been evaluated.[a] (Compare *Chromic acid,* and *Chromium compounds.*)

a. Pitter J, Vyhamek J: The treatment of eye injuries from potassium permanganate crystals. *KLIN MONATSBL AUGENHEILKD* 133:265–267, 1958.
b. Thomson WE: Vesication of cornea by potassium bichromate. *OPHTHALMOSCOPE* 1:214–216, 1903.

Dicloxacillin, a penicillin-type antibacterial, was injected subconjunctivally in rabbits in a dose of 50 mg, resulting in very slight local reaction according to one report,[a] but according to another report causing opacification of the cornea, sloughing of the epithelium, and necrosis of the conjunctiva.[b] In the second report, the authors mentioned that they had also observed severe corneal and conjunctival reactions in dogs and cats, but gave details only on rabbits.[b]

a. Records RE: Intraocular penetration of dicloxacillin in experimental animals. *INVEST OPHTHALMOL* 7:663–667, 1968.
b. Kobetz LE, Bussanich MN, Rootman J: Toxic effects of subconjunctival dicloxacillin. *CAN J OPHTHALMOL* 13:206–209, 1978.

Dicumarol (dicoumarol, dicoumarin, bishydroxycoumarin), an anticoagulant, in overdosage may produce hemorrhages in various tissues. Hemorrhage occurring posteriorly in the eye has been known to cause loss of vision.[a,b] Possibly a similar disturbance has been produced by warfarin. (See *Warfarin* for further information.)

a. Klingensmith W, Oles P: Surgical complications of dicumarol therapy. *AM J SURG* 108:640–644, 1964.
b. Feman SS, et al: Intraocular hemorrhage and blindness associated with systemic anticoagulation. *J AM MED ASSOC* 220:1354–1355, 1972.

Dicyclomine (dicycloverine, Atumin, Bentyl), an anticholinergic antispasmodic used in gastrointestinal disorders, has been tested in normal and glaucomatous patients for mydriatic effect and for influence on ocular pressure when administered systemically in usual doses. Pupil size has been reported to be unaffected.[b,e] This drug has been taken orally by patients known to be subject to angle-closure glaucoma without adverse effect on the pupil or ocular pressure.[a,b,81] However, some patients who have taken this drug without difficulty in the presence of angle-closure glaucoma have been under topical miotic treatment at the same time, and in some evaluations of this drug in patients with chronic glaucoma the type of glaucoma has not been clearly described. There is one report that when patients under treatment for glaucoma of unspecified type were given 10 mg of dicyclomine hydrochloride orally, they had a rise of 3 to 10 mm Hg for two to three hours.[f] In most cases no rise in ocular pressure has been found, regardless of the type of glaucoma.[c,d] In nonglaucomatous patients the ocular pressure has not been elevated.[c] (See also *Anticholinergic drugs.*)

a. Brown DW, Guilbert GD: Acute glaucoma in patient with peptic ulcer. *AM J OPHTHALMOL* 36:1735–1736, 1953.
b. Chalfin JE: Effect of dicyclomine hydrochloride on narrow-angle glaucoma. *NY J MED* 67:917–920, 1967.
c. Cholst M, Goodstein S, Berens C: Glaucoma in medical practice, danger of use of systemic antispasmodic drugs in patients predisposed to or having glaucoma. *J AM MED ASSOC* 166:1276–1280, 1958.
d. Hufford AR: Bentyl hydrochloride: successful administration of a parasympatholytic antispasmodic in glaucoma patients. *AM J DIG DIS* 19:257–258, 1952.
e. McHardy G, Brown DC: Clinical appraisal of gastrointestinal antispasmodics. *SOUTHERN MED J* 45:1139–1144, 1952.
f. Mody MV, Keeney AH: Propantheline (Pro-Banthine) bromide in relation to normal and glaucomatous eyes: effects on intraocular tension and pupillary size. *J AM MED ASSOC* 159:1113–1114, 1955.

Dieffenbachia plants (Dumb cane) are ornamental house plants (of the *Araceae* family) with stems which contain a juice that is very irritating to the eyes. Dieffenbachia plants also have been long known to irritate the skin on contact, and, when pieces of the stem are chewed or eaten, they cause great irritation of the mouth and throat, temporarily disabling the vocal cords, wherefrom came the common name Dumb cane.[b,c]

Reports on people who have suffered from a squirt of the juice in the eye provide a fairly uniform picture.[e-h] Usually the victim had the juice accidentally squirted in one eye when the stalk of the plant was cut, broken, or squeezed. Immediately there was pain, burning sensation, tearing, blepharospasm and photophobia. The conjunctiva became moderately hyperemic. Injury to the corneal epithelium varied from punctate to extensive, with different degrees of edema, but in each case in which slit-lamp biomicroscopy was performed numerous fine needle-like crystals called raphides, were seen in the conjunctiva and cornea. Usually by the next day these were seen at all levels in the cornea, as far back as Descemet's membrane, but not in the anterior chamber. Regularly the epithelium healed and the raphides gradually disappeared. A decrease in number was noticeable in a few days, but some persisted for 3 to 8 weeks. In one case, iritis was present during the first several days, but cleared while the raphides were still present.[e] Usually patients have become comfortable when the epithelium healed, despite continued presence of raphides in the cornea, and in all reported cases the eyes have returned completely to normal.

The composition and properties of the juice have received much attention. The raphides are present suspended in the juice, and having the same appearance as in the conjunctiva and cornea.[h] They are said to be calcium oxalate crystals, and at one time were thought to be responsible for the toxic properties of the juice. However, experimental work in animals has shown this not to be so.

In rabbits several investigators have reproduced the acute keratoconjunctivitis seen in human beings.[a,d,f,g,i] They have determined that a more severe reaction is induced by juice from *D. picta* than from *D. exotica*,[a,d] that less reaction is produced by juice from leaf stems,[f] and that juice pressed from the stalk is required to produce the complete picture with intracorneal raphides.[f] The juice produces equally severe reactions whether it is filtered to remove the raphides, or is applied whole.[f] It becomes less irritating if treated with trypsin,[d] and non-irritating if allowed to stand at room temperature for 24 hours.[a,d] Tests of calcium oxalate, sodium oxalate, and oxalic acid have produced no reaction like that from the plant juice.[a,d,f,81]

These observations indicate that the toxic properties of Dieffenbachia juice are not attributable to the calcium oxalate raphides, but probably to some type of protein.[a-f,i] One report of faster healing in rabbits treated topically with EDTA was based on the aim of solubilizing the raphides, but other mechanisms of action of EDTA are possible.[g]

In general, symptomatic treatment of patients has led to complete recovery.

a. Manno JE, Fochtman FW, et al: Toxicity of plants of the genus Dieffenbachia. *TOXICOL APPL PHARMACOL* 12:405 (abstr. 73), 1967.
b. Pohl RW: Poisoning by Dieffenbachia. *J AM MED ASSOC* 177:812–813, 1961.
c. Pohl RW: Dieffenbachia poisoning: a clarification. *J AM MED ASSOC* 187:963, 1964.
d. Fochtman FW, Manno JE, et al: Toxicity of the genus Dieffenbachia. *TOXICOL APPL PHARMACOL* 15:38–45, 1969.
e. Egerer I: Eye disturbance by the juice of the ornamental Dieffenbachia plant. *KLIN MONATSBL AUGENHEILKD* 170:128–130, 1977. (German)
f. Ellis W, Barfort P, Mastman GJ: Keratoconjunctivitis with corneal crystals caused by the Dieffenbachia plant. *AM J OPHTHALMOL* 76:143–147, 1973.
g. Riede B: Eye injury caused by the juice of the plant Dieffenbachia seguine. *DTSCH GESUNDH WES* 26:73–76, 1971. (German)
h. Roggenkamper P: Keratopathy caused by plant juice. *KLIN MONATSBL AUGENHEILKD* 164:421–423, 1974. (German)
i. Occhion P, Rizzini CT: Cited by Pohl[b,c] and Ellis.[f]

Dieldrin is an insecticide which has caused numerous cases of chronic poisoning in workers who have sprayed the compound for several months. Characteristically there is headache, dizziness, and involuntary muscular movements. In severe cases there are epileptic convulsions with loss of consciousness. The only ocular disturbance so far noted in human beings has been "blurred vision" of undetermined cause, and nystagmus accompanying incoordination and tremor.[c] Experimental feeding of dieldrin to rabbits at 60 to 110 mg/kg weekly for twelve weeks caused convulsions and apparent "blindness". The nature of this "blindness" has not been determined.[a] In mice, retinal photorecpetor electrical responses have been disturbed by 20 mg intraperitoneally.[290]

One case is reported of dense central scotomas 20° in diameter in both eyes with slight congestion of the nerveheads, in a man who had prolonged and recent intensive exposure to a proprietary mixture containing dieldrin, pentachlorophenol, and possibly other unidentified substances in a wood preservative spray.[d] Deterioration of vision occurred during two weeks and did not recover in spite of corticosteroid treatment. Medical and neurological studies were negative. Whether dieldrin itself was responsible could not be proved. A review and discussion of instances of dieldrin poisoning suggest that if dieldrin has serious effects on vision in human beings, this must be rare.[b,e]

a. Bundren J, Howell DE, Heller VG: Absorption and toxicity of dieldrin. *PROC SOC EXP BIOL MED* 79:236, 1952.
b. Committee on Toxicology: Occupational dieldrin poisoning. *J AM MED ASSOC* 172:2077–2080, 1960.
c. Hayes WJ: Dieldrin poisoning in man. *US Public Health Rep* 72:1087–1091, 1957.
d. Jindal HR: Bilateral retrobulbar neuritis due to insecticides. *POSTGRAD MED J* 44:341–342, 1968.
e. Zavon MR: Dieldrin intoxication. *J AM MED ASSOC* 173:1160, 1960.

Diepoxybutane (erythritol anhydride, butadiene diepoxide), has been tested on rabbit eyes. Application of the liquid causes severe injury, graded 9 on a scale of 1 to 10.[226] Exposure to vapor at 3 to 12 ppm in air for four hours is also very injurious, causing loosening and sloughing of the rabbit's corneal epithelium and opacification of the corneal stroma, with permanent scarring and vascularization, but no interference with subsequent regeneration of the epithelium.[114,173] Partial clearing of the cornea has occurred several days after exposure.[114]

Diethanolamine is a strongly basic solid, liquefying readily on contact with moist air. Applied to the rabbit cornea, the liquid may cause moderate injury, graded 5 on a scale of 1 to 10 after twenty-four hours,[27] but if the liquid is washed off with water within a few minutes, the injury is slight and the eyes return to normal within twenty-four hours.[81]

Diethylamine is a strongly alkaline liquid which is severely damaging to rabbit eyes when applied as a drop, causing injury graded 10 on a scale of 1 to 10 after twenty-four hours.[225] Chronic exposure to the vapors at concentrations as low as 50 ppm in air causes conjunctival and pulmonary irritation in rabbits; corneal erosion develops after two weeks of exposure.[a]

People working in an atmosphere containing vapors of amines in plastic manufacturing sometimes develop blue hazy vision at the end of the workday, due generally to a subtle temporary disturbance of the corneal epithelium. Diethylamine is said to be one of the amines that can produce this effect.[c]

a. Brieger H, Hodes WA: Toxic effects of exposure to vapors of aliphatic amines. *ARCH IND HYG OCCUP MED* 3:287–291, 1951.
b. Peyresblanques J: Corneal burn by diethylamine with an endothelial lesion. *BULL SOC OPHTALMOL FRANCE* 731–732, 1963.
c. Munn A: Health hazards in the chemical industry. *TRANS SOC OCCUP MED* 17:8–14, 1967.

3-β-(β-Diethylaminoethoxy) androst-5-en-17-one-methoxime hydrochloride, a steroid which reduces cholesterol in the circulation, has produced cataracts in weanling rats when added to the diet.[75] Experimental investigation has shown a lowering of gamma-crystallin which could be caused by reduction of protein synthesis, and it has been postulated that this is a selective block secondary to alterations of intracellular sodium and potassium.[a]

  a. Cenedella RJ, Bierkamper GG: Mechanism of cataract production by 3-β(2-diethyl-aminoethoxy) androst-5-en-17-one hydrochloride, U18666A: An inhibitor of cholesterol biosynthesis. *EXP EYE RES* 28:673–688, 1979.

4,4'-Diethylaminoethoxyhexestrol administered orally to rats induced storage of lipids in the retina affecting mainly neurons and Mueller cells.[304]

Diethylcarbamazine (Carbamazine, Hetrazan) an antifilarial used mainly in treatment of onchocerciasis, appears to have very low toxicity to uninfected people and no particular toxicity to the eye, but when given orally or transepidermally to people who have onchocerciasis, it may cause severe reactions due to destruction of the microfilariae in the tissues. The reaction in the eye may include appearance of fluffy punctate corneal opacities, anterior uveitis, optic nerve involvement with constriction of visual fields and optic atrophy, and chorioretinal changes. These reactions that are precipitated by the treatment are said to represent the same types of changes which occur at a slow rate in the absence of treatment, and generally have not been attributed to toxic effects of the drug itself on the eye.[a,c,f] Use of corticosteroids and anticholinergic eyedrops may reduce the inflammation, but if the reaction is excessive, the use of diethylcarbamazine may have to be interrupted.

Flubendazole, a newer drug, is reported to kill the microfilariae more slowly, but to cause much less adverse effects in the eyes.[d]

Possible use of diethylcarbamazine in eyedrops for treatment of ocular onchocerciasis has been explored. There has been no toxicologic problem in providing a suitable preparation, well tolerated and providing good penetration of the drug into the eye, but the fundamental problem of reactions to killed organisms was not solved in that way.[b,e]

  a. Anderson J, Fuglsang H: Further studies on the treatment of ocular onchocerciasis with diethylcarbamazine and suramin. *BR J OPHTHALMOL* 62:450–457, 1978.
  b. Ben-Sira I, Aviel E, et al: Topical Hetrazan in the treatment of ocular onchocerciasis. *AM J OPHTHALMOL* 70:741–743, 1970.
  c. Bird AC, El Sheikh H, et al: Changes in visual function and in the posterior segment of the eye during treatment of onchocerciasis with diethylcarbamazine citrate. *BR J OPHTHALMOL* 64:191–200, 1980.
  d. Dominguez-Vazquez A, Taylor RH, et al: Comparison of flubendazole and diethylcarbamazine in treatment of onchocerciasis. *LANCET* 1:139–143, 1983.
  e. Jones BR, Anderson J, Fuglsang H: Effects of various concentrations of diethylcarbamazine citrate applied as eye drops in ocular onchocerciasis. *BR J OPHTHALMOL* 62:428–439, 1978.
  f. Taylor HR, Green BM: Ocular changes with oral and transepidermal diethylcarbamazine therapy of onchocerciasis. *BR J OPHTHALMOL* 65:494–502, 1981.

Diethyl diglycolate as a vapor in air is said to give no warning of irritation and causes no immediate lacrimation, but induces corneal epithelial edema which fogs the vision until spontaneous recovery in twenty-four to forty-eight hours.[a] The dimethyl ester has been reported to have the same effects on the eyes as does the diethyl ester.[a]

> a. Fleming AJ: Chemical health hazards. In Fleming; d'Alonzo; Zapp (Eds.): *Modern Occupational Medicine*, Philadelphia, Lea & Febiger, 1954, p. 324.

Diethyldithiocarbamate sodium (Dithiocarb), a chelating agent for metals, with therapeutic uses in metal poisoning, has been tested on rabbit corneas at 0.01 to 0.05 M concentrations by injection or application to the denuded surface and was found nontoxic.[123] Administered systemically, it is reported to have caused detachment of the retina in dogs, but no damage to the retina in monkeys.[a] In albino rats and beagle dogs, it caused no impairment of vision or structural alteration in the eye after administration daily for ninety days.[c]

A comprehensive review of the pharmacologic properties and therapeutic uses of diethyldithiocarbamate has been published, with eighty-one references.[b]

Diethyldithiocarbamate does not appear to be suitable for treatment of corneal injuries by copper salts. In experimental treatment of a rabbit eye immediately after exposure of bare corneal stroma to *copper nitrate*, it did not prevent opacification, and it caused discoloration of the cornea from precipitation of an insoluble copper compound.[81]

> a. Scholler J, Brown D, Timmens E: Toxicology and pathology of diethyldithiocarbamate. *PHARMACOLOGIST* 3:62, 1961.
> b. Sunderman FW Jr: Diethyldithiocarbamate therapy of thallotoxicosis. *AM J MED SCI* 253:209–220, 1967.
> c. Sunderman FW, Paynter OE, George RB: The effects of the protracted administration of the chelating agent, sodium diethyldithiocarbamate. *AM J MED SCI* 254:24–34, 1967.

Diethylene glycol tested by application of a drop to rabbit corneas is found not injurious, and tests on excised beef corneas have shown that it does not alter the adhesion of epithelium to stroma.[27,107]

Diethylene glycol monoalkoxymethyl ethers (Efirans) of various compositions have been tested by application to eyes of rabbits, and some have been found to be local anesthetics on the cornea, without affecting the pupil, without causing irritation or injury to the surface of the eye, and without raising the intraocular pressure.[a]

> a. Tagdisi DG, Safarov RI, et al: Effect of new anesthetics, alkoxymethyl monoethers of diethylene glycol on the cornea. *DOKL ADAK NAUK SSSR* 24:56–59, 1968. (*Chem Abstr* 70:2194, 1969.)

Diethylene glycol monoethyl ether (Carbitol) is a solvent of low volatility. The liquid is moderately irritating to the eye, but on brief exposure causes no permanent damage.[27] When applied to the eyes of cats, it causes immediate tearing and vigorous rubbing of the eyes, whereas in rabbits the response is less vigorous and the material appears to remain longer in the conjunctival sac. Cats exhibit only slight conjunctival reddening for a day or two, whereas rabbits have been known occasionally to develop conjunctivitis with discharge, iritis, and temporary corneal opacification, with return to normal in a week or two.[b] The response in human eyes may be expected to resemble that in cats.[27]

Dissolved in physiologic salt solution and tested on rabbit eyes, Carbitol was less irritating than glycerol similarly tested. At 30% concentration, Carbitol caused only mild conjunctival vasodilation, no damage.[a]

a. Cranch AG, Smyth HF, Carpenter CP: External contact with monoethylether of diethylene glycol (Carbitol Solvent). *ARCH DERM SYPH* 45:553–559, 1942.
b. Walther R: On the toxicology of the glycols. *ARCH GEWERBEHYG* 11:326–344, 1942.

Diethyleneglycol monoethyl ether acetate ester (Carbitol acetate) has the same effect on rabbit eyes as Carbitol.[3]

Diethylenetriamine (DETA) is a strongly alkaline liquid, having a strong odor of ammonia. It is a potent primary skin irritant, causing edema and sometimes necrosis. The skin irritation is frequently complicated by a high incidence of allergic skin sensitization. The majority of workers chronically exposed to it become sensitized.[a] The liquid is caustic to the eyes. Tests on rabbits have yielded results varying from moderate injury, graded 5 to 8 on a scale of 1 to 10, to severe injury of the degree caused by ammonium hydroxide.[b,27,222,224] Even when diluted to 15% in water it has damaged rabbit corneas severely.[b] The injury caused by a single splash without complications of sensitization appears to be attributable to the highly alkaline character of the material, rather than to some other innate toxicity.

DETA in 0.2 M aqueous solution neutralized with hydrochloric acid has no toxic effect on rabbit corneas although applied for ten minutes to the bare stroma after mechanical removal of the epithelium.[81]

DETA at 1% concentration in water, adjusted with boric acid to between pH 7.2 and 8.5, has been used as an irrigating fluid on the surface of eyes of rabbits, causing no irritation or injury, and is said to be effective as a neutralizing solution in treatment of experimental burns of rabbit eyes with sulfuric acid and hydrochloric acid if started within fifteen minutes after exposure to the acid.[c] In treatment of forty-five patients with burns of the eye from contact with inorganic acids, organic acids, phenols, and aldehydes, this same solution is said to have been helpful if used within ten to fifteen minutes. Some benefit has been claimed even when used within ninety minutes.[d,e] What local side effect this treatment may produce in patients who are allergic or hypersensitive to DETA remains to be seen.

a. Ingberman AL, Pott CF: Low toxicity epoxy "Couplers." *CHEM ENG NEWS* 4815, Oct 1, 1956.
b. Savitt LE: Contact dermatitis encountered in the production of epoxy resins. *ARCH DERM SYPH* 71:212–213, 1955.
c. Krejci L, Obenberg J, et al: Experiences with a new neutralising agent DETA in acid burns of the eye. *CS OFTAL* 20:314–320, 1964. (*ZENTRALBL GES OPHTHALMOL* 95: 84, 1965.)

d. Krejci L: A new neutralizing agent diethylenetriamin (DETA) in the treatment of acid burns of the eye. *CS OFTAL* 23:283–287, 1967.

e. Krejci L, Jansa J: Diethylenetriamine as first aid in eye burns due to phenol and aldehydes. *CS OFTAL* 24: 132–134, 1968. (*Excerpta Med* (Sect. 12), 22:2423, 1968.)

Diethylethanolamine is a strongly alkaline liquid which has the same severity of injurious effect on rabbit eyes as ammonium hydroxide,[222] judged at twenty-four hours.

Diethylpropion (2-diethylaminopropiophenone, Tenuate), an appetite depressant, increases the critical flicker fusion frequency in normal human subjects within three hours after ingestion of 25 mg, similar to other CNS stimulants.[219] Tests of 25 and 50 mg of diethylpropion hydrochloride orally in a young normal patient with active pupils had no detectable effect on the size of the pupils.

1,3-Diethylthiourea has been used as an inhibitor in sulfamic acid scaling solution and as an accelerator in manufacture of synthetic rubber. While it appears to have had no known special toxic effects itself, it has been present in two different episodes of severe superficial keratitis in workmen. In one episode, in manufacture of synthetic rubber, thirty-two patients developed pain, photophobia, and blurring of vision associated with punctate epithelial erosions after working in the presence of a blowing agent known as Genitron C.R. and diethylthiourea.[h] It was postulated that decomposition by heat led to the release of ethyl isothiocyanate and ethylamine. Ethyl isothiocyanate in the air was suspected of being responsible for the eye injuries, but no information was provided on concentrations of any of the substances in the air, nor any information on duration of exposure or time to development of keratitis.

In the other episode of keratitis, which is described in more detail under *sulfamic acid,* men who were exposed to the atmosphere of a large cupronickel evaporator which had been treated with a solution of sulfamic acid containing a small amount of diethylthiourea as an inhibitor developed painful, slow-healing superficial keratitis several hours after exposure. Whether diethylthiourea or its decomposition products could have been responsible was not certain in this episode either. There seems to be no evidence to prove that ethyl isothiocyanate was responsible in either case, though ethyl isothiocyanate is known to be directly irritating to the eye, both as a liquid and as vapor, but whether it can produce delayed, severe superficial keratitis as in the above episodes seems not actually to have been demonstrated.

Diethylthiourea has been shown to be a potent skin sensitizer,[b] but whether this has any relationship to the possible keratitis remains to be determined.

a. Groves JS, Smail JM: Outbreak of superficial keratitis in rubber workers. *BR J OPHTHALMOL* 53:683–687, 1969.

b. White WG, Vickers HR: Diethyl thiourea as cause for dermatitis in car factory. *BR J IND MED* 27:167–169, 1970.

N,N-Diethyl-m-toluamide (Deet, m-Delphene, Detamide, Dieltamid, Flypel, Meta-Delphene, Off) is a liquid insect repellent for application to the skin.[171] Application of pure N,N-diethyl-m-toluamide to rabbit eyes has caused edema of the conjunctiva, lacrimation, discharge, and slight transient cloudiness of the corneas. Injury of the epithelium, indicated by staining with fluorescein, persisted for two days, but the eyes returned to normal in five days.[a] Tests on rabbit eyes by applying a 10% solution in cottonseed oil caused no irritation or discomfort.[b]

One patient who was accidentally sprayed in the eye with Off had immediate smarting sensation which subsided rapidly when he flushed his eye with water. Two hours later the only abnormality was fine gray stippling of the corneal epithlium with tiny gray dots in the palpebral fissure. Vision at that time was reduced from 20/15 to 20/20. The eye returned rapidly to normal.[81]

a. Ambrose AM, Huffman DK, Salamon RT: Pharmacologic and toxicologic studies on N,N-diethyltoluamide. *TOXICOL APPL PHARMACOL* 1:97–115, 1959.
b. Ambrose AM, Yost DH: Pharmacologic and toxicologic studies of N,N-diethyltoluamide. *TOXICOL APPL PHARMACOL* 7: 772–780, 1965.

Difluoro (methylphosphonic difluoride), an intermediate in manufacture of Sarin, in vapor form is extremely irritating to eyes and respiratory tract, resembling hydrogen fluoride, so that people are likely to escape as quickly as possible from threatening concentrations. Monkeys exposed to the vapor showed great distress and kept their eyes closed. However, dogs, though showing similar distress, developed corneal opacity as a result of forced exposure for thirty minutes.[a]

a. Crook JW, Musselman NP, et al: Acute inhalation toxicity of Difluoro vapor in mice, rats, dogs, and monkeys. *TOXICOL APPL PHARMACOL* 15:131–135, 1969.

Digitalis (foxglove, dried leaves of *Digitalis purpurea*) contains digitoxin, digitonin, and digitalin. It has long been employed in treatment of heart failure. Digitalis has been known since the eighteenth century to induce a variety of reversible disturbances of vision. Several derivatives of digitalis and certain pharmacologically related drugs from other sources have similar effects, but among these drugs there are differences enough to make it worthwhile to describe each separately. The description given here is limited to the effects of digitalis itself. The properties of several related drugs are described elsewhere under the separate headings, *Acetyl digitoxin, Digitonin, Digoxin, Lanatoside-C, Ouabain,* and *Strophanthin.* Properties that appear to be common to the whole group are summarized under the title *Cardiac glycosides.*

The earliest descriptions of visual symptoms were reviewed with particular detail and historical interest by Sprague, White, and Kellogg in 1925, adding the symptoms reported by their own patients, but without reporting measurements of the vision or examination of the eyes.[k] The commonest visual complaints from excessive dosage of digitalis have been described many times and in much detail.[b,e,f,h,k,l,n,o,q]

Visual side effects from digitalis include flickering, dazzling, color illusions, reduction of visual acuity, and most rarely temporary blindness. In all cases, return to normal is expected when digitalis is discontinued or the dosage reduced. Patients experiencing visual side effects typically sense shimmering or flickering of light, and may observe that light-colored objects outdoors appear dazzling as though covered with snow. They may see blue-colored borders on objects, or general yellow, orange, or green coloration.

While the glare phenomenon and disturbance of color vision have become most familiar associated with digitalis intoxication, a relatively small but impressive number of cases of reversible reduction of visual acuity have been reported.[a,c,e,f,h,i,m,n,p] In most instances the more common flickering, snow, or disturbances of color vision have been noted before or in association with the reduction of visual acuity. In the most carefully examined patients the reduced visual acuity has been shown to be in the form of bilateral central scotomas. Formerly, there was a tendency to consider that disturbances of color vision probably originated from toxic effect on the cerebral cortex, and that reduction of central vision and central scotomas were probably due to retrobulbar neuritis,[c,f,m,p] but since neither optic neuritis nor optic atrophy has been seen after digitalis intoxication, there has been no sound basis for placing a suspected lesion in the optic nerve, and evidence has been presented particularly by Robertson, Hollenhorst, and Callahan, indicating that it is much more likely that central scotomas are due to actions of digitalis on the receptor cells of the retina.[h,i] They have comprehensively reviewed the literature on the ocular aspects of action of digitalis, and have demonstrated experimentally in normal people that standard dosage of digitalis or digitoxin given for two or four weeks produced a reversible elevation of the dark adaptation threshold in an area $5°$ from fixation. Cone function was affected more than rod function. These reversible functional changes were demonstrable in the absence of any of the ordinary visual symptoms of excessive digitalis dosage. These authors have suspected that a high incidence of visual functional disturbance would be demonstrable in patients being treated with digitalis if tests of sufficient sensitivity were made. Studies on other cardiac glycosides have also added to the evidence pointing to the retina as the probable prime site of action of drugs in this category when they affect vision. (See *Cardiac glycosides*.) However, it is still quite possible that digitalis may also affect vision at higher levels and in central nervous system.

A correlation of distinct reduction of the ERG with bilateral reduced visual acuity, relative central scotomas, and impaired discrimination of colors has been reported in a patient taking digitalis, but without other signs of toxicity.[g] When digitalis was stopped, the ERG, visual acuity, fields and color vision returned to normal within weeks, strongly suggesting that the retina had been the site of toxic action.

Complete temporary blindness was said by Lewin and Guillery to have been known prior to 1913 in numerous cases of digitalis poisoning.[153] The pupils were said sometimes to have been paralyzed and dilated. Blindness was described as lasting as long as three days, but then vision regularly returned to normal. In more recent literature there appears only one case of sudden total blindness related to digitalis glycosides. (This is described under *Digoxin*.)

Increase in size of the pupils has been noted also in less severe digitalis intoxication,[a,d] and has been pointed out as particularly conspicuous in children who have been accidentally poisoned by digitalis.[d]

Diplopia and ptosis have been mentioned as rare and atypical side effects of digitalis, but their occurrence may have been coincidental.[f] Such may have been the case in a patient with monocular ptosis and paresis of the superior rectus in association with hypertensive retinopathy, plus visual side effects from digitalis.j

Inhibition of NaK-ATPase, suppression of formation of aqueous humor, reduction of intraocular pressure, and injurious effects on the cornea have been reported from several glycosides derived from or related to digitalis. (A summary of these effects is given under *Cardiac glycosides.*)

a. Carapancea M: Neuropsychic-ophthalmologic manifestations and mechanisms in digitalis poisoning. *REV OTONEUROOPHTALMOL* 39:433–440, 1967. (French)
b. Carroll F: Visual symptoms caused by digitalis. *AM J OPHTHALMOL* 28:373–376, 1945.
c. Frandsen E: Visual manifestations of digitalis poisoning; two cases of toxic amblyopia. *ACTA MED SCAND* 157:51–59, 1957.
d. Freeman R, Farrar JF, Robertson SEJ: Accidental digitalis poisoning in childhood. *MED J AUST* 2:655, 1961.
e. Gerra V: Contribution to study of the neurophthalmic syndrome of digitalis poisoning. *MINERVA OFTAL* 7:156–160, 1965. (Italian)
f. Gillette DF: Visual disturbances due to digitalis. *TRANS AM OPHTHALMOL SOC* 44:156–164, 1946.
g. Babel J, Stangos N: Retinal intoxication by digitalis. *BULL SOC BELGE OPHTALMOL* 160:558–566, 1972. (French)
h. Robertson DM, Hollenhorst RW, Callahan JA: Ocular manifestations of digitalis toxicity. *ARCH OPHTHALMOL* 76:640–645, 1966.
i. Robertson DM, Hollenhorst RW, Callahan JA: Receptor function in digitalis therapy. *ARCH OPHTHALMOL* 76:852–857, 1966.
j. Ross JVM: Visual disturbances due to the use of digitalis and similar preparations. *AM J OPHTHALMOL* 33:1438–1439, 1950.
k. Sprague HB, White PD, Kellogg JF: Disturbances of vision due to digitalis. *J AM MED ASSOC* 85:716–720, 1925.
l. Strzyzewski K: Disturbance of color vision as a side effect of digitalis. *KLIN OCZNA* 32:45–48, 1962.
m. Sykowski P: Retrobulbar optic neuritis. Case reports. *AM J OPHTHALMOL* 36:976–978, 1953.
n. Turtz CA: Visual toxic symptoms from digitalis. *AM J OPHTHALMOL* 38:400–401, 1954.
o. Ungar L: Chromatopsia from digitalis. *OPHTHALMOLOGICA* 136:326–332, 1958. (German)
p. Wagener HP, Smith HL, Nickeson RW: Retrobulbar neuritis and complete heart block caused by digitalis poisoning: report of a case. *ARCH OPHTHALMOL* 36:478–483, 1946.
q. White PD: An important toxic effect of digitalis overdosage on the vision. *N ENGL J MED* 272:904–906, 1965.

Digitonin (digitin) is a substance extracted from the seeds of *Digitalis purpurea* and employed principally as a chemical reagent in determination of certain steroids, including cholesterol.[171] In contact with the eye, powdered digitonin causes much irritation. Dusted on a guinea pig eye, it caused blepharospasm, chemosis, erosion of the corneal epithelium, and much blue-gray swelling of the corneal stroma, reaching its maximum in two or three days.[81] Commercial digitonin is a mixture containing 5% to 15% saponins in addition to digitonin, and it has not been determined to which of the components the local damaging effect is attributable.

Digitoxin (crystallin digitalin) is a glycoside extracted from digitalis and employed medically for the same purposes as digitalis, but having more rapid onset and shorter duration of action. It has reversible effects on vision, such as have long been familiar in association with the parent digitalis, consisting of illusions of flickering or shimmering lights, appearance as of snow on objects outdoors or in bright light, and disturbances of color vision, particularly causing yellow or green appearance of objects.[a,b,d] Digitoxin also can reduce visual acuity reversibly. This has variously been reported with and without central scotomas and has been attributed variously to effects on the central nervous system, the optic nerve, and the retina. Formerly, there was a tendency to assume a diagnosis of retrobulbar neuritis in patients having central scotomas, but more recent evidences indicate that the retina is more likely the principal site of toxic action.

The following are examples of reports on effects of digitoxin on visual acuity. In one patient vision decreased to 20/100 in each eye during four weeks of digitoxin medication, and pericentral scotomas were found. The patient has no chromatopsia, but the visual impairment appeared to relate to the dosage, and vision returned to 20/25 in the ninth week when the drug was stopped for three days. Sluggishness of pupillary response to light paralleled visual impairment, but ophthalmoscopy was negative. The patient was assumed to have toxic retrobulbar neuritis.[1] Another patient who was assumed to have bilateral retrobulbar neuritis from digitoxin had vision of 1/15 and 1/10 after taking 0.3 mg per day for two months.[k] Visual disturbances disappeared in one week after the digitoxin was discontinued. No evidence was presented to establish the anatomic site of toxic affect on vision. Two cases were presented by Robertson, Hollenhorst, and Callahan with description of bilateral central scotomas and an opinion that these were caused by action of digitoxin on the retinal receptor cells rather than on the optic nerve.[i] The same authors showed experimentally in one normal human volunteer that ordinary dosage of digitoxin elevated the dark adaptation threshold in a manner indicative of a disturbance of cone function.[i] Similarly, color vision measurements and evaluation of dark adaptation curves by Gibson in a patient who saw objects as though covered by frost, and lights with a yellow hue, indicated that digitoxin influenced the red-sensitive color vision system most readily, and made it seem probable that digitoxin had a selective effect probably localized within the retina rather than the optic nerve.[c]

More recently, Grutzner described a patient who had been receiving excessive doses of digitoxin for six weeks, "nearly went blind" within a few days, and complained of an appearance of yellowish flickering light. The patient was found to have normal fundi, but central scotomas and abnormal color vision characterized as an advanced tritan defect. When the digitoxin was discontinued, the visual acuity, visual fields, and color vision all improved rapidly. The optic nerveheads appeared normal at all times, and the author interpreted the findings as indicating that digitoxin more likely caused disturbance of the retina rather than of the optic nerve.[95]

Evidence of action on the retina after systemic administration has been obtained also from tests on guinea pigs, demonstrating by ERG measurements that under the influence of repeated sublethal daily doses of digitoxin the responsiveness of the retina to different portions of the spectrum is altered and that this effect is reversible when administration of digitoxin is discontinued.[e]

Evidences have been obtained not only from observations on digitoxin, but also from studies on digitalis and other cardiac glycosides, increasingly pointing to the receptor cells of the retina, rather than the optic nerve, as the primary site of action of this whole category of drugs. This is summarized separately under the heading *Cardiac glycosides.*

Apart from the visual effects, digitoxin has been suspected of causing monolateral paresis of the superior oblique muscle in two patients. These patients had no other indication of drug toxicity. In both patients the muscle action slowly improved when the drug was stopped, and in one the paresis became worse when the drug was given again.[j]

Inhibition of NaK-ATPase, interference with formation of aqueous humor, reduction of intraocular pressure, and injurious effect when applied to the cornea have been noted in varying degree with different digitalis derivatives and related drugs. (These general effects are summarized under *Cardiac glycosides.*) For digitoxin itself administered systemically there have been varying reports regarding influence on intraocular pressure in glaucoma in human beings, none reporting adverse effect, some describing a reduction of pressure,[g,h] and some finding no reduction.[f,g] Digitoxin applied in eyedrops or ointment in sufficient concentration to reduce intraocular pressure unfortunately tends to cause corneal edema and clouding in human eyes, though apparently not in rabbit eyes.[g]

Digitoxin has been tested by application to the eye, in search for a topical preparation to reduce ocular pressure through inhibition of NaK-ATPase in the secretory epithelium of the ciliary processes. A solution of 0.2 mg/ml of 49% ethyl alcohol was tolerated by rabbit eyes when applied twice a day for several days, but in one human eye it caused severe corneal edema within a day. This preparation also produced corneal edema in dogs' eyes. All corneas returned to normal. The intraocular pressure was reduced 4 to 5 mm Hg during the reaction of the corneas.[220]

a. Cozijnsen M, Pinckers AJLG: Ophthalmological aspects of digitoxin intoxication. *NEDERL T GENEESK* 113:1735–1737, 1969.

b. Gelfand ML: Visual symptoms after digitoxin therapy. *J AM MED ASSOC* 147:1231–1233, 1951.

c. Gibson HC, Smith DM, Alpern M: Specificity in digitoxin toxicity. *ARCH OPHTHAL-MOL* 74:154–158, 1965.

d. Lely AH, van Enter CHJ: Large scale digitoxin intoxication. *BR MED J* 3:737–740, 1970.

e. Muller-Limmroth W, Dimakos C: An electroretinographic contribution to the interpretation of the cornflower phenomenon in digitalis poisoning. *ARZNEIMITTELFORSCHUNG* 20:286–291, 1966. (German)

f. Peczon JD: Clinical evaluation of digitalization in glaucoma. *ARCH OPHTHALMOL* 71:500–504, 1964.

g. Pilz A (1967, 1968)—see references under *Digoxin.*

h. Radzik M (1967)—see reference under *Lanatoside-C.*

i. Robertson DM, Hollenhorst RW, Callahan JA (1966)—see references under *Digitalis.*

j. Ross JVM (1950)—see reference under *Digitalis.*

k. Schliak H, Fischer G, Ruiz-Torres G: Picture of a bilateral retrobulbar optic neuritis associated with digitalis overdosage. *DTSCH MED WOCHENSCHR* 92:973–977, 1967.

l. Sykowski P: Digitoxin intoxication resulting in retrobulbar optic neuritis. *AM J OPHTHALMOL* 32:572–574, 1949.

Diglycidyl ether (bis [2,3-epoxypropyl] ether) is a liquid which causes severe but reversible corneal injury in rabbits when applied as a drop. It is also very irritating to the skin. Its vapors cause eye and respiratory irritation which provide sufficient warning to prevent dangerous industrial exposures. However, rats subjected to high vapor concentrations developed corneal opacities.[115] Rabbits exposed to 20 to 27 ppm of diglycidyl ether in air for four hours showed complete loosening of the corneal epithelium from the stroma, but the epithelium subsequently regenerated normally.[173]

Diglycidyl resorcinol and **Epon 562** are epoxy compounds encountered industrially in the manufacture of epoxy resins. They are highly irritating to the eyes of animals, and instances of eye irritation in workers have been noticed.[a]

a. Hine CH, Kodama JK, et al: Toxicology of epoxy resins. *ARCH IND HEALTH* 17: 129–143, 1958.

Digoxin (Lanoxin), a cardiotonic drug used for the same purposes as digitalis and digitoxin, has become widely used only in recent years, so there has been much less time than in the case of digitalis to accumulate experience with side effects on vision and the eyes. However, this is building, and shows that there is much resemblance to the effects of the other cardiac glycosides. The clinical aspects have been reviewed in 1981 by Duncker.[c] Cases of bilateral central and paracentral scotomas, disturbed color vision, and abnormal ERG have been reported by Robertson, Moore and Weleber.[g,l,m] In each case when the drug was stopped, or dosage reduced, vision and ERG returned to normal. A systematic study by Rietbrock and Alken in 1980 showed that nearly 80% of patients receiving digoxin had a generalized disturbance of color vision, although most patients were unaware of visual disturbance.[k] Digoxin was shown to have a greater tendency to impair color vision than digitoxin or pengitoxin.[h]

Cortical blindness has been reported in one case while digoxin was being used, but the relationship seems questionable; more likely anoxia or cerebrovascular insufficiency in this moribund patient was responsible.[d]

In experimental study of possible site of toxic effect of digitalis glycosides in the eye, a tritiated radioactive form of digoxin as well as unlabeled digoxin, have been utilized to determine the distribution of the drug after it was administered parenterally to cats, dogs, and rats. The retina accumulated much greater concentrations than other tissues examined, contrasting particularly with the optic nerve and brain, which showed no selective uptake.[a,b,e,f] In rats the concentration in the retina, especially in the ganglion cell layer was 50 times that in the brain and 20 times that in the optic nerves.[e] This has been taken as additional indication that the retina is the most likely anatomical site of the toxic actions of cardiac glycosides that cause visual disturbances.

Evidence of action on the retina from systemically administered digoxin has also

been obtained from tests on guinea pigs, demonstrating changes in the ERG measurements in response to stimulation by different parts of the spectrum both acutely
after doses which were lethal in about an hour and after repeated sublethal daily
doses.[h]

Inhibition of NaK-ATPase, interference with formation of aqueous humor, reduction of intraocular pressure, and injurious effects on the cornea have been reported
from digoxin as well as from glycosides derived from digitalis and related drugs.
(These effects are summarized under *Cardiac glycosides.*)

Attempts to use digoxin in eyedrops or ointment to reduce intraocular pressure
have shown that pressure can be reduced in this way, but in human beings the
concentration required (25 mg/100 ml) when applied three times a day caused
injury of the cornea consisting of epithelial edema, swelling of the corneal stroma,
and wrinkling of Descemet's membrane, all of which were reversible when the
medication was discontinued.[i,j]

The effects of drugs related to digoxin are described individually elsewhere and
are summarized under *Cardiac glycosides.*

a. Babel J, Stangos N: Retinal intoxication by digitalis. *BULL SOC BELGE OPHTALMOL*
    160:558–566,
b. Binnion PF, Frazer G: [^{3}H] Digoxin in the optic tract in digoxin intoxication. *J
    CARDIOVASC PHARMACOL* 2:699–706, 1980.
c. Duncker G: Digitalis side effects on the eye. *KLIN MONATSBL AUGENHEILKD*
    178:397–398, 1981.
d. Gelfand ML: Total blindness due to digitalis toxicity. *N ENGL J MED* 254:1181–1182,
    1956.
e. Lissner W, Greenlee JE, et al: Localization of tritiated digoxin in the rat eye. *AM J
    OPHTHALMOL* 72:608–614, 1971.
f. Lufkin MW, Harrison CE JR, et al: Ocular distribution of digoxin-^{3}H in the cat. *AM J
    OPHTHALMOL* 64:1134–1140, 1967.
g. Moore CE, Gilliland JM: Central scotomas due to digoxin toxicity. *AUST J OPHTHAL-
    MOL* 1:76–79, 1973.
h. Muller-Limmeroth W, Dimakos C:—see reference under *Digitoxin.*
i. Pilz A: Pressure-reducing action of digoxin in glaucoma. *KLIN MONATSBL AUGEN-
    HEILKD* 151:492–500, 1967. (German)
j. Pilz A: Basis and possibilities of cardiac glycoside treatment in the eye. *NOVA ACTA
    LEOPOLDINA* 183:1–103, 1968. (German)
k. Ritebrock N, Alken RG: Color vision deficiencies: a common sign of intoxication in
    chronically digoxin-treated patients. *J CARDIOVASC PHARMACOL* 2:93, 1980.
l. Robertson DM, Hollenhorst RW, Callahan JA:—see references under *Digitalis.* 1972.
m. Weleber RG, Shults WT: Digoxin retinal toxicity. *ARCH OPHTHALMOL* 99:1568–1572,
    1981.
n. Haustein KO, Oltmanns G, et al: Differences in color vision impairment caused by
    digoxin, digitoxin, or pengitoxin. J *CARDIOVASC PHARMACOL* 4:536–541, 1982.

1,2-Dihydro-1,2-dihydroxynaphthalene has been found to cause damage to the
retina in rabbits after intravenous injection of 100 mg per day for three days. The
damage appeared to be the same as that produced by feeding naphthalene, but no
abnormalities were produced in the lenses. Application as 1% eyedrops to rabbits

every half hour throughout the day for two to five days did cause biomicroscopically visible abnormalities in the lenses of three out of four animals.[a] This compound has been found to be present in the blood of rabbits fed naphthalene.

a. van Heyningen R, Pirie A: The metabolism of naphthalene and its toxic effect on the eye. *BIOCHEM J* 102:842–852, 1967.

Dihydroergotamine mesylate (DHE-45), an antiadrenergic used in vascular headaches, has been administered many times to patients with migraine or glaucoma with no significant effects on intraocular pressure and no adverse effect on vision or visual fields.[a-d] A noteworthy review (19 references) by Garcia-Gomez lists uses that have been made of dihydroergotamine in treatment of the eye, reporting no adverse side effects except some irritation, hyperemia, and exudate after topical application.[b] However, a case of overdosage (3.5 mg in one day) by a young person with severe headache was followed by occlusion of a branch of a retinal artery.[e] This was considered to be due to vascular spasm. (See also *Ergotamine tartrate* regarding similar side effect.)

a. Carreras M: The post traumatic constriction of retinal arterioles. *ARCH SOC OFTAL HISP-AM* 24:379–399, 1964.
b. Garcia-Gomez S: The use of dihydroergotamine in ophthalmology from its semisynthesis in 1943 to today. *ARCH SOC OFTAL HISP-AM* 25:661–665, 1965.
c. Martin M: Contribution to the use of dihydroergotamine in the treatment of glaucoma. *ARCH SOC OFTAL HISP-AM* 25:139–144, 1965.
d. Persichetti C: Dihydroergotamine (DHE-45) in ophthalmic migraine and glaucoma. *BOLL OCULIST* 29:234–250, 1950.
e. Hanselmayer H, Werner W: Retinal artery spasm after oral overdosage of DHE medication. *KLIN MONATSBL AUGENHEILKD* 162:807–811, 1973. (German)

Dihydrostreptomycin, an antimicrobial known to be toxic to the cochlear branch of the eighth nerve, has been observed to produce green-blindness in patients after daily doses of 1 g for six days or more, regardless of the patient's previous type of color vision. The effect has been reversible.[a] (Compare *Streptomycin.*)

a. Laroche J: Modification of color vision in man under the influence of certain medicinal substances. *ANN PHARMACOL FRANC* 23:313–315, 1965. (*ANN OCULIST* (Paris) 200:275–286, 1967.)

Dihydrotachysterol (AT 10), a substance which raises blood calcium, appears not to have had toxic effect on normal eyes but has been found to promote calcification of the cornea in rabbits and rats when the epithelium has been removed from the corneas experimentally,[a] and after the cornea was made edematous in rabbits by irrigating the anterior chamber with potassium permanganate.

a. Obenberger J, Ocumpaugh DE, Cubberly MG: Experimental corneal calcification in animals treated with dihydrotachysterol. *INVEST OPHTHALMOL* 8:467–474, 1969.
b. Obenberger J, et al: Experimental corneal calcification. *OPHTHALMIC RES* 1:175–192, 1970; 3:174–182, 1972.

Dihydroxyacetone has been widely employed in cosmetic preparations to create a synthetic suntan of the skin. Testing on rabbits eyes by applying 50 mg of the powder to the surface of the cornea under local anesthesia caused no injury to cornea or conjunctiva.[81]

2,3-Dihydroxynaphthalene tested by injection into rabbit cornea in 0.05 M aqueous solution caused moderately severe reaction.[123]

Diisopropenylacetylene and **monoisopropenylacetylene** are irritants of the eyes, skin, and respiratory tract. When tested by application to the eye of rabbits, they are said to have been irritating and damaging, but the eyes recovered and healed without corneal opacity.[a]

    a. Feinsilver L, Rothbert S, et al: Toxicology of mono- and diisopropenylacetylene. *US DEPT COM OFFIC TECH SERV PB REPT* 147:683, 1960. (*Chem Abstr* 55: 25037, 1961.)

Diisopropylamine is a strongly alkaline liquid having an irritating ammonia-like odor. Inhalation may cause nausea and pulmonary edema.[171] Temporary impairment of vision has occurred in men after exposure to vapor concentrations possibly as low as 25 to 50 ppm in air.[a,51] (See also *Amines* for possible similar effects from related compounds.)

Experimental exposures of rabbits, guinea pigs, rats, and cats have established that the vapor is injurious to the corneal epithelium; this presumably is the cause of the visual disturbances observed in men. Exposure of experimental animals to vapor concentrations from 260 to 2,200 ppm in air for several hours causes clouding of the cornea from epithelial injury and stromal swelling.[a] The highest concentrations were lethal in many instances, owing to severe pulmonary damage, but the corneas of surviving animals ultimately returned to normal.

Splash of liquid diisopropylamine in the eye would be potentially serious, as indicated by injury graded 8 on a scale of 1 to 10 in tests in rabbit eyes.[226]

    a. Treon JF, Sigmon H, et al: The physiological response of animals to respiratory exposure to the vapors of diisopropylamine. *J IND HYG* 31:142–145, 1949.

Diisopropylglycerol ether tested by drop application to rabbit eyes caused no serious injury.[116]

Dimercaprol (BAL; 2,3-dimercaptopropanol) as a result of systematic, scientific investigation was selected as a suitable agent for counteracting the effects of lewisite on the eye. Dimercaprol has since proved effective in relieving systemic poisoning from a variety of arsenical compounds, and experimentally has been effective as antidote to certain of the heavy metals. Dimercaprol has most commonly been available for medical use in the form of a 10% solution in a mixture of 20% benzylbenzoate and 80% peanut oil. When administered by intramuscular injection to human beings at a dose of 8 mg/kg, it produces severe burning sensation in the eyes, with tearing, blepharospasm, and conjunctival edema. This may be accompanied by salivation and vomiting.[a] The same ocular reactions can be induced by rubbing 1 ml into the forearm in human beings,[d] and can be induced in animals by giving toxic amounts parenterally.[e] A satisfactory explanation for this effect is yet to be found.

Contact of the same commercial preparation with the human eye causes very severe, persistent stinging sensation, blepharospasm, lacrimation, and photophobia for an hour or two, but no damage to the eye.[c,81] Similarly, several drops applied to the rabbit eye cause prolonged blepharospasm, but no damage.[81] Introduced into the anterior chamber of rabbit eyes a 1% solution of pure dimercaprol in water causes severe iritis, corneal infiltration, vascularization, and permanent scarring. A 0.125% solution, however, is tolerated without significant injury.[b]

   a. Dimercaprol. Council on pharmacy and chemistry. *J AM MED ASSOC* 131:824, 1946.
   b. Newell FW: Effect of BAL (2,3-dimercaptopropanol) on intraocular copper. *AM J OPHTHALMOL* 32:161–167, (part II) 1949.
   c. Scherling SS, Blondis RR: The effect of chemical warfare agents on the human eye. *MILIT SURG* 96:70–78, 1945.
   d. Peters RA, Stocken LA, Thompson RH: British anti-lewisite (BAL). *NATURE* 156:616–619, 1945.
   e. Waters LL, Stock C: BAL (British Anti-Lewisite). *SCIENCE* 102:601–606, 1945.

Dimethoate, an anticholinesterase insecticide, is said not to be an irritant to skin or eyes.[70] In one instance of a splash of an insecticide liquid containing both dimethoate and carbaryl into the eyes no serious damage developed, only transient injury of the corneal epithelium, accompanied by much swelling of the lids, but this all cleared rapidly.[a]

In the manufacture of dimethoate, by-products that cause severe eye irritation have been identified, mainly *bis (dimethoxythiophosphoryl) disulfide,* which in rabbits produced opacity of the cornea, inflammatory reaction and edema in conjunctiva and lids.[b]

   a. Haley, Warren: Personal communication, 1968.
   b. Wenzel KD, Dedek W: Isolation and identification of eye-irritating by-products of dimethoate synthesis. *Z CHEM* 11:461–462, 1971.

2,5-Dimethoxy-4-methyl-amphetamine (4-methyl-2,5-dimethoxy-α-methylphenethylamine; STP; "Speed"), a hallucinogenic drug, produces visual imagery and dilates the pupils when taken systemically.[b] It is related chemically to mescaline and to amphetamine, and has effects similar to LSD. (See also *Hallucinogens.*)

In cats an accumulation of this drug has been found in the visual pathways, and the suggestion has been made that this might explain the mechanism of visual hallucinations in man.[a]

Although this drug dilates the pupil in human beings, it has been found to cause strong constriction of the pupils in cats, whether given intravenously or topically.[a]

   a. Idanpaan-Heikkila JE, McIsaac WM, et al: Relation of pharmacological and behavioral effects of a hallucinogenic amphetamine to distribution in cat brain. *SCIENCE* 164:1085–1087, 1969.
   b. Snyder SH, Faillace L: 2,5-Dimethoxy-4-methyl- amphetamine (STP) a new hallucinogenic drug. *SCIENCE* 158:669–670, 1967.

Dimethylamine forms very alkaline solutions in water. A 5% solution dropped once on a rabbit eye caused hemorrhages in the conjunctiva, corneal edema, and superficial opacities. It is not reported whether these were permanent.[63] A drop of undiluted dimethylamine placed on a rabbit's cornea, with the lids then closed and no irrigation performed, caused the cornea to become whitish blue and translucent within a few seconds, then white as the sclera in a minute, a very severe injury.[170]

Munn reported seeing cases of temporary mistiness of vision after industrial exposure to dimethylamine vapor, the same as from a number of other amines.[363] (See INDEX for *Amines.*)

Dimethylamineborane is one of the boranes which has been employed in high energy rocket fuels. Test of a 10% aqueous solution by application of a drop to a rabbit's eye caused tearing, hyperemia, and edema, but the eye improved in forty-eight hours and returned to normal in eleven days.

   a.   Roush G Jr: The toxicology of the boranes. *J OCCUP MED* 1:46–51, 1959.

3-Dimethylaminopropylamine vapor has caused corneal disturbance and blurred vision. Workers exposed to concentrations thought to be about 30 ppm in air noted during several days that vision became blurred toward the end of the work day, sometimes with appearance of haloes around lights, pain, photophobia, and headache, usually better by the next day. The complaints apparently were due to a disturbance of the corneal epithelium similar to that caused by vapors of certain other amines. In three workers who had symptoms persisting two to three days after exposure, the corneal epithelium was seen to be edematous, but no other ocular abnormalities were observed.[a]

Liquid 3-dimethylaminopropylamine has been tested on rabbit eyes and found to cause severe injury, graded 9 on a scale of 10. A 1:100 aqueous solution at pH 12 also caused severe alkali-type corneal injury in rabbits, but a 1:100,000 solution at pH 7.6 caused almost no injury.[a] Whether alkalinity or some more subtle property is responsible for the toxic effect of the vapor on human corneas remains to be determined. (See INDEX for *Amines.*)

   a.   Spaeth GL, Leopold IH: Ocular toxicity of dimethyl-aminopropylamine. *AM J OPHTHALMOL* 57:632–639, 1964.

4-(p-Dimethylaminostyryl) quinoline (4M20; NSC-4236; NCS-10482), a radiomimetic drug, is cataractogenic in mice, causing lens opacities first detectable eighty-seven days after a single intravenous injection of 0.1 mg/kg.[a] Morphologically the cataracts become indistinguishable from radiation-induced cataracts, but they tend to start at the anterior pole of the lens rather than at the posterior. This compound is reported to be significantly more cataractogenic than busulfan, chlormethine, or tretamine.[a]

   a.   Christenberry KW, Conklin JW, et al: Induction of cataracts in mice by 4-(p-dimethyl-aminostyryl) quinoline. *ARCH OPHTHALMOL* 70:250–252, 1963.

N,N-Dimethylformamide is in widespread use as a solvent. Tested by drop application to rabbit eyes, a 25% solution in water had no effect; 50% solution was slightly irritant; 75% to 100% produced a more severe reaction, but no details of the reaction were reported.[a] A drop of pure dimethylformamide applied to rabbit eyes, followed two minutes later by brief irrigation with water, caused only edema of the corneal epithelium, and the eyes returned to normal within a day or two.[81]

    a. Massmann W: Toxicological investigations on dimethylformamide. *BR J IND MED* 13:51–54, 1957.

Dimethylhydrazine exists as 1,1-dimethylhydrazine (unsymmetrical dimethylhydrazine, UDMH), and 1,2-dimethylhydrazine. Both are fuming, strongly alkaline, moderately volatile liquids having ammoniacal odor. They are highly corrosive and irritating to skin, eyes, and mucous membranes.[171] UDMH has been used in large amounts in rocket fuels, with reportedly only mild irritation of skin and eyes from exposure to small amounts of vapor escaping in this application.[a] However, when UDMH was applied to dogs over a large area of the chest it was absorbed, passed into the aqueous humor, and caused opacity of the corneas.[b]

    a. Boysen JA: Health hazards of selected rocket propellants. *ARCH ENVIRON HEALTH* 7:71–75, 1963.
    b. Smith EB, Castaneda FA: Effect of UDMH (unsymmetrical dimethylhydrazine) on blood coagulation, the blood-aqueous barrier, and the cornea. *AEROSP MED* 41:1240–1243, 1970.

Dimethyl phosphorochloridothionate (DMPCT) industrial exposure has caused superficial punctate lesions of the corneas after a latent period of at least 8 hours in 6 people, but all healed completely.[a]

    a. Hartz WP, Swencicki RE: Keratitis on exposure to dimethyl phosphorochloridothionate (DMPCT). *J OCCUP MED* 17:335–336, 1975.

Dimethyl phthalate (DMP) is employed as an insect repellent for application to the skin.[171] Contact with the eye produces considerable pain, but causes either no damage, or only slight reversible disturbance of the epithelium.[a,27,46,165]

    a. Kuchle 1958—reference under *Peroxides, organic.*

Dimethyl sulfate (methyl sulfate) is a colorless, oily liquid, sufficiently volatile at room temperature to produce poisonous concentrations of vapor. Dimethyl sulfate is widely used as a methylating agent in chemical manufacture, and has been used as a war gas. Both the liquid and the vapor are extremely injurious. After exposure, an asymptomatic latent period is most characteristic before the appearance of signs and symptoms of burns of the skin and eyes and systemic poisoning. In this respect, dimethyl sulfate resembles mustard gas.

On the skin, the liquid may cause no immediate discomfort, but results several hours later in a burning and itching sensation with redness followed by severe blistering and necrosis. Similarly, a drop of pure dimethyl sulfate splashed in the eye causes no immediate discomfort. However, if slightly hydrolyzed from contact with water and thereby contaminated with sulfuric acid, it does cause immediate pain and gray-white opacification. A burn of the eye by liquid dimethyl sulfate under these conditions is a combination of immediate acid-type burn and delayed severe denaturation and necrosis from methylation. The lids become extremely swollen, the anterior chamber may fill with exudate, and the cornea may become almost completely necrotic.[153]

Cases in which the eye has been immediately irrigated with water after splashing with liquid dimethyl sulfate have had a severe reaction beginning in several hours but have been known to recover completely.[81] Testing of the liquid on rabbit corneas has produced an injury graded 8 on a scale of 1 to 10 after twenty-four hours, but if the subsequent course were taken into consideration, it would probably be given a worse score.[27,225]

Injury of the eye by vapor of dimethyl sulfate is a much more common industrial accident than injury by a splash of liquid, which is more easily prevented by goggles. Numerous instances of burns and poisoning from the vapor have been described.[a-d, g-i, q, 46, 61, 153, 253] Also in animal eyes the effects of the vapor have several times been studied and reproduced. Characteristically during exposure to vapor of dimethyl sulfate the patient or experimental animal is not aware of irritation or unpleasant sensation but begins to develop discomfort several hours later.

Moeschlin in his book on poisonings particularly has placed great emphasis on the latent period that is characteristic of the action of dimethyl sulfate vapors on the eyes, giving description of specific cases in which there were latent periods as long as six hours before severe inflammation of the eyes and respiratory tract developed.[177] Browning in her book on toxicology has reviewed several of the reports in the literature of eye involvement from vapor exposure.[21]

Typical industrial exposure occurs when workmen pour dimethyl sulfate from one container to another, with no irritation of eyes or nose, or no unpleasant odor to warn of danger. After several hours the eyes begin to feel irritated and have a sandy sensation. Photophobia and lacrimation develop; the lids become edematous and the conjunctiva hyperemic. The skin of the face and other exposed parts is reddened. The symptoms increase in intensity for several hours, and then superficial clouding and irregularity of the corneal epithelium may be seen. Associated with the ocular symptoms are temporary loss of smell and taste, with horseness and irritation of the respiratory passages which may become severe, and in the worst cases may develop into fatal pneumonia.

The course of the eye injuries in the mildest cases may be spontaneous return to normal in a few days, or, in severe cases, gray necrosis of the epithelium, edema and infiltration of the corneal stroma, and permanent partial opacification may result.

Observations on patients and on experimental animals have indicated that dimethyl sulfate has a selective injurious action on the corneal endothelium which particularly favors development of edema of the corneal stroma.[b,c] Subsidence of corneal edema seems to depend on recovery of the endothelium. After subsidence of the edema a mottled cloudiness of stroma may remain.

The mechanism of poisonous action of dimethyl sulfate on the eye and on other tissues is currently believed to be based on methylation (alkylation), causing denaturation and enzyme inhibition, analogous to poisoning and injury by mustard gas.

A search of the literature has revealed no case presenting unequivocal evidence of damage to the optic nerve or retina from dimethyl sulfate. The vapor has frequently caused blurring of vision attributable to injury and edema of the cornea, but any other type of visual disturbance has rarely been described. Reports of blindness for a few hours,[e] slight transient contraction of the fields,[a] or contraction of fields for colors (in a person admittedly having had poor vision before exposure)[k] appear of little value on close scrutiny. Visual fields and optic nerves have specifically been established as normal in a recent case of severe poisoning.[j] A choroidal melanoma developed in an eye of a worker chronically exposed for 6 years, but whether related is unknown.[272]

For treatment of dimethyl sulfate burns or systemic poisoning, no specific measures are known. Assuming injury to be due to methylation of tissues, a means for demethylation might be beneficial if one were known. On the same assumption, immediately after gross contamination with liquid dimethyl sulfate, protection might, theoretically, be afforded by a compound which would be more readily methylated than tissue proteins and would thereby spare the tissues from injury. The situation is analogous to that encountered with mustard gas, and in that case no practically effective means have been discovered for dealkylation or protection of tissues by competing agents. The standard immediate treatment is the same as for other chemical exposures, consisting of immediate, copious irrigation with water. The subsequent treatment is the same as for other chemical burns of the eye.

a. Adams PH, Cridland B: Effect of fumes of dimethyl sulphate on the eye. *OPHTHALMO-SCOPE* 8:717, 1910.

b. Brina A: Two cases of poisoning by dimethyl sulfate. *MED LAVORO* 37:225–228, 1946. (Italian)

c. Erdmann P: On eye disturbances from dimethyl sulfate. *ARCH AUGENHEILKD* 62:178–227, 1909; and 64:249, 1910. (German)

d. Grosz S de: Dimethyl sulphate poisoning in relation to ophthalmology. *AM J OPHTHALMOL* 20:700–707, 1937.

e. Haswell RW: Dimethyl sulfate poisoning by inhalation. *J OCCUP MED* 2:454–455, 1960.

f. Littler TR, McConnell RB: Dimethyl sulphate poisoning. *BR J IND MED* 12:54–56, 1955.

g. Luthy F: Peripheral neuritis in industrial poisoning and contribution to the question of the exposition. *Z UNFALLMED BERUFSKR* 34:34, 1940. (*Z GEW HYG* 28:27, 1941.)

h. Merkelbach O: Dimethyl sulfate poisoning. *SCHWEIZ MED WOCHENSCHR* 73:481, 1943.

i. Mohlau FD: Report of two cases of dimethyl sulfate poisoning. *J IND HYG* 2:238–240, 1920.

j. Roche L, Robert JM, Paliard P: Poisoning by dimethyl sulfate. *ARCH MAL PROF* 23:391, 1962. (French)

k. Senn HE: Changes in the cornea after burning by dimethyl sulfate. *OPHTHAL-MOLOGICA* 110:307, 1945. (German)

l. Stern HJ: Conjunctivitis due to exposure to dimethyl sulfate. *BR J OPHTHALMOL* 31:373–375, 1947.

m. Strothman H: On poisoning with dimethyl sulfate. *KLIN WOCHENSCHR* 8:493–496, 1929. (German)

n. Tara S: Concerning dimethyl sulfate. *ARCH MAL PROF* 16:368, 1956. (French)

o. Tara S, Cavigneaux A, Delplace Y: Accidents to the eye from dimethyl sulfate. *ARCH MAL PROF* 15:291, 1954. (French)

p. Weber S: On the poisonous nature of dimethyl sulfate. *NAUNYN–SCHMIEDEBERG'S ARCH EXP PATH PHARMAK* 47:113, 1902. (German)

q. Savic S: Eye injuries from the action of dimethyl sulfate. *KLIN MONATSBL AUGENHEILKD* 159:221–223, 1971. (German)

Dimethyl sulfoxide (DMSO) is a hygroscopic liquid having useful solvent properties for a wide variety of substances. Medical applications developed during the 1960's. DMSO became widely used as an analgesic and anti-inflammatory agent in musculoskeletal disorders by application to the skin. It also came into use as a penetrating solvent to aid absorption of drugs, particularly through the skin. By 1969 more than eight hundred articles are said to have been published on the medical uses and related pharmacology and toxicology. Clinically, the principal adverse side effects that became evident were unpleasant odor of the breath and occasional irritation of the skin. However, a major problem arose when laboratory animals receiving large doses developed changes in the nucleus of the crystalline lenses resembling juvenile nuclear sclerosis; although this was not found in human beings or monkeys, this caused the U.S. Food and Drug Administration to ban medical use of DMSO in the United States in 1965. Later, resumption of testing on a very limited scale was permitted. Comprehensive reviews of pharmacology and toxicology for the period up to 1970 were published by David and by Meyer.[d,s]

Here only the ophthalmologic aspects of DMSO action will be outlined, covering first the effects of local application to the eye, then effects of systemic administration. (Note that the effect of dimethyl sulfoxide on the eye is quite different from that of *dimethyl sulfate.*)

Numerous tests for contact toxicity have been made. In anesthetized rabbits when the surface of the eye was flooded with dimethyl sulfoxide and no attempt was made to remove the material, only the epithelium of the cornea was injured. The conjunctival blood vessels immediately became dilated, but circulation was not interrupted and there were no hemorrhages. The corneal epithelium in the course of an hour developed a finely granular, ground-glass appearance by microscopic examination, but remained grossly clear with poor surface luster. Discharge was moderate and mucoid, not purulent. In two days, the eyes returned to normal.[81] Testing on rabbit eyes by Smyth and Carpenter,[228] Conquet and the Draize evaluation gave low scores.[295] The intraocular pressure was not affected.[276]

Water and DMSO mixtures have been tested on both rabbit and human eyes by several investigators in evaluating DMSO as a topical anti-inflammatory agent on the eye or as a solvent and carrier for ophthalmic drugs.[h,q,r,t,j] Generally, aqueous solutions containing 50% to 90% DMSO have proved irritating when applied as eyedrops, causing temporary sensation of stinging and burning. A 10% to 30% solution of DMSO has been well tolerated when applied in eyedrops or by subconjunctival injection.[q,r,j] A 5% solution injected into the anterior chamber did not damage the aqueous outflow system.[n]

DMSO has been used without initial evidence of toxic effect in preservation of frozen corneas. However, studies on bovine and human corneal endothelium have revealed latent injury which becomes evident in culture.[za,zb] Appropriate choice of concentration and composition of the medium has been found to reduce toxic effect significantly.[zb] DMSO binds to the corneal stroma, mostly reversibly, but a very small fraction apparently irreversibly.[g] Permeation of the cornea by sodium ions is not influenced by DMSO when the epithelium and endothelium are intact.[u]

Systemically administered DMSO, mainly given in drinking water or applied to large areas of skin, through which DMSO is absorbed, has been shown to become fairly uniformly distributed in all body tissues, including the eye. As a result of repeated systemic administration, several investigators have described changes in the crystalline lenses of dogs, rabbits, pigs, guinea pigs, and rats.[e, m, o, p, v–z, zf]

In rabbits DMSO given in drinking water 10 g/kg per day showed a change in refractive index of the nucleus of the crystalline lenses detectable by retinoscopy in three to four weeks, also detectable by slit-lamp biomicroscopy as an interface between the nucleus and the anterior cortex. Very good slit-lamp photographs of the characteristic changes in the rabbit nucleus have been published by Wood and Wirth.[zf] Dogs similarly given large doses daily have developed slight opalescence of the nucleus of the crystalline lenses with difference in refractive index between nucleus and cortex, inducing considerable myopia. Beginning development of myopia is detectable within a week on a dosage of 5 ml/kg per day. Even with daily administration continuing for seventeen months the lenses did not become opaque, but the nuclei developed increased opalescence which was very slowly and incompletely reversible.[o, p] It has been pointed out that the total doses to cause these changes in the lenses have been far greater than amounts of DMSO absorbed by patients.[z] In pigs, refractive changes in the lens have been induced, but these have been relatively slight in rats.[v] In guinea pigs, vacuolated areas extending subcapsularly from periphery to center have been described.[w]

In monkeys attempts have been made to induce changes in the lenses such as observed in the lower animals, but apart from a preliminary report by Barnett and Noel of beginning changes in refractive index, these attempts were otherwise negative up to 1970.[a, z, ze]

In human beings incidental to the medical use of DMSO there have been no lens changes attributed to this substance, and no changes in the eyes were detectable by extensive testing in normal people during, and for a year after, daily application of 1 g to the skin for weeks or months.[b, k]

Recapitulations of evidence of lack of significant adverse effect on the lens in human beings from clinical use of DMSO, and reviews of related animal studies have been published by Caldwell, Gordon, Jacob, and others.[c, f, i, l]

Investigations of biochemical changes induced in animals have been carried out to try to find an explanation for the changes in the lens produced by dimethyl sulfoxide.[zd, zg–zi] In rabbits, there has been found a loss of gamma-crystallin and an increase in water insoluble protein, limited to the lens nucleus.[zd] No hydration changes were found.[zh] Lens glutathione reduced some of the dimethyl sulfoxide to dimethyl sulfide,[zh] but experimental lenses maintained normal glutathione content.[zd] Large doses of metabolites of dimethyl sulfoxide, specifically *dimethyl sulfide, dimethyl sulfone, dimethyl sulfate,* failed to produce changes in the lenses of rabbits.[zh] Young rabbit lenses in culture in the presence of dimethyl sulfoxide have been observed to develop changes in refraction similar to those that develop in the course of months in vivo.[zi]

a. Barnett KC, Noel PRB: Dimethyl sulphoxide and lens changes in primates. *NATURE* 214:1115–1116, 1967.

b. Brobyn RD: The human toxicology of dimethyl sulfoxide. *ANN NY ACAD SCI* 243:497–506, 1975.

c. Caldwell AD, Bye PG, Briggs MH: Side effects of dimethyl sulphoxide. *NATURE* 215:1168, 1967.

d. David NA: The pharmacology of dimethyl sulfoxide. *ANN REV PHARMACOL* 12:353–374, 1972.

e. Esila R, Tenhunen T: Dimethyl sulphoxide: Lens changes, composition of the anterior aqueous humour and intraocular pressure in rabbits during oral administration. *ACTA OPHTHALMOL* 45:530–535, 1967.

f. Garcia CA: Ocular toxicology of dimethyl sulfoxide and effects on retinitis pigmentosa. *ANN NY ACAD SCI* 411:48–51, 1983.

g. Gerhards E, Gibian H: The metabolism of dimethyl sulfoxide and its metabolic effects in man and animals. *ANN NY ACAD SCI* 141:65–76, 1967.

h. Gordon DM: Dimethyl sulfoxide in ophthalmology with special reference to possible toxic effects. *ANN NY ACAD SCI* 141:392–401, 1967.

i. Gordon DM, Kleberger KE: The effect of dimethyl sulfoxide (DMSO) on animal and human eyes. *ARCH OPHTHALMOL* 79:423–436, 1968.

j. Hanna C, Fraunfelder FT, Meyer SM: Effects of dimethyl sulfoxide on ocular inflammation. *ANN OPHTHALMOL* 9:61–65, 1977.

k. Hull FW, Wood DC, Brobyn RD: Eye effects of DMSO. Report of negative results. *NORTHWEST MED* 68:39–42, 1969.

l. Jacob SW, Wood DC: Dimethyl sulfoxide (DMSO): Toxicology, pharmacology and current clinical usefulness. *ARZNEIMITTEL-FORSCH* 17:1553–1560, 1967. (*Excerpta Med* (Sect. 2C), 21(10):2860, 1968.)

m. Kamiya S, Wakao T, Nishioka K: Confirmation of the chronic toxicity of DMSO. *FOLIA OPHTHALMOL* JPN 18:387–389, 1967.

n. Kaufman PL, Erickson KA: Cytochalasin B and D dose-outflow facility response relationships in the cynomolgus monkey. *INVEST OPHTHALMOL VIS SCI* 23:646–650, 1982.

o. Kleberger K-E: An ophthalmological evaluation of DMSO. *ANN NY ACAD SCI* 141:381–385, 1967.

p. Kleberger E: Lens with double focal points. *GRAEFES ARCH OPHTHALMOL* 173:269–281, 1967. (German)

q. Kligman AM: Topical pharmacology and toxicology of dimethyl sulfoxide. *J AM MED ASSOC* 193:923–928, 1965.

r. Liegl O, Erhard I: Dimethylsulfoxide (DMSO) and Herpes simplex-virus. *GRAEFES ARCH OPHTHALMOL* 169:75–84, 1966.

s. Meyer SL: Dimethyl sulfoxide (DMSO). *SURVEY OPHTHALMOL* 16:36–42, 1971.

t. Morris RW: Analgesic and local anesthetic activity of dimethyl sulfoxide. *J PHARM SCI* 55:438–440, 1966.

u. Mrzyglod S, Segal P, Plonda A: Experimental investigations on the influence of DMSO on the permeability of the cornea. *KLIN OCZNA* 37:311–314, 1967.

v. Noel PRB, Barnett KC, et al: Toxicity of dimethyl sulfoxide for the dog, pig, rat, and rabbit. *TOXICOLOGY* 3:143–169, 1975.

w. Rengstorff RH, Petrali JP, Sim VM: Cataracts induced in guinea pigs by acetone, cyclohexanone, and dimethyl sulfoxide. *AM J OPTOM* 49:308–319, 1972.

x. Rubin LF, Mattis PA: Dimethyl sulfoxide: Lens changes in dogs during oral administration. *SCIENCE* 153:83–84, 1966.

y. Rubin LF: Toxicity of dimethyl sulfoxide, alone and in combination. *ANN NY ACAD SCI* 243:98–103, 1975.

z. Smith ER, Mason MM, Epstein E: The influence of dimethyl sulfoxide on the dog with emphasis on the ophthalmologic examination. *ANN NY ACAD SCI* 141:386–391, 1967.

za. Sperling S: Toxicity of DMSO to bovine corneal endothelium. *OPHTHALMIC RES* 8:233–240, 1976.

zb. Sperling S, Larsen IG: Toxicity of dimethyl sulfoxide (DMSO) to human corneal endothelium in vitro. *ACTA OPHTHALMOL* 57:891–898, 1979.

zc. Smith ER, Mason MM, Epstein E: Ocular effects of repeated dermal applications of dimethyl sulfoxide to dogs and monkeys. *J PHARMACOL EXP THER* 170:364–370, 1969.

zd. Van Heyningen R, Harding JJ: Some changes in the lens of the dimethylsulfoxide-fed rabbit. *EXP EYE RES* 14:91–98, 1972.

ze. Vogin EE, Carson S, et al: Chronic toxicity of DMSO in primates. *TOXICOL APPL PHARMACOL* 16:606–612, 1970.

zf. Wood DC, Wirth NV: Changes in rabbit lenses following DMSO therapy. *OPHTHAL-MOLOGICA ADDIT AD* 158:488–493, 1969.

zg. Wood DC, Weber FS, Palmquist MA: Toxicology of dimethyl sulfoxide (DMSO). *J PHARMACOL EXP THER* 177:520–527, 1971.

zh. Wood DC, Wirth NV, et al: Mechanism considerations of dimethyl sulfoxide (DMSO) -lenticular changes in rabbits. *J PHARMACOL EXP THER* 177:528–535, 1971.

zi. Wood DC, Palmquist MA, Jacob SW: Eye lens changes with dimethyl sulfoxide; in vitro system. *PHYSIOL CHEM PHYS* 5:43–48, 1973.

3,5-Dimethyltetrahydro-1,3,5,2H-thiadiazine-2-thione (Mylone, UCC-974), a soil fungicide and weed killer, tested on rabbit eyes by application of 0.5 ml of 15% solution, caused temporary loss of a small patch of corneal epithelium from only one of five eyes, and this healed completely.[a]

a. Smyth HF, Carpenter CP, Weil CS: Toxicologic studies on 3,5-dimethyltetrahydro-1,3,5,2H-thiadiazine-2-thione, a soil fungicide and slimicide. *TOXICOL APPL PHARMACOL* 9:521–527, 1966.

Dimidium bromide (Phenanthridinium 1553) used in treatment of trypanosomiasis in cattle, according to Garner's book, Veterinary Toxicology, causes photosensitization, photophobia, and lacrimation associated with dermatitis in animals, but he has not described examinations of the involved eyes.[64]

Dinitrobenzene is a yellowish crystalline solid which has caused poisonings principally in the munitions industry at the end of the nineteenth century and during World War I. Of the three isomers of dinitrobenzene, m-dinitrobenzene was most commonly manufactured.[18] The dust or fumes of this substance may be absorbed through the skin, respiratory, or gastrointestinal tract. Surface contact may cause yellowing of the skin, and purportedly of the conjunctiva and cornea,[61] but no original observations on corneal changes were found in the literature. The skin, conjunctiva, and ocular fundus may show bluish discoloration from formation of methemoglobin.[a, 153]

Chronic poisoning has been observed in numerous cases following exposure for nine to eighteen months to the dust and vapor in munitions plants.[153] Symptoms of poisoning start with headache, and burning pain and parethesias in the feet, ankles, hands, and forearms. The peripheral nerve disturbances have all been sensory with no motor disturbances, ataxia, or intention tremor. Vision has been affected in numerous cases, but the pupils have remained normal unless vision was much reduced, and there has been no nystagmus or disturbance of extraocular muscles.

In cases of chronic poisoning, impairment of vision appears to have been common.[d,153] Typically, the visual fields have been slightly contracted, and visual acuity has been much reduced, with central scotomas, particularly for red and green. These findings are characteristic of retrobulbar neuritis. Usually there has been no abnormality in appearance of the optic nervehead other than slight pallor, but in occasional cases partial optic atrophy has developed. The retinal blood vessels have usually appeared normal, but in one patient retinal hemorrhage was seen.[d] In most instances vision has gradually recovered in the course of several months after exposure to dinitrobenzene has been discontinued. Descriptions of the effect of dinitrobenzene on the eye have been remarkably uniform in numerous case reports.[a-g,24,153]

Teleky in his book on toxicology has observed that visual disturbances from dinitrobenzene usually appear after long industrial exposure and often have been precipitated by a brief increase in intensity of exposure. Teleky has also called attention to the interesting contrast that reduction of vision has not been characteristic of nitrobenzene or trinitrobenzene, but definitely of dinitrobenzene.[239]

However, similar disturbances of vision have been reported from *Dinitrochlorobenzene* and by *Dinitrotoluene*.

a. Blyth AW, Blyth MW: *Poisons, Their Effects and Detection.* London, C Griffin 1920.
b. Capellini A, Zanottin GG: A case of occupational chronic poisoning with dinitrobenzene. *MED LAVORO* 37:265–270, 1946. (*Chem Abstr* 41:1760.)
c. Cords R: Dinitrobenzene and the optic nerve. *ZENTRALBL GEWERBEHYG* 7:6–11, 1919. (German)
d. Hubner AH: On dinitrobenzene poisoning. *MUNCH MED WOCHENSCHR* 65:(ii): 1285–1287, 1918. (German)
e. Nieden A: On amblyopia from Roburit poisoning. *ZENTRALBL PRAKT AUGEN-HEILKD* 12:193, 1888. (German)
f. Pockley FA: A case of amblyopia due to dinitrobenzol. *AUSTRALIAN MED GAZ* 13:340, 1894.
g. Reis: Optic nerve injury by trinitrotoluol. *Z AUGENHEILKD* 47:199–208, 1922. (German)
h. Snell S: Remarks on amblyopia from dinitrobenzene. *BR MED J* 1:449, 1894.

4,6-Dinitro-2-sec-butylphenol (Butofen), a herbicide, tested in the form of a combination preparation containing also 10% to 20% of 2,4-dinitrophenol and 4-nitrodibutylphenol is said to have caused permanent damage to the cornea after application of a drop to the eye. No test was reported of the pure compound.[a]

a. Vinokurova MK, Kharitonova ES: The toxicity of the herbicide 4,6-dinitro-2-sec-butylphenol (Butofen). (*Chem Abstr* 60:12575, 1964.)

Dinitrochlorobenzene (DNCB; chlorodinitrobenzene) is known to cause sensitization and dermatitis. Ocular neuropathologic effects ascribed to dinitrochlorobenzene are essentially the same as those attributed to *dinitrobenzene.*[a,b] Both of these substances and others may be present in manufacture of munitions, and it has been unclear whether the intoxications should be attributed to one or both of these substances.

Typically, chronic poisoning by industrial exposure to these substances has been said to cause gradual development of symptoms of retrobulbar neuritis, with blurring of vision, central scotoma, especially for green, and constriction of visual fields. At first the ophthalmoscopic findings are normal, but optic neuritis may gradually become evident, in exceptional instances leading to optic atrophy.[a,b] Impaired pupillary reaction in accommodation has been noted despite good pupillary response to light. Typically the retrobulbal neuritis has been associated with peripheral neuritis manifest as paresthesias and pains in the legs and burning of the feet. (Compare *Dinitrobenzene* and *Dinitrotoluene.*)

Dinitrochlorobenzene has been used as an adjuvant in immunotherapy of tumors of the skin, and of the conjunctiva.[c,d] This has involved applying 2 mg to the skin to induce a systemic hypersensitivity reaction, and later repeatedly applying much smaller quantities to the tumors themselves to induce local reaction and necrosis. Care has been taken not to allow this very irritating substance to come in contact with the cornea, but there seems to be no observation on what would happen if it did. Also, it apparently is assumed that the quantities of DNCB involved in this treatment are too small to induce optic or peripheral neuropathy such as reported in industry, and there seem to be no clinical experiences to the contrary.

a. Nieden A: On amblyopia from Roburite poisoning. *ZENTRALBL PRAKT AUGEN-HEILKD* 12:193, 1888. (German)
b. Sollier P, Jousset X: Nitrophenol neuritides. *CLIN OPHTHALMOL* 22:78–87, 1917.
c. Ferry AP, Meltzer MA, Taub RN: Immunotherapy with dinitrochlorobenzene (DNCB) for recurrent squamous cell tumor of conjunctiva. *TRANS AM OPHTHALMOL SOC* 74:154–171, 1976.
d. Petrelli R, Cotlier E, et al: Dinitrochlorobenzene immunotherapy of recurrent papilloma of the conjunctiva. *OPHTHALMOLOGY* 88:1221–1225, 1981.

Dinitro-o-cresol (DNOC; 4,6-Dinitro-o-cresol) commonly employed in the form of a sodium salt as a herbicide and insecticide, is irritating to the eyes and skin.[36] At one time it was used medically as a weight-reducing agent similar to dinitrophenol, and cataracts occurred as a result.[a–d] Glaucoma has been known to develop secondary to the cataracts.[a] DNOC poisoning appears to be on the same basis as the poisoning caused by dinitrophenol; the metabolic rate is increased secondary to inhibition of oxidative phosphorylation. (Compare *Dinitrophenol.*)

a. Gilbert-Dreyfus, Onfray R: Poisoning during treatment by dinitrocresol. Cataract followed by glaucoma. *BULL SOC MED HOP PARIS* 53:1073–1078, 1937. (French)
b. Mahlen S: On awareness of cataract in dinitroorthocresol treatment. *ARCH OPHTHALMOL* 16:563–578, 1938. (German)
c. Ploman KG: A case of dinitroorthocresol cataract. *HYGEIA* (Stockholm) 99:688–689, 1937. (*ZENTRALBL GES OPHTHALMOL* 41:691, 1938.)

d. Mahlen S: Table of eye investigations in patients treated with dinitroorthocresol. *ACTA OPHTHALMOL* 17:215, 1939. (German)

2,4-Dinitrofluorobenzene (DNFB), like *2,4-dinitrochlorobenzene* (DNCB), reacts with proteins to form *dinitrobenzene-protein conjugates.* The effects of hypersensitivity to these substances in guinea pigs on the responses to intraocular and extraocular testing have been described by Silverstein.[a] Subtoxic doses of DNFB administered topically or intravitreally to hypersensitized animals produced little inflammatory reaction in conjunctiva, retina, or uvea. Dinitrobenzene-protein conjugates produce anaphylactic-type inflammatory responses.

a. Silverstein AM, Welter S, Zimmerman LE: Studies on experimental ocular hypersensitivity to simple chemicals. *AM J OPHTHALMOL* 50:937–944, 1960.

Dinitronaphthalene many years ago in the munitions industry was thought to cause corneal disturbances. It was always in combination with mono-nitronaphthalene, and it is not clear which was responsible. (See *Nitronaphthalene* for more details.) Exposure of rabbits to sublethal concentrations of vapor for several hours caused no changes in the cornea.[a]

a. Koelsch F: Study on the toxicology of aromatic nitro-compounds. *ZENTRALBL GEWERBEHYG* 5:60, 65, 98, 109, 142, 1917. (German)

2,4-Dinitrophenol (DNP), employed for treating obesity, is toxic, causing increase in metabolism and temperature. In severe poisoning, sweating and collapse and death may result. Chronic poisoning has occurred principally in the use of dinitrophenol for reducing.

The most notorious toxic effect has been the production of cataracts, first noted in 1935 and reported in nearly two hundred cases in the next few years until the sale of the compound for internal use was prohibited. At least seventy articles have been published concerning cataract production by dinitrophenol. More than half of the publications have been case reports, and the remainder have been experimental studies. Several good reviews of the literature are available.[g, k, x, 46, 255] Nearly all the clinical literature appeared in the years 1935 to 1937. The literature on experimental studies is scattered more evenly through the years since 1935.

Estimates of the incidence of cataract among people taking dinitrophenol for reducing varied from 0.1% to 1%. Onset of cataract characteristically occurred several months after the drug had been used. The cataracts were of uniform sort, occurring in both eyes, appearing first in the anterior cortex as fine gray cloudy opacities associated with a spotty lusterless appearance of the anterior lens capsule. In the posterior cortex, golden granular opacities appeared, with polychromatic specular reflections. With rapid progress of the cataract, the lenses became swollen and the embryonic suture lines were separated by dark clefts. Soon the whole lens became opaque with mature cataract.

In numerous cases secondary glaucoma was associated with the mature cataract, but it is not certain whether this was due to a swelling of the lens inducing pupillary block and angle-closure or whether it was due to a phacolytic process inducing secondary open-angle glaucoma. In essentially all cases surgical removal of the cataracts cured the glaucoma and left normal aphakic eyes with good vision and no indication of damage to cornea, retina or optic nerve.

Toxic effects on the eyes other than production of cataract have been rare. In one case, a severe reaction of the skin and mucous membranes involved the conjunctiva, causing symblepharon and leading to the loss of one eye.[n] One case of transient paresis of accommodation has been recorded, associated with taking dinitrophenol, and improving when the drug was discontinued. In acute industrial poisoning, nystagmus was said to be present in cases of moderate poisoning, and dilated pupils were noted in severe cases with poor prognosis.[61]

Dinitrophenol and dinitrocresol, unlike dinitrobenzene or chlorodinitrobenzene, appear not to have caused optic nerve disturbances. Dinitrophenol has been shown to have no effect on the ERG of rabbits.[179] However, in pieces of retina surviving in culture a concentration of 0.005 M 2,4-dinitrophenol causes unselective degeneration of cells.[99]

Dust and vapor of dinitrophenol have been reported to be irritating to mucous membrane in industrial exposure, but no contact injuries seem to have been reported.[61] Tests of aqueous solution of 2,4-dinitrophenol on rabbit corneas by injection into the corneal stroma or application to the eye after removing the corneal epithelium caused no significant reaction at 0.012 M concentration, but at 0.05 M caused a moderate reaction, graded 52 on a scale of 1 to 100.[123] Also a toxic effect on the cornea was indicated by an increase in water uptake by this tissue when dinitrophenol was added to the aqueous humor of rabbits, but this seems to have no clinical counterpart.[198] Both dinitrophenol and dinitrocresol cause loss of cohesion of the epithelial cells of excised beef corneas after several hours of incubation.[e]

Most of the experimental toxicology of dinitrophenol has been concerned with cataract production, and cataracts have been repeatedly induced in ducklings and chickens, less reliably in guinea pigs, only in certain types of mice, and rabbits under special conditions, not in rats, or dogs.[p] Not only are there great species differences in susceptibility, but the type of cataract varies strikingly. In ducklings and chickens the cataracts appear within a few hours after feeding 2,4-dinitrophenol.[a, b, d, q, r] In these animals the cataract consists of microscopic granular and vacuolar changes in the anterior and posterior portions of the lens, but these cataracts spontaneously clear in a week or two, despite continued administration of the poison. In congenitally obese mice, not in ordinary mice, cataracts have been produced after four to eight weeks and have been permanent rather than reversible.[b] In guinea pigs it has been claimed that cataract can be induced, provided the animals are deficient in vitamin C, but this is yet to be confirmed.[o]

In chicks intramuscular injection of 2.5 mg/kg causes appearance of opacities around the suture lines within one-half to one hour, spreading to a maximum involving the whole cortex at three to four hours, and clearing spontaneously by eight to nine hours. Repeated daily doses of the same size do not cause persistent opacity. Histologic examination at the stage of maximum effect indicates edematous changes, but there is no associated gain in total water content. Less opacification develops if glutathione (2 g/kg) is given intramuscularly five to seven minutes before the dinitrophenol, but ascorbic acid and catalin have had no inhibitory effect.[m]

Electron microscopy of lenses of albino rabbits given 2,4-dinitrophenol, according to Watanabe, showed vacuoles that originated from mitochondria and endoplasmic reticulum of the lens epithelial cells at the equator, and the nuclear membranes became destroyed and the cell membranes separated. Vacuoles and opacities were visible and were photographed at the equator of the lens three hours after the administration of dinitrophenol, but these disappeared in twenty-four hours. Similar vacuoles in mitochondria and intracellular spaces were seen in the non-pigmented epithelium of the ciliary body, and these were reversible.[u] It is reported that administering tiopronin prior to dinitrophenol has resulted in some reduction of the ultrastructural changes in the lens.[v]

In rabbits congenital cataracts have been found in the lenses of two offspring of two rabbits that were given repeated intravenous injections of dinitrophenol during pregnancy, but the mother rabbits did not develop cataracts.[t]

Studies of the blood aqueous barrier and differences of penetrability of 2,4-dinitrophenol into the eye from the blood in different species by Gehring and Buerge have shown that dinitrophenol gets into the aqueous humor more readily and reaches a higher concentration in ducks that develop cataracts than in rabbits that do not. Also in immature rabbits, in which cataracts can be produced, dinitrophenol entered the aqueous humor more readily than in mature rabbits which did not develop cataracts. Differences in penetration could be partially accounted for by differences in amount bound by plasma proteins. These observations offered an explanation for apparent species specificity dependent principally on how readily dinitrophenol reached the lenses of the various experimental animals. Evidence to support this explanation has been obtained by the same investigators who have reported that mature rabbits can be caused to develop cataracts when the dinitrophenol is administered locally by way of the conjunctival sac or injected into the eye, whereas mature rabbits do not develop cataracts when given dinitrophenol systemically.[i,j]

The mechanism by which dinitrophenol and related compounds produce cataract has been investigated from several standpoints. Early suppositions that dinitrophenol had a direct denaturing effect on lens proteins seemed to be eliminated by demonstration that no cataract was produced in vitro. It seemed likely to most investigators that it was the uncoupling of oxidative phosphorylation and increase in oxygen consumption which was responsible for changes in metabolism of the lens leading to cataract.[h,n,135] A theory that dinitrophenol changes the permeability of the capsule of the lens was not supported by the results of experiments in vitro on beef lenses and in vivo in rats, testing the permeability to a variety of dyes.[c] Also, the temperature-reversible cation shift of the lens, involving concentration of potassium and excretion of sodium by active transport, is inhibited only by concentrations of dinitrophenol that are higher than are likely in poisoned patients or animals.[k] According to Ikemoto, concentrations of 2,4-dinitrophenol that inhibit cation transport do not inhibit glycolysis in rabbit lenses surviving in culture.[126] In toad lenses, dinitrophenol in the bathing fluid has been shown to enter the lens rapidly, to depolarize the lens membrane, and to markedly increase the membrane conductance.[w]

Secretion of sodium into the eye by the ciliary processes has been shown to be inhibited, and the electric potential and intraocular pressure to be reduced in rabbits by dinitrophenol injected into the arterial blood supply of the eye; related effects can be produced in excised surviving ciliary processes.[f,g,10] What relation these effects on the ciliary body may have to formation of cataracts is not known, and the concentration required to obtain these effects may be considerably greater than is involved in cataractogenesis from systemic intoxication.

Among compounds related to 2,4-dinitrophenol, only *4,6-dinitro-o-cresol* has been known to cause cataracts in human beings. This same compound produced cataracts in the same animals as dinitrophenol, and at lower dosages. Other compounds which have been found to produce the acute transient type of cataract in ducklings or chickens are *2,4-dinitro-6-aminophenol;*[q] *2-sec. butyl-4,6-dinitrophenol;*[r] *2,4-dinitro-anisole; 2,4-dinitrophenetole; 2,6-dibromo-4-nitrophenol; 2-chloro-4,6-dinitrophenol; 2,6-dinitrophenol.*[d] It appears that a phenolic hydroxyl and at least one nitro group, preferably in para position, are essential for cataractogenesis.[d]

a. Bettman JW: Production of cataracts in chicks with dinitrophenol. *ARCH OPHTHALMOL* 36:674–676, 1946.

b. Bettman JW: Experimental dinitrophenol cataract. *AM J OPHTHALMOL* 29:1388–1395, 1946.

c. Borley WF, Tainter ML: Effects of dinitrophenol on the permeability of the capsule of the lens. *ARCH OPHTHALMOL* 18:908–911, 1937.

d. Buschke W: Acute reversible cataract in chickens due to various nitrocompounds. *AM J OPHTHALMOL* 30:1356–1368, 1947.

e. Buschke W: Effects of metabolic poisons and other agents on intercellular cohesion in corneal epithelium. *AM J OPHTHALMOL* 33:59–66, 1950.

f. Cole DF: Electrochemical changes associated with the formation of the aqueous humor. *BR J OPHTHALMOL* 45:202–217, 1961.

g. Cole DF: Electrical potential across the isolated ciliary body observed in vitro. *BR J OPHTHALMOL* 45:641–653, 1961.

h. Field J II, Tainter EG, et al: Studies on the oxygen consumption of the rabbit lens and the effect of 2,4-dinitrophenol thereon. *AM J OPHTHALMOL* 20:7779–794, 1937.

i. Gehring PJ, Buerge JF: The cataractogenic activity of 2,4-dinitrophenol in ducks and rabbits. *TOXICOL APPL PHARMACOL* 14:475–486, 1969.

j. Gehring PJ, Buerge JF: The distribution of 2,4-dinitrophenol relative to its cataractogenic activity in ducklings and rabbits. *TOXICOL APPL PHARMACOL* 15:574–592, 1969.

k. Harris JE: The temperature-reversible cation shift of the lens. *TRANS AM OPHTHAL-MOL SOC* 64:675–699, 1966.

l. Horner WD: Dinitrophenol and its relation to cataract. *ARCH OPHTHALMOL* 27:1097–1121, 1942.

m. Miyata A: Studies on the experimental dinitrophenol cataract. *ACTA SOC OPHTHAL-MOL JPN* 72:2307–2324, 1968.

n. Muller HK, Kleifeld O, et al: The effect of age, poisoning with naphthalene, dinitro-phenol, and alloxan upon the incorporation of phosphorus-32 in the electrophoretically separable phosphate fractions. *GRAEFES ARCH OPHTHALMOL* 156:460–466, 1955.

o. Ogino S, Yasukura K: Biochemical studies on cataract. VI. Production of cataracts in guinea pigs with dinitrophenol. *AM J OPHTHALMOL* 43:936–946, 1957.

p. Rigdon RH, Feldman GL, et al: Cataracts produced by dinitrophenol. *ARCH OPHTHALMOL* 61:249–257, 1959.

q. Robbins BH: Dinitrophenol cataract. *J PHARMACOL EXP THER* 80:264, 1944; and 82:301, 1944.

r. Spencer HC, Rowe VK, et al: Toxicological studies on laboratory animals of certain alkyldinitro phenols used in agriculture. *J IND HYG* 30:10–25, 1948.

s. Swett WF: Eye complications following the use of reducing agents. *AM J OPHTHALMOL* 19:796–797, 1936.

t. Vassilev I, Dabov S, Rankov B: Congenital cataract induced experimentally by dinitrophenol. *ARCH OPHTALMOL (Paris)* 19:13–18, 1959.

u. Watanabe T: Electron microscopic studies of the lens and the ciliary body of rabbits with experimental dinitrophenol cataract. *ACTA SOC OPHTHALMOL JPN* 73:393–411, 1969.

v. Bauchiero L, Dalmas EM et al: Experimental cataract and tiopronin ultrastructural histological evaluation in rabbits. *BOLL OCULIST* 59:253–270, 1980. (Italian)

w. Duncan G, Croghan PC: Effect of changes in external ion concentrations and 2,4-dinitrophenol on the conductance of toad lens membranes. *EXP EYE RES* 10:192–200, 1970.

x. Van Oye R: Slenderizing treatments. *BULL SOC BELGE OPHTALMOL* 160:111–115, 1972. (French)

Dinitrotoluene is an explosive substance which has been known to cause systemic intoxication.[252] A workman employed for a year in nitration of mononitrotoluene to dinitrotoluene developed tingling and numbness in the toes and legs, but no pain. After two years these symptoms became worse, and vision decreased from 20/40 to 6/200 in both eyes. Cursory examination of the fields showed them to be full, but the optic nerveheads appeared atrophic and the retinal arteries were narrow. The work was discontinued, and after a year vision improved to 20/40 and 20/60, but slight paresthesia of the feet persisted.[a] (The signs and symptoms in this case resemble those described under *Dinitrochlorobenzene* and *Dinitrobenzene*.)

a. Hamilton AS, Nixon CE: Optic atrophy and multiple neuritis developed in the manufacture of explosives. (Binitrotoluene.) *J AM MED ASSOC* 70:2004–2006, 1918.

Dinoprost, prostaglandin F2α, a uterine stimulant, has been reported to cause a rise of intraocular pressure of the order of 1 to 12.5 mm Hg within 10 to 15 minutes after intravenous administration to patients, but the pressure then rapidly dropped, and no significant consequences have been reported. The pupils constricted during this reaction. A pressure rise is relatively uncommon after gradual intrauterine administration, but a transient rise of intraocular pressure to the high 20's has been reported in one young woman with open anterior chamber angles and previously normal pressure. Similar pressure responses have been reported in monkeys and lower experimental animals. Transient increase in formation of aqueous humor is believed to be the cause of the rise in pressure.

a. Kelly RGM, Starr MS: Effects of prostaglandins and a prostaglandin-antagonist on intraocular pressure and protein in the monkey eye. *CAN J OPHTHALMOL* 6:205–211, 1971.

b. Ober M, Scharrer A: Changes in intraocular pressure during prostaglandin-induced abortion. *KLIN MONATSBL AUGENHEILKD* 180:230–231, 1982.

c. Zajacz M, Torok M, Mocsary P: Effect on human eye of prostaglandin and a prostaglandin analog used to induce abortion. *IRCS MED SCI: Libr Compend* 4:316, 1976.

d. Zajacz M, Torok M: Glaucoma tolerance test with prostaglandin. *SZEMESZET* 114:220–224, 1977.

Diodone (iodopyracet, Diodrast) is a radiopaque contrast medium for intravascular and renal administration. The patient's conjunctival sac has been utilized for testing for allergy to this material. The instillation of a drop of solution causes no reaction unless there is hypersensitivity.

Ocular complications from intravenous administration have been rare, but there have been reports of mydriasis, conjunctival petechiae, retinal hemorrhages and exudates, and visual loss on the side of the injection. (See also *Radiopaque x-ray media.*)

Diphenhydramine (Benadryl) is an antihistaminic drug which has a slight atropine-like effect on the pupil and on accommodation, particularly when applied in 0.5% aqueous solution to the eye. It seldom causes ocular effects in ordinary doses administered systemically.[a,c]

An instance of severe poisoning and temporary blindness has been reported by Walsh.[225] An eighteen-month-old baby swallowed 350 mg and, despite washing out of the stomach and treatment with barbiturates, had convulsions. Subsequently the baby seemed quite blind and deaf. The pupils were large, but after ten days reacted to light, and in two to three weeks vision and hearing began to return. Recovery was complete in the course of several months. The fundi, cerebrospinal fluid, and EEGs were normal during the intoxication.

In another case of poisoning from overdosage, which occurred in a sixteen-year-old girl who took ten 50 mg capsules, the pupils became dilated and unreactive to light while the patient had visual hallucinations and behavior suggestive of acute schizophrenic reaction, all reversible and resembling atropine poisoning. Presumably the characteristics of this type of poisoning are attributable to the anticholinergic properties of diphenhydramine.[b] (Compare *Anticholinergic agents* and *Antihistamines.*)

Administration of diphenhydramine hydrochloride to weanling rats during twelve weeks produced no opacities in the lenses.[75]

a. Harris R, McGavack TH, Elias H: Action of dimethylaminoethyl benzohydryl ether hydrochloride (Benadryl) effects on the human eye. *J LAB CLIN MED* 31:1148–1152, 1946.

b. Nigro SA: Toxic psychosis due to diphenhydramine hydrochloride. *J AM MED ASSOC* 203:301–302, 1968.

c. Delaney WV: Explained anisocoria. *J AM MED ASSOC* 244:1475, 1980.

Diphenhydramine theoclate (dimenhydrinate, Dramamine), an antiemetic, has been tested for effects on vision at a dose of 300 mg in a day in normal young sailors, and was reported to adversely affect color discrimination, night vision, and stereopsis.[a]

a. Luria SM, Kinney JAS, et al: *BR J CLIN PHARMACOL* 7:585, 1979.

Diphenylcarbazone has been tested in rabbits by intravenous injection of 40 to 50 mg/kg and produced no injury of the retina nor diabetes, unlike the chemically related compound dithizone.[233]

Diphenylchloroarsine (diphenylarsine chloride) is a low-melting solid which when vaporized or dispersed is an irritant military poison.[61,129] It is lacrimogenic, but the mechanism by which it irritates nerve endings in the cornea and respiratory tract is not established. Peters has noted that this compound is an enzyme inhibitor, reacting with a single thiol group, and has inferred that the arsenical may react with an -SH group in nerve endings to produce a stimulus, and has supposed that this reaction may be slowly reversible to account for the fact that the irritation disappears.[195] (See also *Lacrimatory Action.*)

Diphenylcyanoarsine (diphenylarsinecyanide, Clark II), has been of interest as a chemical warfare agent. Its maximum irritating effect on the eyes and skin is said to appear after a latent period of four to six hours. Then there is severe irritation of the eyes with necrosis of corneal epithelium, blistering of the skin, and inflammation of the respiratory tract.[155]

Diphenyl guanidine as a dust in contact with the eye causes punctate corneal epithelial defects, and edema of lids and conjunctiva.[a,b]

   a. Kowalski Z, Bassendowska E: Toxic effects of certain vulcanizing accelerators. *MED PRACY* 16:35–43, 1965. (*Chem Abstr* 63:18930, 1965.)
   b. Tartakovskaya AI: Prophylaxis of occupational lesions of the eyes in the chemical industry. *VESTN OFTAL* 70:47–53, 1957. (*ZENTRALBL GES OPHTHALMOL* 71:258, 1957.)

Diphenylthiocarbazide has been tested in rabbits by intravenous administration of 40 to 50 mg/kg and produced no injury of the retina nor change in blood sugar, unlike dithizone.[233]

Diphenylthiourea has been tested in one rabbit by intravenous administration of 50 mg/kg, and produced no injury of the retina, nor change in blood sugar, unlike dithizone.[233]

Diphtheria toxin produced by the diphtheria bacillus has toxic effects on the eye which are very seldom seen at present, due to the rarity of diphtheria. In 1913, however, the effects of diphtheria and diphtheria toxin on the eye were of such importance that Lewin and Guillery devoted forty-one pages of their book to the subject.[153] The most common effect of diphtheria toxin on the eye was partial paralysis of accommodation. Donders in 1861 first explained that this was the basis for apparent impairment of vision which was often associated with diphtheria.[153]

   Usually disturbance of vision began about the fourth week after the beginning of the disease, although in exceptional cases vision was affected in a few days. Paralysis of accommodation characteristically was slight or moderate rather than complete. As a rule, the disturbance of accommodation affected both eyes, although not always to equal degrees. It came on gradually, and recovery was gradual, with total duration of approximately four weeks. Usually, the pupils were not abnormal, but exceptionally mydriasis and impaired response to light did accompany the paralysis of accommodation.[153]

A model of a focal demyelinating lesion in the optic chiasm and optic nerve has been produced in cats by microinjection of diphtheria toxin directly at this site. Histological observations subsequently showed scarring, but no remyelination.[b]

A high concentration of diphtheria toxin applied to an animal's eye for one hour by means of a conjunctival pack is said to have caused temporary opacification of the cornea, and edema and hyperemia of the conjunctiva.[a]

a. Ross EL, Lederer LG: Influence of some toxic substances on the inner ear. *TRANS AM OTOL SOC* 27:327–344, 1937.
b. Eames RA, Jacobson SG, McDonald WI: Pathological changes in the optic chiasm of the cat following injection of diphtheria toxin. *J NEUROL SCI* 32:381–393, 1977.

Dipivefrin (dipivalyl epinephrine, Propine), an ophthalmic adrenergic used in treatment of glaucoma, was designed to minimize some of the unwanted effects of epinephrine on the anterior segment of the eye. However, a small proportion of patients have been found to develop blepharoconjunctivitis after many months of twice daily use.[b] Fraunfelder's National Registry[312] has reported receiving notification of cases of maculopathy, but whether these and a published case[a] are coincidental or toxic manifestations is uncertain so far.

a. Mehelas TJ, Kollaritis CR, et al: Cystoid macular edema presumably induced by dipivefrin hydrochloride (Propine). *AM J OPHTHALMOL* 94:682, 1982.
b. Wandel T, Spinak M: Toxicity of dipivalyl epinephrine. *OPHTHALMOLOGY* 88:259–260, 1981.

Dipropylene glycol monomethyl ether applied to rabbit eyes caused only slight reaction, graded 2 on a scale of 10,[21,228] yet a 50% solution in water caused a transient 25% rise in intraocular pressure.[276]

Dipyridamole (Persantine), a coronary vasodilator usually taken orally, has been tested for influence on intraocular pressure by injection of 20 mg intravenously in normal human beings. It is said to have reduced resistance to aqueous outflow and to have hastened return of ocular pressure to normal after tonographic compression of the eye.[a] Elevation of ocular pressure above normal has not been reported, but tests in glaucoma are yet to be made. (See also *Vasodilator drugs.*)

a. Magdalena-Castineira J: Persantin as a vasodilator. *ARCH SOC OFTAL HISP-AM* 25:145–149, 1965. (Spanish)

Diquat (1,1'-ethylene-2,2'-dipyridylium dibromide or dichloride) is a widely used herbicide similar to Paraquat. Toxic reactions to commercial preparations containing both substances are described elsewhere under *Paraquat.*

Cataracts have been produced in rats and dogs by feeding diquat for months.[a-c,e] There has been no suggestion of cataract formation in human beings. Cataracts in animals have started at the posterior pole of the lens beginning as vacuoles with lace-like appearance, gradually spreading to involve the whole lens.[b,e] In rats, subsequently anterior and posterior synechias, hemorrhages into the vitreous, and detachment of the retina have been observed.[a] The incidence of cataracts in rats has not been affected by intensity of illumination or by amount of ascorbic acid in the diet.[a] The ascorbic acid concentration in aqueous and vitreous humors falls during cataract development. Studies by Pirie and associates on biochemical changes associated with diquat cataract in rats showed that this type of cataract differed from most other types in that the GSH glutathione concentration in the lens remained at a normal level whereas generally this concentration is diminished in cataracts.[c] Evidence has been presented that diquat as a free radical might reduce GSSG glutathione in the lens.[c] The reduction could involve the enzyme glutathione reductase, and could involve NADPH as an intermediate.[f] This would be a mechanism for the peculiar maintenance of near normal GSH content. Diquat free radicals may also lead to formation of superoxide radicals which in turn may react with lens constituents as part of the cataractogenic mechanism.[g]

Diquat and paraquat have been shown to bind to uveal melanin in competition with other cations by an ionic mechanism,[d] but there appears to have been no attempt to relate this to the retinal detachments already mentioned in cataractous rats.

In rats, subcutaneous injection of a lethal dose of diquat has produced extreme dilation of the pupil after many hours, but this effect on the pupil is not produced by oral administration or application of an eye drop containing 20% solution of diquat.

On rabbit eyes, one drop of a 20% solution of diquat has caused slight irritation and hyperemia of the lids and conjunctivae, persisting for two days, but no serious injury and no dilation of the pupils.[a] (See also *Paraquat* for additional information.)

a. Clark DG, Hurst EW: The toxicity of diquat. *BR J IND MED* 27:51–55, 1970.
b. Conning DM, Fletcher K, Swan AAB: Paraquat and related bipridyls. *BR MED BULL* 25:245–249, 1969.
c. Pirie A, Rees JR, Holmberg NJ: Diquat cataract in the rat. *BIOCHEM J* 114:89P, 1969.
d. Larsson B, Oskarsson A, Tjalve H: Binding of paraquat and diquat on melanin. *EXP EYE RES* 25:353–359, 1977.
e. Pirie A, Rees JR: Diquat cataract in the rat. *EXP EYE RES* 9:198–203, 1970.
f. Pirie A, Rees JR, Holmberg NJ: Diquat cataract: formation of the free radical and its reaction with constituents of the eye. *EXP EYE RES* 9:204–218, 1970.
g. Stancliffe TC, Pirie A: Production of superoxide radicals in reactions of the herbicide diquat. *FED EUR BIOCHEM SOC LETT* 17:297–299, 1971.

Disophenol (2,6-diiodo-4-nitrophenol), an anthelmintic for animals, resembles cataractogenic *dinitrophenol* in pharmacologic and toxicologic properties. In early studies, daily oral administration of very toxic dose to dogs for as long as thirty days caused no eye disturbance evident by external examination or ophthalmoscopy.[a] However, subsequently, dosage somewhat above the therapeutic was found to produce cataracts, especially in puppies.[b,c] At a therapeutic dosage of 10 mg/kg subcutaneously few opacities were produced.

a. Kaiser JA: Studies on the toxicity of disophenol (2,6-diiodo-4-nitrophenol) to dogs and rodents plus some comparisons with 2,4-dinitrophenol. *TOXICOL APPL PHARMACOL* 6:232–244, 1964.

b. Martin CL, Christmas R, Leipold HW: Formation of temporary cataracts in dogs given a disophenol preparation. *J AM VET MED ASSOC* 161:294–301, 1972.

c. Martin CL: Formation of cataracts in dogs with disophenol. *CAN VET J* 16:228–232, 1975.

Disulfiram (tetraethylthiuram disulfide, bis(diethyl thiocarbamoyl) disulfide, Antabuse, Abstensil, Esperal), has been used for treatment for chronic alcoholism. Acetaldehyde, formed normally from ethyl alcohol, reaches excessive concentrations when disulfiram or its breakdown products interfere with acetaldehyde detoxication. Disulfiram itself is broken down to diethyldithiocarbamate and carbon disulfide.[c] Patients who drink alcohol while taking disulfiram suffer vasodilation of the neck and face, increase in heart and respiratory rates, followed by nausea, vomiting, and decreased blood pressure. Reactions may be alarming but rarely fatal.

During the reaction to alcohol induced by disulfiram, there has been described in the eye a complete circulatory arrest in some of the retinal arterioles, with fall in retinal diastolic pressure, and subsequent elevation of the pressure to a level which the observer thought to be dangerous.[b]

Bilateral optic neuritis has been caused by disulfiram in several cases.[a, d-i, k-o, 255] Characteristically after several months of regular dosage of disulfiram, with alcohol intake stopped, but usually with tobacco smoking continuing, visual acuity has greatly decreased due to central or cecocentral scotoma. Color sense is then abnormal. In the fundus, typically no abnormality is seen, but hyperemia of the optic nervehead has been described.[h] The retrobulbar neuritis generally improves when the disulfiram is discontinued, but it can return if the drug is given again. Usually recovery of vision is complete within a few weeks after stopping disulfiram, but in exceptional cases slight impairment of vision has persisted, associated with pallor of the nervehead.[n] Peripheral neuritis, both motor and sensory from axonal degeneration, has also been caused by disulfiram, and may accompany the retrobulbar neuritis.[a, i, j, m, 273]

There are several reviews of the pharmacology and toxicology of disulfiram.[c, j, l, m]

A question has been raised whether the zinc concentration in the serum may be abnormal in optic neuropathy from disulfiram; in one patient tested the concentration was 0.95 mg/l, compared to mean normal of 1.093 mg/l.[k] (Also see INDEX for *Zinc systemic level.*)

a. Corydon L: Optic neuritis and polyneuropathy and disulfiram (Antabuse) therapy. *UGESKR LAEG* 135:1470–1472, 1973. (English abstract)

b. Debrousse JY: Systematic examination of the fundus of the eye in the treatment of alcoholism by tetraethylthiuram disulfide. *SEM HOP PARIS* 26:4132–4133, 1950. (French)

c. Fischer R, Brantner H: Metabolism of disulfiram. *ARZNEIMITTEL-FORSCH* 17:1461–1464, 1967. (German)

d. Humblet M: Chronic retrobulbar neuritis from antabuse. *BULL SOC BELGE OPHTALMOL* 104:297, 1953. (French)

e. Kirk L: Should we continue to use disulfiram (Antabuse). *UGESKR LAEG* 135:1481–1482, 1973.

f. Maugery J, Magnard P, Villon JC: Optic neuritis in the course of treatment with esperal. *BULL SOC OPHTALMOL FRANCE* 74:779–781, 1974. (French)

g. Norton AL, Walsh FB: Disulfiram-induced optic neuritis. *TRANS AM ACAD OPHTHAL-MOL OTOL* 76:1263–1265, 1972.

h. Perdriel G, Chevaleraud J: Concerning a new case of optic neuritis due to disulfiram. *BULL SOC OPHTALMOL FRANCE* 66:159–165; *ANN OCULIST (PARIS)* 199:810–811, 1966. (French)

i. Pommier, Reiss-Byron M: Retrobulbar neuritis from disulfiram. *BULL SOC OPHTAL-MOL FRANCE* 63:254–256, 1963. (French)

j. Rainey JM Jr: Disulfiram toxicity and carbon disulfide poisoning. *AM J PSYCHIATRY* 134:371–378, 1977.

k. Saraux H, Bechetoille A, et al: The decrease in serum zinc concentration in certain toxic optic neuritides. *ANN OCULIST (PARIS)* 208:29–31, 1975. (French)

l. Van Oye R: Disulfiram. *BULL SOC BELGE OPHTALMOL* 160:484–485, 1972. (French)

m. Wise JD: Disulfiram toxicity—a review of the literature. *ARK MED J* 78:87–92, 1981.

n. Woillez M, Asseman R, Blervacque A: Drug-induced toxic neuritis in the course of alcohol detoxification. *BULL SOC FRANC OPHTALMOL* 75:350–355, 1962. (French)

o. Saraux H, Biais B: Optic neuritis from disulfiram. *ANN OCULIST (PARIS)* 203:769–774, 1970. (French)

Dithiazanine iodide (Delvex, Omni-Passin), a green-colored compound used as a broad spectrum anthelmintic, may cause bluish green discoloration of the normally white sclera and the skin, but no harm from this has been reported clinically.[4] Two people pressing powdered drug into tablets were exposed to enough dust in the course of a week to develop faint blue discoloration of the conjunctiva and slight hyperemia and swelling of the plica semilunaris, but with a change in occupation this all cleared in 10 days.[a]

Rabbits exposed to a 1% suspension of dithiazanine iodide in physiologic salt solution applied as an eye drop three times a day developed similar blue discoloration of the conjunctiva.[a] However, with repeated application of the suspension, in 6 days they developed conjunctival inflammation, and a few days later extensive corneal opacification, with ulceration of the cornea in some animals. The corneas were diffusely infiltrated with leucocytes, and the conjunctivae were necrotic. This exposure was far far more severe than anything that might be expected clinically.

a. Eichholtz W, Goebel HH, Muller-Lotz P: Conjunctival and corneal damage from dithiazanine iodide. *KLIN MONATSBL AUGENHEILKD* 165:656–660, 1974.

2,2'-Dithiobis (benzothiazole) (MBTS, Benzothiazyl Disulfide), an accelerator in the rubber industry, is very irritating to the eyes when in the air as a dust.[a]

a. Kowalski Z, Bassendowska E: Toxic effects of certain vulcanization accelerators. *MED PRACY* 16:35–43, 1965. (*CHEM ABSTR* 63:18930, 1965.)

Dithizone (diphenylthiocarbazone) is a substance which chelates metals. Administered experimentally to animals, it induces diabetes and causes changes in the ocular fundus and lens. In rabbits intravenous administration of 50 to 100 mg/kg causes disappearance of the ERG in three to four hours, at which time hypoglycemia is extreme. In the same animals chorioretinal lesions become visible ophthalmoscopically in about twelve hours.[b,f] Changes in the lens epithelium are detectable by electron microscopy in about six hours; and by clinical methods, incipient cataract is recognizable in the region of the equator in about thirty-six to ninety-six hours.[k] Changes in the retina are detectable by light microscopy in forty hours, as degeneration in Muller's cells, then disappearance of rods and cones, migration of pigment cells, and proliferation of glia.[f, 206]

The retinopathy in rabbits can be produced by doses of dithizone too small to cause diabetes, according to Sorsby and Harding.[233] In the damaged retina, Reading and Sorsby have found elevation of the total sulfhydryl content and have postulated an effect on a specific protein.[207] A sulfhydryl compound, thioctic acid, administered by Alagna had partially protective effect.[a] In dithizone-damaged retinas the monoamine oxidase content has been shown to be reduced.[i]

In rats, special attention has been called to unusual osmiophilic inclusion bodies discovered in the retinal pigment epithelium by electron microscopy after intraperitoneal injection of dithizone or 1,10-phenanthroline.[m]

In dogs, intravenous administration of 25 mg/kg per day has caused inflammation of the anterior segment of the eyes in one to five days, and then progressive clouding of the vitreous, retinal edema, retinal hemorrhages, and exudative detachment, occasionally with cataract.[e, g, l] Histologically the eyes show edema and degeneration of the choroid, necrosis and extreme edema of the tapetum, with later migration of pigment into edematous and degenerated retina.[g] The degenerative changes in the tapetum lucidum and in the choroid and retina in dogs have been thought to be related to chelation of zinc in the tapetum by dithizone.[e, g, l]

The eyes of rabbits have less zinc in the tapetum, and less toxic chorioretinal reaction than dogs. The zinc content of the rabbit's eye is not altered by dithizone according to Galin.[e, h]

The eyes of monkeys and human beings, which have no zinc-containing tapetum, seem to have been unaffected by dithizone. In human beings, dithizone has been used medically in treatment of prostatic cancer, and there seem to be no reports of toxic effects on the eyes of patients so treated.

a. Alagna G: Thioctic acid in poisoning by dithizone. *ARCH OTTALMOL* 64:75–86, 1960. (Italian)

b. Babel J, Ziv B: The action of dithizone on the retina of the rabbit. *EXPERIENTIA* 13:122–123, 1957.

c. Bailar JC, Busch DH: *The Chemistry of the Coordination Compounds.* New York, Reinhold, 1056, p. 692.

d. Bietti GB, Porta CF: Investigation of the influence exerted by some poisonous substances on the retinal neuroepithelium and on the cochleo-vestibular apparatus. *RIV OTONEUROOFTAL* 34:249–271, 1959. (Italian)

e. Budinger JM: Diphenylthiocarbazone blindness in dogs. *ARCH PATHOL* 71:304–310, 1961.

f. Butturini U, Grignolo A, Baronchelli A: "Diabetes" from dithizone: metabolic, ocular and histologic aspects. *G CLIN MED* 34:1253–1347, 1953. (Italian)

g. Delahunt CS, Stebbins RB, et al: The cause of blindness in dogs given hydroxypyridinethione. *TOXICOL APPL PHARMACOL* 4:286–291, 1962.

h. Galin MA, Nano HD, Hall T: Ocular zinc concentration. *INVEST OPHTHALMOL* 1:142–147, 1962.

i. Mizuno K: Studies on retinitis pigmentosa. *EYE EAR NOSE THROAT MONTHLY* 39:493–499, 1960.

j. Paganoni C, Manuelli G: Thoughts on the changes in the retina induced by dithizone. *ANN OTTALMOL CLIN OCUL* 88:185–192, 1962. (Italian)

k. Tokunaga T: Studies on early lens changes of experimental cataract. *ACTA SOC OPHTHALMOL JPN* 62B:1383–1399, 1958.

l. Weitzel G, Strecker FJ, et al: Zinc in the tapetum lucidum. *Z PHYSIOL CHEM HOPPE-SEYLER'S* 296:19–30, 1954. (German)

m. Leure-duPree AE: Electron-opaque inclusions in the rat retinal pigment epithelium after treatment with chelators of zinc. *INVEST OPHTHALMOL VIS SCI* 21:1–9, 1981.

Dithranol (1,8,9-anthracenetriol; Anthralin) has been employed in ointment or cream for treatment of chronic dermatoses in a manner similar to chrysarobin. It is very irritating if it comes in contact with the eyes; for this reason it is not recommended to be applied to the scalp or near the eyes.[171] In pharmaceutical manufacture, fumes of dithranol have caused lacrimation and photophobia.[176] (See also, *Dithranol triacetate*).

Dithranol triacetate (1,8,9-triacetoxyanthracene; Exolan) has been used as a substitute for dithranol to reduce the incidence of burning and staining of the skin, but this derivative also is very irritating to the eyes.[e] In three cases in which apparently there was unintended contamination of the eyes with Exolan ointment or cream a strikingly severe edema of the epithelium and stroma of the cornea developed, but with surprisingly little discomfort in two of the cases.[a,c] The third patient had pain and blurring of vision to 20/200 owing to edema of the corneal epithelium and stroma, with folds in Descemet's membrane, flare, but no cells in the aqueous humor, and tension elevated to 29 mm Hg in both eyes.[a] The condition of the angles of the anterior chambers was obscured by the corneal edema, but it was thought that the glaucoma was secondary to the iritis. The corneas and the anterior chambers cleared in nineteen days.

On rabbit eyes, application of a drop of a suspension of Exolan, containing the equivalent of 2% dithranol triacetate, caused no immediate signs of injury, but three hours later, superficial staining with fluorescein, fine folds in Descemet's membrane, and an appreciable increase in thickness of the cornea were noted. Gross edema and opacity of the cornea developed in six days and cleared slowly, beginning sixteen days from exposure. Vascularization developed both superficially and in the corneal stroma, but the corneas grossly cleared in about five weeks. Surprisingly, histologic studies suggested no significant injury to the endothelium.[b,d] In rabbit tests of Exolan comparing the effects of the whole preparation and of the vehicle alone have demonstrated that the chemical rather than the vehicle has been responsible for the toxic effects.[b]

The manufacturer of Exolan has pointed out that the triacetate hydrolyzes to release a therapeutically active intermediate, *1,8-diacetoxy-9-anthranol*, forming a small amount of acetic acid in the process.[f] The characteristics of the corneal injury suggest that it is not the acetic acid that is responsible for the injury, but rather an anthranol derivative. This is also consistent with the fact that dithranol itself, which does not release any acetic acid, is also very irritating to the eye.

New evidence has been presented that skin inflammation from dithranol is induced by a mechanism involving free radicals.[g] This has, however, been contested.[h]

a. Brodkin RH, Bleiberg J: Ophthalmologic side effects of a new topical psoriatic medication. *ARCH DERMATOL* 98:525, 1968.
b. Easty DL, Mathalone MBR: Toxicity of 1,8,9-triacetoxyanthracene to the cornea in rabbits. *BR J OPHTHALMOL* 53:819–823, 1969.
c. Mathalone MBR, Easty DL: Acute keratitis in psoriatic patients using triacetoxyanthracene. *LANCET* 2:195, 1967.
d. Mathalone MBR, MacFaul PA: Toxic effects of drugs on the cornea. In Pigott PV (Ed.): *Evaluation of Drug Effects on the Eye.* London, F.J. Parsons, 1968.
e. Today's drugs: Triacetoxyanthracene. *BR MED J* 1:682, 1967.
f. Yarrow H: Keratitis from triacetoxyanthracene. *LANCET* 2:311, 1967.
g. Finnen MJ, Lawrence CM, Shuster S: Inhibition of dithranol inflammation by free-radical scavengers. *LANCET* 2:1129–1130, 1984.
h. Whitefield M, Leeder GMA, Mosedale AR: Inhibition of dithranol inflammation by free-radical scavengers. *LANCET* 1:173, 1985.

Diving mask defogger, chemical mixtures which are applied to the inside of scuba divers' masks to prevent fogging, have caused transient injury of the corneal epithelium in two cases in which they were not used according to manufacturer's instructions.[a] An excessive amount was applied, and was not adequately buffed, or allowed to dry sufficiently before wearing. One patient, using a preparation composed of 70% isopropyl alcohol, ammonium lauryl sulfate and neutral methoxy phenols, had no immediate discomfort, but for about 30 minutes had blurring with haloes, and after an hour had burning sensation, photophobia and blepharospasm. This was attributable to diffuse superficial punctate keratitis (keratitis epithelialis). The patient was completely well by the next day. The other patient, using a preparation composed of surface-active agents and polyglycols, had no symptoms until about 3 hours after surfacing he developed the same symptoms and disturbance of the cornea as the first patient, with the same complete recovery by the next day.

a. Wright WL: Scuba diver's delayed toxic epithelial keratopathy from commercial mask defogging agents. *AM J OPHTHALMOL* 93:470–472, 1982.

Divinyl sulfone can be derived from mustard gas and can cause burns of the skin and eyes similar to those from mustard gas, but divinyl sulfone differs in having no chlorine and liberating no acid. Divinyl sulfone can cause injury and enzyme inhibition by condensing with amino and other groups.[a,b] This knowledge has helped establish that mustard gas owes its toxicity to its alkylating properties rather than to liberation of acid as postulated in pre-World War II concepts.)

Little has been published concerning wartime investigations of divinyl sulfone, but information made public in 1960 indicates that in industrial use the substance is a lacrimator and that animal experiments show it can cause severe skin and eye burns. Its toxicity by oral administration compares with that of acrylonitrile.[c]

Under the name "vinyl sulfone", tests on rabbit eyes have shown injuriousness graded greater than 5 on a scale of 10, indicating severe burn from 0.005 ml.[228]

In treatment of skin or eyes contaminated with divinyl sulfone the usual immediate copious irrigation with water is appropriate. Attempts to counteract with oxidizing agents are useless. Studies on an isolated enzyme system[b] suggest that competing agents with highly reactive sulfhydryl groups, such as dimercaprol or mercaptoethanol, applied immediately after exposure may provide partial protection from injury. These agents, would, however, be of no use after a few minutes, once the divinyl sulfone had reacted with the tissue.

Evidences of burns of eyes and skin may be expected after a latent period, as with alkylating agents. Late treatment is nonspecific.

a. Boursnell JC, Francis GE, Wormall A: The action of mustard gas, β,β'-dichlorodiethyl sulfone and divinyl sulfone on amino acids. *BIOCHEM J* 40:737, 1946.
b. Grant WM, Kinsey VE: Factors influencing the inactivation of urease by alkylating agents. *J BIOL CHEM* 165:485–493, 1946.
c. Union Carbide Chemicals Company. Information sheet F-40351, June 1960.

Dixyrazine (Esucos), a phenothiazine tranquilizer available in Europe, has caused severe blepharo-conjunctivitis in four reported cases, associated with ichthyosis, hair loss and depigmentation, but recovery when use of the drug was discontinued.[a]

a. Poulsen J: Hair loss, depigmentation of hair, ichthyosis, and blepharoconjunctivitis produced by dixyrazine. *ACTA DERM VENEREOL* 61:85–88, 1981.

Dodine (dodecylguanidine acetate, Cyprex), an agricultural fungicide, has been reported by a manufacturer to cause severe irritation of the skin and eyes when there is contact with strong solutions, but that usual spray concentrations have little effect.[70]

Dopamine, closely related to levodopa has been tested for effects on the pupil by applying eyedrops containing 10% dopamine hydrochloride and has produced mydriasis without affecting accommodation. (The influence on intraocular pressure was not measured.) The mydriatic effect was blocked by topical guanethidine. This supports the belief that dopamine acts indirectly by releasing noradrenalin from adrenergic nerve endings.[a] Large doses systemically have also produced mydriasis.[c]

Studies of retinal activity in cats have shown a decrease in amplitude of electric potential in the optic tract evoked by exposure of the eye to light flashes, after intravenous administration of levodopa, and also a depressant effect on retinal ganglion cell activity from dopamine hydrochloride applied directly.[b] No visual effects in human beings have been reported so far from either compound. (See also *Levodopa.*)

a. Spiers ASD, Calne DB: Action of dopamine on the human iris. *BR MED J* Nov. 8, 1969, pp. 333–335.
b. Straschill M, Perwin J: Inhibition of retinal ganglion cells by catechol amines. *PFLUEGER ARCH* 312:42–54, 1969. (*Chem Abstr* 72:2038, 1970.)
c. Bruining HA, Ong GL: Dilated pupils not responding to light observed in five patients during administration of dopamine. *MED TIJDSCHR GENEESKD* 124:838–839, 1980. (Dutch)

Dowtherm-A is a mixture of diphenyloxide (75%) and diphenyl (25%). It has a high boiling point and low vapor pressure. When concentrations of 3 or 4 ppm in air are reached, there is irritation of the eyes, nose, and throat.[a] In one instance a man received in the eyes a spray of fine droplets of Dowtherm under pressure. He felt no immediate discomfort, but within five minutes he began to feel stinging and burning of the eyes and also of the skin about his eyes; his discomfort was relieved immediately when the eyes and skin were washed with a bland oil. Slit-lamp biomicroscopic examination shortly thereafter revealed no corneal injury.[81] In four other cases listed as corneal burns from diphenyl oxide, recovery was complete within forty-eight hours.[165]

    a. Dowtherm-A. *AM PETROL INST TOXIC REV,* September, 1948.

Doxapram (Dopream), a CNS stimulant for respiratory depression, has been examined toxicologically in dogs. Overdosage caused constriction of cerebral vessels and reduced cerebral blood flow and produced tissue anoxia secondary to respiratory stimulation and loss of carbon dioxide. Petechial and perivascular hemorrhages were found throughout the brain, but, surprisingly, histologic examination showed no abnormality in the eyes or optic nerves.[a,b]

    a. Funderburk WH, Oliver KL, Ward JW: Modification of cerebral blood flow in dogs with doxapram hydrochloride. *TOXICOL APPL PHARMACOL* 13:67–75, 1968.

    b. Ward JW, Gilbert DL, et al: Toxicologic studies of doxapram hydrochloride. *TOXICOL APPL PHARMACOL* 13:242–250, 1968.

Doxorubicin (adriamycin), an antineoplastic, has been tested for toxicity in the vitreous cavity of rabbit eyes.[277,369] After extracapsular lens extraction and vitrectomy, 5 μg/ml of infusion fluid was non-toxic to the retina.

Drano® is the proprietary name for a drain cleaner available in two different forms, a granular solid and a liquid. These have vastly different effects on the eye. Drano in granular solid form consists mainly of sodium hydroxide, which can produce devastating damage to the eye. (See *Alkalies* and *Sodium hydroxide*.) Liquid Drano consists mainly of 1,1,1-trichloroethane, which, though irritating on contact with the eye, does not produce serious damage. (See *1,1,1-Trichloroethane*.)

Drazoxolon, a fungicide, has been tested on rabbit eyes by application of a 10% suspension. This caused only slight immediate irritation. The eyes were normal within an hour and remained normal during seven days observation.[a]

    a. Clark DG, McElligott TF: Acute and short-term toxicity of Drazoxolon (4-(2-Chl orophenylhydrazone)-3-methyl-5-isoxazolone). *FOOD COSMET TOXIC* 7:481–491, 1969.

Droperidol (Inapsine; component of Innovar), an antipsychotic, has produced oculogyric crises, effects similar to those associated with phenothiazine tranquilizers.[a,d] It has not raised ocular pressure in nonglaucomatous patients when used as an adjuvant in general anesthesia.[b] In rabbits it is reported to cause a preliminary small rise of ocular pressure, then a reduction.[c] It does have some anticholinergic activity. (See *Anticholinergics*.)

    a. Freeman JE, Robertson AC, Ngan H: Oculogyric crises due to phenothiazines. *BR MED J* Sept. 16, 1967, p. 738.

b. Pontinen PJ, Miettinen P, Reinikainen M: Neuroleptanalgesia in cataract surgery. *ACTA OPHTHALMOL SUPPL* 80:10–36, 1966.

c. Ramos L, Ramos AO: Influence of tranquilizers derived from butyrophenone on the intraocular pressure of the rabbit. *REV FAC FARM BIOQUIM S PAULO* 4:259–263, 1966.

d. Patton CM Jr: Rapid induction of acute dyskinesia by droperidol. *ANESTHESIOLOGY* 43:126, 1975.

Duraluminum, an aluminum alloy containing small amounts of copper and magnesium, has been tested by insertion of fragments into eyes of rabbits. In the vitreous body it often was without adverse effect, and in the anterior chamber caused less reaction than bronze.[a]

a. Afaunov AL: Characteristics of the reaction of eye tissues to some fragments of nonferrous metals. *MATER NAUCHNO-PRAKT KONF OFTALMOL SEV KAVK* 5th:38–40, 40–43, 1974. (*Chem Abstr* 85:73062, 73063).

Dusts of very great variety have been discussed in detail by Jaensch (1958) concerning their effects on the eye.[129] Dusts having chemical or toxic effect on the eye are described in the present work under individual subject headings, but those having purely physical action are not included. (See INDEX).

Dyes—*(1) Introduction.* There is a voluminous history dating from 1888 concerning contact injury of the eye by the so-called aniline dyes which are used in dyeing fabrics, in staining tissues in histology, and in manufacture of colored pencils. This was particularly well reviewed by Wagenmann in 1913.[253] Early in the manufacture of aniline dyes, people who worked in their preparation, or their use in dyeing cloth, suffered injuries principally from accidental contamination of the eyes with the powdered material, more rarely from splashed solution. Often the powder caused severe conjunctival inflammation, and in numerous cases it caused injury of the cornea, which was superficial in most instances, but sometimes involved the deeper layers. This was accompanied by swelling of the lids, hyperemia, and swelling of the conjunctiva, with much tearing.

When the cornea was affected, it had a lusterless appearance with erosions of the epithelium and faint superficial opacity and vascularization. In more severe cases, corneal infiltrates, ulceration, and scarring occurred. In the majority of cases the eyes recovered, but in some patients recovery was slow, and in the severe cases corneal opacities and visual disturbance remained.

A peculiar brownish discoloration of the cornea and conjunctivae developed in people who worked for long periods over steaming vats of dyes, due to the action of oxidation products, quinones, in the steam from the vats. This sometimes had serious late consequences. (The characteristics are described elsewhere under *Quinones,* and under *Hydroquinone;* see INDEX for page numbers.)

Classic studies on ocular toxicity of dyes performed by Graeflin in 1903 and Vogt in 1905 and 1906 included reports on a total of ninety-four cases of injury in human beings and presented results of extensive experiments on rabbits.[78,250,251] Experimental studies were also published by Kuwahara in 1903.[141] The conclusions from these studies was that the injurious dyes were the so-called basic or cationic dyes, and that the so-called acid or anionic dyes were noninjurious. Since that time many more dyes have been tested on rabbit eyes.[81] The results generally have supported the earlier fundamental distinction that was made between cationic and anionic dyes, the cationic regularly showing the greater toxicity to the eye.

Dyes—*(2) Tests on the Eyes.* Most commonly, dyes have been tested on the eyes of rabbits, either by application of 4 to 8 mg of powdered dye to the conjunctival sac[78,250,251] or by irrigating the surface of the eye for ten minutes with 0.02 M solution near neutrality after the epithelium has been removed to facilitate penetration.[81] The results have been observed usually during several weeks. The effects on the eyes have generally not been reported according to any numerical system of grading, but rather in terms of clinical description. In a few instances tests have been made on human eyes after tests on rabbits demonstrated lack of injury. More information on effects on human eyes has come from accidental contamination.

Dyes—*(3) Information on Individual Dyes.* In the following alphabetical list of dyes I have tried to summarize information on ocular toxicity for each from tests on rabbits and human beings, and from reported accidental contaminations. When the statement is made that a dye was "not damaging in rabbit eye test," which is usual in the case of anionic dyes, this means that it caused no more than slight transient irritation when tested as described in foregoing subsection *(2) Tests on the Eyes.* When the statement is made that a dye is "moderately injurious" or "injurious", which is more usual in the case of cationic dyes, this means that it caused injury ranging in severity from conjunctival edema, hyperemia, and purulent discharge to total opacification and even necrosis and sloughing of the corneal stroma. The type of severe damage often produced by cationic dyes is described further, and its possible mechanism is discussed, in subsection *(4) Mechanisms of Injury.*

Acid Fuchsin; anionic; not damaging in rabbit eye test.[81,250,251]

Acid green; anionic; not damaging in rabbit eye test.[250,251]

Acid rhodamin 3R; anionic; not damaging in rabbit eye test.[250,251]

Acridine red; cationic; moderately injurious to rabbit eye.[81]

Acridine yellow; cationic; moderately injurious to rabbit eye.[81,250,251]

Acridine orange; cationic; 0.1% applied 3 times in 2 hours to eyes with herpes of the cornea produced no adverse effect.[zj]

Acriflavine; cationic; injurious to rabbit eye.[81]

Alcian blue; cationic dye of varied composition containing copper; injurious to rabbit eye in standardized testing,[81] but not damaging at 0.25% concentration applied once,[zf] and clinically useful at this concentration for staining and studying mucous on the surface of the eye, not staining normal epithelial cells.[t, u, z] In several instances 0.25% to 1% solution applied to corneas with areas lacking a covering of epithelium caused discoloration deep in the cornea lasting as long as six months.[t, u, za]

Alizarin red S; anionic; not damaging in rabbit eye test;[81] has been used as 1% single-instillation eye drop for vital staining of outer surface of cornea and conjunctiva in a series of patients without adverse effect.[zd]

Alkali violet; cationic; injurious to rabbit and human eye.[250, 251]

Amaranth; anionic; not damaging in rabbit eye test.[81]

Amethyst violet; cationic; injurious to rabbit eye.[81]

Aniline blue W.S.; anionic; not damaging in rabbit eye test.[78, 81]

Anisolin conc.; cationic; injurious to rabbit eye.[250, 251]

Anthracene red; anionic; not damaging in rabbit eye test.[81]

Auramine; cationic; injurious to rabbit and human eye.[78, 81, 153, 250, 251]

Aurin tricarboxylate; anionic; not damaging in rabbit eye test.[81] (See also *Beryllium* injury treatment.)

Azocarmine B; anionic; not damaging in rabbit eye test.[81]

Benzidine yellow; was introduced accidentally through the skin into the upper lid by injury with the tip of a yellow pencil, producing a persistent granuloma, which was reproduced and studied histologically in mice.[o]

Benzyl green; anionic; not damaging in rabbit eye test.[250, 251]

Biebrich scarlet; anionic; not damaging in rabbit eye test.[81]

Bindschedler's green; cationic; injurious to rabbit eye.[81] A trial therapeutic application has been made of sodium hydrosulfite to reduce and bleach Bindschedler's Green. After removal of the corneal epithelium, 0.01 M solution of the dye at pH 4.5 was applied to rabbit eyes for ten minutes, followed by irrigation with 1% neutral sodium hydrosulfite for ten minutes, which caused immediate bleaching of the green-stained cornea to light yellow, but this did not prevent subsequent development of severe opacification and vascularization. The degree of injury was the same as in control green-stained eyes irrigated only with saline.[81]

Bismarck brown; cationic; moderately injurious to rabbit eye.[250, 251]

Brilliant cresyl blue; cationic; injurious to rabbit eye.[81]

Brilliantfirnblau; cationic; injurious to rabbit eye.[250,251]

Brilliant green; cationic; injurious to rabbit and human eye.[m,250,251] In one patient an attempt to treat conjunctivitis with 1% solution of this dye resulted in destructive keratitis with hypopyon and terminated in bilateral blindness due to corneal opacification.[m]

Brilliant green disulfonic acid; anionic; not damaging in rabbit eye test.[250,251]

Brilliant phosphin 5G; cationic; injurious to rabbit eye.[250,251]

Brilliant Victoria blue RB; cationic; injurious to rabbit eye.[250,251]

Brilliant yellow; anionic; not damaging in rabbit eye test.[81]

Bromcresol green; anionic; not damaging in rabbit eye test.[81]

Bromthymol blue; anionic; a drop of 0.2% solution on human eyes caused no damage detectable with the slit-lamp biomicroscope.[w]

Chrysoidine; cationic; moderately injurious to rabbit eye.[250,251]

Chrysoidine Y; anionic; not damaging in rabbit eye test.[81]

Chrysophenin; anionic; not damaging in rabbit eye test.[250,251]

Clematin; cationic; injurious to rabbit eye.[250,251]

Congo red; anionic; not damaging in rabbit eye test,[78,81,123] and it has been applied as a drop of 1% solution to human eyes as a vital stain, without toxic effects.[ze]

Coriphosphine; cationic; injurious to rabbit eye.[81]

Crystal violet; cationic; injurious to rabbit and human eye.[78,123,153,250,251] Ballantyne has provided detailed dose-response information and description of the characteristics of injury in rabbit eyes, with measurement of rise and fall of intraocular pressure.[c,276] It can produce severe permanent damage to the cornea.[c] (See closely related *Gentian violet* for description of injuries to human eyes.)

Delphine blue conc.; anionic; not damaging in rabbit eye test.[250,251]

Diamond fuchsin; cationic; injurious to rabbit eye.[250,251]

Diphenyl blue; anionic; not damaging in rabbit eye test.[78]

Direct black; anionic; not damaging in rabbit eye test.[78]

Echtblau 2B; cationic; injurious to rabbit eye.[250,251]

Eosin; anionic; not damaging in rabbit eye test.[250,251]

Eosin Y; anionic; not damaging in rabbit eye test.[78,81]

Erioglaucin A; anionic; not damaging in rabbit eye test.[250,251]

Erioviolet; anionic; not damaging in rabbit eye test.[250,251]

Erythrosin; anionic; not damaging in rabbit eye test.[250,251]

Erythrosin bluish; anionic; not damaging in rabbit eye test.[81]

Ethyl violet; cationic; injurious to rabbit eye.[141,250,251]

Evans blue; anionic; not damaging in rabbit eye test.[81]

Fast green FCT; anionic; not damaging in rabbit eye test.[81]

Fluorescein; anionic; not damaging in rabbit and human eye test.[81,123] (Additional information on *fluorescein* is given separately elsewhere; see INDEX for page number.)

Fuchsin, basic; cationic; moderately injurious to rabbit eye.[250,251]

Gentian violet; cationic; closely related to crystal violet, injurious to rabbit and human eyes.[zh,141,153] (Details of two cases of injury of human eyes are given elsewhere under another heading for *Gentian violet;* see INDEX for page number.)

Hair dyes and their components are described elsewhere under separate heading for *Hair dyes;* see INDEX for page number.)

Helianthin G; anionic; not damaging in rabbit eye test.[250,251]

Henna is described separately elsewhere; see INDEX for page number.

Homacridine yellow; cationic; injurious to rabbit eye.[250,251]

Indelible pencils are described separately elsewhere; see INDEX for page number.

Indigo; cationic; injurious to rabbit eye.[153]

Indocyanine green (Cardio-Green); anionic; used clinically in angiography, has been tested at 1% in rabbit anterior chamber as vital stain for the corneal endothelium without causing abnormal swelling of the cornea,[l,p] but when injected into the vitreous cavity it caused a decrease in the number of ganglion cells.[l]

Indoin; cationic; injurious to rabbit eye.[250,251]

Iodonitrotetrazolium; cationic; not damaging to rabbit eyes or to human eyes as a vital stain,[y,zf] but in several instances when applied in combination with *Acian blue* to eyes with areas of cornea lacking a covering epithelium it has produced long-persisting discoloration.[za]

Janus black; cationic; injurious to rabbit eye.[81]

Janus green B; cationic; injurious to rabbit eye.[81] The acid mucopolysaccharides of rabbit corneas are altered after induction of corneal edema by injection into the anterior chamber. This dye has also proved very toxic to the endothelium of the cornea.[s]

Jasmin; anionic; not damaging in rabbit eye test.[250,251]

Lissamine green; anionic; as single-application 1% eye drops has been utilized clinically as a vital stain for cornea and conjunctiva, with no evident toxicity.[zb]

Malachite green; cationic; injurious to rabbit and human eye.[78,123,153,250,251]

Meldola blue; cationic; injurious to rabbit eye.[81]

Mepacrin (Quinacrine); cationic; injurious to rabbit eye.[81]

Merbromin; anionic; not damaging in rabbit and human eye tests.[186]

Metanil yellow; anionic; not damaging in rabbit eye test.[250,251]

Methyl blue; anionic; either slightly[81] or not damaging in rabbit eye test.[250,251]

Methyl green; cationic; injurious to rabbit and human eye.[81,250,251]

Methyl orange; anionic; not damaging in rabbit eye test.[81]

Methyl rosaniline; cationic; injurious to rabbit eye.[h]

Methyl violet; cationic; injurious to rabbit and human eye.[81,141,153,250,251] In rabbit eyes after staining with 1% *methyl violet* solution slight benefit appears to have been obtained in occasional animals by irrigation with 10% alcohol or 1% acetic acid.[e] Stronger solutions of alcohol or acetic acid actually had detrimental effect. More information on this dye is given separately elsewhere; see *Methyl violet* in the INDEX for page number.)

Methylene blue; cationic; injurious to rabbit and human eyes.[78,81,123,250,251] In the anterior chamber of rabbits has caused reversible anterior subcapsular cataract.[d] Applied chronically in dilute form in eyedrops it has been known to discolor the eye.[r,zi] (More information on this dye is given separately elsewhere; see *Methylene blue* in the INDEX for page number.)

Methylene green; cationic; injurious to rabbit eye.[250,251]

Mimosa; anionic; not damaging in rabbit eye test.[250,251]

Naphtho yellow S; anionic; not damaging in rabbit eye test.[250,251]

Neutral red vital stain; cationic, but not damaging in rabbit eye test,[81] and tested as 0.1% eye drop in photodynamic treatment of corneal herpes simplex in rabbits without evident toxicity.[a] However, in vitro the treatment caused significant changes in stromal and epithelial corneal cells.[n]

New blue R; cationic; injurious to rabbit eye.[250,251]

New fuchsin; cationic; injurious to rabbit eye.[81]

Niagara sky blue 6B; administered intraperitoneally to pregnant rats caused eye anomalies in the offspring, including anophthalmia and microphthalmia.[b]

Night blue; cationic; injurious to rabbit and human eye.[250,251]

Orange II; anionic; not damaging in rabbit eye test.[250,251]

Orange G; anionic; not damaging in rabbit eye test.[81]

Paraphenylenediamine is described separately elsewhere; see INDEX for page number.)

Pararosanilin; cationic; injurious to rabbit eye.[81]

Patentphosphin G; cationic; injurious to rabbit eye.[250,251]

Pheno-safranin; cationic; injurious to rabbit eye.[81,123]

p-Phenylenediamine is described separately elsewhere; see INDEX for page number.

Phloxine; anionic; not damaging in rabbit eye test.[250,251]

Phloxine B; anionic; but an apparent exception to the general rule of lack of toxicity among the anionic dyes; moderate injury with irregular opacity was produced in several rabbits by exposure for ten minutes to 0.02 M (pH 7 to 7.8) solution.[81] Chromatographically purified *Phloxine B* exhibited this unusual toxicity to the same degree as did the commercial dye.

Phosphine; cationic; moderately injurious to rabbit eye.[81]

Polyphenyl black; anionic; not damaging in rabbit eye test.[250,251]

Ponceau R, 3R; anionic; not damaging in rabbit eye test.[250,251]

Prune pure; cationic; injurious to rabbit eye.[78,153,250,251]

Quinoline yellow conc.; anionic; not damaging in rabbit eye test.[250,251]

Rhodamine B; weakly cationic; injurious to rabbit and human eye by some reports,[78,81,250,251] but not in a careful study after topical, intravitreal, or intravenous administration,[zm] also, unlike other cationic dyes, not inhibitory to corneal turgescence.[81]

Rhodamine 6G; cationic; injurious to rabbit eye.[78]

Rhodamine S; cationic; moderately injurious to rabbit eye.[250,251]

Rose Bengal; anionic; not damaging in rabbit and human eye tests,[t,u,81,123,186,250,251] including 1% concentration.[zg] This concentration injected into the interior chamber of patients undergoing surgery did not cause clinically evident injury, but when mixed with trypan blue at 0.25% it did cause corneal edema.[x] In vitro tests showed abnormally high corneal swelling rates when the endothelial cells were subjected to light in addition to very dilute rose bengal, probably due to formation of hydrogen peroxide.[j]

Safranin O; cationic; injurious to rabbit and human eye.[78,81,157]

Scarlet red O; anionic; not damaging in rabbit and human eye tests.[186]

Setocyanin; cationic; injurious to rabbit eye.[250,251]

Setoglaucin; cationic; injurious to rabbit eye.[250,251]

Spirit blue; cationic; injurious to rabbit and human eye.[78,153]

Sun yellow; anionic; not damaging in rabbit eye test.[250,251]

Tartrazine; anionic; not damaging in rabbit eye test.[153]

Thiazin blue; cationic; injurious to rabbit eye.[250,251]

Thionin; cationic; injurious to rabbit eye.[81]

Titan yellow; anionic; not damaging in rabbit eye test.[81]

Toluidine blue; cationic; injurious to rabbit eye.[81,123] Chemical analyses of corneas of rabbit eyes with swelling inhibited by 0.5% *Toluidine Blue* have shown that the hexosamine of the mucoid stays in the cornea with only slight loss in six days, in contrast to rapid disappearance of hexosamine following chemical injuries in which turgescence is not prevented.[i] This suggests that there is fixation or denaturation of corneal mucoprotein by this dye.

Trypan blue; anionic; tested by injection of 0.2 ml of 1% solution subconjunctivally in patients caused no injury.[e] A small drop at the same concentration applied to the surface of the eye in patients caused practically no irritation, and though it stained superficial tissues, especially degenerating epithelial cells and mucous, it caused no damage.[v] Filling the anterior chamber of patients undergoing cataract extraction with a 1% solution as a vital stain for the corneal endothelium appeared to have no injurious effect immediately, or in a follow-up of 8 years, and caused no abnormal increase in thickness of the cornea.[x,zc,zg] (More information on this dye is given separately elsewhere; see *Trypan blue* in the INDEX for page number.)

Victoria blue R; cationic; injurious to rabbit and human eye.[78,153,250,251]

Victoria pure blue BO; Dupont FDL 306, caused an eye injury in a patient described to me by McFadden when a large amount of solution used in paper manufacture splashed in the eyes causing intense blue staining of the lids and conjunctivae, still conspicuous the next day, also diffuse stippling of the corneal epithelium at that time, but no evidence of deeper disturbance. Hydrocortisone ointment was applied frequently and appeared fortuitously to dissolve the dye and remove it rapidly from the conjunctiva. The epithelium was lost from the center of the cornea within the next two days but soon healed completely.[q]

Victoria R.B.; cationic; injurious to rabbit and human eye.[250,251]

Violet 4RN; cationic; injurious to rabbit eye.[250,251]

Wool green; anionic; not damaging in rabbit eye test.[250,251]

Dyes—(4) Mechanisms of Injury. The typical course following exposure of rabbit eyes to toxic amounts of cationic dyes involves the following phases. Initially, during exposure, the cornea and conjunctiva become deeply colored and the stain is not removable even by copious irrigation with water. Nevertheless, by the next day most of the stain is gone spontaneously, and the cornea appears translucent grayish and only slightly tinted. Thereafter there may be increasing opacity, and within two weeks the cornea may become softened, greatly bulging and weak, sometimes necrotic and sloughing. The result is usually permanent opacification from scarring and vascularization. The stages appear to consist of initial chemical alteration and probable denaturation of the tissue, then biologic reaction to this abnormality.

The chemical basis for the toxicity of cationic dyes is not connected with any single dye type, since the list of those which are injurious to the eye includes several different structural types, such as xanthene, acridine, thiazin, azin, triphenylmethane, and indamin types. All owe their basicity or cationic nature to their amino groups. However, the toxicity of these dyes to the cornea and conjunctiva is a property peculiar to them, not shared by non-dye colorless cationic mono-, di-, and tri-amino compounds which have also been tested on rabbit cornea near neutrality in the same manner as the dyes.

For example, I have found that test applications of 0.02 M solutions at pH 5 to 7 for ten minutes to rabbit eyes from which the corneal epilthelium has been removed produced relatively slight or no injury with the following substances; *o-toluidine; p-aminoacetophenone; 2-amino-pyridine; p-phenylenediamine; 1,4-bis(aminoethyl) cyclohexane; 1,3-bis(dimethylamino)-2-propanol; pyridine;* all three *toluenediamines,* and a series of *alkyl quaternary ammonium salts from tetramethyl to tetrabutyl.*[81] Cationic dyes tested under the same conditions cause severe injury.[i]

It appears that the structural characteristics of the cationic dye molecule which endows it with color and basicity is intimately connected with production of biologic injury. The toxicity of certain cationic dyes is significantly lessened when they are reversibly reduced to colorless bases. For instance, I have observed that 0.01 M near-neutral solutions of **pararosaniline** and **thionin** after they have been reduced and rendered practically colorless by addition of 1% to 2% sodium hydrosulfite ($Na_2S_2O_4$) cause relatively slight corneal opacification when tested on rabbit eyes, whereas the same dye solutions without reduction cause severe opacification and vascularization. The cationic dyes appear to have a special attribute of a nitrogen atom which is part of the resonant system responsible for color, and which appears to be associated with a propensity to very strong binding to carboxyl groups of the corneal mucoproteins.

The evidence that cationic dyes are bound to the mucoprotein of the cornea has been obtained by chemical and histological comparison of the binding of dyes by corneas from which various amounts of mucoprotein have been removed.[g,k] These studies have shown that both cationic and anionic dyes react principally with the mucoproteins of the cornea and only slightly with collagen.[k] Examination of the relationship of binding to pH has shown that the cationic dyes interact with the carboxyl groups of the mucoproteins but not the sulfate groups. Chemical competition studies by Kern have shown that the binding of cationic dyes to the carboxyl groups of the mucoproteins is very strong, quantitatively comparable to the very strong binding of toxic trivalent rare-earth cations.[k]

Denaturation of the mucoproteins of the cornea as a consequence of the strong chemical attachment of cationic dyes may be responsible, at least in part, for disturbance of the biologic properties. Denaturation may lead to the opacification, infiltration, and necrosis of the cornea which develop sometime later than the initial chemical interaction. (Kern and I have postulated an analogous mechanism for injuries of the cornea by other cationic substances, such as metal and rare-earth ions.)

Kern and I have obtained evidence of a denaturing effect by studying the influence of test substances on the turgescence properties of the cornea. Normally, pieces of cornea placed in water swell to several times their original size, but after reaction with fixatives or other recognized denaturing agents, including many substances clinically injurious to the cornea, this tissue loses some of its capacity to absorb water and to swell. Our tests on eleven of the cationic dyes which have been found injurious to the eyes of rabbits, showed that all, *with the exception of rhodamine B,* markedly inhibited absorption of water by the cornea.[81] By contrast we found that twenty anionic dyes which were noninjurious *in vivo* caused little or no interference with *in vitro* swelling of cornea in water.[81] Pieces of cornea placed in solutions of the two types of dyes were seen to be stained by both, but only the cationic dyes significantly denatured the cornea, as evaluated by alteration of turgescence properties.

Besides reacting with extracellular mucoprotein and causing denaturation, cationic dyes penetrate into cells and stain cell nuclei more readily than do anionic dyes.[250, 251] Cationic dyes are well known to bind to nucleic acids. This may account for injurious effects on the epithelium of the cornea and conjunctiva and on bacteria, but seems less likely to account for corneal opacification than the denaturant effect on the extracellular mucoproteins of the cornea.

Chemical analyses of corneas of rabbit eyes exposed to 0.5% *toluidine blue* have shown that the hexosamine of the mucoid stays in the cornea with only slight loss in six days, in contrast to its rapid disappearance following types of chemical injury in which turgescence is not prevented.[i] This too suggests fixation or denaturation of corneal mucoprotein by cationic dyes. The acid mucopolysaccharides of rabbit corneas have also been shown by histochemical procedures to be altered after induction of corneal edema by injection of the cationic dye *Janus green B* into the anterior chamber.[s]

Among other reactions of cationic dyes of interest in relation to the eye is a strong *binding to uveal pigment granules in vitro* by certain of these dyes, demonstrated by Potts (1964) to be comparable to the binding of *chloroquine* and *chlorpromazine.*[203] The dyes *acridine orange, neutral red,* and *methylene blue* are taken up by the pigment granules to a greater extent than chlorpromazine. *Alizarin red,* an anionic dye, is taken up similarly. Whether there may be toxic effects *in vivo* related to these interactions remains to be explored.

Dyes—*(5) Antidotes and Treatments.* In treatment of eyes contaminated with cationic dyes, first aid measures are aimed at getting rid of dye which has not yet reacted with the tissues. This includes copious irrigation, mechanical removal of particles, and in the case of imbedded colored pencil may necessitate surgical exploration and careful removal of the particles.

Solutions of tannin or tannic acid precipitate cationic dyes and render them essentially noninjurious, but this disposes of only that portion of the dye which has not already reacted with the tissues. Vogt determined experimentally that a 5% to 10% solution of tannin was effective essentially in a prophylactic sense if applied within three minutes following application of powdered basic dyes to the eyes of rabbits, but that the effectiveness of this treatment rapidly diminished after three minutes.[250, 251] Other forms of chemical treatment have been aimed at removing both combined and excess dye. However, studies of the reaction of cationic dyes with cornea *in vitro* have shown these dyes to bind very tenaciously and to be very difficult to remove from combination with the tissue.[k]

Clinical trials have been made of various acids, such as acetic acid, ascorbic acid, and hydrochloric acid, as well as hydrogen peroxide solutions and alcohol in various strengths, but none of these treatments has proven very effective. In rabbit eyes, after staining with 1% *methyl violet* solution slight benefit appears to have been obtained in occasional animals by irrigation with 10% alcohol or 1% acetic acid.[f] Stronger solutions of alcohol or acetic acid actually had detrimental effect. Swabbing with 95% alcohol has been claimed to be helpful in treatment of eyes contaminated with particles of indelible pencil containing this type of dye, but in the one patient and in all rabbits in which good results were reported, the particles were all removed surgically, and the beneficial action which was ascribed to the alcohol was not clearly established.[zk]

Frequent irrigation with 2% solution of sodium fluorescein at pH 8.5 has been recommended on the basis of clinical impression in one case.[h] Unfortunately, controlled tests which I have made of this treatment on rabbit eyes contaminated with *methyl violet* or *crystal violet* have shown no beneficial effect, even when applied immediately following exposure to the dyes.[81] Furthermore, tests on rabbit corneas *in vitro* have shown no reversal of the antiturgescent denaturant effect of the cationic dyes by treatment with fluorescein.[81]

Trial therapeutic application of sodium hydrosulfite solution to the eye to reduce and bleach a cationic dye after it has had an opportunity to react with the cornea in its normal colored form also appears not to lessen the degree of injury. I have tested this with *Bindschedler's green,* applying approximately 0.01 M solution at pH 4.5 to rabbit eyes for ten minutes (after removal of corneal epithelium), then irrigating with 1% neutral sodium hydrosulfite for ten minutes. This treatment caused immediate bleaching of the green-stained cornea to light yellow, but did not prevent subsequent development of severe opacification and vascularization. The degree of injury was the same as in control green-stained eyes irrigated only with saline.[81]

It appears that the best that can be offered for immediate treatment of eyes contaminated with cationic dyes is copious irrigation and meticulous mechanical or surgical removal of all particles. Irrigation with water or saline solution is recommended, unless in the future more definite evidence is obtained of benefit from 10% ethyl alcohol, 1% acetic acid, or other special solutions. Later treatment of severely burned eyes may follow the general procedures under *Treatment of Chemical Burns.*

a. Allen JC, Szjnader E: Neutral red treatment of herpes simplex in rabbits. *INVEST OPHTHALMOL VIS SCI* 15:142–143, 1976.
b. Amels D, Checiu M, Sandor S: Contributions to the study of bisazo dyes induced eye anomalies in rats. *REV ROUM MEP SER MORPHOL* 23:93–101, 1977.
c. Ballantyne B, Gazzard MF, Swanston DW: Eye damage caused by crystal violet. *BR J PHARMACOL* 49:181–182, 1973.
d. Briggs RC, Wainwright N, Rothstein H: Biochemical events associated with healing of a chemical injury in the rabbit lens. *EXP EYE RES* 24:523–529, 1977.
e. Busacca A: The lymphatic vessels of the human bulbar conjunctiva studied by the

method of *in vivo* injections of trypan blue. *ARCH OPHTALMOL (Paris)* 8:10–32, 1948. (French)

f. Comberg: Evidence on the question of acid-alcohol effect on dye burns of the eye. *KLIN MONATSBL AUGENHEILKD* 80:685–686, 1928. (German)

g. Francois J, Rabaey M: New physical and histochemical researches on the mucoid of the cornea. *ACTA OPHTHALMOL* 34:45–62, 1956. (French)

h. Hosford BN, Smith JG: Treatment of ocular methylrosaniline poisoning with fluorescein. *J AM MED ASSOC* 150:1482–1484, 1952.

i. Hughes WF: Alkali burns of the eye. *ARCH OPHTHALMOL* 35:423–449, 1946.

j. Hull DS, Strickland ED, Green K: Photodynamically induced alteration of cornea endothelial cell function. *INVEST OPHTHALMOL* 18:1226–1231, 1979; *also, BIOCHEM BIOPHYS ACTA* 640:231–239, 1981; *also, CURR EYE RES* 1:487–490, 1981.

k. Kern HL, Grant WM: Interaction of acidic and basic dyes and beef corneal stroma. *J HISTOCHEM CYTOCHEM* 9:380–384, 1961.

l. Kobayashi N, Tamaki R, et al: Studies on aqueous outlets. II. *ACTA SOC OPHTHALMOL JPN* 80:1526, 1976. (English summary)

m. Kruckels H: On Brilliant green burn of the eye. *KLIN MONATSBL AUGENHEILKD* 106:571–574, 1941. (German)

n. Lahav M, Albert DM, et al: The effect of photodynamic action on corneal cells in tissue culture. *EXP EYE RES* 20:571–583, 1975.

o. Matsuo N, Okabe S, Yamamoto K: A case of lid granuloma induced by a yellow pencil. *JPN J CLIN OPHTHALMOL* 26:113–121, 1972. (English summary)

p. McEnerney JK, Peyman GA: Indocyanine green. *ARCH OPHTHALMOL* 96:1445–1447, 1978.

q. McFadden WM: Personal communication, 1969.

r. Morax S, Limon S, Forest A: Exogenous conjunctival pigmentation from methylene blue. *ARCH OPHTALMOL* (Paris) 37:708–709, 1977. (French)

s. Nicholas JP: Mucopolysaccharide staining in experimental corneal edema. *ARCH OPHTHALMOL* 76:238–243, 1966.

t. Norn MS: Specific double vital staining of the cornea and conjunctiva with rose bengal and alcian blue. *ACTA OPHTHALMOL* 42:84–96, 1964.

u. Norn MS: Vital staining in practice. *ACTA OPHTHALMOL* 42:1046–1053, 1964.

v. Norn MS: Trypan blue, vital staining of cornea and conjunctiva. *ACTA OPHTHALMOL* 45:380–389, 1967.

w. Norn MS: Bromthymol blue: Vital staining of conjunctiva and cornea. *ACTA OPHTHALMOL* 46:231–242, 1968.

x. Norn MS: Vital staining of corneal endothelium in cataract extraction. *ACTA OPHTHALMOL* 49:725–733, 1971.

y. Norn MS: Iodonitrotetrazolium vital staining of cornea and conjunctiva. *ACTA OPHTHALMOL* 49:90–102, 1971.

z. Norn MS: Tetrazolium-alcian blue mixture. I. *ACTA OPHTHALMOL* 50:277–285, 1972.

za. Norn MS: Side-effects of vital staining with tetrazolium-alcian blue. *ACTA OPHTHALMOL* 51:159–164, 1973.

zb. Norn MS: Lissamine green. *ACTA OPHTHALMOL* 51:483–491, 1973.

zc. Norn MS: Pachometric study on the influence of corneal endothelial vital staining. *ACTA OPHTHALMOL* 51:679–686, 1973.

zd. Norn MS: Alizarin red. *ACTA OPHTHALMOL* 52:468–476, 1974.

ze. Norn MS: Congo red vital staining of cornea and conjunctiva. *ACTA OPHTHALMOL* 54:601–610, 1976.

zf. Norn MS: Peroperative trypan blue vital staining of corneal endothelium. *ACTA OPHTHALMOL* 58:550–555, 1980.

zg. Norn MS: Vital staining of external eye of rabbit by fluorescein, rose bengal, tetrazolium, and alcian blue. *ACTA OPHTHALMOL* 58:454–458, 1980.

zh. Parker WT, Binder PS: Gentian violet keratoconjunctivitis. *AM J OPHTHALMOL* 87:340–343, 1979.

zi. Pasticier-Florquin, Boski, et al: Ocular tattooing from overuse of methylene blue collyrium. *BULL SOC OPHTALMOL FRANCE* 77:147–148, 1977. (French)

zj. Pinter L, Biro A, Berencsi G: Treatment of herpes of the cornea with a photosensitizing dye. *KLIN MONATSBL AUGENHEILKD* 163:600–604, 1973. (German)

zk. Sedan J: On alcohol treatment of injuries of the cornea by aniline dye pencils. *ANN OCULIST (Paris)* 177:65–77, 1940. (French)

zl. Ubels JL, Edelhauser HF, Austin KH: A comparison of healing of corneal epithelial wounds stained with fluorescein or Richardson's stain. *INVEST OPHTHALMOL VIS SCI* 23:127–130, 1982.

zm. Guss R, Johnson F, Maurice D: Rhodamine B as a test molecule in intraocular dynamics. *INVEST OPHTHALMOL VIS SCI* 25:758–762, 1984.

Dyes for fluorescence angiography of the retina. Fluorescein and *indocyanine green* administered intravenously has been very widely used in patients, without significant toxicity to the eye.[b] *Acridine orange* has similarly been used in rabbits.[a] All three have been well tolerated when tested on rabbit corneas; see foregoing section *(3) Information on Individual Dyes.*

A series of dyes have been tested in animals for retinal and choroidal angiography, and reported not injurious to the retina according to histologic findings. This has included the following:

Eosin-Y; Erythrosin-B; Phloxine-B; 4,5-Dichlorofluorescein; NK 1460; NK 1639; Resazurin; Rhodamine-S; Phloxine; Rhodamine 3-Hydroxy-1,3,6-pyrene trisulfonate; Brilliant sulfoflavin; Patent blue; Congo red derivatives

Similarly, *Disulphine blue* and *Evans blue* given intravenously to rabbits have colored normal retina only briefly, but experimental lesions of the retina have shown more persistent coloration.[e]

a. Kuwamoto K: Studies on the blood retinal barrier. *ACTA SOC OPHTHALMOL JPN* 72:1244–1252, 1968.

b. Hochheimer BF: Angiography of the retina with indocyanine green. *ARCH OPHTHALMOL* 86:564–567, 1971.

c. Hochheimer BF, D'Anna SA: Angiography with new dyes. *EXP EYE RES* 27:1–16, 1978.

d. Zenatti C: Performance of synthetic derivatives of Congo red in an angiographic study. *ANN OCULIST (Paris)* 204:257–270, 1971.

Dyes for vital staining of the ocular fundus. In rabbits and patients, intravenous administration of dyes has been explored in an effort to aid diagnosis and study of pathology of the ocular fundus by vital staining, intending to differentiate pathologic from normal. Among the dyes that have not had excessive systemic toxicity for this purpose are *fast acid violet; kiton fast green 5; light green SF;* and *xylene fast green B.* No

toxicity to ocular structures has been mentioned as a result of intravenous administration of these dyes.[b,c,d]

Kutschera in 1969 reviewed retinal vital staining and described experimental
staining of the retina by intravitreal injection of dyes in rabbit and human eyes to
show up breaks in the retina in retinoscopy.[a] The dye *patent blue* was found to be
particularly useful. It stained the retina when injected intravenously as well as
intravitreally, and did not disturb the morphology or metabolism of the retina in
rabbits.[a]

a. Kutschera E: Vital staining of the detached retina and its defects. *GRAEFES ARCH
OPHTHALMOL* 178:72–87, 1969. (German)
b. Sorsby A, Elkeles A, et al: Experimental staining of the retina in life. *PROC ROY SOC
MED* 30:1271–1272, 1937.
c. Sorsby A: Vital staining of the retina. *BR J OPHTHALMOL* 23:20–24, 1939.
d. Sorsby A: Vital staining of the fundus. *TRANS OPHTHALMOL SOC UK* 59:727–729,
1939.
e. Oliver M, Lauberman H, Ivry M: Staining of experimentally-induced chorioretinal
lesions with Disulphine blue and Evans blue. *BR J OPHTHALMOL* 54:569–571, 1970.

Dynamite fundamentally consists of nitroglycerin absorbed by woodpulp or diato-
maceous earth. In the literature are three cases in which visual disturbances followed
exposure to the fumes from explosion of dynamite in excavations.[a,b,153,247] These
poisonings have been attributed to carbon monoxide.

Two men became unconscious and then experienced a period of confusion during
recovery. One was said to be blind for thirty-two hours, but soon recovered completely.
The other had only light perception. His pupils were said initially to be semidilated
but reactive to light, and the fundi were not definitely abnormal. After eighteen months
his vision remained reduced to counting fingers close before his eyes. His pupillary
reflexes were then normal, but the temporal halves of the discs were thought to be pale.[a]

A third man exposed to fumes from explosion of dynamite suffered severe
headache the next day but did not lose consciousness. He seemed to have recovered,
but two weeks later his vision rapidly decreased to finger-counting. Pronounced
papilledema was observed, progressing to optic atrophy.[b] (See also *Carbon monoxide.*)

a. Brose LD: Amaurosis following the entrance of a well after use of dynamite. *ARCH
OPHTHALMOL* 28:402–406, 1899.
b. Lindemann K: A case of blindness from breathing residual fumes from dynamite
blasting in excavating. *Z AUGENHEILKD* 61:72–79, 1927. (German)

Dysprosium chloride, one of the rare earth or lanthanide salts, has been tested on
intact rabbit eyes by application of 0.1 ml of a 1:1 aqueous solution at approximately
pH 4. No damage to cornea or iris was seen, but considerable conjunctival reaction
with some ulceration occurred, with very slow healing. The conjunctival reaction
was more severe than that from hydrochloric acid at pH 1.[98] (For comparison of
effect of related compounds, also see *Rare-earth salts.*)

Ecballium elaterium (squirting cucumber [in German, *Eselgurke*]) is a fruit or
vegetable having a juice which in two instances is known to have caused swelling of

the lids, inflammation of the conjunctiva, and slight reversible corneal clouding from accidental contact with the eye.[253] The active principle is *elaterin*, which has been used as a drastic cathartic.[171]

Edetate (EDTA, edathamil, ethylenediamine tetraacetate, Versene, Sequestrene, Endrate) is a chelating agent which binds metals. Edetate is available principally as either sodium edetate or calcium edetate, which have different uses.

Disodium edetate has been used therapeutically on the cornea for removal of the superficial calcific opacities that occur in band keratopathy or that result from calcium hydroxide burns of the eye. Disodium edetate has also been used as an aid in decontaminating the eye after a splash of calcium hydroxide or lime in its various forms. In rabbits, irrigation of the surface of the eye with 0.01 M solution at pH 7 to 8 for fifteen minutes either on the intact cornea or after removal of the epithelium has caused no damage (Grant). Injected into the stroma of the cornea, it has produced a localized faint opacity which disappeared at approximately two weeks (Grant). (Opacity from injection of 0.9% sodium chloride solution clears in 24 to 48 hours.) A similar result is obtained with 0.03 M edetate at pH 7.2 injected into the cornea; subsequently the cornea is found histologically normal (Sallai[213]). A 0.1 M solution dropped continuously for fifteen minutes on rabbit eyes from which the corneal epithelium has been removed induces mild corneal edema, chemosis, and hyperemia of the iris, but no persistent damage (Grant). Sodium edetate increases permeability of the cornea (Grass).

In excised corneas, permeability, cytotoxicity and ion flux studies have shown sodium edetate at low concentrations to have little effect other than what can be attributed to loss of calcium (Krejci; Takeda; Green[320]).

In normal human eyes, a near-neutral 0.1 M solution of disodium edetate applied as eyedrops or as an eye bath causes only mild stinging sensation. Bathing or irrigating human eyes with solutions ranging in concentration from 0.01 to 0.1 M at pH 8 for fifteen minutes after a burn by calcium hydroxide or after mechanical removal of the epithelium for treatment of calcific deposits of band keratopathy has, so far as is known, caused no damage and has been therapeutically helpful (Abel; Alexandridis; Bloomfield; Breinin; Frezzotti; Garcia; Grant; Gunderova; Konig; Oosterhuis; Scherz; Feller[58]; Giesecke[67]; Glasmacher[69]; Gorska[76]; Lohse[156]; Oosterhuis[185]; Sallai[213]; Szeghy[237]; Thiel[241]).

A 10% (0.3M) solution, which has been reported irritating and injurious to lime-burned rabbit eyes (Giesecke[67]; Lohse[156]), has been evaluated clinically (Moon). When the 10% solution was applied to lime-burned eyes it caused pain, required local anesthetic, and was associated with longer hospital stay than required by patients without this treatment. It seems clear that lower concentrations are preferable.

A suitable solution for 15 minute treatment of human eyes that have had lime burns or have band keratopathy can be prepared conveniently by diluting a 20 ml ampule of Endrate disodium (Abbott Laboratories) with 180 ml sterile 0.9% sodium chloride solution. The ampule contains 150 mg disodium edetate per ml, which when diluted in this way provides a 1.5%, approximately 0.05 M sterile neutral solution suitable for use on the human eye. (This is for use on the outer surface of the eye, not for introduction into the anterior chamber.)

Alternative methods of utilizing edetate for treatment of corneal calcification have involved irrigation with 0.007 M edetate for 3 hours at a time (Vidal), or application by means of a hydrophilic gel contact lens pre-soaked in edetate (Praus).

Tetrasodium edetate used industrially as a sequestering agent should not be applied to the eye unless first neutralized, because it forms solutions sufficiently alkaline to be injurious to the eye. A 1% solution has a pH of 11.8.[171]

In treatment of chemically burned eyes, for decontaminating the eye, disodium edetate irrigating solutions have been most widely applied and evaluated in calcium hydroxide ("lime") burns. (This is discussed under *Calcium hydroxide* and in Chapter III.) Also this form of treatment has been evaluated in rabbit eyes experimentally contaminated with *toxic metal salts*. Edetate treatment has been found particularly effective for eyes contaminated with salts of *rare earths*, principally *lanthanum chloride* and *yttrium chloride*. It has been found significantly more effective than sodium chloride solution in decontaminating rabbit eyes to which 50% *zinc chloride* has been applied, but significant benefit in ultimate result has been observed only if the treatment was started within a minute or two after exposure.

In treatment of chemically burned and otherwise ulcerated corneas, sodium and calcium edetate solution have also been applied as collagenase inhibitors. This use has been based on experimental and clinical evidences that collagenase is released from injured corneal epithelial cells and is damaging to the stroma of the cornea (Henck; Itoi; Robertson; Slansky; Brown[18]; Itoi[128]). It is believed that it is through chelation of a metal that is necessary to collagenase activity, probably zinc, that edetate stops the enzyme action. *Calcium edetate* is effective for this purpose, and reported to be virtually non-toxic to the human cornea at a concentration of 0.2M (Slansky). (Also, see Chapter III, *Treatment of Chemical Burns of the Eye.*)

In solutions for external ophthalmic application, edetates have been used not only for the therapeutic purposes already described but also have been incorporated in low concentration in many eyedrops, to inactivate trace amounts of heavy metals to aid in preservation of the solutions. Edetates have been found capable of causing allergic contact sensitivity, though tests in guinea pigs and clinical observations suggest that it is rare (Raymond).

Injection into the rabbit anterior chamber of 0.03 M sodium edetate at pH 7.2 causes diffuse edema of the cornea and hyperemia of the iris and conjunctiva, from which the eyes recover in two or three weeks (Grant). Perfusion of the monkey's anterior chamber with 0.005 M concentration for 40 to 80 minutes causes separation of corneal endothelial cells and trabecular meshwork cells with loss of extracellular material and disintegration of trabecular cores (Bill). This is attended by a large increase in facility of aqueous outflow (Bill; Kaufman; Warner).

Intravitreal injection can cause destruction of the vitreous body and damage to all layers of the retina (Roll). Intravitreal injection of 1 mg in rabbits has produced reversible posterior subcapsular cataracts (Sanders[375]).

Disodium edetate administered intravenously to patients in treatment of sclero-derma has incidentally been noted to cause transient diplopia, but it is not apparent whether this side effect is related to hypocalcemia (Downing). Systemic administration of sodium edetate by subcutaneous injection in dogs and rats has been evaluated for effect on the crystalline lens, but this treatment has caused no abnormality of the lens detectable ophthalmoscopically or histologically, either during the period of administration or subsequent observation (Bruckner).

Calcium disodium edetate is used systemically in treatment of poisoning by lead and other heavy metals. When evaluated as a possible agent for treatment of ocular siderosis, a neutral 0.15 M solution of this salt injected subconjunctivally in rabbits was found to be irritating to the external tissues, but did not produce signs of intraocular damage (Wise).

In dogs, edetate is one of a series of *derivatives of ethylenediamine* that has been studied in connection with the peculiar effect of *ethambutol* on the zinc-containing dog's tapetum. Edetate is one of a series that decolorizes the tapetum when administered systemically. (See *Ethambutol* for further information.)

Teratogenic effects have been discovered when edetate was administered systemically to animals, but when administered as eye drops to rabbits 6 times a day from the 6th to 18th day of gestation neither 0.1% nor 3% solution had teratogenic effect, though with the higher concentration only 30% of the progeny survived (Gasset).

Abel S: Experiences with EDTA. *TRANS OPHTHALMOL SOC S AFRICA* 81–83, 1962. (*AM J OPHTHALMOL* 57:528, 1964.)

Alexandridis A, Stefani FH: Treatment of band keratopathy. *KLIN MONATSBL AUGENHEILKD* 176:968–971, 1980.

Bill A, Lutjen-Drecoll E, Svedbergh B: Effects of intracameral disodium EDTA and EGTA on aqueous outflow routes in the monkey eye. *INVEST OPHTHALMOL VIS SCI* 19:492–504, 1980.

Bloomfield SE, David DS, Rubin AL: Acute corneal calcification. *ANNALS OPHTHALMOL* 10:355–360, 1978.

Breinin GM, DeVoe AG: Chelation of calcium with edathamil calcium disodium in band keratopathy. *ARCH OPHTHALMOL* 52:846–851, 1954.

Bruckner R, Hess R, et al: Pathologic lens changes in experimental animals after long-term administration of high doses of Desferal. *HELV PHYSIOL ACTA* 25:62–77, 1967.

Downing JG: Dermatology. *N ENGL J MED* 260:1271–1277, 1959.

Frezzotti R, Bardelli AM: On a case of calcareous band keratopathy, treated with sodium EDTA, with unique course. *ANN OTTALMOL CLIN OCUL* 102:377–384, 1976. (Italian)

Garcia F, Brini A, Risse JF: Local treatment of band keratopathy with EDTA. *BULL SOC OPHTALMOL FRANCE* 80:635–637, 1980.

Gasset AR, Akaboshi T: Embryopathic effect of ophthalmic EDTA. *INVEST OPHTHALMOL VIS SCI* 16:652–654, 1977.

Grant WM: New treatment for calcific corneal opacities. *ARCH OPHTHALMOL* 48:681–685, 1952.

Grass GM, Wood RW, et al: Effects of calcium chelating agents on corneal permeability. *INVEST OPHTHALMOL VIS SCI* 26:110–113, 1985.

Gunderova RA, Lenkevich MM, Tartakovskaya AI: Treatment of lime burns of the cornea with EDTA. *VESTN OFTALMOL* 80:42–45, 1967. (*Chem Abstr* 67:20545, 1967.)

Henck JW, Lockwood DD, Olson KJ: Skin sensitization potential of trisodium ethylenediaminetetraacetate. *DRUG CHEM TOXICOL* 3:99–103, 1980.

Itoi M, Gnadinger MC, et al: Collagenase in the cornea. *EXP EYE RES* 8:369–373, 1969.

Kaufman PL, Svedbergh B, Lutjen-Drecoll E: Medical trabeculocanalotomy in monkeys with cytochalasin B or EDTA. *ANNALS OPHTHALMOL* 11:795–796, 1979.

Konig H, Marty F: A new disolver for calcareous deposits of the cornea. *OPHTHALMOLOGICA* 129:219–224, 1955.

Krejci L, Harrison R: Antiglaucoma drug effects on corneal epithelium. *THER HUNG* 18:766–769, 1970.

Moon MEL, Robertson IF: Retrospective study of alkali burns of the eye. *AUST J OPHTHALMOL* 11:281–286, 1983.

Oosterhuis JA: Treatment of calcium deposits in the cornea by irrigation and by application of EDTA. *OPHTHALMOLOGICA* 145:161–174, 1963. (*SURVEY OPHTHALMOL* 9:275–277, 1964.)

Praus R, Brettschneider I, Krejci L: Ethylenediamine tetraacetate: its release from hydrophilic gel contact lenses, intraocular penetration and effect on calcium in the cornea after lime burns. *OPHTHALMIC RES* 8:161–168, 1976.

Raymond JZ, Gross PR: EDTA: Preservative dermatitis. *ARCH DERM* 11:436–440, 1969.

Robertson IF: Indolent corneal ulceration: a systematic method of management. *AUST J OPHTHALMOL* 5:169–173, 1977.

Roll P, Schmut O, et al: The effect of ethylenediaminetetraacetic acid on the retina. *GRAEFES ARCH OPHTHALMOL* 202:205–212, 1977. (German)

Scherz W, Vogel M: Medical treatment of band keratopathy with EDTA. *KLIN MONATSBL AUGENHEILKD* 172:371–378, 1978.

Slansky HH, Freeman MI: Collagenolytic activity in bovine corneal eplithelium. *ARCH OPHTHALMOL* 80:496–498, 1968.

Slansky HH, Gnadinger MC, et al: Collagenase in corneal ulcerations. *ARCH OPHTHALMOL* 82:108–111, 1969.

Slansky HH, Dohlman CH, Berman MB: Presentation of corneal ulcers. *TRANS AM ACAD OPHTHALMOL OTOL* 6:1208–1211, 1971.

Takeda H: Effect of Ca-free EDTA solution on sodium transport of the isolated rabbit cornea. *FOLIA OPHTHALMOL JPN* 25:473, 1974. (English summary)

Vidal RF, Duros D, Hamard H: Use of disodium tetracemate in calcific impregnations of the cornea after burning by liquid tear gas. *ANN OCULIST* (Paris) 210:855–859, 1977.

Warner DM, Chu EB: The role of ionic calcium in the resistance to aqueous outflow in the cat. *CAN J OPHTHALMOL* 2:226–232, 1967.

Wise JB: Treatment of experimental siderosis bulbi, vitreous hemorrhage, and corneal bloodstaining with deferoxamine. *ARCH OPHTHALMOL* 75:698–707, 1966.

Eel blood has occasionally come in contact with the eyes of fishhandlers and has caused a severe burning sensation, conjunctival inflammation and chemosis, purulent discharge, swelling of the lids, keratitis epithelialis, and photophobia. There have been no serious sequelae.[129,214,253] An *ichthyotoxin* in eel blood is said to be responsible for these effects.[253] The same type of injury has been produced experimentally by dropping eel blood on the eyes of rabbits, cats, and human beings. Dogs appear to be more resistant than other species.[253]

Emetine hydrochloride is an alkaloid extracted from ipecac and employed in treatment of acute amebiasis, usually injected subcutaneously, never taken by mouth. Many reports describe the results of accidental contact of this substance with the eye, from splash of 2% to 6% aqueous solution, or from contact with dust of emetine or ipecac.[b,c]

The response of human eyes has been remarkably uniform in a large number of cases; no discomfort is felt at the time of exposure; but after a latent period of four to ten hours, there is severe discomfort consisting of a scratchy feeling in the eye, accompanied by much tearing and blepharospasm, photophobia, edema of the lids, and hyperemia of the conjunctiva. There is irregularity and roughening of the corneal epithelium or, in more severe cases, actual erosion of the corneal epithelium. Discomfort persists for a day or two and then subsides, with rapid, complete recovery. The reaction is similar to that induced by ultraviolet, hydrogen sulfide, or osmic acid vapor.

The same reactions as seen in human beings have been reproduced by many investigators experimentally in rabbit eyes.[b] In dog eyes a more severe reaction has been described, consisting of deep keratitis with lymphocytic infiltration of the cornea, iris, and ciliary body, and eventual interstitial vascularization of the cornea.[f]

An extensive review and bibliography was published in 1948 by Fontana.[b] No specific treatment is known. Treatment is the same as for corneal abrasion or ultraviolet keratitis, consisting of sterile dressings and avoidance of local anesthetics.

In none of the cases of local toxic effect has any damage of the retina or optic nerve been described, but following systemic administration of exceptionally large doses of emetine (100 to 300 mg per day) to a large group of soldiers in World War I, 22 percent of them were described as having lacrimation and photophobia with hyperemic conjunctivae like those who have had local contact with the drug. In addition, many of these patients were said to have had transient mydriasis with loss of pupillary reaction to light and accommodation; some were said to have had diminution of vision to light perception, with constriction of visual fields; seven patients were found to have central scotoma.[d] Hyperemia of the optic nervehead and retina was described, followed in a day or two by ischemia, then return to normal in a week or two. No information was given on the condition of the corneas in these patients. Symptoms were relieved promptly when emetine was discontinued.[d]

An attempt was made to reproduce this reaction in rabbits, but no damage to the optic nerve could be demonstrated; however, transient mydriasis was induced by near-lethal (110 mg) systemic doses or by subconjunctival injections of emetine hydrochloride.[a] A definite elevation of intraocular pressure (as high as 50 mm Hg) lasting many hours followed both systemic and local injection in rabbits. Also photophobia developed and the vitreous became turbid. Subconjunctival injection caused permanent corneal damage and vascularization.[a]

In only one patient has a secondary glaucoma been reported, and this was associated with ulcerative keratitis.[e]

a. Alajmo B: Ocular reactions to emetine (Experimental study). *G ITAL OFTALMOL* 5:113–118, 1924. (Italian)
b. Fontana G: The effect of emetine on the cornea. *ARCH OTTALMOL* 52:115–132, 1948. (Italian)
c. Gallet M, Durix C: Keratoconjunctivitis from squirt of emetine hydrochloride in the eyes. *ACTA XVII CONCILIUM OPHTALMOL (1954)* 3:1797–1805, 1955. (French)

d. Jacovides: Visual difficulties as a consequence of large injections of emetine. *ARCH OPHTALMOL (Paris)* 40:657–660, 1923. (French)

e. Lasky MA: Corneal response to emetine hydrochloride. *ARCH OPHTHALMOL* 44:47–52, 1950.

f. Torres Estrada A: Ocular lesions caused by emetine. *BOL HOSP OFTAL NS LUZ* (Mex) 2:145, 1944. (*AM J OPHTHALMOL* 28:1060, 1945.)

Endothal (disodium 3,6-endoxohexahydrophthalic acid), a defoliant and herbicide, is said to be very irritating to the skin, eyes, and mucous membranes,[70,171] but original observations were not found.

Epichlorohydrin (1-chloro-2,3-epoxypropane) vapor is known to be highly irritating to the respiratory passages, skin, and eyes, and a maximal allowable concentration of 5 ppm has been recommended.[51] Test by application of a drop of rabbit eyes has caused mild and presumably reversible injury, graded 4 on a scale of 1 to 10 after twenty-four hours.[27,223]

After systemic administration to rabbits by daily intraperitoneal injection of 60 mg/kg for one week in two animals and for four weeks in two other animals, I found no ocular abnormality with the ophthalmoscope or slit-lamp biomicroscope. One of the rabbits was examined seven months later and still had normal eyes.[81]

Epinephrine (adrenaline) has many noteworthy side effects when administered in eyedrops for glaucoma, when injected into the anterior chamber, and when given systemically to experimental animals. Adverse effects will be described under the following headings: (1) *Epithelial disturbances in conjunctiva and cornea*, (2) *Corneal endothelial disturbances*, (3) *Retinopathy and choroidopathy*, (4) *Lens changes*, (5) *Intraocular pressure*, and (6) *Systemic effects from use in the eye.*

(1) Epithelial disturbances: Allergy or contact sensitivity develops in many patients (Becker; Fechner). This is characterized by itching and burning sensation, epiphora, and hyperemia of conjunctiva and lids. Follicular conjunctivitis has been described in one case of this sort, but more commonly follicular hyperplasia is caused by miotic drugs employed in treatment of glaucoma (Byron). With or without contact sensitivity associated with epinephrine eyedrops, reactive hyperemia of the superficial vessels is a common complaint, blanching each time a drop is applied, but reappearing in half an hour or less (Becker).

Tiny black or dark brown deposits in the conjunctiva have been very commonly produced by chronic use of epinephrine eyedrops. Deposits in the conjunctiva consist of tiny dark specks, usually 1 mm or less in diameter. They generally cause no symptoms or inflammation and most commonly are found in the conjunctiva of the lower lid, discovered only when the lower lid is pulled down.

They appear to have been described first in 1927 by Lowenstein (Lipovetskaya; Marchesani). Since then, they have been redescribed and investigated many times (Becker; Von Burstin; Corwin; Hansen; Marchesani; Rutllan; Veirs; Bietti; Cashwell; Mooney; Paufique; Paul; Ramos; Sanchez-Macho; Schmitt; Schuster; Spiers; Zolog). They consist of melanin-like oxidation products of epinephrine accumulated in conjunctival cysts. They are quite innocuous and require no treatment (Von Burstin; Marchesani), with rare exceptions (Pardos). A large proportion of patients who are under long-term treatment with epinephrine eyedrops have them. Many publications in their titles or in their text have referred to these deposits as "adrenochrome", but this must be an error, for, as pointed out by Ramos and Urquiaga (Ramos), adrenochrome is brilliant red and very water-soluble,[171] unlike the conjunctival inclusions, which are brown and water-insoluble. Since the material is produced by oxidation and polymerization of epinephrine, and chemically is related to melanin, yet somewhat different from natural melanin, the terms *adrenomelanin*, (Ramos) or *adrenomelanosis* seem preferable.

"Black cornea", apparently caused by the same material as accumulates in the conjunctival cysts, appears as a black plaque of amorphous material covering most of the cornea. This has been described several times (Blobner; Calmettes; Donaldson; Ferry; Green; Krejci; Von Domarus; Madge; McCarthy). In all cases the corneal epithelium has been abnormal before development of the black plaque, typically with edema and bullous keratopathy from advanced glaucoma. Histologically, Ferry and Zimmerman have found the pigment at various levels below the epithelium, in Bowman's membrane, and below Bowman's membrane in the stroma after it has entered through breaks in the epithelial surface (Ferry). The material was shown by Reinecke and Kuwabara to have the properties of oxidized epinephrine (Reinecke). Attempts to induce pigmentation of the cornea in rabbits by intensive application of epinephrine eyedrops have been shown by Krejci and Harrison to succeed only when the corneal epithelium has been injured, such as by elevation of the intraocular pressure and scraping of the cornea. They found that the pigmentation could be enhanced by using epinephrine preparations that had become discolored by oxidation (Krejci).

An actual toxic effect on the corneal epithelium, rather than discoloration, is seen very rarely. Chandler and Grant have described rare instances in which eyes, usually aphakic, with functionally poor corneal endothelium have had a tendency to develop epithelial edema, which may be aggravated by topical epinephrine, and improves when this medication is stopped.[291] Four cases of this sort have been reported from France (Valiere-Vialeix). I have seen a young woman with Chandler's syndrome[291] who had remarkable improvement in the corneal epithelial edema in her affected eye after epinephrine eyedrops were stopped, but pilocarpine, timolol and methazolamide were continued, suggesting a potential for toxic influence on either the epithelium or the endothelium in this condition. In tissue culture, toxic effects on corneal epithelium have been demonstrated, but have required many hours of continuous exposure (Krejci).

The conjunctival epithelium in rare cases develops white keratinized plaques under epinephrine treatment.[291] If the keratinized plaque involves the conjunctiva of the lower lid and rubs on the cornea, there may be loss of epithelium and development of vascularization in the lower part of the cornea. The drops must be stopped, but recovery tends to be very slow and incomplete.

Ocular pemphigoid has been ascribed to long-term treatment with epinephrine in several cases, with usually a tendency to arrest or improvement when the drops are stopped (Hoffer; Kristensen; Norn; Vadot).

Loss of eyelashes, reversibly, is reported in one case in one eye (Kass). Epinephrine was being used only in that eye.

Obstruction of nasolacrimal ducts by epidermalization and accumulation of oxidation products of epinephrine has been described in a few cases (Barishak; Hansen; Spaeth). The symptoms have been epiphora, or excessive tearing. Two patients described by Spaeth had their symptoms relieved when black casts of material were irrigated out of the nasolacrimal ducts (Spaeth). In one case obstruction has been caused by occlusion of the puncta by keratinization (Romano).

Persistent meibomianitis has been ascribed to epinephrine eyedrops in rare instances by Kaufman.[336]

(2) Corneal endothelial disturbances: Injection of epinephrine into the anterior chamber during surgery has been used to dilate the pupil, and in occasional cases corneal edema has developed, raising the question of toxicity to the corneal endothelium (Edelhauser). Results of animal tests have varied, probably in part due to different testing techniques. Olson and associates working with cats have replaced an equal volume of aqueous humor with 0.1 to 0.5 ml of a solution containing 0.1% epinephrine hydrochloride, 0.1% sodium bisulfite and 0.5% chlorobutanol, and by specular microscopy found no abnormality of the corneal endothelium.[366] Others, working with rabbits, replacing the aqueous humor, or perfusing the anterior chamber with test solutions, and measuring corneal swelling and examining histologic morphology for assessment of toxicity, conclude that 0.1% epinephrine salts themselves are not significantly damaging, but that bisulfite at acid pH is, and that the more effectively the buffer system maintains a low pH the more damage is produced (Edelhauser; Hull). A question whether commercial epinephrine eyedrops, that usually include bisulfite and other preservatives, may cause changes in the endothelium during long-term treatment of glaucoma has been addressed by examining corneal thickness and cell counts in a group of patients using epinephrine drops in only one of their eyes, and finding a slightly but significantly lower count in the treated eyes, which remained nevertheless within a normal range (Waltman).

(3) Retinopathy and choroidopathy: Reduction of visual acuity from toxic effect of epinephrine eyedrops on the retina seems not to have been recognized until the 1960's, when a small number of cases were described by Kolker, Becker, and Goldmann. Maculopathy from chronic use of epinephrine eyedrops on aphakic glaucomatous eyes was described by Kolker and Becker (1968) in fifteen patients (22 eyes), documenting subnormal vision (20/40 to 20/400) while epinephrine eyedrops were being administered, and a significant improvement, almost to normal, in most cases when epinephrine was discontinued (Kolker). In most of these cases epinephrine eyedrops had been used for several months, but duration of use of epinephrine in extreme cases ranged from one or two weeks to six years before reversible reduction of visual acuity was demonstrated. The time for recovery of vision after discontinuing the medication was several months in most cases, but the extreme range was one week to sixteen months. In four cases a second impairment and recovery of vision was demonstrated by giving and then withholding epinephrine a second time after the first cycle of impairment and recovery. Permanent reduction

of vision was said to have been observed occasionally when epinephrine was not stopped early enough. The macular region of the patients was described as appearing slightly edematous, occasionally with small flameshaped hemorrhages, or with pale gray or yellow cysts close to the fovea, accompanied by central or paracentral scotomas.

Several observers have provided additional case reports, corroborating the clinical findings, and adding information obtained by retinal fluorescein angiography (Caffi; Ito; Mackool; Michels; Thomas). It was remarkable that in some cases showing leakage identical with what is found in other types of optic macular edema, the visual acuity was not necessarily very much impaired, typically ranging for 20/30 to 20/100 (Mackool; Michels). Thomas and his colleagues found macular edema by angiography in 28% of 56 aphakic eyes under treatment with epinephrine drops for glaucoma, which was significantly more than the 13% incidence in aphakic eyes not receiving epinephrine (Thomas). Reversibility upon stopping epinephrine has been a characteristic in most cases.

The hypothesis that epinephrine applied in eyedrops might reach the retina in aphakic eyes in larger amount than in normal eyes was investigated by Kramer, using radioactively labeled epinephrine in rabbits and cats, showing this was indeed so (Kramer). The drug was localized at the junction of inner nuclear and inner plexiform layers of the retina, essentially at the same site at which others found edema fluid. Morgan also showed in rabbits that removal of the lens led to an increased vasoconstrictive response at the posterior pole after application of epinephrine eyedrops.

In rabbits, daily intravenous injections of near-lethal doses have caused choroidal hemorrhages and exudates, with degenerative changes in the retina, also hemorrhages in the conjunctiva, and opacity of the cornea (Chen; Komi; Sunada). In monkeys, repeated intravenous injections of epinephrine have produced a central serous chorioretinopathy with angiographic findings similar to those of spontaneous central serous maculopathy in human beings (Yoshioka). Similar lesions have been produced in rabbits by injection of epinephrine close to Bruch's membrane.

The ERG in rabbits which have been given epinephrine intravenously has shown selective change in the c-wave, suggesting to Francois and associates a toxic effect on the pigment epithelium of the retina (Francois). Normal human beings have shown no significant changes in the a- and b-waves after injection of 1 mg of epinephrine, according to Wirth, Palombi, and Stirpe, who have carried out ERG studies and reviewed relevant literature (Wirth).

(4) Lens changes: Effects of a toxic nature appear to have been described only in experimental animals. In rats and mice, lens opacities have been seen to appear rapidly, and then to disappear, after systemic administration of very large doses of epinephrine (Scullica; Smith; Suden).[62] This appears to have been the same phenomenon as has been induced by several other drugs which have caused temporary decrease in blinking, allowing exposure of the cornea, increased evaporation, and dehydration of the lens. These conditions and the development of the lens opacities are preventable by keeping the lids closed.[62] Cataracts in the rat fetus have been produced by giving near-lethal doses of epinephrine at a critical period in pregnancy,

possibly affecting the developing lens by constricting the hyaloid arteries and causing anoxia (Pitel). Localized posterior cortical opacities are said to have been produced by intravitreal or retrobulbar injection of epinephrine in animals. In rabbits a reduction in mitoses in the lens epithelium has been demonstrated from subconjunctival injections (Scullica). There seems to have been no allegation of lens opacities in human beings from epinephrine.

(5) Intraocular pressure: Reactions to epinephrine consist of a reduction of pressure most often, but in a very small proportion of cases the pressure may be raised transiently, with the angle remaining open. An idea of the incidence is given by observations by Fechner (1969) in which 24 out of 427 open-angle glaucomatous eyes showed a tension rise averaging 3.9 mm Hg, but a maximum of only 7.7 mm Hg (Fechner). In very unusual cases I, and others, have seen transient elevations to between 30 and 40 mm Hg. Generally the brief elevations of pressure by epinephrine eyedrops in open-angle glaucomatous eyes are prevented if miotic antiglaucoma eyedrops are being administered.

In eyes with abnormally shallow anterior chambers and narrow angles, the intraocular pressure can be raised if sufficient mydriasis is induced to cause closure of the angle, resulting in angle-closure glaucoma, but if the angle does not close or is prevented from doing so by concomitant use of miotic eyedrops, the epinephrine may cause reduction of pressure (Fechner).

In rats given intravenous infusion of epinephrine, the intraocular pressure has been described by Ohnesorge and associates as rising in association with rising blood pressure, but continuing to rise after the blood pressure had leveled off (Ohnesorge). This confirmed an observation reported by Wesseley in 1908. Slow, continuous rise of intraocular pressure was observed during twenty minutes of epinephrine infusion, but was thought not to be related to contraction of orbital smooth muscle, contrary to what had been postulated by Wesseley.

An experimentally induced glaucoma in rabbits has been reported by Lipovetskaya, produced by multiple intravenous injections of epinephrine (Lipovetskaya).

(6) Systemic effects from use on or in the eye: Systemic reactions to epinephrine eyedrops have been rare. The few recorded cases have been reviewed by Becker and Lansche (Becker; Lansche). Lansche described two cases in which within a minute after administration of local anesthetic and epinephrine eyedrops the patient felt faint, became pale, trembling and perspiring (Lansche). These reactions were accompanied by severe headache and probably transient elevation of systemic blood pressure. However, the reactions were transitory. In a three-year survey by Hillsdorf and Marxer no systemic side effects were noted (Hilsdorf). Kerr found most glaucoma patients had no cardiovascular side effects, but in exceptional patients a transitory rise of systolic pressure of 20 or more mm Hg occurred, and ventricular ectopic beats were more frequent (Kerr). Others have reported extrasystoles to be more common (Ballin; Becker).

In patients undergoing ocular surgery under halothane anesthesia there is believed to be a special risk of cardiac disturbance if too much epinephrine reaches the circulation from eye drops, from supplementary injection of local anesthetic solution containing epinephrine, or from injection of epinephrine into the anterior chamber. Francois has reported on one patient in this situation who developed transient ventricular fibrillation after one eye drop containing 1 mg of epinephrine was instilled (Francois). However, in a series of 19 patients having cataract operation under halothane anesthesia, Smith and colleagues found that injecting 0.04 to 0.7 mg of epinephrine into the anterior chamber caused no significant difference in incidence of cardiac arrythmias than occurred in a control group without epinephrine (Smith).

In patients using epinephrine in addition to timolol eyedrops Blondeau and Cote report a slight transitory rise of diastolic pressure and slightly more frequent arrythmias (Blondeau).

Ballin N, Becker B, Goldman ML: Systemic effects of epinephrine applied topically to the eye. *INVEST OPHTHALMOL* 5:125–129, 1966.

Barishak R, Romano A, Stein R: Obstruction of lacrimal sac caused by topical epinephrine. *OPHTHALMOLOGICA* 159:373–379, 1969.

Becker B: Topical epinephrine in the treatment of the glaucomas. *Symposium on Glaucoma.* (TRANS. NEW ORLEANS ACAD. OPHTHALMOL.) St. Louis, Mosby, 1967, pp. 152–169.

Becker B, Morton, WR: Topical epinephrine in glaucoma suspects. *AM J OPHTHALMOL* 62:272–277, 1966.

Bietti G: Melanotic conjunctival concretions as a result of prolonged instillations of adrenaline. *BOLL OCULIST* 17:65–79, 1938. (Italian)

Blobner F: Corneal discoloration from an epinephrine preparation. *KLIN MONATSBL AUGENHEILKD* 100:758, 1938. (German)

Blondeau P, Cote M: Cardiovascular effects of epinephrine and dipivefrin in patients using timolol. *CAN J OPHTHALMOL* 19:29–32, 1984.

Byron HM: Conjunctival reaction due to 1-epinephrine bitartrate. *ARCH OPHTHALMOL* 63:567–570, 1960.

Caffi M: Maculopathy from topical application of epinephrine. *ANN OTTALMOL CLIN OCUL* 95:591–595, 1969. (Italian)

Calmettes L, Deodati F, Bechac G: Corneal pigmentation by epinephrine bitartrate. *ARCH OPHTHALMOL (Paris)* 28:303–305, 1968. (French)

Cashwell LF, Shields MB, Reed RW: Adrenochrome pigmentation. *ARCH OPHTHALMOL* 95:514–515, 1977.

Chen SH: Experimental study of retinopathy caused by intravenous injections of adrenalin. *VESTN OFTAL* 1:33–34, 1957. (Abstr. *AM J OPHTHALMOL* 43:997, 1957.)

Corwin ME, Spencer WH: Conjunctival melanin depositions. *ARCH OPHTHALMOL* 79:317–321, 1963.

Donaldson DD: Epinephrine pigmentation of the cornea. (photo). *ARCH OPHTHALMOL* 72:74–75, 1967.

Edelhauser HF, Hyndiuk RA, et al: Corneal edema and the intraocular use of epinephrine. *AM J OPHTHALMOL* 93:327–333, 1982.

Fechner PU: Report on further experiences with epinephrine-eyedrops in glaucoma therapy. *KLIN MONATSBL AUGENHEILKD* 154:19–31, 1969. (German)

Ferry AP, Zimmerman LE: Black cornea: A complication of topical use of epinephrine. *AM J OPHTHALMOL* 58:205–210, 1964.

Francois J, Jonsas C, DeRouck A: Studies of the effect of levorenine on the electroretinogram and the electrooculogram in rabbits. *AM J OPHTHALMOL* 68:119–122, 1969.

Francois J, Verbraeken H: Danger of collyrium with 2% levorenone. *BULL SOC BELGE OPHTALMOL* 185:99–102, 1979. (French)

Goldmann H: Is epinephrine treatment of glaucoma simplex harmless? *ARCH PORT OFTAL SUPPL.* 165, 1966. (Cited by Meyer and Herxheimer, 1968.)[174]

Green WR, Kaufer GJ, Dubroff S: Black cornea, a complication of topical use of epinephrine. *OPHTHALMOLOGICA* 154:88–95, 1967.

Hansen E: Conjunctival deposits after topical administration of epinephrine. *T NORSK LAEGEFOREN* 84:678–679, 1964. (*Zentralbl Ges Ophthalmol* 92:13, 1964.)

Hilsdorf C, Marxer J: Epinephrine eyedrops in management of glaucoma. *KLIN MONATSBL AUGENHEILKD* 152:398–404, 1968. (German)

Hoffer KJ: Pemphigoid related to epinephrine treatment (Letter). *AM J OPHTHALMOL* 83:601, 1977.

Hull DS, Chemotti MT, et al: Effect of epinephrine on the corneal endothelium. *AM J OPHTHALMOL* 79:245–250, 1975.

Ito R, Yoshizumi M, Futa R: A case of epinephrine maculopathy. *JPN J CLIN OPHTHALMOL* 30:809, 1976.

Kass MA, Stamper RL, Becker B: Madarosis in chronic epinephrine therapy. *ARCH OPHTHALMOL* 88:429–431, 1972.

Kerr CR, Hass I, et al: Cardiovascular effects of epinephrine and dipivalyl epinephrine. *BR J OPHTHALMOL* 66:109–114, 1982.

Kolker AE, Becker B: Epinephrine maculopathy. *ARCH OPHTHALMOL* 79:552–562, 1968.

Komi T: Ocular changes in rabbits caused by repeated intravenous injections of adrenaline. *ACTA SOC OPHTHALMOL JPN* 59:313–315, 1955. (*AM J OPHTHALMOL* 40:141, 1955.)

Kramer SG: Epinephrine distribution after topical administration to phakic and aphakic eyes. *TRANS AM OPHTHALMOL SOC* 78:947–982, 1980.

Krejci L, Harrison R: Corneal pigment deposits from topically administered epinephrine. *ARCH OPHTHALMOL* 82:836–839, 1969.

Krejci L, Harrison R: Epinephrine effects on corneal cells in tissue culture. *ARCH OPHTHALMOL* 83:451–454, 1970.

Kristensen EB, Norn MS: Benign mucous membrane pemphigoid. *ACTA OPHTHALMOL* 52:266–281, 1974.

Lansche RK: Systemic reactions to topical epinephrine and phenylephrine. *AM J OPHTHALMOL* 61:95–98, 1966.

Lee PF: The influence of epinephrine and phenylephrine on intraocular pressure. *ARCH OPHTHALMOL* 60:863–867, 1958.

Lipovetskaya EM: Morphologic peculiarities of tissue structures which form the anterior chamber angle in experimental glaucoma. *OFTAL Z (Kiev)* 23:607–611, 1968. (English summary)

Lipovetskaya EM, Zbandut IS: The significance of scleral rigidity in the development of experimental glaucoma. *OFTAL Z (Kiev)* 24:306–309, 1969.(English summary)

Lowenstein A: Artificially induced melanotic little tumors in the conjunctiva. *BER DTSCH OPHTHALMOL GESELLSCH* 46:439–441, 1927. (German)

Mackool RJ, Muldoon T, et al: Epinephrine-induced cystoid macular edema in aphakic eyes. *ARCH OPHTHALMOL* 95:791–793, 1977.

Madge GE, Geeraets WJ, Guerry D III: Black cornea secondary to topical epinephrine. *AM J OPHTHALMOL* 71:402–405, 1971.

Marchesani O, Ullerich K: Pigmented bodies in the conjunctiva after use of epinephrine. *DTSCH OPHTHALMOL GESELLSCH* 56:312–315, 1950. (German)

McCarthy RW, LeBlanc R: A "black cornea" secondary to topical epinephrine. *CAN J OPHTHALMOL* 11:336–340, 1976.

Michels RG, Maumenee AE: Cystoid macular edema associated with topically applied epinephrine in aphakic eyes. *AM J OPHTHALMOL* 80:379–388, 1975.

Mooney D: Pigmentation after long-term topical use of adrenalin compounds. *BR J OPHTHALMOL* 54:823–826, 1970.

Morgan TR, Mirate DJ, et al: Topical epinephrine and regional ocular blood flow. *ARCH OPHTHALMOL* 101:112–116, 1983.

Norn MS: Pemphigoid related to epinephrine treatment. *AM J OPHTHALMOL* 83:183, 1977.

Ohnesorge FL, Soyka H, van Zwieten PA: On the influence of systemically administered catecholamine on the intraocular pressure of rats. *GRAEFES ARCH OPHTHALMOL* 173:241–249, 1967. (German)

Pardos GJ, Krachmer JH, Mannis MJ: Persistent corneal erosion secondary to tarsal adrenochrome deposit. *AM J OPHTHALMOL* 90:870–871, 1980.

Paufique L, Audibert J, Ravault MP: A curious case of black cornea. *BULL SOC OPHTALMOL FRANCE* 408–409, 1960. (French)

Paul H, Schmitt-Graff A: Pigmented conjunctival inclusions after topical adrenaline administration. *GRAEFES ARCH OPHTHALMOL* 216:69–75, 1981. (German)

Pitel M, Lerman S: Studies on the fetal rat lens. *INVEST OPHTHALMOL* 1:406–412, 1962.

Ramos JA, Urquiaga AM: Adrenomelanic deposits in the conjunctiva. *J FR OPHTALMOL* 4:45–48, 1981. (French)

Reinecke RD, Kuwabara T: Corneal deposits secondary to topical epinephrine. *ARCH OPHTHALMOL* 70:170–172, 1963.

Romano A, Barishak R, Stein R: Obstruction of lacrimal puncta caused by topical epinephrine. *OPHTHALMOLOGICA* 166:301–305, 1973.

Rutllan J: Effects secondary to the local administration of epinephrine. *AN INST BARRAQUER* 8:272–275, 1968. (Spanish)

Sakata H: Studies on experimental serous choroidopathy. *ACTA SOC OPHTHALMOL JPN* 79:1845, 1975.

Sandez-Macho M, Carbajo Vincente M, Sanchez Saloria M: Pigmented conjunctival deposits produced by epinephrine. *ARCH SOC ESP OFTALMOL* 33:537, 1973. (Spanish)

Schmitt H, Remler O: Adrenochrome conjunctival inclusions as a consequence of topical adrenaline therapy. *KLIN MONATSBL AUGENHEILKD* 165:332–336, 1974. (German)

Schuster H: On an infrequent side effect of adrenaline drops. *KLIN MONATSBL AUGENHEILKD* 165:517–519, 1974. (German)

Scullica L, Bisantis C, Pezzi PP: Effects of epinephrine on the mitotic activity of the lens epithelium. *BOLL OCULIST* 47:561–567, 1968. (Italian)

Smith A, Gavitt J, Kaplan M: Some relationships between catecholamines and morphine-like drugs. Recent advances. *BIOL PSYCHIATR* 6:208–213, 1963.

Smith RB, Douglas H, et al: Safety of intraocular adrenaline with halothane anesthesia. *BR J ANAESTH* 44:1314–1317, 1972.

Spaeth GL: Nasolacrimal duct obstruction by topical epinephrine. *ARCH OPHTHALMOL* 77:355–357, 1967.

Spiers F, Eldrup-Jorgensen P: External side-effects of Eppy. *TRANS OPHTHALMOL SOC UK* 86:255–260, 1966.

Suden CT: Opacities of the lens induced by adrenaline in the mouse. *AM J PHYSIOL* 130:543–548, 1940.

Suden CT, Wyman LC: Adrenaline induced opacities in the lens of the rat. *ENDOCRINOLOGY* 27:628–632, 1940.

Sunada I, Mii T, et al: Electron microscopic studies of epinephrine choroiditis in rabbits. *ACTA SOC OPHTHALMOL JPN* 79:1608, 1975.

Thomas JV, Gragoudas ES, et al: Correlation of epinephrine use and macular edema in aphakic glaucomatous eyes. *ARCH OPHTHALMOL* 96:625–628, 1978.

Vadot E, Etienne R: Cicatricial pemphigoid following long-term instillation of adrenaline. *BULL SOC OPHTALMOL FRANCE* 81:693–695, 1981. (French)

Valiere-Vialeix JP, Lehner MA, Couderc JL: Four observations on unusual effects of epinephrine. *BULL SOC OPHTALMOL FRANCE* 80:1153–1155, 1980. (French)

Veirs ER, McGrew JC: Ocular complications from topical epinephrine therapy of glaucoma. *EYE EAR NOSE THROAT MONTHLY* 42:46–52, 1963.

Von Domarus D: Adrenochrome deposits in the cornea ("Black Cornea"). *OPHTHALMOLOGICA* 175:166–170, 1977. (German)

Von Burstin D: On the question of melanoma production by epinephrine. *KLIN MONATSBL AUGENHEILKD* 132:329–344, 1958. (German)

Waltman SR, Yarian D, et al: Corneal endothelial changes with long-term topical epinephrine therapy. *ARCH OPHTHALMOL* 95:1357–1358, 1977.

Wirth A, Palombi R, Stirpe M: The electroretinogram after administration of epinephrine in man. *BOLL OCULIST* 44:696–703, 1965. (Italian)

Yoshioka H, Katsume Y, Akune H: Experimental central serous chorioretinopathy. *JPN J OPHTHALMOL* 25:112–118, 1981.

Zolog N, Leibovici M: Conjunctival "melanosis" from epinephrine. *BULL SOC FRANCE OPHTALMOL* 86:198–200, 1973. (French)

Ergot (*Secale cornutum*, [in German, *Mutterkorn*]) is a substance formed by a fungus which is parasitic on rye. Epidemics of ergotism from eating the contaminated grain have a long history. In most epidemics, convulsive reactions have been common and gangrenous changes relatively rare.

The convulsive form of ergotism begins from one day to three weeks after contamination of the daily food supply. A feeling of numbness and tingling begins in the fingers and spreads over the whole body, finally to the tongue and throat. Next, painful cramp-like contractions of the muscles begin. These may affect the voice and respiration. Very commonly diplopia and scintillating scotomas are said to occur.[194] A second stage following the period of muscular contractions is characterized by psychic and neurologic disturbances, particularly ataxia, lack of coordination, and disturbance of patellar and Achilles reflexes. Nystagmus is said to be a frequent accompaniment.[194]

Cataracts following convulsive ergotism have been noted by several writers since they were first mentioned by Taube in 1782.[194] It has been estimated that 2 to 9 per cent of patients having convulsive ergotism have developed cataracts. The cataracts in all cases have been bilateral. They have become complete in one to three months in children or in eight to eleven months in adults. Women have most commonly been affected.

Ergot used medically is said never to have caused cataract. Scott in 1962 pointed out that all reports of cataract from ergot poisoning originated in the eighteenth and nineteenth centuries in association with epidemics of poisoning from eating infected grain, and that for more than a century there had been no report of cataract following medical use of ergot.[d] Scott also doubted that cataract had been produced in experimental animals by means of ergot or its alkaloids.

In rare instances cycloplegia and slight hyperopia have been observed following ingestion of medications containing ergot.[b,c] In a few instances acute poisoning by extract of ergot, usually used postpartum or for abortion, has caused blindness or serious bilateral decrease of vision. This as a rule has been completely reversible. Characteristically during the acute phase the pupils are wide and poorly reactive to light. The fundi appear normal or show slight edema and narrowing of the arteries.[153,214,247] No specific or uniform abnormality of visual fields has been recognized in these cases.

In one exceptional case ergot poisoning has been held responsible for secondary optic atrophy, with concentric contraction of the fields and small central scotomas. This case was also exceptional in that the dosage of *ergotin* taken daily for six days was not excessive, and vision failed gradually in the course of several weeks after discontinuance of the medication. The optic nervehead and surrounding retina were described as edematous, but no hemorrhages were observed. Vision was permanently reduced to 20/200 and 20/50.[a]

Experimental poisoning of animals with ergot many years ago was found to induce narrowing of retinal arteries, mydriasis with absence of pupillary reflex to light, degeneration of retinal ganglion cells, changes in the pigment epithelium of the ciliary processes, and cataracts.[214] Which of the many constituents of ergot are responsible for the toxic effects on the eye has not been determined.

Ergot alkaloids have presented no problem in the presence of glaucoma, and at one time were tried in the treatment of glaucoma, but with little effect.

(See also *Ergotamine, Dihydroergotamine, and Dihydroergotoxine.*) (See INDEX for page numbers.)

a. Kravitz D: Neuroretinitis associated with symptoms of ergot poisoning. Report of a case. *ARCH OPHTHALMOL* 13:201–206, 1935.
b. Schneider: Bilateral ophthalmoplegia interna induced by extract of ergot. *MUNCHEN MED WOCHENSCHR* 5:1602, 1902. (German)
c. Stepka J: Accommodation paresis after ergot extract. *CAS LEK CESK* 1:305–307, 1929. (*ZENTRALBL GES OPHTHALMOL* 21:845, 1929.)
d. Scott JG: Does ergot cause cataract? *MED PROC* 8:4–8, 1962.

Ergotamine tartrate (Gynergen, Ergomar, Ergostate, component of Cafergot), employed mainly in treatment of migraine, is one of several purified medically useful compounds derived from ergot. These derivatives differ among themselves in their pharmacologic and toxic properties. Ergotamine retains the vasoconstricting action of ergot, and in overdosage has caused peripheral vasculopathy and neuropathy secondary to ischemia. At standard therapeutic dosage apparently ergotamine can be taken over long periods without harm to the eyes.[d] An example of seeming relative immunity of the eye to toxic effects from ergotamine was given by Gastaldi, describing a forty-three-year-old woman who began taking intramuscular injections of ergotamine tartrate at age nineteen years because of severe migraine, gradually increasing the dosage from 0.25 mg per week to as much as 2 mg per day in later years, until she developed evidence of peripheral vascular alterations with acroparesthesias and difficulties in walking. Despite this, a thorough eye examination showed no detectable abnormality of vision, dark adaptation, or ERG. Ophthalmoscopically the retinal vessels appeared entirely normal. Also immediately after large doses of ergotamine they showed no change.[h]

However, one case, which is apparently unique, has been mentioned by Crews (1963) in which a 19-year-old girl developed an occlusion of a central retinal artery after an injection of ergotamine tartrate was given for a headache.[a]

Overdosage with ergotamine has led to a small number of cases of disturbance of retinal arteries or optic nerves, as reported by Gupta (1972), Merhoff (1974), Wollensak (1978) and Mindel (1981).

Gupta described a young woman with previously normal fundi who took 104 Cafergot tablets in 13 days for headache and developed blurring in one eye, vision 20/60 right, 20/30 left, withl bilateral papilledema and partial ring scotomas. Although the retinal vessels were not described, it was postulated that there was ischemia of the nerveheads. The medication was stopped, and in 2½ weeks the vision and fundi had returned to normal.

Merhoff reported on a young man who took Cafergot suppositories for headache, 8 to 10 a week for two years, then 2 to 3 a day for several months, and developed ischemia in one leg, sudden blur and decrease of vision in the left eye to 20/400, associated with central scotoma, retinal vasospasm and retinal pallor. The medication was stopped, and in 24 hours the vision had returned to normal. The leg also recovered completely, but more slowly.

In Wollensak's case a young woman had regularly taken ergotamine-containing suppositories for some years, apparently excessively, and developed vascular papillitis and retinal edema, first in one eye and then both, with central scotomas, decreased visual acuity, and star-figure in the macula of the worse eye. The ERG remained normal. After the suppositories were stopped, there was rapid improvement of the fundi and vision, but permanent partial optic atrophy in one eye.

These cases seem significantly different from the case of neuroretinitis from an extract of ergot described by Kravitz (1935), summarized in the foregoing section on *Ergot.*

Mindel's case was more complex, concerned with a woman who attempted suicide by taking *Vacor* (N-(4-nitrophenyl)-N'-(3-pyridinylmethyl) urea), a rodenticide, which induced diabetes, severe orthostatic hypotension, and apparently a right occipital cortical infarct, with left homonymous hemianopia, but normal fundi and visual acuity. Thirty months after the suicide attempt, in order to relieve the orthostatic hypotension, she was given 6 mg of ergotamine tartrate per day for 3 weeks, until vision began to blur. There was some macular edema, and the ERG was extinguished in both eyes, but whether the ERG was normal before ergotamine was unknown. The retinal arterioles were seen to have become attenuated, appearing thread-like on angiography. Three months after the medication was discontinued, the vessels were still abnormal, but retinal edema was gone, and visual acuity was normal.

Treatment with ergotamine has presented no problem in patients with glaucoma.[b,f]

There has been no evidence of production of cataracts by ergotamine in patients.[e]

a. Crews SJ: Toxic effects on the eye and visual apparatus resulting from the systemic absorption of recently introduced chemical agents. *TRANS OPHTHALMOL SOC UK* 82:387–406, 1963.

b. Friedenwald JS: In discussion of Christensen L, Swan KC: Adrenergic blocking agents in the treatment of glaucoma. *TRANS AM ACAD OPHTHALMOL OTOLARYNG* 53:489–497, 1949.

c. Panter H: Tabetic symptoms after Gynergen injections. *MED KLIN* 22:880–881, 1926. (German)

d. Peters GS, Horton BT: Headache: With special reference to the excessive use of ergotamine preparations and withdrawal effects. *PROC STAFF MEET MAYO CLIN* 26:153, 1951.

e. Scott JG: Does ergot cause cataract? *MED PROC* 8:4–8, 1962.

f. Thiel R: Experimental and clinical investigations on the influence of Ergotamine (Gynergen) on the intraocular pressure in glaucoma. *KLIN MONATSBL AUGENHEILKD* 77:753, 1926. (*ZENTRALBL GES OPHTHALMOL* 18:236.) (German)

h. Gastaldi GM: Ophthalmologic findings in a case of intoxication by ergotamine. *MINERVA OFTAL* 11:176–178, 1969. (Italian)

i. Gupta DR, Strobos RJ: Bilateral papillitis associated with Cafergot therapy. *NEUROLOGY* 22:793–797, 1972.

j. Merhoff GC, Porter JM: Ergot intoxication. *ANN SURG* 180:773–779, 1974.

k. Mindel JS, Rubenstein AE, Franklin B: Ocular ergotamine tartrate toxicity during treatment of Vacor-induced orthostatic hypotension. *AM J OPHTHALMOL* 92:492–496, 1981.

l. Wollensak J, Grajewski O: Bilateral vascular papillitis after ergotamine medication. *KLIN MONATSBL AUGENHEILKD* 173:731–737, 1978. (German)

Erythrophleum alkaloids from *Erythrophleum guineense* include *erythrophleine* and *cassaine* (Nervocidine), which are known to have digitalis-like activity.[171] When applied to the eye they are irritating and injurious to the cornea, conjunctiva, and iris.[253] After subconjunctival injection they lower the intraocular pressure for several days, presumably by poisoning the aqueous secretory mechanism, but chemosis and corneal edema are too much for antiglaucoma therapeutic use.[a,b] (Compare *Cardiac glycosides* and *Toad poisons.*)

a. Ascher KW: Long-lasting reduction of intraocular pressure by a local anesthetic. *BER DTSCH OPHTHALMOL GESELLSCH* 47:207–213, 1928. (German)

b. Ascher KW: Experimental analysis of drug-induced reduction of intraocular pressure by erythrophleine. *BER DTSCH OPHTHALMOL GESELLSCH* 49:136–147, 1930. (German)

Ethambutol (Myambutol), a tuberculostatic antibacterial, has generally been well tolerated by human beings except for occasional reduction of central or peripheral vision, sometimes to a serious degree. When originally investigated clinically, it was employed as a mixture of D and L-isomers, but soon it was found that the L-isomer had little antituberculous effect and was more toxic than the antituberculous D-isomer.

In an early clinical report by Carr and Henkind (1962) concerning the DL-mixture a significant disturbance of vision was reported in 8 out of 18 patients. An apparently representative patient who was studied in detail had reduction of visual acuity after receiving 6 g of DL-mixture per day for 10 weeks. The patient had paracentral scotomas, impaired color vision, and hyperemia of the optic nerve heads. After the drug was discontinued the vision became worse during two weeks, as large centrocecal scotomas developed, the retinal veins became dilated, the discs blurred, and a flame-shaped hemorrhage appeared in the fundus. Subsequently during five months after the drug was stopped, the vision, the fields, and the fundi all returned spontaneously to normal.

A thorough functional and neuranatomic study of toxicity in monkeys by Schmidt and Schmidt showed that the D-isomer and the DL-racemic mixture had qualitatively the same toxic properties, but that quantitatively the DL-racemate was more severely toxic than the D-isomer. In either case, the first lesion to develop in poisoned monkeys was located centrally in the optic chiasm, spreading into the optic tracts, creating necrotic areas. Lesions in the optic nerves tended to develop later, and characteristically were centrally located near the midportion of the nerves. There was no definite retinal pathology. The monkeys behaved as though blind. Lessell, in rats, similarly demonstrated chiasmal lesions, but no changes in the retina or in the immediately retrobulbar portion of the optic nerves. Matsuoko, in rabbits, found demyelination and axonal fragmentation in the optic nerves.

Autopsy findings in patients have been rarely reported, but Pahlitzsch and Tiburtius described a patient who had developed unilateral retrobulbar neuritis with absolute central scotoma after receiving ethambutol 25 mg/kg for six weeks, then died from heart failure, and showed in the affected optic nerve diffuse edema without cellular infiltration or myelin changes. Shiraki reported on a patient who had impaired vision for seven months from ethambutol before dying in uremia. This patient at autopsy had demyelination in the chiasm, comparable to the findings in poisoned monkeys.

In dogs and cats, the findings have been different than in other species, apparently due to the presence of a tapetum lucidum. Dogs and cats that have been given ethambutol (and several related compounds) have shown decoloration of their tapetum lucidum (Capiello; Kaiser; Place; Vogel). Cats have also had detachment of the retina (Diermeier). In dogs, after a single intravenous dose of 100 mg/kg decoloration is noticeable in 15 to 30 minutes and is complete in four hours. After this, the color begins to return to normal in two or three days. Electron microscopy showed bundles of parallel rods in tapetal cells became swollen and disoriented, but this was reversible (Vogel). Because the tapetum is known to have a high zinc content and because ethambutol is a derivative of ethylenediamine, known to chelate zinc and other metals, it was suspected that the loss of color might be due to the removal of zinc, and some decrease in zinc content was demonstrated (Place). Tests of a series of other ethylenediamine derivatives chemically related to ethambutol, including sodium edetate, established that several of these compounds which also have chelating properties cause temporary decoloration of the tapetum (Kaiser). What this may have to do with effects of ethambutol on vision in primates remains to be seen.

Clinically, since the mid-1960's ethambutol has been employed exclusively as the D-isomer, and the incidence of disturbances of vision has been low. However, ethambutol has been so widely used that, despite the low incidence, there have been many instances of visual disturbance, and numerous case reports and clinical studies have been published. (The bibliography at the end of this synopsis is limited to selected references representing fundamental as well as recent works.)

The incidence of disturbance of vision by ethambutol is dose-related, though some people are more susceptible than others. A survey of approximately 2000 patients by Derka in 1975 indicated that optic neuropathy occurred in 10% of those who received 30 mg/kg daily, in 5% at 25 mg/kg, and in 0% at 20 mg/kg. These figures are inevitably complicated by the fact that patients tend to be started at a higher dose (e.g. 25 mg/kg) and then to be maintained at a lower dose. An overall incidence of 1% has been a common estimate. It is recognized that patients with kidney disease may have toxic effects at lower dosage than people with normal kidneys (Bronte-Stewart), and in such cases it is desirable to regulate dosage according to serum levels.

The most characteristic disturbance of vision is bilateral reduction of acuity due to development of central scotomas (Pau; Toth), but in a small proportion of cases there is constriction of the visual fields with normal visual acuity (Barron; Toth). It has been suggested that this depends on whether involvement of the optic nerves, chiasm and tracts is axial or paraxial. Occasional bitemporal hemianopic features are found in the field defects, pointing to chiasmal involvement (Bronte-Stewart; Karmon; Toth). Rarely, retinal hemorrhages or fine pigmentation between disc and macula have been described (Pau; Toth).

Onset of visual disturbances is usually not until several months after starting ethambutol. In most cases if the ethambutol is promptly stopped, or the dosage is reduced, the vision very slowly returns, sometimes taking many months, and sometimes with a period of worsening before improving. Exceptionally, loss of vision of varying degree has been permanent, with varying degrees of optic atrophy (Bronte-Stewart; Pau; Takeuchi; Toth).

Color vision disturbances by ethambutol have received much attention, particularly with a view to a potential means of early diagnosis before decrease of visual acuity (Arruga; Jaeger; Trusiewicz; Zrenner). Ethambutol causes changes in red-green color vision which may be detectible when there is little or no decrease in visual acuity. In certain cases a different desaturation of red in the right and left fields of each eye has suggested a disturbance located after decussation of optic nerve fibers in the chiasm (Arruga).

The possible role of the retina in visual disturbance from ethambutol has intrigued a number of investigators despite the fact that retinal abnormalities have seldom been seen clinically, in poisoned monkeys, or in autopsies. Electroretinographic findings have been controversial, some reporting reversible abnormalities of the ERG even in the absence of visual disturbances (Bourquin; Gigon), and others reporting normal ERG despite reduced vision (Weder), or abnormality of ERG only when vision is seriously reduced (Hennekes). *In vitro*, rabbit retina ERG has been irreversibly reduced by ethambutol, but at concentrations higher than would be encountered clinically (Okada).

The visual evoked cortical response in ethambutol intoxication has been studied as a potential means of early diagnosis, and has been found to be altered in association with visual disturbance (Adachi-Usami; Trau; Van Lith; Weder). As an objective method of evaluation and diagnosis it has been held to be useful clinically (Trau; Van Lith).

Intriguing though rather nebulous studies on visual disturbances associated with ethambutol have sought to find a role for zinc, stemming in part from the observations on dogs and cats mentioned earlier. Treatment of patients with ethambutol 25 mg/kg for 8 weeks has caused no change in plasma-zinc or blood-copper levels (Campbell), but in rabbits given 1200 mg/kg/day for 15 days the mean plasma-zinc was 0.9 mg/l compared to 1.71 mg/l in controls; microscopically the optic nerves of the rabbits were interpreted as showing dilated axons with vacuoles (Grignolo). Particular attention has been given to plasma-zinc levels before the start of treatment with ethambutol, and some investigators have concluded that patients with 0.7 mg/l are at greater risk of developing visual disturbance than patients with 0.8 to 1 mg/l (Delacoux; Fioretti; Saraux). (Also see INDEX for *Zinc systemic level.*)

Ethambutol has been shown in monkeys to affect parts of the central nervous system in addition to the visual system, but clinically only occasional mention has been made of other induced neurologic problems. Peripheral mixed, but predominantly sensory, neuropathy has been noted (Takeuchi).[273]

Adachi-Usami E, Kellerman FJ, Makabe R: Visual evoked responses in patients with ethambutol damage. *DEUTSCH OPHTHALMOL GESELLSCH* 72:181–185, 1974. (German)

Arruga J: Test of subjective desaturation of color in diagnosis of effect of ethambutol on anterior optic pathway. *BULL SOC OPHTALMOL FRANCE* 82:182–192, 1982. (French)

Barron GJ, Tepper L, Iovine G: Ocular toxicity from ethambutol. *AM J OPHTHALMOL* 77:265–260, 1974.

Bourquin C, Korol S: Ocular toxicity of Myambutol. *OPHTHALMOLOGICA* 172:264–265, 1976.

Bronte-Stewart J, Pettigrew AR, Foulds WS: Toxic optic neuropathy and its experimental production. *TRANS OPHTHALMOL SOC UK* 96:355, 1976.

Campbell IA, et al: Ethambutol and the eye; zinc and copper. *LANCET* 2:711, 1975.

Capiello VP, Layton WM Jr: A one-year study of the toxicity of ethambutol in dogs; results of gross and histopathologic examinations. *TOXICOL APPL PHARMACOL* 7:844–849, 1965.

Carr RE, Henkind P: Ocular manifestations of ethambutol. *ARCH OPHTHALMOL* 67:566–571, 1962.

Delacoux E, Moreau Y, et al: Prevention of ocular toxicity of ethambutol; study of zincemia and chromatic analysis. *J FR OPHTALMOL* 1:191–196, 1978. (French)

Derka H: Does a correlation exist between the level of the Myambutol dosage and the frequency of optic neuritis? *OPHTHALMOLOGICA* 171:123–131, 1975.

Diermeier HF, Kaiser JA, Yuda N: Safety evaluation of ethambutol. *ANN NY ACAD SCI* 135:732–746, 1966.

Fioretti F, Minervino M: Zincemia as a clue to the ocular toxicity of ethambutol. *ANN OTTALMOL CLIN OCUL* 106:543–548, 1980. (Italian)

Gigon S, de Haller R: Retinal lesions due to ethambutol and serum levels of zinc and vitamin A. *KLIN MONATSBL AUGENHEILKD* 182:469–473, 1983. (French)

Grignolo FM, LaRosa G, et al: Evaluation of plasma zinc in retrobulbar optic neuritis. *BOLL OCULIST* 59:813–821, 1980. (Italian)

Hennekes R: Clinical ERG findings in ethambutol intoxication. *GRAEFES ARCH OPHTHALMOL* 218:319–321, 1982.

Jaeger W: Acquired disturbances of color vision as side effect of medications. *KLIN MONATSBL AUGENHEILKD* 170:453–460, 1977. (German)

Kaiser JA: Toxicology of ethambutol: long term studies in dogs. *PHARMACOLOGIST* 4:176, 1962.

Kaiser JA: Tapetal depigmentation in dogs produced by ethylenediamines. *FED PROC* 22:369, 1963. (*FOOD COSMET TOXICOL* 2:134, 1964.)

Kaiser JA, Paino AF: A one-year study of the toxicity of ethambutol in dogs; results during life. *TOXICOL APPL PHARMACOL* 6:557–567, 1964.

Karmon G, Savir H, et al: Bilateral optic neuropathy due to combined ethambutol and isoniazid treatment. *ANNALS OPHTHALMOL* 11:1013–1017, 1979.

Lessell S: Histopathology of experimental ethambutol intoxication. *INVEST OPHTHAL-MOL* 15:765–769, 1976; *AM J MED SCI* 272:765–769, 1976.

Matsuoka Y, Mukoyama M, Sobue I: Histopathological study of experimental ethambutol neuropathy. *CLIN NEUROL* 12:453–459, 1972.

Okada K, Honda Y: Experimental studies on the mode and site of action of antituberculous agent, ethambutol, in the visual system. *ACTA SOC OPHTHALMOL JPN* 79:783–789, 1975.

Pahlitzsch H, Tiburtius H: Eye studies in treatment with the new tuberculostatic ethambutol-dihydrochloride Lederle (Myambutol). *KLIN MONATSBL AUGENHEILKD* 154:228–232, 1969. (German)

Pau H, Wahl M: Myambutol-injury of th eyes. *BER DTSCH OPHTHALMOL GESELLSCH* 72:176–181, 1974; *KLIN MONATSBL AUGENHEILKD* 165:121–126, 1974. (German)

Place VA: Personal communication, 1963.

Place VA, Peets EA, et al: Metabolic and special studies of ethambutol. *ANN NY ACAD SCI* 135:775–795, 1966.

Saraux H, Bechetoille A, et al: Reduction of serum zinc level in certain toxic optic neuritides. *ANN OCULIST (Paris)* 208:29–31, 1975. (French)

Schmidt IG: Central nervous system effects of ethambutol in monkeys. *ANN NY ACAD SCI* 135:759–774, 1966.

Schmidt IG, Schmidt LH: Studies of the neurotoxicity of ethambutol and its racemate for the rhesus monkey. *J NEUROPATHOL EXP NEUROL* 25:40–67, 1966.

Shiraki H: Neuropathy due to intoxication with antituberculous drugs from neuro-pathological viewpoint. *ADV NEUROL SCI* 17:120–125, 1973.

Takeuchi H, Takahashi M, et al: Ethambutol neuropathy. *FOLIA PYSCHIATR NEUROL JPN* 34:45–55, 1980.

Toth LC, Hermans G, Berthelon S: Optic neuritis and ethambutol. *BULL SOC BELGE OPHTALMOL* 165:382–394, 1973. (French)

Trau R, Salu R, et al: Early diagnosis of Myambutol (ethambutol) ocular toxicity by electrophysiological examination. *BULL SOC BELGE OPHTALMOL* 193:201–212, 1981.

Trusiewicz D: Farnsworth 100-hue test in diagnosis of ethambutol-induced damage to optic nerve. *OPHTHALMOLOGICA* 171:425–431, 1975.

Van Lith GHM: Electro-ophthalmology and side-effects of drugs. *DOC OPHTHALMOL* 44:19–21, 1977.

Vogel A, Kaiser J: Ethambutol induced transient change and reconstitution (*in vivo*) of the tapetum lucidum color in the dog. *EXP MOL PATHOL* (Suppl)2:136–149, 1963.

Weder W: Myambutol-injury of the optic nerve. *BER DTSCH OPHTHALMOL GESELLSCH* 72:172–175, 1974. (German)

Zrenner E, Kruger CJ, Baier M: The toxic effects of ethambutol on spectral sensitivity. *BER DTSCH OPHTHALMOL GESELLSCH* 78:1031–1037, 1981. (German)

Ethanolamine (2-aminoethanol, monoethanolamine) is a liquid having an unpleasant fishy ammoniacal odor which serves as a warning against inadvertent vapor exposure.[a] A drop of ethanolamine applied to rabbit eyes causes injury similar to that caused by ammonia, but slightly less severe; graded 9 on a scale of 10 after twenty-four hours.[a,27,161] However, if ethanolamine is neutralized to pH 5.5 with hydrochloric acid (to form ethanolamine hydrochloride), one drop of 30% solution causes only transient smarting and hyperemia, like soap, but no injury to either rabbit or human eyes.[317]

    a. Hygienic guide series. Ethanolamines. *AM IND HYG ASSOC J* 29:312–315, 1968.

Ethanolamine oleate has been used as a sclerosing agent. In rabbits subconjunctival injection of 1% aqueous solution caused a severe local reaction, but did not prove satisfactory for inducing glaucoma experimentally.[a] Injected into cavernous hemangiomas of the lid a 5% solution has been found therapeutically satisfactory.[b]

    a. Luntz MH: Experimental glaucoma in the rabbit. *AM J OPHTHALMOL* 61:665–680, 1966.
    b. Hassan AM: The effect of ethanolamine injections on haemangioma of the lid. *BULL OPHTHALMOL SOC EGYPT* 66:433–442, 1973.

Ethchlorvynol (Placidyl), a sedative, was suspected by Haining and Beveridge (1964) of producing toxic amblyopia in a man who took 0.5 to 1 g orally each night for three months and then noted disturbance of color vision and difficulty in reading.[b] He had normal fundi but bilateral central scotomas and visual acuity of 6/18 in both eyes. Within six weeks after the drug was discontinued, the vision returned nearly to normal, with some abnormalities of color vision remaining.

Two additional cases of optic neuritis in patients taking ethchlorvynol have been mentioned by Walsh and Hoyt (1969), who had been told about them by J. Lawton Smith, but they gave no details or place of publication.[256] Another case has been reported by Brown and Meyer (1969), who have described in some detail a man who earlier had electroconvulsive treatment for recurrent depression and who for five years had been taking ethchlorvynol in increasing dosage up to 2500 mg each night in addition to 50 mg of promazine hydrochloride, with gradual loss of weight and impairment of vision.[a] Visual acuity was reduced to counting fingers at two to three feet because of central and cecocentral scotomas. The patient also had signs of slight peripheral neuropathy indicated by weakness of foot dorsiflexion, wasting and weakness and sensory loss in the hands, but otherwise essentially normal ophthalmogic and neurologic examinations and no indications of vitamin deficiencies. The vision returned essentially to normal in five months after the medication was changed.

Hudson and Walker described transient blurred vision, diplopia, and difference in size of the pupils during an acute intoxication by ethchlorvynol in one patient.[c] This resembled a case reported by Millhouse et al. in which a woman developed diplopia, coarse nystagmus on looking to the side, gross ataxia, slurring of speech, drowsiness, and confusion while taking 1,000 to 2,000 mg each night, but improved within three days when the drug was discontinued.[d] Nystagmus has also been described by Ropper.[e]

a. Brown E, Meyer GC: Toxic amblyopia and peripheral neuropathy with ethchlorvynol abuse. *AM J PSYCHIATR* 126:882–884, 1969.

b. Haining WM, Beveridge GW: Toxic amblyopia in a patient receiving ethchlorvynol as a hypnotic. *BR J OPHTHALMOL* 48:598–600, 1964.

c. Hudson HS, Walker HI: Withdrawal symptoms following ethchlorovynol, (Placidyl) dependence. *AM J PSYCHIATR* 118:361, 1961.

d. Millhouse J, Davies DM, Wraith SR: Chronic ethchlorvynol intoxication. *LANCET* 2:1251–1252, 1966.

e. Ropper AH: Unusual nystagmus after ethchlorvynol use. *J AM MED ASSOC* 232:907, 1975.

Ether (ethyl ether) causes a transitory smarting sensation if splashed in the eye or if a high vapor concentration contacts the eye, but momentary exposure generally does not cause injury. Prolonged exposure of the cornea to high concentration of ether vapor, such as employed in general anesthesia, does cause superficial epithelial injury, from which recovery is usually prompt. Corneal opacification from injury by ether in the course of general anesthesia has apparently occurred rarely.[249] However, slight injury by ether vapor appears to render the corneal epithelium abnormally vulnerable to mechanical injury and to injury with substances such as alcohol or isopropyl alcohol.[81,317]

Ether tested in a standard manner on rabbit eyes has caused slight reversible injury, graded 2 on a scale of 1 to 10.[228]

Ethionamide, a tuberculostatic, has been mentioned in reviews as a very rare possible cause of polyneuritis and optic neuritis.[273,359] Ethionine has been studied mainly in connection with experimental carcinogenesis. Tumor of the iris has been observed in a rat's eyes after repeated systemic administration of both ethionine and *N-2-fluorenylacetamide.*[a] Ethionine has been found not to affect the glucose uptake of rats' retinas.[137]

a. Benson WR: Intraocular tumor after ethionine and N-2-fluorenylacetamide. *ARCH PATHOL* 73:404–406, 1962.

Ethopropazine (Profenamine, Parsidol), an antiparkinsonian drug, has anticholinergic properties, and can cause mydriasis and cycloplegia. In one patient acute angle-closure glaucoma developed after the drug was administered.[a]

a. Liebman SD: personal communication, 1972.

Ethotoin, an anticonvulsant, has caused diplopia and nystagmus.[171]

Ethoxolamide (ethoxyzolamide, ethoxzolamide, Cardrase, Ethamide), a carbonic anhydrase inhibitor employed in reducing ocular pressure in glaucoma and as a diuretic, has been reported in rare instances to induce acute transient myopia, similar to acetazolamide and many other drugs.[a,b] (Compare *Acetazolamide* and *Myopia, acute transient*—See INDEX for page numbers.)

a. Halpern AE, Kulvin MM: Transient myopia during treatment with carbonic anhydrase inhibitors. *AM J OPHTHALMOL* 48:534–535, 1959.

    b. Beasley FJ: Transient myopia and retinal edema during ethoxzolamide (Cardrase) therapy. *ARCH OPHTHALMOL* 68:490–491, 1962.

2-Ethoxyethanol (Cellosolve, ethylene glycol monoethyl ether) when dropped on rabbit eyes causes discomfort, but only slight reversible injury, graded 3 on a scale of 10 after twenty-four hours.[27,151] Exposure of rabbits to high vapor concentrations causes symptoms of ocular and respiratory irritation, but even at concentrations which are probably lethal, causes no significant ocular injury.[151,230]

Ethoxytrimethyl silane tested by application of 0.02 ml to rabbit eyes causes immediate symptoms of irritation but no corneal damage; the eyes were completely normal in twenty-four hours.[211]

Ethyl acetate at a concentration of 400 ppm in air causes a sensation of irritation in human eyes.[183] However, exposure of rabbits to concentrations which would be scarcely tolerable to human beings caused no corneal damage despite exposure for eight hours a day, five days a week, for periods up to seven weeks. Only the conjunctivae gave indications of irritation.[230] Exposure of cats to ethyl acetate vapor has produced vacuoles in the corneal epithelium of the type described under *Solvent vapors,*[216] but this has not been observed in human beings. A study of thirty workers exposed chronically to 15 to 50 mg of ethyl acetate in addition to 20 to 80 mg of amyl acetate per liter of air showed no vacuoles or other abnormalities in the cornea, merely hyperemia of the bulbar conjunctiva.[a] Prolonged inhalation may be damaging to lungs, liver, kidney, and heart,[171] but no effect on the eyes has been known from systemic absorption.

    Application of two drops of liquid ethyl acetate to the corneas of rabbits, followed two minutes later by irrigation with water, caused immediate fine optical irregularity of the corneal epithelium, but the eyes were nearly normal the next day and completely normal in two days.[81] Standard testing on rabbit eyes has resulted in a rating of 2 on a scale of 10.[228]

    a. Valvo A, Spagna C, Parlato G: Ocular pathology of industrial solvents. *ANN OTTALMOL CLIN OCUL* 93:799–807, 1967. (Italian)

Ethyl acrylate vapor is irritating to the eyes, nose and respiratory passages.[b] The liquid applied to rabbit corneas causes injury similar to that caused by ethyl alcohol, limited to damage of the corneal epithelium.[a] The degree of recovery has not been reported, but if similar to ethyl alcohol, presumably recovery would be complete.

    a. Pozanni UC, Weil CS, Carpenter CP: Sub-acute vapor toxicity and range-finding data for ethyl acrylate. *J IND HYG* 31:311–315, 1949.
    b. Treon JF, Sigmon H, et al: The toxicity of methyl and ethyl acrylate. *J IND HYG* 31:317–325, 1949.

Ethylamine is a gas, having a strong fishy ammonia odor. In water it forms strongly alkaline solutions. Experimental exposure of rabbits to 50 ppm of the gas in air for six weeks is reported to have caused erosions of the cornea, conjunctiva, and lungs, but it is not reported how soon the ocular damage appeared.[a] Tested on rabbit eyes, it has been shown to be severely damaging, graded 9 on a scale of 10.[226]

There have been reports of temporary blue hazy vision from subtle disturbance of the corneal epithelium in people exposed to "ethyl amines". This term could include *diethylamine* and *triethylamine* as well as ethylamine itself. *Diethylamine* has been identified as having this effect, but it is not clear whether *ethylamine* and *triethylamine* also have this action.[b,c] (See the INDEX for page numbers of *Amines, Diethylamine,* and *Triethylamine.*)

a. Brieger H, Hodes WA: Toxic effects of exposure to vapors of aliphatic amines. *ARCH IND HYG* 3:287–289, 1951.
b. Amor A: The toxicity of solvents. *MANUFACTURING CHEMIST* 20:540–544, 1949.
c. Jones WT, Kipling MD: Glaucopsia—blue-gray vision. *BR J IND MED* 29:460–461, 1972.

Ethylarsine dichloride (ethyl dichloroarsine) is an extremely poisonous liquid with vapor that is a powerful lacrimatory irritant of the eyes and nose, also very irritating to the skin and respiratory tract. The vapor is said to cause necrosis of the corneal epithelium. It has been studied primarily as a potential war gas.[61, 155]

Ethyl benzene (phenyl ethane) vapor has a transient irritant effect on human eyes at 200 ppm in air. At 1,000 ppm on the first exposure it is very irritating and causes tearing, but tolerance rapidly develops. At 2,000 ppm eye irritation and lacrimation are immediate and severe; 5,000 ppm causes intolerable irritation of the eyes and nose.[188] Drop application to rabbit eyes caused slight irritation and no corneal injury demonstrable by fluorescein staining.[27, 265] Standard testing on rabbit eyes gave an injury grade of 2 on a scale of 10.[228]

Ethyl bromoacetate has been employed as a tear gas. The vapors are irritant to all the mucous membranes, especially to the eyes, and are unbearable for more than a minute at a concentration of 8 ppm in air.[61] Exposure of human eyes to high concentration of vapor from tear gas shells has caused corneal edema with wrinkling of Descemet's membrane, but in most patients the eyes have eventually returned to normal. Direct contact with the liquid, according to one report, has caused permanent corneal scarring and opacification.[a] However, another report has indicated that usually the outcome is less serious, even after liquid splash. This observation comes from a study of 19 people who were all injured by the same material on the same evening.[b] Explosive grenades containing approximately 100 ml of liquid exploded close to the victims, and all those with serious effects were splashed with the liquid into their open eyes. The reactions were different from those of commoner tear gases. Even after splashing with liquid ethyl bromoacetate, tearing and pain was brief, and was followed by complete corneal anesthesia. In general the patients were not aware of the seriousness of their eye injuries, because of lack of pain, and commonly did not seek medical attention until about four days later because of decrease in vision. Typically they had extensive loss of corneal epithelium and edema of the corneal stroma, which sometimes took weeks or months to clear, in association with slow recovery of corneal sensation. Despite the initial seriousness of the appearance of the corneas in some of these patients, all eventually recovered most of their vision, without serious sequelae. (See also *Tear gas weapons,* and *Lacrimatory Action.*)

a. Durix C, Gallet M: Severe ocular lesions caused by tear gas. *BULL SOC FRANCE OPHTALMOL* 69:125–137, 1956. (French)
b. Royer J, Gainet F: Ocular effects of ethyl bromoacetate tear gas. *BULL SOC OPHTALMOL FRANCE* 73:1165–1171, 1973. (French)

Ethyl chloride liquefied under moderate pressure and sprayed on rabbit corneas has caused epithelial damage, not attributable to temperature lowering, but to solvent or chemical action. The degree and rate of recovery was not recorded.[b] The gas at a concentration of 4% in air has been noted to cause slight irritation of the eyes in human beings.[a]

a. Sayers RR, Yant WP, et al: Acute response of guinea pigs to vapors of some new commercial organic compounds; ethylene dichloride. *PUBLIC HEALTH REP* 45:225–239, 1930.
b. Vannas S: Experimental examination of the freezing of the anterior parts of the eye for the purpose of operation. *ACTA OPHTHALMOL* 32:631–632, 1954.

Ethyl chloroacetate vapors irritate the eyes.[171] The liquid tested by drop application to rabbit eyes caused severe damage similar to that caused by ammonia, graded 9 on a scale of 10 after twenty-four hours.[27] The liquid is also said to have caused severe injury of human eyes, but no details appear to have been reported.[27]

Ethylenediamine (1,2-diaminoethane) is a strongly alkaline liquid, having an odor of ammonia. The vapor is slightly irritating to the nose at 200 ppm in air, and strongly irritating at 400 ppm.[a] Workmen exposed to ethylenediamine are said occasionally to see haloes around objects and to have some blurring of vision, presumably attributable to an effect on the corneal epithelium.[b] (See also *Amines—* see INDEX for page number.)

Splashes in the eye cause acute pain and potentially can cause serious injury. Applied to rabbit eyes ethylenediamine causes severe injury, graded 8 on a scale of 10 after twenty-four hours, but not as severe as ammonium hydroxide.[a, b, 27, 225] Even when ethylenediamine is diluted with water to 15%, it seriously damages rabbit corneas, but at 5% it induces minor injury.[b] When neutralized, as ethylenediamine hydrochloride, it was found not to injure rabbit eyes which were irrigated with a 0.02 M solution for ten minutes after mechanical removal of the epithelium to facilitate penetration.[81] The injuriousness of the free base seems to be attributable principally to its strong alkalinity.

Ethylenediamine is a frequent cause of contact dermatitis, but there is little information concerning possible ocular sensitization.[c, d]

a. Boas-Traube SG, Dresel EM, Dryden IGC: *NATURE* 162:960, 1948. (Quoted by Bourne LB, et al: *BR J IND MED* 16:81–97, 1959.)
b. Savitt IE: Contact dermatitis encountered in the production of epoxy resins. *ARCH DERM SYPH* 71:212–213, 1955.

c. White MI, Douglas WS, Main RA: Contact dermatitis attributed to ethylenediamine. *BR MED J* 1:415–416, 1978.

d. Bernstein JE, Lorincz AL: Ethylenediamine-induced exfoliative erythroderma. *ARCH DERM* 115:360–361, 1979.

Ethylenediamine derivatives in which both nitrogen atoms have additional organic groups attached have remarkable and often valuably enhanced chelating action toward metal ions. *Edetate* (ethylenediaminetetraacetate) is a prime example. Certain other derivatives have shown remarkable selective ocular toxic effects. These include the drug *ethambutol,* and a series of *N,N'-alkyl substituted ethylenediamines.*

N,N'-alkyl substituted ethylenediamines have been examined for ocular toxicity in the beagle dog by Kaiser, who has systematically studied a series of compounds with alkyl chains ranging from C_1 to C_4. All caused depigmentation of the tapetum lucidum in these dogs after single oral dose of 400 mg/kg. This was presumably due to removal of zinc, which is known to be a significant element in the normal green reflecting material in the back of the eye of these dogs. This effect was partially antagonized by administration of zinc sulfate, cysteine hydrochloride, or ascorbic acid in large doses.[a] (See also *Ethambutol* and compare *Dithizone and Pyrithione*—see INDEX for page numbers.)

a. Kaiser JA: Tapetal depigmentation in dogs produced by ethylenediamines. *FED PROC* 22:369, Abstr #1247, 1963.

Ethylene glycol is widely used as an antifreeze in automobiles, and therefore is easily available. Many cases of fatal or near-fatal poisoning have resulted from drinking it, either accidentally or suicidally. Poisoning of animals also is not uncommon.[b] For adult human beings the lethal dose is said to be 100 ml, though more than 900 ml has been survived.[za] Ingestion is followed in some cases by nausea, vomiting and abdominal pain. Within hours a characteristic sequence of cerebral, cardio-pulmonary, and renal complications begins to evolve.[c] In the first stage there is stupor or coma. In the second stage there may be cardiac failure or pulmonary edema, and in the third stage, reached in one to several days by survivors of the preceding stages, there is renal failure. Death may occur at any stage, or there may be remarkable recovery, despite severe involvement at each stage.[b] Those who die within the first three days usually have cerebral edema with engorgement of capillaries, scattered small hemorrhages in all parts of the brain, and toxic meningoencephalitis. Later, there has been loss of cells from the cerebral cortex and cerebellum.[i, v, za]

The biochemical aspects of the intoxication have been well reviewed by Vale[za] (1979) and Beasley[b] (1980). There are similarities to poisoning by methanol. Both substances are converted in the liver to aldehydes and acids, and these metabolic products are held to be responsible for the toxic effects, rather than the original unoxidized ethylene glycol or methanol. Both chemicals characteristically induce severe acidosis, which is accounted for by formation of glycolic acid from ethylene glycol, and formic acid from methanol.[g] (A relatively small amount of oxalic acid is produced by ethylene glycol, giving rise to calcium oxalate crystals in tissues and urine, but this is considered to be of more diagnostic than toxic significance.) Administration of ethanol interferes with the first step of metabolism of both ethylene glycol and methanol, and is helpful in treatment of poisoning by either. Also, administration of sodium bicarbonate has proven valuable to neutralize the acidosis produced by either chemical. There are, however, some noteworthy differences between ethylene glycol and methanol. Ethylene glycol is excreted in the urine, or is metabolized, much more rapidly than is methanol. Ethylene glycol has a greater tendency to cause renal failure. And, of particular interest here, ethylene glycol is not so notorious as methanol for causing toxic effects on the eyes and on vision.

Many case reports and a number of reviews of ethylene glycol poisoning do not even mention involvement of the eyes or of vision. This has been well pointed out by Berger and Ayyar[c], supplying a table and review of reported neurologic and ophthalmologic toxic complications. There are in fact a number of reports that mention dilated unreactive or poorly reactive pupils in association with coma[i,k,l,p,q,zz,zc], blurred or edematous optic discs[a,c,i,n,t,z], or decrease of vision.[a,c,l,w] Also, numerous reports mention strabismus from oculomotor nerve palsies,[d,f,i,j,m,q,u,z] and nystagmus, presumably from toxic effects on the cerebellum.[m,u,v,zc,zd]

Joly has described cases of poisoning in children from ingestion of ethylene glycol.[n,o] Ophthalmoscopically, papilledema was evident, with indistinct borders to the optic nerve head and dark dilated retinal veins, owing to cerebral edema and very high cerebrospinal fluid pressure.

Vainshtein has reported a series of poisonings in adults.[z] Drinking of 400 to 600 g resulted in severe poisoning, which in five out of six cases was lethal within seventy-two hours. In these severely poisoned patients, who presumably were comatose, the pupils were large and poorly reactive to light, and four were said to have pallor of the temporal half of the optic nervehead. Weakness of the eye muscles and disturbed eye movements were also noted.

Effects on the eyes from severe poisoning by ethylene glycol in four cases were also described by Friedman.[i] In one young patient who died forty-seven hours after drinking 100 to 120 ml of ethylene glycol, both eyes had dilated and unreactive pupils, and bilateral papilledema without retinal hemorrhages or exudates, when the patient was comatose and convulsing. A second young patient, who drank about the same amount and died after seventeen days, was described at forty-eight hours as having "confusion, ocular palsy, and anuria," also "headache and blurred vision" and "bilateral ophthalmoplegia" with "medial strabismus of the left eye." In both eyes "disc blurring" was noted, but no hemorrhages or exudates were seen. No measurements of vision were made.

Hagstam reported on a boy who was severely poisoned by ethylene glycol, with brain involvement manifested by convulsions, varying levels of consciousness paralleling electroencephalographic abnormality, and kidney involvement producing anuria and uremia.[l] From days 5 to 18 the pupils were large, and visual acuity seemed to be reduced to 0.7–0.5 right, 0.5–0.4 left, but difficult to evaluate because of poor cooperation. Comments on the fundi indicated slight retinal edema on day 5, but none on day 18. Following repeated hemodialysis, the boy made a remarkable recovery during the fourth week, and was "recovered completely" within 3 months, presumably including vision, though this was not specifically mentioned.

Smith mentioned in one fatal case that after the first day following poisoning the patient was lethargic and complained of blurred vision as he became anuric.[w]

Ahmed has described a man who drank antifreeze, not clearly identified as ethylene glycol, and temporarily had loss of vision to no light perception, then gradually improving to 4/60 at best.[a] The optic discs were said to be normal when vision was first lost, but to show bilateral optic atrophy 5 months later. Practically no information was given on the patient's general condition or treatment, which, together with lack of chemical identification of the responsible substance, suggests that this should not be accepted without question as an authentic case of ethylene glycol poisoning.

Berger has described a patient who had acute ethylene glycol poisoning, then 6 days later in renal failure, requiring hemodialysis, developed dysarthria, dysphagia, and bilateral facial nerve paralysis.[c] By 12 days the patient's visual acuity dropped to 20/100 right, 20/200 left, with blurring of the disc margins, inequality and subnormal reactivity of the pupils, but peripheral fields intact to confrontation testing. There was also nystagmus and clumsy gait. With more hemodialysis, the patient improved, and in a month the visual acuity increased to 20/60 in both eyes, and the pupils became normal.

The mechanism of impairment of vision in ethylene glycol poisoning has not been definitively studied, but the clinical observations suggest that disturbance of the optic nerves is important. However, whether ethylene glycol poisoning may in rare cases produce partial optic atrophy is difficult to say from the published evidence.[a,z] In a case of fatal poisoning in a human being ethylene glycol has been demonstrated to be present in the vitreous humor,[e] but there appears to have been no attempt to examine the effect of this on retinal function.

In animals, including rats, cats, dogs and monkeys, little attention has been given to ocular or visual effects from experimental or accidental systemic poisoning.[b,g]

A most unusual type of intoxication affecting eye movement occurred in a group of women working in the presence of vapor from ethylene glycol that was heated in open containers. Of thirty-eight women exposed, nine were subject to attacks of unconsciousness of five to ten minutes' duration, occurring two or three times a week while at work. These patients, and an additional five who were exposed but not subject to attacks of unconsciousness, had nystagmus, usually horizontal, but definitely rotatory in two cases. The nystagmus appeared to be of supranuclear origin without participation of the vestibular nuclei. The attacks ceased on discontinuing exposure.[y]

Experimental exposure to vapor or spray of ethylene glycol in air at a concentration of 17 mg/cu m is said to have produced no ill effects in human beings during 4 weeks, and 265 mg/cu m produced no ocular damage in a chimpanzee, but in rabbits and rats exposure for several days to 12 mg/cu m induced severe eye irritation, edema of the lids, and corneal opacity.[h]

The effect of splash contact of ethylene glycol with the eye has been found without exception in tests on rabbits to result in immediate moderate symptoms of discomfort with mild temporary conjunctival reaction, but no significant corneal damage.[h,zb,27,45,123] In one accident to a human eye the conjunctiva became inflamed, but there was no permanent damage.[x] Experiments in which aqueous solutions of ethylene glycol were dropped repeatedly on eyes of rabbits for hours or days showed the maximal non-damaging concentration to be 4% for the conjunctiva, but 20 to 40% for the cornea.[s]

Replacement of the aqueous humor in eyes of rabbits with aqueous solutions of ethylene glycol showed the maximal non-damaging concentration to be 2% for the iris, but 20 to 40% for the cornea and lens.[s] Significantly more reaction was produced by daily repeated injections into the anterior chamber.[r]

a. Ahmed MM: Ocular effects of antifreeze poisoning. *BR J OPHTHALMOL* 55:854–855, 1971.

b. Beasley VR, Buck WB: Acute ethylene glycol toxicosis: a review. *VET HUM TOXICOL* 22:255–263, 1980.

c. Berger JR, Ayyar DR: Neurological complications of ethylene glycol intoxication. *ARCH NEUROL* 38:724–726, 1981.

d. Berman LB, Schreiner GE, Feys J: The nephrotic lesion of ethylene glycol. *ANN INTERN MED* 46:611–619, 1957.

e. Bogusz M: Vitreous humor as reliable material for ethylene glycol determination. *FORENSIC SCI INT* 16:75–76, 1980.

f. Brekke A: Two cases of poisoning with ethylene glycol. *NORSK MAG LAEGEVID* 91:318–388, 1930.

g. Clay KL, Murphy RC: On the metabolic acidosis of ethylene glycol intoxication. *TOXICOL APPL PHARMACOL* 39:39–49, 1977.

h. Coon RA, Jones RA, et al: Animal inhalation studies. *TOXICOL APPL PHARMACOL* 16:646–655, 1970.

i. Friedman EA, Greenberg JB, et al: Consequences of ethylene glycol poisonings. *AM J MED* 32:891–892, 1962.

j. Grant AP: Acute ethylene glycol poisoning treated with calcium salts. *LANCET* 2:1252–1253, 1952.

k. Hagemann PO, Chiffelle TR: Ethylene glycol poisoning. *J LAB CLIN MED* 33:573–784, 1948.

l. Hagstam KE, Ingvar DH, et al: Ethylene glycol poisoning treated by hemodialysis. *ACTA MED SCAND* 178:599–606, 1965.

m. Hansen K: Ethylene glycol poisoning. *SAMML VERGIFTUNGSF* 1:175–176, 1930. (German)

n. Joly JB, Hauault G, et al: Severe poisoning by ethylene glycol in a child of six years. *PRESSE MED* 75:2041–2044, 1967. (French)

o. Joly JB, et al: Acute poisoning by ethylene glycol (apropos of 4 cases in young children.) *BULL SOC MED HOSP PARIS* 119:27–45, 1968. (French)

p. Levinsky NG, Robert NJ, et al: Severe metabolic acidosis in a young man (CPC 38-1979). *N ENGL J MED* 301:650–657, 1979.

q. McDonald SF: Poisoning from drinking glycolethylene. *MED J AUST* 1:204–205, 1947.

r. McDonald TO, Roberts MD, Borgmann AR: Ocular toxicity of ethylene chlorohydrin and ethylene glycol in rabbit eyes. *TOXICOL APPL PHARMACOL* 21:143–150, 1972.

s. McDonald TO, Kasten K, et al: Acute ocular toxicity of ethylene oxide, ethylene glycol, and ethylene chlorohydrin. *BULL PARENTER DRUG ASSOC* 27:153–164, 1973; and 31:25–32, 1977.

t. Nadeau G, Delaney FJ: Two cases of ethylene glycol poisoning. *CAN MED ASSOC J* 70:69–70, 1954.

u. Parry MF, Wallach R: Ethylene glycol poisoning. *AM J MED* 57:143–150, 1974.

v. Pons CA, Custer RP: Acute ethylene glycol poisoning. *AM J MED SCI* 211:544–552, 1946.

w. Smith DE: Morphologic lesions due to acute and subacute poisoning with antifreeze (ethylene glycol). *ARCH PATHOL LAB MED* 51:423–433, 1951.

x. Sykowsky P: Ethylene glycol toxicity. *AM J OPHTHALMOL* 34:1599–1600, 1951.

y. Troisi FM: Chronic intoxication by ethylene glycol vapor. *BR J IND MED* 7:65–69, 1950.

z. Vainshtein VI: Ophthalmological diagnosis of acute poisoning with antifreezes. *VESTN OFTALMOL* 80:62–63, 1967. (English summary)

za. Vale JA: Ethylene glycol poisoning. *VET HUM TOXICOL* 21(Suppl):118–120, 1979.

zb. Walther R: On the toxicology of glycols. *ARCH GEWERBEPATH* 11:326, 1942. (German)

zc. Widman C: A few cases of ethylene glycol intoxication. *ACTA MED SCAND* 126:295–306, 1946.

zd. Zehrer G: Fatal poisoning by a glycerin substitute (diethylene glycol). *MED KLIN* 43:369–371, 1948. (German)

Ethylene oxide (1,2-epoxyethane; oxirane) is a liquid below 12° and a gas at room temperature, having no particularly characteristic or unpleasant odor. Exposure of animals to high concentration of the gas has caused lacrimation in cats, and inflammation of the conjunctiva and clouding of the cornea in dogs, cats, rabbits, and especially guinea pigs.[a,k]

Thiess has published an authoritative report of his own observations in forty-one cases of excessive industrial exposure to ethylene oxide, mainly in accidents.[j] The principal characteristic effect after excessive exposure to the vapor was vomiting, recurring periodically for hours, accompanied by nausea and headache. Thiess observed that protracted contact of the vapor or the liquid with the skin caused toxic dermatitis with large bullae. The eyes of workers excessively exposed to ethylene oxide vapor occasionally showed slight irritation, but there were no injuries of the cornea. Thiess observed no lacrimatory effect that could be considered a warning symptom.

Accidental exposure of a person to an estimated 500 ppm in air for 2 or 3 minutes was enough to cause temporary unconsciousness and seizures, but apparently did not produce ocular symptoms.[g]

I have observed the effects of an accidental forceful blast of ethylene oxide vapor that struck a nurse in the eye, nose and mouth, from a gas sterilizer that employed a cartridge of ethylene oxide. This caused no immediate discomfort, but within two hours one eye became mildly uncomfortable and one nostril felt sore and obstructed. The only abnormality in the eye at that time was fine gray dots in the corneal epithelium in the palpebral fissure, staining with fluorescein. In three hours the foreign-body type irritation in the affected eye and soreness in one nostril were enough to interfere with her working. The foreign-body type discomfort reached the maximum nine to ten hours after the exposure, but by fifteen hours began to subside, and in twenty-four hours the eye was entirely normal. Soreness in the nose persisted a little longer, but at no time was there respiratory distress or alteration of taste or sensation in the mouth.

Thiess has reported an instance of a squirt of pure ethylene oxide into one eye of a patient, treated immediately with copious irrigation with water; this resulted only in irritation of the conjunctiva lasting for one day.[j] Thiess quoted Hollingsworth and associates as having observed in rabbit eyes after application of a drop of ethylene oxide only intense conjunctivitis which cleared in four days.[c] A corneal burn from ethylene oxide in a workman has been listed by McLaughlin, as also having prompt recovery, but no details of the type of exposure were recorded.[165]

In aqueous solution in prolonged contact with the skin, ethylene oxide is well known to be vesicant,[h,j] but probably the volatility of ethylene oxide and the fact that there are rarely circumstances in which considerable concentrations are kept in protracted contact with the eye account for the mildness of ocular injuries which have been observed clinically so far.

McDonald performed tests on rabbits showing that in aqueous solution the maximum concentration that could be applied externally to the eye, one drop every 10 minutes for 6 hours, without causing damage to the conjunctiva was 0.1%, to the cornea was 1%, and to the lens or retina was 20%.[f] (This was the same whether the eyes were normal at the start or had been irritated by an application of diluted commercial shampoo.) McDonald also showed in rabbits that if the aqueous humor was replaced once with an aqueous solution of ethylene oxide the maximum non-damaging concentration for the iris and lens was 0.1%, and for the cornea was 1%.[f] At higher concentrations, damage consisted of irreversible opacities of cornea and lens.

These observations relate particularly to clinical problems that have been attributed to intraocular ethylene oxide, or its reaction products, ethylene glycol and ethylene chlorohydrin.

As mentioned elsewhere under the heading "Acetylcholine", Leibowitz has reported on corneal edema, corneal opacity, and lens opacities, retinal vascular toxicity, and optic atrophy that developed in a small group of patients who had Miochol injected into the anterior chamber after it had been inadvertently contaminated by attempted sterilization with ethylene oxide.[e] Also, Stark has reported that in a series of patients in whom ethylene-oxide-sterilized intraocular lenses were implanted there was an impressively higher incidence of sterile hypopyon, and recurrent or persistent iritis than in a series of patients who received lenses that had been sterilized and cleaned by sodium hydroxide.[i] While ethylene oxide was suspect in the case of the intraocular lenses, other possible factors were also considered.

A possibility that systemic intoxication with ethylene oxide may lead to cataract formation has been raised. Gross described four patients, aged 27 to 31, who were exposed for 2 weeks to 2 months to a leaky sterilizer with detectible odor. One had irritation of the eyes and blunting of smell and taste, then a series of motor seizures. The others had no eye symptoms, but developed evidence of sensorimotor polyneuropathy.[b] All recovered, but a follow-up of these same patients four years later reported by Jay, revealed that one had developed cataracts, which has been extracted, one had posterior subcapsular opacities, and one had anterior vacuoles with posterior subcapsular opacities, but both had visual acuities of 20/20 or 20/25.[d] None of the four patients had symptoms of corneal disturbance, but 2 had slightly thicker than normal corneas, with normal number of endothelial cells. An additional 8 people, ages 22 to 48, who had worked with ethylene oxide, with no known over-exposures, had normal eyes and no neurologic abnormalities.[d]

a. Flury F: On ethylene oxide. *NAUNYN-SCHMIED ARCH EXP PATHOL PHARMAKOL* 157:107–108, 1931. (German)

b. Gross JA, Haas ML, Swift TR: Ethylene oxide neurotoxicity. *NEUROLOGY* 29:978–983, 1979.

c. Hollingsworth RL, Rowe VK, et al: Toxicity of ethylene oxide determined on experimental animals. *ARCH IND HEALTH* 13:217, 1956.

d. Jay WM, Swift TR, Hull DS: Possible relationship of ethylene oxide exposure to cataract formation. *AM J OPHTHALMOL* 93:727–732, 1982.

e. Leibowitz HM: Unexpected problems with intraocular acetylcholine. In Fraunfelder (1979).[311]

f. McDonald TO, Kasten K, et al: Acute ocular toxicity of ethylene oxide, ethylene glycol, and ethylene chlorohydrin. *BULL PARENTER DRUG ASSOC* 27:153–164, 1973; and 31:25–32, 1977.

g. Salina E, Sasich L, et al: Acute ethylene oxide intoxication. *DRUG INTEL CLIN PHARMACOL* 15:384–386, 1981.

h. Sexton R, Henson EV: Experimental ethylene oxide human skin injuries. *ARCH IND HYG* 2:549–564, 1950.

i. Stark WJ, Rosenblum P, et al: Postoperative inflammatory reactions to intraocular lenses sterilized with ethylene oxide. *OPHTHALMOLOGY* 87:385–389, 1980.

j. Thiess AM: Observations on injuries to health under the influence of ethylene oxide. *ARCH TOXIKOL* 20:127–140, 1963. (German)

k. Waite CP, Patty Fa, Yant WP: Acute responses of guinea pigs. IV. Ethylene oxide. *PUB HEALTH REP* 45:1832–1843, 1930.

Ethylenimine (ethylene imine, aziridine) is an alkylating agent, particularly reactive with sulfhydryl groups. It is considered to be in the same hazard class with volatile cyanides from the standpoint of systemic poisoning.[b] It is believed to be analogous in structure and reactivity to the cyclic intermediates formed in the reaction of nitrogen mustards.

Remarkably selective atrophy of rods and cones and their nuclei is produced in cats by a single dose of 5 to 20 mg/kg, but not in dogs, rabbits, guinea pigs, or rats.[g] In cats, mydriasis and blindness become evident in one to six days, with progressive narrowing and sometimes disappearance of retinal vessels. In higher doses ethylenimine characteristically causes death in experimental animals in a day or two.[c] No instance of damage to the retina is known in human beings.[g]

An authoritative report by Thiess in 1965 based on review of the literature and medical examination of seventy-three patients after industrial contact with ethylenimine established the characteristics of both immediate and delayed injurious effect.[f] The effects on the eyes in several cases in this report were from exposure to the vapors, resulting in severe irritation and reddening of the eyes with increased tearing, all getting worse during several hours after exposure, during the same time that severe effects in the respiratory passages were developing. Recovery from the conjunctivitis or possibly keratoconjunctivitis was slow, requiring at least several days and in some cases several weeks. No permanent eye disturbances were encountered. No specialized eye examinations were described. No instance of splash of liquid ethylenimine in the eye was observed.[f]

One example of the effects of excessive exposure to the vapor has been recorded in the case of five students who were exposed for two hours to vapors of *ethylenimine* and *N-ethylethylenimine*. After a latent period of three to seven and one-half hours they developed severe irritation of the eyes and respiratory tract, but eventually recovered.[h] In addition to being immediately irritating, ethylenimine apparently has the same characteristic latent period before onset of more serious poisoning that is associated with other alkylating agents such as dimethyl sulfate and mustard gas.[e-h]

Though human beings have apparently been fortunate in escaping injury from splashes of ethylenimine, this must be regarded as potentially extremely dangerous in liquid form. Patty has reported application of 0.005 ml of liquid ethylenimine or 0.5 ml of a 15% aqueous solution to the eye of a rabbit caused destruction of the cornea and death of the animal.[d]

A chloroderivative of ethylenimine, *1-chloroaziridine*, is said to be strongly lacrimogenic.[a]

a. Anonymous. *CHEM ENGIN NEWS* Oct. 27, 1958, p. 52.
b. Carpenter CP, Smyth HF, Shaffer CB: The acute toxicity of ethylene imine to small animals. *J IND HYG* 30:1–6, 1948.
c. Danehy JP, Pflaum DJ: Toxicity of ethylene imine. *IND ENGIN CHEM* 30:778, 1938.
d. Patty FA: *INDUSTRIAL HYGIENE AND TOXICOLOGY.* New York, Interscience, 1962, vol. 2, pp. 2172–2175.
e. Silver SD, McGrath FP: A comparison of acute toxicities of ethylene imine and ammonia to mice. *J IND HYG* 30:7–9, 1948.
f. Thiess AM: Injuries to health and poisonings through the action of ethylenimine. *ARCH TOXIKOL* 21:67–82, 1965. (German)
g. von Canstatt BS, Hofmann HT, et al: Disturbances of the cat retina by poisoning with perorally or percutaneously administered chemicals. *VERH DTSCH GES PATH* 50:429–435, 1966. (German)
h. Weightman J, Hoyle JP: Accidental exposure to ethylenimine and N-ethylethylenimine vapors. *J AM MED ASSOC* 189:543–545, 1964.

Ethyl formate vapor at a concentration of 330 ppm in air causes irritation of the eyes which subsides only after several hours.[61] It has been assumed, but not proved, that hydrolysis and release of formic acid on the moist surfaces are responsible for the irritant action of ethyl formate.[56] Ethyl formate liquid tested in a standard way by application to rabbit eyes has caused moderate reversible injury graded 4 on a scale of 10.[226]

Ethylhydrocupreine hydrochloride (Optochin, Numoquin), a derivative of quinine, formerly was employed systemically in treatment of pneumonia, and topically for pneumococcal infections of the eye,[171] though it could induce corneal anesthesia and clouding of the corneal epithelium.[48] There seem to have been no cases of blindness following local application to the eye,[a,b,214,247] but visual disturbances from systemic administration have been described in at least fifty articles. The first observations of visual disturbance were made in 1915 and 1916.

A dose of 2 to 4 g/day caused visual disturbances in 3 to 4 per cent of patients. The toxic effects on the eye were remarkably uniform, and closely resembled the effects of quinine. Usually clouding of vision developed rapidly, going to complete blindness in a few hours. This was commonly associated with tinnitus and impairment of hearing. During the acute blindness, the pupils were dilated and unreactive to light but still responsive to attempted accommodation. The refractive media of the eyes were never affected, and commonly the fundi appeared normal. However, in many cases retinal edema and narrowing of the retinal arteries were observed. With discontinuance of medication, vision usually returned within a few hours or days. A small proportion of patients recovered more slowly and incompletely. A smaller proportion remained blind and developed optic atrophy.

The visual fields characteristically remained concentrically constricted for white, and especially for colors, even though visual acuity returned to normal. The optic nervehead usually appeared normal at first, but subsequently became pale, and in cases of optic atrophy became white. Pigmentary changes in the retina occurred rarely. Postmortem examination of poisoned patients showed degeneration of retinal ganglion cells and optic nerve fibers.

Experimental poisoning in animals was found to cause not only injury of the retinal ganglion cells but also degeneration in the outer nuclear layer and disappearance of peripheral rods, sometimes accompanied by choroidal atrophy, but usually without narrowing or abnormality of the retinal blood vessels.

Ethylhydrocupreine is no longer employed medically, and accordingly poisonings from it are no longer seen. (Compare *Cinchona derivatives, Quinine,* and *Quinoline derivatives.*)

   a. Birch-Hirschfeld A: On the subject of toxic amblyopias from methanol, optochin, and granugenol. *ZENTRALBL AUGENHEILKD* 35:1–12, 1916. (German)
   b. Jess A: The dangers of chemotherapy for the eye. *GRAEFES ARCH OPHTHALMOL* 104:48–74, 1921. (German)

Ethyl iodoacetate, a lacrimogenic substance, has been investigated as a potential poison to the retina, because of its relationship to *sodium iodoacetate,* particularly its similarity in inhibiting respiration and glycolysis, and its activity as a thiol poison. Unlike *sodium iodoacetate,* ethyl iodoacetate was found not to be damaging to the retina in rabbits and rats,[231] although it did prove damaging to surviving rabbit retina *in vitro.*[157]

Ethyl iodoacetate has been shown to have the same type of powerful inhibitory effects as a number of other well-known lacrimators on a series of thiol enzymes *in vitro.*[160] (See also *Lacrimatory Action.*)

Ethyl isothiocyanate (ethyl mustard oil) vapors are irritating to the eyes. The liquid blisters the skin.[171]

A speculation has been recorded that ethyl isothiocyanate might be involved as a decomposition product of diethylthiourea in production of painful keratitis. (See *Diethylthiourea* for more details.)

N-Ethylmaleimide is a strongly irritant substance, melting at 45°, a lacrimator when liquid.[171] In cultures of retina it has been shown at 0.0005 M concentration to cause unselective degeneration of retinal cells.[99] Injected intravitreally in rats, it alters the ERG.[a] In the anterior chamber it inhibits glycolysis in the trabecular meshwork, and increases facility of aqueous outflow in excised calf and monkey eyes.[b]

a. Buckser S: Effect on the ERG of injecting N-ethyl maleimide into the eye after light adaptation. *OPHTHALMOLOGICA ADDIT AD* 158:633–646, 1969.

b. Epstein DL, Patterson MM, et al: N-ethylmaleimide increases the facility of aqueous outflow of excised monkey and calf eyes. *INVEST OPHTHALMOL VIS SCI* 22:752–756, 1982.

Ethyl mercury compounds resemble *methyl mercury* compounds, but the effects on vision have not been so extensively studied. The following ethyl mercury salts and diethyl mercury salts have been reported to impair vision seriously.

Ethyl mercury chloride, ethyl mercury sulfate, and *diethyl mercury* have been administered subcutaneously to frogs, rabbits, cats, and dogs.[a] Also, small amounts of these compounds were administered briefly to human beings in treatment of syphilis before their toxicity was recognized, but apparently no poisoning of the human beings resulted. Blindness has been described in one dog and one cat given *diethyl mercury,* and another cat given *ethyl mercury sulfate* similarly seemed blind, but the pupils continued to react to light. Unfortunately, at autopsy little attention was paid to the brain, and none to the eyes.[a]

Ethylmercuric chloride (chloroethyl mercury, Ceresan), a fungicide for treating seeds, is highly toxic to the skin and brain.[171] In cultures of retina it has been shown to cause selective degeneration of the rod cells at 5×10^{-6} M concentration.[99]

N-(Ethylmercuri)-p-toluenesulfonanilide (ethyl mercury toluene sulphonanilide, Ceresan-M), a fungicide, is reported to have caused at least twenty-six cases of poisoning in Iraq in 1956 and 1960 from eating of treated seeds.[b] Constriction of visual fields or marked loss of central vision with optic atrophy, along with kidney damage, skin lesions, and motor disturbances in the legs, was said to be not infrequent. In one such case a patient who had severe ataxia and was almost blind appeared to respond well to treatment with dimercaprol. In five other cases the treatment with dimercaprol was, however, apparently of no value.[b] (See *Methyl mercury compounds* for description of closely related substances.)

a. Hepp P: On ethylmercury compounds and on the relationship of ethyl mercury to mercury poisoning. *NAUNYN-SCHMIEDEBERG'S ARCH EXP PATH PHARMAKOL* 23:91–128, 1887. (German)

b. Jalili MA, Abbasi AH: Poisoning by ethyl mercury toluene sulphonanilide. *BR J IND MED* 18:303–308, 1961.

Ethylmorphine hydrochloride (Codethyline, Dionin), formerly used in eyedrops for analgesia, produced conjunctival vasodilation and edema. Local application to glaucomatous patients or intravenous administration to rabbits has variously been reported to raise, or reduce the intraocular pressure, but careful, controlled clinical studies with adequate documentation have yet to be done.

Ethyl morpholine (N-ethylmorpholine, 4-ethylmorpholine), a moderately volatile liquid, has peculiarly disturbing action on the cornea, like certain other volatile amines, causing transient edema of the corneal epithelium in workers exposed to 40 ppm or more in air during the work day, causing onset of blue-grey vision or colored haloes around lights a few hours after exposure, without discomfort.[40,164,170,334] Tested in liquid form, a drop to a rabbit's eye causes the cornea to become hazy in about five minutes and the epithelium to slough from the surface, grade 7 injury on a scale of 10.[226] (See also *Amines.*)

N-Ethylpiperidine has been tested by applying one drop to a rabbit's cornea. In five minutes the cornea became hazy and the epithelium sloughed from the surface[170] Exposure of the human eye to the vapor is reported to have caused "grey haziness" of vision, similar to the effect of ethyl morpholine.[334] (See also *Amines* and *Ethyl morpholine.*)

Ethylpyridine has been suspected of causing amblyopia in one instance in the manufacture of isoniazid.[a] A man engaged in distilling ethylpyridine developed central scotomas in both eyes. When work was discontinued and B vitamins were administered, vision returned to 5/6 in several weeks. Similar disturbances have been caused by isoniazid. (Compare *Isoniazid.*)

   a. Planten JT: Toxic amblyopia from ethylpyridine. *NEDERL T GENEESK* 97:540–542, 1953.

Ethyl silicate (tetraethyl silicate) is insoluble in water, but is slowly hydrolysed to release ethyl alcohol and deposit silica. It is employed as a waterproofing agent on masonry. A drop applied to rabbit eyes caused immediate signs of discomfort, but the eyes were found to be normal in twenty-four hours and the corneas took no fluorescein stain.[211,224]

   Exposure of albino rabbits and guinea pigs to vapor of ethyl silicate caused no disturbance of the eyes at concentrations of 700 ppm or less, but at all concentrations over 1,000 ppm irritation of the eyes and nose occurred at once. Exposure to 2,500 ppm caused opacities of the cornea if carried out for at least two hours.[a] The human experiments found: 3,000 ppm is extremely irritating to the eyes and nose; 1,200 ppm stings eyes and nose and produces tears; 700 ppm mildly stings eyes and nose; 250 ppm makes the eyes and nose tingle slightly; 85 ppm can be detected only by odor. It appeared that 700 ppm would be intolerable to human beings for more than half an hour.[a]

   Ethyl silicate is much less toxic to the eyes than *methyl silicate.*

   a. Smyth HF Jr, Seaton J: Acute response of guinea pigs and rats to inhalation of the vapors of tetraethyl orthosilicate (ethyl silicate). *J IND HYG* 22:288–296, 1940.

Etidronate disodium, a pharmaceutical calcium regulator, evaluated on rabbit eyes as a constituent of mouth wash or dentrifice, caused transient moderate conjunctival irritation at 3% concentration, and only slight conjunctivitis at 1%.[a]

   a. Nixon GA, Buehler EV, Newmann EA: Preliminary safety assessment of disodium etidronate as an additive to experimental oral hygiene products. *TOXICOL APPL PHARMACOL* 22:661–671, 1972.

Etomidate, hypnotic, has lowered the intraocular pressure when given intravenously in non-glaucomatous patients,[b] and when applied as drops to eyes of rabbits.[c] However, in animals an hour of anesthesia with etomidate was followed by ultrastructural changes in the retina, which gradually improved during the next two days.[a]

  a. Antal M: Etomidate induced retinal changes. *GRAEFES ARCH OPHTHALMOL* 215:193–201, 1981.
  b. Famewo CE, Odugbesari CO, Osuntokun OO: Effect of etomidate on intraocular pressure. *CAN ANAESTH SOC J* 24:712–716, 1977.
  c. Oji EO, Holdcroft A: Comparison of the ocular effects of topical etomidate and pilocarpine in rabbits. *INT OPHTHALMOL* 2:71–76, 1980.

Eucatropine (euphthalmine hydrochloride), used in eye drops for short duration mydriasis, has been known to precipitate acute glaucoma in predisposed eyes. Most cases have been reported without benefit of gonioscopy,[b,83] but one study has been published in which eyes with normal tensions were separated into categories according to whether they had normal angles or narrow angles before testing with topical 5% eucatropine hydrochloride.[a] In the normal eyes there was no increase in pressure or change in tonographic facility of outflow, but in a considerable proportion of eyes with narrow angles the pressure rose at least 8 mm Hg and facility of outflow decreased at least 25 per cent. A comparison in eyes with open-angle glaucoma remains to be made.

  a. Becker B, Thompson HE: Tonography and angle-closure glaucoma: diagnosis and therapy. *AM J OPHTHALMOL* 46:305–310, 1958.
  b. Gradle HS: Effects of mydriatics upon intraocular tension. *TRANS AM OPHTHALMOL SOC* 33:175–184, 1935.

Eucupine (isoamylhydrocupreine) formerly was employed as an antibacterial agent. In the influenza epidemic of World War I three instances of visual disturbance were reported by one author.[a,214] One patient received 5 g in four days, and twenty-five days later complained of visual disturbance; vision was 6/12 and 6/8, with central scotoma for green. The fundi appeared normal. It is not known whether vision improved subsequently. The second patient received 6 g, and on the third day had rapid complete loss of vision with almost unreactive pupils but normal fundi. Eleven days later the retinal arteries appeared narrowed and the nerveheads pale. Nevertheless in the course of three months the vision improved to 6/10 in both eyes. The visual fields remained constricted to white. The third patient took 3.6 g in two days, and became suddenly completely blind, with widely dilated unreactive pupils but normal fundi. This patient died a day later. The posterior segment of the eyes and the optic nerves were examined histologically but showed no degeneration.[a]

Related compounds have caused serious visual loss characterized by narrowing of retinal vessels, whitening of the optic nerveheads, and constriction of visual fields. Compare *Ethylhydrocuprein, Quinine, Cinchona derivatives,* and *Quinoline derivatives.*

  a. Franke: On injuries of the eye by Eukupin. *BER DTSCH OPHTHALMOL GESELLSCH* 42:177–182, 1920. (German)

Euphorbia (*Euphorbiaceae*) is a plant genus embracing some 1500 species, mostly spurge or cactus-like. Many *Euphorbia* plants contain a sap or latex which is irritating to the skin, and in contact with the eyes causes severe inflammation, both external and intraocular.[153,214,249,253] The juices of some of these plants have been used in treatment of warts and malignant tumors.

There have been numerous case reports describing the experiences of patients who have accidentally squirted sap into their eyes when cutting the plants, or who have contaminated their eyes when attempting to treat warts on the eyelids.[a-g,i-k] A typical case is as follows. A patient cutting *E.peplus* felt something squirt into one eye, causing immediate smarting and pain and headache. Marked swelling of the lids, diffuse corneal epithelial defects, blepharospasm, and iritis developed in an hour or two and progressed to severe keratitis with corneal edema, bedewing of the posterior surface with fine deposits, and folds in Descemet's membrane. A thick serofibrinous exudate formed in the anterior chamber. Photophobia, tearing, lid swelling, and hyperemia reached a maximum in three days; recovery was gradual but complete, taking ten to twelve days.[g] Less fortunate outcome has occurred in occasional patients, particularly after contamination with latex from *E. royleana*, which has produced corneal ulceration and scarring, and left posterior synechias.[j,k]

Investigations on the eyes of animals by Lewin and Guillery in 1905 showed that *Euphorbia* latex tended to cause severe inflammation when fresh; but when allowed to age the latex lost some of its irritancy. Differences in irritancy were noted among various *Euphorbias*.[153] Also striking variations have been noted among different animal species in the nature of the reaction of their eyes to contact with *Euphorbia* latex. Generally rabbits and guinea pigs have responded with conjunctivitis, but not with keratitis or iridocyclitis. This has particularly been pointed out in a literature review and in experiments by Angius.[a] Experiments on the eyes of animals have given remarkably variable results.

Euphorbias which have sap irritating to human eyes are *E. candelabrum, E. resinifera, E. cyparissias, E. lathyris, E. esula, E. helioscopa, E. nerifolia, E. lactea* (candelabra cactus), *E. peplus, E. antiquorum, E. canariense, E. dendroides, E. royaleana,* and *E. tirucalli* (pencil cactus, milk bush); also *Pedilanthus tithymaloides* (Christmas candle, redbird cactus, slipper flower, Jew bush) and *Hura crepitans* (sandbox tree, monkey pistol).[142]

Euphorbia lathyris in contact with human eyes characteristically causes miosis with transient conjunctivitis and keratitis but without iritis, according to Geidel.[e] The same author experimented on rabbits and dogs, but could provoke little or no inflammatory reaction with *Euphorbia lathyris* even though in the rabbits the corneal epithelium was abraded before the material was applied. However, in guinea pigs, Geidel did obtain a severe but mostly reversible swelling of the lids, conjunctivitis and keratitis. *Euphorbia lactea* and *Euphorbia tirucalli* (candelabra cactus and pencil tree) saps produce keratoconjunctivitis, according to Crowder and Sexton, characterized by immediate burning sensation, lacrimation, and photophobia, followed in eight to twelve hours by chemosis, increased pain, loss of corneal epithelium, and corneal edema, but with subsequent slow, complete recovery.[d] The same authors experimented on rabbits without obtaining uniform responses, but in dogs succeeded in regularly provoking reaction similar to the human response, consisting of a severe reaction with corneal opacification developing after a delay of twenty-four to thirty-six hours with subsequent clearing during one to three weeks. Histology showed infiltration with inflammatory cells and probable endothelial damage. The same report by Crowder and Sexton also has provided a good review and bibliography of *Euphorbia* toxicity in general.[d]

There has been much chemical investigation of the constituents of *euphorbia* latex because of interest in antineoplastic action in experimental animals,[h] but so far no discovery of a specific antidote for the irritancy. Ocular reactions seem best treated by standard anti-inflammatory measures, including topical corticosteroid.

a. Angius T: Eye injuries from Euphorbia sap. *RASS ITAL OTTAL* 7:649–660, 1938. (Italian)

b. Biedner BZ, Sacks U, Witztun A: Euphorbia peplus latex keratoconjunctivitis. *ANN OPHTHALMOL* 13:739–740, 1981.

c. Boiman R, Savir H: Chemical eye injury by Euphorbia dendroides. *HAREFUAH* 87:308–309, 337, 1974. (Hebrew)

d. Crowder JI, Sexton RR: Keratoconjunctivitis resulting from sap of candelabra cactus and the pencil tree. *ARCH OPHTHALMOL* 72:476–484, 1964.

e. Geidel K: Clinical observation and experimental animal investigations on the action of the sap of Euphorbia lathyris on the eye. *KLIN MONATSBL AUGENHEILKD* 141:374–379, 1962. (German)

f. Guggenheim I: Keratoconjunctivitis from the sap of Euphorbia helioscopa. *KLIN MONATSBL AUGENHEILKD* 77:521–523, 1926. (German)

g. Hartmann K: Eye injuries from the sap of Euphorbia peplus. *KLIN MONATSBL AUGENHEILKD* 104:324–325, 1940. (German)

h. Kupchan SM, Uchida I, et al: Antileukemic principles isolated from Euphorbiaceae plants. *SCIENCE* 191:571–572, 1976.

i. Lisch K: The effect of the latex of Euphorbias on the eye. *KLIN MONATSBL AUGENHEILKD* 176:469–471, 1980. (German)

j. Sofat BK, Sood GC, et al: Euphorbia royaleana latex keratitis. *AM J OPHTHALMOL* 74:634–637, 1972.

k. Sood GC, Sofat BK, Chandel RD: Injury to the eye by the sap of Euphorbia royaleana. *BR J OPHTHALMOL* 55:856–857, 1971.

Eye cosmetics consist mainly of *mascara, eye liners,* and *eye shadows.* As coloring materials, carbon black, iron oxide and other inorganic pigments may be present. Details have been published by Thorne.[s] Eye cosmetics sometimes cause dermatitis of the eyelids,[p] as well as conjunctival and corneal discoloration. ***Mascara,*** containing carbon black or a variety of other inorganic pigments, is used in the form of liquid cream, cake or pencil. Daily application to the lid margin over considerable periods has produced a pigmentation of the palpebral conjunctiva that has been the subject of several reports in the ophthalmic literature.[b,d,e,h,j,l,m,n,q,r,w] Typically brown or black punctate pigment deposits are found at the upper margin of the tarsus when the upper lid is everted. This is accompanied in some cases by slight irregularity of the surface of the conjunctiva in this area, due to formation of lymph follicles. Microscopically an infiltration with lymphocytes and macrophages containing pigment have been observed.[l] As a rule the bulbar conjunctiva and cornea remain normal, and no serious consequences have been recognized. Usually the deposits cause no symptoms and are discovered incidentally during examination of the eye, but may occasionally be associated with mild burning or foreign-body sensation and tearing.[e] Attempts to reproduce the condition in guinea pigs and rabbits have not been successful, but reactions to injected pigments have been studied.[k] In human beings, no blue or other light-colored deposits have been reported, only brown or black. (See also *Carbon*.)

Wearers of contact lenses have some special problems with eye cosmetics, such as irritation when caught under contact lenses, but these appear to constitute mechanical rather than toxic problems.[g]

Surma is an eye cosmetic from Asia that is centuries old, consisting of a mineral powder that is applied to the eyelids beginning in infancy. It has been known to cause minute conjunctival abrasions, but no toxic effect to the eye.[i] However, the fact that surma may contain from 5 to 85% *lead sulfide* has attracted considerable interest in the British Isles, because of the possibility that this might contribute to systemic lead poisoning in Asiatic immigrant children who rub their eyes and suck their fingers. There has been controversy over whether the danger is real or theoretical, but steps have been taken to try to limit the use of surma.[a,c,k,o,t]

Compounds of *arsenic, barium, chromium, silver,* and heavy metals that were formerly sometimes incorporated in cosmetics were capable of harm to the eyes.[f] Also, *eyelash dyes* were a problem at an earlier period. Prior to the United States Federal Food, Drug, and Cosmetic Act of 1938, which barred further use of coal tar dyes and para-phenylenediamine for the eyelashes and eyebrows, there were many severe reactions of lids, conjunctiva, and cornea. A preparation known as Lash-Lure was notoriously injurious. (Further information is given under *Hair dyes* and *Paraphenylenediamine*.)

A *silver lactate* preparation used for darkening the eyelashes was used for 20–35 years by two women without precautions to keep it out of the conjunctival sac. Their eyes were unharmed, but by slit-lamp examination Descemet's membrane was seen to have greenish discoloration, presumably from taking up silver, as in argyria from various causes.[u]

Bacteria and fungi in eye cosmetics are a threat to the eye, but not a toxicologic problem, and are mentioned here only as a possible source of confusion in differential diagnosis of eye disturbances from cosmetics.[v]

a. Attenburrow AA, Campbell S, et al: Surma and blood lead levels in Asian children in Glasgow. *LANCET* 1:323, 1980.
b. Donaldson DD: Mascara pigmentation of the conjunctiva. *ARCH OPHTHALMOL* 81:124–125, 1969.
c. Editorial: Surma and lead poisoning. *LANCET* 1:28, 1979.
d. Fernandez FM: Conjunctival pigmentation from use of cosmetics. *ARCH SOC OFTAL HISP AM* 30:464, 1970. (Spanish)
e. Franguelli R: Exogenous pigmentation of the conjunctiva from eye cosmetics. *ANN OTTALMOL CLIN OCUL* 92:1012–1016, 1966. (Italian)
f. Fuller JW: Report on mascaras, eyebrow pencils and eye shadows. *J ASSOC AGRIC CHEM* 26:317–324, 1943.
g. Gustafson JC: The dangers of cosmetics in contact lens wearing. *J CONTACT LENS SOC AM* 1:5–8, 1967.

h. Haddad R, Zehetbauer G: Problems arising from use of cosmetics on the lid margins. *KLIN MONATSBL AUGENHEILKD* 177:829–831, 1980.

i. Howells CHL, Johnson L, et al: Changing incidence of trachoma in the West Midlands. *BR MED J* 2:127–129, 1969.

j. Jervey JW: Mascara pigmentation of the conjunctiva. *ARCH OPHTHALMOL* 81:124–125, 1969.

k. Marzulli FN, Davis KJ, Yoder PD: Evaluation of a new test for eye area cosmetics. *CTFA COSMETIC J* 3:42–45, 1971.

l. Platia EV, Michels RG, Green WR: Eye cosmetic induced conjunctival pigmentation. *ANN OPHTHALMOL* 10:501–504, 1978.

m. Reese AB: Pigmentation of the palpebral conjunctiva resulting from mascara. *AM J OPHTHALMOL* 30:1352–1355, 1947.

n. Remler O: Use of cosmetics on the eye and its side effects on the conjunctiva. *KLIN MONATSBL AUGENHEILKD* 156:119–122, 1970. (German)

o. Snodgrass GJAI, Zideman DA, et al: Cosmetic plumbism. *BR MED J* 230, 1973.

p. Spoor HJ: Eye glamour-products, predictions and problems. *CUTIS* 8:458–462, 1971.

q. Stewart CR: Conjunctival absorption of pigment from eye makeup. *AM J OPTOM* 50:571–574, 1973.

r. Sugar HS, Kobernick S: Subconjunctival pigmentation associated with the use of eye cosmetics containing carbon black. *AM J OPHTHALMOL* 62:146–149, 1966.

s. Thorne N: Cosmetics and the dermatologist. *BR J CLIN PRACT* 20:275–277, 1966.

t. Warley MA, Blackledge P, O'Gorman P: Lead poisoning in eye cosmetic. *BR MED J* 117, 1968.

u. Weiler HH, Llemp MA, et al: Argyria of the cornea due to self-administration of eyelash dye. *ANN OPHTHALMOL* 14:822–823, 1982.

v. Wilson LA, Ahearn DG: Pseudomonas-induced corneal ulcers associated with contaminated eye mascaras. *AM J OPHTHALMOL* 84:112–119, 1977.

w. Zuckerman BD: Conjunctival pigmentation due to cosmetics. *AM J OPHTHALMOL* 62:672–676, 1966.

Fava beans produce favism in people who have a genetic deficiency of glucose-6-phosphate dehydrogenase, mainly people in Mediterranean countries. The ocular side effects of the hemolytic reaction have been summarized by Walsh and Hoyt.[256] They indicate that hemorrhages in the retina tend to have good prognosis, but that optic atrophy has been known to follow severe hemolytic reactions with blurring of disc margins and attenuation of retinal arteries. Also, hemorrhage into the vitreous humor has been described.[a] Cataractous lenses from people with G-6-PD deficiency lack this enzyme, but it is obscure whether this has anything to do with development of cataract, since cataract occurs no more frequently than in non-deficient people.[b]

a. Sorcinelli R, Guiso G: Vitreoretinal hemorrhages after ingestion of fava beans in G-6-PD-deficient subject. *OPHTHALMOLOGICA* 178:259–262, 1979.

b. Orzalesi N, Sorcinelli R, Binaghi F: Glucose-6-phosphate dehydrogenase in cataracts of subjects suffering from favism. *OPHTHALMIC RES* 8:192–194, 1976.

Fenfluramine (Ponderax), an amphetamine-like appetite-suppressant, may produce mydriasis,[298] and overdosage, which may be lethal, has featured widely dilated pupils reacting poorly to light.[a] Rotary nystagmus has been noted.[b]

a. Veltri JC, Temple AR: Fenfluramine poisoning. *J PEDIATR* 87:119–121, 1975.
b. Riley I, Corson J: Fenfluramine overdosage. *LANCET* 1:1162–1163, 1969.

Ferric dimethyldithiocarbamate (Ferbam) is a fungicide, the dust of which is irritating to the eye, nose, throat, and skin.[5,36]

Ferricyanide, potassium, is a water-soluble salt having little toxicity to the eye either in rabbits or human beings. Injections of 0.07 M aqueous solution into the cornea of rabbits caused only a grade 5 reaction on a scale of 0 to 100.[123] As 0.25% aqueous solution in combination with 6% sodium thiosulfate this substance has been injected subconjunctivally and has been employed for irrigation of the cornea in treatment of argyrosis in patients, without evident injurious effect.[a,81]

a. Stillians, AW, Lawless TK, (1929): — see *Silver* for reference.

Ferritin is an iron-storage protein that is widely distributed in animals and plants. Injection of ferritin from horse spleen into the vitreous body of rabbits induces uveitis, with the ferritin acting as an antigen, rather than as a primarily toxic substance.[a]

a. Gnad HD, Schimmelpfennig B, Witmer R: Observations on the effect of steroids on experimental uveitis. *OPHTHALMIC RES* 5:204–214, 1973.

Fibrinolysin (Plasmin, Actase, Thrombolysin), a proteolytic enzyme used in treatment of clotted hyphema, has been evaluated for toxicity in the anterior chamber of eyes of rabbits, with particular attention to the corneal endothelium. A concentration of 1,250 units/ml, which was effective in removing clotted human blood, caused slight disturbance of the endothelium, with complete recovery in seven days. However, 5,000 to 10,000 units/ml caused severe damage to the corneal endothelium persisting more than six months.[a]

a. Morton WR, Turnbull W: The effect of intracameral fibrinolysin on the rabbit cornea. *AM J OPHTHALMOL* 57:280–287, 1964.

Ficin is a proteolytic enzyme obtained from the latex of tropical trees of the genus *Ficus.* Commercially, ficin is available as a powder having an acrid odor and involving hazards in handling, owing to tissue-dissolving properties. The enzyme is employed industrially in preparation of food, leather, and wool. On the skin, the powder or concentrated solutions may cause irritation and dermatitis. Applied to rabbit eyes, the powder has been found injurious within eighty seconds.[171] (Also see *Fig, wild.*)

Fig, wild (*Ficus tumila*) grows in Australia and is reported to have a sap which causes blistering of the skin, intense conjunctivitis, and nasopharyngeal irritation. Four cases of eye injury have been described in detail.[a] Two had defects of the corneal epithelium. One developed a small corneal ulcer, and vision was no better than 6/9 three weeks later, but the others returned to normal in a few days. The enzyme *ficin* presumably is responsible for these injurious effects. (See *Ficin.*)

a. English PB: Sap-dermatitis and conjunctivitis caused by the wild fig (*Ficus tumila*). *MED J AUST* 1:578–579, 1943.

Fish or **Shellfish poisoning** may occur in several forms, from eating poisonous fish, from eating material contaminated with poisonous micro-organisms, or from exposure to products of decomposition. The fish poisoning known as *Ciguatera*, ascribed to eating various species of tropical fish that have ingested blue-green algae, has been said to cause redness and sandy sensation in the eyes, occasionally diplopia, in association with vomiting, prostration, numbness and tingling of the face and hands, and profuse sweating.[a-c] In one outbreak of *Ciguatera* poisoning, 24 men on a cargo ship ate meat from a barracuda, and within 30 minutes to 6 hours developed acute gastro-intestinal reactions, then tingling and burning sensation of the tongue.[c] Seven of the men had "transient blindness or blurred vision lasting three to ten minutes in the first 3 hours of illness." All recovered. There is no information on the basis for the transient losses of vision.

Poisoning from eating *red whelks* has caused temporary blurring of vision, said to be from impaired accommodation.[d]

Decomposing fish have evolved gases that have induced keratitis epithelialis in fishermen working in confined quarters.[66] The victims developed severe discomfort in their eyes several hours after exposure, but all recovered spontaneously, except for two who had deep keratitis and scarring. The gases present were principally *ammonia, hydrogen sulfide*, and *methyl amines*. As a result of testing of a variety of nitrogenous compounds on the eyes of rabbits, suspicion has been cast primarily on the methyl amines.[66] However, the reaction may have been caused by hydrogen sulfide, which is well known to induce a keratitis epithelialis that develops several hours after exposure.

Fish handlers have in rare instances suffered irritation of the eyes from a squirt of the *blood from eels*. (See INDEX).

A dinoflagellate, *Gy. breve*, which causes *red tides* on the east coast of the United States and contaminates shellfish with its neurotoxins, can be disrupted by surf, and its toxins can become airborne. People who are exposed are reported to develop transient acute irritation of the eyes and respiratory tract.[b]

a. Tonge JI, Battey Y, et al: Ciguatera poisoning: a report of two outbreaks and a probable fatal case in Queensland. *MED J AUST* 54(II)24:1088–1090, 1967.
b. Hughes JT, Merson MH: Fish and shellfish poisoning. *N ENGL J MED* 295:1117–1120, 1976.
c. Barkin RM: Ciguatera poisoning. *SOUTH MED J* 67:13–16, 1974.
d. Fleming C: Case of poisoning from red whelk. *BR MED J* 3:520–521, 1971.

Flaxseeds in the conjunctival sac may produce erythema, edema and abrasions, but by mechanical rather than toxic action.[a]

a. Humphrey WT: Flaxseeds in ophthalmic folk medicine. *AM J OPHTHALMOL* 70:287–290, 1970.

Flumequine, an antibacterial, is reported to have caused bilateral positive scotomas, bilateral symmetrical macular bullae and reduction of visual acuity to 4/10 in 3 patients after administration of 1.2 g/day for 3 days for infection of the urinary tract.[a] Each of the patients had prior chronic renal failure. When flumequine was discontinued, visual acuity became normal in 2 days, and the bullae were gone in 5 days. A direct cytotoxic affect on the retina has been considered a possibility.

a. Sirbat D, Saudax E, et al: Serous detachment of macular neuro-epithelium and flumequine. *J FR OPHTALMOL* 6:829–836, 1983. (French)

Flunitrazepam (Rohypnol), a hypnotic, has an affinity for retinal melanin and cells,[a,b] similar to chloroquine, but despite treating mice and cats for 6 to 12 months with dosage equivalent to hundreds or thousands of times human dosage no structural alterations were induced, quite different from serious retinotoxic effects obtained with chloroquine.[a]

a. Kuhn H, Keller P, et al: Lack of correlation between melanin affinity and retinopathy in mice and cats treated with chloroquine or flunitrazepam. *GRAEFES ARCH OPHTHALMOL* 216:177–190, 1981.
b. Sieghart W, Drexler G, et al: Properties of benzodiazepine receptors in rat retina. *EXP EYE RES* 34:961–967, 1982.

Fluorescein, an anionic dye, usually used as sodium fluoresceinate, has been very widely applied for testing corneas for epithelial injuries or abnormal permeability, and has been essentially without toxic effect in this application. Maurice provided an excellent review of this and many other uses which have been made of fluorescein in ophthalmic research.[r] In clinical studies of the retina by fluorescein angiography, 5 or 10 ml of a 10% solution, or 2 to 3 ml of 25%,[zb] have been injected rapidly intravenously in many patients without toxic effects on the eyes. However, experimentally it has been demonstrated that in albino mice fluorescein can act as a photosensitizer in the retina, causing marked degeneration of visual cells under artificial illumination.[t]

In patients, there have been no indications of adverse effects on vision, but side-effects of nausea, urticaria, sneezing, bitter taste, or dizziness have been common. Plasma histamine has been found elevated in 66% of patients with these symptoms, though also elevated in 15% without symptoms.[b] Administration of diphenhydramine reduced the incidence of minor side effects, but because of its own side effects, was thought to be indicated only in patients with a strong history of allergies.[g] Antibodies to fluorescein have not been demonstrated in patients with systemic reactions.[y] Diabetic patients show essentially the same types of reactions as nondiabetics.[c] Young men appear to have a special tendency to react.[k]

In addition to the minor side-effects, there is a low incidence of serious, life-threatening, or fatal reactions. These have included instances of respiratory embarassment,[k] pulmonary edema,[l,w] pharyngeal edema,[q] cardiac arrest,[e] myocardial infarction,[f,q,w,z,za] shock and hypotension,[r,q] with some deaths.[j,y,z] These more serious reactions have been reviewed.[h,w,y,ze] Enzmann has provided a well organized synopsis on management for these emergencies.[h]

No specific basis for any of these adverse side effects has been established, but the purity of the fluorescein involved has been looked into on occasion, and in two series of cases there has been reason to suspect greater severity and frequency in association with contaminants,[m,zd] identified in one series as residual *dimethyl formamide* from the manufacturing process.[m]

No evidence of teratogenicity has been found in rats[u] or rabbits.[s]

Extravasation of sodium fluorescein into subcutaneous tissues from leaking intravenous connections have produced skin reactions ranging from transient eczematous dermatitis to skin necrosis requiring grafting.[i,o,x,zc]

Lumbar puncture and intrathecal injection of a small amount of 5% sodium fluorescein in study of pit of the optic disc in one case caused anesthesia and paralysis of the legs for 45 minutes, with no sequelae.[n]

a. Amalric P, Biau C, Fenies MT: Side effects and accidents in the course of fluorescein angiography. *BULL SOC OPHTALMOL FRANCE* 68:968–973, 1968. (French)

b. Arroyave CM, Wolbers R, Ellis PP: Plasma complement and histamine changes after intravenous administration of sodium fluorescein. *AM J OPHTHALMOL* 87:474–479, 1979.

c. Chazan BI, Balodimos MC, Koncz L: Untoward effects of fluorescein retinal angiography in diabetic patients. *ANN OPHTHALMOL* 3:42–49, 1971.

d. Cohn HC, Jocson VL: A unique case of grand mal seizure after Fluress. *ANN OPHTHALMOL* 13:1379–1380, 1981.

e. Cunningham EE, Balu V: Cardiac arrest following fluorescein angiography. *J AM MED ASSOC* 242:2431, 1979.

f. Deglin SM, Deglin EA, Chung EK: Acute myocardial infarction following fluorescein angiography. *HEART LUNG* 6:505–509, 1977.

g. Ellis PP, Schoenberger M, Rendi MA: Antihistamines as prophylaxis against side reactions to intravenous fluorescein. *TRANS AM OPHTHALMOL SOC* 78:190–205, 1980.

h. Enzmann V, Ruprecht KW: Side effects of fluorescein angiography of the retina. *KLIN MONATSBL AUGENHEILKD* 181:235–239, 1982. (German)

i. Francois JH, Poletti J, Stecken M: Regional impregnation of the skin after an injection of fluorescein. *BULL SOC OPHTALMOL FRANCE* 81:671–673, 1981. (French)

j. Fujita K, Suzuki H, Amano K: A case of death after fluorescein angiography. *JPN J CLIN OPHTHALMOL* 31:575–577, 1977.

k. Greene GS, Bell LM, et al: Adverse reaction to intravenous fluorescein. *ANN OPHTHALMOL* 8:533–536, 1976.

l. Hess JB, Pacurariu RI: Acute pulmonary edema following intravenous fluorescein angiography. *AM J OPHTHALMOL* 82:567–570, 1976.

m. Jacob JSH, Rosen ES, Young E: Report of the presence of a toxic substance, dimethyl formamide, in sodium fluorescein used for fluorescein angiography. *BR J OPHTHALMOL* 66:567–568, 1982.

n. Kalina RE, Conrad WC: Intrathecal fluorescein for serous macular detachment. *ARCH OPHTHALMOL* 94:1421, 1976.

o. Krata RP, Mazzocco TR, Davidson B: A case report of skin necrosis following infiltration of I.V. fluourescein. *ANN OPHTHALMOL* 12:654–656, 1980.

p. La Piana FG, Penner R: Anaphylactoid reaction to intravenously administered fluorescein. *ARCH OPHTHALMOL* 79:161–162, 1968.

q. Marcus DF, Etienne C: Adverse effects of sodium fluorescein as used in fluorescein angiography.[311]

r. Maurice DM: The use of fluorescein in ophthalmological research. *INVEST OPHTHAL-MOL* 6:464–477, 1967.

s. McEnerney JK, Wong P, Peyman GA: Evaluation of the teratogenicity of fluorescein sodium. *AM J OPHTHALMOL* 84:847–850, 1977.

t. Miyata M, Tanaka K, Mizuno K: Toxicology of fluorescein. *ACTA SOC OPHTHALMOL JPN* 76:1601–1607, 1972. (English summary)

u. Nichols CW: Toxicology and teratogenicity of sodium fluorescein in fetal rats.[311]

w. Pacurariu RI: Low incidence of side effects following intravenous fluorescein angiography. *ANN OPHTHALMOL* 14:32–36, 1982.

x. Schatz H: Sloughing of skin following fluorescein. *ANN OPHTHALMOL* 10:625, 1978.

y. Stein MR, Parker CW: Reactions following intravenous fluroescein. *AM J OPHTHAL-MOL* 72:861–868, 1971.

z. Tamaki Y: A fatal reaction to intravenous fluorescein. *JPN J LEG MED* 28:453–454, 1974.

za. Wesley RE, Blount WC, Arterberry JF: Acute myocardial infarction after fluorescein angiography. *AM J OPHTHALMOL* 87:834–835, 1979.

zb. Willerson D, Tate GW, et al: Clinical evaluation of fluorescein 25%. *ANN OPHTHAL-MOL* 8:833–842, 1976.

zc. Wing GL, Weiter JJ: Eczematous dermatitis following fluorescein extravasation. *ANN OPHTHALMOL* 12:825–826, 1980.

zd. Yannuzzi LA, Justice J Jr, Baldwin HA: Effective differences in the formulation of intravenous fluorescein and related side effects. *AM J OPHTHALMOL* 78:217–221, 1974.

ze. Zografos L: International investigation on the incidence of serious or fatal accidents potentially associated with fluorescein angiography. *J FR OPHTALMOL* 6:495–506, 1983. (French)

Fluorides are salts of hydrofluoric acid. They owe their injurious properties to the innate toxicity of the fluoride ion rather than to acidity or basicity.

Industrially, irritation of the eyes and nose has been reported when fluoride concentration has reached 5 mg/cu m of air.[51]

Experimentally, sodium fluoride has been tested on rabbit eyes in several different ways. Application of a 2% aqueous solution to the eye caused corneal epithelial defects and necrotic areas in the conjunctiva. Injection subconjunctivally or into the anterior chamber caused corneal edema and a severe inflammatory reaction in the eye with hemorrhages in the iris.[153,198] Injection of 0.084% solution into the stroma of the cornea caused only moderate reaction. In excised beef corneas, injection of a similar amount (0.1 to 0.3 mg) into the stroma caused loosening of the epithelium after six to ten hours.[h,107]

In chronic fluoride poisoning of human beings it has been said that changes in the bones of the skull have sometimes led to optic atrophy through compression of the optic nerves, but no direct toxic effect on these nerves is known.[33]

In human beings sodium fluoride has been used for prevention of caries by addition of 0.7 to 1 ppm to drinking water (so called fluoridation), also by application of 1 to 2% solution or gel to the teeth, and it has been given orally in treatment of osteoporosis, multiple myeloma, and otosclerosis in doses of 0.5 to 1.5 mg/kg per day.

I have found no documented evidence of injury to the eyes or disturbance of vision in human beings from the small amounts of fluoride that have been added to drinking water to prevent caries. From a presumed higher level of chronic fluoride exposure to dusts in the neighborhood of fertilizer factories, but insufficient to cause dental or skeletal fluorosis, Waldbott and Cecilioni have spoken of ten patients who "complained of visual disturbances (scotomata, blurred vision) which were not corrected by glasses," and they mentioned that two had "evidence of incipient retinitis." They reported no ophthalmologic examination to support this extremely vague statement.[x] Bernstein recorded an occurrence of bilateral pigmentary macular degeneration in two 15-year-old patients 6 to 8 weeks after a single application of a commonly used dental fluoride gel to prevent caries, but recognized that it was uncertain whether there was a connection.[e]

At higher levels of fluoride intake such as used in treatment of osteoporosis I know of only one documented case of apparent toxic eye involvement. In this case, reported by Geall and Beilin, osteoporosis was treated with calcium salts, calciferol, and 60 mg of sodium fluoride per day until vision was affected in both eyes. After six weeks of this treatment both optic nerveheads and one macula were observed to be edematous. Subsequently, vision was recovered in one eye, but optic atrophy developed in the other.[k] In five other patients studied carefully by Guerra and Medaglini under treatment for osteoporosis with ordinary dosage for three months, then unusually high dosage of 2.58 mg/kg per day for a year, no disturbance of vision, no abnormality of the ERG, and no pigmentary retinopathy were found.[m] Also in other series no ocular involvement has been found.[f,j,u] Lessell has suggested that the case reported by Geall and Beilin in which there was pain and visual failure in one eye could be interpreted as ischemic optic neuropathy from some cause other than fluoride.[344]

Acute human poisonings by fluoride have been comprehensively reviewed by Waldbott with no mention of effects on vision or of ophthalmologic examinations in the acutely poisoned patients.[w]

In rabbits, administration of sodium fluoride at doses approximately twenty times those used in treatment of osteoporosis in human beings during three to five months produced no significant abnormalities of the ERG, or changes in the ocular fundi detectable by ophthalmoscopy, fluorescein angiography, or histology in a careful study by Bloome and Burian.[q]

However, the retina can be injured by administering fluoride in near-lethal doses, but only a small proportion of animals develop retinopathy unless the fluoride is injected intravenously or directly into the carotid artery to reach the eye on that side in very high concentration. After intracarotid injection, complete atrophy of the retina and choroid on the same side was described by De Berardinis and associates, with no damage to the other eye.[i]

Babel and associates demonstrated retinal degeneration in rabbits, evident by ophthalmoscopy, ERG, and histology, from doses of 40 to 60 mg/kg given intravenously.[c,d] Sorsby and Harding described the characteristic ophthalmoscopic appearance of retinopathy induced in this manner in rabbits, describing localized retinal edema in two or three days, changing to patches of round black dots in pigmented animals in two weeks, associated with destruction of pigment epithelium and photoreceptor layer. The retinotoxic effect of fluoride was potentiated by oxidizing agents, especially permanganate.[t, 133, 207, 234]

Vanyseck and associates demonstrated that repeated near-lethal intravenous doses induced changes in retinal metabolism and gradually destroyed the retina, with degeneration beginning in the outer parts of the photoreceptors, leading finally to extinction of the ERG.[v] According to Grignolo, Orzalesi, and others, structural changes were first detectable in the retinal pigment epithelium, and necrosis of these cells was followed by degeneration of the outer segments of the visual cells. Rhodopsin resynthesis was found to be interfered with when the pigment cells showed injury.[a, p, q, 49]

In rabbits intravitreal injection by Ponte and Lauricella caused changes in inner layers preceding those of the outer layers.[s] In kittens Pedlar found intravitreal injection of fluoride to cause swelling of the inner layers of immature retinas, but not in mature retinas.[r]

In vitro in experimental studies on metabolism of the lens and of the retina sodium fluoride has been employed as an enzyme inhibitor.[b, l, o] Rabbit retina surviving in culture has shown nonselective cell destruction when exposed to sodium fluoride.[99] In rat lenses surviving in culture, cataractous changes have been induced by adding fluoride to the medium.[n]

a. Anton M, Hrachovina V, Moster M: Experimental degeneration of the retina from the electrophysiological, histological and biochemical point of view. *CESK OFTALMOL* 26:299–303, 1970.

b. Ashton N, Graymore C, Pedlar C: Studies on developing retinal vessels. *BR J OPHTHALMOL* 41:449–460, 1957.

c. Babel J, Ziv B: Researchs on experimental retinal degenerations. *OPHTHALMOLOGICA* 132:65–75, 1956. (French)

d. Babel J, Avanza C: Experimental retinal degeneration provoked by sodium fluoride. *EXPERIENTIA* 17:180–181, 1961.

e. Bernstein HN: Possible retinotoxicity of sodium fluoride in children.[311]

f. Black MM, Kleiner IS, Bolker H: The toxicity of sodium fluoride in man. *NEW YORK MED J* 49:1187–1188, 1949.

g. Bloome MA, Burian HM: Chronic fluoride ingestion in rabbits: absence of ocular effects. *ARCH OPHTHALMOL* 83:354–356, 1970.

h. Buschke W: Effects of metabolic poisons and of some other agents on intercellular cohesion in corneal epithelium. *AM J OPHTHALMOL* 33:59–66, 1950.

i. DeBerardinis E, Tierei O, Vecchione L: Monolateral retinal degeneration due to sodium fluoride. *ACTA OPHTHALMOL* 40:65–68, 1962.

j. Deuxchaisnes CN de, Krane SM: Paget's disease of bone. *MEDICINE* (BALT) 43:223–266, 1964.

k. Geall MG, Beilin LJ: Sodium fluoride and optic neuritis. *BR MED J* 5404:355–356, 1964.

l. Graymore C: In vitro swelling of the kitten retina induced by sodium fluoride inhibition. *BR J OPHTHALMOL* 43:40–41, 1959.

m. Guerra R, Medaglini E: Clinical and electroretinographic findings in a sodium fluoride long treated group of patients. *ANN OTTALMOL* 94:327–333, 1968.

n. Hammar H: The formation of amino acids in vitro from glucose in the eye lens of rats and the influence of sodium fluoride and alloxan diabetes. *ACTA OPHTHALMOL* 43:543–556, 1965.

o. Kleifeld O, Hockwin O, Ayberk N: The effect of sodium fluoride on the metabolism of the lens. *GRAEFES ARCH OPHTHALMOL* 158:39–46, 1956.

p. Orzalesi N, Grignolo A, Calabria A: Experimental degeneration of the rabbit retina induced by sodium fluoride. *EXP EYE RES* 6:165–170, 1967.

q. Orzalesi N: The effect of sodium fluoride upon the retina. *FLUORIDE QUART REP* 3:114–120, 1970.

r. Pedlar C: Studies on developing retina vessels. *BR J OPHTHALMOL* 43:559–565, 1959.

s. Ponte F, Lauricella M: The intravitreal route of administration in study of experimental physiopathology of the retina. *ANN OTTALMOL CLIN OCUL* 94:1049–1062, 1968. (Italian)

t. Sorsby A, Harding R: Experimental degeneration of the retina. *BR J OPHTHALMOL* 44:213–224, 1960.

u. Taylor WH: Osteoporosis and fluoride therapy. *BR MED J* 2:304–305, 1970.

v. Vanysek J, Anton M, et al: Some metabolic disturbances of the retina due to the effect of natrium fluoride. *OPHTHALMOLOGICA ADDIT AD* 158:684–690, 1969.

w. Waldbott GL: Acute fluoride intoxication. *ACTA MED SCAND, SUPPL* 400, 1963.

x. Waldbott GL, Cecilioni VA: "Neighborhood" fluorosis. *CLIN TOXICOL* 2:387–396, 1969.

Fluorine is a gas having notorious corrosive and toxic properties. Small amounts of the gas in air have been reported to be strongly irritating to the eyes and respiratory tract.[b,33] Exposure of human volunteers to fluorine in air showed that although it caused very little irritation up to 25 ppm, it caused much irritation of the eyes and nose at 100 ppm. However, there were no aftereffects from exposure to 100 ppm for one-half minute.[a] Contact with high concentration of fluorine gas or liquified fluorine would presumably be extremely destructive. (See also *Hydrofluoric acid.*)

a. Keplinger ML, Suissa LW: Toxicity of fluorine short-term inhalation. *AM IND HYG ASSOC* 29:10–18, 1968.

b. Ricca PM: Exposure criteria for fluorine rocket propellants, occupational and nonoccupational considerations. *ARCH ENVIRON HEALTH* 12:399–407, 1966.

Fluoroacetate (1080) is manufactured, mostly in the form of sodium fluoroacetate, for use as a rat poison, and it is a highly poisonous component of a South African plant, *Gifblaar.*

In human beings, fluoroacetate is known to have caused sixteen deaths and thirty poisonings. Characteristically, nausea and vomiting occur soon after ingestion; then, usually after a relatively asymptomatic period of as much as six hours, numbness, tingling, epigastric pain, and apprehension begin. Subsequently, muscular twitching or convulsions, low blood pressure, and blurred vision may develop.[a]

The nature and basis of blurring of vision has not been established either clinically or experimentally. There have been no known instances of permanent visual impairment in patients or animals that have recovered from poisoning, but a transient disturbance of vision appears definite in certain cases. In severely poisoned cattle it is reported that vision has been so impaired that the animals have not avoided objects, but walked into them. In human poisonings, reviewed in 1959 by Pattison, transient failure of the pupils to react to light appears to have been associated only with periods of coma or convulsions.

In one unusual case a person was working with sodium fluoroacetate when a gust of wind blew the powder into his face, and some of it was inhaled. This caused an almost immediate tingling sensation around the corners of the mouth and in the nasal passages, and soon the entire face became numb. This was accompanied by salivation and loss of speech. Vision was blurred from the outset, with an inability to focus on objects. Although the parethesias spread to the arms and legs, and violent convulsions and coma followed, the patient ultimately recovered completely.[a]

Numerous toxic *aliphatic fluorine compounds* with fluorine in a terminal position owe their toxicity to metabolic conversion to fluoroacetate in the body; this includes *fluoroethanol, fluorohydrocarbons, higher fluorocarboxylic acids,* and others. Conversion of a higher fluorocarboxylic acid to fluoroacetate is believed to be responsible for the poisonous properties of the plant *Ratsbane,* and in instances of poisoning of human beings by this plant it was noted long ago that the pupils remained normal, but the patient's vision was not acute.[a]

Sodium fluoroacetate has been found to injure surviving retina at a concentration of 0.005 M or greater,[157] and at 0.05 M causes unselective degeneration of cells in cultured retina.[99] Whether poisoning of the retina is involved in the ill-defined visual disturbances observed in poisoned human beings and animals is not known.

The toxicity of fluoroacetate is attributable to an entirely different mechanism from that of iodoacetate or bromoacetate. In fluoroacetate the fluorine atom is essentially unreactive and the whole molecule closely resembles normal acetate, for which it successfully substitutes in metabolic processes, as far as conversion to fluorocitrate. The fluorocitrate is accepted by the enzyme aconitase as if it were citrate, but unlike normal citrate it is not further metabolized, and at this point it blocks the tricarboxylic acid cycle.

a. Pattison FLM: *Toxic Aliphatic Fluorine Compounds.* Amsterdam, Elsevier, 1959.

1-Fluoro-2,4-dinitrobenzene has been tested in rabbits and rats at near-lethal doses for toxic effects on the fundus of the eye, but none was detected ophthalmoscopically or histologically.[231] Surviving rabbit retina is damaged in vitro at a concentration of 0.05 M.[157]

p-Fluorophenylalanine, an antiviral agent used on the eye in treatment of dendritic keratitis from herpes simplex, has prolonged the time for regeneration of corneal epithelium in experimental lesions in noninfected rabbits,[a] but a 0.1% solution or ointment has been well tolerated and effective in use by patients.

a. Wollensak J, Kypke W: Retardation of epithelial regeneration and corneal wound healing by antimetabolites in rabbits. *GRAEFES ARCH OPHTHALMOL* 168:102–115, 1965.

Fluorouracil (5-fluorouracil, Fluoroplex, Efudex, Adrucil), an antineoplastic, may be applied to the skin, be injected into or about the eye, or be given intravenously. Williams reported on application to the face and neck in 700 patients, with only rare erythema or swelling of the lids. Dillaha reported dermatitis and edema of the lids with conjunctival inflammation but without ectropion, while Galentine described an extraordinary case in which a patient developed a severe eythematous reaction involving the whole face after applying a 5% cream twice a day for 2 weeks. In this case the conjunctivae were chemotic, and the lower lids began to evert. After a month the ectropion of both lower lids was severe, with some corneal exposure. However, in 3 months the whole reaction had resolved.

Injection into a kerato-acanthoma of the upper lid in one patient was therapeutically effective without notable adverse effect (Hochart). However, Fraunfelder has recorded that in two cases reported to his Registry injection into skin tumors on the lids did cause ectropion requiring surgical correction.[313]

Systemic administration of fluorouracil has also had adverse effects on the lids, lacrimal system and eyes, producing excessive tearing and discomfort from obstruction of the lacrimal system (Caravella; Christophidis; Haidak; Hamersley), from ectropion of the lower lids (Straus), or from blepharoconjunctivitis.[333] Fortunately, there has been a strong tendency to recovery from these side effects when fluorouracil has been discontinued.

Central nervous system dysfunction has been a complication of fluorouracil treatment, and has been associated with oculomotor disturbance (diplopia from weakness of convergence and divergence) in two patients (Bixenman), nystagmus from cerebella involvement (Moertel), and blindness in one cat (Harvey). (The cause of blindness in the cat was not determined.)

Optic neuritis was mentioned by Weiss in 1961 in one out of a series of 149 patients studied during and after intravenous fluorouracil, noting that there were two episodes coincidental with the treatment, but there was no suggestion of optic nerve disturbance in the other patients, and no way to establish whether the fluorouracil was actually to blame.

In treatment of neoplasms which subjects the eye to supervoltage irradiation it has been reported that added systemic treatment with fluorouracil has caused a large increase in complications such as cataract, keratopathy, conjunctivitis or blindness within two years (Chan).

Because of interest in using fluorouracil within the globe in treatment of proliferative vitreoretinopathy, there have been several experiments on rabbits. Blumenkranz et al injected 1 mg into the vitreous body and found no evidence of retinal toxicity by microscopy or electrophysiologic measurements. Stern et al found after pars plana lensectomy and vitrectomy that 0.5 mg could be injected daily for 7 days without causing change in the ERG, but that 1.25 mg once or twice a day for 7 days caused extinction of the b-wave of the ERG, loss of outer segments of the photoreceptors, and corneal opacification. Barrada et al on the basis of histology and ERG studies concluded that 0.25 mg/ml was a "non-toxic" concentration for use in infusion fluid.[277] Nao-I and Honda determined *in vitro* the effects of various concentrations on the ERG of rabbit retinas.

In a series of patients given subconjunctival and intraocular injections of fluorouracil, in addition to surgery for proliferative vitreoretinopathy, Blumenkranz found no serious complications, but noted slow healing of corneal epithelial defects.

Fluorouracil has been used to inhibit proliferation of fibroblasts and consequent scarring and failure of filtration blebs. Gressel and Parrish developed an owl-monkey model in which subconjunctival injections of the drug were given once or twice daily after standard filtering surgery. Complications noted were persistent corneal epithelial defects, delayed healing conjunctival wounds, hyphemas, and flat anterior chambers more frequent than in controls, yet a higher success rate in formation of filtering blebs in the fluorouracil-treated animals. In a follow-up clinical study by Heuer and Parrish, human glaucomatous eyes of types notoriously prone to failure similarly had subconjunctival injections of 3 to 5 mg of the drug once or twice daily for two weeks after standard filtering surgery. Complications, occurring in nearly half of the eyes, consisted of corneal epithelial defects and leakage from conjunctival wounds or needle tracts, but most healed in a few days to two weeks from the end of fluorouracil treatment, and encouraging results were obtained in reducing intraocular pressure by formation of the desired filtration blebs. No problems with the lacrimal system and no cicatricial entropion was encountered in this series, and no systemic complications.

Bixenman WW, Nicholls JVV, Warwick OH: Oculomotor disturbances associated with 5-fluorouracil chemotherapy. *AM J OPHTHALMOL* 83:789–793, 1977.

Blumenkranz MS, Ophir A, et al: Fluorouracil for the treatment of massive periretinal proliferation. *AM J OPHTHALMOL* 94:458–467, 1982.

Blumenkranz M, Hernandez E, et al: 5-Fluorouracil: New applications in complicated retinal detachment for an established antimetabolite. *OPHTHALMOLOGY* 91:122–130, 1984.

Caravella LP Jr, Burns JA, Zangmeister M: Punctal canalicular stenosis related to systemic fluorouracil therapy. *ARCH OPHTHALMOL* 99:284–286, 1981.

Chan RC, Shukorsksy LJ: Effects of irradiation on the eye. *RADIOLOGY* 120:673–675, 1976.

Christophidis N, Lucas I, et al: Lacrimation and 5-fluorouracil. *ANN INTERN MED* 89:574–575, 1978.

Dillaha CJ, Jansen GT, et al: Further studies with 5-fluorouracil. *ARCH DERMATOL* 92:410–415, 1965.

Galentine P, Sloas H, et al: Bilateral cicatricial ectropion following topical administration of 5-fluorouracil. *ANN OPHTHALMOL* 13:573–577, 1981.

Gressel MG, Parrish RK II, Folberg R: 5-Fluorouracil and glaucoma filtering surgery. Part I. Animal model. *OPHTHALMOLOGY* 91:378–383, 1984.

Haidak DJ, Hurwitz BS, et al: Tear duct fibrosis (dacryostenosis) due to 5-fluorouracil. *ANN INTERN MED* 88:657, 1978.

Hamersley J, Luce JK, et al: Excessive lacrimation from fluorouracil treatment. *J AM MED ASSOC* 225:747–748, 1973.

Harvey HJ, MacEwen GG, Hayes AA: Neurotoxicosis associated with use of 5-fluorouracil in five dogs and one cat. *J AM VET MED ASSOC* 171:277–278, 1977.

Heuer DK, Parrish RK II, et al: 5-Fluorouracil and glaucoma filtering surgery. II. A pilot study. *OPHTHALMOLOGY* 91:384–394, 1984.

Hochart G, Piette F: Treatment of a kerato-acanthoma of the upper lid by injection of fluorouracil into the lesion. *BULL SOC OPHTALMOL FRANCE* 82:269–270, 1982. (French)

Moertel GG: Cerebellar ataxia associated with fluorinated pyrimidine therapy. *CANCER CHEMOTHER REP* 41:15–18, 1964.

Nao-I N, Honda Y: Toxic effect of fluorouracil on the rabbit retina. *AM J OPHTHALMOL* 96:641–643, 1983.

Stern WH, Guerin JC, et al: Ocular toxicity of fluorouracil after vitrectomy. *AM J OPHTHALMOL* 96:43–51, 1983.

Straus DJ, Mausolf FA, et al: Cicatricial ectropion secondary to 5-fluorouracil therapy. *MED PEDIATR ONCOL* 3:15–19, 1977.

Weiss AJ, Jackson LG, Carabasi R: An evaluation of 5-fluorouracil in malignant disease. *ANN INTERN MED* 55:731–741, 1961.

Williams AC, Klein E: Experience with local chemotherapy and immunotherapy in premalignant and malignant skin lesions. *CANCER* 25:450–462, 1970.

Fluphenazine hydrochloride (Permitil, Prolixin), a phenothiazine antipsychotic, appears not to have unusual ocular toxicity. Production of deposits in cornea and lens, as from chlorpromazine, has been suspected but has been difficult to prove, because affected patients generally have also taken chlorpromazine and other phenothiazine derivatives.[a,b] One patient who took only fluphenazine has been reported to have developed brown anterior subcapsular lens deposits.[c]

Oculogyric crises in association with the acute head-neck syndrome have been induced by fluphenazine, as by other phenothiazine derivatives.[a]

Intraocular pressure has been reduced slightly by fluphenazine in normal patients without changing facility of outflow.[d] It should be safe to use in the presence of glaucoma.

a. Ayd FJ Jr: Fluphenazine: Twelve years experience. *DIS NERV SYST* 29:744–747, 1968.
b. Barsa JA, Newton JS, Saunders J: Lenticular and corneal opacities during phenothiazine therapy. *J AM MED ASSOC* 193:98–100, 1965.
c. Calluaud JL, DiBattista, et al: Ocular pigmentation and phenothiazine derivatives. *BULL SOC OPHTALMOL FRANCE* 77:661–664, 1977. (French)
d. Petrosillo O, Beccaria F: Tonography and tranquilizers. *ARCH OTTALMOL* 67:135–152, 1963. (Italian)

FMLP (N-formyl-methionyl-leucyl-phenylalanine), a synthetic peptide which induces superoxide production, release of lysosomal enzymes, phagocytosis, and aggregation of polymorphonuclear leukocytes, has been tested by injection into the cornea and vitreous body of rabbit eyes. It has been shown to produce acute inflammatory responses that have promise for exploitation in study of ocular inflammations and anti-inflammatory mechanisms.

a. Ben-Zvi A, Rodriques MM, et al: Induction of ocular inflammation by synthetic mediators. *ARCH OPHTHALMOL* 99:1436–1444, 1981.

Formaldehyde is a gas, having a pungent suffocating odor, usually supplied as formalin, a 40% solution in water, or in solution in organic solvents. Gaseous formaldehyde in the air is irritating to the eyes and respiratory tract at 1 to 2 ppm.[o,r] Even at concentrations from 0.5 to 0.05 ppm a sensation of eye irritation is detectable by some people. Irritation of human eyes has been ascribed to formaldehyde liberated from urea-formaldehyde and phenol-formaldehyde resins, and formaldehyde has been considered as a possible factor in smog irritation. (See also *Plastics and Smog.*)

Experimental exposure of rabbits and guinea pigs to 40 to 70 ppm in air for ten days has caused slight tearing and discharge from the eyes but no injury of the corneas, and no disturbance of corneal sensation.[81] However, exposure of cats to a lethal concentration of 4,900 ppm in air for three hours has produced necrotic lesions in the corneas as well as the lungs. At a concentration of 8,150 ppm for three and one-half hours bloody discoloration of the aqueous humor was observed, associated with hemolysis.[g]

Aqueous solutions of formaldehyde splashed or dropped on human eyes have caused injuries ranging from severe permanent corneal opacification and loss of vision to minor transient injury or discomfort, depending upon whether the solutions were of high or low concentrations.

Guillery, from his experiments on rabbits in 1910, emphasized that clouding of the cornea after contact with formaldehyde is a delayed phenomenon.[96] Even the most concentrated commercial solution takes several minutes to produce a faint clouding of the epithelium. Early injury of the corneal stroma is masked by the denaturation and histologic fixing action of formaldehyde which reduces the swelling potential of the stroma and masks the severity of injury until later infiltration and rejection of the devitalized tissue occur.

A splash of 40% solution in human eyes is immediately painful but characteristically leaves the eye looking deceptively normal for at least an hour or two after exposure, seemingly little injured, but in the course of the next twelve hours all layers of the cornea may show obvious damage and edema, and the anterior segment may subsequently undergo devastating degeneration. Corneal hypesthesia and pericorneal ischemia seem to be particularly bad prognostic signs.

A splash of 40% solution of formaldehyde has had severe consequences in several cases. In one accident, well described by Kelecom, the faces of two workmen were sprayed by heated 40% solution.[j] One immediately washed his eyes with water, but the other did not. Two hours later the conjunctivae were hyperemic but the corneas transparent, with smooth surface reflex and no abnormal staining by fluorescein. Vision was normal. Despite treatment by irrigation and application of mydriatics and chloramphenicol, the next day the lids had become swollen, the corneas edematous with wrinkling of Descemet's membranes and loss of epithelium, and areas of conjunctivae appeared ischemic. The corneas were then definitely hypesthetic. The eyes of the workman who had not immediately washed his eyes with water after the accident had progressive degeneration and opacification of the cornea, evidence of damage to the irides, and gradual development of cataract. Despite all treatment, including repeated keratoplasty, one eye perforated and was exenterated; the other developed glaucoma with hemorrhages in the anterior chamber and ultimately became atrophic. The second workman, who had immediately washed his eyes, had persistent opacification and vascularization of one cornea, but the other eventually became clear.

In two other cases of injury from 40% solution, this was applied at room temperature accidentally as eyedrops and resulted in permanent corneal opacification and reduction of vision to 6-20/200.[f,253]

Still another patient whose eye was accidentally contaminated with one drop of 40% solution at room temperature had the eye washed with water within fifteen seconds, and then had little further pain or inconvenience for three to four hours.

However, within six hours this patient began to have great and increasing pain. In five days his cornea had become opaque, and he had much photophobia, epiphora, swelling of the lids, chemosis, and echymosis. After six months his cornea still had a steamy or fine opalescent appearance, and vision varied between 6/12 and 6/36.[m]

A splash of 26% solution of formaldehyde is reported in one patient to have caused severe inflammatory reaction, thickening of the cornea, wrinkling of Descemet's membrane, and iritis, but the eye recovered completely, in the course of two months.[g]

A splash of 4% solution of formaldehyde in one eye of a nurse caused immediate strong smarting discomfort. In approximately fifteen seconds the eye was washed with water. The eye appeared normal and the cornea transparent thirty minutes later, but it had optical irregularity, distorting the ophthalmoscopic view of the fundus. Slit-lamp examination showed no abnormality. Optical clarity and normal vision returned the next day without need for treatment. (Personal observation.)

A splash of 0.2% solution of formaldehyde has been reported to cause irritation with stinging and hyperemia in human eyes, but no permanent injury from brief contact.[253]

An accidental orbital injection of formalin in one patient caused loss of both upper and lower lids, requiring extensive reconstructive surgery; the eye itself apparently escaped serious injury.[p]

Experimental application of a drop of formalin to rabbit and guinea pig eyes has been observed to cause severe reaction, with edema of the cornea and conjunctiva, and iritis, graded 8 on a scale of 10 at twenty-four hours but with a tendency to recovery in the course of a month or two.[27,81,161] A 0.05% solution applied to rabbit eyes caused complete loss of the top layer of corneal epithelial cells.[300] Injected into the stroma of the cornea, even a 1% solution has caused severe reaction.[123] Keratitis induced by intracorneal injection of 0.35% solution is associated with biochemically demonstrable marked degradation of tissue glycosaminoglycans.[q]

Guillery, in his experiments on rabbits in 1910, found that after fifteen minutes' contact with concentrated commercial formaldehyde there was moderate haze and loss of part of the epithelium of the cornea, leaving the stroma clear beneath. In such severely exposed eyes, histologic studies on subsequent days showed severe damage not only of epithelium but also of endothelium, lens, iris, and ciliary body.[96]

Biomicroscopic study of corneas after contact with a small amount of 40% formaldehyde solution in rabbits has shown changes differing appreciably from those produced by other chemicals.[161] After three hours the corneal corpuscles became visible as minute opaque white dots, having slightly stellate shape, but the remainder of the stroma remained clear until swelling became evident the next day. Swelling then lasted for two weeks and was succeeded by an appearance of long swirling fibriles in the cornea. These in turn disappeared, leaving the stroma clear in about a month.

The intraocular pressure rises rapidly in rabbits when formaldehyde is applied to the surface or injected into the anterior chamber. This is accompanied by miosis and increase in protein in the aqueous humor. The possibilities have been considered that this might involve a prostaglandin or a neural mechanism. Most evidence points to a sensory antidromic or axonal reflex mechanism, since the reaction can be blocked by local anesthetic or pharmacologic denervation, but probably not by indomethacin.[b] Prostaglandin concentration is reported not to be raised.[b] The reaction involves uveal vasodilation, and this aspect can be antagonized by polyphloretin phosphate[d] and by vasoconstrictors.[b,c]

The question of ocular injury from formaldehyde possibly reaching the eye by way of the bloodstream has received considerable attention. However, despite reports in the literature of two or three dozen cases of poisoning from drinking of formaldehyde, there appear to have been no observations of visual or ocular disturbance.[a,21,225] Although formaldehyde has been shown to be highly toxic to the retina in vitro and produces neovascularization and membrane-formation when injected into the vitreous in rabbits,[e,s] parenteral administration to rats and rabbits has failed to induce blindness or to alter the glucose uptake of the retina.[81,137] However, in mice chronic oral administration has caused structural changes in the retinal pigment epithelium that are detectable by electron microscopy.[i]

I do not know of any case in human beings or animals in which inhaled or ingested formaldehyde has been shown to have affected the vision from action on the retina, optic nerve, or central nervous system, nor do I know of a demonstration in animals of injury to retina or optic nerve from intravenous administration. However, in animals the methods used for vision testing have so far mostly been limited to simple observations of behavior and of pupillary response to light. More refined measurement by means of ERG has been made by Potts (1955) in monkeys showing an immediate change in the ERG from intravenous formaldehyde, but not blindness. (This is discussed under *Methanol.*)

One patient has been described in whom the question as raised of exposure to small amounts of formaldehyde vapor as a factor in development of bilateral optic atrophy.[n] However, considering all the circumstances, it would be very difficult to consider seriously a suggestion that formaldehyde vapors were responsible for the papillitis and optic atrophy in this case.[h]

A possible reason for failure to induce ocular injury by systemic administration either in human beings or animals is that formaldehyde reacts very rapidly either with the tissues or with components of the blood itself. I have been able to detect free formaldehyde in rabbits in the circulation or in the eye only with doses that were lethal.[81]

At low concentrations formaldehyde in the eye may be at least partially eliminated by retinal hexokinase,[e] or by formaldehyde dehydrogenase with glutathione as coenzyme, converting formaldehyde to formate. This latter enzyme system has been demonstrated by Kinoshita to be present in the retinas of cattle, human, and rabbit eyes.[k,l] The reaction is of interest not only in relation to formaldehyde but also in relation to methanol poisoning.

a. Bohmer K: Formalin poisoning. *DTSCH Z GES GERICHT MED* 23:7–18, 1934.
b. Butler JM, Unger WG, Hammond BR: Sensory mediation of the ocular response to neutral formaldehyde. *EXP EYE RES* 28:577–589, 1979.
c. Chiang TS, Leaders FE: Antagonism of formaldehyde-induced ocular hypertension by phenylethylamines. *PROC SOC EXP BIOL MED* 135:249–252, 1970.
d. Cole DF: Formaldehyde-induced ocular hypertension. *EXP EYE RES* 19:533–542, 1974.

e. Cooper JR, Marchesi VT: The possible biochemical lesion in blindness due to methanol poisoning. *BIOCHEM PHARMACOL* 2:213–215, 1959.

f. Fortenberry B, Kagawa CM, Leaders FE, Jr: Chemically induced experimental ocular hypertension for evaluating drug effects in albino rabbits. *PROC SOC EXP BIOL MED* 131:637–641, 1969.

g. Hisatomi Y: An unusual case of an eye burn from formalin solution. *ZENTRALBL GES OPHTHALMOL* 44:671–672, 1940. (German)

h. Iwanoff N: Experimental investigations of the effects of industrially and hygienically important gases and vapors. *ARCH HYG* 73:307–340, 1911. (German)

i. Kawano M: The effect of orally administered formaldehyde on the mouse retina. *FOLIA OPHTHALMOL JPN* 26:529, 1975. (English summary)

j. Kelecom J: Ocular burns from formaldehyde. *ARCH OPHTALMOL* (PARIS) 22:259–262, 1962. (French) (*SURVEY OPHTHALMOL* 8:165–166, 1963.)

k. Kini MM, Cooper JR: Methanol poisoning. *BIOCHIM BIOPHYS ACTA* 44:599–601, 1960.

l. Kinoshita JH, Masurat T: The effect of glutathione on formaldehyde oxidation in the retina. *AM J OPHTHALMOL* 46:42–46, 1958.

m. Sager DS: The effect of formaldehyde upon the cornea. *OPHTHALMOSCOPE* 4:63–64, 1906.

n. Saury A, Revault M–P, Vincent V: Optic atrophy manifest after exposure to formaldehyde vapors. *BULL MED LEGALE* 8:466–469, 1965. (French)

o. Schuck EA, Stephens ER, Middleton JT: Eye irritation response at low concentrations of irritants. *ARCH ENVIRON HEALTH* 13:570–575, 1966.

p. Smith BC, Nesi FA: Upper lid loss due to formalin injection. *OPHTHALMOLOGY* 86:1951–1955, 1979.

q. Thiel H–J, Parwaresch MR, Hartmann G: Use of polyacrylamide gel for the estimation of the degradation products of glycosaminoglycans in formalin-induced keratitis. *GRAEFES ARCH OPHTHALMOL* 190:133–143, 1974. (German)

r. Weber-Tschopp A, Fischer T, Grandjean E: Irritating effects of formaldehyde on men. *INT ARCH OCCUP ENVIRON HEALTH* 39:207–218, 1977. (German)

s. Weiss H: A simple method of producing neovascularization and vitreous membranes in the rabbit eye. *GRAEFES ARCH OPHTHALMOL* 190:267–274, 1974.

Formic acid is a colorless liquid, dangerously caustic to the skin.[171] The vapors are irritating to the eyes and respiratory passages.[46,252] In experiments on excised corneas, formic acid is one of the most rapidly penetrating acids.[79] In a live rabbit, pure liquid formic acid applied with a brush to part of the cornea in an experiment by Guillery in 1910 was seen to cause immediate local opacity. This began to clear slightly in five days, but by that time there was hypopyon, posterior subcapsular lens opacity, absence of portions of corneal endothelium, infiltration, and growth of new blood vessels at the limbus. The iris was also infiltrated and hyperemic. In another rabbit a five-minute application of formic acid diluted to 10% also caused dense white local opacity, and at five days the reaction in the cornea was similar to that of the eye exposed to concentrated acid, but hypopyon was absent.[96] Experiments that seem to give a different impression of the toxicity of formic acid were published by Strebel in 1931, when investigating the effect of bee venom on the eye. Strebel replaced the aqueous humor with solutions of formic acid, and reported that even as much as 10% formic acid caused no opacity of the lens, although it did produce protracted iritis. He did not mention the effect on the cornea. He concluded that there was not nearly enough formic acid in bee venom to account for the severe reactions produced by bee venom in the eye.[i] In a patient described by Sudarsky in 1965, a drop of a reaction mixture composed of 0.8 ml 90% formic acid and 0.2 ml 30% hydrogen peroxide splashed in one eye. The eye was quickly irrigated with water, but an area of swelling of the epithelium and anterior stroma of the cornea, and cells and flare in the anterior chamber were observable half an hour later. However, in twelve hours the aqueous and cornea had become clear except for an area of loss of epithelium, and in thirty-six to sixty hours recovery was complete.[j] A more serious injury to the eye occurred in a farm worker who was spraying silage with formic acid (concentration unstated), and accidentally was struck in the eye by a jet of the liquid. Despite immediate irrigation with water, the cornea became infiltrated with blood vessels. Dense symblepharon formed between the upper lid and limbus. This was separated surgically, but because of clouding of the cornea the vision remained 3/10 at best.[f]

In Finland, accidents in treatment of silage with "AIV solution", composed of 80% formic acid and 2% orthophosphoric acid, have recently caused about half of all acid eye burns there. Most eyes irrigated for 1 to 2 hours with physiologic saline have had good final visual acuity, despite initial damage to the corneal epithelium and chemosis, but one eye with less irrigation had corneal stromal and scleral damage, leading to perforation and enucleation.[h]

The systemic effects of formic acid and formate are of considerable interest, because formic acid is one of the products of metabolism of methanol, which is notorious for its severe toxicity, particularly to the eye. Neutral formate is known to be an inhibitor of certain enzymes, e.g., catalase, and has been investigated for potential injuriousness to the retina and optic nerve. However no evidence has been obtained of retinal toxicity in experimental animals, and 0.02 M formate has not been found to affect the metabolism of the retina in vitro.[b] Sodium formate, has been fed to various animals and administered parenterally without ocular disturbance. Also it has been employed in the form of potassium formate as a substitute for sodium chloride for patients who need to limit their sodium intake, and this apparently has caused no disturbance of vision. However, Fink in 1943 claimed that formic acid administered in unspecified quantity to rabbits and dogs produced the same histopathology in the retina and optic nerve as did methanol.[a] Presumably, acidosis was induced by the formic acid in these experiments in which the eyes were found to be injured, whereas acidosis would not be produced by feeding neutral formates. Acidosis has been a prominent feature of poisoning by methanol in primates in which blindness may occur. In this connection, in a series of studies in dogs, Herken and Rietbrock concluded that metabolism of methanol to formic acid could produce generalized acidosis. Furthermore, they postulated that as the tissue pH was lowered in acidosis, the toxicity attributable to this metabolite increased, owing to a greater proportion being present as formic acid and a smaller proportion as relatively innocuous formate ion.[c,g] An important series of studies has shown that in monkeys there is a marked increase in formic acid in the blood, with metabolic acidosis, after administration of methanol, and that the accumulation of formic acid can be accentuated by deficiency of folate. The same type of toxicity to the optic nerves has been demonstrated by administration of formic acid to monkeys as by administration of methanol, and it now appears that the accumulation of formic acid and the associated metabolic acidosis is the actual mechanism underlying the blindness notoriously produced by methanol.[d,e] (See *Methanol* for further description.)

a. Fink WH: The ocular pathology of methyl alcohol poisoning. *AM J OPHTHALMOL* 26:694–709; 802–815, 1943.
b. Greig ME, Munro MP, Elliott KAC: The metabolism of lactic and pyruvic acids in normal and tumor tissues. *BIOCHEM J* 33:443–453, 1939.
c. Herken W (1969):—reference in *Methanol* bibliography.
d. McMartin KE, Martin-Amat G, et al: Methanol poisoning. V. Role of formate metabolism in the monkey. *J PHARMACOL EXP THER* 201:564–572, 1977.
e. McMartin KE, Martin-Amat G, et al: Lack of a role for formaldehyde in methanol poisoning in the monkey. *BIOCHEM PHARMACOL* 28:645–649, 1979.
f. Peyresblanques J: Ocular burn by formic acid in agriculture. *BULL SOC OPHTALMOL FRANCE* 81:679–680, 1981. (French)
g. Rietbrock N (1968, 1969):—references in *Methanol* bibliography.
h. Saari KM, Leinonen J, Aine E: Management of chemical eye injuries with prolonged irrigation. *ACTA OPHTHALMOL Suppl* 161:52–59, 1984.
i. Strebel J: Bee and wasp sting injuries of the eye. *KLIN MONATSBL AUGENHEILKD* 86:657–662, 1931. (German)
j. Sudarsky DR: Ocular injury due to formic acid. *ARCH OPHTHALMOL* 74:805–806, 1965.

Framycetin sulfate (neomycin B; Soframycin), an antibiotic, when injected subconjunctivally produces the same blood concentrations as intramuscular injection. However, standard subconjunctival dosage had produced no systemic toxic effects according to a 10 year review.[b] An odd local effect has been reported in one instance in which 50 mg in 0.25 ml was injected subconjunctivally after goniotomy.[c] Superficial dense white corneal opacities formed, but were gone by the next day. It was thought that alcohol which had been used in removal of corneal epithelium before the goniotomy was still present after the operation in sufficient concentration to precipitate the antibiotic.

Injection of 0.5% solution into the anterior chamber has been "well tolerated".[a]

a. Bharadwaj PC, Shrivastava KN, et al: Intracameral injections of framycetin sulphate. *BR J OPHTHALMOL* 53:185–187, 1969.
b. Bron AJ, Richards AB, et al: Systemic absorption of Soframycin after subconjunctival injection. *BR J OPHTHALMOL* 54:615–620, 1970.
c. Hamilton AM: Unusual complication associated with a subconjunctival injection of Soframycin. *BR J OPHTHALMOL* 56:637–638, 1972.

Fructose, a natural sugar, when administered to rats as 68% of the diet, has induced retinopathy.[a]

a. Boot-Handford RP, Heath H: Fructose as a retinopathic agent. *IRCS MED SCI: LIBR COMPEND* 5:583, 1977.

Fuel for model airplanes is commonly a mixture of methyl alcohol (methanol), nitromethane or nitropropane, and castor oil. An accidental squirt of this type of fuel into a boy's eye has been observed to cause immediate pain, loss of corneal epithelium, and much swelling of the lids. However, the corneal stroma remained clear and the eye healed promptly and completely.[a]

a. Haley W: Personal communication, 1960.

Furfural (2-furaldehyde) vapor at concentrations of 13.5 ppm in air is reported to cause reddening of the eyes, tearing, and irritation of the throat in workers.[a,c] Test application of 10% aqueous solution of furfural on the eyes of animals has caused immediate pain, lasting for a minute or two, followed by complete anesthesia of cornea and conjunctiva. At the same time the lids and conjunctivae became red and swollen, but in twenty-four hours the eyes returned to normal.[c,d] When applied full strength to rabbit eyes a drop caused immediate edema of the corneal epithelium followed by loss of the epithelium in sheets. Small hemorrhages appeared in the nictitating membrane, and edema in the conjunctiva, but the eyes rapidly returned to normal.[81]

a. Clinton M: Furfural. *AM PETROL INST TOXIC REV,* Mar. 1948.
b. Cohn A: On the toxic action of furfural. *NAUNYN-SCHMIEDEBERG'S ARCH EXP PATH PHARMAK* 31:40–48, 1893. (German)
c. Korenmann JN, Resnik JB: Furfural as an industrial poison and its determination in air. *ARCH HYG* 104:344–357, 1930. (German)
d. Lepine: On the action of furfural. *C R SOC BIOL PARIS* 1887, p. 437. (French)

Furmethonol (Furaltadone, Altafur), an antibacterial, was withdrawn in 1961 because of neurotoxic and other side effects.[b] Neurotoxicity was the principal adverse effect, but its incidence appears to have been low, consisting of sixty-nine known cases among 900,000 estimated courses of treatment. In sixty-one out of the sixty-nine cases the patients were said to have completely recovered.[h] All published reports were summarized in tabular form in a survey edited by Michiels in 1972.[359]

The first twenty-five cases of neurologic disturbance included diplopia, paresis of individual extraocular muscles, nystagmus, and blurring of vision. Also ten of the patients had impaired hearing, peripheral neuritis, and difficulty in swallowing and speaking. Such side effects appeared after the drug was administered for about thirty-eight days.[g] A subsequent compilation indicated that disturbance of eyes or vision consisted of diplopia in 68 per cent, "blurring" in 29 per cent, rotary nystagmus in 14 per cent, lateral rectus palsy in 7 per cent, and scotomas in 4 per cent.[c]

Several of the instances of diplopia caused by lateral rectus muscle paresis have been described in separate reports.[a,f,j,m] Usually the diplopia disappeared within two weeks after discontinuing furmethonol, but some cases took months.[a,e] One woman developed severe burning sensation in the hands and feet, aphonia, and long-lasting diplopia associated with paresis of the lateral rectus, the facial and other cranial nerves.[i]

One patient was found by Jacobson to have cone blindness with dayblindness and nystagmus.[d] This patient was known to have had entirely normal vision previously. Detailed analysis has been published.[k,l]

One other case of reduced visual acuity in bright light is reported to have developed after treatment, but in this case no special measurements were made to determine the basis for the visual change. This patient also had paresis of a lateral rectus muscle, but pupillary reactions and fundi were normal, and later the patient developed peripheral polyneuritis, which recovered after the furmethonol was discontinued.[j]

a. Bell DM, Freehafer AA: Neuropathy associated with Furaltadone. *J AM MED ASSOC* 176:806–807, 1961.
b. Council on Drugs: Furaltadone (Altafur). *J AM MED ASSOC* 172:1932–1933, 1960.
c. Fajardo RV, Pryor J, Leopold IH: Furaltadone in ophthalmology. *AM J OPHTHALMOL* 54:114–119, 1962.
d. Jacobson J: Personal communication. May 1966.
e. Lee MLH: Toxic effects of prolonged treatment with Furaltadone. *LANCET* 2:374–375, 1960. (*SURVEY OPHTHALMOL* 7:73, 1962.)
f. Loftus LR: New allergic reaction for Furaltadone. *J AM MED ASSOC* 173:362, 1960.
g. MacLeod PF: Eaton Laboratories, Norwich N.Y. 1960.
h. MacLeod PF: Regarding Furaltadone. (Correspondence.) *N ENGL J MED* 264:517–518, 1961.
i. Mast WH: Neuropathy due to Furaltadone. *N ENGL J MED* 263:963, 1960.
j. Pereyra KJ, Poch GF, Herskovita E: *REV ASS MED ARGENT* 76:574–577, 1962.
k. Siegel IM, Smith BF: Acquired cone dysfunction. *ARCH OPHTHALMOL* 77:8, 1967.
l. Siegel IM, Arden GB: The effect of drugs on colour vision. In Herxheimer, A. (Ed.): *Drugs and Sensory Functions.* Boston, Little, 1968, pp.210–228.
m. Smith JL, Creighton JB, Jr: Sixth nerve palsy due to Furaltadone (Altafur). *ARCH OPHTHALMOL* 65:61–62, 1961.

Furtrethonium iodide (Furfuryltrimethyl ammonium iodide, Furmethide) is a potent parasympathomimetic agent employed for several years as a miotic eyedrop in treatment of glaucoma, until discovery that it induced abnormalities in the conjunctival epithelium resulting in deforming membranes and stenosis of the tear ducts.[a] For this reason it is no longer used on the eye.

a. Shaffer RN, Ridgway WL: Furmethide iodide in the production of dacryostenosis. *AM J OPHTHALMOL* 34:718–720, 1951.

Fusidic acid, an antimicrobial, came under some suspicion because it was being administered to a patient who developed optic neuritis and blindness, but the patient was also under treatment with cephaloridine and cloxacillin.[a,b] Since then, rare cases of retinopathy have been ascribed to cephaloridine. (See INDEX for more on *Cephaloridine.*)

a. Ballingall DLK, Turpie AGG: Cephaloridine toxicity. *LANCET* 2:835–836, 1967.
b. Crosbie RB: Cephaloridine toxicity. *LANCET* 1:422, 1968.

G1047 (N-(p-amido-sulpho-phenyl)-alpha methyl alpha ethyl succinimide), an investigational antiepileptic drug, has been associated in one case with optic neuritis that improved when the drug was discontinued.[a]

a. Mikkelsen B: Optic neuritis ascribed to our antiepileptic drug. *UGESKR LAEG* 134:391–392, 1972. (English abstract)

Gadolinium chloride, a water soluble rare-earth salt, has been tested for toxicity on rabbit corneas and has been found to have properties essentially the same as lanthanum chloride, the prototype of the rare-earth group. The cornea is seriously damaged only by prolonged contact after the epithelial barrier has been injured or removed.[88,90] Applying 1 mg to intact rabbit eyes causes only transitory irritation.[a]

a. Haley TJ, Raymond et al: Toxicological and pharmacological effects of gadolinium and samarium chlorides. *BR J PHARMACOL* 17:526–532, 1961.

Galactose is a natural sugar, a component of lactose. In normal adult human beings, no significant ocular toxicity from galactose has been detected, even from 100 g daily for more than four months (Hartstein). However, certain individuals have a congenital abnormality in galactose metabolism which renders them susceptible to poisoning by galactose and leads to formation of cataracts in infancy. In animals, cataracts can be produced by feeding large amounts of galactose.

The clinical aspects of hereditary galactosemia in human beings and the responsible metabolic disorders have been summarized by Hansen, Nordmann, Wilson, and others (Hansen; Nordmann; Wilson). In a review concerning human galactosemic cataract, Cordes estimated that cataracts occurred in about 75 percent of cases of galactosemia (Cordes), but Nordmann thought that the incidence might approach 100 percent (Nordmann). Cordes gave particular attention to the morphology of human galactose cataracts, the age of development, and the reversibility. The earliest change in the lens, noted as early as three weeks of age, is an increase in refractive power around the fetal nucleus, giving the ophthalmoscopic appearance of a drop of oil or central refractile ring. This has usually been followed by either zonular or nuclear cataracts, plus faint striate and dust-like opacities in the anterior cortex, also posterior subcapsular star-shaped opacities (Scheibenreiter). The cataracts may disappear wholly or in part when milk or other sources of galactose are eliminated from the diet, particularly if this is done before three months of age (Cordes; Ritter).

Most cases of galactosemia with cataracts very early in life are due to congenital deficiency of the enzyme galactose-1-phosphate uridyl transferase, and this deficiency also causes life-threatening, often lethal, systemic complications, unless milk is promptly removed from the diet (Beutler). A smaller number of cases of galactosemia with cataracts are caused by a congenital deficiency of the enzyme galactokinase, which as a rule is not life-threatening (Beutler; Schuette). Whether partial lack of galactokinase may also cause infantile cataracts is uncertain, but in one child a simultaneous partial lack of both enzymes has been associated with cataracts early in life (Winder). Winder has given particular attention to the genetics of these conditions (Winder). It is unlikely that galactosemic cataracts ever make their appearance after the first year of life. Histologic abnormalities, but no gross opacities, have been found in a 5 month human fetus with transferase enzyme deficiency, suggesting that some opacities might be present at birth, but go unnoticed (Vannas).

Galactose cataracts in experimental animals and in lenses surviving in culture have received a great deal of attention. Cataracts were first induced in animals by feeding excessive galactose in 1935. In 1959 van Heyningen made an important observation that galactose was partially converted to a sugar alcohol which accumulated in the lenses of animals to which excessive galactose was fed (Van Heyningen). Kinoshita and his associates soon thereafter began reporting an intensive series of studies demonstrating many significances of this accumulation of sugar alcohol in the lens and elucidated a number of important features of the cataractogenic mechanism, not only in galactose cataracts but also in sugar cataracts in general, with ramifications into pathogenetic mechanisms of diabetes (Chylack; Hayman; Holt; Kador; Kinoshita; Kuwabara; Thoft). These advances attracted many investigators and produced a large literature concerning many aspects of galactose cataracts, especially the biochemical aspects. Series of papers appeared in symposia on bio-chemistry of the eye in 1968 and 1970 (Dardenne).[319] Chylack and Cheng reviewed the carbohydrate biochemistry of sugar cataracts in 1978 (Chylack). Kinoshita reviewed the role of aldose reductase in sugar cataracts in 1981 (Kinoshita).

Experimentally, galactose cataracts have most often been produced in the lenses of normal young rats by feeding large amounts of galactose. Cataracts can similarly be produced in gerbils (El-Aguizy). The type of cataract produced is morphologically somewhat different from that in human galactosemia. Rats are not as subject to severe systemic abnormalities as human patients.

In development of galactose cataracts in rats, vacuoles consisting of accumulations of sugar alcohol dulcitol (galactitol) and water appear first in the equatorial region of the lens, proceeding to dense nuclear opacities. Species, age, and state of develop-ment are significant factors in determining the morphology. It has been suggested by Talman that young rats and hamsters may be particularly susceptible because of special enzymic inadequacies in their erythrocytes and livers which permit large amounts of galactose to reach the lens (Talman). When pregnant rats have been maintained on a galactose diet, the newly born rat has developed a nuclear lamellar type of cataract, more closely resembling the type seen in the human infants (Segal).

The details of experimental galactose cataract in rats have been described in several reports (Grimes; Kinoshita; Kuwabara; Philipson; Schrader). Kuwabara, Kinoshita, and Cogan by electron microscopy found these changes to be very similar to changes observed in cataracts due to diabetes, the first morphologic alteration being the appearance of hydropic lens fibers (Kuwabara). Grimes and von Sallmann have observed that as some cells and lens fibers swell and degenerate, other lens cells proliferate more rapidly than normal, as though in a compensatory way (Grimes). Reversal of lens opacification in rats by eliminating galactose from the diet after exposure to excessive galactose, has been an intriguing phenomenon that has been studied both morphologically (Unakar) and biochemically (Kador; Shinohara). During development of opacity the synthesis of lens crystallins by lens cortical fiber cells is depressed, and some leaks out of the lens, but during regression of opacity the synthetic process recovers (Kador; Shinohara). Similarly, Na-K-ATPase activity of the lens is depressed, and then recovers when galactose is withdrawn (Unakar).

As the key to explaining the mechanism of sugar cataracts, Kinoshita and his associates obtained a great deal of evidence for an osmotic mechanism that accounts for the morphologic changes observed in the lenses and also accounts for a series of secondary biochemical derangements (Kinoshita). The crux of the osmotic mechanism, which is believed to apply to all sugar cataracts, is the fact that while sugars readily enter the lens, the corresponding sugar alcohols to which they may be converted in the lens have solubility characteristics that are different and prevent the sugar alcohols from escaping from the lens. The sugar alcohols that are trapped and accumulate in the lens have an osmotic effect, causing water to enter the lens, and causing lens cells and fibers to swell and become disrupted. These changes reduce the transparency of the lens, and they lead to a series of biochemical disturbances which further contribute to formation of cataract (Kinoshita; Schuette).

The amount of sugar alcohol that forms and accumulates in the lens, and consequently the amount of change in transparency and biochemical derangement, is influenced by the amount of sugar presented to the lens, but varies from one sugar to another. Aldose reductase is responsible for the reduction of the sugars to their corresponding alcohols (galactose to dulcitol or galactitol, glucose to sorbitol, and xylose to xylitol) (Hayman; Jedziniak). Reduction of the sugars by this enzyme proceeds at an important rate only when the concentrations of the sugars are considerably elevated. At the concentrations at which these sugars are normally present in the aqueous humor or lens there is negligible reduction to the sugar alcohols by aldose reductase, and the sugars are metabolized by other paths to noninjurious metabolites. This is true for galactose as for other sugars. When sugars are presented to the lens in abnormally high concentrations sufficient to induce significant conversion to the corresponding sugar alcohols by the action of aldose reductase, the amount of each that accumulates in the lens varies considerably from one sugar alcohol to another. This appears to be governed primarily by the effectiveness of a second enzyme, polyol dehydrogenase, which tends to eliminate the sugar alcohols. This enzyme eliminates sorbitol, the sugar alcohol of glucose, much more effectively than the dulcitol from galactose. Because of these differences, sugar cataract can be produced by galactose in a few days in rats or in incubated rabbit lenses, but to produce sugar cataract with glucose requires a longer time and a high concentration (Chylack).

The first effect of accumulation of a sugar alcohol such as dulcitol in the lens is an osmotic movement of water into the lens, both into the cells and between the cells. Secondarily, the lens becomes abnormally permeable to potassium and sodium so that sodium begins to leak in, and potassium to leak out (Thoft). Initially the cation pump of the lens increases its rate of pumping potassium into the lens, but before long the lens becomes excessively leaky. Sodium and chloride both diffuse into the lens, and the lens proteins then undergo Donnan swelling. Ultimately the lens cells and fibers disintegrate. The lens proteins are fundamentally altered in the process (Holt; Sinha). The amount of reduced glutathione in the lens decreases, as in most other cataracts (Sippel).[12]

The key role of aldose reductase in formation of sugar alcohols and production of sugar cataracts by an excess of galactose or of glucose has been further demonstrated by Kinoshita and his associates through use of inhibitors of this enzyme, which they and others have shown to prevent formation of sugar cataracts in animals (Beyer-Mears; Datiles; Parmar). One of these inhibitors, sorbinil, has reached the stage of clinical evaluation for toxicity and inhibitory effect on aldose reductase in the lenses of human beings, with a view to examining potential therapeutic action in sugar-induced complications of diabetes (Datiles; Kinoshita). In animals, sorbinil can prevent or reverse cataract formation (Datiles; Beyer-Mears; Hu).

Prolactin can accentuate galactose-induced cataract formation in rats (Gona).

There has been no indication that the sugar alcohols, dulcitol, sorbitol, or xylitol, are themselves toxic to the lens. The principal evidence that their effect in the lens is osmotic rather than toxic has been the repeated demonstration in lenses surviving in vitro that swelling of the lens and all the secondary results of swelling have been preventable by adjustment of the tonicity of the bathing fluid to compensate for the accumulation of sugar alcohol in the lens. Additional evidence concerning the toxicity of sugar alcohols has been sought by feeding experiments. No cataract has been produced by feeding large amounts of dulcitol to animals (Wilson).

Ocular disturbances from galactose other than cataract formation have included interference with healing of corneal epithelial wounds in rats (Datiles), and thickening of basement membrane of retinal capillaries (Frank; Robinson). Both of these effects are of special interest because they resemble disturbances that occur in diabetes mellitus in human beings. Both effects can be prevented in rats by administering sorbinil.

Beutler E, Matsumoto F, et al: Galactokinase deficiency as a cause of cataracts. *N ENGL J MED* 288:1203–1239, 1973; and *LANCET* 1:1161, 1978.

Beyer-Mears A, Farnsworth PN: Diminished sugar cataractogenesis by quercetin. *EXP EYE RES* 28:709–716, 1979.

Beyer-Mears A, Cruz E, et al: Sorbinil protection of lens protein components and cell hydration during diabetic cataract formation. *PHARMACOLOGY* 24:193–200, 1982.

Chylack LT, Kinoshita JH: Biochemical evaluation of a cataract induced in high glucose medium. *INVEST OPHTHALMOL* 8:401, 1969.

Chylack LT, Cheng HM: Sugar metabolism in the crystalline lens. *SURVEY OPHTHALMOL* 23:26–34, 1978.

Cordes FC: Galactosemia cataract: A review. *AM J OPHTHALMOL* 50:1151–1157, 1960.

Dardenne MU and Nordmann JB (eds.): *Biochemistry of the Eye*. New York, Karger, 1968.

Datiles M, Fukui H, et al: Galactose cataract prevention with sorbinil, an aldose reductase inhibitor. *INVEST OPHTHALMOL VIS SCI* 22:174–179, 1982.

Datiles MB, Kador PF, et al: Corneal re-epithelialization in galactosemic rats. *INVEST OPHTHALMOL VIS SCI* 24:563–565, 1983.

El-Aguizy HK, Richards RD, Varma SD: Sugar cataracts in Mongolian gerbil. *EXP EYE RES* 36:839–844, 1983.

Frank RN, Keirn RJ, et al: Galactose-induced retinal capillary basement membrane thickening. *INVEST OPHTHALMOL VIS SCI* 24:1519–1524, 1983.

Gona O, Fu SCJ: Effect of prolactin on galactose-induced cataractogenesis in the rat. *PROC SOC EXP BIOL MED* 171:285–288, 1982.

Grimes P, von Sallmann L: Lens epithelium proliferation in sugar cataracts. *INVEST OPHTHALMOL* 7(5):535–543, 1968.

Hansen RG: Hereditary galactosemia. *J AM MED ASSOC* 208:2077–2082, 1969.

Hartstein J: Studies of the crystalline lens in humans receiving galactose over prolonged periods. *ARCH OPHTHALMOL* 59:406, 1958.

Hu TS, Datiles M, Kinoshita JH: Reversal of galactose cataract with sorbinil in rats. *INVEST OPHTHALMOL VIS SCI* 24:640–644, 1983.

Hayman S, Kinoshita JH: Isolation and properties of lens aldose reductase. *J BIOL CHEM* 240:877, 1965.

Hayman S, Lou MF, et al: Aldose reductase activity in the lens and other tissues. *BIOCHIM BIOPHYS ACTA* 128:474, 1966.

Holt WS, Kinoshita JH: Starch gel electrophoresis of the soluble lens proteins from normal and galactosemic animals. *INVEST OPHTHALMOL* 7:169–178, 1968.

Jedziniak JA, Kinoshita JH: Lens aldose reductase. *EXP EYE RES* 8:232, 1969.

Kador PF, Zigler JS, Kinoshita JH: Alterations of lens protein synthesis in galactosemic rats. *INVEST OPHTHALMOL VIS SCI* 18:696–702, 1979.

Kinoshita JH: Cataracts in galactosemia. The Jonas S. Friedenwald Memorial Lecture. *INVEST OPHTHALMOL* 4:786, 1965.

Kinoshita JH, Kador P, Catiles M: Aldose reductase in diabetic cataracts. *J AM MED ASSOC* 246:257–261, 1981.

Kuwabara T, Kinoshita JH, Cogan DG: Electron microscopic study of galactose-induced cataract. *INVEST OPHTHALMOL* 8:133–149, 1969.

Nordmann J: Concerning relationships between galactose and the crystalin lens. *DOCUM OPHTHALMOL* 26:334–348, 1969.

Parmar NS, Ghosh MN: Effect of gossypin, a flavonoid, on the formation of galactose-induced cataracts in rats. *EXP EYE RES* 29:229–232, 1979.

Philipson B: Galactose cataract: Changes in protein distribution during development. *INVEST OPHTHALMOL* 8:281–289, 1969.

Ritter JH, Cannon EJ: Galactosemia with cataracts. Report of a case with notes on physiopathology. *N ENGL J MED* 252:747–751, 1955.

Robinson WG Jr, Kador PF, Kinoshita JH: Retinal capillaries; basement membrane thickening by galactosemia prevented with aldose reductase inhibitor. *SCIENCE* 1177–1179, 1983.

Scheibenreiter S, Zehetbauer G: On the morphology of galactosemic cataracts. *KLIN MONATSBL AUGENHEILKD* 162:665–669, 1973. (German)

Schrader KE, Beneke G: Morphologic and histochemical studies of galactose cataract in albino rats. *GRAEFES ARCH OPHTHALMOL* 168:341–357, 1965. (German)

Schuette E, Reim M: Lens opacities in galactokinase deficiency. *KLIN MONATSBL AUGENHEILKD* 166:553–556, 1975. (German)

Segal S, Bernstein H: Observation on cataract formation in the newborn offspring of rats fed on high galactose diet. *J PEDIATR* 62:363–370, 1963.

Shinohara T, Piatigorsky J: Crystallin synthesis and crystallin mRNAs in galactosemic rat lenses. *EXP EYE RES* 34:39–48, 1982.

Sinha BN: Electrophoresis of soluble protein fraction in normal and cataractous lens (galactose fed) of albino rats. *INDIAN J MED RES* 57:348–390, 1969. (*CHEM ABSTR* 71:36905, 1969.)

Sippel TO: Changes in the water, protein, and glutathione contents of the lens in the course of galactose cataract development in rats. *INVEST OPHTHALMOL* 5:568–575, 1966.

Sippel TO: Enzymes of carbohydrate metabolism in developing galactose cataracts of rats. *INVEST OPHTHALMOL* 6:59–63, 1967.

Talman EL: Mechanism for galactose 1-phosphate accrual in galactose cataract. *PHYSIOL CHEM PHYS* 1:131–140, 1969.

Thoft RA, Merola LO, Kinoshita JH: The rate of potassium exchange of galactosemic rat lenses. See pages 383–387 in Dardenne reference.

Unakar NJ, Smart T, et al: Regression of cataract in the offspring of galactose fed rats. *OPHTHALMIC RES* 11:52–64, 1979.

Unakar NJ, Tsui J: Sodium-potassium-dependent ATPase. II. *INVEST OPHTHALMOL VIS SCI* 19:378–385, 1980.

Van Heyningen R: Metabolism of xylose by the lens. *BIOCHEM J* 73:197–207, 1959.

Vannas A, Hogan MJ, et al: Lens changes in a galactosemic fetus. *AM J OPHTHALMOL* 80:726–733, 1975.

Wilson WA: Cataracts and galactose metabolism. *TRANS AM OPHTHALMOL SOC* 65:661–704, 1967.

Wilson WA: Failure to produce cataracts in rats with galactitol diet. *AM J OPHTHALMOL* 67:224–229, 1969.

Winder AF, Fells P, et al: Galactose intolerance and the risk of cataract. *BR J OPHTHALMOL* 66:438–441, 1982.

Gallium salts given in lethal amounts to rats appeared to cause photophobia and then blindness two to four days prior to death.[a] However, rabbits, dogs, and goats that were lethally poisoned did not have photophobia and did not appear blind.[b]

a. Dudley HC, Levine MD: Studies of the toxic action of gallium. *J PHARMACOL EXP THER* 95:487–493, 1949.

b. Dudley HC, Henry KE, Lindsley BF: Studies of toxic action of gallium II. *J PHARMACOL EXP THER* 98:409–417, 1950.

Gamboge is a gum resin from an East Indian plant. It is intensely irritating. Tests on rabbits long ago showed that contact with the eye could cause purulent keratitis.[46]

Gelatin has been tested as an intrascleral implant in cats and rabbits, shown to be absorbed with very little inflammatory reaction,[a] and has been used clinically.[b,c]

a. Daniele S, Jacklin HN, et al: Gelatin as an absorbable implant in scleral buckling procedures. *ARCH OPHTHALMOL* 80:115–119, 1968.

b. King LM Jr, Margherio RR, Schepens CL: Gelatin implants in scleral buckling. *ARCH OPHTHALMOL* 93:807–811, 1975.

c. Ray GS, van Heuven AJ, Patel D: Gelatin implants in scleral buckling procedures. *ARCH OPHTHALMOL* 93:799–802, 1975.

Gelsemium sempervirens (Carolina yellow jessamine,[142] yellow jasmine, wild woodbine) yields a mixture of alkaloids which formerly had some use in treatment for neuralgia. Overdosage has been reported to cause mydriasis and paralysis of accommodation. Also, severe systemic reactions, characterized by slow pulse, low temperature, great weakness, and difficulty in swallowing, have occasionally been accompanied by ocular motor palsies, especially of the lateral recti, with diplopia and ptosis.[153,171,246,252] In nonfatal cases the ocular symptoms have always disappeared in a day or two.

Gentamicin sulfate (Genoptic, Garamycin), an antibacterial, is not injurious to the eye when applied as eye drops at a concentration of 1%, or as 0.3% ointment.[a] However, experimentally 1% solution can retard healing of corneal epithelium.[368] Subconjunctival injection of 20 to 40 mg is not injurious from a clinical viewpoint, but may cause slight irritation and chemosis,[b,d,f] and in the immediate area of injection has been shown by electron microscopy to cause lysosomal storage of phospholipid character, similar to what gentamicin can induce in kidney proximal tubules.[e] This has been observed in rat, rabbit, and human eyes, limited to the conjunctiva.

Effects of injection of gentamicin sulfate solutions into the anterior chamber, replacing the aqueous humor after paracentesis, are dependent on amount injected. Hanselmayer reported 0.2% solution in human beings, and 0.4% in rabbits to be well tolerated; 1% in rabbits caused temporary irritation.[c] However, Mester reported that in 2 human eyes with infected blebs, irrigation of the anterior chamber with 0.5% solution caused marked swelling of the corneas.[h] A study in rabbits utilizing vital staining with dyes showed that 0.5% and 1% solutions killed many corneal endothelial cells, but 0.25% appeared to be tolerable.[h] Scanning and transmission electron microscopy also showed damage to these cells at higher concentrations.[270,271] Peyman reported that rabbit eyes with a concentration as high as approximately 2.6% in the anterior chamber could eventually recover.[j] A lower concentration of 0.04% caused microscopically visible edema and dilation of endoplasmic reticulum of corneal endothelium, but return to normal in two days.[341]

Intravitreal injections have been reported, usually expressing the dose in μg or mg per injection, rather than as % concentration, because of the undetermined degree of dilution by mixing with vitreous humor. Usually a volume of 0.1 ml has been injected. Bennett (1974) found no ocular toxicity in owl monkeys from a dose of 0.5 mg.[280] Peyman reported that 3 mg or more consistently produced cataracts in rabbits, beginning as posterior vacuoles in 2 days, and maturing in five weeks.[j] (More will be said about effects on the lens below.) Injection of 2 mg or more into the vitreous body consistently produced diffuse retinal degeneration, affecting first the outer half of the retina, then causing complete degeneration. Intravitreal 8 mg caused, in addition, iritis, posterior synechias, and band keratopathy. When the dose was reduced to 0.5 mg, the eyes remained histologically normal.[j] Zachary (1976) and Palimeris (1979) found that 4 mg caused the vitreous to become cloudy, and caused pigmentary retinopathy to develop, with extinction of the E R G. in a week.[i] With decreasing doses the E R G changes took longer to develop, and histologic changes were less, until below 0.1 or 0.05 mg there was no longer evidence of toxicity.[i,l] Morgan (1979) reported that 0.8 μg/ml in combination with other antibacterials could be used in vitrectomy replacement fluid without undue change in the E R G in rabbits.[361]

In rabbits, treatment of experimental bacterial endophthalmitis with injections of 0.125 to 0.5 mg into the vitreous body caused minute vacuoles to become visible at the posterior pole of the lens by direct ophthalmoscopy, but these cleared in 4 to 5 weeks.[g]

The effect of gentamicin sulfate on bovine lens cells has been investigated in culture by Mayer (1982)[355] who found that 8 mg/100 ml caused their death and destruction, while 2 mg/100 ml appeared to be well tolerated.

Gentamicin is both ototoxic and nephrotoxic, but customary repeated eye drops or subconjunctival injections have not produced sufficient plasma concentrations to cause these complications.[k]

a. Furgiuele FP: Ocular penetration and tolerance of gentamicin. *AM J OPHTHALMOL* 64:421–426, 1967.

b. Goulstein DB, Marmion VJ: Subconjunctival gentamicin. *BR J OPHTHALMOL* 55:478–480, 1971.

c. Hanselmayer H: On tolerance of intraocularly administered gentamicin. *GRAEFES ARCH OPHTHALMOL* 181:277–280, 1971. (German)

d. Kuming BS, Tonkin M: Use of gentamicin sulphate in ophthalmology. *BR J OPHTHAL-MOL* 58:609–612, 1974.

e. Libert J, Ketelbant-Balasse PE, et al: Cellular toxicity of gentamicin. *AM J OPHTHAL-MOL* 87:405–411, 1979.

f. Litwack KD, Pettit T, Johnson BL: Penetration of gentamicin. *ARCH OPHTHALMOL* 82:687–693, 1969.

g. May DR, Ericson ES, et al: Intraocular injection of gentamicin. *ARCH OPHTHALMOL* 91:487–489, 1974.

h. Mester U, Stein HJ: Investigations of the injurious action of intraocularly administered gentamicin. *KLIN MONATSBL AUGENHEILKD* 168:221–223, 1976. (German)

i. Palimeris G, Moschos M, et al: Intravitreal injection of gentamicin—own findings. *KLIN MONATSBL AUGENHEILKD* 175:216–219, 1979. (German)

j. Peyman GA, May DR, et al: Intraocular injection of gentamicin. *ARCH OPHTHALMOL* 92:42–47, 1974.

k. Trope GE, Lawrence JR, et al: Systemic absorption of topical and subconjunctival gentamicin. *BR J OPHTHALMOL* 63:692–693, 1979.

l. Zachary IG, Forster RK: Experimental intravitreal gentamicin. *AM J OPHTHALMOL* 82:604–611, 1976.

Gentian violet (methyl rosaniline chloride) is a basic cationic dye, closely related to but not identical to *crystal violet* and *methyl violet.* Experimentally in rabbits it can be severely injurious to cornea and conjunctiva.[150, 153] Ballantyne has found that an aqueous solution of 0.025% is the maximum concentration that can be applied to rabbit eyes without causing injury,[a] similar to the 0.01% maximum reported by Thompson.[d] Slightly higher concentration causes transient rise of intraocular pressure, and 2% causes necrosis of conjunctiva, and opacification, distortion and vascularization of the cornea, with iritis.[a]

In one instance of human eye injury a drop of gentian violet solution intended for use on the skin was applied to a boy's eye, causing immediate severe pain, blepharospasm, and dark purple staining of cornea and conjunctiva. By the next day most of the color was gone, but the corneal epithelium was absent and the corneal stroma slightly cloudy. Healing was slow. The stroma was still hazy on the fifth day. On the tenth day the corneal epithelium was still irregular, and the eye was hyperemic and uncomfortable. In five weeks the eye had returned to normal. Local corticosteroids and atropine were included in the treatment.[b]

Parker and Binder have reported a second and more severe case in good clinical detail.[c] In their case a patient self-administered a 1% solution to both eyes, and after six months was left with some corneal scarring and vascularization, despite months of appropriate treatment for keratoconjunctivitis, uveitis, and bacterial conjunctivitis.

(See also the INDEX for *Dyes, cationic* and *Pencils, indelible,* for similar injuries.)

a. Ballantyne B, Gazzard MF, Swanston DW: Eye damage caused by crystal violet. *BR J PHARMACOL* 49:181–182, 1973.

b. Haley W: Personal communication, 1960.

c. Parker WT, Binder PS: Gentian violet keratoconjunctivitis. *AM J OPHTHALMOL* 87:340–343, 1979.

d. Thompson R, Isaacs ML, Khorazo D: A laboratory study of some antiseptics with reference to ocular application. *AM J OPHTHALMOL* 20:1087, 1937.

Germanium tetrachloride is a volatile liquid, and ***Germanium tetrafluoride*** is a gas, both said to be highly irritating to the eyes and respiratory tract.[171]

Ginger (Jamaica ginger) has been used in foods and beverages, without toxic action on the eyes. However, alcoholic essence or extract of ginger has been notoriously connected with poisonings, owing to adulteration. From 1901 to 1903 several cases were reported in which loss of vision occurred, characterized by central scotoma and optic atrophy, after ingestion of ginger essence adulterated with methanol.[a,153] In the early 1930's there were many cases of poisoning from adulteration with tricresylphosphate, resulting in the so-called Jake Paralysis, but in none of these was there involvement of the eyes.

a. Burnett SM: An additional case of amblyopia with central scotoma and general defective color perception following the ingestion of Jamaica Ginger. *OPHTHALMOL REC* 11:309–313, 1902.

Gitalin (Gitaligin), extracted from *Digitalis purpurea*,[171] has been tested on the human eye by application of a solution containing 0.1 mg/ml and found to cause corneal edema, with a slight reduction of ocular pressure.[220]

Glass in any part of the eye appears not to have toxic effects but to cause irritation and injury mechanically.[a,189] However, in one case intracorneal glass fragments have caused corneal haze and pannus, without edema.[c] In the anterior chamber, glass typically causes corneal edema from mechanical injury of the endothelium, and this may be reversible when the foreign body is removed.[c,d,81] In the vitreous humor of one patient, glass caused no reaction during five years of observation,[d] but in the vitreous humor of rabbits it has eventually caused degenerative changes in the retina.[150] Testing in tissue culture for cytotoxicity has been negative for both crown glass and photosensitive spectacle lenses.[d]

a. Archer DB, Davies MS, Kanski JJ: Non-metallic foreign bodies in the anterior chamber. *BR J OPHTHALMOL* 53:453–456, 1969.

b. Kronenfeld M, Worthen DM: Toxicity of photosensitive lenses. *ANN OPHTHALMOL* 12:274–276, 1980.

c. Mannis MJ, Krachmer JH, et al: Keratopathy associated with intracorneal glass. *ARCH OPHTHALMOL* 99:850–852, 1981.

d. Mitchell B, Wolkowicz MI: A case of migratory intraocular foreign body. *AM J OPHTHALMOL* 65:620–622, 1968.

Glibenclamide (glyburide), an anti-diabetic, led to optic atrophy in a 2-year old child who took about 45 mg and had severe hypoglycemia. It was thought that the optic atrophy was analogous to the child's posthypoglycemic encephalopathy, a result of circulatory disturbance, rather than a toxic effect on the nerve.

> a. Simon G: Optic atrophy after glibenclamide. *DTSCH GESUNDH WES* 30:898–901, 1975. (German)

Glucose (dextrose) is innocuous to the eye in physiologic concentrations and probably innocuous on the surface of the eye in concentrated (30 to 50%) solution,[a] but in two instances injection of a 5% solution into a superficial temporal artery caused severe damage to the eye on the same side. In one of the eyes, extensive atrophy of the temporal half of the choroid was observed ophthalmoscopically.[c]

Glucose at abnormally high concentration in culture medium for incubation of rabbit lenses, or in the blood of animals made diabetic, has been shown to induce gradual accumulation of sorbitol and water, causing the lens to swell and the cell membranes to become abnormally permeable. This effect can be blocked by inhibiting aldose reductase in the lens,[b] and by adding anti-oxidants to the culture medium.[d]

Also in relation to diabetes, it has been shown that elevated glucose concentration has toxic effect on human retinal vascular cells in culture.[e]

> a. Bietti GB, Pecori-Giraldi J: Topical osmotherapy of corneal edema. *ANN OPHTHAL-MOL* 1:40–49, 1969.
> b. Kinoshita JH, Kador P, Catiles M: Aldose reductase in diabetic cataracts. *J AM MED ASSOC* 246:257–261, 1981.
> c. Goldberg FP, Chutko SM: Eye changes in acute occlusion of the temporal artery after injection of glucose thereto. *VESTN OFTALMOL* 81:43–45, 1968.
> d. Trevithick JR, Creighton MO, et al: Modelling cortical cataractogenesis. *CAN J OPHTHALMOL* 16:32–38, 1981.
> e. Tripathi BJ, Tripathi RC: Human retinal vessels in tissue culture. *OPHTHALMOLOGY* 89:858–864, 1982.

Glucosulfone (Promin) in treatment of ocular leprosy has been well tolerated as a 40% eyedrop applied 2 to 4 times a day for months or years, except when a corneal erosion or ulcer is present it causes excessive pain.

> Bouzas A: Long-term observations on local application of promin in ocular leprosy. *ARCH OPHTALMOL (PARIS)* 31:629–636, 1971. (French)

Glutamate, or L-glutamic acid, is one of the natural amino acids widely present in food. It also has been added to foods, usually as monosodium glutamate (Accent), to enhance flavor. Glutamate has been administered medically in treatment of epilepsy and mental deficiency. Metabolically, glutamate can be derived from aspartate, as well as from proteins. Both glutamate and aspartate belong to a group of aminoacids that are neuroexcitatory, and are known as neuroexcitatory toxins, or excitotoxins.[n] In human beings no ocular toxic effects have been reported, but in animals there have been many reports of injury to the retina and to the embryonic lens. Brain damage in animals has been the most frequently noted toxic effect of glutamate, and there has been much debate about potential risk to human beings.[d,n,o]

The specificity of site of action of glutamate in the rodent retina is remarkable. In newborn mice, administration of sublethal amounts caused necrotic changes in the ganglion cells and inner nuclear layer, and the ERG was abolished except for the a-wave.[l] With lower dosage some intermediate cell layer persisted and the b-wave was present.[q] The retinotoxic effect in mice has been examined with light and electron microscopy.[f,o] Studies by Olney made particularly clear that the retinotoxic effect of glutamate in the mouse was related to the age at which the glutamate was administered.[o] The severity of damage to the ganglion cells and to cells of the inner nuclear layer increased with age up to the tenth postnatal day, but after the tenth to eleventh days it was difficult to produce significant lesions in the retina even with lethal doses. At the tenth postnatal day, the retina showed a rapid response and progression of changes. Within thirty minutes of a single subcutaneous injection, morphologic changes were evident, and massive edema of the inner portions of the retina developed within ninety minutes, increasing the thickness of the whole retina by 40 to 60 percent in several hours. Within the first day most of the cells of the inner layers became necrotic and degenerated, and within forty-eight hours the fragments mostly disappeared, thinning the retina to about 65 per cent of normal. No primary effect on photoreceptor cells was found either by light or electron microscopy, while most of the neurons of the ganglion cell layer were destroyed. Changes in nerve fibers at a distance from ganglion cells in the optic nerve and tracts occurred later.

Similarly in young rats, glutamate in sublethal doses destroyed nerve cells in the ganglion cell layer and the inner nuclear layer, causing disappearance of the b-wave, and causing reduction of myelinated axons in the optic nerves to 1% of normal.[g,h] The retina in rats becomes resistant to toxic action of glutamate at 10 days after birth, but this does not appear to be related to development of the blood-retina barrier.[c]

In rabbits, retinotoxicity has been reported even at adult age.[i,j,m] Prolonged treatment has caused degeneration of the ganglion cell layer and inner nuclear layer, but without great change in ERG or EOG.

In chick embryos glutamate has caused damage in the inner layers of the retina, including the ganglion cells.[e] Concentrations that killed about half of the embryos caused cataracts in 77% of those that survived, and total destruction of the lens at the highest concentration used.[k]

In young frog retinas in vitro, glutamate caused decrease in protein synthesis in the inner retina, but increase in synthesis in the photoreceptors.[a]

In monkeys and human beings there appear to be no reports of damage to the retina or disturbance of vision by glutamate. No neurological changes were detected in adult humans who were fed high doses for 14–42 days.[b] However, there seems to be as yet no systematic study with sophisticated methods to test retinal and visual functions when large amounts of glutamate are added to the human diet.[318]

a. Anderson RE, Hollyfield JE, Verner GE: Regional effects of sodium aspartate and sodium glutamate on protein synthesis in the retina. *INVEST OPHTHALMOL VIS SCI* 21:554–562, 1981.

b. Bazzano G, D'Elia JA, Olson RE: Monosodium glutamate: feeding of large amounts in man and gerbils. *SCIENCE* 169:1208–1209, 1970.

c. Bellhorn RW, Lipman DA, et al: Effect of monosodium glutamate on retinal vessel development and permeability in rats. *INVEST OPHTHALMOL VIS SCI* 21:237–247, 1981.

d. Bigwood EJ: L–Glutamic and L-aspartic acids—a question of hazard? *FOOD COSMET TOXICOL* 13:300–301, 1975.

e. Blanks JC, Reif-Lehrer L, Casper D: Effects of monosodium glutamate on the isolated retina of the chick embryo as a function of age. *EXP EYE RES* 32:105–124, 1981.

f. Cohen AI: An electron microscopic study of the modification by monosodium glutamate of the retinas of normal and "rodless" mice. *AM J ANAT* 120:319, 1967.

g. Freedman JK, Potts AM: Repression of glutaminase I in the rat retina by administration of sodium-L-glutamate. *INVEST OPHTHALMOL* 1:118–120, 1962; 2:252–258, 1963.

h. Hansson HA: Ultrastructural studies on the long term effects of sodium glutamate on the rat retina. *VIRCHOWS ARCH B ZELL PATH* 6:1–11, 1970.

i. Imaizumi K, Takahashi R, et al: Histological findings of retina in adult albino rabbits treated with sodium-L-glutamate. *ACTA SOC OPHTHALMOL JPN* 69:2150–2154, 1965.

j. Kobayaski H: Electron miccroscopic observation on the rabbit retina treated with long term daily administration of small dose of sodium iodate or sodium L-glutamate. *ACTA SOC OPHTHALMOL JPN* 74:902, 1970. (English summary)

k. Laszczyk WA: Development of cataract as the effect of glutamic acid administration to chick embryo. *OPHTHALMIC RES* 7:432–439, 1975.

l. Lucas DR, Newhouse JP: The toxic effect of sodium L-glutamate on the inner layers of the retina. *ARCH OPHTHALMOL* 58:193–201, 1957.

m. Ogawa K: Experimental studies on the EOG of the rabbit's eyes affected with administration of sodium L-glutamate. *ACTA SOC OPHTHALMOL JPN* 71:1466–1476, 1967.

n. Olney JW: Excitatory neurotoxins as food additives: an evaluation of risk. *NEUROTOXICOLOGY* 2:163–192, 1980.

o. Olney JW: Glutamate-induced retinal degeneration in neonatal mice. *J NEUROPATH EXP NEUROL* 28:455–474, 1969.

p. Oser BL, Morgareidge K, Carson S: Monosodium glutamate studies in four species of neonatal and infant animals. *FOOD COSMET TOXICOL* 13:7–14, 1975.

q. Potts AM, Modrell RW, Kingsbury C: Permanent fractionation of the electroretinogram by sodium glutamate. *AM J OPHTHALMOL* 50:900–906, 1960.

Glutaraldehyde a histologic fixative, tested as a 25% aqueous solution on rabbit eyes, caused severe injury, graded 9 on a scale of 10.[228] A 1% solution quickly abolishes the b-wave of the rabbit retina in vitro.[a]

a. Honda Y, Hope MG: Effects of glutaraldehyde upon some physiological properties of rabbit retinas in vitro. *JPN J OPHTHALMOL* 21:72–77, 1977.

Glutathione has been applied repeatedly as a 2% aqueous solution to the eyes of numerous patients with normal and diseased corneas, and no toxic effect has been noted.[317]

Glutethimide (Doriden, Noxyron), a sedative and hypnotic, when taken in excessive amount, has caused cerebellar ataxia with horizontal and vertical nystagmus, and widely dilated poorly reactive pupils.[b] Also in coma from over-dosage the pupils have been dilated and unreactive to light,[a,359] asymmetrically in one case.[c]

a. DeMyttenaere M, Schoenfeld L, Maher JF: Treatment of glutethimide poisoning. *J AM MED ASSOC* 203:885–887, 1968.

b. Huttenlocher PR: Accidental glutethimide intoxication in children. *N ENGL J MED* 269:38–39, 1963.

c. Brown DG, Hammill JF: Glutethimide poisoning. *N ENGL J MED* 285:806, 1971.

Glyceraldehyde tested as a 40% aqueous solution by dropping on rabbit eyes, and washing off with water two minutes later, caused no injury.[81] After parenteral administration of glyceraldehyde to rabbits, no retinal histologic or electroretinographic abnormality was found.[a,179] However, in vitro 5 mM or higher concentration is mildly injurious to surviving rabbit retina.[157]

a. Babel J, Ziv B: Researchs on experimental retinal degenerations. *OPHTHALMOLOGICA* 132:65–75, 1956. (French)

Glycerin or **Glycerol,** dropped on the human eye causes a strong stinging and burning sensation, with tearing and dilation of the conjunctival vessels, but no obvious injury. In fact, full strength glycerin has been employed to clear the haze of corneal epithelial edema by its hydroscopic action, to permit examination of the interior of the eye, and this has been without known damaging effect.[a] Application full strength to rabbit eyes likewise has produced no significant injury as judged by ordinary clinical means.[d,27] Glycerin diluted with water to 43% and applied for 30 minutes to rabbit eyes with mechanically damaged corneal endothelium has apparently produced only edema of conjunctiva and nictitating membrane lasting a few hours, even when repeated daily for 20 days.[e] However, when the specular corneal microscope has been used to evaluate the effect of glycerin solutions on rabbit corneas, it has been seen that some of the endothelial cells can be lost.[j] Enough rabbit corneal endothelial cells have survived to maintain normal deturgescence function after exposure of the *epithelium* to 30% glycerin for 20 minutes, 50% for 10 minutes, or 92% for 4 minutes, but 92% was observed to destroy the endothelium if exposure extended to 30 minutes.[j] Endothelial damage in these circumstances can be explained on the basis of an osmotic, rather than a toxic, mechanism. In human eyes, specular microscopy has shown that repeated application of 100% glycerin to the surface of the eye causes extensive changes in the appearance of the endothelium, but most of these changes disappear within 90 minutes after exposure is ended.[c] Some changes may be permanent.

When introduced into the anterior chamber of the rabbit eye, full strength glycerin causes an inflammatory reaction and edema of the cornea with wrinkling of the posterior surface and damage of endothelial cells.[h,i,m,o] The intensity of the reaction can be reduced by corticosteroid or phenylbutazone, but not by salicylate.[h,n,o] Without treatment the eyes have returned to normal in eight to ten days, as judged by slit-lamp examination and histology.[m,o] Aqueous 50% glycerin in the anterior chamber of rabbits causes significantly less reaction, though within five minutes it visibly dehydrates the lens, causing its capsule to become wrinkled. In a few patients with intumescent or hypermature cataracts this effect has been exploited to make the lens easier to grasp with forceps for extraction after 50% glycerin has been allowed to remain in the anterior chamber for 5 minutes at the time of operation.[g] It is claimed that reaction to this procedure is slight if a mydriatic, rather than a miotic, is used afterwards. When injected into the vitreous humor close to the retina in rabbits, glycerin damages the endothelial cells of the retinal vessels and renders them permeable to colloidal carbon.[b] With smaller amounts it has been observed that localized edema of the retina can be produced without increasing permeability of retinal vessels to trypan blue, and the edema clears spontaneously in about a week.[l]

Orally administered glycerin has come into widespread use as an osmotic agent for reducing ocular pressure in patients. To a minor extent glycerin has been administered intravenously for the same purpose. This type of treatment appears as a rule to be innocuous to the eye, although glycerin enters the intraocular fluids at a moderate rate from the bloodstream. However, Fraunfelder has discussed the possibility of retinal tear from shrinkage of the vitreous body.[312] Serious systemic side-effects occur occasionally when glycerin is given systemically in treating glaucoma, particularly in patients with renal failure, or previous gastrectomy.[f,k]

a. Cogan DG: Clearing of edematous corneas by glycerine. *AM J OPHTHALMOL* 26:551, 1943.

b. Cunha-Vaz JG: Studies on the permeability of the blood-retinal barrier. *BR J OPHTHALMOL* 50:454–462, 1966.

c. Goldberg MH, Koffler BH, et al: The effect of topically applied glycerin on the human corneal endothelium. *CORNEA* 1:39–44, 1982.

d. Hine CH, Anderson HH, et al: Comparative toxicity of synthetic and natural glycerine. *ARCH IND HYG* 7:282, 1953.

e. Meyer W, Reinhardt H: Experimental studies on influencing corneal edema with glycerin and glucose solutions. *GRAEFES ARCH OPHTHALMOL* 181:216–227, 1971. (German)

f. Oakley DE, Ellis PP: Glycerol and hyperosmolar nonketotic coma. *AM J OPHTHALMOL* 81:469–472, 1976.

g. Polzella A, Tieri O, Iura V: Dehydration of the crystalline lens. *ACTA OPHTHALMOL* 50:144–146, 1972.

h. Scassellati-Sforzolini G: Sodium salicylate in experimental ophthalmology. *RASS ITAL OTTAL* 26:429–435, 1957. (Italian)

i. Seegal D, Seegal BC: Local organ hypersensitiveness. *J EXP MED* 54:249, 1931.

j. Sherrard ES: The corneal endothelium in vivo. *EXP EYE RES* 22:347–357, 1976.

k. Sollom AW: Dangers of glycerol therapy for acute glaucoma after a partial gastrectomy. *BR J OPHTHALMOL* 56:506–507, 1972.

l. Tieri O, Iura V, et al: Rupture of the blood-retina barrier as a basis for disclosure of the retinotoxic property of a substance. *BOLL SOC ITAL BIOL SPER* 43:1117–1119, 1967. (Italian)

m. Vass Z, Katona J: The effect of glycerol on the eye lens of experimental animals. *ACTA OPHTHALMOL* 44:843–845, 1966.

n. Woods AC: ACTH and cortisone in ocular disease. *AM J OPHTHALMOL* 33:1325–1348, 1950.

o. Yourish N, Paton B, et al: Effect of phenylbutazone (Butazolidin) on experimentally induced ocular inflammation. *ARCH OPHTHALMOL* 53:264–266, 1955.

Glyceryl methacrylate polymer is a synthetic material that forms a hydrogel which has been found to cause very little inflammatory reaction within the cornea and within the vitreous humor of rabbits.[a,b] It has retained its transparency in the vitreous humor. It has caused no change in the ERG nor elevation of intraocular pressure.

a. Daniele S, Refojo MF, et al: Glyceryl methacrylate hydrogel as a vitreous implant. *ARCH OPHTHALMOL* 80:120–127, 1968.
b. Dohlman CH, Refojo MJ, Rose J: Synthetic polymers in corneal surgery. I. Glyceryl methacrylate. *ARCH OPHTHALMOL* 77:252–257, 1967.

Glycidaldehyde tested by dropping on the eyes of rabbits and washing off with water two minutes later caused immediate extensive loss of corneal epithelium followed within an hour by great chemosis. Severe corneal damage, intense iritis, and hypopyon resulted, and there was much necrosis of tissue and permanent corneal opacity.[81] The vapor is irritating to the eyes, nose, and throat of human beings at 1 to 5 ppm in air.[a]

a. Hine CH, Guzman JR, et al: Toxicity of glycidaldehyde. *ARCH ENVIRON HEALTH* 2:23–30, 1961.

Glycidol (1,2-epoxypropanol) applied as a drop to eyes of rabbits has caused severe but reversible corneal injury. For human beings the vapor has adequate warning properties, consisting of eye and respiratory irritation, to preclude excessive industrial exposure.[115]

Glycine is a natural amino acid, which when fed in large amount to chicks has caused peculiar enlargement of the eyeballs.[a] When injected intravitreally in rabbits it causes temporary loss of the oscillatory potentials of the b-wave of the ERG, and temporary changes in cell membranes of retinal amacrine cells.[b]

a. Groschke AD, Anderson JO, Briggs GM: Peculiar enlargement of eyeballs in chicks caused by feeding a high level of glycine. *PROC SOC EXP BIOL MED* 69:488–491, 1948.
b. Korol S, Leuenberger PM, et al: In vivo effects of glycine on retinal ultrastructure and averaged electroretinogram. *BRAIN RES* 97:235–251, 1975.

Glyoxal, a dialdehyde, tested by application of a drop to eyes of rabbits has caused moderate injury, graded 3 to 5 on a scale of 1 to 10 after twenty-four hours.[27,228] Glyoxal vapor has been reacted with excised corneas to make them non-swelling for use as bandage grafts, but postoperative inflammation has been excessive, due to free aldehyde groups. Treatment with basic amino acids after reaction with glyoxal corrects this problem.[a]

a. Payrau P, Moczar M, et al: Studies of non-swelling corneas. *ANN OCULIST (PARIS)* 204:583–594, 1971.

Gold may affect the eyes as a result of systemic administration of gold-containing medications, or from local contact with the metal or its salts. The effects of systemic medications will be described first. Following chronic parenteral administration of gold compounds it has been repeatedly observed that gold accumulates in the cornea in various forms observable with the slit-lamp biomicroscope. This condition, known as ocular chryseosis or chrysiasis, has most commonly resulted from treatment of arthritis, or formerly tuberculosis, with *gold thiosulfate* or *thiomalate*. There appears to be a considerable spectrum of changes in the cornea, probably related to total dose and length of treatment. Usually from 0.5 to 1.5 g of gold must be administered over several months before corneal changes are noted. The slightest abnormality appears to consist of deposits deep in the corneal epithelium, described by Bron (1979)[f] as "tiny, punctate, glittering golden-yellow crystal-like opacities," and reported in several series of cases.[k,l,s,w] These may disappear several months after treatment is discontinued. At a somewhat more advanced stage, fine deposits may be seen in the stroma in front of Descemet's membrane.[c-e,j,p,t] In the most advanced stage, usually after enough gold has been administered to give the skin a violet tint, changes are seen throughout the corneal stroma.[j,n,o] By slit-lamp examination there is a myriad of fine distinct dust-like granules varying in color from gold to violet, throughout the stroma, with greatest density in the deepest layers. Granules may be seen in Descemet's membrane and endothelium, but probably there is no special affinity for Descemet's membrane itself. More granules are present near the limbus than in the axial portions of the cornea. By transillumination with the slit-lamp the cornea appears purple or violaceous, like colloidal gold. In some reports describing characteristic changes in the corneal stroma there is mention that no deposits were seen in the epithelium. It may be that in these cases the treatment had been discontinued long enough to allow epithelial deposits to disappear, and that the stromal deposits were more persistent.

Besides deposits in the cornea, in a few cases deposits have been noted in the conjunctiva, and in rare instances particles have been seen in or on the lens, with the same appearance as those seen in the corneal stroma.[j,q] No interference with vision and no symptoms are associated with the deposits in cornea, conjunctiva, or lens.

Chemical, spectroscopic and other analytical methods have established that deposits in the cornea, conjunctiva and lens do contain gold, and that it is both extracellular and intracellular, within the cytoplasm of corneal stromal cells, sometimes within lysosomes.[j,n] Characteristically there is no histologic evidence of inflammation or foreign-body reaction.[q,n]

In rabbits and rats an apparently identical type of gold deposition in eye tissues has been induced by chronic systemic administration of gold salts.[d,e,i,m]

Although clinically gold deposition in the anterior segment of the eye is regarded as innocuous, there have been possible rare exceptions. A unique case of bilateral severe open-angle glaucoma has been described by Segawa (1981)[u] in a patient who had received during 8 years 11,700 mg of *gold thiomalate,* and had gold in lysosomes of endothelial cells of the trabecular meshwork in surgical trabeculectomy specimens. Otherwise the histopathology was described as resembling that of corticosteroid glaucoma, but the patient had received no corticosteroid. Whether other cases will be found in which gold and glaucoma are associated remains to be seen.

In very rare cases, marginal ulcerative keratitis has occurred, presumably as a manifestation of intolerance to gold. A white crescent-shaped ulcer 2 to 3 mm long, following the limbus, has been described associated witih conjunctival hyperemia and moderate pain, but with no evidence of infection. In two cases the ulcer healed within ten days without use of antibiotics.[h] Review of the literature by Azzolini in 1946 and personal observations by Mylius in 1950 suggested that limbal ulcerative keratitis and infiltration might not be a rare complication.[a,p] Walsh estimated that it occurred in less than 1 per cent of patients treated with gold.[255] Rodenhauser described one of these rare cases.[b,r,s] Ulcerative gold keratitis has not yet been reproduced in animals. Dimercaprol in one case appeared to give rapid relief of pain and to bring about prompt healing of ulcerative keratitis ascribed to gold.[g] D–Penicillamine appears subsequently to have replaced dimercaprol as the most effective systemic treatment for gold toxicity.

Metallic gold has been tested in rabbit eyes;[150] introduced as dust into the corneal stroma, it has persisted for many months but has caused invasion by leukocytes, vascularization, and accumulation of giant cells. In the conjunctiva it is rapidly taken up by leukocytes and removed. In the anterior chamber its effect depends on the size of the particles; the finest dust is rapidly taken up and removed by leukocytes, but particles too big to be ingested by these cells become encapsulated by endothelium and giant cells. A small particle of 22 carat gold was observed for 9.5 years in a patient's anterior chamber without irritation.[v] In the vitreous body of rabbits, gold particles have remained shiny and uncoated for months, but eventually have caused atrophic changes in the retina.[150]

Numerous attempts have been made to introduce gold into the cornea in soluble form and to cause it to precipitate there for the purpose of tatooing the cornea, but no satisfactory persistent darkening has been obtained.[199] Tests on albino rabbit eyes applying 2% to 5% solutions of *gold chloride* for ten to twenty-five minutes caused only slight irritation and no staining of normal eyes, but if the epithelium was removed from the cornea before exposure, a brown stain appeared and gradually deepened. However, this was accompanied by considerable iritis, and the brown stain was replaced by a nebula or leukoma with vascularization.[199] Clinical experiences have been similar.

Gold cyanide solution is irritating to intact eyes, and when applied to corneas from which the epithelium was removed, induced corneal clouding and severe iritis, but no darkening of the cornea.[153,199]

Injection of 2 mg *gold sodium thiosulfate* into the anterior chamber of a rabbit caused injury of the endothelium, corneal edema, and vascularization. The same injected into the corneal stroma caused transient local edema and vascularization, but the cornea did not ulcerate or become opaque.[81]

a. Azzolini V: Serious corneal and dermal manifestations in the course of gold therapy. *RIV OFTAL* 1:361–373, 1946. (Italian)
b. von Behrend T, Rodenhauser JH: Eye disturbances in parenteral gold treatment of chronic polyarthritis. *Z RHEUMAFORSCHUNG* 28:441–447, 1969. (German)
c. Bonnet P, Bonamour G: Bilateral keratitis from gold impregnation in the course of treatment with gold salts for pulmonary tuberculosis. *BULL SOC OPHTALMOL PARIS* 528–530, 1936. (French)
d. Bonnet P, Bonamour G: Ocular manifestations of ocular intolerance toward gold salts. *BULL SOC OPHTALMOL PARIS* 438–439, 1939. (French)
e. Bonnet P, Bonamour G, Khalifah ME: Chryseosis of the eye. *ARCH OPHTHALMOL (PARIS)* 3:385–394, 1939. (French)
f. Bron AJ, McLendon BF, Camp AV: Epithelial deposition of gold in the cornea in patients receiving systemic therapy. *AM J OPHTHALMOL* 88:354–360, 1979.

g. Contardo R: Auric keratitis-treatment with BAL. *OPHTH IBERO–AMER* 11:111–122, 1949.

h. d'Autrevaux JE: Two cases of marginal keratitis in the course of chryso-therapy. *BULL SOC OPHTALMOL PARIS* 767–770, 1931. (French)

i. Esente I, Petronios G: Experimental chryseosis of the eye. *G ITAL OFTAL* 3:133–145, 1950. (Italian)

j. Gottlieb NL, Major JC: Ocular chrysiasis correlated with gold concentrations in the crystalline lens during chrysotherapy. *ARTHRITIS RHEUM* 21:704–708, 1978.

k. Hashimoto A, Maeda Y, et al: Corneal chrysiasis. *ARTHRITIS RHEUM* 15:309–312, 1972.

l. Jahne M, Becker S: On chrysiasis corneae in parenteral gold therapy. *FOLIA OPHTHAL-MOL* 3:172–178, 1978. (German)

m. Kameyama K, Otsuka S, et al: Study of experimental corneal chrysiasis. *ACTA SOC OPHTHALMOL JPN* 84:233–239, 1980. (English summary)

n. Kincaid MC, Green WR, et al: Ocular chrysiasis. *ARCH OPHTHALMOL* 100:1791–1794, 1982.

o. Lisch K: On involvement of the eye in generalized chrysosis. *KLIN MONATSBL AUGENHEILKD* 102:103–106, 1939.

p. Mylius K: On a toxic keratitis. *DTSCH OPHTHALMOL GES* 56:265–269, 1950. (German)

q. Roberts WH, Wolter JR: Ocular chrysiasis. *ARCH OPHTHALMOL* 56:48–52, 1956.

r. Rodenhauser JH: On eye changes after parenteral gold treatment. *KLIN MONATSBL AUGENHEILKD* 155:61–65, 1969. (German)

s. Rodenhauser JH, von Behrend T: Type and incidence of eye involvement after parenteral gold therapy. *DTSCH MED WOCHENSCHR* 94:2389–2392, 1969. (German)

t. von Sallmann L: On eye changes in human chrysosis after Sanocrysin treatment. *ZENTRALB AUGENHEILKD* 79:208–212, 1933; also *GRAEFES ARCH OPHTHALMOL* 128:245–264, 1932.[374] (German)

u. Segawa K: Electron microscopy of the trabecular meshwork in open-angle glaucoma associated with gold therapy. *GLAUCOMA* 3:257–258, 1981.

v. Sen SC, Ghosh A: Gold as an intraocular foreign body. *BR J OPHTHALMOL* 67:398–399, 1983.

w. Thiel HJ, Langness U: Eye symptoms in parenteral gold therapy of chronic polyarthritis. *MED KLIN* 65:29–30, 1970. (German)

Golf ball contents are encapsulated in the rubber core of the ball under pressure from many tight wrappings of elastic cord. The composition of the contents has undergone significant modifications over the years. Since the 1960's, formerly caustic contents appear to have been replaced by a non-caustic paste containing barium sulfate, with or without zinc sulfide. Since the 1960's this new preparation has been involved in most recorded injuries from incised or disrupted liquid center golf balls.[a–k] When the paste is suddenly ejected under great pressure, it can penetrate through the conjunctiva, or into the skin of the eyelids and, less often, into the cornea. Injection into the conjunctiva and lids can be painless, but characteristically a white plaque of injected material is visible beneath the surface. This evokes a non-purulent inflammatory reaction with swelling of the tissues, followed in a few weeks by tissue fibrosis. In the foreign-body granuloma are found macrophages and foreign-body giant cells associated with aggregations of doubly-refracting crystals. Surgical evacuation of this material usually results in complete or nearly complete recovery. Even when the cornea has been struck, and when hypema with traumatic mydriasis have occurred, the end results have usually been good.[f,i] In one case fine deposits were visible in the cornea nine months after injury, but they appeared to be well tolerated, and visual acuity was normal.

Several histological studies have been reported,[a,c,e,g-j] and analyses have been performed on material in excised tissues, as well as on samples of material removed from golf balls, showing most commonly the mineral *barytes*, composed mainly of barium sulfate, and less commonly the mineral *lithopone*, which contains barium sulfate and zinc sulfide, and least often the mineral *muscovite*.[c,e,g]

Lucas (1976) has provided a tabular review of 12 of the reported cases of eye injury from 1965 to 1973, and an original clinical and histological study of 9 new cases.[e]

In earlier times when liquid core golf balls contained strongly caustic chemicals, many severe burns of the eyes occurred, with loss of some eyes. A considerable number of such cases were reported in the years 1912 to 1914.[46] The liquids or pastes utilized in golf-ball cores at that time were selected primarily for appropriate physical properties of density and viscosity, with little consideration for chemical or toxic properties. A great variety of substances were employed, and in most instances manufacturers were secretive about their composition. However, it appears that the most serious injuries have been attributable to sodium hydroxide. A historical bibliography of this subject was compiled by Duke-Elder in 1954.[46]

a. Berkman N, Dhermy P, Moubri M: Eye accidents from golf balls. *BULL SOC OPHTALMOL FRANCE* 80:139–143, 1980.

b. Editorial: Eye injuries from disrupted golf balls. *LANCET* 1:181, 1977.

c. Johnson FB, Zimmerman LE: Barium sulfate and zinc sulfide deposits resulting from golf-ball injury to the conjunctiva and eyelid. *AM J CLIN PATHOL* 44:533–538, 1965.

d. Lim KH: eye injury from an exploding golf ball. *SINGAPORE MED J* 16:78–80, 1975.

e. Lucas DR, Dunham AC, et al: Ocular injuries from liquid golf ball cores. *BR J OPHTHALMOL* 60:740–747, 1976.

f. Nelson C: Eye injury from exploding golf balls. *BR J OPHTHALMOL* 54:670–671, 1970.

g. O'Grady R, Shoch D: Golf ball granuloma of the eyelids and conjunctiva. *AM J OPHTHALMOL* 76:148–151, 1973.

h. Penner R: The liquid center golf ball. *ARCH OPHTHALMOL* 75:68–71, 1966.

i. Slusher MM, Jaegers KR, Annesley WH Jr: Liquid center golf balls and ocular injury. *AM J OPHTHALMOL* 64:736–740, 1967.

j. Taylor JN, Greer CH: Ocular injuries by explosion of the liquid centers of golf balls. *MED J AUST* 1:632–633, 1969.

k. Yamaki K, Hayakawa M, Sakuragi S: Eye injury from exploding golf balls. *FOLIA OPHTHALMOL JPN* 29:1538, 1978. (English summary)

Grease, when injected forcefully into tissues, causes compression and displacement, with low-grade granulomatous foreign-body type reaction. In the orbit it has caused displacement of the globe, congestion of retinal vessels and optic nervehead with loss of part of the visual field.[a] Surgical evacuation and treatment with corticosteroid has been employed, but treatment is difficult and not very satisfactory.

a. Dallas NL: Chronic granuloma of the orbit caused by grease-gun injury. *BR J OPHTHALMOL* 48:158–159, 1964.

Grisein, (albomycin), an antimicrobial, is reported from Russia to cause inflammation and necrosis of the cornea when applied at 30% concentration to animal eyes.[a]

    a. Melnikova EA, Rodionov GA: Experimental pathology of the rabbit and guinea pig eye caused by the antibiotic grisein. *VRACH DELO* (6)85–88, 1979.

Griseofulvin (Fulvicin), an antifungal antibiotic taken by mouth, has been tested for toxicity by administration to piebald rats with special attention to the retina.[a] The rats were fed a diet containing 0.1% griseofulvin. The eyes were then examined histologically and found to be normal. Similar feeding of a special strain of weanling albino rats which were subject to spontaneous retinal atrophy caused no increase in incidence or severity of retinal abnormality compared to controls that did not receive griseofulvin. However, one patient while receiving 1 g griseofulvin per day is reported to have noted slight blur and greenish tint with one of his eyes after ten days, the other eye remaining normal.[a] The symptomatic eye had 20/25 vision but discernible edema of the macula area. The findings remained unchanged during ten days after griseofulvin was stopped. Systemic corticosteroid was then started, and in a week the eye was normal except for slight residual pigment disturbance in the macula area. In the absence of other cases, it would be difficult to implicate griseofulvin.

Walsh and Hoyt have reported seeing a patient who had papilledema associated with the pseudo-tumor cerebri syndrome seemingly due to treatment with griseofulvin, and which cleared when the treatment was discontinued.[256]

    a. Delman M, Leubuscher K: Transient macular edema due to griseofulvin. *AM J OPHTHALMOL* 56:658, 1963.

    b. Sharpe HM, Tomich EG: Studies in the toxicology of griseofulvin. *TOXICOL APPL PHARMACOL* 2:44–53, 1960.

Guanethidine (Ismelin), an antihypertensive, also is used in eyedrops for glaucoma and for reducing lid retraction in thyroid disease. Toxic effects on the eye have been slight. Application of 5% to 10% guanethidine sulfate solution to the eyes of patients has induced slight miosis, noticeable ptosis and hyperemia from antiadrenergic action. About 50 per cent of patients with thyroid dysfunction and exophthalmos have developed burning and redness of the eyes. Some have had superficial changes in the corneal epithelium, less from 5% than 10% eyedrops. Sensitization and contact dermatitis in the course of several weeks has been observed several times.[a,c,d]

In one group of thirty patients given an average oral dose of 70 mg per day for systemic hypertension, an incidence of "blurring of vision" in 17 per cent has been reported as a symptom, with no investigation of the basis for it.[b]

    a. Bonomi L: On the effectiveness of prolonged treatment with guanethidine on intraocular pressure. *BOLL OCULIST* 45:338–344, 1966. (Italian)

    b. Brest AN, Novack P, et al: Guanethidine. *DIS CHEST* 42:359–363, 1962.

    c. Crombie AL, Lawson AAH: Long-term trial of local guanethidine in treatment of eye signs of thyroid dysfunction and idiopathic lid retraction. *BR MED J* 4:592–595, 1967.

    d. Cant JS, Lewis DRH: Unwanted pharmacological effects of local guanethidine in the treatment of dysthyroid upper lid retraction. *BR J OPHTHALMOL* 53:239–245, 1969.

Guanidine has been noted to cause mydriasis in animals after local or systemic administration. (*Methyl guanidine* has the same effect.)[153] Guanidine hydrochloride is known to deaggregate complex proteins, and in vitro it has been shown to aid in dissolution of lacerated cataractous human lenses. However, when 1 molar solution was tested in rabbit eyes by injection into the anterior chamber it caused corneal opacities, reversible in some eyes, but permanent in others.[a]

  a. Klein J, Cotlier E: Chemical and mechanical dissolution of human senile cataracts in vitro. *ACTA OPHTHALMOL* 50:215–228, 1972.

Gun powder, either black or smokeless, ignited or exploded close to the eyes has occasionally caused corneal injury. The injuries are primarily physical from heat and force of contact of particles with the eye. The products do not appear to be toxic. The corneal epithelium may be coagulated and stippled with black particles, but normal epithelium soon replaces it after the foreign material and dead cells are removed. Black particulate products of combustion have been driven into the cornea, and even into the vitreous body, but have been inert and well tolerated.

  a. Belkin M, Ivry M: Explosive intraocular foreign bodies. *AM J OPHTHALMOL* 85:676–678, 1978.
  b. Runyan TE, Ewald RA: Blank cartridge injury of the cornea. *ARCH OPHTHALMOL* 84:690–691, 1970.
  c. Sheppard LB: Gun powder injury to the eyes. *VIRGINIA MED MONTHLY* 65:152–154, 1938.

Hair dyes have been held responsible for irritation or injury to corneas, conjunctivae, and lids. Hair dyes are of several different chemical types.[70] The *metallic type hair dyes* contain salts of various metals commonly in combination with pyrogallol. The *vegetable type hair dyes* consists of henna and indigo. The *oxidizing type hair dyes* most often contains paraphenylenediamine, sometimes with diaminophenol. In general, hair dyes other than those containing indigo and henna do not contain dyes in a strict sense, but rather contain compounds which oxidize and polymerize in the presence of air or hydrogen peroxide, sometimes catalyzed by metal salts, to form dark-colored substances which stain the hairs.

In almost all instances, ocular injuries have been attributable to the paraphenylenediamine type of hair dye, and in a great majority of instances the injury resulted from application of the coloring material to the eyelashes. For this reason the compound is no longer permitted to be used in the United States in cosmetics to be used in the region of the eyes. (See *Paraphenylenediamine* for details of its ocular toxicity, also *Eye cosmetics.*)

A unique report from India by Jain in 1979 describes a clinical and experimental study undertaken because of a clinical impression that users of hair dyes had cataractous changes more often than non-users.[a] Systematic examination of 200 eye-clinic patients who used hair dyes for more than a year disclosed lenticular changes in 89%, discernible by slit-lamp examination, but not affecting the visual acuity in most cases. Similar changes were described in 23% of non-users. (It was not stated whether the examiners knew which patients were users and which were not.) In the report the only substance mentioned was paraphenylenediamine, as though this was the only substance involved. Similarly, experiments in rats and rabbits were done only with this substance, and production of eye injuries in the animals was interpreted as supporting the clinical conclusion. (See *Paraphenylenediamine* for description of the experiments.)

    a. Jain IS, Jain GC, et al: Cataractogenous effect of hair dyes. *ANN OPHTHALMOL* 11:1681–1686, 1979.

Hair sprays and lacquers typically are composed of polyvinyl pyrrolidone, polyvinyl acetate, shellac, or other resins, dissolved in alcohol, pressurized for spraying. An occasional accidental misdirection of the spray into the open eye has caused a transient stinging sensation and a temporary fine keratitis epithelialis composed of microscopic gray dots in the corneal epithelium.[81] It has been suggested that dried particles from the spray might be driven into the corneal epithelium, becoming embedded and giving rise to irritation.[a-c] Apparently this suggestion has been based on interpretation of slit-lamp appearance and is yet to be proven by experiment. In any case, recovery has generally been spontaneous and rapid, usually in one to three days.[a-d,81] A report from Egypt on severe effects of hair spray on corneas of rabbits provides no information on the manner of application or the composition of the spray.[e] (Among household sprays that have caused injury of the corneal epithelium are *Oven cleaners, Deodorants, and Perfumes.*)

    a. Carella G, Trimarchi F, Asperti G: Keratopathy from sprays. *ANN OTTALMOL CLIN OCUL* 94:571–583, 1968. (Italian)
    b. MacLean A: Spray keratitis. *TRANS AM ACAD OPHTHALMOL OTOL* 71:330–339, 1967.
    c. MacLean AL: Aerosol keratitis: a common epithelial foreign-body reaction to household chemical sprays. *AM J OPHTHALMOL* 63:1709–1719, 1967.
    d. Bonnet I: Bilateral corneal lesions from spraying beauty and hygiene products from aerosol cans. *BULL SOC OPHTALMOL FRANCE* 73:767–768, 1973. (French)
    e. El-Gammal MY, Soliman AM, Mostafa MSE: The effect of sprayed material on the cornea and the eye. *BULL OPHTHALMOL SOC EGYPT* 66:121–125, 1973.

Hair straighteners sometimes contain sodium hydroxide, and are sufficiently alkaline to burn the human cornea, as well as rabbit corneas.[a] The less alkaline preparations, which have a composition similar to *Hair-waving preparations,* cause little or no injury.

    a. Smith RS, Shear G: Corneal alkali burns arising from accidental instillation of a hair straightener. *AM J OPHTHALMOL* 79:602–605, 1975.

Hair-waving preparations (cold wave permanent wave preparations) are usually composed of a perfumed, slightly alkaline solution (e.g., pH 9.5) of ammonium thioglycolate plus wetting agents and other adjuvants. This solution is applied to reduce and break the disulfide bonds of the keratin, to permit physical rearrangement to a new form. A second solution containing an oxidizing agent such as sodium or potassium bromate or sodium perborate is applied subsequently to induce reformation of disulfide cross-links in the new arrangement in which the hair has been placed.

The chemistry of preparations used for hair waving have been reviewed by Rieger, and the toxicity of these preparations when taken orally or in contact with the skin has been reviewed by Norris, but without considering effects on the eye.[a,b]

The toxic effects of *thioglycolates,* which are described in more detail elsewhere under that heading, consist of rare and poorly founded suspicions of optic neuritis from use on the hair, and one instance of reversible keratitis which was attributed to a splash in the eye, although application of a typical hair-waving preparation to a rabbit's eye had no similar effect. No toxic effects on the eyes have been reported from external application of neutralizers, *sodium or potassium bromate.* Also, hydrogen peroxide has not been significantly injurious to human or monkey eyes at the concentrations employed. The rabbit eye is peculiarly more vulnerable. (See *Hydrogen peroxide.*)

a. Norris JA: Toxicity of home permanent waving and neutralizer solutions. *FOOD COSMET TOXICOL* 3:93–97, 1965.
b. Rieger MM: Recent developments in permanent waving. *AM PERFUMER AROMAT* 75:33–37, 1960.

Haloperidol (Haldol), an antipsychotic, has so far shown no significant toxic effect on the eye.[a] It appears safe to use in the presence of glaucoma, since no elevation, but instead a slight reduction, in ocular pressure has been observed in patients after parenteral administration.[b,c] Mydriasis and cycloplegia have been reported, but, at least in some instances, this has been attributable to simultaneous administration of anticholinergic antiparkinsonian drugs.[a] Haloperidol tends to produce extrapyramidal side effects; neuromuscular disturbances involving the neck and face may include oculogyric crises.

a. Laties AM: Ocular toxicology of haloperidol. In *Symposium on Ocular Therapy,* ed. by Leopold IH, Burns RP: New York, John Wiley and Sons, 9:87–95, 1976.
b. Graziano FM: The pressure lowering effect of Serenase in ocular surgery. *ANN OTTALMOL CLIN OCUL* 91:979–983, 1965. (Italian)
c. Pontinen PJ, Miettinen P: Neuroleptanalgesia in cataract surgery. *ACTA OPHTHALMOL SUPPL* 80, 1964.

Halothane (Fluothane), an inhalation anesthetic, has numerous time been reported to lower the intraocular pressure, probably associated with acute systemic hypotension and disturbance of blood supply to the eye, as seen in fainting.[31] Dark adaptation in monkeys and human beings, determined by electroretinography, is retarded by halothane anesthesia, but this is reversible, and without known clinical significance.[a,b] The visual evoked response similarly shows increase in latency under halothane anesthesia.[c] A sensation of irritation of the eyes upon exposure to operating room atmosphere containing halothane was developed by one anesthetist after repeated contact, an apparently unique case.[e]

Epinephrine eye drops administered during halothane anesthesia are known to have precipitated ventricular fibrillation.[d]

a. Norren DV, Padmos P: Cone dark adaptation: the influence of halothane anesthesia. *INVEST OPHTHALMOL* 14:212–227, 1975.

b. Norren DV, Padmos P: The effect of halothane anesthesia on retinal processes. *OPHTHALMOLOGICA* 173:286–289, 1976.

c. Uhl RR, Squires KC, et al: Effect of halothane anesthesia on the human cortical visual evoked response. *ANESTHESIOLOGY* 53:273–276, 1980.

d. Janssens ML, Cockx F: A case of ventricular fibrillation during halothane anesthesia caused by eye drops. *ACTA ANESTHESIOL BELG* 20:273–275, 1979.

e. Boyd CH: Ophthalmic hyper-sensitivity to anesthetic vapour. *ANESTHESIA* 27:456–457, 1972.

Halquinols, a mixture from chlorination of 8-quinolinol, used as an anti-infective, has been reported to have caused blindness from optic atrophy in two patients. In one case this was associated with tingling and numbness in the legs, with difficulty in walking. It is also said to have produced blindness in calves. (A similarity to *iodochlorhydroxyquin,* or *clioquinol,* has been noted.)

a. Hansson O, Herxheimer A: Neuropathy and optic atrophy associated with halquinol. *LANCET* 1:450, 1981.

Harmaline is an amine oxidase inhibitor and CNS stimulant which produces visual hallucinations that are said to be different from those of a number of other hallucinogens in that harmaline does not distort the appearance of the environment but causes imaginary scenes to appear superimposed on the undistorted view of real objects. Images, often vividly colored, are also said to be seen with the eyes closed.[a] Harmaline also causes changes in the electroretinogram of rats.[b]

a. Naranjo C: Psychotropic properties of the Harmala alkaloids. In Efron, DH (Ed.): *ETHNOPHARMACOLOGIC SEARCH FOR PSYCHOACTIVE DRUGS.* U.S. Pub. Health Service Publ. No. 1645, pp. 385–391, 1967.

b. Rojas A, Herrera J: Effects of harmaline on the visual system of the rat. *VISION RES SUPPL* 3:437–445, 1972.

Helichrysum is a plant genus with at least one toxic species, *Helichrysum argyrosphaerum DC,* which has caused blindness in grazing sheep, and occasionally cattle, in South Africa.[a] It has also caused general paresis and paralysis of the legs. Two types of blindness have been described. One is an amaurosis with dilated pupils, papilledema, retinal edema and congestion of retinal vessels, retinal photoreceptor degeneration, swelling of the optic nerves and chiasm, with hemorrhages in the optic nerves in some animals. Bilateral *status spongiosus* has been evident histologically in the optic nerves, chiasm, lateral geniculate bodies, optic tracts, and various other portions of the brain and spinal chord. The other type of blindness is associated with formation of cataracts, not necessarily associated with dilated pupils or amaurosis. When the plant was gathered from grazing areas and was fed to normal animals, paresis and paralysis were reproduced, with the same, but milder, histologic abnormalities in the visual neural system and brain as in the grazing animals. However, signs of blindness and retinopathy were not reproduced, and it was thought that the feeding experiments probably were not of sufficiently long duration.

Another species of the plant, *Helichrysum bracteatum,* has caused a reaction resembling *ophthalmia nodosa* in the conjunctiva of a child, probably a physical rather than toxic effect.[b]

a. Basson PA, Kellerman TS, et al: Blindness and encephalopathy caused by *Helichrysum argyrosphaerum DC.* (*Compositae*) in sheep and cattle. *ONDERSTEPOORT J VET RES* 42:135–147, 1975.
b. Karbe M: A case of ophthalmia nodosa of the conjunctiva of a child, caused by playing with everlasting flowers. *ARCH AUGENHEILKD* 93:160–164, 1923. (German)

Helvella esculenta is a poisonous fungus mentioned to have caused pupillary dilation in human poisoning, but no disturbances of vision or accommodation.[a, 153] In one patient the pupils appeared dilated but reacted well to light.[a] This patient also had spasmodic movements of his eyes associated with generalized clonic convulsioins, but recovered completely.

a. Jung J, Stuhlfauth J: Poisoning with Lorcheln. *KLIN WOCHENSCHR* 19/20:312–315, 1947. (German)

Hematoporphyrin is a substance prepared from hemin, and formerly employed under the name Sensibon in depressive psychosis. Photophobia has been noted in white mice injected with lethal amounts of this compound.[a] A comprehensive review with bibliography concerning ocular disturbances in porphyria has been published in connection with a series of observations on rats and rabbits given subcutaneous injections of hematoporphyrin.[b] In these animals exposure to bright lights caused hyperemia and edema of the lids and conjunctiva, sometimes with moderate edema of the corneal stroma, and a low incidence of small round opacities in the anterior cortex of the crystalline lens.[b] Also after exposure to strong light the blood aqueous barrier in the rabbits became abnormally permeable to fluorescein.[b] In pigmented rabbits given hematoporphyrin intraperitoneally, exposure to bright light caused a high incidence of damage to the retina.[c]

Hematoporphyrin derivative, prepared from hematoporphyrin dihydrochloride, used in treatment of malignant tumors, has been tested for injurious effects on normal mouse retina. Injury was produced only when combined with light irradiation. The outer layers of the retina were most sensitive.[d]

a. Francesco De L: Photosensitization by blood porphyrins in general blood diagnosis. *FOLIA MED NAPLES* 35:1026–1033, 1952. (*CHEM ABSTR* 47:7179).
b. Del Buono G, Artifoni E: Behavior of the ocular apparatus in the course of photosensitization. *G ITAL OFTAL* 15:283–309, 337–347, 437–445, 488–491, 1962. (Italian)
c. Freeman RG, Troll D: Hematoporphyrin photosensitization of rabbit eye to visible light. *ARCH OPHTHALMOL* 78:766–768, 1967.
d. Winther J, Ehlers N: The combined effect of haematoporphyrin derivative and light. *ACTA OPHTHALMOL* 62:112–122, 1984.

Hemoglobin has been studied for toxicity to the vitreous humor and retina in relation to the injurious effects of blood. Regnault has provided a review of the toxic effects of blood, iron, and hemoglobin on the vitreous body and retina, and has reported animal experiments in which labeled hemoglobin was injected into the vitreous and its rate of disappearance was determined.[a] The hemoglobin appeared to begin to break down in about seven days, but about 25% of the iron content still remained in the eye after 2 months. Most of the organic portions of the hemoglobin appeared to be gone by that time. Regnault showed that when a hemoglobin solution was injected into the vitreous it produced histologically demonstrable damage to the rods in three days, and the injurious effect progressed until all visual cells disappeared in fifteen days. It was not ascertained whether this toxic effect was from the hemoglobin itself or from its degradation products. Injections of hemoglobin into the vitreous in rabbits has been reported by Burke to stimulate proliferation of cells throughout the retina in the first 3 or 4 days, and also to stimulate a transient multiplication of vitreous cells and migration of phagocytic cells into the vitreous humor.[b,c]

a. Regnault FR: Vitreous hemorrhage: an experimental study. *ARCH OPHTHALMOL* 83:458–474, 1970.
b. Burke JM, Sipos E, Cross HE: Cell proliferation in response to vitreous hemoglobin. *INVEST OPHTHALMOL VIS SCI* 20:575–581, 1981.
c. Burke JM, Smith JM: Retinal proliferation in response to vitreous hemoglobin or iron. *INVEST OPHTHALMOL VIS SCI* 20:582–592, 1981.

Hemosiderin, a breakdown product of hemoglobin, demonstrable histologically in eyes that have had intraocular hemorrhages, has been suspected of having toxic effects. A review with discussion and presentation of histologic specimens by Babel has given the interpretation that excessive residue of hemosiderin from repeated hemorrhages can be deleterious to the retina, the ciliary epithelium, and the aqueous outflow channels.[a] It is implied that hemosiderin has something to do with producing glaucoma, and possibly with causing neovascular glaucoma. However, the evidence to support this thesis does not yet seem convincing.

In this connection, in a case of neovascular glaucoma reported by Winter, one eye was examined histologically and was seen to have a fibrovascular membrane in addition to iron staining in the trabecular meshwork and in other ocular tissues, all secondary to occlusion of central retinal vessels, but these findings, though suggestive, do not seem to provide definitive evidence concerning the role of hemosiderin in the process.[c]

Sugar and colleagues have described seven cases which they considered to be examples of hemosiderosis in which anterior subcapsular rust-like deposits or siderotic discoloration of the iris developed in eyes in which there had been hemorrhage in the posterior portion of the globe from various causes, including diabetes, occlusion of the central retinal vessels, sickle cell disease, and trauma.[b] Glaucoma was present in two of the seven cases. In one, painful glaucoma was evident two and one-half years after occlusion of the central retinal vein. In the other case, glaucoma developed also after occlusion of the central retinal vein in an eye that previously had been under treatment for chronic open-angle glaucoma. Whether these were cases of neovascular glaucoma such as commonly develop after occlusion of central retinal vessels without clinical evidence of hemosiderosis was not made clear. Sugar postulated, as have the other authors mentioned, that iron had toxic effects on the corneoscleral meshwork. Clear evidence to establish this as a special toxic effect of either iron or hemosiderin remains to be obtained.

Glaucoma has been reported in association with intraocular iron foreign bodies. The mechanism in that association is also not yet clearly established. (For further related details, see INDEX for *Iron*.)

a. Babel J: The toxic action of hemosiderin on ocular tissues. *ARCH OPHTALMOL (PARIS)* 24:405–416, 1964. (French)

b. Sugar HS, Kobernick SD, Weingarten JE: Hematogenous ocular siderosis of local cause. *AM J OPHTHALMOL* 64:749–756, 1967.

c. Winter FC: Ocular hemosiderosis. *TRANS AM ACAD OPHTHALMOL OTOL* 71:813–819, 1967.

Henna is a natural dye used for tinting the hair a dark reddish color. There appears to be no case of ocular injury unequivocally caused by henna. However, two groups of cases have been described in which eye injury was attributed to henna. The patients, mostly blondes, used a hair coloring material to darken their eyebrows and eyelashes, and twelve to twenty-four hours later began to have swelling of the lids, tearing, discharge, and much pain.[a,b] In a small proportion of these cases corneal erosions and opacity developed.

In one of these groups of cases the hair coloring material contained *paraphenylenediamine* in addition to henna,[a] and in the other group the coloring material was not accurately identified, merely said to contain henna. There is a strong probability that henna itself was not responsible for the injuries. (Compare *Hair dyes* and *paraphenylenediamine*.)

a. Abramowicz I: Clinical and experimental investigations of eye injuries from the hair dye henna. *KLIN OCZNA* 8:153–158, 1930. (*ZENTRALB GES OPHTHALMOL* 25:674, 1931.) (German abstract)

b. Bab WL: Injury of the eyes by eyelash coloring. *DTSCH MED WOCHENSCHR* 59:1041, 1933. (German)

Heparin, an anticoagulant, when tested on rabbits as a 5% heparin sodium solution applied repeatedly to the surface of the eye, was not injurious,[a] but 30% heparin sodium solution injured the corneal epithelium slightly, demonstrable only by staining with fluorescein.[b] Heparin was then detectable in the anterior chamber, but there were no overt signs of irritation. The same concentration injected subconjunctivally caused chemosis, but no serious injury.[b] Injection of 30% solution into the anterior chamber of rabbits caused edema and reversible opacification of the cornea, conjunctival chemosis, hyperemia of the iris, and inflammatory cells in the aqueous humor.[b] Milder reactions were induced by 2% to 15% solutions. Intraocular pressure was raised transiently. There is one report of hyphema after intravenous heparin.[c]

a. Fumarola D, Balacco-Gabrieli C: On passage of 5% heparin collyrium into the anterior chamber. *ANN OTTALMOL CLIN OCUL* 93:808–816, 1967. (Italian)

b. Vannas S: Experimental and clinical investigations into the effect of locally administered heparin on the eye. *ACTA OPHTHALMOL* (SUPPL 40), 1953.

c. Slusher MM, Hamilton RW: Spontaneous hyphema during hemodialysis. *N ENGL J MED* 293:561, 1975.

Heptachlor, an insecticide, is reported to cause cataracts in offspring of rats after long-term feeding.[a]

a. Mestitzova M: On reproduction studies and the occurrence of cataracts in rats after long-term feeding of the insecticide heptachlor. *EXPERIENTIA* 23:42–43, 1967.

2-Heptadecyl-2-imidazoline (2-heptadecyl glyoxalidine, glyoxalidine, glyodin) is a fungicide applied to fruit as a wettable powder or spray. It is insoluble in water and not readily absorbed unless dissolved in a solvent such as propylene glycol. Tested in such a solvent, this compound and its acetate were found to be severely injurious to rabbit eyes, graded 9 on a scale of 1 to 10 after twenty-four hours.[27, 36] There seems to be no firsthand report of injury to human eyes.

n-Heptanol (1-heptanol, n-heptyl alcohol) has been found effective in removing epithelium from rabbit corneas, with advantages over other alcohols having chains of 5 to 10 carbons, and advantages over mechanical scraping.[a] Application of a disc of filter paper soaked with heptanol to the cornea for 1 minute removes the epithelium without damaging extracellular components of the cornea, but it does penetrate enough to destroy keratocytes near the anterior surface. Healing occurs essentially the same as after mechanical scraping of the epithelium. This is also true in monkeys' eyes, with good adhesion of epithelium to basement membrane promptly re-established.[329]

a. Cintron C, Hassinger L, et al: A simple method for the removal of rabbit corneal epithelium utilizing n-heptanol. *OPHTHALMIC RES* 11:90–96, 1979.

Herbatox, a herbicide composed of 2,4-dichlorophenoxypropionic and 2,4-dichlorophenoxyacetic acids, has caused systemic poisonings, in some cases involving long-lasting polyneuritis, and in one case impairment of memory and alterations of color vision.[a]

a. Herbatox poisoning; a brief review and report of a new case. *UGESKRIFT LAEGER* 133:500–503, 1971. (Danish; English abstract)

Heroin (diacetyl morphine) appears to have no established toxic effect on the eyes,[255] but in one instance it was blamed for causing a temporary central scotoma.[b] In addiction to heroin, within two to three hours after injection, there may be contraction of the pupils, photophobia, but little blinking.[a] The pupils remain reactive to light. During withdrawal from heroin addiction the pupils enlarge, and may become temporarily unequal.[c, d] Addicts taking intravenous injections are prone to effects of contaminants, bacteria causing endophthalmitis, and particulate material causing retinal emboli.[e] A series of 34 cases of blindness from Candida albicans contamination has been reported from France.[f]

a. Rathod NH, de Alarcon R, Thompson IG: Signs of heroin usage detected by drug users and their parents. *LANCET* 2:1411–1414, 1967.
b. Stieren E: Blindness from heroin in the nostrum "Habitana". *J AM MED ASSOC* 54:869, 1910.
c. Cosgriff TM: Anisocoria in heroin withdrawal. *ARCH NEUROL* 29:200–201, 1973.

   d. Robinson MG, Howe RC, et al: Assessment of pupil size during acute heroin with-
      drawal in Viet Nam. *NEUROLOGY* 24:729–732, 1974.

   e. Siepser SB, Magargal LE, Augsburger JJ: Acute bilateral microembolization in a
      heroin addict. *ANN OPHTHALMOL* 13:699–702, 1981.

   f. Dally S, Thomas G, Mellinger M: Loss of hair, blindness and skin rash in heroin
      addicts. *VET HUM TOXICOL* 24(Suppl):62, 1982.

Hexachlorobenzene, a fungicide, not to be confused with *benzenehexachloride* or *Lindane,* and not intended for human use, has been reported in one incident of accidental contamination of food in Turkey, to have caused numerous cases of porphyria cutanea tarda which frequently involved the face around the eyes, and in one instance was associated with corneal opacities.[a]

   a. Cam C, Nigogosyan G: Acquired toxic porphyria cutanea tarda due to hexachlorobenzene.
      J AM MED ASSOC 183:88–91, 1963.

Hexachlorocyclopentadiene is an intermediate in the manufacture of the insecticide *Chlordane.* This intermediate has been noted to cause irritation of the eyes of workers in the laboratory and in a sewage treatment plant.[a,b] In mice exposed experimentally to the vapors it has caused "apparent blindness". Pure *Chlordane* had no such toxicity.[a]

   a. Ingle L: The toxicity of chlordane vapors. *SCIENCE* 118:213, 1953.

   b. Norse DL, Kominsky JR, et al: Occupational exposure to hexachlorocyclopentadiene. *J*
      AM MED ASSOC 241:2177–2179, 1979.

Hexachloroethane has been employed in military smoke candles. Exposure of workmen to fumes from hot hexachlorethane has caused blepharospasm, photophobia, lacrimation, and reddening of the conjunctivae, but no corneal injury and no permanent damage.[a,165] Crystalline hexachloroethane applied to the corneas of rabbits (following topical anesthesia) and allowed to remain for several minutes, caused no injury.[81]

   a. Scherling SS, Blondis RR: The effect of chemical warfare agents on the human eye.
      MIL SURGEON 96:70–78, 1945.

Hexachloronaphthalene has caused hyperkeratosis in cattle, sheep, and swine, with excessive lacrimation, but the nature of eye involvement seems not to have been described in detail.[a]

   a. Huber WG, Link RP: Toxic effects of hexachloronaphthalene on swine. *TOXICOL*
      APPL PHARMACOL 4:257–262, 1962.

Hexachlorophene (hexachlorophane), a topical anti-infective, and a variable component of detergents such as "pHisohex", and of soaps and medicated talcum powders, was formerly widely used without prescription and without awareness of its potential toxicity. Now that a number of accidental poisonings of human beings have occurred, and toxicity has also been demonstrated in animals, hexachlorophene is available only by prescription in the United States. Hexachlorophene has been used as a veterinary anthelmintic, but by 1970 was known to have adverse effects on sheep and calves, producing cerebral edema, papilledema, mydriasis and unresponsiveness of the pupils to light, associated with flattening and atrophy of the intracranial portions of the optic nerves.[o] A good review of the toxicity of hexachlorophene was provided by Towfighi in 1980, particularly concerning effects on the visual system from retina to cerebral cortex.[n]

Human beings have been poisoned as follows. In 1972 in France a talcum powder which accidentally contained higher than ordinary concentration of hexachlorophene was applied repeatedly to small children, mostly in the presence of severe diaper rash, causing severe illness in 204, and death in 36.[c] The victims had intracranial hypertension, papilledema and retinal hemorrhages. Histologically they showed widespread "status spongiosus", vacuolation of the white matter of the central nervous system. A more detailed study was reported of 18 children age 3 months to 3 years who were poisoned in this way, with 4 deaths and 2 paraplegic, with intracranial hypertension, also swelling of the spinal cord from intramyelinic edema.[a] Ocular abnormalities among these 18 children consisted of papilledema in 6, "ocular jerks" in 4, mydriasis in 1, and sixth nerve palsy in one. In nearly all cases the victims of this epidemic were inadvertently poisoned at home, and many improved while hospitalized and separated from the poisonous batch of talcum powder, only to relapse upon returning home and being exposed to the same material again. As example, the sixth nerve palsy mentioned in one case above, disappeared during hospitalization, but, after the child returned home, papilledema and "blindness" developed.[a]

In 1974 a 7-year-old boy was mistakenly given 45 ml of a 3% hexachlorophene emulsion orally in 3 days, causing him to become severely ill.[d] On the 3rd day he was alert and well oriented, but "totally unable to see and could not distinguish light from dark." A day later, before respiratory arrest, "pupils were constricted and unreacting to light." At autopsy there was severe cerebral edema ("status spongiosus"), but most remarkably there was widespread severe disintegration and necrosis of myelin sheaths and axon cylinders of optic nerves, optic chiasm, and optic tracts. Although the lateral geniculate bodies did not show significant abnormality, the deepest layers of the calcarine fissure showed severe degeneration, and optic pathways anterior to the geniculate bodies "were frankly necrotic."

Bilateral optic atrophy developed in a 31-year-old woman who daily swallowed 10–15 ml of a 3% emulsion of hexachlorophene ("pHisohex") during a period of ten months.[i] Her vision decreased to hand movements in one eye and 6/90 in the other, from optic atrophy. She had no other signs of neurotoxicity. Fourteen months after having stopped taking hexachlorophene emulsion her vision was 6/120 and 6/7.5 respectively.

In monkeys, visual evoked cortical responses were reduced by orally administered doses of hexachlorophene even though the amount was too small to cause microscopic abnormalities of the brain.[h] Subcutaneously injected hexachlorophene caused both "status spongiosis" of the brain white matter and reduction of the visual evoked response.[h] Newborn monkeys washed daily with 3% hexachlorophene emulsion for 3 months also showed extensive myelin vacuolation, and 2 out of 5 had blurred optic discs.[b]

Beagle dogs to which hexachlorophene ointment of various concentrations was applied for 12 weeks had irreversible loss of vision, permanent mydriasis, and peripapillary exudates in the retina.[j]

In rats, in which most of the experimental work on hexachlorophene toxicity has been done, characteristically there has been vacuolation of the white matter of the brain, with degeneration of myelin and axons, with predilection for optic pathways at all levels, and consequent impaired vision.[e-g,k-n,p] Optic atrophy and gliosis have been common findings.[f,l-n,p] In the retina, disappearance of ganglion cells probably secondary to optic atrophy has been observed,[m,n] but there has been more attention to changes in the photoreceptors, which can be severely disrupted.[g,k,m,n] Vacuolar degeneration of the outer segments of photoreceptors has involved separation of inner aspects of the discs, and has been suggested to be analogous to the formation of myelin vacuoles elsewhere in the nervous system.[g,k]

Clearly many observations give evidence that hexachlorophene has special toxicity for the whole visual system, from retina to cerebral cortex. (For comparable neurotoxins, see INDEX for *Myelin vacuolation* and *Status spongiosus of the white matter.*)

Topically on the cornea, hexachlorophene (0.3%) and "pHisoHex" (3%) cause reversible loss of some of the epithelial cells.[300,350]

a. Goutieres F, Aicardi J: Accidental percutaneous hexachlorophene intoxication in children. *BR MED J* 2:663–665, 1977.

b. Lockhart JD: How toxic is hexachlorophene? *PEDIATRICS* 50:229, 1972.

c. Martin-Bouyer G, Lebreton R, et al: Outbreak of accidental hexachlorophene poisoning in France. *LANCET* 1:91–95, 1982.

d. Martinez AJ, Boehm R, Hadfield MG: Acute hexachlorophene encephalopathy. *ACTA NEUROPATHOL* 28:93–103, 1974.

e. Rose AL, Wisniewski HM, Cammer W: New observations on hexachlorophene neurotoxicity in rats. *J NEUROPATHOL EXP NEUROL* 33:176, 1974.

f. Rose AL, Wisniewski HM, Cammer W: Neurotoxicity of hexachlorophene. *J NEUROL SCI* 24:425–435, 1975.

g. Rose AL, Wen GY, Cammer W: Hexachlorophene retinopathy in suckling rats. *J NEUROL SCI* 52:163–178, 1981.

h. Santolucito JA: Electroencephalograms and visual evoked potential of the squirrel monkey fed hexachlorophene. *TOXICOL APPL PHARMACOL* 22:276, 1972.

i. Slamovits TL, Burde RM, Klingele TG: Bilateral optic atrophy caused by chronic oral ingestion and topical application of hexachlorophene. *AM J OPHTHALMOL* 89:676–679, 1980.

j. Staben P: The effect of hexachlorophene on the optic nerve and visual faculty in beagle dogs after prolonged dermal application. *TOXICOL LETT* 5:77–82, 1980.

k. Towfighi J, Gonatos NK, McCree L: Hexachlorophene neuropathy in rats. *LAB INVEST* 29:428, 1973.

l. Towfighi J, Gonatos NK, McCree L: Hexachlorophene induced changes in central and peripheral myelinated axons of developing and adult rats. *LAB INVEST* 31:712, 1974.

m. Towfighi J, Gonatos NK, McCree L: Hexachlorophene retinopathy in rats. *LAB INVEST* 32:330, 1975.

n. Towfighi J: Hexachlorophene. Chapter in Spencer and Schaumburg (1980).[378]

o. Udall V, Malone JC: Optic nerve atrophy after drug treatment. *PROC EUROP SOC STUDY DRUG TOXICITY* 11:244–248, 1970.

p. Udall V: Drug-induced blindness in some experimental animals and its relevance to toxicology. *PROC ROY SOC MED* 65:197, 1972.

Hexafluoroisopropanol (HFIP) is a volatile liquid which causes lacrimation at 300 ppm as a vapor in air. When applied as liquid to rabbit eyes, it causes severe permanent injury, which is not made less by washing the eye within twenty seconds after exposure.[37]

Hexamethonium, a ganglion blocking agent, has been involved in loss of vision. In the first such case, hexamethonium was administered during general anesthesia. Loss of vision in one eye was noted on return to consciousness. The visual acuity gradually returned to normal, but the visual field remained contracted.[b] In the second case, four minutes after intramuscular injection of 6 mg in a hypertensive woman, the vision blurred, and in a few more minutes decreased to complete blindness in one eye and light perception in the other. The color of the discs was normal at that time, but the arteries were narrowed. Subsequently optic atrophy developed in both eyes, along with an appearance of hypertensive retinopathy with hemorrhages and exudates.[a] Two additional cases, one with transient macular edema, have been reported in less detail.[a, 255]

a. Bruce GM: Permanent bilateral blindness following use of hexamethonium chloride. *ARCH OPHTHALMOL* 54:422–424, 1955.
b. Goldsmith AJ, Hewer AJ: Unilateral amaurosis with partial recovery after using hexamethonium iodide. *BR MED J* 2:759–760, 1952.

n-Hexane, a widely used volatile solvent, is a well-established cause of peripheral polyneuropathy.[h] Repeated prolonged inhalation of air containing at least 60 to 240 ppm is required. This characteristically causes gradual development of paresthesias of hands and feet in glove and stocking distribution, followed by weakness in the hands and feet, without ataxia or spasticity. This has occurred mostly in manufacturing, such as shoemaking, and in "glue sniffers." Pathologically, there are giant neuronal swellings, due to collections of neurofilaments, along the nerve fibers. The nerve fibers may degenerate and myelin may be lost, a "dying back" process.

n-Hexane's toxic properties are shared by certain other *hexacarbon neurotoxins,* particularly by *2-hexanone (methyl n-butyl ketone)* and by *2,5-hexanedione,* the latter being a toxic metabolite of both *n-hexane* and *2-hexanone.* In descriptions of toxic properties, it seems to have been common to assume that what is found for one of these substances applies equally to the others. For the neurotoxic hexacarbons in general, it appears that the vulnerability of nerve fibers is proportional to length of fibers and diameter of axons in either peripheral or central nervous systems. Long tracts of the spinal cord are especially vulnerable. Shorter and smaller fibers such as in the optic nerves and tracts may be affected at a later phase.[h]

Effects of n-hexane itself on the visual system have received relatively little attention.[318] "Blurred vision", without explanation for its basis, and without further characterization has been mentioned in association with hexane polyneuropathy by Wada (1 case),[i] Gonzalez (1 case),[c] Korobkin (1 case),[d] and Yamamura (13 cases).[j] Among 39 ophthalmologically examined patients, Yamamura listed 8 cases with eye findings, including 7 cases of "constriction of visual field", 2 cases of "optic nerve atrophy", and 1 case of "retrobulbar neuritis", but said they tended to be "mild", with normal ocular fundi, and no correlation with the severity of peripheral neuropathy.[j]

Documentation is also limited in a report of a patient who noted difficulty in recognizing colors in dim light, but had normal visual acuity, normal Goldmann perimetry, and no sign of optic atrophy, leaving open a question whether there was an acquired change in color vision associated with exposure to hexane.[b]

Two reports have indicated that changes in the macula, particularly macular edema, may be produced by solvent vapors from shoemaker's cement, such as n-hexane.[e,f] Fifteen people who were exposed industrially to hexane for a mean of 12 years, but with no mention of peripheral neuropathy, had normal visual acuity and visual fields, but only three were thought to have normal color discrimination. Ophthalmoscopically there seemed to be vague disturbances in the appearance of the macula areas in eleven of the patients, and vague abnormalities were suspected in retinal fluoroangiograms in some patients.[f] Visual evoked potentials in industrial workers are said to have been found abnormal.[g]

Electroretinograms in guinea pigs have been temporarily extinguished by breathing hexane vapor.[a]

(For a more comprehensive picture of hexacarbon neurotoxicity, see also *hexanedione, hexanol,* and *hexanone.*)

a. Barlotta F, Malfitano D, et al: Electroretinographic study of experimental hexane intoxication. *BOLL SOC ITAL BIOL SPER* 48:115–117, 1972. (Italian)

b. Davenport JE, Farrell DF, Sumi SM: "Giant axonal neuropathy" caused by industrial chemicals. *NEUROLOGY* 26:919, 1976.

c. Gonzalez E, Downey J: Polyneuropathy in a glue sniffer. *ARCH PHYS MED* 53:333–337, 1972.

d. Korobkin R, Asbury AK, et al: Glue-sniffing neuropathy. *ARCH NEUROL* 32:158–162, 1975.

e. Loffredo A, Sammartino A, De Luca M: Observations on edematous maculopathy in people affected by "polyneuritis of industrial adhesive." *ANN OTTALMOL CLIN OCUL* 103:533–542, 1977.

f. Raitta C, Seppalainen A–M, Huuskonen MS: n-Hexane maculopathy in industrial workers. *GRAEFES ARCH OPHTHALMOL.* 209:99–110, 1978.

g. Seppalainen AM, Raitta C, Huuskonen MS: n-Hexane-induced visual-evoked potentials and electroretinograms of industrial workers. *ELECTROENCEPHALOGRAPHY AND CLINICAL NEUROPHYSIOLOGY,* referred to as in print by Spencer PS.[g]

h. Spencer PS, Couri D, Schaumburg HH: n-Hexane and methyl n-butyl ketone. Chapter 32 in Spencer and Schaumburg (1980).[378]

i. Wada Y, Okamoto S, Takagi S: Intoxication polyneuropathy following exposure to n-hexane. *CLIN NEUROL* 5:591–598, 1965.

j. Yamamura Y: n-Hexane polyneuropathy. *FOLIA PSYCHIATR NEUROL JPN* 23:45–57, 1969.

2,5-Hexanedione is a water-soluble neurotoxic metabolite of *n-hexane, 2-hexanone* (*methyl n-butyl ketone*), and *2-hexanol.* In experimental animals it produces the same type of peripheral neuropathy.[a,b] A study on cats by Schaumburg and Spencer has been of particular interest, showing that 2,5-hexanedione produced axonal swellings "throughout the mammilary bodies, the lateral geniculate body and distal optic tract, and the superior colliculus." Since axonal swellings developed in the distal optic tract while the more proximal optic nerve was preserved, the findings were interpreted as distal (dying back) axonopathy.[a] Further, it was concluded that the vulnerability of nerve tracts is related to length and diameter of the axons, with spinal cord pathways suffering earlier and more severely, while the retina-geniculate fibers might be expected to be less affected because of their shortness and small size. In the intoxicated cats no visual loss or abnormal pupillary reflexes were observed. If similar changes occur in the visual nuclei or tracts in human beings who are exposed to *n-hexane* or *2-hexanone*, special tests might be required to detect resulting functional changes. More severe intoxication presumably could affect the optic nerves, and more obvious disturbance of vision might result, but clinical observations have as yet provided meager documentation. (See INDEX for *n-Hexane* and *2-Hexanone* for further information.)

a. Schaumburg HH, Spencer PS: Environmental hydrocarbons produce degeneration in cat hypothalamus and optic tract. *SCIENCE* 199:199–200, 1978.
b. Krinke G, Schaumburg HH, et al: Clioquinol and 2,5-hexanedione induced different types of distal axonopathy in the dog. *ACTA NEUROPATHOL* 47:213–221, 1979.

1-Hexanol (n-hexanol), unlike *2-hexanol,* probably has low neurotoxicity, but by drop application to rabbit eyes causes injury graded 9 on a scale of 10 after 24 hours.[225] However, in 4 instances of corneal burns in workmen, recovery was complete in 48 hours.[165]

2-Hexanol has been reported to produce in rats the same type of peripheral polyneuritis as produced by *n-hexane, 2,5-hexanedione,* and *2-hexanone,* and is probably a metabolic intermediate.[a] By analogy some effect on the visual system might be anticipated, but appears not yet to have been described.

a. Perbellini L, DeGrandis D, et al: An experimental study on the neurotoxicity of n-hexane metabolites: hexanol-1 and hexanol-2. *TOXICOL APPL PHARMACOL* 46:421–427, 1978.

2-Hexanone (methyl n-butyl ketone, MBK), a widely used solvent, has been clearly shown to cause peripheral polyneuropathy in people and experimental animals exposed for long periods to its vapors. Its effects are similar to those of *n-hexane,* and both substances are believed to act through formation of the same toxic metabolites, *2,5-hexanedione* and *2-hexanol.* There is little clinical or experimental evidence of disturbance of the eyes or the visual system by *2-hexanone,* though the metabolite *2,5-hexanedione* has been shown in cats to produce axonal swellings in the distal optic tract and lateral geniculate body. It has been shown that 2-hexanone, like the metabolites, can impair the pupillary responses to flashes of light in guinea pigs,[a] and in monkeys can increase the latent time of visually evoked cortical potentials, which has been interpreted as the functional counterpart of damage in the optic tracts and hypothalamus produced in cats given *2,5-hexanedione.*[c–e] However, in a series of 86 cases of peripheral polyneuropathy from 2-hexanone in human beings no impairment of visual fields or loss of visual acuity was reported which could be attributed to abnormality of optic nerves or retina.[b]

(See INDEX for descriptions of the related hexacarbon neurotoxins, *n-Hexane, 2,5-Hexanedione,* and *2-Hexanol.*)

a. Abdel-Rahman MS, Saladin JJ, et al: The effect of 2-hexanone and 2-hexanone metabolites on pupillomotor activity and growth. *J AM IND HYG ASSOC* 39:94–99, 1978.

b. Allen N, Mendell JR, et al: Toxic neuropathy due to methyl n-butyl ketone. *ARCH NEUROL* 32:209, 1975.

c. Johnson BL, Setzer JV, et al: Effects of methyl n-butyl ketone on behavior and the nervous system. *J AM IND HYG ASSOC* 38:567–579, 1977.

d. Johnson BL, Anger WK, et al: Neurobehavioral effects of methyl n-butyl ketone and methyl n-amyl ketone in rats and monkeys. *J ENVIRON PATHOL TOXICOL* 2:113–133, 1979.

e. Johnson BL: Electrophysiological methods in neurotoxicity testing. Chapter 49 in Spencer and Schaumburg (1980).[378]

Hexylresorcinol tests on rabbit eyes have shown that the surface of the cornea can be irrigated for five minutes with a 1:10,000 solution without injury, but that irrigation with a 1:1,000 solution for one to five minutes causes diffuse edema of the epithelium, followed in two or three hours by bluish stromal edema and hyperemia of the iris. The corneas gradually clear, even after five minutes irrigation, approaching normal in several weeks.[81]

Hirudin, the anticoagulant secreted by leeches, can cause profuse and prolonged bleeding from the conjunctiva, without significant damage to the eye. When a leech enters the conjunctival sac and attaches to the conjunctiva it causes burning discomfort, then itching, blepharospasm and awareness of a motile and gradually enlarging foreign body. The leech should not be roughly pulled from the eye, or the hirudin-secreting head may remain behind, prolonging the trickling of uncoagulable blood from the eye. Instead, 20% sodium chloride solution is applied with an applicator to the leech, after topical anesthesia, and the parasite is gently removed.[a]

a. Verin P, Sekkat A, Morax S: Eye and leech. *ANN OCULIST (PARIS)* 206:21–35, 1973. (French)

Histamine applied in concentrations from 0.1% to 10% of the phosphate or dihydrochloride salts causes no significant injury to human or rabbit eyes, but it does cause vasodilation and edema of the conjunctiva.[f,53,123] A low concentration can cause tickling and sneezing.[c] Intraocular injection of histamine in animals has been shown to cause vasodilation and edema in the ciliary body, increase in permeability of the blood vessels[292], and transitory rise of intraocular pressure.[d] In rats, histamine increases the permeability of venules, permitting colloidal carbon and thorotrast to come through the walls of blood vessels of the ciliary processes, iris, and choriocapillaris, but not through retinal vessels. The increase in permeability is most easily demonstrated when ocular pressure is reduced.[b,h]

In some human glaucomatous eyes, application of 3% histamine hydrochloride eyedrops has been said to cause a rise in ocular pressure, particularly in cases of acute glaucoma.[a]

Experiments on excised beef corneas have demonstrated that histamine at a concentration as low as 5×10^{-6}M loosens the superficial epithelial cells from the basal cells of the cornea after several hours of incubation.[g] However, exposure of excised cornea to 10^{-5}M for 2 minutes does not alter the permeability.[321]

a. Alajmo B: The effect of "Istamine" on normal and glaucomatous eyes. *RASS ITAL OTTAL* 2:1–31, 1933. (Italian)

b. Ashton N, Cunha-Vaz JG: Effect of histamine on the permeability of the ocular vessels. *ARCH OPHTHALMOL* 73:221–223, 1965.

c. Kirkegaard J, Secker C, Mygind N: Effect of the H_1 antihistamine chlorpheniramine maleate on histamine-induced symptoms in the human conjunctiva. *ALLERGY* 37:203–208, 1982.

d. Friedenwald JS, Pierce HF: Pathogenesis of acute glaucoma; experimental study. *ARCH OPHTHALMOL* 3:574–582, 1930.

f. Hagedoorn WG, Maas ER: The effect of histamine on the rabbit's cornea. *AM J OPHTHALMOL* 42:89–93, 1956.

g. Herrmann H: The effect of histamine and related substances on the cohesion of the corneal epithelium. *BULL JOHNS HOPKINS HOSP* 82:208–212, 1948.

h. Sakuragi S: An electron microscopic observation of the leaking vessels of the eye. *ACTA SOC OPHTHALMOL JPN* 72:1920–1935, 1968.

Homatropine hydrobromide and hydrochloride have long been used in eyedrops (1% to 2% solution) as an anticholinergic mydriatic and cycloplegic. Fortuitous clinical observations as well as systematic tests of the influence of topical homatropine on intraocular pressure have been made in patients with various types of eyes. In nonglaucomatous eyes with wide anterior chamber angles, homatropine rarely causes a rise of pressure, but in open-angle glaucoma it commonly raises pressure and reduces facility of aqueous outflow. This rise of pressure occurs with the angles remaining open. In eyes with narrow angles subject to angle-closure glaucoma, homatropine can provoke a rise of pressure by closing the angle.[83] (See also *Anticholinergic drugs.*)

Hura crepitans (sandbox tree, monkey pistol), a tree of the *Euphorbiaceae* family, said to have toxic substances *hurin* and *crepitan* in the sap, with the juice from all parts of the tree said to be very irritating to the skin and eyes.[142] (See also *Euphorbias.*)

Hyacinth bulbs many years ago were noted to cause reddening of the skin of the face and arms, conjunctivitis, photophobia, epiphora, and itching among bulb growers in Holland. This seems to have come from the dust from dried bulbs,[214,246] and may have been a manifestation of hypersensitivity rather than a toxic effect.

Hyaluronic acid sulfate injected into the vitreous humor is reported to have caused contraction of the vitreous with detachment of the retina in dogs and rabbits, also occasionally to have caused cataract and dislocation of the lens.[44,259] (Also see INDEX for *Sodium hyaluronate.*)

Hyaluronidase, an enzyme that depolymerizes hyaluronic acid and other mucopolysaccharides of connective tissue, is used medically to promote diffusion of local anesthetic agents. Toxic effects have been attributed to insufficient purification of the enzyme or to immune reaction to impurities. Rohen (1965) reported inducing changes in the trabecular meshwork and producing glaucoma in monkeys by repeated injection into the vitreous humor, but attributed this to an immune reaction to impurities.[d] Intravitreal injection of hyaluronidase produced iritis and formation of strands or sheets between lens and optic nervehead.[a,c] In guinea pigs intravitreal injection produced plasmoid aqueous and hazy, liquefied vitreous humor.[b] Refractile particles appeared four days later, resembling asteroid bodies clinically and microscopically. After six weeks the particles became fewer and finer, as viscous, polymerized vitreous humor was being formed.

Glaucomatous patients who were given subconjunctival injections of hyaluronidase developed redness and irritation of the eyes, accompanied by myopia and astigmatism, but the reaction gradually disappeared.[f] The same effect has been obtained in nonglaucomatous patients who were given subconjunctival injections of hyaluronidase (1,500 IU in 0.5 ml saline), with astigmatism and myopia of as much as 3 diopters reaching a maximum in ten days and lasting several weeks.[g] The effect has also been observed in patients with aphakic eyes.[g] In rabbits it has been shown to be due to changes in corneal curvature, which develops in about a week and disappears several weeks later.[g,h]

The possibility that hyaluronidase mixed with local anesthetic injected behind the eye prior to cataract extraction may induce cystoid macular edema has been raised by a study in which maculopathy developed in 6 out of 24 patients who were given this type of injection, but in none of 16 who were given the local anesthetic without hyaluronidase.[e] Analysis of more data is needed.

a. Agarwal LP, Dhiri S, et al: Experimental retinal detachment. *MOD PROB OPHTHALMOL* 8:106–110, 1969.
b. Lamba PA, Shukla KN: Experimental asteroid hyalopathy. *BR J OPHTHALMOL* 55:279–283, 1971.
c. Machemer R, Norton EWD: Experimental retinal detachment and reattachment. *MOD PROBL OPHTHALMOL* 8:80–90, 1969.
d. Rohen JW: On the reactive alterations of the corneoscleral trabeculum in primate eyes after action of hyaluronidase. *Z ZELLFORSCH* 65:627–645, 1965. (German)
e. Roper DL, Nisbet RM: Effect of hyaluronidase on the incidence of cystoid macular edema. *ANN OPHTHALMOL* 10:1673–1678, 1978.
f. Stanworth A: The ocular effects of local corticosteroid and hyaluronidase. In Paterson; Miller; Paterson (Eds.); *DRUG MECHANISMS IN GLAUCOMA*. London, Churchill, 1966, pp. 231–246.
g. Treister G, Romano A, Stein A: The effect of subconjunctivally injected hyaluronidase on corneal refraction. *ARCH OPHTHALMOL* 81:645–649, 1969.
h. Turan S, Slem G, et al: An experiment on the effect of hyaluronidase on corneal refraction. *ANN OPHTHALMOL* 4:403–419, 1972.

Hydralazine hydrochloride (Apresoline hydrochloride, Lopress), an antihypertensive, is said occasionally to have caused flushing of the face, headache and stuffy nose, edema of the eyelids and extremities, with lacrimation and blurring of vision.[252,255]

The intraocular pressure after administration orally or intramuscularly has usually been unaffected.[a, 266] However, after retrobulbar injection the intraocular pressure has been found raised, despite lowering of blood pressure.[a, c] (See also *Vasodilator drugs.*)

Uveitis and keratitis are reported to have been induced in a few guinea pigs by systemic administration of hydralazine in combination with Freund's adjuvant.[b]

   a. Eberhartinger W, Schenk H: Investigation of the intraocular pressure under medication with hydralazine. *OPHTHALMOLOGICA* 133:406–413, 1957. (German)
   b. Leovey A, Alberth B, Szegedi G: Experimentally produced (autoimmune?) uveitis and keratitis. *GRAEFES ARCH OPHTHALMOL* 169:294–298, 1966. (German)
   c. Schenk H, Eberhartinger W: Investigation of the intraocular pressure after administration of blood-pressure lowering agent. *OPHTHALMOLOGICA* 130:312–320, 1955. (German)

Hydrargaphen (phenylmercuric dinaphthyl-methanedisulfonate), an antibacterial and antifungal, has been used in 0.033% concentration in treatment of blepharitis, but questions have been raised concerning the incidence of irritation to the eye and the possible equal therapeutic effectiveness of the vehicle without hydrargaphen. Side effects have not been severe.[a–c] Discoloration of the lens such as induced by prolonged use of phenylmercuric nitrate in eyedrops has not been encountered with hydrargaphen. In rats and guinea pigs 0.1% eyedrops have induced corneal opacities and vascularization.[6]

In guinea pigs, applying hydrargaphen eyedrops for 5 weeks and measuring the mercury levels in the ocular tissues showed that simultaneous treatment with melanocyte-stimulating hormone caused a significant increase in the levels in the aqueous humor, retina, and lens; however, no toxic effects were identified.[d]

   a. Jackson B: The use of Penotrane in ophthalmology. *BR J OPHTHALMOL* 49:307–311, 1965.
   b. Marmion VJ, Silva M: Side effects of topical therapy with Optrane. *BR J OPHTHALMOL* 51:142, 1967.
   c. More BM: Penotrane in blepharitis. A double blind controlled trial. *BR J OPHTHALMOL* 52:383–387, 1968.
   d. Ancill RJ, Richens ER: The effect of various hormones on the uptake and distribution of an organic mercurial compound in the guinea pig eye. *TOXICOL APPL PHARMACOL* 20:206–215, 1971.

Hydrazine vapor is very irritating to the eyes, nose, throat, and lungs. Contact of the liquid with the skin produces burns, and presumably would be severely injurious to the eyes.[a]

Similar to anhydrous hydrazine is *hydrazine hydrate*, a strong corrosive alkali which presumably would be seriously damaging on contact with the eye.

A neutral salt, *hydrazine sulfate* has been found not to be injurious to the rabbit eye when applied at 0.02 M concentration for ten minutes after mechanical removal of the corneal epithelium to facilitate penetration.[81]

Choroidal malignant melanoma developed in one person who worked with aqueous solution of hydrazine for 6 years.[b]

a. Montgomery V, Reeves JL: Toxicity of chemicals. *LECTURES IN AEROSPACE MED,* Jan. 11–15, 1960, pp. 1–22. (School of Aviation Medicine, Brooks Air Force Base, Texas)

b. Albert DM, Puliafito CA: Choroidal melanoma. *N ENGL J MED* 296:634–635, 1977.

Hydrochloric acid (muriatic acid) is a solution of hydrogen chloride in water. Hydrogen chloride gas which escapes from the aqueous solution is immediately irritating to the eyes and respiratory passages. The protective response is so strong that human beings have rarely submitted to damaging concentrations. However, in animals a concentration of 1,350 ppm in air for one and one-half hours has been found to cause clouding of the cornea; 300 ppm for six hours caused slight erosion of the corneal epithelium, but 100 ppm for six hours daily for fifty days caused only slight unrest and irritation of the eyes, but no injury.[188]

Hydrochloric is one of the most common acids, and for more than a century reports have been appearing of injuries of the eye from splashes of this substance. The severity has varied according to the quantity, concentration, and time of contact, and has ranged from inconsequential redness and irritation of the conjunctiva to total corneal opacification and loss of the eye. In rare instances opacities of the lens have been produced in human and rabbit eyes.[153]

Most commonly a drop splashed in the eye and immediately washed out with water causes white coagulation of corneal and conjunctival epithelium, but does no significant damage to the corneal stroma or deeper parts of the eye. Usually the injured epithelium comes loose in a day or two and is replaced in a few days by new epithelium, and the eye returns to normal.

In treatment of band calcification of human corneas 2% hydrochloric acid has been applied for a few seconds with a swab without significant injury.[b]

The reactions of rabbit eyes to hydrochloric acid have been studied in great detail.[a-f,161] Hydrochloric acid is injurious only below pH 3.[123] Contact with 0.25N to 1N acid for twenty seconds results in some scarring of rabbit corneas.[101] In rabbit eyes after contact with hydrochloric acid, assays have been made of ascorbic acid, phosphatase, glycolytic activity, and oxygen uptake of the cornea.

Considerable ascorbic acid is lost when the epithelium is lost but in the stroma the ascorbic acid merely becomes temporarily diluted by edema fluid. The concentration in the aqueous humor decreases in association with iritis. Phosphatase, which is normally abundant in the blood serum, but not in the aqueous or cornea, has not been found to be increased in the cornea after acid burn. Stromal edema fluid appears to consist of accumulated water and salt, but not of whole aqueous humor nor of blood serum. Both glycolysis and oxygen uptake are greatly inhibited immediately after acid burn, probably owing to severe damage of the corneal epithelium.

Studies by Tartakovskaya on the chemical composition of rabbit corneas after exposure to 10% hydrochloric acid have indicated that at three days after exposure, when the cornea was swollen and collagen structure disorganized, the hydroxyproline content was reduced but tryosine was increased. Hexosamine, hexose, and total nitrogen were also decreased. From the third to the fifteenth day, when vascularization was taking place, there was an increase in collagen, with increase in hydroxyproline, and accumulation of mucoproteins. Also from the fifteenth to the sixtieth day, when the corneas were becoming scarred and fibroblasts were active, the total collagen and acid mucopolysaccharides were increased.[f]

Additional observations on the effects of hydrochloric acid on the eyes of experimental animals can be found in several publications in which hydrochloric acid was the agent employed for producing a standard burn of the eye, but in which the prime interest was in studying the effects of various treatments.[30,57,140,182,238,254] (Also see INDEX for *Acids,* and for *Treatment of Chemical Burns of the Eye.*

a. Allen JH, Manning JW, et al: Changes in aqueous flow and bloodaqueous barrier after hydrochloric acid burns to the eye. *ARCH OPHTHALMOL* 57:1–6, 1957.
b. Francois J: *BULL SOC OPHTHALMOL PARIS* Dec. 15, 1934, pp. 1–7.
c. Friedenwald JS, Hughes WF, Herrmann H: Acid burns of the eye. *ARCH OPHTHALMOL* 35:98–108, 1946.
d. Guidry AM, Allen JH, Kelly JB: Some biochemical characteristics of acid injury of the cornea. *AM J OPHTHALMOL* 40:111–119, 1955.
e. Guidry MA, Allen JH, Kelly JB: Some biochemical characteristics of hydrochloric-acid injury of the cornea. *AM J OPHTHALMOL* 44:243–248, 1957.
f. Tartakovskaya AI: Changes in the protein-polysaccharide composition of the cornea in various phases of connective tissue disorganization during chemical injury. *SOEDIN TKAN NORME PATOL, MATER SOVESHCH* 1966, pp. 202–205. (*CHEM ABSTR* 71:28722, 1969.)

Hydrochlorothiazide (Hydro-Diuril, Esidrix, Oretic, Thiuretic), a diuretic, has no consistent pattern of ocular toxicity.[312] As a rare but recognized type of side effect, a young woman under treatment for edema of the legs associated with pregnancy developed acute bilateral myopia of about 3 diopters after taking 100 mg.[a] In three to four days the myopia cleared after the drug was discontinued. (Also see the Index for *Myopia, acute transient,* for discussion of this type of drug reaction.)

Intraocular pressure in glaucomatous patients has not been adversely affected by hydrochlorothiazide.[b] However, when given in association with carbonic anhydrase inhibitors, attention should be paid to the possibility of inducing hypokalemia.

a. Beasley FJ: Transient myopia and retinal edema during hydrochlorothiazide (Hydro-Diuril) therapy. *ARCH OPHTHALMOL* 65:212–213, 1961.
b. Fajardo RV, Hamilton R, Leopold IH: The effect of hydrochlorothiazide (Esidrex) on intraocular pressure in man. *AM J OPHTHALMOL* 49:1321–1324, 1960.

Hydrofluoric acid (HF) is a solution of hydrogen fluoride in water. Both the gas and the liquid are extremely poisonous and injurious. Hydrogen fluoride causes irritation of all mucous membranes, including the conjunctiva. Air containing as little as 5 ppm causes irritation of the eyes and nose.[188] Chronic exposure of guinea pigs and rabbits has caused injury of the cornea as well as of the mucous membranes.[61] Industrial experience in chemical manufacturing where a mixture of fluorine, fluorides, and hydrogen fluoride may be present in the air indicates that conjunctival hyperemia in the palpebral fissure occurs commonly, irritation of the eyelids occurs occasionally, but corneal disturbance is rare.[c]

On the skin, hydrofluoric acid causes pain, with a notorious peculiar tendency to become gradually more severe, especially in the fingertips. In some cases pain is said to have developed after a latent period of an hour or so, followed by vesication and destruction of tissue, with slow tendency to heal.[171,252] The type of injury produced is different from injuries produced by hydrochloric acid, and it is generally held that it is the toxicity of the fluoride ion that is to blame.

Burns of the eye by hydrofluoric acid can be devastating. Anhydrous hydrogen fluoride has been known to destroy the eye and to require enucleation, according to Trevino.[e] The danger of hydrofluoric acid solutions depends upon the concentration. Experimental splash burns in rabbits by McCulley and colleagues have shown 20% solution to cause immediate damage with total corneal opacification with conjunctival ischemia, and with corneal stromal edema within an hour, followed by necrosis of anterior ocular structures.[d] An 8% solution produced ischemia and corneal stromal edema persisting for 40 to 65 days, accompanied by corneal vascularization. Even 2% solution caused mild persistent stromal edema and vascularization, but after 0.5% solution there was recovery in 10 days.

Human eye injuries have rarely been reported. McCulley has described a severe one in detail.[d] Both eyes were splashed in this case. The corneal epithelium immediately became moderately opaque, and within the first day separated from the stroma. The conjunctiva was entirely ischemic. Because of severe pain this patient was treated with repeated subconjunctival injections of 10% calcium gluconate, which eased the pain. However, re-epithelization of the cornea took 20 days, and during the following year keratitis sicca and recurrent corneal epithelial erosions were a problem. Corneal pannus vascularization progressed for more than 3 years, and vision stabilized only after 4 years, at 20/80 in one eye, 20/30 in the other.

One case of eye burns from a fine spray of hydrofluoric acid has been described in considerable detail by Bertuna.[a] In this case a fine spray of concentrated acid struck the victim's face, causing immediate severe pain. Irrigation with water was started immediately. After ten minutes, considerable loss of epithelium from cornea and conjunctiva was observed, and small white spots of burns on the skin were evident. On the basis of the previous experience in which HF burns of the skin appeared to be benefited by treatment with a quaternary ammonium surfactant, this patient's eyes were then irrigated with 0.5% solution of benzethonium chloride for three hours. After that, there was seen to be extensive edema of the lids, conjunctivae, and corneas. However, three days later the corneal epithelium was regenerating, and within nineteen days the corneas had recovered so well that normal vision was regained in both eyes.

It is noteworthy that irrigation with 0.5% benzethonium chloride solution for nearly three hours was itself tolerated by the eyes. At this concentration, even with brief surface exposure, this compound has been considered to be potentially damaging, at least to the epithelium of the cornea. This type of compound is also potentially injurious to the corneal endothelium. (See INDEX for *Benzalkonium, Benzethonium,* and *Surfactants.*)

Treatments of hydrofluoric acid burns of the *skin* are designed to inactivate free fluoride ions by chemical binding of fluoride with calcium or with quaternary ammonium compounds.[b] Some experts recommend local treatment with calcium gluconate solution,[e] which may be injected into the skin, or soaking the burns with

0.2% benzethonium chloride (Hyamine) solution.[f] Both treatments are effective in relieving pain, but there appears to be disagreement on which is better.[b]

In treatment of hydrofluoric acid burns of the *eye* there has similarly been the possibility of treatment with calcium gluconate or with benzethonium hydrochloride, as in the two cases described above. Trevino and associates, with an impressive industrial background have recommended immediate copious washing of the eyes, followed by application of ice packs until a medical facility is reached, then 1% calcium gluconate irrigation for 5 to 10 minutes, and drop instillation every 2 to 3 hours for 2 to 3 days.[e] However, they warn that while some eyes may recover in 4 to 5 days, others may have corneal scarring or perforation, or may require long-term monitoring.

McCulley and associates have performed an extensive experimental evaluation of possible treatments of hydrofluoric acid burns of rabbit eyes, which, to the extent that rabbit and human eyes are comparable, appears to provide a sound scientific basis for a choice.[d] In essence, they substantiated that fluoride ion is toxic when it gains access to the corneal stroma through damage of the corneal epithelium by low acid pH. They compared the results of irrigating burned eyes for 30 minutes with one liter each of a series of substances designed to inactivate fluoride ion, and separately evaluated the toxicity of these substances themselves. They also tested subconjunctival injections. They concluded that subconjunctival 10% calcium gluconate or irrigation with 0.2% benzethionum chloride or 0.05% benzalkonium chloride were themselves too injurious to normal rabbit eyes to recommend for clinical use. They found the only non-toxic treatment with therapeutic value was a single irrigation with isotonic sodium chloride or magnesium chloride. They found that repeated irrigation was inadvisable because it strikingly increased the frequency of corneal ulceration in burned eyes. Finally, they concluded that the simplest and most effective first-aid treatment was copious irrigation with water or saline.

a. Bertuna S: quoted by de Treville RTP: Hydrofluoric acid burn management. *MEDICAL SERIES BULLETIN* NO. 17–70 (1970). Industrial Hygiene Foundation of America.
b. Carney SA, Hall M, et al: Rationale of the treatment of hydrofluoric acid burns. *BR J IND MED* 31:317–321, 1974.
c. Mathis G: Direct ocular lesions from vapors of fluorine and derivatives. *RASS ITAL OTTALMOL* 10:327–337, 1941. (Italian)
d. McCulley JP, Whiting DW, et al: Hydrofluoric acid burns of the eye. *J OCCUP MED* 25:447–450, 1983.
e. Trevino MA, Herrmann GH, Sprout WL: Treatment of severe hydrofluoric acid exposures. *J OCCUP MED* 25:861–863, 1983.
f. Wetherhold JM, Shepherd FP: Treatment of hydrofluoric acid burns. *J OCCUP MED* 7:193–195, 1965.

Hydrogen peroxide is a strongly oxidizing liquid which is employed almost always in aqueous solution. Injuries of human eyes have been rare. Workers exposed to vapors from 90% hydrogen peroxide have noted primarily respiratory irritation, but splash of such high concentration is generally feared as a potential cause of severe corneal damage.[i,227] In treatment of corneal ulcerations, particularly in herpetic dendritic keratitis, 20% solution has been applied, after local anesthetic, every two hours as a localized cautery to the ulcer, and has been reported to have had good effect in numerous patients.[1] In one instance a 10% solution was dropped on one eye of a patient after application of cocaine, and this eye was normal by the next day.[153]

Dropping 1 to 3% hydrogen peroxide solution on the human eye causes severe pain, but this soon subsides.[f,153] Historically, 1 to 3% solution was utilized as an antibacterial agent, dropped 3 to 5 times a day on the eye without causing significant injury. Even a 0.5% solution caused pain and conjunctival hyperemia, however.

Koster (1921) described a patient who had iridocyclitis in one eye, with a recollection of having once applied 3% hydrogen peroxide 8 to 10 days before the onset.[h] However, the cornea was normal, and from general experience with hydrogen peroxide it seems quite doubtful that it was responsible. Knopf (1984) has described an extraordinary incident in which a soft contact lens of 55% water content had inadvertently been stored in 3% hydrogen peroxide and then was placed on a patient's eye, causing immediate pain, tearing, and spasm of the eyelids. The contact lens was removed, and a local anesthetic was applied. At that time no corneal injury was evident, and vision was normal. However, during the next 48 hours, despite treatment with 0.1% dexamethasone, the eye became intensely painful, there was punctate staining of the cornea, and vision decreased to 20/40. However, recovery was rapid, and after several days only minimal punctate keratopathy and mild discomfort remained.[g]

Experiments on rabbit eyes by Huss (1902) showed corneal injury from drop application to depend not only on the concentration of hydrogen peroxide, but also on the integrity of the corneal epithelium, which had a protective influence.[f] Application of a drop of 10 to 30% caused superficial corneal haze, and, if there were defects in the epithelium, could cause localized swelling and opacities in the corneal stroma. Also, 5% solution caused superficial corneal haze and much conjunctival reaction, but these effects were gone in 24 hours. The effects of 10% solution usually took longer to disappear, and occasionally could result in lasting localized opacities.

Miller (1958) reported rabbit eyes returned to normal within 24 hours after a drop of 0.5% solution.[175]

Mann (1948) described the reaction of rabbit eyes after application of 5% hydrogen peroxide as corneal edema, flare in the aqueous humor, congestion of the iris, and vascularization of the cornea, with only partial improvement in 4 to 5 months.[161]

Koster (1921) examined the effects of applying several drops one after another on rabbits' eyes, finding 2 to 5% solutions caused much clouding of the cornea, inflammation of the conjunctiva, and in the worst examples cyclitis and atrophy of the globe.[h] A 1% solution applied repeatedly caused conjunctival hyperemia and slight corneal haze, followed by recovery.

Intracorneal injection of 0.1% to 0.3% solution in rabbits caused rather severe reactions.[123] Intracorneal 0.001 to 1% solution caused dose-related infiltration with PMN leukocytes in guinea pigs.[a] Subconjunctival injections of hydrogen peroxide caused oxygen bubbles to appear in the corneal stroma and in the anterior chamber.[153]

Hydrogen peroxide is normally present in the aqueous humor in a higher concentration than in other body fluids, and any increase that might occur has been considered a potential threat to the lens, cornea, and aqueous outflow system.[c] Hydrogen peroxide has been shown in cultured lenses to affect the uptake of rubidium adversely.[b] The proteins of cataractous lenses that have non-diabetic senile nuclear sclerosis have been found to be oxidized, particularly their thiol groups. Patients with this type of cataract have been found to have an abnormally high concentration of hydrogen peroxide in their aqueous humor.[k] The corneal endothelium has been shown to be damaged by abnormally high concentrations of hydrogen peroxide in the aqueous humor, with resulting swelling of the cornea.[d,e,j,k] The possibility of some similar toxic action on the aqueous outflow system in glaucoma is being investigated.

Because of these and other observations, there is much interest in the potential toxic role of endogenous chronically high levels of hydrogen peroxide in the aqueous humor, which might arise from excessive formation or impaired detoxication. Its formation is believed to start with generation of superoxide ions when aerobic cells utilize molecular oxygen, possibly in oxidation of ascorbic acid in the aqueous humor, followed by conversion of the superoxide to hydrogen peroxide by superoxide dismutase.[c,d] Detoxication may be accomplished by at least two mechanisms, one relying on catalase, and the other on a glutathione peroxidase-reductase pathway, which depends on the hexose monophosphate shunt for recycling glutathione.[c] These and other pathways for formation and detoxication of endogenous hydrogen peroxide, and their possible significance in relation to degenerative eye diseases are being intensively investigated. Metals act as catalysts in generation of free radicals. Accordingly the role of hydrogen peroxide in toxicity of iron and copper is under study. (See INDEX for *Iron* and *Copper.*)

a. Chusid MJ, Starkey DD: Polymorphonuclear leukocyte kinetics in experimentally induced keratitis. *ARCH OPHTHALMOL* 103:270–274, 1985.
b. Fukui HN: The effect of hydrogen peroxide on the rubidium transport of rat lens. *EXP EYE RES* 23:595–599, 1976.
c. Giblin FJ, McCready JP, Reddy VN: The role of glutathione metabolism in the detoxication of H_2O^2 in rabbit lens. *INVEST OPHTHALMOL VIS SCI* 22:330–335, 1982.
d. Hull DS, Scukas S, et al: Hydrogen peroxide and corneal endothelium. *ACTA OPHTHALMOL* 59:409–421, 1981.
e. Hull DS, Green K, et al: Hydrogen-peroxide mediated corneal endothelial damage. *INVEST OPHTHALMOL VIS SCI* 25:1246–1253, 1984.
f. Huss H: On the influence of hydrogen peroxide (Merck) on the eye. *KLIN MONATSBL AUGENHEILKD* 40:333–347, 1902. (German)
g. Knopf HLS: Reaction to hydrogen peroxide in a contact-lens wearer. *AM J OPHTHALMOL* 97:796, 1984.
h. Koster GW: Injury of the eye by hydrogen peroxide (H_2O_2). *GRAEFES ARCH OPHTHALMOL* 105:538–541, 1921. (German)
i. Krachkow EH: Preliminary data on the acute toxicity of 90% hydrogen peroxide. *US NAVY MED NEWS LETTER* 15:23, 1950.
j. Riley MV, Giblin FJ: Toxic effects of hydrogen peroxide on corneal endothelium. *CURR EYE RES* 2:451–458, 1982/1983.
k. Spector A, Garner WH: Hydrogen peroxide and human cataract. *EXP EYE RES* 33:673–681, 1981.
l. Vala M: Treatment of corneal diseases with 20% solution of peroxide of hydrogen. *CESK OFTALMOL* 21:357–359, 1965. (*EXCERPTA MED* (SECT. XII) 20:1244, 1966.)

Hydrogen sulfide is an extremely poisonous gas with an odor characteristic of rotten eggs, recognizable at 1 to 5 ppm in air. Inhalation of a high concentration of hydrogen sulfide may within seconds cause collapse, coma, and death from respiratory failure.

Effects of hydrogen sulfide on the eyes are notable only at sublethal concentrations, most commonly at concentrations so low that they have no discernible systemic effect. At least 120 articles have been published describing a highly characteristic superficial injury of the cornea and conjunctiva occurring in workmen exposed to low concentrations of hydrogen sulfide in sewers, caissons, tunnels, sugar beet refineries, rayon or artificial silk manufacture, sulfur baths, refining of sulfur-containing petroleum, tanneries, and sulfur mining.

Irritation and inflammation of the eyes in workers in cesspools and sewers were noted by the Romans, and again by Ramazzini in 1700. In 1913 Lewin and Guillery recorded clinical observations and the results of experiments on themselves and on animals, noting that after exposure for two and one-half hour to an atmosphere containing 200 ppm of hydrogen sulfide there developed pain in the eyes, and blurring of vision, reaching a maximum the next day.[153] They also noted superficial corneal turbidity when the eye was examined with focal illumination. Since then the characteristic signs and symptoms have been repeatedly described.[33,46,61,129]

Typically, workmen exposed to low concentrations of hydrogen sulfide gas are initially aware of the unpleasant odor, but soon become accustomed to it, and usually have no sensation of irritation or discomfort for at least several hours, or sometimes for several days while working in the presence of low concentrations. Ocular symptoms generally start after several hours exposure, and may not appear until the patient has finished work for the day. There is then gradual onset of scratchy irritated sensation in the eyes, with tearing and burning.

At the onset little may be seen on examination of the eyes other than conjunctival hyperemia and scattered fine gray dots of keratitis epithelialis visible only by slit-lamp biomicroscopy. Recovery may be spontaneous from this stage, or the symptoms may increase in the next few hours to greater burning discomfort and photophobia. The patient may observe colored haloes or rings about lights. At this stage, hyperemia of the conjunctivae and redness and swelling of the lids are more marked than earlier, and the fine gray stippling of the corneal epithelium and optical irregularity of the corneal epithelium are more evident.

In the most severe cases the corneal surface may become lusterless and eroded from loss of epithelial cells. As a rule the only sign of iritis is constriction of the pupils. The aqueous humor remains clear. The layers of the cornea deeper than the epithelium are rarely involved unless there is a secondary infection.

Almost always recovery is spontaneous and complete. In the mildest cases the eyes may be essentially normal by the next day, and most commonly they are normal within two or three days.

Experimentally it is demonstrable that at a concentration of 100 ppm in air an immediate irritation of the eyes and respiratory tract is produced, but conditions responsible for the vast majority of cases of hydrogen sulfide keratoconjunctivitis are those in which concentration is too low to cause immediate irritation, and has toxic effect only after several hours or days of exposure. However, in industries where the concentration is regularly kept below 10 ppm in air, it is rare to have any irritation of the eyes.[m] In quite rare cases, an intense keratoconjunctivitis has been induced by a brief spurt of concentrated gas into the eyes, the symptoms and signs reaching a maximum twelve to twenty-four hours later.[a] The injurious effect upon the eye appears in either case to be a direct and local one, selectively affecting the cornea and conjunctiva in the exposed palpebral fissure.[h] Some workmen are more resistant to the effect than others.

Concentrations of hydrogen sulfide sufficient to cause ocular disturbances are generally enough to discolor metals, such as coins in the pockets of the workmen, and it is helpful in establishing the diagnosis to inspect the coins they have been carrying at work. The history of smell of hydrogen sulfide obtained from the victims is not very dependable, because with continued exposure the sense of smell rapidly fatigues. However, the odor may be detectable on their clothes.[81]

In animal experiments the temporary damaging effect of hydrogen sulfide on the corneal epithelium has several times been demonstrated in dogs, cats, rabbits, and guinea pigs,[b,e,f,81] usually by exposure to 50 to 100 ppm for several hours or days. Animals possibly are less sensitive to the ocular effects of hydrogen sulfide than are human beings and appear to be more prone to develop respiratory disturbances.

The toxic action of hydrogen sulfide on the corneal epithelium has been postulated to be due to enzyme inhibition.[p] It appears reasonable to suppose that hydrogen sulfide may poison a metal-dependent enzyme or coenzyme in the epithelium, but so far there seems to have been no specific biochemical investigation of its effect on corneal enzymes. It is remarkable how this question that is seemingly so accessible to investigation has been neglected experimentally, while clinical descriptions have piled up for centuries. Studies of mechanisms which may be involved in the acute systemic poisoning produced by sulfide have pointed out that sulfide can inhibit cytochrome oxidase by formation of a complex with the iron in the molecule or it can split the disulfide bond upon which this enzyme also is dependent, in either case reducing the oxygen uptake of cells. The inhibition of cytochrome oxidase by either of these mechanisms is reversible. Detoxication of hydrosulfide ion formed by dissociation of hydrogen sulfide and protection from systemic poisoning can be provided experimentally by glutathione in its disulfide form, also by disulfiram, and by methemoglobin.[c,r] How much of this information on mechanism of systemic toxicity can eventually be applied to explaining the special toxic action of hydrogen sulfide on the corneal epithelium, and to local detoxification remains to be seen.

For treatment of keratoconjunctivitis from hydrogen sulfide, there is at present no specific antidote. When the biochemical basis for the epithelial poisoning is eventually elucidated, a specific remedy may well be found. At present the patient is merely provided with as good an opportunity as possible for the spontaneous healing of the epithelium. A brief-acting mydriatic-cycloplegic, a bland antibiotic ointment, bedrest with the eyes closed, and systemic medication such as aspirin for discomfort are all that is required. No local anesthetic should be used except at the initial examination.

Experimental injection of 0.5 to 1 ml of hydrogen sulfide gas into the vitreous humor of rabbits has been noted not to have injurious effect on the eye.[j] In view of the great toxicity of hydrogen sulfide, this seems surprising. Possibly closer examination would reveal intraocular toxic effects.

Abnormal appearance of the fundus of the eye in a patient who had an acute exposure and subsequent typical keratitis epithelialis has been described in only one case.[u] The first day after poisoning, the retinal veins seemed turgescent. After two days there was moderate papilledema, more on the right than the left, and there were a few retinal hemorrhages not far from the optic discs. After five days there was not much change in the fundi, but the corneas had returned to normal. Investigations disclosed no reason for the fundus abnormalities other than the poisoning, and soon they cleared completely.

a. Ahlberg G: Hydrogen sulfide poisoning in whale oil industry. *ARCH IND HYG* 3:247–266, 1951.
b. Beasley RWR: The eye and hydrogen sulfide. *BR J IND MED* 20:32–34, 1963.
c. Evans CL: The toxicity of hydrogen sulphide and other sulphides. *Q J EXP PHYSIOL* 52:231–248, 1967.
d. Frankisek MV: Lesions of the eye due to hydrogen sulfide. *CS OFTAL* 6:5–8, 1950. (*EXCERPTA MED* 4:1214.)
e. Hartmann K: To the question of eye injuries from hydrogen sulfide gas. *KLIN MONATSBL AUGENHEILKD* 101:510–515, 1938. (German)
f. Hoppe: On secondary eye inflammation from hydrogen sulfide. *Z AUGENHEILKD* 43:195–201, 1920. (German)
h. Karsch J: Chemical keratoconjunctivitis in the Saxon artificial silk factory Pirna. *KLIN MONATSBL AUGENHEILKD* 123:440–449, 1953. (German)
j. Krwawicz T, Zagorski K, Szwarc B: Experimental investigations on the possibility of stopping the chemical activity of copper splinter in the vitreous body. *KLIN OCZNA* 36:1–5, 1966. (*ZENTRALBL GES OPHTHALMOL* 96:578, 1966.)
k. Mita H: On eye injuries of sulfur miners. *KLIN MONATSBL AUGENHEILKD* 83:797–806, 1929. (German)
l. Moser P: On chronic hydrogen sulfide inhalation by dogs. *NAUNYNSCHMIEDEBERGS ARCH EXP PATH PHARMAK* 196:446–454, 1940. (German)
m. Poda GA: Hydrogen sulfide can be handled safely. *ARCH ENVIRON HEALTH* 12:795–800, 1966.
n. Rankine D: Artificial silk keratitis. *BR MED J* 2:6–9, 1936.
o. Rochat GF: Injury of the cornea by hydrogen sulfide. *KLIN MONATSBL AUGENHEILKD* 70:152–154, 1923. (German)
p. Rodenacker G: The chemical industrial diseases and their management. Volume 12 *Occupational Medicine: Discussions of Occupational Diseases and their Prevention,* Johann Ambrosius Barth, Leipzig, 1940. (German)
q. Sjogren H: Contribution to our knowledge of ocular changes induced by sulfuretted hydrogen. *ACTA OPHTHALMOL* 17:166–171, 1939.
r. Smith RP, Abbanat RA: Protective effect of oxidized glutathione in acute sulfide poisoning. *TOXICOL APPL PHARMACOL* 9:209–217, 1966.
t. Weill G: Keratitis in artificial silk factories. *BULL SOC OPHTALMOL PARIS* 9:567–568, 1927. (French)
u. Berkman N, Moubri M: Ophthalmologic manifestations during subsidence of a poisoning by hydrogen sulfide. *BULL SOC OPHTALMOL FRANCE* 80:369–372, 1980. (French)

Hydroquinone (p-dihydroxybenzene; 1,4-bezenediol) in aqueous solution is oxidized by air, forming a brown color, partly due to conversion of hydroquinone to *1,4-benzoquinone.* (See *Quinones.*) Acute exposure to the dust causes eye irritation, and chronic, low-grade long-time exposure has caused discoloration, distortion, and opacification of the corneas of workmen.

The clinical characteristics of eye lesions in workers manufacturing hydroquinone have several times been described.[a,b,h,j,k,m–t] A particularly thorough exposition has been given by Anderson and his associates from a survey of workers exposed for several years to *benzoquinone* vapor in air from oxidation of hydroquinone ranging from 0.01 to 3.2 ppm, with the exposure limited only by the degree of ocular irritation the workers could tolerate.[a,b,q]

Acute exposure to high concentrations of vapor was observed to cause immediate irritation, photophobia, lacrimation, injury of the corneal epithelium, and even frank corneal ulceration without discoloring the eye. In some instances after an acute inflammatory reaction of this character, the corneas healed without aftereffect, but in other instances the cornea developed superficial opacities in the palpebral fissure, accompanied by folds in the posterior surface. A similar acute reaction has been noted in several instances in which the eyes were contaminated with particles of hydroquinone.

A different type of ocular disturbance without acute reaction was observed in numerous workers who were exposed chronically to vapors of benzoquinone or dust of hydroquinone. These workers developed in the course of two years a brownish tinge overlying the sclera in the palpebral fissure. At this stage, the conjunctival surface appeared slightly dry, and the deeper layers of the conjunctiva had a light brownish stain visible biomicroscopically, but no discrete colored particles.

After another two or three years, the conjunctiva appeared more thickened and more dry, with superficial white flecks and brown stain. In the deeper layers, the brown discoloration was then seen biomicroscopically as discrete brown granules or globules. Pigment was observed to begin to migrate from the limbus into the cornea.

After five or more years of exposure, the staining in the conjunctiva was more intense and the number of granules was greater. Also the cornea was diffusely stained brown, and gray refractile dots and gray-white areas of scarring were seen beneath the corneal epithelium. These opacities were associated with an irregular beaten-silver sheen, a homogeneous greenish-yellow staining of the anterior layers of the cornea, and fine vertical wrinkles in Descemet's membrane. The cornea was characteristically hypesthetic.

Finally, in several cases vision became seriously reduced from permanent fine opacities and much astigmatism and irregularity in the cornea. After exposure to quinone vapors was discontinued, the discoloration decreased, but the visual disturbance was permanent. Many years later in such cases a Hudson-Stahli pigment line in the epithelium and severe astigmatism from formation of facets in the cornea have been observed.[b]

Late changes with severe progressive corneal flattening and astigmatism have been described in a series of cases by Gernet.[h] An extensive study by Naumann and Rossman, including follow-up examinations as long as twenty years after patients had been employed in manufacture of hydroquinone, showed that in twenty-one out of twenty-five workers the eyes were affected, in most instances only by brown discoloration of the conjunctiva near the limbus in the palpebral fissure, but eight out of the twenty-five workers developed corneal abnormalities after latent periods of three to eleven years. The corneas developed discoloration, then hypesthesia, then astigmatism, flattening, and irregularity. Finally they became clouded, ulcerated, and had folds in Descemet's membrane. The severe irregular astigmatism disturbed vision worse than the discoloration or turbidity. Penetrating corneal transplant gave improvement in vision, but grafts that were initially clear gradually developed pigmentation, and there was indication of migration of pigment from the conjunctival pigment deposits. The severe morphologic histologic changes in the excised corneal buttons have been studied and described in detail.[n,o]

Hydroquinone and benzoquinone seem to act directly on the eyes, but the resemblence of the resultant discoloration to that seen in endogenous ochronosis has given rise to a discussion of possible respiratory and systemic routes of absorption.[s,t] The dark brown material deposited in the conjunctiva and cornea most probably is polymerized benzoquinone or hydroxyquinone.[q] Biopsy of the conjunctiva of patients has shown the pigment to be deposited as small granules in the superficial epithelium and as large granules in the basal epithelial cells. Attention has been called to the fact that the pigment is distributed in regions of the cornea and conjunctiva where fat is most common.[a]

Experimental exposure of rabbit eyes to high concentrations of *benzoquinone* vapor or direct contact with powder or concentrated solutions has caused severe reactions with conjunctivitis, corneal edema, and necrosis.[q,53] Immediately after exposure to a high concentration of *benzoquinone* vapors, a superficial brownish discoloration has been observed in the exposed surfaces of a rabbit's eye,[i] but chronic exposure of rabbits to low concentrations of *benzoquinone* vapor which were not acutely injurious has failed to induce corneal or conjunctival pigmentation or opacities like those seen in workmen.[f,q]

Application of powdered hydroquinone to rabbit eyes has induced a pigment accumulation in conjunctiva and cornea similar to that in human beings, but only when daily applications have been carried on for two to four months.[g,s,t] Earlier, gray opacification and scarring has appeared, apparently also similar to the fine gray opacities seen in the corneas of workmen. Not all rabbits developed pigmentation; the tendency to pigment formation appeared to be related to amount of exposure to light, and older animals seemed more prone to develop pigment than the younger. Pigment was deposited in albino rabbit eyes as well as in the normally pigmented.[g]

Experiments with excised bovine corneas have shown that hydroquinone can be oxidized by this tissue, presumably by cytochrome oxidase.[108] Also it has been shown that *benzoquinone* causes a loss of intercellular cohesion of the corneal epithelium upon incubation for several hours, in a manner similar to other metabolic poisons.[e]

No disturbance of the inner parts of the eye is known to have been produced by exposure to hydroquinone or benzoquinone, although experimentally *benzoquinone* has been shown to be damaging to isolated rabbit retinas at a concentration of 0.05 mM.[157]

Tests on rabbit lens surviving in culture in vitro have shown hydroquinone to have very little effect on cation transport or glycolysis of the lens, but showed *benzoquinone* to be inhibitory to both activities, despite potent antagonism to the action of *benzoquinone* by the ascorbic acid of the lens.[126]

a. Anderson B: Corneal and conjunctival pigmentation among workers engaged in manufacture of hydroquinone. *ARCH OPHTHALMOL* 38:812–826, 1947.

b. Anderson B, Oglesby F: Corneal changes from quinone-hydroquinone exposure. *ARCH OPHTHALMOL* 59:495–501, 1958.

c. Bachsetz E: Aniline injuries of the cornea. *KLIN MONATSBL AUGENHEILKD* 63:240, 1919. (German)

d. Bruckner R von: Scarring and contraction of the conjunctiva as a result of industrial injury in dyers' occupation. *OPHTHALMOLOGICA* 102:221–225, 1941. (German)

e. Buschke W: Effects of metabolic poisons and of some other agents on intercellular cohesion in corneal epithelium. *AM J OPHTHALMOL* 33:59–66, 1950.

f. Cogan DG, Grant WM: Corneal and conjunctival pigmentation in workers in hydroquinone. *ARCH OPHTHALMOL* 38:847, 1947.

g. Ferraris de Gaspare PF: Experimental studies on the keratoconjunctivitis from hydroquinone. *BOLL OCULIST* 28:361–367, 1949. (Italian)

h. Gernet H: Late sequelae of disturbances of the cornea by hydroquinone. *BULL SOC FRANC OPHTALMOL* 75:527–529, 1962. (French)

i. Koll C: Brown coloration of the cornea by chromium. *Z AUGENHEILKD* 13:220–225, 1905. (German)

j. Krahnstover M: Severe corneal and conjunctival injuries of the palpebral fissure area in hydroquinone workers. *ZENTRALBL ARBEITSMED* 1:75–78, 1951. (Abstr: *ARCH IND HYG* 5:595, 1952.)

k. Krahnstover M: Late damages to the eye with hydroquinone. *KLIN MONATSBL AUGENHEILKD* 126:340–341, 1955. (Abstr: *AM J OPHTHALMOL* 40:310, 1955.)

l. Mackinlay JG: Intense pigmentation of corneas and conjunctiva. *TRANS OPHTHALMOL SOC UK* 6:144, 1886.

m. Miller SJH: Ocular ochronosis (hydroquinone—its properties and uses). *TRANS OPHTHALMOL SOC UK* 74:349–366, 1954.

n. Naumann G: Corneal damage in hydroquinone workers. *ARCH OPHTHALMOL* 76:189–194, 1966.

o. Naumann G, Rossman H: Injuries of the cornea in hydroquinone-workers. *OPHTHALMOLOGICA ADDIT AD* 158:371–375, 1969. (German)

p. Senn A: Corneal disease from aniline dyes. *KORRESP-BL SCHWEIZ ARZ* 27:161–164, 1897. (German)

q. Sterner JH, Oglesby FL, Anderson B: Quinone vapors and their harmful effects. *J IND HYG* 29:60–73, 74–84, 1947.

r. Straub W: Disturbances of the human eye by hydroquinone. *BULL SOC FRANC OPHTALMOL* 72:231–235, 1959. (French)

s. Velhagen K: The occupational eye diseases of hydroquinone-workers. *KLIN MONATSBL AUGENHEILKD* 86:391, 1931. (German)

t. Velhagen K: Quinone discoloration in the palpebral fissure as an industrial disease in hydroquinone manufacture. *KLIN MONATSBL AUGENHEILKD* 86:739–752, 1931. (German)

Hydroxychloroquine sulfate (Plaquenil), related to chloroquine, is used in treatment of malaria, lupus erythematosus, and rheumatoid arthritis. After chloroquine was discovered to produce retinopathy, hydroxychloroquine was suspected of having the same effect, but initially this was uncertain because patients commonly had taken both drugs. Then a survey of ninety-four patients and review of the literature by Shearer and Dubois established that hydroxychloroquine, like chloroquine, could produce retinopathy and deposits in the corneal epithelium, but in much lower incidence.[h] The patients in this series had taken 800 mg a day for as long as 54 months, and only one developed retinopathy, but this was definite, with chloroquine-like bilateral bull's eye pigment disturbance and reduction of visual acuity to 20/50. This same series of patients developed corneal deposits similar to deposits from chloroquine, with an incidence of 32% at six months, and 100% at four years.

A report from a clinic in Cardiff which was established to screen rheumatology and dermatology patients receiving hydroxychloroquine has provided information on 347 patients who received this drug during the period 1969 to 1980, and had never received chloroquine.[c] The maximum daily dose of hydroxychloroquine sulfate was 600 mg, approximately 200 g per year. The most consistent abnormality found in the eyes was granularity of macular pigment with loss of foveal reflex, much like the changes found in senile macular pigmentary degeneration. This was observed in 29% of those who had received a total of 800 g or more. A mild bull's eye retinopathy was found in only 3 eyes. Visual acuity tended to be slightly poorer in those with retinopathy, but most retained normal vision. It was concluded that a total dose of 200 g was unlikely to produce retinopathy, but that a total of 800 g should not be exceeded, especially in patients who started treatment at age 40 years or older.

In another series of 99 patients receiving hydroxychloroquine, but no chloroquine, after a median length of treatment of 57 months, 65 patients were still taking the drug.[e,i] No patient took more than 400 mg hydroxychloroquine sulfate per day, and the median total was 657 g. Three had taken more than 1000 g. In the whole series of 99 patients, mild toxic effects were detected in only four, consisting of paracentral scotomas, or constricted fields to a red test object, not to a white test object. These abnormalities regressed when the drug was stopped. Corneal deposits were not found in any patient. It was concluded that 400 mg hydroxychloroquine sulfate per day presents little risk to the eyes of most patients, but eye examinations at 6-month intervals were advised.

In a group of 5 patients who had received only 200 mg daily for 1.5 to 7 years (totally 108 to 336 g) tests of vision and fields were normal, but slight abnormalities in the electroretinograms and in the appearance of the macula area after intravenous injection of fluorescein were suspected. As in the larger series, no serious abnormality was found at this dosage in these patients.[g] In 20 other patients who had received total doses mostly over 200 g, but not enough to produce clinical evidence of retinopathy or keratopathy, foveal electroretinograms were reported to be slightly, but not significantly, subnormal.[f]

In rats, very large daily doses of hydroxychloroquine have been shown to cause changes in the ERG in albino, as well as in pigmented, animals, and the effect on the ERG is enhanced by increased illumination.[a,b]

In dogs, feeding hydroxychloroquine produced no deposits in the corneas, but did cause reversible changes in the ERG and subtle changes in the appearance of the fundi.[d] There was a loss of color and brightness of the tapetum lucidum, but the behavior of the dogs did not suggest impairment of vision.

a. Legros J, Rosner I: Electroretinographic changes after administration of large doses of hydroxychloroquine. *ARCH OPHTALMOL (PARIS)* 31:165–180, 1971. (French)

b. Legros J, Rosner I, Berger C: Influence of the ambient light level on the ocular changes induced by hydroxychloroquine in the rat. *ARCH OPHTALMOL (PARIS)* 33:417–428, 1973. (French)

c. Mills PV, Beck M, Power BJ: Assessment of the retinal toxicity of hydroxychloroquine. *TRANS OPHTHALMOL SOC UK* 101:109–113, 1981.

d. Rosner I, Legros J: Experimental study of the ocular effects of two 7-chloro-4-amino-quinolines in the dog. *ARCH OPHTALMOL (PARIS)* 30:865–882, 1970. (French)

e. Rynes RI, Krohel G, et al: Ophthalmologic safety of long-term hydroxychloroquine treatment. *ARTHRITIS RHEUM* 22:832–836, 1979.

f. Sassaman FW, Cassidy JT, et al: Electroretinography in patients with connective tissue diseases treated with hydroxychloroquine. *AM J OPHTHALMOL* 70:515–523, 1970.

g. Sebastiani A, DePalma P, et al: Hydroxychloroquine retinopathy in patients with rheumatoid arthritis. *ARCH RASS ITAL OTTAL* 3:36–49, 1973. (Italian)

h. Shearer RV, Dubois EL: Ocular changes induced by long-term hyddroxychloroquine (Plaquenil) therapy. *AM J OPHTHALMOL* 64:245–252, 1967.

i. Tobin DR, Krohel GB, Rynes RI: Hydroxychloroquine. Seven year experience. *ARCH OPHTHALMOL* 100:81–83, 1982.

6-Hydroxydopamine has been shown to destroy adrenergic terminal fibers in the eye without causing the adrenergic ganglion to degenerate.[b] Chemical sympathectomy in the eye by subconjunctival injection has been utilized as an investigative therapeutic aid in glaucomatous patients.[c] In rabbits this has caused some depigmentation of the iris stroma.[a] In chick embryos adding 6-hydroxydopamine during incubation has interfered with development of the rods and cones,[e] and in goldfish intravitreal injection has been shown to destroy dopaminergic cells of the retina.[d]

a. Brini A: Hypochromia of the rabbit iris induced by 6-hydroxydopamine. *INVEST OPHTHALMOL* 12:312–313, 1973.

b. DeChamplain J: Degeneration and regrowth of adrenergic nerve fibers in the rat peripheral tissues after 6-hydroxydopamine. *CAN J PHYSIOL* 49:345–355, 1971.

c. Holland MG, Mims JL III: Anterior segment chemical sympathectomy with 6-hydroxydopamine. *INVEST OPHTHALMOL* 10:120–143, 1971.

d. Negishi K, Teranishi T, Kato S: New dopaminergic and indoleamine accumulating cells in the growth zone of goldfish retinas after neurotoxic destruction. *SCIENCE* 216:747–749, 1982.

e. Yew DT, Ho AKS, Meyer DB: Effect of 6-hydroxydopamine on retinal development in the chick. *EXPERIENTIA* 30:1320–1322, 1974.

Hydroxylamine is an alkaline, water-soluble reducing substance, an inhibitor of catalase. Local application of a 10% solution of hydroxylamine to rabbit eyes has caused moderate inflammation of the conjunctiva.[a]

On the other hand, an 8% solution of hydroxylamine hydrochloride made neutral with ammonia and dropped continuously for five minutes on a rabbit eye caused no corneal injury, although it markedly inhibited the catalase in the cornea.[79,81] The same solution dropped for thirty minutes on rabbit eyes caused extreme chemosis, mydriasis, and passage of protein into the aqueous humor. The cornea did not become opaque, but by the next day became bluish and markedly edematous.[81]

a. Binz C: *VIRCHOW ARCH PATH ANAT* 113:1, 1888.

2-Hydroxy-1-naphthyl sulfate has been examined for toxicity to the eye because it has been found in the blood of rabbits that have been fed *naphthalene,* a known cataractogenic compound. However, it has been applied as 1% eyedrops to rabbits frequently during five to six days without causing observable changes in the lenses, and injection of 50 mg intravenously has produced no abnormality of lens or retina.[a] (See also *Naphthalene.*)

a. van Heyningen R, Pirie A: The metabolism of naphthalene and its toxic effect on the eye. *BIOCHEM J* 102:842–852, 1967.

8-Hydroxyquinoline (8-quinolinol, oxyquinoline, oxine) is a chelating agent for metals, and a fungistat and antiseptic. Tests by injection of 0.01 M solution into the rabbit cornea caused very slight reaction, graded 5 on a scale of 0 to 100.[123]

Intravenous injections in rabbits caused prompt and transient proptosis associated with venous engorgement, hyperpnea, rapid pulse, and salivation. Cervical sympathectomy had no influence on the degree of proptosis.[a] This is probably not a selective ocular effect, since transient bulging of the eyes not uncommonly occurs in rabbits in association with convulsions or severe venous congestion from other causes. (See also *Quinoline derivatives,* and particularly *Clioquinol.*)

a. Miller HR, Taub H: Exophthalmos in rabbits produced by oxyquinoline sulphate. *PROC SOC EXP BIOL* 32:1207, 1935.

Hydroxystilbamidine isothionate, an antileishmanial, has affected the sensory portion of the trigeminal nerve bilaterally in seven patients, causing numbness and paresthesias, sometimes with pain, in both sides of the face in all divisions of the nerve.[a]

a. Goldstein NP, Cibilisco JA, Ruston JG: Trigeminal neuropathy and neuritis. *J AM MED ASSOC* 184:458–462, 1963.

Hygromycin B (Hygromix), an anthelmintic used in swine and poultry, has produced cataracts when fed to dogs and pigs.[a,b,c] Mature sows have developed posterior subcapsular cataracts, characterized by swelling of lens fibers, and vacuolation and globular degeneration in areas of opacity, bearing a resemblance to human posterior subcapsular cataracts. (Boars given the same diet did not develop cataracts, but this probably is explained by a much higher food intake by the sows.) Incubated rat lenses have developed similar morphologic changes and opacities in the presence of very low concentrations of hygromycin B.[a]

a. Creighton MO, Trevithick JR, et al: Modelling cortical cataractogenesis. IV. Induction by hygromycin B in vivo (swine) and in vitro (rat lens). *EXP EYE RES* 34:467–476, 1982.
b. Sanford SE, Dukes TW: Acquired bilateral cortical cataracts in mature sows. *J AM VET MED ASSOC* 173:852–853, 1979.
c. Sanford SE, Dukes TW, et al: Cortical cataracts induced by hygromycin B in swine. *AM J VET RES* 42:1534–1537, 1981.

Hyoscyamus niger (henbane) contains hyoscyamine and scopolamine. Poisoning from ingestion or chewing the leaves or seeds causes the same type of mydriasis and paralysis of accommodation as does atropine.[a,171,214]

  a. Renard, Surugue: Three cases of paralysis of accommodation associated with henbane poisoning. *ANN OCULIST (PARIS)* 179:449, 1946. (French)

Hypericum (St. John's wort) is reported by Garner in his book on veterinary toxicology to cause photosensitized dermatitis and conjunctivitis, known as *hypericism,* in animals that have eaten it. This is said to be particularly well known in New Zealand, and to be more common in cattle than sheep.[64]

Hypochlorites in the form of calcium hypochlorite, sodium hypochlorite, or potassium hypochlorite have long been employed as bleaching and disinfecting agents. (Descriptions of the actions of high concentration on the eye are to be found under the headings *Calcium hypochlorite, Chlorine, Potassium hypochlorite,* and *Sodium hypochlorite.*)

At low concentration in water all have the same effect upon the eyes. Their action is influenced principally by the pH of the solution rather than by the concentration of calcium, sodium, or potassium which may be present. Hypochlorite in low concentration most commonly contacts the eye in swimming pools, where it is the most widely employed disinfectant. Up to a concentration equivalent to 1 ppm of chlorine in water, this is not irritating to the eyes if the pH is kept higher than pH 7.2. However, at slightly lower pH a sensation of smarting and stinging of the eyes may be experienced, and slight hyperemia of the conjunctiva may result, but no injury. (See *Swimming pool water.*)

Hypochlorites react with acids to release chlorine, and react with ammonia to produce chloramines that are toxic and irritating to the eyes. (See *Hypochlorite and acid mixtures,* and *Hypochlorite and ammonia mixtures,* below.)

Hypochlorite and acid mixtures, such as a mixture of household bleach and an acid toilet bowl cleaner, can release chlorine gas into the air, causing burning sensation in eyes, nose, and throat. However, these effects are much less of a danger than pulmonary edema, which may be produced. This is illustrated by a case in which Clorox (sodium hypochlorite solution) and Sani-Flush (sodium bisulfate) were mixed in a bathtub.[a]

  a. Jones FL Jr: Chlorine poisoning from mixing household cleaners. *J AM MED ASSOC* 222:1312, 1972.

Hypochlorite and ammonia mixtures, such as a mixture of household bleach and household ammonia, can produce irritating and poisonous substances that affect the respiratory tract and eyes. As an example, a young woman closed the door of her small bathroom and cleaned the bath tub with household ammonia mixed with Clorox (a commercial hypochlorite bleach solution) and a detergent. She worked for about an hour, during which she was quite aware of the strong penetrating smell, but did not find it too disagreeable, though it made her cough. She then went to bed feeling all right. About four hours later she awoke coughing, with irritation of her respiratory tract and eyes. She found it very difficult to open her eyes, but managed to irrigate them with water before coming to the hospital, where examination showed bilateral keratitis epithelialis, which was evident as a diffuse stippling of both corneas, mostly in the palpebral fissures. This was associated with conjunctival hyperemia and much tearing. With no special treatment, the patient's eyes and respiratory irritation completely cleared by the next day.[a]

A similar case has been reported by Dunn and Ozere (1966) who described the reaction of a woman who cleaned a floor with a mixture of a hypochlorite cleaner and ammonia cleaner.[c] Within half an hour after her exposure, this patient developed burning sensation in her eyes, mouth, and throat, continuous uncontrollable coughing and flushing of the face. She too recovered within twenty-four hours. In this patient, respiratory distress was more of a problem than was involvement of the eyes. Eye examination was not described.

Other cases of poisoning by gaseous products from the reaction of hypochlorite and ammonia which have been described by Faigel and by Gellman have also stressed the irritating effects on the respiratory tract and the systemic reactions of nausea and vomiting, but have not mentioned involvement of the eyes.[d,e]

The probable chemical basis for the peculiarly irritating and noxious effects of mixing hypochlorite and ammonia solutions has been discussed by Pinkus, offering the explanation that *monochloramine* is produced, and that this is a volatile substance having sufficiently irritating effects on the eyes and respiratory tract to account for the reactions that have been observed clinically.[f] Pinkus relayed personal communications from Henderson and Pfitzer that less than 10 ppm of *monochloramine* in air would likely cause irritation of eyes and respiratory tract after a few minutes exposure, and that animal experiments had established the fact that vapors from mixtures of sodium hypochlorite and ammonium hydroxide had produced much more discomfort and respiratory embarrassment than either substance separately. Observations on the eyes of these animals were not mentioned.

A related problem is encountered in swimming pool water where chlorine or hypochlorites are used for purification. Urea in the water decomposes to ammonia, which then reacts to produce chloramines. Reaction of chlorine or hypochlorite with ammonia replaces one, two, or three of the hydrogens of ammonia with chlorine, depending upon relative concentrations and pH. The resulting chloramines are all irritating to the eyes, and may account for some of the eye irritation noted in swimming pools. Conditions influencing chloramine formation have been reviewed by Brown, pointing out that the formation of dichloramine (nitrogen dichloride) and trichloramine (nitrogen trichloride) become less as the pH is raised in the pH range 7.0 to 9.0.[b] (See also *Chlorine, Nitrogen trichloride,* and *Swimming pool water.*)

a. Aiello L: Personal communication, Sept. 1962.
b. Brown JG: A higher chlorine system is urged. *SWIMMING POOL AGE,* Aug. 1964, pp. 20–21, 41.
c. Dunn S, Ozere RL: Ammonia inhalation poisoning—household variety. *CAN MED ASSOC J* 94:401, 1966.
d. Faigel HC: Mixtures of household cleaning agents. *N ENGL J MED* 271:618, 1964.

e. Gellman V: The mixture of household bleach and ammonia. (Case report.) *MANITOBA MED REV* 46:441–442, 1966.

f. Pinkus JL: Monochloramine hazard from a mixture of household cleaning solutions. *N ENGL J MED* 272:1133, 1965.

Hypoglycemic oral agent therapy in diabetes mellitus has been reported in one clinical study to be significantly associated with formation of posterior subcapsular cataracts.[a] (The agents were not identified by name.) Whether there is cause and effect, or some other explanation for the seeming association, remains to be seen.

a. Skalka HW, Prchal JT: The effect of diabetes mellitus and diabetic therapy on cataract formation. *OPHTHALMOLOGY* 88:117–125, 1981.

Ibotenic acid a structural analog of glutamate, isolated from *Amanita muscaria* mushrooms, is a neurotoxin which on direct contact destroys nerve cells, but not axons. It probably would be toxic to the retina like glutamate, if brought into direct contact. A human being who took 20 mg orally noticed no disturbance of vision until a day later, when migraine with "one-sided visual disturbance" developed for the first time in the person's life.[a]

a. Waser PG: *The pharmacology of Amanita muscaria.* U.S. Public Health Service Publ. 1645, 1967, pp. 419–439.

Ibuprofen (Motrin, Brufen) an anti-inflammatory phenylpropionic derivative, was reported in 1971 to have caused reversible centrocecal field defects and reduced visual acuity in two patients, and a reversible "moving mosaic of colored lights in front of both eyes" in another.[b] In the next year, one patient was reported to have a drastic impairment of color vision and decrease in visual acuity, which were largely reversible on discontinuing ibuprofen.[f] Another patient on two occasions after taking ibuprofen has complained of seeing streaks shooting from lateral to central field of vision; eye examinations were normal.[h] In one case transient, promptly reversible diplopia has been reported.[a] Cortical visual evoked potentials were evaluated in a patient who had 20/50, 20/60 vision with decreased brightness of colors after taking ibuprofen for 2 months, showing decreased amplitudes and increased conduction times, but these became normal six days after the drug was stopped; vision became normal later.[d]

On the contrary, in a series of 293 patients treated during a five-year period no visual symptoms were detected that were thought attributable to the drug,[g] and in another series of 247 patients there was no evidence of toxic amblyopia or maculopathy attributable to ibuprofen.[i] A prospective study in 1975 reported no evidence of eye toxicity in 45 healthy volunteers treated for 3 months, or in 78 patients with osteoarthritis during 6 months.[e]

Ibuprofen has been a very widely used medication, and Fraunfelder has recorded that many and varied reports of suspected ocular effects have been received by his National Registry.[312] Surveying these reports, he believed that there were enough similar instance to recognize a rare but typical adverse side effect consisting of unilateral decrease in visual acuity to 20/80-20/100, with central scotoma, after one to three weeks of medication; recovery might require one to three months after stopping ibuprofen.[312]

a. Asherov J, Schoenberg A, Weinberger A: Diplopia following ibuprofen administration. *J AM MED ASSOC* 248:649, 1982.

b. Collum LMT, Bowen DI: Ocular side-effects of ibuprofen. *BR J OPHTHALMOL* 55:472–477, 1971.

c. Filipowicz M: Visual disorders following Brufen administration. *KLIN OCZNA* 46:339–340, 1976. (Polish)

d. Hamburger HA, Beckman H, Thompson R: Visual evoked potentials and ibuprofen (Motrin) toxicity. *ANN OPHTHALMOL* 16:328–329, 1984.

e. Melluish JW, Brooks CD, et al: Ibuprofen and visual function. *ARCH OPHTHALMOL* 93:781–782, 1975.

f. Palmer CAL: Toxic amblyopia from ibuprofen. *BR MED J* 3:765, 1972.

g. Thompson M: Toxic amblyopia from ibuprofen. *BR MED J* 4:550, 1972.

h. Tullio CJ: Ibuprofen-induced visual disturbances. *AM J HOSP PHARM* 38:1362, 1981.

i. Williamson J: An ophthalmic study of ibuprofen in rheumatoid conditions. *CURR MED RES OPIN* 4:128–131, 1976.

Idoxuridine (Dendrid, Herplex Liquifilm, Stoxil), an ophthalmic antiviral, has been tested for ocular toxicity by repeated application to the eyes of rabbits, with and without preliminary wounding of corneal epithelium or stroma. Most investigators have found that when part of the corneal epithelium is removed the defect is filled in as rapidly during treatment with idoxuridine as without.[c,e,g,i,o] However, application in ointment has caused delay.[j] After healing, the epithelium may temporarily be edematous, and the cell layers may be irregular.[c,i] Wounds that involve the corneal stroma, in addition to the epithelium, heal abnormally slowly and have subnormal strength in the presence of idoxuridine.[e,i,m,o,p] Evidence of cytotoxicity has been observed microscopically in cultures of corneal epithelial cells to which idoxuridine was added, and this was made worse when corticosteroids were added along with the idoxuridine, though the growth rate was not affected.[d,h]

Clinically, repeated applications of idoxuridine in treatment of herpes simplex keratitis not uncommonly cause punctate epithelial erosions and epithelial edema, and sometimes persistent epithelial defects.[b,i,l] Follicular conjunctivitis and contact dermatitis also occur.[k] Rarely, occlusion of the lacrimal puncta has caused persistent watering of the eye.[b,l] Cicatricial conjunctival disease resembling pemphigoid has been reported in 4 patients under treatment for 1 to 3.5 years.[k]

Idoxuridine has been tested for teratogenicity in animals. Although when fed to newborn rats it has caused developmental defects in the eye, cerebellum, and kidney,[n] it is reported not to be teratogenic in rats.[f] However, in rabbits it has produced fetal malformations, including exophthalmos, retinal proliferation, and abnormalities of iris and ciliary body.[a,f]

a. Alfieri G, Brovarone FV, Rolla AG: Ocular changes in newborn rabbits following idoxuridine administration to the mother during pregnancy. *ARCH RASS ITAL OTTALMOL* 3:225–234, 1973. (Italian)

b. Collum LMT, Benedict-Smith A, Hillary IB: Randomized double-blind trial of acyclovir and idoxuridine in dendritic corneal ulceration. *BR J OPHTHALMOL* 64:766–769, 1980.

c. Foster CS, Pavan-Langston D: Corneal wound healing and antiviral medication. *ARCH OPHTHALMOL* 95:2062–2067, 1977.

d. Gnadinger M: Experiments on cultures of cells from the rabbit cornea. *OPHTHAL-MOLOGICA* 152:435–443, 1966. (German)

e. Hanna C: Effect of IDU on DNA synthesis during corneal wound healing. *AM J OPHTHALMOL* 61:279–282, 1966.

f. Itoi M, Gefter JW, et al: Teratogenicities of ophthalmic drugs. *ARCH OPHTHALMOL* 93:46–51, 1975.

g. Kilp H, Walzer P, Hardke W: Influence of rate of epithelisation of the rabbit eye by eye ointments containing IDU and tromantadin. *KLIN MONATSBL AUGENHEILKD* 168:354–361, 1976. (German)

h. Krejci L, Krejcova MD: Effects of I.D.U. and corticosteroids on corneal epithelium. *CAN J OPHTHALMOL* 9:221–224, 1974.

i. Langston RHS, Pavan-Langston D, Dohlman CH: Antiviral medication and corneal wound healing. *ARCH OPHTHALMOL* 92:509–513, 1974.

j. Lass JH, Pavan-Langston D, Park NH: Aciclovir and corneal wound healing. *AM J OPHTHALMOL* 88:102–108, 1979.

k. Lass JH, Thoft RA, Dohlman CH: Idoxuridine-induced conjunctival cicatrization. *ARCH OPHTHALMOL* 101:747–750, 1983.

l. Patterson A, Jones BR: The management of ocular herpes. *TRANS OPHTHALMOL SOC UK* 87:59–84, 1967.

m. Payrau P, Dohlman CH: IDU in corneal wound healing. *AM J OPHTHALMOL* 57:999–1002, 1964.

n. Percy DH, Albert DM, Amamiya T: Ocular defects in newborn rats treated with 5-iododeoxyuridine (IUDR). *PROC SOC EXP BIOL MED* 142:1272–1276, 1973.

o. Polack FM, Rose J: The effect of 5-iodo-2-deoxyuridine (IDU) in corneal healing. *ARCH OPHTHALMOL* 71:520–530, 1964.

p. Puelhorn G, Sosath G, Thiel HJ: The effect of 5-iodo-2-deoxyuridine (IDU) and dexamethasone on corneal wound healing in the rabbit. *ACTA OPHTHALMOL* 56:40–52, 1978.

Imidazo quinazoline (7-chloro-2-methyl-5-phenylimidazoline (5.1-b)-5H-quinazoline) administered orally to beagle dogs caused invasion of the tapetum lucidum by pigment, and elevation of the retina by hemorrhage, but not blindness such as produced by *dithizone, diethyldithiocarbamate,* or *hydroxypyridinethione,* which have similar site of action.[a] Red-eyed beagle dogs and monkeys that have no tapetum lucidum were unaffected.

a. Schiavo DM: Retinopathy from administration of an imidazo quinazoline to beagles. *TOXICOL APPL PHARMACOL* 23:782–783, 1972.

Iminodipropionitrile (β,β-iminodipropionitrile; di(2-cyanoethyl) amine) has been investigated principally in connection with lathyrism, a form of spastic paraparesis with paresthesias in the feet induced in human beings by eating the seeds of *Lathyrus sativus* as the principal nourishment. It is characterized by paralysis of the extremities, particularly of the legs, rather than ocular involvement.[b,194]

There are two aspects of lathyrism, the neuronal disease already mentioned, and a non-neuronal "osteo-lathyrism" in which there are changes in collagen in experimental animals induced by several lathyrogenic chemicals.[b] Iminodipropionitrile has produced the neuronal disease as well as changes in tissue collagen in experimental animals. The neuronal abnormalities consist of interference with slow axonal transport, resulting in accumulation of material in the proximal portion of axons, causing them to swell, without injuring the ganglion cells. This process is widespread, involving brain, spinal chord, and optic nerve fibes in the retina and at the optic disc.[b]

Iminodipropionitrile administered subcutaneously to monkeys, guinea pigs, rats, rabbits, cats, dogs, and hamsters induces ocular lesions varying with the species.[i,j] In monkeys, orbital and palpebral edema are always pronounced, but retinal changes are exceptional. In guinea pigs, striking enlargement of axons of the optic nerve head have been shown.[b]

In rats, systemic poisoning has caused opacification of the cornea, exudates and hemorrhages in the anterior chamber, shallowing and disappearance of the anterior chamber, vascularization of the cornea, and perforation.[a] Changes produced in the cornea by less damaging doses have been studied chemically and histologically.[k,m] In rats, iminodipropionitrile also induces retinal angiopathy characterized by endothelial proliferation, development of microaneurysms, and deposition of periodic acid Schiff positive material in the retina, with extinction of the ERG within a few days.[c-h,l] Edema of the retina develops in association with degenerative changes in the inner and outer nuclear layers and retinal detachment. Thyroxine has been reported to have a remarkable protective action against the poisoning in rats, completely preventing all toxic effects upon the eyes.[j]

In rabbits, subcutaneous injection has caused reduction of intraocular pressure within a day, reversibly or irreversibly, depending on the dose. Later there is a gradual reduction of the ERG.[e] (Also see INDEX for page number of *Lathyrism,* and *Lathyrogens.*)

a. Forgacs J: Ocular disturbances in experimental lathyrism from iminodipropionitrile. *ARCH OPHTALMOL* (PARIS) 20:275–284, 1960. (French)

b. Griffin JW, Price DL: Proximal axonopathies induced by toxic chemicals. Chapter 11 in Spencer and Schaumburg (1980).[378]

c. Heath H, Rutter AC: Retinal angiography in the iminodipropionitrile-treated alloxan-diabetic rat. *BR J EXP PATHOL* 47:116–120, 1966.

d. Heath H, Paterson RA, Hart JCD: Changes in the hydroxyproline, hexosamine, and sialic acid of the diabetic human and β,β-iminodipropionitrile treated rat retinal vascular systems. *DIABETOLOGIA* 3:515–518, 1967.

e. Heath H, Wang MK: Changes in the intraocular pressure and the electroretinogram in the β,β-iminodipropionitrile treated rabbit. *EXP EYE RES* 7:332–334, 1968.

f. Paterson RA, Heath H: Chemical changes in human diabetic, cataractous and β,β-iminodipropionitrile-treated rat lens capsules. *EXP EYE RES* 6:233–238, 1967.

g. Paterson RA, Heath H: The effect of β,β-iminodipropionitrile treatment and alloxan diabetes on the glycosaminoglycans of the rat retina and aorta. *BIOCHIM BIOPHYS ACTA* 148:207–214, 1967.

h. Paterson RA: The effect of hydroxyethyl-substituted rutosides on the β,β-iminodipropionitrile-induced retinopathy in the rat. *BR J EXP PATH* 49:283–287, 1968.

i. Selye H: Lathyrism. *REV CAN BIOL* 16:1–82, 1957.

j. Selye H: Prevention by thyroxine of the ocular changes normally produced by β,β-iminodipropionitrile (IDNP). *AM J OPHTHALMOL* 44:763–765, 1957.

k. Takaku I, Yamashita S: Changes of the rat cornea treated by β,β-iminodipropionitrile. *BIOCHEM PATH CONNECT TISSUE* 277–287, 1974, edited by Otaka Y, Igoku Shoin Ltd. Tokyo.

l. Wang MK, Heath H: Effect of β,β-iminodipropionitrile and related compounds on the electroretinogram and the retinal vascular system of the rat. *EXP EYE RES* 7:56–61, 1968.

m. Yamashita S: Studies on the ocular changes of experimental lathyrism. *ACTA SOC OPHTHALMOL JPN* 77:834–837, 1973.

Imipramine (Imavate, Janimine, Presamine, SK–Pramine, Togranil), an anti-depressant, has atropine-like side effects, manifested in a small proportion of patients by dryness of the mouth, mydriasis, and blurring of vision from interference with accommodation.[a-d] Imipramine has been reported also to cause dysarthria, diplopia, and tremors similar to parkinsonism.[a,b]

There is potential hazard of inducing angle-closure glaucoma by mydriasis in elderly patients with small eyes and shallow anterior chambers,[210] but in patients with chronic open-angle glaucoma with iridocorneal angles of safe width, ordinary dosage of imipramine probably has no adverse effect on intraocular pressure in the presence of standard antiglaucoma treatment. (See also *Anticholinergic drugs.*)

Davidson and Fraunfelder in their national reporting systems for adverse reactions have recorded a wide variety of suspected or possible ocular side-effects, but with no clear pattern emerging other than mentioned above.[298,312]

Imipramine is one of many substances that can produce retinal lipidosis when force-fed to rats, but no clinical implication is yet evident.[348] (See INDEX for page numbers of *Lipidosis, drug induced* and *Retinal lipidosis.*)

a. English HL: Alarming side-effect of Tofranil. *LANCET* 1:1231, 1959.

b. Foster AR, Lancaster NP: Disturbance of motor function during treatment with imipramine. *BR MED J* 2:1452, 1959.

c. Garrison HF, Moffitt EM: Imipramine hydrochloride intoxication. *J AM MED ASSOC* 179:456–458, 1962.

d. Steel CM, O'Duffy J, Brown SS: Clinical effects and treatment of imipramine and amitriptyline poisoning in children. *BR MED J* 2:663–667, 1967.

Indarsol (methylindolarsinate) in tests on cats and rabbits was found to damage the retina and optic nerve in the same manner as arsanilate.[a]

a. Birch-Hirschfeld A, Inouye N: Experimental investigation of the effect of indarsol on the optic nerve and retina. *GRAEFES ARCH OPHTHALMOL* 79:81–95, 1911. (German)

Indigo (indigotin, indigo blue) is a dye which is essentially insoluble in water in its colored oxidized form, but is soluble when reduced to a colorless form. A man accidentally splashed his eyes with a 7% alkaline solution of the reduced form. The conjunctiva appeared blue several hours later; the cornea was somewhat turbid but not stained.[a] In the course of ten days the cornea cleared. Some fine blue dots were seen in the stroma and along the conjunctival blood vessels, appearing rather inert and nontoxic. On rabbit eyes indigo has been reported to be mildly toxic.[153]

a. Kramer R: Indigo blue staining of the living eye, a noteworthy dye injury. *KLIN MONATSBL AUGENHEILKD* 73:155–158, 1924. (German)

Indomethacin (Indocin, Amuno), an antiinflammatory, has been associated with a variety of rather vague ocular complaints, such as "blurred vision." However, one careful evaluation showed that while 20.4 per cent of arthritic patients receiving this drug claimed to have "blurred vision", 18.3 per cent of patients of the same type receiving a placebo reported the same symptom.[m] In another series, only 3 out of 122 had this complaint.[g] In an ophthalmologic study reported in 1968 on thirty-four patients who were taking indomethacin, six had an appearance in the cornea consisting of fine speckled opacities in the stroma resembling chloroquine keratopathy, and these disappeared when the medication was stopped.[b,c] A variety of abnormalities were described in the fundi of these same patients, including paramacular depigmentation, macula edema, central serous retinopathy, and pallor of the disc, but there was no uniform type of abnormality. A decrease in retinal sensitivity was shown by electroretinography, by measurements of dark adaptation, and by visual field tests. In some of these patients the functional abnormalities improved when the medication was discontinued. The ocular pressures were not abnormal. This was followed by controversy among those who did not find these changes in their patients and those who found some abnormalities similar to those described in the corneas or retinas of their patients.

Disagreeing was one clinical ophthalmological study in 1972 of 147 patients, among whom the most intensively treated 30 had received daily doses up to 200 mg for 6 months to 3 years, but no abnormality attributable to the drug was found.[h] Also disagreeing were the results of an investigation in 1973 in which 18 patients who had been receiving indomethacin for some time were compared with 10 un-medicated controls by electroretinography and retinal sensitivity profiles, disclosing no significant difference attributable to retinotoxic effects.[d] Differences in dosage and in measuring techniques were held out as possible grounds for negative versus positive results.[c]

Support for a belief in retinotoxic effects from indomethacin have consisted of the following. In 1972 a patient was described who had arthritis, mild myopic retinal degeneration, and had been on a low dosage of this medication for several years, showing slight changes in vision, ERG, EOG, and possible pigment disturbance in the fundi; there was some improvement after the medication was stopped.[f] The same year in a group of 18 patients who had been receiving 75 to 200 mg of indomethacin per day for 1 to 1.5 years, and who were examined after treatment was started and also after discontinuation, 3 had pigment disturbance in the macula region, 3 had abnormality of ERG or EOG, 3 had abnormal dark adaptation, and 2 had abnormal color vision; these were found to improve during a year off treatment.[l] Again in 1972, among 11 patients treated for 1.5 years with indomethacin for arthritis, 3 had defects of color vision, associated with pigment disturbance in the macula area in two; a year after discontinuing the medication, color vision became almost normal.[i] In 1978, a patient who had taken 100 g of indomethacin during 4 years was reported to have an appearance of white stippling abnormality of the retinal pigment layer and abnormal EOG.[a]

Occasional occurrence of deposits in the cornea have been more clearly substantiated, though only rarely reported since the first description.[l,n]

In rare instances, pseudotumor cerebri has been induced by indomethacin, and has caused transient papilledema and sixth nerve paralysis.[j,312]

Also rarely, hemorrhage into the vitreous body, or occlusion of the central retinal vein have been reported in patients taking indomethacin.[g,o]

Indomethacin in eyedrops applied to the eyes of rabbits have not altered the healing of experimental wounds.[e] Comprehensive clinical examinations in 10 normal people have shown no abnormality after 1% eyedrops were used 4 times a day for 2 weeks.[k]

a. Buchanan T, Archer D: Indomethacin retinopathy. *IRISH J MED SCI* 147:255–256, 1978.

b. Burns CA: Indomethacin, reduced retinal sensitivity, and corneal deposits. *AM J OPHTHALMOL* 66:825–835, 1968.

c. Burns CA: Indomethacin induced ocular toxicity. *AM J OPHTHALMOL* 76:312–313, 1973.

d. Carr RE, Siegel IM: Retinal function in patients treated with indomethacin. *AM J OPHTHALMOL* 75:302–306, 1973.

e. Hanna C, Keatts HC: Indomethacin in ocular inflammation in rabbits. *ARCH OPHTHALMOL* 77:554–558, 1967.

f. Henkes HE, van Lith GHM, Canta LR: Indomethacin retinopathy. *AM J OPHTHALMOL* 73:846–856, 1972.

g. Kelly M: Treatment of 193 rheumatic patients with indomethacin. *J AM GERIATR SOC* 14:48–55, 1966.

h. Klein G, Fellner S, Fellner R: Indomethacin in rheumatic diseases. *MED KLIN* 67:250–254, 1972. (German)

i. Koliopoulos J, Palimeris G: On acquired colour vision disturbances during treatment with ethambutol and indomethacin. *MOD PROBL OPHTHALMOL* 11:178–184, 1972.

j. Konomi H, Imai M, et al: Indomethacin causing pseudotumor cerebri in Bartter's syndrome. *N ENGL J MED* 298:855, 1978.

k. Krogh E, Henning V, Gluud B: Local application of indomethacin in healthy eyes. *ACTA OPHTHALMOL* 62:96–103, 1984.

l. Palimeris G, Koliopoulos J, Velissaropoulos P: Ocular side effects of indomethacin. *OPHTHALMOLOGICA* 164:339–353, 1972; *ADV EXP MED BIOL* 24:323–329, 1972.

m. Schindel L: Placebo-induced side effects. In Meyler L, Peck HM, (Eds.): *DRUG INDUCED DISEASES.* Amsterdam Excerpta Med Foundation 1968, vol. 3.

n. Tillmann W, Keitel L: Corneal disturbance from indomethacin (Amuno). *KLIN MONATSBL AUGENHEILKD* 170:756–759, 1977. (German)

o. Zucchini G, Vannozzi G, Capobianco W: On the possibility of eye injuries from indomethacin. *ANN OTTALMOL CLIN OCUL* 103:279–286, 1977. (Italian)

Insect parts or fragments have been described as superficial foreign bodies in or on the cornea in numerous cases, causing local ulceration until removed, but generally no toxic action has been indicated from parts other than the actual stinger.[a] The same was true of an *insect egg* located superficially in the cornea, and identified microscopically as from the order *Hemiptera.*[b]

a. Zaubereman H, Neumann E: Superficial corneal foreign bodies of organic origin. *AM J OPHTHALMOL* 60:467–469, 1965.

b. Bullock JD, Albert DM, Richman SJ: Insect egg keratitis. *AM J OPHTHALMOL* 78:339–341, 1974.

Insulin is not known to be directly toxic to the eye, though it may cause functional changes secondary to its influence on blood glucose concentration. A monkey model of diabetic retinopathy, in which there are progressive proliferative changes in retinal vessels, has been based on intravitreal injection of insulin in sensitized animals.[a] In non-sensitized rabbits it has been shown that insulin can be injected subconjunctivally and retrobulbarly without causing abnormalities recognizable by light microscopy in any part of the eye.[b]

a. Shabo AL, Maxwell DS: Insulin-induced immunogenic retinopathy resembling the retinitis proliferans of diabetes. *TRANS AM ACAD OPHTHALMOL OTOL* 81:OP497–508, 1976.
b. Polychroniadis F, Livanou T: Research concerning the effect of locally administered insulin on ocular tissues. *ANN OCULIST (PARIS)* 208:787–793, 1975. (French)

Intraocular solutions, i.e. solutions that are injected into the eye, or that are used to irrigate within the eye during ocular surgery, fall into two categories. The first category includes solutions of antimicrobials, fibrinolytics, miotics, mydriatics, and viscous substances intended to have therapeutic or protective effects. The medications or preservatives which these solutions contain may, however, have toxic effects within the eye. Descriptions of unwanted effects can be found under the names of the specific medications or preservatives. (See INDEX.)

Intraocular solutions belonging to the second category do not contain medications, but are used for postoperative replacement of the aqueous or vitreous humor, or for intraocular irrigation during vitrectomy or phacoemulsification. A considerable literature details the efforts that have been and are being made to make these solutions as nearly physiologic as possible. In general this does not involve trying to eliminate a toxic substance, but rather consists of trying to supply adequately the various substances needed for normal functioning of ocular tissues, despite the rigors imposed by surgery. To compare how well artificial solutions of varied compositions support normal functioning of ocular tissues, tests have been made on animal and human eyes *in vivo,* and on excised tissues, particularly corneas which have been either immersed or clamped in a chamber and exposed to perfusion with test solutions. Methods that have been used to compare how well the structure and function of ocular tissues hold up in the artificial environment of the test solutions have included transmission and scanning electron microscopy, specular microscopy, measurement of corneal thickness and rate of swelling, measurement of electrical resistance and cellular potentials, observation of staining with nitroblue tetrazolium, determination of lens clarity, and examination of the electroretinogram.

While most of these studies have been concerned primarily with improving the physiologic qualities of the intraocular irrigating fluids, it has been clearly pointed out that actual damage can be caused if the osmotic pressure or the pH of the solutions are made excessively abnormal. Marmor has shown that retinal detachment can be produced by intravitreal injection of hyperosmotic solutions.[d] The cornea, however, can tolerate considerable abnormality of osmotic pressure, according to Edelhauser et al.[a]

Toxic effects of abnormal pH on the corneal endothelium of rabbit and human eyes have been examined by Gonnering et al, showing that at pH 3.5 there was destruction of endothelial cells and rapid swelling of the cornea; at pH 5.5 there was less damage and slower swelling; while at pH 6.5 to 8.5 swelling was minimal, and slight morphologic abnormality was detectable only by electron microscopy.[b] Similarly, Malinverni and Bosio showed that when most of the aqueous humor in rabbits' eyes was replaced by buffer solution of varied pH (but uniform osmotic pressure), specular microscopy showed much damage of corneal endothelium at pH 3.5 and pH 9, none at pH 6 to 7.5, and intermediate degrees at intermediate pH levels.[c] Within 48 hours the corneas of the eyes with pH 9 buffer were edematous and were not transparent, but those with pH 3.5 buffer did not lose their transparency.

a. Edelhauser HF, Hanneken AM, et al: Osmotic tolerance of rabbit and human corneal endothelium. *ARCH OPHTHALMOL* 99:1281–1287, 1981.
b. Gonnering R, Edelhauser HF, et al: the pH tolerance of rabbit and human corneal endothelium. *INVEST OPHTHALMOL VIS SCI* 18:373–390, 1979.
c. Malinverni W, Bosio P: Changes in the corneal endothelium induced experimentally by introducing substances of varied pH into the anterior chamber. *BOLL OCULIST* 59:127–138, 1980. (Italian)
d. Marmor MF: Retinal detachment from hyperosmotic intravitreal injection. *INVEST OPHTHALMOL VIS SCI* 18:1237–1244, 1979.

Iodate, usually in the form of sodium iodate, has remarkable toxic effects on the retina. Ocular injury from iodate was observed in 1925 in two patients who temporarily lost vision as the result of intravenous injection of an anti-infective solution known as Septojod.[c,g] In the next few years several other patients who were given Septojod intravenously or intraperitoneally also had marked reduction of vision within twenty-four hours. Initially in some patients there appeared to be no ophthalmoscopic change, but retinal edema was evident in others. Subsequently the victims of this medication developed a disturbance of the retinal pigment epithelium resembling retinitis pigmentosa. In most patients, vision eventually improved, returning to normal in some, despite persistent disseminated pigmentation of the retina, but in the majority a central scotoma or constriction of the visual fields remained.[zc,214]

Septojod contained iodide, hypoiodite, and iodate ions.[g] In 1935 Vito established that it was the *iodate* in the mixture which was responsible for the ocular injuries.[zl] Once the toxic effect of iodate on the retina became well known, its use in patients was terminated and clinical reports ceased.

Despite the elimination of iodate as a poison to patients, interest in the mechanism of toxic actions on the retina increased, and a large number of fundamental experimental studies have been published.

Investigations of the chemical aspects of the poisoning of the retina have indicated that iodate acts directly on the eye. Injection into the carotid artery damages the retina only on the same side as the injection.[k,w] When iodate containing isotopes of iodine has been given intravenously, iodine has been found to pass into the aqueous and vitreous humors in rabbits, but iodate itself was not found.[f,x,w] Presumably in the eye iodate reacts rapidly and is reduced to iodide. Injected into the vitreous, sodium iodate causes changes in retinal histology and ERG similar to the effects after systemic administration.[y]

The toxic action of iodate in the eye appears not to be attributable simply to its oxidizing properties, since other oxidizing agents, such as *perborate* and *potassium permanganate* have been shown not to have comparable toxic effect.[ze,234] Sorsby reported that intravenous *bromate* had effects similar to iodate in rabbits,[ze] but Cima was unable to cause the characteristic changes either by means of *bromate* or *periodate*.[d]

Studies of the effect of iodate on enzymatic and metabolic processes in rabbits *in vivo* and *in vitro* have so far revealed no striking effect on respiration, glycolysis, pentosephosphate cycle, or transamination in the retina in the initial phase of poisoning,[167] though numerous enzymes have been shown to be inhibited at concentrations of iodate considerably higher than those calculated to be attained in the eyes of animals, and alterations of enzyme activities are found after degeneration of the cells is morphologically evident. No specific effect on sulfhydryl groups of retinal enzymes or other proteins has been demonstrated, though a slight transient decrease of total retinal sulfhydryl has been detected.[zf]

The electrophysiologic, histologic, and ophthalmoscopic sequence of changes in the retina after systemic administration of iodate has been described in rabbits[b,d,m,o,p,v,zb,zg,zj,zk,zl,94,167] dogs,[zm] rats,[a] and sheep.[u] It is widely agreed that the prime injury is specifically to the retinal pigment epithelium, and that other, later changes are secondary, including degeneration of rods and cones, with pigment migration and clumping. For unknown reasons, the juxtapapillary portion of the retinal pigment epithelium has a greater resistance to iodate than the rest of the pigment epithelium.[y]

Electrical activity of the eye in iodate poisoning has been extensively studied, showing rapid reduction of the corneoretinal standing potential and the c-wave of the ERG, attributable to damage to the retinal pigment epithelium.[u,x,zk,zn,zo] The a- and b-waves of the ERG show little or no change during the first hour, but as the photoreceptors degenerate secondary to the poisoning of the retinal pigment epithelium the a- and b-waves begin to disappear.[o,q,u,v,zh,zi]

Increase in permeability or "breakdown" of the blood-retina or blood-vitreous barrier is an outstanding feature of the toxic action of iodate on the retinal pigment epithelium. Protein-free fluid injected beneath the retina is absorbed much faster after the barrier properties of the RPE are destroyed by iodate.[t] Normal transport of organic anions from the vitreous humor to the blood is disrupted, and tracer substances, such as fluorescein, diffuse with abnormal ease from blood to vitreous body.[a,j,m,r,s,zb,zd] Histologically, there is marked destruction of the retinal pigment epithelium, followed by replacement with a new layer of a different sort of cell in subsequent weeks. This new layer has been variously described as leaky,[zg] or tight.[zb]

The intraocular pressure in rabbits rapidly becomes low after systemic administration of iodate, and may remain low for 10 to 14 days. Originally this was thought to be attributable to interference with formation of aqueous humor from poisoning of the ciliary body,[f] but more recent evidence shows little effect on the morphology or function of the ciliary body,[j,za] except some edema of iridial processes.[za] It seems that the hypotony may be caused by abnormal leakage of fluid from the vitreous humor through the broken-down blood-retinal barrier to the vessels of the choroid, which carries the fluid away.[zb]

Adhesion of the retina to the retinal pigment epithelium is weakened to a minimum with an hour, presumably due to rapid metabolic changes induced by iodate, before structural changes are evident.[b]

The lens remains clear and the anterior segment without inflammation from parenteral or intravitreal injections of doses of sodium iodate sufficient to cause severe damage to the retina.[z] The mitotic activity of the cells of the lens in rabbits decreases to a minimum in 3 days, but then recovers, with no residual abnormality of transparency or histology, apparently not involving a direct toxic effect of iodate on the lens, but presumably some factor such as hypoxia or abnormality of the blood-vitreous barrier.[e]

The cornea is apparently not damaged in systemic iodate poisoning, and even intracorneal injection of 0.16 M solution causes slight reaction.[123]

a. Anstadt B, Blair NP, et al: Alteration of the blood-retinal barrier by sodium iodate. *EXP EYE RES* 3:653–662, 1982.

b. Ashburn FS Jr, Pilkerton AR, et al: The effects of iodate and iodacetate on the retinal adhesion. *INVEST OPHTHALMOL VIS SCI* 19:1427–1432, 1980.

c. Auricchio G, DeVincentiis: Experimental investigations of the pathogenesis of pigmentary degenerations of the retina. *G ITAL OFTAL* 3:118–127, 1950. (Italian)

d. Babel J, Ziv B: Research on experimental retinal degenerations. *OPHTHALMOLOGICA* 132:65–75, 1956. (French)

e. Bisantis C, Broccio D, Vaccaro F: Alterations of the lens epithelium in the course of experimental chorio-retinal degenerations. *BOLL OCULIST* 52:329–336, 1973.

f. Calabria GA, Orzalesi N: The distribution of labeled sodium iodate in the rabbit after intravenous administration. *BOLL SOC ITAL BIOL SPER* 41:1153–1156, 1965.

g. Cima V: Research on the retinitis pigmentosa from iodate. *BOLL OCULIST* 28:614–620, 1949. (Italian)

h. Clifton L, Makous W: Iodate poisoning: early effect on regeneration of rhodopsin and the ERG. *VISION RES* 13:919–924, 1973.

i. Cole DF: Reduction in aqueous humor formation as caused by iodate, spirolactone, and polyphloretin phosphate. *BR J OPHTHALMOL* 46:291–303, 1962.

j. Davson H, Hollingsworth JR: The effects of iodate on the blood-vitreous barrier. *EXP EYE RES* 14:21–28, 1972.

k. DeBerardinis E, Vecchione L, Tieri O: Studies of the mechanism of the action of the sodium iodate on the rabbit retina. *ACTA OPHTHALMOL* 42:713–718, 1964.

l. DeCrecchio G, Menna F, et al: Experimental degenerative retinopathy. *ANN OTTALMOL CLIN OCUL* 103:311–322, 1977. (Italian)

m. Flage T, Ringvold A: The retinal pigment epithelium diffusion barrier in the rabbit eye after sodium iodate injection. *EXP EYE RES* 34:933–940, 1982.

n. Flage T: Changes in the juxtapapillary retinal pigment epithelium following intravenous injection of sodium iodate. *ACTA OPHTHALMOL* 61:20–28, 1983.

o. Francois J, et al: Electrophysiologic and histologic study of experimental tapetoretinal degeneration from sodium iodate. *OPHTHALMOLOGICA* 152:131–148, 1966; 152:219–240, 1966. (French)

p. Grignolo A, Orzalesi N, Calabria GA: The fine structure and the rhodopsin cycle of the rabbit retina in experimental degeneration induced by sodium iodate. *EXP EYE RES* 5:86–97, 1966.

q. Hamatsu T: Experimental studies on the effect of sodium iodate and sodium L-glutamate on the ERG and histological structure of the retina in adult rabbits. *ACTA SOC OPHTHALMOL JPN* 68:1621–1636, 1964.

r. Krupin T, Waltman SR, et al: Fluorometric studies on the blood-retinal barrier in experimental animals. *ARCH OPHTHALMOL* 100:631–634, 1982.

s. Kuwamoto K: Studies on the blood retinal barrier. *ACTA SOC OPHTHALMOL JPN* 72:1244–1252, 1968.

t. Negi A, Marmor MF: The resorption of subretinal fluid after diffuse damage to the retinal pigment epithelium. *INVEST OPHTHALMOL VIS SCI* 24:1475–1479, 1983.

u. Nilsson SEG, Knave B, Persson HE: Changes in ultrastructure and function of the sheep pigment epithelium and retina induced by sodium iodate. *ACTA OPHTHALMOL* 55:994–1043, 1977.

v. Noell WK: Experimentally induced toxic effects on structure and function of visual cells and pigment epithelium. *AM J OPHTHALMOL* 36:103, 1953.

w. Olsen KJ, Ehlers N, Schoenheyder F: Studies on the handling of retinotoxic doses of iodate in rabbits. *ACTA PHARMACOL TOXICOL* 44:241–250, 1979.

x. Orzalesi N, Calabria GA: The penetration of I^{131} labeled sodium iodate into the ocular tissues and fluids. *OPHTHALMOLOGICA* 153:229–238, 1967.

y. Orzalesi N, Calabria GA, Vittone P: The behavior of rhodopsin in the retina of rabbits treated with $NaIO_3$. *BOLL SOC ITAL BIOL SPER* 40:1679–81, 1964.

z. Ponte F, Lauricella M: The intravitreal route of administration in the study of experimental physiopathology of the retina. *ANN OTTALMOL CLIN OCUL* 94:1037–1048, 1968. (Italian)

za. Ringvold A: The effect of sodium iodate on the ciliary body/iris in rabbits. *EXP EYE RES* 27:87–100, 1978.

zb. Ringvold A, Olsen EG, Flage T: Transient breakdown of retinal pigment epithelium diffusion barrier after sodium iodate. *EXP EYE RES* 33:361–369, 1981.

zc. Roggenkamper W: Acute retinal pigment disintegration from Septojod poisoning. *KLIN MONATSBL AUGENHEILKD* 79:827–828, 1927. (German)

zd. Shimotori S: Fluorescein angiographic study of the experimental retinal degeneration with sodium iodate in rabbits. *ACTA SOC OPHTHALMOL JPN* 71:2030–2036, 1967.

ze. Sorsby A: Nature of experimental degeneration of retina. *BR J OPHTHALMOL* 25:62–65, 1941.

zf. Sorsby A, Reading HW: Experimental degeneration of the retina. *VISION RES* 4:511–514, 1964.

zg. Suyama T: Electron microscopic study on experimental retinal degeneration induced by sodium iodate injection. *ACTA SOC OPHTHALMOL JPN* 69:440–460, 1965.

zh. Tajima Y, Sato T: Studies on experimental pigmentary degeneration of the retina. *ACTA SOC OPHTHALMOL JPN* 68:1645–1655, 1964.

zi. Takase A: Studies on ERG of experimental retinal degeneration produced by $NaIO_3$. *ACTA SOC OPHTHALMOL JPN* 70:161–175, 1966.

zj. Tamaki S: The influence of sodium iodate on ERG of rats. *FOLIA OPHTHALMOL JPN* 19:566–571, 1968.

zk. Textorius O, Welinder E: Early effects of sodium iodate on the directly recorded standing potential of the eye and on the c-wave. *ACTA OPHTHALMOL* 59:359–368, 1981.

zl. Vito P: Contribution to the study of the retinal pigmentary degeneration induced by Pregl's iodized solution. *BOLL OCULIST* 14:945–959, 1935. (Italian) zm. Webster SH, Stohlman EF, Highman B: The toxicology of potassium and sodium iodates. *TOXICOL APPL PHARMACOL* 8:185–192, 1966.

zn. Welinder E, Textorius O: Early effects of sodium iodate on the slow off-effects, particularly on the h-wave and on the c-wave. *ACTA OPHTHALMOL* 60:305–312, 1982.

zo. Yoshida G: Experimental studies on the EOG of the rabbit's eyes affected with administration of sodium iodate. *ACTA SOC OPHTHALMOL JPN* 69:1249–1262, 1965.

Iodides, usually as sodium or potassium iodide, given systemically are not intrinsically toxic to the eyes. However, in individuals hypersensitive to iodide a state of *iodism* may be precipitated by small doses, and not uncommonly the lids and conjunctivae are involved. In this condition there is a watery rhinitis, lacrimation, edema of the eyelids, and conjunctival hyperemia.

A skin manifestation of delayed-type hypersensitivity to iodide, *iododerma*, may develop gradually from tender pustules or vesicles to nodular lesions; in one case there was also conjunctivitis with a tender nodule of the conjunctiva due to intense inflammatory cell infiltration.[f] Improvement was rapid when the patient stopped taking potassium iodide.

Serious involvement of the eyes in iodism or iododerma is rare, but in four patients severe keratoconjunctivitis has been reported.[c-e] In one of these there were hemorrhagic iritis and vitreous opacities, but the eyes recovered when iodides were discontinued.[c] In another there was destruction of the scleral with threatened rupture of the globes.[e]

In so-called pseudotumor of the orbit there is occasionally an exacerbation of exophthalmos shortly after very small doses of iodides by mouth. Also a rare instance of severe reaction to iodide has been reported in a case of syphilitic osteoperiostitis of the orbit resulting in acute orbital edema and exophthalmos, leading to bilateral optic atrophy.[a]

Sodium iodide injected into the vitreous in rabbits is reported not to have altered the ERG.[g]

Testing of potassium iodide on rabbit eyes by injection of 3% solution into the cornea has caused only slight reaction, graded 17 on a scale of 0 to 100.[123] Bathing the cornea with 12 M solution of sodium iodide for a minute after removal of the epithelium caused no permanent change.[h]

Long ago when dusting the eyes with calomel was practiced medically, it was observed that taking iodides by mouth simultaneously caused the eyes to become irritated, and the conjunctivae to become swollen and covered by a fine yellowish membrane, which resolved when treatment was discontinued.[b] It was supposed that irritation was caused by an iodide of mercury formed by local interaction of calomel and iodide. (Also see *Mercurous chloride.*)

a. Besso MG: On a case of acute bilateral edema of the orbit and secondary atrophy of the optic nerves from administration of potassium iodide. *RASS ITAL OTTALMOL* 6:381–401, 1937. (Italian)

b. Doljenkoff: Burn of the conjunctiva from use of iodide and of mercury. *RECUEIL OPHTALMOL* 7:634, 1885. (French)

c. Gerber M: Ocular reactions following iodide therapy. *AM J OPHTHALMOL* 43:879–881, 1957.

d. Goldberg HK: Iodism with severe ocular involvement. *AM J OPHTHALMOL* 22:65–68, 1939.

e. Inman P: Iododerma. *BR J DERMATOL* 91:709–711, 1974.

f. Kincaid MC, Green WR, et al: Iododerma of the conjunctiva and skin. *OPHTHAL-MOLOGY* 88:1216–1220, 1981.

g. Ponte F, Lauricella M: The intravitreal route of administration in study of the experimental physiopathology of the retina. *ANN OTTALMOL CLIN OCUL* 94:466–476, 1968. (Italian)

h. Cress J, Maurice DM: An attempt at a chemical treatment of myopia. *ARCH OPHTHAL-MOL* 86:692–693, 1971.

Iodine is a solid which vaporizes readily in air. Iodine vapor is irritating to the eye but causes no permanent damage in human beings. In the treatment of dendritic keratitis from herpes simplex virus, the corneas of patients have been locally exposed to air practically saturated with iodine vapor for periods of three to four minutes, resulting in brown staining of the corneal epithelium and subsequent spontaneous loss of this layer, but complete recovery in two or three days.[b] The same procedure has been applied to eyes of rabbits to remove a standard disc of epithelium in study of healing of corneal epithelium.[d,e] Tincture of iodine, swabbed on the cornea, has been employed in treatment of dendritic keratitis in patients. The epithelium dies and is sloughed off, but it is rapidly replaced.[184] Although the eye is temporarily painful and inflamed, it regularly recovers from the injury.[249] In rabbits, 2% tincture causes loss of corneal epithelial cells, but with return to normal in a week.[350] However, 7% solution of iodine causes severe damage to the corneal stroma in rabbit and squirrel monkey eyes.[330]

Injection of tincture of iodine into the vitreous humor of dogs has produced severe damage to the retina, choroid, ciliary body, and lens,[153] but in patients tincture of iodine has been applied by careful injection in treatment of detached retinas to promote adherent scarring, and in treatment of epithelial implantation cysts in the anterior chamber to cause these cysts to shrink and disappear. It was early advised that one should dilute the tincture of iodine with dilute alcohol and inject carefully into the cyst, trying to avoid leakage into the anterior chamber, particularly if the lens was present. This is said to have been effective and to have caused only moderate inflammation, with only local clouding of the cornea. If undiluted tincture was injected and leaked into the anterior chamber, it was observed to cause white opacity of the anterior lens capsule and moderate injury of the cornea.[c]

Iodine has been used in low concentration in swimming pools in the same manner as chlorine. Based on examination of swimmers exposed daily for a month, it has been reported that effective disinfectant action can be obtained with concentrations which are safe, and possibly superior to chlorine with respect to eye discomfort and irritation.[a]

a. Byrd OE, et al: Safety of iodine as a disinfectant in swimming pools. *PUBLIC HEALTH REP* 78:393–397, 1963.

b. Grant WM: An iodine vapor applicator for treatment of dendritic keratitis. *ARCH OPHTHALMOL* 48:749–751, 1952.

c. Schoeler F: On treatment of serous iris cysts. *KLIN MONATSBL AUGENHEILKD* 49:703–709, 1911. (German)

d. Moses RA, Parkinson G, Schuchardt R: A standard large wound of the corneal eplithelium in the rabbit. *INVEST OPHTHALMOL VIS SCI* 18:103–106, 1979.

e. Moses RA, Parkinson G, Schuchardt R: Healing of the corneal eplithelium after repeated iodine cautery. *ANN OPHTHALMOL* 12:630–631, 1980.

Iodoacetamide is damaging to rat and rabbit retina surviving in culture, but it has not induced retinal injury upon intravenous administration in animals.[157,231] In the anterior chamber of enucleated eyes, a low concentration of iodoacetamide inhibits glycolysis in the trabecular meshwork, but a higher concentration is required to influence (raise) facility of aqueous outflow.[a]

a. Epstein DL, Hashimoto JM, et al: Effect of iodoacetamide perfusion on outflow facility and metabolism of the trabecular meshwork. *INVEST OPHTHALMOL VIS SCI* 20:625–631, 1981.

Iodoacetic acid or **Iodoacetate,** most often as sodium iodoacetate, is toxic to essentially all parts of the eye, when either applied directly or administered systemically. Iodoacetate has been shown to be toxic to the cornea, iris, lens, ciliary body, and retina.

When applied externally to the eyes of rabbits, iodoacetate at concentrations from 0.01 M to 1 M has produced marked conjunctivitis but no injury of the cornea, providing the epithelium is intact.[101] When applied to eyes from which the corneal epithelium has been removed, or when injected into the corneal stroma, solutions from 0.001 M to 0.1 M cause severe to devastating injury.[101,123] Addition of iodoacetate to the aqueous humor causes corneal edema.[198] Injection of 0.03 mg into the stroma of excised beef corneas results in marked loosening of the epithelium after incubation for six to ten hours.[107]

Iodoacetate injected intravenously in rabbits or cats causes almost immediate drop in the electric action potentials of the retina, owing to injury of the visual cells.[d,w] It also causes proteins and cells to appear in the aqueous humor two to three days later, and induces cellular exudation into the vitreous body in five days. Intraocular pressure does not fall immediately, but is reduced after two to three days, and returns to normal in five to seven days.[j] Histologic changes are observable in the corneal endothelium and ciliary epithelium.[j] Mitosis of lens epithelium is inhibited after two days, but after a single dose may recover by sixteen days. In subsequent months posterior cortical cataracts resembling those produced by radiation usually develop.[i,j,zd] Also the iris, ciliary body, and choroid become atrophic and fibrosed. The outer layers of the retina and pigment epithelium degenerate.[i]

Cataract produced by iodoacetate in rabbits has been studied by systemic administration and by direct injection into the anterior chamber of the eye. Injection into the anterior chamber caused severe damage to the cornea and iris as well as cataract.[zk] Some have thought that iodoacetate acted directly on the lens. Others have thought that opacification in the lens was secondary to changes in the retina.[zg]

There is evidence from studies on rabbit lens *in vitro* that iodoacetate inhibits glycolysis, and thereby stops active transport of sodium, potassium and calcium.[zl]

Although the effects of systemically administered iodoacetate on the eye resemble the effects of ionizing radiation, differences have been pointed out.[q]

Retinal injury by iodoacetate has been produced in experimental animals by intravenous, intracarotid, and intravitreal injections. Also retinal poisoning has been demonstrated and studied *in vitro*. Reviews of experimental work on retinal degeneration in animals have been provided by Karli and by Meier-Ruge and Werthemann.[133,167]

Intravenous administration of sodium iodoacetate to rabbits causes the retina to appear grayish and edematous the next day; this appearance persists for about a week, at which time the retinal pigment appears to be clumped.[d] Lesions of the outer segments of the rods in rabbit retinas are apparent by electron microscopy as early as three hours after administration of iodoacetate, and the changes are marked after six hours. The cones are more resistant to damage.[s] The earliest ultrastructural changes may be seen in the Muller cells.[f] The DNA of retinal cells has been shown to be altered even while the ERG and morphology was still normal.[z] The cone cells of ground squirrels have shown disruption of cyclic nucleotide metabolism prior to morphological abnormality.[zk]

Intracarotid injections produce toxic effects on the eye on the same side, with doses of considerably smaller size, producing less systemic toxicity than if given in the general circulation.[o,zf] The ERG on the same side disappears in a few minutes after the injection. The effects on the retina otherwise appear to be the same as after intravenous injection.

Intravitreal injection of iodoacetate in rabbits rapidly affects the ERG, as by other routes of administration, but in still lower dosage.[h,za] However, when injected into the vitreous body, iodoacetate causes histologic changes in the ganglion and bipolar cells before the outer layers of the retina, presumably because of proximity to the vitreous.[za]

Excised or isolated rabbit retina has been shown by several investigators to be directly poisoned by iodoacetate, abolishing the ERG and causing selective destruction of rod cells at low concentrations.[99,119,158]

The histology and histochemistry of iodoacetate retinopathy in rabbits has received increasing attention by investigators interested in determining the site and nature of the earliest points of attack of the poison.[a,e,g,k,u,y,zi,94] Vanysek and colleagues have provided evidence that iodoacetate is selectively more injurious to the rods than to the cones.[zh] Francois and associates, examining both the ERG and EOG, have also interpreted these as indicating selective toxic effect of iodoacetate on retinal receptors.[n]

Very early signs of degeneration have been observed as swelling of the mitochondria in the inner segment of the visual cells.[94] Some of the decreases in enzyme activity have been observed to develop after morphologic changes are evident.[g] It has been postulated that alteration of membrane permeability of visual cells may be a primary action preceding enzyme inhibition.

Adhesion of the retina to the retinal pigment epithelium becomes reduced 8 to 12 hours after exposure to iodoacetate, at a time when structural changes in the photoreceptor outer segments are appearing.[zb]

Studies with special attention to the influence of iodoacetate on the retinal blood vessels and the water content of the retina have substantiated that poisoning with this substance causes the retina to become edematous and causes closure of the vessels.[c,p] Degeneration of retinal vessels has been studied both in flat digested preparations and fluorescence angiograms, demonstrating onset of vessel changes to be among the secondary phenomena.[k,r]

The optic nerve does not escape the toxic action of iodoacetate, according to findings of reduced phosphorous metabolism reported by Maruyama.[t]

The retina has an unusually high affinity for systemically administered iodoacetate compared to other tissues, but the significance in the mechanism of poisoning remains to be elucidated.[y]

Metabolic studies on the retina subjected to poisoning by iodoacetate *in vivo* and *in vitro* have shown this substance to have high antiglycolytic action and moderate antirespiratory action.[v] In rat retina from animals with inherited retinal degeneration, glycolysis is inhibited more readily than in retina from normal animals.[zb] Apparently, the toxic effect of iodoacetate on the retina is not attributable to a general thiol poisoning, since investigation of numerous other known thiol poisons has shown only *bromoacetate* to have similar effects on the retina.[231] Retinal sulfhydryl groups have been reported by Reading and Sorsby to increase after damage to the retina by iodoacetate, and they have postulated that this may represent a denaturing effect of the poison on some specific protein.[207]

Sodium iodate, which has also been much studied for its effect on the retina, has notably different action from iodoacetate. Iodoacetate given systemically almost immediately reduces or abolishes the ERG response to illumination, while the steady potential across the eye may remain unchanged. *Iodate* on the other hand causes only slight change in the ERG within the first few hours after injection, but causes a rapid decline in the steady potential of the eye.[x]

a. Anton M: A few remarks on the histological picture of experimental pigmentary degeneration. *SCR MED FAC MED BRUN* 41:123–128, 1968.

b. Ashburn FS Jr, Pilkerton AR, et al: The effects of iodate and iodoacetate on the retinal adhesion. *INVEST OPHTHALMOL VIS SCI* 19:1427–1432, 1980.

c. Ashton N: Retinal vascularization in health and disease. *AM J OPHTHALMOL* 44:7–17, 1957.

d. Babel J, Englert U: Early alterations of retinal ultrastructures in experimental degenerations. *OPHTHALMOLOGICA* 156:286, 1968. (French)

e. Babel J, Stangos N: Attempt at correlation of electroretinography with retinal ultrastructure. *ARCH OPHTALMOL (PARIS)* 33:297–312, 1973. (French)

f. Babel J, Ziv B: Researches on experimental degenerations. *OPHTHALMOLOGICA* 132:65–75, 1956. (French)

g. Birrer L: On histochemistry of sodium iodate and sodium iodoacetate retinopathy. *OPHTHALMOLOGICA* 160:176–194, 1970. (German)

h. Bock J, Bornschein H, Hommer K: Experimental investigations of a transvitreal influence on the electroretinogram. *DOC OPHTHALMOL* 16:35–52, 1962. (German)

i. Cibis PA, Noell WK: Iodoacetic acid cataract. *AM J OPHTHALMOL* 40:379–382, 1955.

j. Cibis PA, et al: Ocular lesions produced by iodoacetate. *ARCH OPHTHALMOL* 57:509–519, 1957.

k. Dantzker DR, Gerstein DD: Retinal vascular changes following toxic effects on visual cells and pigment epithelium. *ARCH OPHTHALMOL* 81:106–114, 1969.

l. Delamere NA, Paterson CA: Lens permeability changes associated with metabolic inhibition by iodoacetate. *EXP EYE RES* 34:797–802, 1982.

m. Farber DB, Souza DW, Chase DG: Cone visual cell degeneration in ground squirrel retina. *INVEST OPHTHALMOL VIS SCI* 24:1236–1249, 1983.

n. Francois J, Jonsas C, deRouck A: Experimental study on the effect of sodium iodoacetate on the electroretinogram and the electro-oculogram of the rabbit. *ANN OCULIST (PARIS)* 202:637–642, 1969. (French)

o. Gaipa M, et al: Studies on the metabolism and function of the visual cells. *VISION RES* 3:285–288, 1963. (French)

p. Graymore C: Swelling of the rat retina induced by metabolic inhibition. *BR J OPHTHALMOL* 42:348–354, 1958.

q. Hong SM, Cibis PA, Constant M: Effects of iodoacetic acid on ocular inflammatory responses. *ARCH OPHTHALMOL* 58:632–640, 1957.

r. Kuwamoto K: Studies on the blood-retinal barrier. *ACTA SOC OPHTHALMOL JPN* 73:659–665, 1969.

s. Lasansky A, DeRobertis E: Submicroscopic changes in visual cells of the rabbit induced by iodoacetate. *J BIOPHYS BIOCHEM CYTOL* 5:245–250, 1959.

t. Maruyama K: Experimental studies on phosphorus metabolism in the retina and optic nerve using radioisotope P^{32}. *ACTA SOC OPHTHALMOL JPN* 70:1622–1630, 1966.

u. Matsuo N: Studies on the elementary particles of the lamella of the visual cell outer segments. *ACTA SOC OPHTHALMOL JPN* 71:1380–1390, 1967.

v. Newhouse JP, Lucas DR: Effects of parenteral iodoacetate and other thiol reagents on the rabbit retina. *BR J OPHTHALMOL* 43:528–539, 1959.

w. Noell WK: Electrophysiologic study of the retina during metabolic impairment. *AM J OPHTHALMOL* 35:127–133, 1952.

x. Noell WK: Experimentally induced toxic effects on structure and function of visual cells and pigment epithelium. *AM J OPHTHALMOL* 36:103, 1953.

y. Orzalesi N, Calabria GA, Grignolo A: Experimental degeneration of the rabbit retina induced by iodoacetic acid. *EXP EYE RES* 9:246–253, 1970.

z. Pautler EL, Wheeler KT, et al: The effect of iodoacetate on the retinal cell DNA in rabbit. *EXP EYE RES* 14:183–188, 1972.

za. Ponte F, Lauricella M: The intravitreal route of administration in study of the physiopathology of the retina. *ANN OTTALMOL CLIN OCUL* 94:477–489, 1968. (Italian)

zb. Ponte F, Lauricella M, Auricchio G: Iodoacetic acid influence on the aerobic glycolysis in surviving retinae of normal rats and of carriers of inherited retinal degeneration. *OPHTHALMOLOGICA* 168:475–480, 1974.

zc. Proeger TS, Dawson WW: Iodoacetate poisoning in fish retinas with broadly distributed cones. *PHYSIOL ZOOL* 48:130–141, 1975.

zd. Ricci A: Further researches on experimental iodoacetic acid cataracts. *ARCH OTTALMOL* 61:411–431, 1957.

ze. Schubert G, Bornschein H: A reflex action property of iodoacetate miosis. *EXPERIENTIA* 14:149–151, 1958.

zf. Tieri O, et al: Studies on the metabolism and function of visual cells. *VISION RES* 2:373–382, 1962. (French)

zg. Tieri O, Vecchione L: Monolateral cataract provoked with iodoacetic acid. *ACTA OPHTHALMOL* 41:205–211, 1963.

zh. Vanysek J, et al: *SCR MED FAC MED BRUN* 41:69–78, 79–87, 89–102, 103–108, 109–114, 117–121, 1968. (*CHEM ABSTR* 70:56189–56191, 1970.)

zi. Vrabec F, Bolkova A: Changes in the rabbit's retina. *CS OFTAL* 25:10–14, 1969.

zk. Vsevolodov EB, Golichenkov VA, Popov VV: Pathogenesis of iodoacetate cataract and its similarity to radiation cataract. *VESTN MOSK UNIV SERIYA VI VIOLOGIYA, POCHVOVEDEMIE* 19:3, 1964. (*FED PRO TRANS (SUPPL)* 25:II:T111–T117, 1966.)

Iodoform; triiodomethane, formerly was employed as a topical and intravitreal antiseptic. Systemic intoxication and visual disturbances resulted from absorption of excessive amounts applied to wounds or abscesses, or from ingestion of large quantities, but not from application to the eye. Numerous cases of visual disturbance were reported early in the present century, but probably none has been observed since then.

Most characteristically vision was impaired by retrobulbar neuritis with accompanying central scotoma. In rare instances transitory complete blindness occurred. In some cases the bulbar portion of the optic nerve was involved, with neuroretinitis and occasional retinal hemorrhages. As a rule, recovery was slow, requiring many months. In most cases vision was completely or partially recovered, but residual pallor of the temporal part of the optic nervehead was common. Exceptionally the whole nervehead became atrophic and white and little vision was recovered.[153,247]

Iodoquinol (diiodohydroxyquinoline, Diodoquin, Ioquin, Quinadome, Yodoxin), an anti-amebic, has caused bilateral optic atrophy in several young children.[a-e,g,h] Iodoquinol was used in treating children with "acrodermatitis enteropathica" before administration of zinc was discovered to be the specific, far more effective treatment. In the first suspected case, a young boy treated with 3.2 g per day for more than two years had obvious deterioration of vision, some improvement when the dosage was reduced, and deterioration when the dose was again raised. He was found to have pallor of the optic nerveheads, edema and pigmentary degeneration of the retinas, vision 20/200 in each eye, and nystagmus.[b] Others treated for the same disease early in life with dosage of approximately 1.5 g per day similarly developed bilateral optic atrophy.[d,e]

A diagnosis of acrodermatitis enteropathica was not essential for optic nerve involvement, since several children treated for non-specific diarrhea with iodoquinol also had severe permanent loss of vision and optic atrophy.[a,c,g,h] Some had received daily dosage of 2 to 3 g for a year or two before loss of vision became obvious,[a,c] but others had severe permanent loss in 8 to 22 weeks on 2 g daily.[a,g,h] In some cases the only abnormality noted in the fundi was pallor of the optic discs,[d,e,g,h] but in one child with vision reduced to finger counting in one eye, and to nil in the other, there has been described generalized fine granular irregularity of the retinal pigment epithelium, narrowing of retinal arterioles, with the electroretinogram markedly reduced in one eye, nil in the other.[c]

Similar loss of vision has been caused by chemically related drugs, *broxyquinoline* and *clioquinol.*[294] (See the INDEX for page numbers.) Symptoms of peripheral neuropathy consisting of dysesthesia and weakness have been reported in some of these cases along with the optic neuropathy.[294]

Fine linear subepithelial corneal opacities have been described, but it was unsure whether to attribute them to acrodermatitis enteropathica, or to iodoquinol.[f]

a. Behrens MM: Optic atrophy in children after diiodohydroxyquin therapy. *J AM MED ASSOC* 228:693–694, 1974.

b. Etheridge JE Jr, Stewart GT: Treating acrodermatitis enteropathica. *LANCET* 1:261–262, 1966.

c. Fleisher DI, Hepler RS, Landau JW: Blindness during diiodohydroxyquin (Diodoquin) therapy. *PEDIATRICS* 54:106–108, 1974.

d. Hache JC, Woillez M, et al: Optic neuritis from the iodoquinolines. *BULL SOC OPHTALMOL FRANCE* 73:501–503, 1973.

e. Idriss ZH, Der Kakoustian VM: Acrodermatitis enteropathica. *CLIN PEDIATR* 12:393, 1973.

f. Matta CS, Felker GV, Ide CH: Eye manifestations in acrodermatitis enteropathica. *ARCH OPHTHALMOL* 93:140–142, 1975.

g. Pittman FE, Westphal MC: S.M.O.N. and inflammation of the colon. *LANCET* 2:566, 1973.

h. Pittman FE, Westphal MC: Optic atrophy following treatment with diiodohydroxyquin. *PEDIATRICS* 54:81–83, 1974.

o-Iodosobenzoate has been found not to be toxic to the retina in animals when given intravenously in sublethal doses, although at 0.05 mM concentration it is injurious to retinas surviving *in vitro*.[157,231]

α-Iodotoluene (benzyl iodide) resembles α-bromotoluene, but is more irritating and lacrimogenic. It was at one time used as a tear gas. A concentration of 3 ppm of vapor in air is unbearable for more than a minute.[61]

Ipecac (ipecacuanha) is a dried and powdered plant material which has been employed medically as an emetic and formerly in treatment of amoebic dysentery. Its most active alkaloid is *emetine*. Individuals exposed to ipecac dust, or malingerers who apply it to the conjunctival sac, have little immediate discomfort, but in the course of half an hour develop burning and smarting sensation which becomes intense and is accompanied by much tearing, photophobia, blurring of vision, conjunctival hyperemia, miosis, and roughness of the corneal surface due to injury of the corneal epithelium. Recovery is gradual and spontaneous in the course of several days.[46,153,253] Particles of ipecac have distinctive microscopic appearance which permits their identification in the conjunctival sac when malingering is suspected.[a]

Emetine is probably responsible for most of the irritant effect of ipecac on the eyes. (Also see INDEX for *Emetine*).

a. Cosse, Delord: Conjunctivitis provoked by powdered ipecac, pepper, and tobacco. Microscopic diagnosis. *ANN OCULIST (PARIS)* 153–162, 1917. (French)

Iprindole (Tertran), an antidepressant, is one of numerous amphiphilic cationic drugs that induce generalized lipidosis with characteristic cytoplasmic lamellated inclusions. In rats, high doses have caused conspicuous inclusions in the lens, with subcapsular and sutural opacities attributable to the light-scattering effect of the inclusions.[303] Also in rats, cytoplasmic inclusions in the retinal pigment epithelial cells have caused a doubling in height of these cells, and this was reversible on stopping the drug.[348] The retinal ganglion cells also accumulated numerous inclusions, reversibly. What the functional or clinical significance may be remains to be seen.

Iron metal and **Iron compounds** have important toxic actions upon the eye. These have been studied for more than a century, and have been the subject of an extensive literature. An alphabetic bibliography which is to be found at the end of the present synopsis represents an important portion of this literature, but not all. Early reports of historical interest have been reviewed by Ballantyne, and are not included here.

The present synopsis of effects of iron on the eye is organized as follows:
1. Clinical observations on iron foreign bodies.
2. Diagnosis and evaluation of iron foreign bodies.
3. Clinical histopathology of intraocular iron from foreign bodies or blood.
4. Animal experiments on effects of iron on the posterior segment.
5. Chemical mechanism for toxicity of iron to vitreous body and retina.
6. Medical treatment of intraocular iron.
7. Iron and iron compounds outside of the eye.
8. Systemic iron.

The terms "siderosis" or "siderosis bulbi" are customary to describe impregnation of eye tissues with iron. "Direct siderosis" indicates impregnation of tissues in close contact with iron-containing foreign body. "Indirect siderosis" indicates impregnation of tissues with iron at a distance from a foreign body. "Hemosiderosis" designates iron deposition in the form of hemosiderin derived from break-down of hemoglobin from intraocular hemorrhage.

1. Clinical observations on iron foreign bodies

Fragments of metallic iron or steel that can rust are notorious for producing ocular siderosis. By contrast, fragments of so-called stainless or inoxidizable steel that do not rust have little tendency to produce siderosis, and are much better tolerated (Ballantyne; Dollfuss).

The extent and intensity of the spread of siderosis is influenced by the site of the foreign body. Iron particles in the cornea or sclera principally have local effects. Particles in the anterior chamber may slowly rust and slowly be washed away by the flow of aqueous humor, causing siderosis only in the anterior chamber.[253] In the lens, metallic iron causes lenticular siderosis, but may have little effect on the posterior portions of the eye (Wolter). The most widespread and serious spread of iron comes from particles in the posterior part of the globe, in the vitreous humor, or in the neighborhood of the ciliary body. The larger the particle and the less encapsulated by dense tissue, the more rapid and extensive the siderosis. The rate at which siderosis develops varies greatly, but signs are usually evident within a few weeks or months. In some cases iron foreign bodies are so small or so unreactive that no significant toxic effects develops over many years.

In the cornea, iron particles very rapidly produce a "rust ring" staining the immediately surrounding cornea the color of rust. This is often associated with irritation and discomfort, hyperemia of the conjunctiva, and inflammatory cells in the anterior chamber. Rust rings have been reproduced experimentally by implanting iron particles in the corneas of guinea pigs and rabbits (Kyung Hwan; Thiel; Zuckerman). In these animals, softening of the cornea about the rust ring, such as is noted to occur in patients in a day or two, was found to be attributable to infiltration of phagocytic leukocytes (Kyung Hwan; Zuckerman). Iron tends not to persist for long in the cornea, as shown by old unsuccessful attempts to tatoo the cornea with ferric hydrate.[199] Corneal rust rings, if not removed mechanically or surgically, are usually absorbed or sloughed off as a result of phagocytic reaction and softening of surrounding cornea. Disappearance of superficial rust rings from the cornea can be hastened by applying deferoxamine, a chelating agent, several times a day as eyedrops or 10% ophthalmic ointment (Cornand; Galin; Harris; North; Valvo).

Ocular siderosis from intraocular iron foreign bodies have the following clinical characteristics. The cornea is seldom discolored by iron from within the eye, though staining with iron-containing products from intraocular hemorrhage is well known. When iron does enter the cornea from the anterior chamber, it is seen as rust-brown dots in the stroma. The iris readily becomes discolored, and this provides one of the earliest and commonest signs of siderosis. Blue irides become yellowish-green to brown, and the pattern of the iris stroma may become indistinct (Cleasby). Discoloration of the iris may remain for years after a foreign body is extracted, but in some cases the color has gradually returned to normal (Gnad; Verin; Welch).[253] Siderosis of the iris commonly causes the pupil to be larger than normal, with poor reaction to light, accommodation, or atropine. This is attributed to impregnation of the iris muscles with iron.[253] Sometimes the pupil gradually recovers normal size and reactivity after removal of a piece of iron from the eye (Francois).

The lens develops a special type of discoloration either from a particle of iron embedded in it, or indirectly from iron in the posterior segment. If the foreign particle has entered the lens, the lens usually becomes cataractous and develops yellowish-brownish discoloration in the neighborhood of the piece of iron; small round dots of the same color are arranged in a ring under the anterior lens capsule (Cleasby). Early, many fine brown dots may be seen immediately beneath the anterior lens capsule by slit-lamp biomicroscope, each dot being a discolored lens epithelial cell (Koby). Later, an accumulation and fusion of brown dots forms a rust-colored subcapsular ring or wreath close to the pupillary margin (Hamai; Pau).[253] Fluorescence has been reported to be reduced in siderotic lenses, but present in normal or ordinary cataractous lenses (Haruta).

The vitreous body in siderosis bulbi tends to become liquified (by mechanisms to be discussed) and to contain floating opacities, but in some cases the vitreous body develops membranes and becomes contracted. Eventually this may lead to retinal detachment, but this does not occur so readily in human eyes as has been found experimentally in rabbits.[150,253]

Although good visual acuity may be retained for a long time in the presence of intraocular iron, the retina is subject to severe injury and eventual destruction from the toxic action of iron, even in cases where the foreign body appears to be causing no irritation. Clinically it has long been recognized that in ocular siderosis there may be a gradual decrease in visual acuity, ending ultimately in blindness. The time of onset of retinal degeneration varies greatly but may occur within months, and can lead to blindness in one or two years. Earlier the visual field may be found constricted, and a proliferation of peripheral pigment epithelium may be observed similar to that of retinitis pigmentosa (Karpe).[253] In exceptional cases the macula of the retina may be injured early and irreversibly, and by ophthalmoscope there may be fine irregular pigmentation and loss of macular reflex.[253]

Glaucoma occurs in some cases of ocular siderosis, but its incidence is uncertain. Jess found only four cases in the literature up to 1924. In three of these four cases the glaucoma developed sixteen to twenty years after entrance of an iron foreign body into the eye. However, a report by Woillez in 1961 on forty cases of siderosis recorded a diagnosis of glaucoma in fourteen cases (35%). In these cases the diagnosis of siderosis and glaucoma appear to have been well established. In all fourteen cases the iron foreign body was in the posterior segment or in the lens, not in the anterior chamber in any case, and it had been present for one to twenty years. The intraocular pressure in most instances was around 50 mm Hg. The glaucoma tended to be chronic and to be unresponsive to the usual medical treatments for glaucoma, except carbonic anhydrase inhibitors, which were helpful. Gonioscopy showed the angles generally to be open, although in some eyes there were peripheral anterior synechias, which were noted postoperatively, but no statement was made on how extensive. In the angle of the anterior chamber on the root of the iris and on the trabecular meshwork were described little tufts or fine disseminated pigment that was interpreted as a siderotic deposit, but this did not seem to be very impressive and was mainly in the dependent portion of the angle. The mechanism of the glaucoma in these cases was not elucidated, and no clear conclusion was given whether the initial physical trauma, attempts to remove the foreign body, or the siderosis itself was of principal importance in causing the glaucoma. In eyes enucleated because of siderosis, Ballantyne found a history of elevated pressure in 3 out of 20, and Yamashita obtained such a history in 6 out of 15.

Occasional additional cases of glaucoma have been reported associated with siderosis from intraocular foreign bodies, generally similar to those described by Woillez (Anderson; Appel; Brasnu; Hochart; Kearns). Typically the anterior chamber angles have been open, and occasionally pigmentation or darker coloration of the angle than in the contralateral eye has been mentioned. Histologically, nothing distinctive has been described in the aqueous outflow system other than a common presence of iron-containing macrophages in the trabecular meshwork, but these have also been present in non-glaucomatous eyes, and are found widely distributed in siderotic eyes (Appel; Ballantyne; Brasnu; Yamashita). Besides the possibility of obstruction of aqueous outflow by the macrophages or by degeneration of trabecular endothelium, the possibility has been considered that iron complexes of intertrabecular mucopolysaccharides might interfere with aqueous outflow (Yamashita).

Elevation of intraocular pressure has been induced in rabbits by injection of a suspension of iron hydroxide or saccharated iron oxide into the anterior chamber (Erdmann; Yamashita), or by putting iron filings in the vitreous humor (Wise), but the conditions produced may have been quite different from those leading to glaucoma in clinical siderosis.

2. Diagnosis and evaluation of iron foreign bodies

Diagnosis of iron intraocular foreign body has usually been based on x-ray demonstration of an opaque foreign body and by establishing that the foreign body can be made to move with a magnet, but in some instances either one or both of these diagnostic measures are inconclusive, yet clinical findings suggestive of siderosis indicate that there may be an intraocular iron foreign body. To help establish the diagnosis, analysis of the aqueous humor for iron, to detect an abnormally high content, has proven useful in a few cases (Baron; Chechan; Francois; Leuenberger). Also as a help in diagnosis, particularly in eyes in which surgery for cataract is required, histologic staining of an excised piece of iris or analysis of the lens for iron has been helpful diagnostically. However, to make a definite diagnosis on the basis of histologic examination it is essential to rule out hemosiderosis, which can be produced by persistent intraocular hemorrhage, because the histologic findings and iron staining are indistinguishable in these two conditions (Calmettes).

Evaluation of how much toxic effect is being produced by intraocular iron may be important in weighing the risks of surgical and medical treatment against the danger of loss of vision from toxic action, particularly on the retina. For this reason, the ERG has received great attention in siderosis, with numerous case reports indicating that the ERG provides a valuable means for early diagnosis of toxic effects of iron on the retina. Abnormalities of the ERG may be detectable before abnormalities of vision and before other clinical signs of siderosis, though in some cases clinical signs of siderosis may be detected at about the same time as abnormality of the ERG. The ERG can become depressed or negative even when good central vision is still present (Cibis; Cleasby).

Analysis of early receptor potentials (ERP) and ERG's has shown that typical progression, first reduction of b-wave, then a-wave, while the ERP is still normal, has suggested that the toxic action of siderosis moves outward from the vitreoretinal interface (Sieving).

A particularly noteworthy clinical study was published by Knave, giving a review with numerous references on the effects of intraocular iron (also copper and aluminum), with a clinical and electroretinographic study of sixty-eight human eyes with intraocular foreign bodies of these metals. Knave regarded the ERG as "of prime importance in the clinical dealing with all cases of retained intraocular metal particles." The ERG can be a valuable indicator of the need for treatment. If the ERG shows beginning abnormality, this is believed to indicate serious danger to vision unless the foreign body is removed. If the ERG already is very abnormal, the changes may be irreversible, even if the foreign body is removed (Calmettes; Franchino; Kozousek; Liuzzi). However, cases of good recovery have been reported after surgical extraction, with or without treatment with deferoxamine (Constantinides; Gnad; Uchino; Verin).

3. Clinical histopathology of intraocular iron from foreign bodies or blood

Cibis provided particularly noteworthy observations and reviews on the anatomic and histologic changes in siderosis. By special staining, iron is demonstrable in the retina, especially in the external limiting membrane and in perivascular tissue. It causes narrowing of the retinal blood vessels, degeneration of the internal and external nuclear layers, and proliferation of pigment epithelium. Ultimately complete degeneration of the retina, atrophy of the optic nerve, and gliosis may result. The inflammatory cellular response is slight. It appears likely that reaction of iron with perivascular tissue and components of the vitreous humor may lead to the formation of contraction bands, and to proliferation and obliteration of blood vessels on the surface of the retina, going on in some cases to retinal detachment.

The choroid and the ciliary muscle appear to be relatively protected from intraocular iron, although in severe siderosis obstruction of capillaries in the choriocapillaris has been observed. Relative freedom of the ciliary muscle from involvement is evident histologically and by the fact that accommodation is usually not affected, even when motion of the pupil has been much reduced.

After intraocular hemorrhage with long persistence of iron-containing siderin or hemosiderin granules from break-down of hemoglobin, the changes in the eye and the distribution of iron are found to the same as in siderosis from intraocular metallic iron (Cibis). This is described further under "Blood". (See INDEX for page number.)

4. Animal experiments on effects of iron on the posterior segment

Experiments on the effects of introducing iron or iron compounds into the eye have been concerned mainly with histologic and biochemical abnormalities in the retina and vitreous body. A small number of experiments have been done introducing iron via the blood stream. Toxic effects on the retina have been demonstrated from repeated systemic administration of iron to rabbits and dogs (Cibis). In most experiments, however, iron or its compounds have been introduced directly into the vitreous humor. The results and the interpretations of different investigators have been influenced by the amount and type of material introduced. The greater the amount, the more conspicuous have been the disturbances of the vitreous body, and the smaller the amount, the more selective the effect has seemed to be on the retina.

Iron fragments, iron dextran, iron oxide, iron hydroxide, or ferrous salts have been introduced into the vitreous body in experimental animals (mainly rabbits) by many investigators to study effects on histology, electroretinography, and the physical properties of the vitreous humor (Asseman; Babel; Barber; Blatt; Brunette; Burger; Burke; Declerc; Gnad; Gunderova; Hasegawa; Kumagi; Masciulli; Matsuo; Moschos; Nakano; Palimeris; Quere; Runyan; Schmidt; Watanabe; Wise; Yamashita; Yoo). Change in the ERG has generally paralleled histologic changes in the retina. Severe damage can be produced in the retina, and the vitreous humor can be caused to liquefy, or to form bands which retract and detach the retina.

An important comparison of the toxicity of metallic iron, of ferrous iron, and of ferric iron when introduced into the vitreous body was reported by Masciulli in 1972, confirmed by Gardner. Ferric chloride proved to be such less damaging to the retina and vitreous body than were ferrous chloride or iron. The latter two caused severe gross and histologic changes in the retina, especially in the photoreceptor outer segments, outer nuclear layer, and pigment epithelium, with rapid deterioration of the ERG, whereas the ferric salt caused little change. This observation fits well with subsequent explanations of the chemical basis of toxicity of iron to the eye. The chemical properties of iron and its ferrous salts in the eye have gained a new significance (Declerc).

5. Chemical mechanism for toxicity of iron to vitreous body and retina

It appears that normally respiring cells of eye tissues reduce molecular oxygen to water through intermediary steps involving superoxide radicals, hydrogen peroxide, and hydroxyl radicals. These intermediates are highly reactive, and are damaging if they are produced at a rate that is greater than the rate at which they can be detoxified by a series of protective enzymes. Experiments on vitreous humor and sodium hyaluronate have shown that addition of ferrous ions promotes liquefaction. Ferrous ions promote reduction of molecular oxygen. The hydrogen peroxide and hydroxyl radicals that result are found to depolymerize the hyaluronate and attack the collagen of the vitreous humor. This destructive effect can be prevented by the enzyme catalase, which catalyzes breakdown of hydrogen peroxide, but is not prevented by superoxide dismutase, which catalyzes conversion of superoxide ions to hydrogen peroxide (Hofmann; Schmut). Catalase and glutathione peroxidase are normally present in the vitreous humor and protect against ordinary levels of hydrogen peroxide, but when ferrous ions are added, or when ferrous ions are generated by oxidation of a metallic iron foreign body, too much of the toxic free radicals from oxygen are produced for these enzymes to handle (Hofmann).

The finding in animal experiments, already mentioned, that ferric ions are less toxic than metallic iron or ferrous ions in the eye is explained on the basis that ferric ions, being already fully oxidized, cannot promote the reduction of molecular oxygen to form toxic intermediates. However, ascorbate, which is normally present in high concentration in aqueous and vitreous humor, is believed to reduce ferric ions to ferrous ions at a sufficient rate to produce some toxic effect (Schmut).

Experiments on the retina provide evidence of injury by an excess of intermediates of reduction of molecular oxygen produced by reaction with ferrous ions. Abnormal amounts of lipoperoxides are found in exposed retinas, and there is a parallel reduction of the ERG (Hiramitsu).

6. Medical treatment of intraocular iron

In medical treatment of intraocular iron, deferoxamine, a specific chelator of iron, has received considerable attention. It is believed that deferoxamine can chelate only ionic iron or iron that is loosely bound, but that it cannot remove iron from the pigments such as siderin or hemosiderin. Wise showed experimentally in rabbits that subconjunctival injections of deferoxamine repeated every three days for months were prophylactic against siderosis from intraocular iron foreign bodies, but this treatment could not reverse established siderosis.

Declerc found slight, and Gardner very little, benefit from treatment with deferoxamine in rabbits. Clinical reports on results of treatment with deferoxamine are difficult to interpret because of the inevitable lack of controls and because some signs of siderosis are spontaneously reversible after an intraocular foreign body has been removed surgically or after a very small foreign body has completely dissolved. Several cases have been reported in which deferoxamine was given repeatedly systemically and some improvement followed (Bessiere; Chevanne; Luongo; Valvo). Decrease in discoloration of the iris has been reported in treatment of siderosis by a combination of intramuscular injections and application of 5% eye ointment for many months (Falbe-Hansen). However, there appear to have been no dramatic results.

Edetate has been evaluated in rabbits, but with slight evidence of benefit (Duntze; Gunderova). Desvignes described two patients in whom the signs of siderosis and the vision gradually improved after removal of intraocular iron foreign bodies and daily intravenous injection of calcium edetate.

7. Iron and iron compounds outside of the eye

Intraorbital implantation of small iron foreign bodies has been performed in rabbits and rats (Burch; Sinovich). Iron staining was detectible within the eyes, with some toxic effect in rats, but in rabbits no histologic evidence of damage within the eye except in the immediate vicinity of extra-scleral particles. Clinically it has generally been thought that iron foreign bodies in the orbit are not likely to produce ocular siderosis.

External contact of the eye with acidic iron salts such as the sulfate or chloride has caused transient irritation and inflammation, owing principally to their acidity. On prolonged contact with the conjunctiva they have been known to cause a local brown discoloration (Salminen).[46,249,253]

In the conjunctiva, chronic exposure to iron-containing mineral dust has produced fine dark deposits at the upper border of the tarsal plate of the upper lid. These seem to be analogous to the carbon and pigment deposits in the same location produced by chronic use of mascara (Chisholm). They appear to be innocuous.

8. Systemic iron

Ocular siderosis from systemic iron is extremely rare, but has been described in one patient after 150 blood transfusions for aplastic anemia (Cibis). In a study of the retinas of forty eyes from patients with systemic siderosis no evidence of injury was found, and deposits of hemosiderin were located mostly external to the retina in choroid and sclera (Duke). In a patient with hemochromatosis a sudden loss of vision in both eyes has been described, with rapid recovery during treatment with deferoxamine, but with no clinical evidence of siderosis bulbi (Sakic).

Another unusual patient was found to have bilateral tapetoretinal degeneration with reduced visual acuity and constricted visual fields, but normal ERG, after weekly intramuscular injections of iron-dextran and cyanocobalamine for 20 years for pernicious anemia (Syversen). However, there was no clinical evidence of systemic siderosis.

Anderson DM: Ocular siderosis; an unsuspected case. *CAN J OPHTHALMOL* 6:227–229, 1971.

Appel I, Barishak YR: Histopathologic changes in siderosis bulbi. *OPHTHALMOLOGICA* 176:205–210, 1978.

Asseman M, Marchand JM, Dupont A: New study of experimental siderosis in rabbits. *BULL SOC OPHTALMOL FRANCE* 70:582–588, 1970. (French)

Babel J: Experimental siderosis. *EXCERPTA MEDICA INTERNATIONAL CONGRESS* 222:574–582, 1970.

Ballantyne JF: Siderosis bulbi. *BR J OPHTHALMOL* 38:727–733, 1954.

Barber AN, Catsulis C, Cangelosi RJ: Studies on experimental retinitis. *BR J OPHTHALMOL* 55:91–105, 1971.

Baron A, Michel G: On two observations on siderosis. *BULL SOC OPHTALMOL FRANCE* 69:93–95, 1969. (French)

Bessiere E, Verin P, et al: On a case of ocular siderosis improved by deferoxamine. *BULL SOC OPHTALMOL FRANCE* 67:1039–1044, 1967. (French)

Blatt N: Biochemical and experimental clinical investigations on the question of tolerance of intraocular iron splinters. *GRAEFES ARCH OPHTHALMOL* 163:501–517, 1961. (German)

Brasnu C, Dufier JL, et al: Generalised ocular siderosis. *J FR OPHTALMOL* 2:747–748, 1979. (French)

Brunette JR, Wagdi S, Lafond G: Electroretinographic alterations in retinal metallosis. *CAN J OPHTHALMOL* 15:176–178, 1980.

Burch PG, Albert DM: Transcleral ocular siderosis. *AM J OPHTHALMOL* 84:90–97, 1977.

Burger PC, Klintworth GK: Experimental retinal degeneration in the rabbit produced by intraocular iron. *LAB INVEST* 30:9–19, 1974.

Burke JM, Smith JM: Retinal proliferation in response to vitreous hemoglobin or iron. *INVEST OPHTHALMOL VIS SCI* 20:582–592, 1981.

Calmettes L, Deodati F, Bec P: Biopsy of the iris in diagnosis of ocular siderosis. *BULL SOC FR OPHTALMOL* 77:413–421, 1964.

Calmettes L, Deodati F, et al: Ocular siderosis and ERG. *BULL SOC OPHTALMOL FRANCE* 65:816–819, 1965. (French)

Chechan C, Francois P, Hache JC: Application of atomic absorption spectrometry to the assay of metals in the aqueous humor. *BULL SOC OPHTALMOL FRANCE* 68:113–120, 1968. (French)

Chevanne H, Demilliere B: Trial of a new chelator of iron, deferoxamine B, in a case of ocular siderosis. *BULL SOC OPHTALMOL FRANCE* 64:810–814, 1964. (French)

Chisholm JF: Iron pigmentation of the palpebral conjunctiva. *AM J OPHTHALMOL* 33:1108–1110, 1950.

Cibis PA, Brown EB, Hong SM: Ocular effects of systemic siderosis. *AM J OPHTHALMOL* 44:158–172, 1957.

Cibis PA, Yamashita T, Rodrigues F: Clinical aspects of ocular siderosis and hemosiderosis. *ARCH OPHTHALMOL* 62:180–1887, 1959.

Cleasby GW: Siderosis iridis (photograph). *ARCH OPHTHALMOL* 75:576, 1966.

Constantinides G, Asseman R, et al: Siderosis from an intralenticular foreign body. *BULL SOC OPHTALMOL FRANCE* 71:765–766, 1971. (French)

Cornand G, Segalen D, et al: Deferoxamine in local treatment of superficial metal foreign bodies in the cornea. *ARCH OPHTALMOL (PARIS)* 34:105–114, 1974. (French)

Declerc SS, Meredith PCA, Rosenthal AR: Experimental siderosis in the rabbit. *ARCH OPHTHALMOL* 95:1051–1058, 1977.

Declerc SS: Desferrioxamine in ocular siderosis. *BR J OPHTHALMOL* 64:626–629, 1980.

Desvignes P, Haut J: Chelators in siderosis. *BULL SOC OPHTALMOL FRANCE* 62:349–351, 1962. (French)

Dollfuss AB, Borsotti J: Experimental study of tolerance of intraocular foreign bodies of stainless steel or non-magnetic alloy. *ARCH OPHTALMOL (PARIS)* 2:911–923, 1938.

Duke JR: Ocular effects of systemic siderosis in the human. *AM J OPHTHALMOL* 48:628–633, 1959.

Duntze J: On therapy of experimental siderosis bulbi. *BER DTSCH OPHTHALMOL GESELLSCH* 62:269–271, 1959. (German)

Erdmann: On experimental glaucoma with studies of glaucomatous animal eyes. *GRAEFES ARCH OPHTHALMOL* 66:325–391, 1907. (German)

Falbe-Hansen I: Treatment of ocular siderosis and haemochromatosis with desferrioxamine. *ACTA OPHTHALMOL* 44:95–99, 1966.

Franchino M: Evolution of the electroretinography of siderosis bulbi. *RASS ITAL OTTALMOL* 35:356–363, 1967. (Italian)

Francois P, Asseman R, Doise P: Four cases of mydriasis from intraocular foreign bodies. *BULL SOC OPHTALMOL FRANCE* 58:13–19, 1958. (French)

Francois P, Hache JC, Turut P: Electro-oculogram in siderosis. *BULL SOC OPHTALMOL FRANCE* 71:928–931, 1971. (French)

Galin MA, Harris LS, Papariello GJ: Nonsurgical removal of corneal rust stains. *ARCH OPHTHALMOL* 74:674–678, 1965.

Gardner HB: Deferoxamine; effects on intravitreal iron. *EXP EYE RES* 23:333–339, 1976.

Gnad HD, Nichorlis S, Fulmek R: On siderosis bulbi. *KLIN MONATSBL AUGEN-HEILKD* 166:65–68, 1975. (German)

Gnad H, Freyler H, Weiss H: Experimental siderosis bulbi. pp 64–72, in *1976 SYMPOSIUM.*[364]

Gunderova RA: Clinical and biochemical changes involving the vitreous body in the presence of iron and copper foreign bodies. *VESTN OFTALMOL* 79:21–26, 1966. (English summary)

Hamai Y, Takahashi S, et al: Electron microscopic studies of siderotic cataract. *JPN J CLIN OPHTHALMOL* 32:119–127, 1978. (English summary)

Harris LS, Galin MA, Mittag TW: Nonsurgical removal of corneal rust stains. *AM J OPHTHALMOL* 71:854–856, 1971.

Haruta C, et al: The fluorescence of the crystalline lens in siderosis bulbi. *JPN J CLIN OPHTHALMOL* 20:555–558, 1966. (English summary)

Hasegawa E: Studies on experimental retinal siderosis. *FOLIA OPHTHALMOL JPN* 20:169–177, 305–309, 421–427, 1969. (English summary)

Hiramitsu T, Majima Y, et al: Role of lipid peroxide in the induction of retinal siderosis. *ACTA OPHTHALMOL JPN* 79:1468–1473, 1975. (English summary)

Hiramitsu T, Majima Y, et al: Formation of lipoperoxide in the retina in ocular siderosis. pp 89–93 in *1976 SYMPOSIUM.*[364]

Hochart G, Asseman R, Francois P: Glaucoma from unrecognized foreign body. *BULL SOC OPHTALMOL FRANCE* 82:1309–1310, 1982. (French)

Hofmann H, Schmut O: The inability of superoxide dismutase to inhibit the depolymerization of hyaluronic acid by ferrous ions and ascorbate. *GRAEFES ARCH OPHTHALMOL* 214:181–185, 1980.

Hofmann H, Khan MAH, Schmut O: The influence of catalase and superoxide dimutase on the change in viscosity of hyaluronic acid solutions from cattle vitreous after addition of iron ions. *KLIN MONATSBL AUGENHEILKD* 182:214–217, 1983. (German)

Jess A: Glaucoma in copper impregnation of the eye. *KLIN MONATSBL AUGENHEILKD* 72:128–133, 1924. (German)

Karpe G: Early diagnosis of siderosis retinae by the use of electroretinography. *DOC OPHTHALMOL* 2:277–296, 1948.

Kearns M, McDonald R: Generalized siderosis from an iris foreign body. *AUST J OPHTHALMOL* 8:311–313, 1980.

Knave B: Electroretinography in eyes with retained intraocular metallic foreign bodies. *ACTA OPHTHALMOL* (Suppl 100), 1969.

Koby: Microscopy of the Living Eye. London, 1930.

Kozousek V: Electroretinography and electron microscopy in the metalloses. *ANN OCULIST (PARIS)* 198:694–702, 1965.

Kumagi S: The EOG and ERG in experimental retinal siderosis. *ACTA SOC OPHTHAL-MOL JPN* 71:1528–1539, 1967.

Kyung Hwan S, Saburo H: Corneal rust ring. *FOLIA OPHTHALMOL JPN* 29:187, 1978. (English summary)

Leuenberger PM: Ultrastructure of retina, ERG, and aqueous humor studies in metalloses. pp 141–149, *1976 SYMPOSIUM.*[364]

Liuzzi L: Electroretinographic aspects of siderosis bulbi. *RASS ITAL OTTALMOL* 33:209, 1964. (Italian)

Luongo E: Treatment of ocular siderosis with deferoxamine. *ANN OTTAL CLIN OCULIST* 94:518–530, 1968. (Italian)

Masciulli L, Anderson DR, Charles S: Experimental ocular siderosis in the squirrel monkey. *AM J OPHTHALMOL* 74:638–661, 1972.

Matsuo N, Hasegawa E: Histochemical and electronmicroscopical studies on retinal siderosis. *ACTA SOC OPHTHALMOL JPN* 68:1702–1717, 1964. (English summary)

Moschos M, Panagakis E, et al: Alterations of the ERG in experimental metalloses. *ARCH OPHTALMOL (PARIS)* 37:285–294, 1977. (French)

Nakano M: Studies of the cause of retinal edema due to a retained intraocular iron foreign body. *ACTA SOC OPHTHALMOL JPN* 78:760–775, 1972. (English summary)

North PJ: Treatment of corneal rust rings with desferrioxamine. *BR J OPHTHALMOL* 54:498–499, 1970.

Palimeris G, Moschos M, et al: ERG-findings in clinical and experimental metallosis. pp 127–135, *1976 SYMPOSIUM.*[364]

Pau H: Siderosis lentis. *KLIN MONATSBL AUGENHEILKD* 168:478–482, 1976.

Quere MA: Pathogenetic and therapeutic value of study of experimental siderosis. *BULL SOC OPHTALMOL FRANCE* 67:756–758, 1967. (French)

Runyan TE, Levri EA: Vitreous analysis in eyes containing copper and iron intraocular foreign bodies. *AM J OPHTHALMOL* 69:1053–1057, 1970.

Sakic D, Zlatar P: Transitory blindness in hemochromatosis. *OPHTHALMOLOGICA* 168:253–260, 1974.

Salminen L, Paasio P, Ekfors T: Epibulbar siderosis induced by iron tablets. *AM J OPHTHALMOL* 93:660–661, 1982.

Schmidt JGH, Stute A, Weber E: Electroretinographic and ophthalmoscopic findings after introducing foreign metal particles into the eye of the rat. pp 391–397, *1976 SYMPOSIUM.*[364]

Schmoeger E: Electroretinography in siderosis and chalcosis. *KLIN MONATSBL AUGENHEILKD* 128:158–166, 1956.

Schmut O, Hofmann H: Liquefaction of the vitreous body. pp 73–75, *1976 SYMPOSIUM.*[364]

Sieving PA, Fishman GA, et al: Early receptor potential measurements in human ocular siderosis. *ARCH OPHTHALMOL* 101:1716–1720, 1983.

Sinovich VA, Gudlova EV: The effect of foreign metal bodies in the orbit on the eyeball coats. *VESTN OFTALMOL* 82:10–13, 1969. (English summary)

Syversen K: Intramuscular iron therapy and tapetoretinal degeneration. *ACTA OPHTHALMOL* 57:358–361, 1979.

Thiel HJ, Puelhorn G: Clinical and morphological aspects of corneal damage after metal implantation. pp 16–19, *1976 SYMPOSIUM.*[364]

Uchino M, Hirata H: Treatment of ophthalmic siderosis. *FOLIA OPHTHALMOL JPN* 29:103–109, 1978. (English summary)

Valvo A: Desferrioxamine B in ophthalmology. *AM J OPHTHALMOL* 63:98–103, 1967.

Verin P: Latency of a large intraocular foreign body. *ARCH OPHTALMOL (PARIS)* 30:661–663, 1970. (French)

Watanabe C, Yamasowa K, et al: Studies on experimental intraocular siderosis. *JPN J CLIN OPHTHALMOL* 26:495–501, 1972. (English summary)

Welch RB: Two remarkable events in the field of intraocular foreign body. *TRANS AM OPHTHALMOL SOC* 73:187–203, 1976.

Wise JB: Treatment of siderosis bulbi, vitreous hemorrhage, and corneal blood staining with deferoxamine. *ARCH OPHTHALMOL* 75:689–707, 1966.

Woillez M, Asseman R, et al: Siderotic glaucoma. *BULL SOC FR OPHTALMOL* 74:711–728, 1961. (French)

Wolter JR: The lens as a barrier against foreign body reaction. *OPHTHALMIC SURG* 12:42–45, 1981.

Yamashita T, Becker B, Johnston G: Histologic and clinical studies of the glaucoma secondary to retained intraocular iron foreign body. *AM J OPHTHALMOL* 50:169 (abstract), 1960.

Yamashita T, Cibis P: Experimental retinitis proliferans in the rabbit. *ARCH OPHTHALMOL* 65:73–82, 1961.

Yoo JH: Responses of Muller cells of rabbit retina in experimental siderosis. *JPN J OPHTHALMOL* 20:149–158, 1976.

Zuckerman BD, Lieberman TW: Corneal rust ring. *ARCH OPHTHALMOL* 63:254–265, 1960.

Isoamyl alcohol (3-methyl-1-butanol) vapors have been found irritating to human eyes at a concentration of 150 ppm in air.[183]

Isobutyl alcohol (isobutanol), tested by application of a drop of rabbit eyes, caused moderate but probably reversible injury to the cornea.[27,226] Industrial exposure to mixed vapor of butyl acetate and isobutyl alcohol has caused vacuolar keratitis in several workers, but it is not known which of the substances was responsible.[a] (Also see *Butanol, Butyl acetate,* and *Solvent vapors.*)

    a. Busing KH (1952):—see reference under *Butyl acetate.*

Isocarboxazid (Marplan), an antidepressant has vaguely been said in reviews or synopses to cause "blurred vision" or "amblyopia", but I found no evidence in the literature of any serious effect on vision.[4] Possibly these statements originated from an article listing in a table one patient as having "blurred vision" out of fifty-one patients treated, with no comments in the text.[a]

    a. Holt JP, Wright ER, Hecker AO: Comparative clinical experience with five antidepressants. *AM J PSYCHIATR* 117-533–538, 1960.

Isocil (Bromacil, Hyvar, 5-bromo-3-isopropyl-6-methyluracil), a weed control agent, is reported when tested on rabbit eyes to cause only slight transient irritation of the conjunctiva without injury of the cornea.[70,171]

Isoniazid (isonicotinic acid hydrazid, INH) an antibacterial employed in treatment of tuberculosis, has caused various neurotoxic side effects, particularly peripheral neuritis with paresthesias and burning of the feet, more rarely optic neuritis and optic atrophy. Injury of the optic nerves has been reported in patients receiving the drug orally or intramuscularly, and in a small number who received it by intrathecal injection for tuberculous meningitis.[b,f,m] A good survey of the basic toxicology of isoniazid has been prepared by Blakemore,[a] and a review of neuro-ophthalmic aspects by Dralands.[e]

Several reports describe reduction of central vision from isoniazid administered orally in treatment of tuberculosis, but most reports are of single cases.[c,g,h,j,l,q] Fewer reports each describe two cases.[d,i,p]

The length of time to beginning loss of vision has usually been a month to several months. Rare cases in which rapid loss of vision with ocular pain has occurred within days are atypical and may represent unrelated disease, such as giant cell arteritis.[i]

Characteristically the fundi have appeared normal early in the course of loss of vision, though occasionally papilledema has been noted. In most cases vision has recovered after isoniazid was stopped,[c,g-i,p] but in some cases there has been little recovery,[d,i,q] sometimes with later development of optic atrophy.[d,q]

In some cases optic neuritis has developed when isoniazid was apparently the only antibacterial given,[c,g,i,l] but in most instances it was being administered in combination with other antibacterials, e.g. with streptomycin and aminosalicylic acid,[d,j,q] or with ethambutol.[h,p] Generally, decrease of visual acuity in these cases has been associated with central scotomas. This type of visual disturbance has been reported very rarely from streptomycin or aminosalicylic acid themselves, but not rarely from ethambutol. In three cases in which isoniazid was administered in combination with ethambutol vision did not improve much after the ethambutol was stopped but improved dramatically later when the isoniazid was stopped.[h,p] In other cases there has been recovery when isoniazid was stopped but streptomycin and aminosalicylic acid were continued.[j]

Administration of pyridoxine 25 to 100 mg daily is said to prevent peripheral neuritis from isoniazid, and this has been recommended also to prevent optic nerve disturbance,[d] but at least one instance of optic neuritis in spite of pyridoxine has been reported.[i]

The factors which seem to have increased the likelihood of optic nerve injury and other neurotoxic effects are high dosage of isoniazid, simultaneous administration of aminosalicylic acid, and malnutrition or chronic alcoholism with vitamin deficiencies. Preexisting eye disease does not appear to have been a disposing factor, since no significant evidence of ocular toxicity was found in a series of patients who were treated systemically with isoniazid for various kinds of inflammatory conditions of the eye.[k]

In rabbits isoniazid penetrates readily into the eye either following topical or systemic administration but without notable toxic effect.[k] Massive doses injected subcutaneously in rabbits have been shown to cause hemorrhages in the meninges at the base of the brain and in the region of the optic nerves, but no inflammatory or degenerative changes in the nerves themselves. Intrathecal injection of isoniazid in rabbits was more seriously damaging, and it is felt that the route of administration was a critical factor in causing optic neuritis in a series of patients who were treated by intrathecal administration of isoniazid for tuberculous meningitis.[b]

In dogs chronic feeding of isoniazid has been reported by Noel and by Tateishi to have caused no histologic abnormalities of the retina, but to have produced mild pathologic changes in the optic nerves and tracts.[o, 384] No ophthalmoscopic examinations were reported. Histologic damage was found in the brains, and in both motor and sensory nerves in these animals.[384]

Impairment of accommodation has been reported in thirty-three out of ninety-five patients receiving isoniazid in combination with other drugs, mainly streptomycin and aminosalicylic acid, tending to relate to the dosage of isoniazid. The effect on accommodation was transient and reversible.[121]

A unique case of bilateral transitory keratopathy has been reported in a patient who was hypersensitive to oral isoniazid.[n] On two occasions subepithelial brownish infiltrates in the cornea and cells in the anterior chamber were associated with slight haziness of vision, resolving completely within weeks after the drug was discontinued.

a. Blakemore WF: Isoniazid. Chapter 33 in Spencer and Schaumburg (1980).[378]
b. Boke W: Investigations into the question of optic nerve injury during treatment with INH. *BER DTSCH OPHTHALMOL GESELLSCH* 59:282–283, 1955; *GRAEFES ARCH OPHTHALMOL* 158:334–345, 1957. (German)
c. Clavel A: Retrobulbar optic neuritis in the course of treatment with isoniazid. *BULL SOC OPHTALMOL FRANCE* 61:786–787, 1961. (French)
d. Dixon GJ, Roberts GBS, Tyrrell WF: The relationship of neuropathy to the treatment of tuberculosis with isoniazid. *SCOTT MED J* 1:350–354, 1956.
e. Dralands L, Garin P: Isoniazid. Chapter 17 in Michiels (1972).[359]
f. Janssen G, Boke W: On the increase in optic nerve involvement in tuberculous meningitis under INH and streptomycin treatment. *KLIN WOCHENSCHR* 33:477–479, 1955. (German)
g. Kalinowski SZ, Lloyd TW, Moyes EN: Complications in the chemotherapy of tuberculosis. *AM REV RESP DIS* 83:359–371, 1961.
h. Karmon G, Savir H, et al: Bilateral optic neuropathy due to combined ethambutol and isoniazid treatment. *ANN OPHTHALMOL* 11:1013–1017, 1979.
i. Kass I, Mandel W, et al: Isoniazid as a cause of optic neuritis and atrophy. *J AM MED ASSOC* 164:1740–1743, 1957.
j. Keeping JA, Searle CWA: Optic neuritis following isoniazid therapy. *LANCET* 2:278, 1955.
k. Kratka W: Isoniazid and ocular tuberculosis. *ARCH OPHTHALMOL* 54:330–344, 1955.
l. Money GL: Isoniazid neuropathies in malnourished tuberculous patients. *J TROP MED HYG* 62:198–202, 1959.
m. Nair KG: Optic neuritis due to INH complicating tuberculous meningitis. *J ASSOC PHYSICIANS INDIA* 24:263–264, 1976.
n. Neff TA: Isoniazid toxicity—lactic acidosis and keratitis. *CHEST* 59:245–248, 1971.
o. Noel PRB, Worden AN, Palmer AC: Neuropathologic effects and comparative toxicity for dogs of isonicotinic acid hydrazide and its methanosulfonate derivatives. *TOXICOL APPL PHARMACOL* 10:183–198, 1967.
p. Renard G, Morax PV: Optic neuritis in the course of treatment of tuberculosis. *ANN OCULIST* 210:53–61, 1977. (French)
q. Sutton PH, Beattie PH: Optic atrophy after administration of isoniazid with PAS. *LANCET* 1:650–651, 1955.

Isopentaquine experimental poisoning of monkeys has damaged the nuclei of the third, fourth, and sixth cranial nerves.[a] (Compare *Quinoline derivatives.*)

a. Moe GK, Peralta B, Seevers MH: Central impairment of sympathetic reflexes by 8-aminoquinolines. *J PHARMACOL EXP THER* 95:407–413, 1949.

Isophorone tested by application of a drop to rabbit corneas causes transient injury, graded 4 on a scale of 1 to 10 after twenty-four hours.[27] Although corneal opacity has been produced in rabbits, it has been reversible.[b] One instance of corneal burn in a human being recovered rapidly.[165]

Human beings can detect eye irritation at a concentration as low as 25 ppm[217] but have no persistent discomfort at 40 to 80 ppm.[a] Objectionable irritation of the eyes and nose is experienced at 200 to 400 ppm, and the conjunctiva appears irritated.[a] It appears that isophorone has adequate warning properties, since objectionable sensation of irritation is experienced at concentrations which are not definitely injurious.

a. Smyth HF, Seaton JJ: Acute response of guinea pigs and rats to inhalation of the vapors of isophorone. *J IND HYG* 22:477–483, 1940.
b. Truhaut R, et al: Toxicity of an industrial solvent, isophorone; its irritant action on the skin and mucous membranes. *EUR J TOXICOL* 5:31–37, 1972.

Isopropyl acetate splashes on human eyes have been noted to result in "slow healing" in two cases, but no details have been published.[165] Tests of vapor on human eyes show that sensation of irritation is detectable at 200 ppm in air, but no injuries from the vapor have been reported.[217]

Isopropyl alcohol (isopropanol, 2-propanol) has been used as a standard for comparison in testing substances for eye irritation or injury by local application to eyes of rabbits.[324, 352] Isopropyl alcohol causes mild transitory injury, graded 4 on a scale of 1 to 10 after twenty-four hours.[27, 223] Irrigation of rabbit eyes for 3 minutes with 50% isopropyl alcohol caused reaction graded 50 on a scale of 0 to 100.[123]

On human eyes very commonly 70% isopropyl alcohol has been employed in cleaning the skin of the lids in preparation for ocular surgery. Often it has entered the conjunctival sac and come in contact with the cornea and conjunctiva for several seconds before being washed away with sodium chloride solution. Usually the patient has felt uncomfortable burning and stinging despite previous application of 0.5% tetracaine or proparacaine, but no damage is observed unless contact has been prolonged. After prolonged contact with 70% solution or high concentration of the vapor the corneal epithelium may become irregular and may be lost in patches, but healing has been prompt.[c, 81] Splash of a drop on the eye in the absence of local anesthetic causes immediate smarting and tearing, but no significant injury.

Vapor of isopropyl alcohol causes sensation of irritation of the eyes in human beings in three to five minutes at concentration of 800 ppm in air.[183]

Apparently, systemically administered isopropyl alcohol has not injured the eyes or affected vision.[a, b] One study, in 1927, specifically on the effects of orally administered isopropyl alcohol on eyes and vision, reported on seven healthy human beings who had careful eye examinations before and after drinking 20 to 30 ml of 50% isopropyl alcohol on three or four occasions during two weeks.[a] The visual fields, ocular fundi, and visual acuity with glasses remained normal.

    a. Fuller HC, Hunter OB: Isopropyl alcohol. *J LAB CLIN MED* 12:326–349, 1927.
    b. Wills JH, Jameson EM, Coulston F: Effects on man of daily ingestion of small doses of isopropyl alcohol. *TOXICOL APPL PHARMACOL* 15:560–565, 1969.
    c. Osborn LM, Rosales TO: Corneal abrasion during alcohol sponging. *CLIN PEDIATR* 20:782, 1981.

Isopropyl ether vapor causes a sensation of ocular irritation to human beings only when a concentration of 300 ppm in air is exceeded.[217]

Isopropyl glyceryl ether tested by application of a drop to rabbit eyes caused slight irritation but no injury.[116]

Isopropyl glycidyl ether tested by application of a drop to rabbit eyes caused moderate reversible corneal injury. The vapor is a moderate eye and respiratory irritant.[115]

1-Isopropyl-4-hydroxy-6-benzyl-pyrazolo(3,4-d)pyrimidine (Ba-24650), a vasodilator, was evaluated clinically in patients with coronary disease, but caused a complaint of "visual disorders" in about 3 percent of patients.[a,b] These disorders consisted of "transient color sensations" which were "of very brief duration," definitely dose-dependent. The cause was not determinable by ophthalmoscopic examination, and the disturbance ceased when medication was discontinued.[a] Experiments in dogs induced "signs of blindness" and histologic abnormalities in the retina in a few days at high dosage (250 mg/kg per day), but at lower doses produced only an appearance of dilated retinal vessels with no histologic abnormality. In rats, administration of 1,000 mg/kg caused gradual progressive "damage of outer nuclear layer of the retina, disintegration of the rods and cones, and focal proliferation of the pigmented epithelial cells." The mechanism is yet to be explained.

    a. Bein HJ: Rational and irrational numbers in toxicology. *PROC EUROP SOC STUDY DRUG TOXICITY* 2:15–26, 1963. (Excerpta Med Foundation.)
    b. Bruckner R: Early diagnosis of drug-induced injury of the retina and optic nerve. *OPHTHALMOLOGICA* 158:245–272, 1969. (German)

Isoproterenol hydrochloride (isoprenaline, N-isopropylnoradrenaline, Aleudrine, Isuprel), a β-adrenergic drug, has been extensively investigated in eyes of animals and of normal and glaucomatous human beings for effects on intraocular pressure and hydrodynamics. When 5% solution is applied to the eye, it reduces intraocular pressure in man. It dilates blood vessels that are visible on the surface of the eye, but has no effect on the pupil. Its potential usefulness in treatment of glaucoma has been limited by a tendency to produce allergy and irritation of the eye upon repeated administration. Also when 5% solution is applied to the eyes enough is absorbed systemically to increase heart rate and cause systemic hypotension, which some patients find unpleasant.[a,d]

In guinea pigs, massive doses of isoprenaline have caused changes in the eyes, but the clinical implication is unknown. Histologically there has been described spreading of spaces in the substantia propria of the corneas and focal lysis of rods and cones, but no abnormality of the optic nerves.[c]

In rats, isoproterenol given either systemically or locally inhibits cell division in the lens epithelium.[b] This effect is potentiated by systemic administration of theophylline, and is completely eliminated by propranolol. It appears that the effect of isoproterenol on lens cell division is through action on a beta adrenergic receptor. Propranolol alone had no effect.

a. Bucci MG, Pescosolido N: On the possibility of reducing systemic side-effects of isoproterenol eyedrops by means of propranolol. *KLIN MONATSBL AUGENHEILKD* 170:586–589, 1977. (German)

b. Grimes P, von Sallmann L: Possible cyclic adenine monophosphate mediation in isoproterenol-induced suppression of cell division in rat lens epithelium. *INVEST OPHTHALMOL* 11:231–235, 1972.

c. Pellegrini N, Ronchieri M: Ocular changes induced experimentally in guinea pigs treated with isoproterenol. *ATTI ACCAD FISIOCR SIENA (MEDICOFIS)* 15:1085–1096, 1966. (Italian)

d. Quaranta CA, Bucci MG, Pescosolido N: Systemic effects from administration orally (propranolol) and locally (isoproterenol) of ocular hypotensive drugs. *ANN OTTALMOL CLIN OCUL* 104:575–582, 1978. (Italian)

Isosorbide dinitrate, a coronary vasodilator, formerly was advertised with an admonition to administer with caution to patients having glaucoma, but this was based on a misapprehension, not on actual published observations of adverse effects in glaucoma.[83] In fact, administration of 40 mg orally twice a day has been reported to reduce intraocular pressure in open-angle glaucoma and in normal eyes.[a]

A single case of unilateral ptosis and miosis with ipsilateral headache has been attributed to pericarotid compression of oculosympathetic fibers by vasodilation induced by isosorbide dinitrate.[b] In another unique case, each time this drug was taken the patient experienced myopia, without miosis, and this could be counteracted by cycloplegic eyedrops.

a. Wizemann AJS, Wizemann V: Organic nitrate therapy in glaucoma. *AM J OPHTHAL-MOL* 90:106–109, 1980.

b. Mueller RA, Meienberg O: Hemicrania from oculosympathetic paresis from isosorbide dinitrate. *N ENGL J MED* 308:458–459, 1983.

c. Dangel ME, Weber PA, Leier CB: Transient myopia following isosorbide dinitrate. *ANN OPHTHALMOL* 15:1156–1158, 1983.

Isotretinoin (13-cis-retinoic acid; Accutane) a keratolytic taken orally for acne, causes blepharo-conjunctivitis in more than 40% of patients, associated with dryness and itching of the skin.[a, e, j] Some patients with positive cultures for Staph aureus and a clinically consistent appearance have responded well to erythromycin ointment while continuing to take isotretinoin. Some patients who took isotretinoin for a disorder of keratinization developed reversible corneal opacities, and some dogs receiving very high dosage developed corneal ulcers and opacities.[i, f] Electroretinography and dark adaptation studies in patients have been reported normal.[j]

Pseudotumor cerebri with papilledema has developed in some patients taking isotretinoin, but some have also been taking tetracyclines or minocycline, which are themselves known to have this effect.[b,c,f] Retinal hemorrhages have accompanied papilledema in a minority of cases.[c]

Acute transient myopia is reported in one case in which the myopia could be repeatedly induced by giving the drug, and each time was relieved within a day or two by stopping the drug.[h] (See *Myopia, acute transient* in INDEX for other drugs with this effect.)

Isotretinoin is recognized as a potent teratogen in man. In addition to many non-ocular malformations, microphthalmia and maldevelopment of visual pathways have been reported.[d,g]

a. Anonymous: Isotretinoin (Accutane) for acne. *THE MEDICAL LETTER* 24:79–81, 1982.
b. Anonymous: Update on isotretinoin (Accutane) for acne. *THE MEDICAL LETTER* 25:105–106, 1983.
c. Anonymous: Adverse effects with isotretinoin. *FDA DRUG BULLETIN* 13:Number 3, 1983.
d. Benke PJ: The isotretinoin teratogen syndrome. *J AM MED ASSOC* 251:3267–3269, 1984.
e. Blackman HJ, Peck GL, et al: Blepharoconjunctivitis: a side effect of 13-cis-retinoic acid therapy for dermatologic diseases. *OPHTHALMOLOGY* 86:753–758, 1979.
f. Fraunfelder FT: Ocular side effects of isotretinoin therapy. *J AM MED ASSOC* 250:2545, 1983.
g. Hill RM: Isotretinoin teratogenicity. *LANCET* 1:1465, 1984.
h. Palestine AG: Transient acute myopia resulting from isotretinoin (Accutane) therapy. *ANN OPHTHALMOL* 16:660–662, 1984.
i. Weiss J, Degnan M, et al: Bilateral corneal opacities: Occurrence in a patient treated with oral isotretinoin. *ARCH DERMATOL* 117:182, 1981.
j. Windhorst DB, Nigra T: General clinical toxicology of oral retinoids. *J AM ACAD DERMATOL* 6:675–682, 1982.

Isoxsuprine (Duvadilan, Vasodilan), a vasodilator, when injected subconjunctivally in human beings causes several mm Hg transient elevation of ocular pressure, maximum in an hour or two, associated with edema and hyperemia of the episcleral tissues. In glaucomatous eyes with abnormally high resistance to aqueous outflow, the elevation of ocular pressure may be greater, and this may be used as a test for glaucoma.[a] The intraocular pressure is not raised when isoxsuprine is given systemically.[b,c]

a. Khosla PK, Agarwal L, Angra S: Duvadilan (isoxsuprine hydrochloride) in ophthalmology. *ORIENT ARCH OPHTHALMOL* 3:193–203, 1965. (*EXCERPTA MED* (Sect XII), 20:1355, 1966).
b. Kitazawa Y, Takeuchi T, Kawanishi K, Nakamura C: The effect of adrenergic β-active compound on aqueous humor dynamics in man. *ACTA SOC OPHTHALMOL JPN* 72:287–292, 1968.
c. Miura M: A new functional test for aqueous outflow with vasodilators. *FOLIA OPHTHALMOL JPN* 18:396–409, 1967.

Jellyfish of certain types have poisonous stings in their tentacles which cause painful irritation of the skin and eyes.[a–c] From Australia have been reported four cases of injury to the eye believed due to *Cyanea annaskala*, occuring in patients who swam with their eyes open beneath the water.[a] They had immediate severe pain, photophobia, and blepharospasm. Injuries of the corneal epithelium resembled abrasions, and multiple fine puncture tracts into the anterior third of the stroma contained refractile threads visible by slit-lamp biomicroscope. There was no complete perforation of the cornea. The lids became moderately swollen, but the eyes became only slightly or mildly hyperemic. All healed without damage to vision in a week with no special treatment. It was suspected that the injuries were caused by forceful ejection of threadlike tubes from the capsule of the stinging cells of the jellyfish and that an unidentified toxin was probably carried through the tubes.[a]

In France, swelling and redness of the lids, without involvement of the cornea is reported from contact with *Physalia pelagica*, and responds within 2 or 3 days to topical corticosteroid treatment.[b]

Composition of the venom of nematocysts of *Cnidaria* has been investigated in much detail, but without reference to effects on the eye.[212]

   a. Mitchell JH: Eye injuries due to jellyfish (*Cyanea annaskala*). *MED J AUST* 2:303–305, 1962; *TRANS AUST COLL OPHTHALMOL* 11:96–99, 1970.
   b. Peyresblanques J: Medusa eye. *BULL SOC OPHTALMOL FRANCE* 77:215, 1977. (French)
   c. Vick HP, Wild H: Eye lesions due to wheal-producing jelly fish. *Z ARZTL FORTBILD* 67:1040–1041, 1973. (German)

Jequirity bean, the seed of *Abrus precatorius,* has many synonyms, including crabs-eye, precatory bean, rosary pea, prayer bead, Buddhist rosary bead, Mienie-mienie Indian bead, Seminole bead, weather plant, and lucky bean.[142] The seed is about 5 mm long, scarlet color, smooth and glossy, with a black spot surrounding the hilum.[142] Imported necklaces and jewelry ornamented with the attractive beans from the West Indies and other tropical areas have been the principal source in North America.[a,f,g] Jequirity bean contains material that is highly irritating when eaten or when in contact with the eye.

When inserted in the conjunctival sac, the beans cause conjunctival inflammation and discharge. In most instances the beans have been inserted as an aid to malingering. Characteristically in such cases a pseudomembrane forms on the lower palpebral conjunctiva. This membrane can be peeled off. Typically also a localized necrotic area is found in the lower bulbar conjunctiva associated with swelling of the preauricular gland. The cornea is rarely involved. Recovery is usually prompt, but a localized obliteration of the lower fornix may persist.

There is a large clinical literature on the effects of jequirity bean and its derivatives on the human eye,[b,c,253] because for a period after 1882, substances extractible from the beans were employed in treatment of trachoma to induce a purulent conjunctivitis which was thought to help heal granulations. However, in some instances the cornea became injured, and this treatment is no longer employed. Materials extractible from the seeds include *Jequiritol,* and the active principal, *Abrin,* a toxalbumin.

Experimentally applied to rabbit eyes, jequirity and its derivatives cause more severe reaction than in human eyes. Corneal infiltration, hypopyon and loss of the eye may occur in rabbits.[253] Introduced into the anterior chamber, jequirity causes very severe inflammatory reaction, and in excessive amount has been known to cause death of the animal in a few hours, before the onset of inflammatory reaction in the eye.[150] Also, the effect of injecting infusions of jequirity bean into the anterior chamber of rabbit eyes has been studied in some detail, showing a range of reactions, depending upon dilution, from mild transient iritis to violent inflammation, necrosis, and rupture of the globe. Cortisone or ACTH administered systemically, or cortisone put into the anterior chamber, has been shown to block the effect of dilute jequirity infusions that would otherwise damage the endothelium and cause opacification of the cornea, but this treatment does not prevent devastating injury by higher concentrations.[d,e]

a. Hart M: Hazards to health (Jequirity bean poisoning). *N ENGL J MED* 268:885–886, 1963.
b. Somerset EJ: Self-inflicted conjunctivitis. *BR J OPHTHALMOL* 29:196–204, 1945.
c. Somerville-Large LB: Self-inflicted eye injuries. *TRANS OPHTHALMOL SOC UK* 67:185–201, 1947.
d. Woods AC: ACTH and cortisone in ocular disease. *AM J OPHTHALMOL* 33:1325–1348, 1950.
e. Woods AC, Wood RM: Effect of cortisone and ACTH on ocular inflammation secondary to the injection of irritant substances. *BULL JOHNS HOPKINS HOSP* 90:134–148, 1952.
f. Poisonous jequirity beans. *CAN MED ASSOC J* 100:21, 1969.
g. Poison beans turn up throughout the U.S. in alarming numbers. *WALL STREET JOURNAL* Jan. 21, 1969, p. 18.

Kainic acid, an analogue of glutamic acid is an excitotoxic amino acid that is more potent than glutamic acid itself as a neurotoxin in retina.[e,g] Intraocular injection in chicks causes rapid degeneration of the inner nuclear layer of the retina, and less damage to all other layers.[g] Only mature neurons are affected.[c] In rats, intravitreal injection causes severe and extensive retinal cell damage, loss of the b-wave of the electroretinogram, and marked decrease in the GABA content of the retina.[a,b,d] Besides causing degeneration of inner laminae of the rat it causes mitoses to appear in the amacrine cells.[d] Intravitreal low doses in cats and rabbits may induce a form of growth of retina horizontal cells.[f]

No human poisoning has been reported from taking kainic acid-containing seaweed orally for treatment of intestinal worms.[e]

a. Goto M, Inomata N, et al: Changes of electroretinogram and neurochemical aspects of gabaergic neurons of retina after intraocular injection of kainic acid in rats. *BRAIN RES* 211:305–314, 1981.
b. Guarneri P, Corda MG, et al: Kainic acid-induced lesion of rat retina. *BRAIN RES* 209:216–220, 1981.
c. Hyndman AG: The effects of glutamate and kainate on cell proliferation in retinal cultures. *INVEST OPHTHALMOL VIS SCI* 25:558–563, 1984.
d. Lessell S, Craft JL, Albert DM: Kainic acid induces mitoses in mature retinal neurones in rats. *EXP EYE RES* 30:731–738, 1980.
e. Olney JW: Excitotoxic mechanisms of neurotoxicity. Chapter 19 in Spencer and Schaumburg (1980).[378]

f. Peickl L, Bolz J: Kainic acid induces sprouting of retinal neurons. *SCIENCE* 223:503–504, 1984.

g. Schwarcz R, Coyle JT: Kainic acid, neurotoxic effects after intraocular injection. *INVEST OPHTHALMOL* 16:141–148, 1977.

Kanamycin sulfate, an antimicrobial administered parenterally, has been reported to have caused "blurring of vision" in four patients, and tinnitus or deafness in a larger number, but the nature of the visual disturbances is not more precisely known.[a–c] Intravitreal injection in rabbits and owl monkeys was tolerated at a dose of 0.5 mg, but 1.5 to 6.0 mg produced cataracts in rabbits.[d,280]

a. Finegold SM, et al: Clinical experience with kanamycin. *ANN NY ACAD SCI* 76:319–347, 1958.

b. Finegold SM: Toxicity of kanamycin in adults. *ANN NY ACAD SCI* 132:949–956, 1966.

c. Freeman FR, Parker RL Jr, Greer M: Unusual neurotoxicity of kanamycin. *J AM MED ASSOC* 200:410–411, 1967.

d. Peyman GA, Nelsen P, Bennett TO: Intravitreal injection of kanamycin in experimentally induced endophthalmitis. *CAN J OPHTHALMOL* 9:322–327, 1974.

Kerosene (kerosine, Deo-Base), a mixture of petroleum hydrocarbons less volatile than gasoline, when applied to the human eye causes no discomfort or injury.[81]

Ketamine (Ketalar), a short-acting general anesthetic administered intravenously, has no adverse effect on the eyes themselves, except occasionally to raise the intraocular pressure transiently.[c,e] However, visual hallucinations during recovery are known,[c] and three cases of blindness lasting about 25 minutes have been described.[b] The locus of the disturbance was believed to be at the lateral geniculate body or at some higher level. Recovery was complete.

What relationship these clinical cases of transient blindness may have to animal experiments which have been reported is unclear, but in rabbits subjected to ketamine anesthesia for one hour almost all layers and types of retinal cells showed ultrastructural abnormalities.[a] These abnormalities were considered characteristic of the effects of hypoxia.

a. Antal M: Ketamine-induced ultrastructural changes in the retina. *GRAEFES ARCH OPHTHALMOL* 210:43–53, 1979.

b. Fine J, Weissmann J, Finestone SC: Side effects after ketamine anesthesia: transient blindness. *ANESTH ANALG CURR RES* 53:72–74, 1974.

c. Harris JE, Letson RD, Buckley JJ: The use of CI-581 a new parenteral anesthetic, in ophthalmic practice. *TRANS AM OPHTHALMOL SOC* 66:207–213, 1968.

d. Hawks WN Jr, Levin KJ, Lowe E: Some side effects of ketamine hydrochloride during ophthalmologic examination. *J PEDIATR OPHTHALMOL* 8:171–172, 1971.

e. Podlesch I, Gortz H, Quint K: On indications, methods and complications of general anesthesia in ophthalmology. *KLIN MONATSBL AUGENHEILKD* 152:405–417, 1968. (German)

Ketoconazole, an antifungal, does not retard healing of standard corneal epithelial defects in rabbits when applied as 1% eye drops in oil, and it causes only transient faint superficial stainable disturbances of the epithelium.[309] Only slight conjunctival hyperemia resulted from applying 5% solution for 2 weeks.[a]

    a. Oji EO: Study of ketoconazole toxicity in rabbit ,cornea and conjunctiva. *INT OPHTHALMOL* 5:169–174, 1982.

Ketoprofen, an anti-inflammatory phenylpropionic acid derivative, administered orally, showed no toxic effect on the eyes or vision in a prospective ophthalmologic study of twelve patients under treatment for arthritis during an average of 21 months.[c] Separately, a single case of painful swollen eyes was associated with treatment of nephrotic syndrome, subsiding during 2 weeks after the medication was stopped; no ophthalmologic details were given, but it was called conjunctivitis.[b] Also separately, an instance of pseudotumor cerebri, with reversible bilateral papilledema and abducens palsy, was reported in a child with Bartter's syndrome, similar to a case of the same complication attributed to a related drug, indomethacin.[a] (Also see INDEX for list of other *Phenylpropionates.*)

    a. Larizza D, Colombo A, et al: Ketoprofen causing pseudotumor cerebri in Bartter's syndrome. *N ENGL J MED* 300:796, 1979.
    b. Umez-Eronini EM: Conjunctivitis due to ketoprofen. *LANCET* 2:737, 1978.
    c. Williams H, Zutshi D, Mushin A: Ophthalmic screening of patients receiving ketoprofen or flurbiprofen medication for inflammatory or degenerative joint disease. *SCAND J RHEUMATOL SUPPL* 14:85–92, 1976.

Lactic acid in concentrated form is caustic to the skin, eyes, and mucous membranes.[46,101,153] Its effect on the eye is similar to that of other acids of moderate strength, causing initial epithelial coagulation on cornea and conjunctiva, but having good prognosis if promptly washed off with water. Compared to other acids, lactic acid has no unusual capacity to penetrate the cornea.[79] Its injurious effect is presumably attributable to its acidity, since the lactate ion is a normal, nontoxic constituent of body fluids. Applied to rabbit eyes in an standard manner, the reaction at twenty-four hours has been graded 8 on a scale of 1 to 10.[27,222] If allowed to remain on rabbit eyes, both the full strength acid and a 50% solution in water have caused corneal necrosis and persistent stromal scarring.[96,101] Lactic acid 0.1% injected into the corneal stroma induces intense vascularization.[a,127] On guinea pig eyes 30% lactic acid has produced slight corneal clouding.[b]

Imre has reported stimulating corneal vascularization by injection of lactate into the stroma, postulating that endogenous lactate was a factor in corneal vascularization from various causes.[a]

    a. Imre G: Mechanism of corneal vascularization. *ACTA MORPHOL* 14:99–104, 1966; 17:171–173, 1969.
    b. Wilhelm G, Gdynia R: On the inflammatory properties of lactic acid in animal experimentation. *ARZNEIMITTELFORSCHUNG* 18, Dec. 1968, pp 1525–1529. (German)

Laminaria digitata, a seaweed, has been found to produce long-lasting glaucoma in rabbits eyes when it is finely powdered and put into the anterior chamber.[a]

a. Priestly BS, Pecori Giraldi J, Valvo A: Experimental glaucoma from *Laminaria digitata*. *BOLL OCULIST* 47:652–668, 1968. (Italian)

Lanolin (wool fat, lanum) has been employed as a base for ointments and creams.[171] It is nonirritating when applied to the eye, but tests on rats showed that application of U.S.P. lanolin following experimental pinprick injuries of the cornea caused the epithelium to heal less rapidly than in untreated eyes. However, if the lanolin was further purified, this retardant effect was eliminated.[c] Following abrasions or burns of the corneas of rats and rabbits, lanolin caused very slight or no delay in healing.[b,d,e] Lanolin was approximately as innocuous as petrolatum in these tests. However, certain ethoxylated lanolin derivatives have caused corneal clouding in animals.[a]

a. Guillot JP, Giauffret JY, et al: Animal toxicological study of various samples of anhydrous lanolin and lanolin derivatives. *INT J COSMET SCI* 2:1–38, 1980. (French)

b. Leopold IH, Steele WA: Influence of local application of sulfonamide compounds and their vehicles on regeneration of corneal epithelium. *ARCH OPHTHALMOL* 33:463–467, 1945.

c. Heerema JC, Freidenwald JS: Retardation of wound healing in the corneal epithelium by lanolin. *AM J OPHTHALMOL* 33:1421–1427, 1950.

d. Smelser GK, Ozanics MS: Effect of chemotherapeutic agents on cell division and healing of corneal burns and abrasions in the rat. *AM J OPHTHALMOL* 27:1063–1072, 1944.

e. Smelser GK: The influence of vehicles and form of penicillin and sulfonamides on mitosis and healing of corneal burns. *AM J OPHTHALMOL* 29:541–550, 1946.

Lantana (*Lantana camara*) is a shrub that grows in most warm countries. Four children who ate green berries from the lantana plant were quite ill with gastrointestinal reaction and depressed respiration and reflexes. One died in coma. The child that died had pinpoint pupils which did not respond to light, but the other three, who were not comatose and recovered, had dilated pupils.[a]

Sheep, cattle, and other grazing animals that have been poisoned by eating the whole plant, with gastrointestinal disturbance and weakness, are said to have also had conjunctivitis, corneal opacities, and blindness, plus ulcerations of the mucous membranes and photosensitization of the skin. Information on these effects on the eyes of animals appears to have been published principally in agricultural periodicals.[142] In the cases of human poisoning there appears to have been no comparable involvement of conjunctiva or cornea, or blindness.

a. Wolfson SL, Solomons TWG: Poisoning by fruit of *Lantana camara*. *AM J DIS CHILD* 107:173–176, 1964.

Lathyrism is a term that has been applied in a confusing way to two different toxic conditions, one a neurotoxic disease, and the other a connective tissue disease. Griffin and Price in 1980 have clearly pointed out that neurotoxic lathyrism ("neurolathyrism") has been known for centuries in various parts of the world, affecting both man and animals, occurring at times of famine when the seeds or beans of *Lathyrus sativus* have been eaten.[b] Paresthesias of the feet may be the first symptom, followed acutely or subacutely by spastic paraparesis, from which there is little recovery. Griffin and Price mention no eye involvement.[b]

The other type of lathyrism is "osteolathyrism", in which abnormalities of connective tissue are most prominent; this is caused by a related plant, *Lathyrus odoratus.*

Several chemicals, known as "lathyrogens", have been identified which can cause one or the other, or both types of lathyrism. A synopsis of effects of various lathyrogens on the eyes follows.

β-Aminopropionitrile has adverse effects related to osteolathyrism, interfering with formation of mucopolysaccharides in the corneas of rats. (Details are given elsewhere; see INDEX for *β-Aminopropionitrile.*)

Iminodipropionitrile in experimental animals produces neuronal disease of the nerve fibers of optic nerve and retina, with retinal angiopathy, and it also causes connective tissue disease in rats, manifested as opacification of the cornea. (Details are given elsewhere; see INDEX for *Iminodipropionitrile.*)

Oxalyldiaminopropionic acid, which has been isolated from the neurotoxic seeds of *Lathyrus sativus,* when administered parenterally to immature mice causes damage to the retina, similar to that produced by glutamic acid.[c]

Methylenaminoacetonitrile, *β-mercaptoethylamine,* and *thiosemicarbazide* have been shown to inhibit the normal sulfation of galactosaminoglycans in incubated bovine corneas.[a]

3-(2-Phenyl)hydrazopropionitrile, an osteolathyrogenic compound, has produced cataracts when fed to weanling rats.[d]

   a. Brettschneider I, Praus R: Effect of lathyrogens on glycosaminoglycans of bovine
      cornea *in vitro.* OPHTHALMIC RES 1:220–227, 1970.
   b. Griffin JW, Price DL: Proximal axonopathies induced by toxic chemicals. Chapter 11
      in Spencer and Schaumburg (1980).[378]
   c. Olney JW, Chandra HM, Rhee V: Brain and retinal damage from lathyrus excitotoxin,
      β-N-oxalyl-L-δ,B -diaminopropionic acid. *NATURE* 264:659–661, 1976.
   d. Dasler W, Wang HLS: Studies on cataracts induced in rats by N-phenyl–β-
      hydrazinopropionitrile. *INVEST OPHTHALMOL* 11:236–240, 1972.

Lead metal foreign bodies in the eye or in the orbit in human beings have been considered to cause little reaction and rarely any toxic effect. Clinical experiences with various intraocular foreign bodies presented in detail with histologic studies by Pau indicated that lead metallic foreign bodies caused minimal inflammatory reaction, mainly mechanical injury.[189] Similarly, Francois and associates concluded that lead fragments in patients were well tolerated in the eye and in the orbit and that they should not be removed unless they were in the anterior chamber. They described one case in which, though a small lead shot was allowed to remain in the vitreous, the vision returned to normal as blood in the vitreous absorbed or settled in the course of a year. In two other cases they reported also good recovery of vision though fragments of bullets were allowed to remain in the orbit.[c] Similar experiences and conclusions have been presented by Maugery[e] and by Skrzypczak.[h] Hinken described a case in which an intraocular foreign body of lead appeared by clinical standards to excite little or no reaction, but migrated from the posterior pole to the anterior chamber (through an aphakic pupil) and was therefore removed.[d] Bohm, concerned with particles in the eye mainly from splashes of molten lead, similarly indicated that eye tissues generally showed little reaction to lead particles.[a] Lead particles have been well tolerated in the eyes of dogs[f] and rats.[g]

In one case, which appears to have been quite exceptional, Dambite reported a patient with a lead shot behind one globe had impaired vision in that eye. This was assumed to be due to a toxic effect of the lead. Whether this interpretation was correct or not, a significant improvement of vision was reported when systemic and topical treatment with 2,3-dimercaptopropansulfonate sodium was started five years after the injury.[b]

From experiments on rabbit eyes, Leber reported more reaction to particles of metallic lead than have been described in human beings.[150] Lead particles in the anterior chamber in rabbits became coated with purulent exudate and sometimes were extruded through the cornea at the limbus. In the vitreous humor in rabbits a similar purulent reaction was observed, causing the vitreous to shrink and the retina to separate.

a. Bohm K: On injuries of eye by splashes of lead. *KLIN MONATSBL AUGENHEILKD* 57:82–109, 1916. (German)

b. Dambite GR: A successful treatment of a lead atrophy of the optic nerve. *OFTALMOL ZH* 21:329–331, 1966.

c. Francois P, Blervacque A, et al: Perforations of the eye by lead. *BULL SOC OPHTALMOL FRANCE* 68:1059–1062, 1968. (French)

d. Hinken MV: Migration of intraocular nonmagnetic foreign body. *ARCH OPHTHALMOL* 74:485–486, 1965.

e. Maugery J, Goudot D: Concerning some observations on well tolerated intraocular foreign bodies of lead. *BULL SOC OPHTALMOL FRANCE* 73:785–787, 1973. (French)

f. Schmidt GM, Dice PF, Koch SA: Intraocular lead foreign bodies in four canine eyes. *J SMALL ANIM PRACT* 16:33–39, 1975.

g. Schmidt JGH, Stute A, Weber E: Electroretinographic and ophthalmoscopic findings after introducing foreign metal particles into the eye of the rat. *BER DTSCH OPHTHAL-MOL GES* 71:391–397, 1972. (German)

h. Skrzypczak KE: On treatment of intraorbital metallic foreign bodies. *KLIN MONATSBL AUGENHEILKD* 149:211–219, 1966. (German)

Lead salts: local effects

Lead chloride and *lead sulfate* placed in the anterior chamber of rabbits have caused a moderate purulent reaction and general inflammation of the eye.[150]

Lead arsenate used in an insecticidal spray was alleged by two patients to have caused conjunctival injury, in one resembling pemphigus, but this compound is practically insoluble in water, and testing topically on rabbit eyes showed it to cause no injury.[d]

Lead acetate (sugar of lead) is of historical interest, because it was formerly applied in aqueous solutions to the eye for astringent effect, but induced opacities and lead encrustation of the cornea and conjunctiva, appearing as whitish chalky areas, assumed to be composed largely of lead carbonate.[b,c,e,46,253] Such opacities occurred in patients when the corneal epithelium had been previously injured, allowing the lead solution to penetrate. The epithelium normally presents a barrier to penetration of lead salts into the cornea, but the epithelium may be injured by high concentrations.[81,253] Lead encrustations could cause long-lasting irritation. They sometimes extruded as a sequestrum, and sometimes became covered by the epithelium, and remained an obstruction to vision. Lead encrustation of the cornea has been removed surgically,[253] or through local use of solutions of ammonium tartrate or ammonium chloride, which dissolve lead salts by formation of complexes.[c,e]

Experimental tests of *lead acetate* in slightly acidic solution, from pH 6.0 to pH 4.2, applying the solution to rabbit eyes after removal of the corneal epithelium or injecting into the corneal stroma, has produced devastating injury at a concentration of 0.08 M, but little or no reaction at 0.001 M.[123] Both *lead acetate* and *lead chloride* if given access in sufficient amount to the corneal stroma of rabbit eyes can cause total and permanent opacification, which is a far worse injury than has commonly been encountered in patients.[81,90,123,253]

The *lead water* or *lead acetate solutions* formerly used on patients apparently were sufficiently dilute to cause only superficial injury and encrustation, usually from prolonged use. The severe deep type of opacity which can be produced in rabbits responds little if at all to treatment with edetate disodium,[81,90] but the superficial encrustation historically described in patients would have been amenable to treatment with this chelating agent, as with the ammonium salts already mentioned.

   a. Bohm K: On injuries of the eye by splashes of lead. *KLIN MONATSBL AUGENHEILKD* 57:82–109, 1916. (German)
   b. Mejer F: A case of artifactual conjunctivitis induced by lead acetate. *OPHTHAL-MOLOGICA* 119:221–251, 1950. (German)
   c. Scheffels: Recent lead encrustation of the cornea after lead water application that was completely cleared by ammonium chloride and ammonium tartrate. *KLIN MONATSBL AUGENHEILKD* 74:511–512, 1925. (German)
   d. Verhoeff FH: Verbal communication.
   e. Zur Nedden M: On the etiology and therapy of lime and lead opacities of the cornea. *ARCH AUGENHEILKD* 57:37–55, 1907. (German)

Lead systemic poisoning can cause a wide variety of visual and ocular disturbances according to many case reports during the past three and a half centuries.

Much of what we know of the clinical aspects of ocular effects comes from early literature which has been condensed in several reviews.[46,129,153,194,214,239,247,255,264] Especially notable are a chronological bibliography of the period from 1611 to 1900 by Uhthoff with a general review of ideas concerning ocular toxicology of lead during that period, and a comprehensive seventy-eight-page discussion of the subject by Lewin and Guillery in 1913, including summaries of 172 case reports.[153] Of the 172 eye cases surveyed by Lewin and Guillery, seventy-nine had colic, fifty-two had headache, forty-seven had convulsions, delirium, stupor, or coma, and twenty-seven had paralysis of extensor muscles. In general ocular disturbances appeared most commonly after many months or years of chronic poisoning, and at least after several weeks of poisoning. As a rule, ocular involvement was not among the early symptoms in adults, although it could be one of the first symptoms, especially in children.

On the basis of clinical and experimental observations, it has been possible to recognize disturbances of the following sites in the visual system: visual cortex and suprageniculate pathways; optic nerve, both retrobulbar and bulbar; retina; intraocular muscles; and extraocular muscles. Unfortunately many reports describing visual symptoms provide insufficient information for determination of site or mechanism.

Numerous monkeys in zoos have been known since the 1930's to have developed a usually fatal condition known as "acute amaurotic epilepsy", later shown by Sauer and by Zook to be an acute encephalopathy from lead paint chewed from the bars of cages. Zook's report provides the evidence, and a historical review with bibliography, but does not discuss the mechanism of loss of vision. Houser has described one rhesus monkey which was accidentally lead-poisoned and developed convulsions, loss of coordination and blindness, but recovered completely, including its sight, after the source of lead was removed. (However, no examination of the eyes was reported.) Lead encephalopathy has been produced experimentally in monkeys (Allen; Clasen; Hopkins). Hopkins recorded cerebral edema and focal cortical necroses, but normal optic nerves. Brown examined Clasen's newborn monkeys with lead encephalopathy and found no papilledema. Apparently the sometimes reversible blindness in monkeys is a manifestation of disturbance of the brain itself.

Blindness has been noted in poisoned calves, mechanism unknown (Harbourne).

In rats, visual evoked cortical responses have remained abnormal long after discontinuation of exposure to lead, suggesting long persisting effect on the brain (Cooper; Feeney).

In lead-poisoned human beings there is a rare type of brain involvement in which the disturbance of vision appears to have been exclusively suprageniculate or cortical. There has been complete loss of vision, but the pupils continued to react to light, and the ocular fundi remained normal. At least ten instances of this type have been reported, occurring mostly in persons suffering an acute exacerbation of lead poisoning, usually with colic (Bihler; Evans; Hertel; Neuman; Pal; Pincus; Posey; Westphal; Williams). The blindness has been bilateral and of sudden onset, persisting variously for hours, days, or months, but mostly for only a few days. During recovery from such an attack, visual hallucinations and temporary alterations of color vision have been noted, but homonymous hemianopsia has been most characteristic. In this particular group of cases, there has been no indication of increased intracranial pressure and no disturbance of the extraocular muscles. It is not known whether the function of the visual cortex or radiation is altered by direct toxic action of lead in these cases, or whether lead causes vasoconstriction of the regional blood vessels and ischemia of the visual pathways.

More commonly in human beings when the brain is affected in lead poisoning, the intracranial pressure is raised and the cranial nerves may be affected. The optic nerves may be injured either by increased intracranial pressure or by direct toxic action of lead on the nerve. In blindness due to involvement of the optic nerve, the pupils are unreactive to light.

Encephalopathy with cerebral edema has been well studied by neuropathologists, who have described swelling of the brain with indications of vascular damage and increased permeability of the blood brain barrier as a factor (Pentschew; Popoff; Smith).

Most characteristically, encephalopathy or meningoencephalitis, with increased intracranial pressure, injury of the optic nerves, and palsies of extraocular motor nerves, occurs in children between the ages of two and eight years. Typically in these patients the poisoning results from eating lead from painted woodwork over a period of several months. The disturbance first to attract attention has been convergent strabismus from paralysis or paresis of one or both external recti, sometimes accompanied by paresis of other extraocular muscles. Rather constantly bilateral papilledema has been found, usually from 5 to 6 diopters, seldom less than 3 diopters. Visual acuity has usually not been appreciably affected despite considerable papilledema. There have been no characteristic abnormalities of color vision, nor central scotoma (Gibson; Gibson; Good).[194]

The evidences of meningoencephalopathy which have usually, but not invariably, been present are headache with rigidity and pain in the neck. Also, symmetrical brain atrophy with hydrocephaly externa and interna or one-sided hemisphere atrophy occurs. Lead encephalopathy in small children can cause permanent cerebral injury, most often of the hemiplegic sort, with mental retardation, tremor of the extremities, and occasional epileptic attacks, in addition to cranial nerve palsies affecting the extraocular muscles and causing strabismus, ptosis, or facial paralysis (Bradley).[194] In some reports of follow-up studies of children who survived lead poisoning there has been mention of residual impairment of "visual-motor" coordination or functioning, but this does not necessarily signify impairment of visual acuity, which often has not even been tested. Rather it refers to results of psychological evaluation of drawing or copying abilities with crayon and paper, which, in the presence of brain damage, may be poorer than expected for the child's mental age (Bradley).

In adults, particularly in young adults, disturbances resembling those associated with encephalopathy in children have been described in several instances, but with some noteworthy differences (Hay). In young adult cases, lead colic has been a prominent symptom, and headache, vomiting, and occasional coma or convulsions have been the evidences of encephalopathy. Confusion and psychosis or epileptic convulsions have occurred more commonly in adults than in children.[194] Increased intracranial pressure has been manifested by papilledema and ocular motor nerve palsies, especially of the sixth nerve. Loss of vision has characteristically occurred more acutely and completely than in children. The pupils have been dilated and unreactive to light. Lewin and Guillery have described cases in which loss of vision occurred almost instantly. More commonly the visual disturbance reached a peak of complete loss of light perception in the course of a few hours, and lasted five or six days.[153]

The usual course has been recovery of vision, often complete, the attacks of colic usually getting better at the same time as the vision. In rare cases various degrees of optic atrophy have resulted. Many cases of this acute and transitory amaurosis were described before the advent of ophthalmoscopy, but in more recent cases blurring of the borders of the optic nervehead, slight turbidity of the surrounding retina, and abnormal distension of the retinal veins have been described. In many cases it is impossible to say whether the visual effects were due to pressure or to a retrobulbar neuritis affecting the nerve directly.

Apparently distinct from disturbances of the optic nerve caused by increased intracranial pressure are cases in which true optic neuritis, either retrobulbar or bulbar, has occurred without hydrocephaly and without involvement of extraocular muscles. Optic neuritis was believed by Lewin and Guillery to be the commonest form of visual disturbance from lead, and many of the cases that they reported were thought to be in this category.[153] They concluded that decrease of vision in optic neuritis was gradual, and that either recovery or transition to permanent blindness was slow. The onset in some cases appeared to be similar to that of "tobacco-alcohol" amblyopia. The visual fields in some cases had normal extent, but in many cases peripheral constriction was found, and in numerous others there was central scotoma. Ring-type scotoma was relatively rare. There seemed to be no one type of field defect typical of lead optic neuritis. A clinical survey by Schuttmann (1971) suggests that optic neuritis as the sole manifestation of lead poisoning has become rare.

Optic neuropathy has been attributed to lead in many cases in which there was no other indication of lead poisoning and in which the main reasons for suspecting lead were a history of exposure to lead or laboratory findings of lead absorption. This has often made it very difficult to be sure whether the diagnosis was correct and whether lead poisoning was in fact responsible for the optic neuropathy. For example, Belova described a person who developed optic atrophy after exposure to lead for twenty-nine years in a printing plant, but had no evidence of lead poisoning according to blood and urine and neurologic examinations. Unseld gave a brief report of three cases with very little information about the eyes except mention of narrowed fields and diagnosis of optic nerve injury from lead, associated with lead encephalopathy in one and disturbances of radial and tibial nerves in another. Stronger presumptive evidence of the role of lead has been given by Baghdassarian, who documented a gradual decrease in visual acuity in a forty-nine-year-old painter to 20/400 and 10/400 due to dense central scotomas involving 5° around the fixation point, but with no discernible abnormality in the fundi. The blood had basophilic stippling of the erythrocytes and lead concentration of 0.08 mg%. Under treatment with penicillamine the visual acuity gradually became normal within four months and the blood lead concentration dropped to 0.04 mg%.

It is not known whether optic neuritis is due to direct toxic action of lead on the optic nerve fibers or whether there is primarily a vascular disturbance leading to optic nerve damage. Optic neuritis can be induced experimentally in animals by administration of lead, but this has not established the mechanism (Giannantoni). In mice, development of the optic nerves can be interfered with by administering lead (Tennekoon).

There has been much discussion of the role of the blood vessels in the retina and optic nerve as well as in the brain, but without substantial conclusions.[194] Uhthoff was particularly impressed with the severity of abnormalities which were visible ophthalmoscopically in the retinal vessels in some cases (narrowing of the vessels, vasculitis, white ensheathing, changes in the walls, and vasoconstriction), but he pointed out that in instances in which histologic examination had been carried out, there were associated inflammatory degenerative changes in the optic nerve.[247] Soos has reported a high incidence of retinal angiosclerosis in lead workers. Lobeck noted that in some instances retinal vascular abnormalities with hemorrhages and exudates dominated the clinical picture, and suspected that the vascular disturbances were indirect manifestations of damage to the kidneys.

The end result of optic nerve disturbance in lead poisoning has been optic atrophy in many cases, whether the disturbance initially was due to increased intracranial pressure or to retrobulbar neuritis or to optic neuritis. Of ninety-seven cases of optic neuritis from lead surveyed by Lewin and Guillery, optic atrophy occurred in thirty-six.[153] Uhthoff at a later date estimated an incidence of only 10% of optic atrophy in cases of lead optic neuritis.[247] In cases of optic atrophy which have not been seen until the late stage, it has commonly been difficult or impossible to determine the primary site of disturbance. In most instances the atrophy of the optic nerves has been of the postneuritic type.[247] However, following retrobulbar neuritis, simple atrophic degeneration may occur (Snell).

Odd ophthalmoscopic findings have occasionally been described in and around the optic nerve head in people exposed to excessive absorption of lead but without disturbances of vision. Imre described an appearance of glial proliferation about the blood vessels on the optic nervehead in forty-two out of 197 workers exposed to excessive absorption of lead, an incidence of 21.3 per cent compared to 8.6 per cent in a control group of unexposed workers. Vints also has described a veiling of the physiologic cup of the optic disc as a common sign. Sonkin described "glistening gray discrete spots" and "stippling around the optic disc" as a characteristic early sign of lead poisoning in people without other ocular disturbance. Mathot described a somewhat similar finding, but questioned its diagnostic value, because it did not correlate with clinical evidence of poisoning. Others (Guiliano; Montoya-Cabrera; Pearce; Savic) were unable to find this sign when looking for it in their own series of individuals with various degrees of lead poisoning. The significance of "stippling of the retina" therefore remains in doubt.

The retina in lead poisoning in experimental animals has held considerable interest. In rabbits the retinal pigment epithelium has been seen to become greatly swollen by accumulation of granules of lipofuscin, and this can occur without change in the visual cells, in the ERG, EOG, or ophthalmoscopic appearance (Brown; Hass; Hughes). However, degeneration of photoreceptors has occurred after development of very advanced changes in the retinal pigment epithelium (Hughes). This phenomenon may be species specific for rabbits, since unsuccessful efforts have been made to induce it in guinea pigs, rats, and monkeys (Hughes).

Experiments investigating influences of the level of illumination on visual functions have revealed that lead affects rods, with little effect on cones, and that lead causes some disturbances of visual function that are detectible in conditions of dark, but not in light, adaptation. Effects on rods in bullfrog retinas are described by Fox and by Sillman. Defective vision in poisoned monkeys in dim illumination has been studied by Bowman and by Bushnell. Human beings chronically exposed to lead similarly have been found by Cavalleri to show abnormalities in their central visual fields under mesopic adaptation, though normal in photopic illumination.

Electroretinographic and electrooculographic abnormalities in patients with early stages of lead poisoning have been reported by Guguchkova. The influence of state of adaptation should be of interest.

The pupils in lead poisoning do not seem to be affected in any specific way. The reactivities of the pupils to light seems principally to reflect the functional state of the retina and optic nerve, the pupils being dilated and unreactive to light when there is blindness due to involvement of the visual pathways below the suprageniculate synapse. Likewise, accommodation does not seem to be selectively impaired (Blatt). There is a rare report of ophthalmoplegia interna by Brose.

The extraocular muscles have been noted to be paretic in a large portion of cases of ocular disturbance by lead, but almost always in association with some involvement of the optic nerves or visual pathways in the central nervous system. Most characteristically the sixth nerves have been affected by increased intracranial pressure, but there are also numerous instances of paralysis of third and fourth nerves, usually in association with optic neuritis. Bilateral limitation of lateral gaze has been reported by Power in 60 per cent of a group of seventy-five soldiers who had acute lead poisoning from eating chile powder contaminated with lead chromate.

Involvement of extraocular muscles without other ocular disturbance has occurred in a small exceptional group of cases.[153] Grogg reported finding swelling and degeneration of the muscle fibers.[194] No special association of peripheral motor neuritis, such as is manifested in wrist drop, is seen with extraocular muscle palsies, but they not uncommonly occur together.

A study of eye movements in lead workers by Baloh has shown accuracy of saccades to be diminished, but not sufficiently to be a reliable indicator of early poisoning.

Treatment of lead poisoning aims to lower the concentration of lead in the circulation and to remove lead from the body, based mainly on use of calcium edetate administered parenterally.

Allen JR, McWey PJ, Suomi SJ: Pathobiological and behavioral effects of lead intoxication in the infant rhesus monkey. *ENVIRON HEALTH PERSPECT* 2:239–245, 1974.

Baghdassarian SA: Optic neuropathy due to lead poisoning. *ARCH OPHTHALMOL* 80:721–723, 1968.

Baloh RW, Landhofer L, et al: Quantitative eye tracking tests in lead workers. *AM J IND MED* 1:109–113, 1980.

Belova SF: The toxic effect of lead on the optic nerve. *VESTN OFTALMOL* 78:43–44, 1965.

Bihler W: A case of lead amblyopia. *ARCH AUGENHEILKD* 40:274–279, 1900. (German)

Blatt A: Paralysis of accommodation and disturbances of the pupil after lead poisoning. *KLIN MONATSBL AUGENHEILKD* 86:482–491, 1931. (German)

Bowman RE, Bushnell PJ: Scotopic visual deficits in young monkeys given chronic daily low levels of lead. pp. 219–231 in Merigan (1980).[358]

Bradley JE, Baumgartner RJ: Subsequent mental development of children with lead encephalopathy. *J PEDIATR* 53:311–315, 1958.

Brose LD: Ophthalmoplegia interna, results of lead poisoning. *ARCH OPHTHALMOL* 44:26, 1915.

Brown DVL: Reaction of the rabbit retinal pigment epithelium to systemic lead poisoning. *TRANS AM OPHTHALMOL SOC* 72:404–447, 1974.

Bushnell PJ, Bowman RE, et al: Scotopic vision deficits in young monkeys exposed to lead. *SCIENCE* 196:333–335, 1977.

Cavalleri A, Trimarchi F, et al: Effects of lead on the visual system of occupationally exposed subjects. *SCAND J WORK ENVIRON HEALTH* 8(Suppl 1) 148–151, 1982.

Clasen RA, Pandolfi S, et al: Experimental lead encephalopathy in the rhesus monkey. *J NEUROPATHOL EXP NEUROL* 32:176, 1973.

Clasen RA, Hartmann JF: Experimental acute lead encephalopathy in the juvenile rhesus monkey. *ENVIRON HEALTH PERSPECT* 7:175–185, 1974.

Cooper GP, Fox DA, et al: Visual evoked responses in rats exposed to heavy metals. pp. 203–218 in Merigan (1980).[358]

Evans TS: Encephalopathy due to chronic plumbism. *ARCH INTERN MED* 49:735–743, 1932.

Feeney DM, Longo JF, et al: Detection of the effects of lead exposure by visual evoked response latency. *PHYSIOL PSYCHOL* 7:143–145, 1979.

Fox DA, Sillman AJ: Heavy metals affect rod, but not cone, photoreceptors. *SCIENCE* 206:78–80, 1979.

Giannantoni C: Experimental research on toxic amblyopia from lead. *BOLL OCULIST* 12:89–128, 1933.

Gibson JL: Plumbic ocular neuritis in Queensland children. *BR MED J* 2:1488–1490, 1908.

Gibson JL: Ocular plumbism in children. *BR J OPHTHALMOL* 16:637–643, 1931.

Guiliano G, Marras O, et al: Peripapillary retinal pigmentation as a presumed sign of saturnism. *ANN OTTALMOL CLIN OCUL* 95:913–920, 1969. (Italian)

Good P: Choked discs in lead encephalopathy. *AM J OPHTHALMOL* 24:794–797, 1942.

Guguchkova PT: Electroretinographic and electrooculographic examinations of persons occupationally exposed for a long time to the effect of lead. *VESTN OFTALMOL* 1:60–65, 1972.

Hass GM, Brown DVL, et al: Relations between lead poisoning in rabbit and man. *AM J PATHOL* 45:691–727, 1964.

Harbourne JF, McCrea CT, Watkinson J: An unusual outbreak of lead poisoning in calves. *VET REC* 83:515–517, 1968.

Hay W: Lead encephalopathy in a cooperage. *BR J IND MED* 7:177–184, 1950.

Hertel: Chronic lead poisoning with left homonymous hemianopsia. *CHARITE ANN* 15:220, 1890. (French)

Hopkins AP, Dayan AD: The pathology of experimental lead encephalopathy in the baboon. *BR J IND MED* 31:128–133, 1974.

Houser WD, Frank N: Accidental lead poisoning in a rhesus monkey. *J AM VET MED ASSOC* 157:1919–1922, 1970.

Hughes WF, Coogan P: Pathology of the pigment epithelium and retina in rabbits poisoned with lead. *AM J PATHOL* 77:237–254, 1974.

Imre G: Glia proliferation on the papillar surface in workers exposed to lead intoxication. *SZEMESZET* 104:133–135, 1967.

Lobeck E: On knowledge of retinal changes in chronic lead poisoning. *GRAEFES ARCH OPHTHALMOL* 135:165–168, 1936.

Mathot J: On the value of examining the ocular fundus in lead poisoning. *MAROC MED* 44:462, 1965. (French)

Montoya-Cabrera M, Cano-Villareal O: Stippling of the retina; a precursor sign of lead poisoning? *ARCH INVEST MED* 8:193–197, 1977. (English summary)

Neuman L: A case of blindness on the basis of lead poisoning. *KLIN OCZNA* 14:408–414, 1936.

Pal: On the pathogenesis of acute transitory amaurosis with lead colic. *ZENTRALB INN MED 17,* 1903. (German)

Pearce WG, Reynard WA: An early sign of lead poisoning. *BR J IND MED* 21:247, 1964.

Pearce WG, Sonkin N: More on retinal stippling. *N ENGL J MED* 270:533–534, 1964.

Pentschew A: Morphology and morphogenesis of lead encephalopathy. *ACTA NEURO-PATH (BERLIN)* 5:133–160, 1965. (Cited by Walsh and Hoyt.[256])

Pincus: A case of transitory lead amaurosis. *MUNCH MED WOCHENSCHR* 1316:1901. (German)

Popoff N, Weinberg S, Feigin I: Pathological observations in lead encephalopathy with special reference to the vascular changes. *NEUROLOGY* 13:101, 1963.

Posey WC, Farr CB: Left homonymous hemianopsia in worker in lead. *UNIV PENNSYLVANIA MED BULL,* Mar. 1910.

Power JG, Barnes RM, Nash WN, Robinson JD: Lead poisoning in Gurkha soldiers in Hong Kong. *BR MED J* 2:336–337, 1969.

Sauer RM, Zook BC, Garner FM: Demyelinating encephalopathy associated with lead poisoning in non-human primates. *SCIENCE* 169:1091–1093, 1970.

Savic S, Kalic-Filipovic D, et al: Studies of the ocular fundus in lead-exposed workers. *ARBEITSMED FRAGEN IN DER OPHTHALMOLOGIE,* Vol 1, 1 Symp Munchen 1966, pp. 187–189, (Karger, Basel, New York 1969.)

Schuttman W, Bohm E, Hager G: Optic neuritis as a monosymptomatic form of lead poisoning. *Z GESAMTE HYG* 17:342–348, 1971. (German)

Sillman AJ, Bolnick DA, et al: The effects of lead and of cadmium on the mass photoreceptor potential. *NEURO TOXICOLOGY* 3:179–194, 1982.

Smith JF, McLaurin RL, Nichols JB, Asbury A: Studies in cerebral oedema and cerebral swelling. *BRAIN* 83:411–424, 1960.

Snell S: A case of optic atrophy (primary) due to lead. *TRANS OPHTHALMOL SOC UK* 24:184–186, 1904.

Sonkin N: Stippling of the retina. *N ENGL J MED* 269:779–780, 1963.

Soos G, Domokos M, et al: Ophthalmological investigation of patients with saturnism. *ORV HETIL* 111:747–750, 1970. (Hungarian)

Tennekoon G, Aitchison CS, et al: Chronic lead intoxication; effects on developing optic nerve. *ANN NEUROL* 5:558–564, 1979.

Uhthoff W: Eye disturbances from poisoning. *GRAEFE-SAMISCHE HANDB DER AUGENHEILKD,* 2nd ed. 1911, vol. 11, pp. 62–75. (German)

Unseld DW: Optic nerve injuries by lead. *MED WELT* 9:444–445, 1966. (German)

Vints LA: Optic nerve changes in workers of lead industry. *OFTALMOL ZH* 28:88–90, 1973. (English summary)

Westphal A: On lead encephalopathy. *ARCH PSYCHIATR* 19:620, 1888. (German)

Williams C: Lead amblyopia, presentation of left homonymous lateral hemianopsia. *ANN OPHTHALMOL* 20:718, 1912.

Zook BC, Sauer RM, Garner FM: Acute amaurotic epilepsy caused by lead poisoning in nonhuman primates. *J AM VET MED ASSOC* 161:683–686, 1972.

Levallorphan tartrate (Lorfan), an antagonist to narcotics, constricts the pupils when given systemically to normal people, but it causes the pupils to dilate in those who are dependent upon opioid drugs.[a,b] This is the basis for a clinical test for opioid dependency.

a. Jasinski DR, Martin WR, Haertzen C: The human pharmacology and abuse potential of N-allylnoroxymorphone (naloxone). *J PHARMACOL EXP THER* 157:420–426, 1967.

b. Martin WR: Opiod antagonists. *PHARMACOL REV* 19:463–506, 1967.

Levodopa (Bendopa, Dopar, Larodopa, Levopa), an antiparkinsonian drug, has had side effects on movements of lids and eyes, and on the pupils. Martin noted "painful eyelid retraction" in 4 out of 60 patients under this treatment.[e] Barbeau and Cotzias reported lifting of the eyebrows, rapid blinking, blepharospasm, strabismus and conjugate deviation of the eyes.[a,b] Shimizu found 8 out 27 patients under treatment had abnormal involuntary ocular movements, different from the oculomotor manifestations of Parkinson's disease itself, and consisting of smooth "to and fro" eye movements behind closed lids with the patient alert.[f] This could be inhibited by voluntary fixation of gaze. Most often involuntary eye movements have been associated with prolonged treatment and bodily dyskinesia from levodopa. Fraunfelder's national registry has also received reports of ptosis, blepharospasm, oculogyric crises, and visual hallucinations.[312]

Brief mydriasis was noted by Yahr occurring occasionally within an hour of a dose of levodopa,[l] but other observers have not observed mydriasis in patients under prolonged treatment with ordinary dosage.[c,d]

Miosis has been reported in patients receiving levodopa for several weeks.[g,h]

Experimental application of levodopa to the eyes of normal people has shown that it can induce mydriasis at sufficiently high concentrations,[g,i] and this can be inhibited by an alpha-adrenergic antagonist, thymoxamine.[i] Further studies, especially of a patient with latent post-ganglionic Horner's syndrome, has provided evidence that when oral levodopa induces mydriasis it is attributable to dopamine-induced increase in sympathetic nerve activity.[k]

The question of mydriasis from levodopa given systemically in treatment of parkinsonism, apart from its pharmacologic interest would have practical implications for patients who might be prone to angle-closure glaucoma on account of abnormally shallow anterior chambers and narrow angles, but if in practice the mydriatic effect is slight, inconstant, short-lasting, and sometimes superseded by miosis, it seems that it may be of very little practical importance. (See also *Dopamine*.)

Testing for cataractogenesis in rabbits has given negative results.[j]

a. Barbeau A: L-Dopa therapy in Parkinson's disease; a critical review of nine years' experience. *CAN MED ASSOC J* 101:791–800, 1969.

b. Cotzias GC, Papavasilliou PS, Gellene R: Modifications of parkinsonism—chronic treatment with L-dopa. *N ENGL J MED* 280:337–345, 1969.

c. Godwin-Austen RB, Lind NA, Turner P: Mydriatic responses to sympathomimetic amines in patients treated with L-dopa. *LANCET* 2:1043–1044, 1969.

d. Kanter P, Koenig S, Lipsich M: Ophthalmic findings in patients using levodopa. *ANN OPHTHALMOL* 5:457–460, 1973.

e. Martin WE: Adverse reactions during treatment of Parkinson's disease with levodopa. *J AM MED ASSOC* 216:1979–1983, 1971.

f. Shimizu N, Cohen B, et al: Ocular dyskinesias in patients with Parkinson's disease treated with levodopa. *ANN NEUROL* 1:167–171, 1977.

g. Spiers ASD: Mydriatic responses to sympathomimetic amines in patients treated with L-dopa. *LANCET* 2:1301, 1969.

h. Spiers ASD, Calne DB, Fayers PM: Miosis during l-dopa therapy. *BR MED J* 2:639–640, 1970.

i. Spiers ASD, Calne DB, et al: Action of thymoxamine on mydriasis induced by levodopa and dopamine. *BR MED J* 2:438–439, 1971.

j. Srivastava SK, Beutter E: Effect of L-dopa administration on rabbit lens and erythrocytes. *BIOCHEM MED* 5:317–324, 1971.

k. Weintraub MI, Gaasterland D, Van Woert M: L-dopa-induced anisocoria in latent Horner's syndrome. *NEUROLOGY* 20:417, 1970.

l. Yahr MD, Duvoisin RC, et al: Treatment of parkinsonism with levodopa. *ARCH NEUROL* 21:343–354, 1969.

Levorphanol tartrate (Levo-Dromoran), an analgesic, narcotic, when administered systemically to mice in 1961 was noted to cause rapid appearance of opacity of the front of the lens as from opaque deposits. These opacities cleared spontaneously.[d,e] A possibility of interaction of catecholamines and levorphanol to produce the opacities was investigated extensively.[b,c] Systemic reserpine was found to block the formation of the opacities, and the effect of reserpine could in turn be antagonized by administering certain adrenergic substances. Also mice given levorphanol repeatedly were shown to develop a tolerance indicated by less formation of opacity.[b,c] Intracerebral injection of levorphanol was also effective in producing lens opacities in mice, although very little of the tritium-labeled drug was found to reach the lens.[b,c] A relatively simple explanation has been advanced that the opacities of the front of the lens produced by levorphanol, as well as by several other drugs, are merely a result of decreased rate of blinking and exposure of the cornea to evaporation, with consequent reversible dehydration and change in transparency of the lens. This effect was shown to be completely preventable by keeping the lids closed. Furthermore reversible lens opacities of the same type as produced by levorphanol could be induced by artificial exposure of the eye without use of drugs, simply by mechanically preventing closure of the lids.[a]

a. Fraunfelder FT, Burns RP: Effects of lid closure in drug-induced experimental cataracts. *ARCH OPHTHALMOL* 76:599–601, 1966.

b. Smith A, Karmin M, Gavitt JA: Central origin of the lenticular opacities induced in mice by opiates. *J PHARM PHARMACOL* 18:545–546, 1966.

c. Smith A, Karmin M, Gavitt JA: Interaction of catecholamines with levorphanol and morphine in the mouse eye. *J PHARMACOL EXP THER* 151:103–109, 1966.

d. Weinstock M: Similarity between receptors responsible for the production of analgesia and lenticular opacity. *BR J PHARMACOL* 17:433–441, 1961.

e. Weinstock M, Stewart HC: Occurrence in rodents of reversible drug-induced opacities of the lens. *BR J OPHTHALMOL* 45:408–414, 1961.

Levothyroxine (Levothroid, Synthroid), a thyroid hormone, has caused reversible pseudotumor cerebri with headache and bilateral papilledema in children treated for hypothyroidism.[a] Treatment with dexamethasone and acetazolamide was helpful.

a. Van Dop C, Conte FA, et al: Pseudotumor cerebri associated with initiation of levothyroxine therapy for juvenile hypothyroidism. *N ENGL J MED* 308:1076–1080, 1983.

Levulinic acid, according to Deichmann and Gerarde,[37] in contact with the eye as concentrated acid "results in severe burns similar to those from glacial acetic acid."

Lewisite (chlorovinyldichloroarsine) is an extremely toxic and vesicant liquid which received considerable attention in World Wars I and II as a potential war gas. A small number of accidental injuries to human beings occurred, and considerable experimental data were obtained on animals. Both the vapor and liquid cause immediate pain in the eyes, resulting in profuse tearing and blepharospasm; this serves as a protection for the eye against serious exposure to vapor, but not against severe damage by splashes of liquid.

Very fine droplet spray, such as produced by dispersal of lewisite in air by a bursting charge of explosive has been observed in human eyes to cause transient corneal epithelial erosions which have healed spontaneously.[a] Experimental application of droplets of lewisite to rabbit eyes has, however, been seen by several experimenters to cause severe and even completely destructive damage to the eye; these observations have been well reviewed in 1954 by Duke-Elder.[46] Little of note has appeared since then, and the compound appears to have no peace-time uses.

A classic series of investigations by Stocken and Thompson revealed the nature of the reaction of lewisite with thiol groups of tissue proteins, and in a triumph of scientific method produced an effective antidote, BAL (British anti-lewisite), or dimercaprol.[b] Experiments in rabbits have demonstrated the effectiveness of dimercaprol in preventing or reducing lewisite damage to the eye if instilled within minutes, but the effectiveness decreases rapidly with time following exposure. Probably an hour is the maximum period in which any benefit can be achieved.[46]

a. Cogan DG: Lewisite burns of the eye. *J AM MED ASSOC* 122:435, 1943.
b. Stocken LA, Thompson RHS: British anti-lewisite. *BIOCHEM J* 40:529–554, 1946.

Librax, a preparation containing *chlordiazepoxide hydrochloride* and *clidinium bromide,* used in treatment of gastrointestinal disorders, has theoretical potentiality of slight anticholinergic effects on the eye, but only during one brief period in 1965 has blurring of vision from mydriasis and impaired accommodation been noteworthy, and this was attributed to an analog of clidinium having greater atropine-like effect, inadvertently present in one batch as an impurity, an episode primarily of historical interest.[a]

Rosselet and Faggioni reported two cases of glaucoma in patients using Librax, which the authors assume to be responsible, but they did not present clear or conclusive evidence or adequate information on the type of glaucoma involved.[210]

a. Roche Laboratories: Drug Warning Letter. Nov. 19, 1965.

Licorice (glycyrrhiza, from *Glycyrrhiza glabra*) can cause severe reversible systemic hypertension when extraordinarily large amounts are ingested, owing principally to its content of a steroid-like compound, glycyrrhetinic acid.[a,b] One young woman developed severe vascular retinopathy associated with severe systemic hypertension after eating about 100 g of licorice candy per day for more than a year, but when this was stopped, her blood pressure returned to normal and the retinopathy resolved in about three weeks.[a]

a. Koster M, David GK: Reversible severe hypertension due to licorice ingestion. *N ENGL J MED* 278:1381–1383, 1968.
b. Rausch-Strooman JG: Reversible severe hypertension due to licorice ingestion. *N ENGL J MED* 279:606, 1968.

Lincomycin hydrochloride (Lincocin hydrochloride), an antibacterial, was accidentally injected (300 mg in 1 ml) through a peripheral iridectomy into the posterior chamber in the eye of a patient undergoing cataract extraction. This was followed by irrigation with 2.5 ml of balanced saline solution, and the operation was completed in a customary manner, utilizing alpha-chymotrypsin to lyse the lens zonules. Postoperatively there was no extraordinary reaction, and in 2 weeks the eye was considered normal.

Tabbara KF, Salamoun SG: Accidental intraocular injection of lincomycin. *AM J OPHTHALMOL* 73:596–597, 1972.

Lindane (1,2,3,4,5,6-hexachlorocyclohexane; gamma isomer of benzene hexachloride, [not to be confused with *hexachlorobenzene*]) is a scabicide and pediculicide usually applied as a 1% lotion, cream, or shampoo, e.g., under the name Kwell or Scabene.

In patients, attempts to apply lindane to treat blepharitis from Demodex folliculorum infestation of the lids are reported to have caused excessive irritation of the eyes, even when concentrations as low as 0.1% were employed in combination with a topical corticosteroid. Kwell ointment containing 1% lindane caused conjunctivitis when applied to the eyelashes.[g] However, clinical experience with use of lindane in topical treatment of *phthiriasis palpebrarum,* an infestation of the eyelashes and lid margin with crab lice (*Phthirus pubis*),[b] has shown that 1% lindane cream or lotion when applied carefully in small amount to lid margins and lashes, and then washed off after several minutes, is very effective and not excessively irritating.[a,e] A single treatment of this sort, repeated in 5 or 6 days if necessary, appears to have caused no harm.

When eyes have been subjected to effects of lindane in other ways, toxic effects have been reported. When applied directly to the eyes of mice, it caused changes in the electrogram.[289] When administered intratracheally for 6 months to rabbits it caused corneal and retinal edema.[d] However, applications of a 3% dust mixture with talc on the eyes of rabbits produced no irritation,[f] and application of a solution of 2 mg in 0.01 ml of acetone caused only slightly more hyperemia than acetone alone.[h]

Systemic poisoning by lindane occurred in seventy-nine patients in Greece in the course of a month through intimate contact with the material in the home and on bedclothing.[c] Gastrointestinal disturbances appeared first, then severe CNS involvement manifested principally by cerebellar derangement and muscle spasm. Blindness from optic atrophy was observed in one patient. A second patient complained of diminution of vision, but nothing abnormal was found in the fundus.

A third patient purportedly had temporary diminution of vision but was not examined medically.

a. Awan KJ: Cryotherapy in phthiriasis palpebrarum. *AM J OPHTHALMOL* 83:906–907, 1977.

b. Couch JM, Green WR, et al: Diagnosing and treating *Phthirus pubis palpebrarum. SURV OPHTHALMOL* 26:219–225, 1982.

c. Danopoulos E, Mellisinos K, Katsas G: Serious poisoning by hexachlorocyclohexane, clinical and laboratory observations on five cases. *ARCH IND HYG* 7:582–587, 1953.

d. El'kind LA, Nuritdinova FN: Morphological data studies on the rabbit eye after chronic intoxication with several pesticides. *MED ZH UZB* (12):37–40, 1974.

e. Kirschner MH: Phthirus pubis infestation of the eyelashes. *J AM MED ASSOC* 248:428, 1982; 249:590, 1983.

f. Letard H, DeSacy G: Toxicology of hexachlorocyclohexane. *C R SOC BIOL* 139:353–354, 1945.

g. Post CF, Juhlin E: Demodex folliculorum and blepharitis. *ARCH DERM* 88:292–302, 1963.

h. Tareeva AI: Results of exploratory toxicity studies of commercial mixtures of hexachlorocyclohexane isomers. *FARMAKOL TOXIK* 16:45–47, 1947. (*CHEM ABSTR* 41:7535.)

Linoleic acid peroxide has been of interest as a probable constituent of lipoperoxides which may be produced in tissues by irradiation with visible light, ultraviolet, and probably x-rays. Opacity has been observed to develop in excised rat lenses placed in contact with linoleic acid peroxide during twenty-four hours, while the ordinary nonperoxide form of linoleic acid under the same circumstances caused essentially no change in transparency.[c] Addition of linoleic acid peroxide to the incubated rabbit retina homogenate has inhibited oxygen consumption and oxidative phosphorylation. When injected into the vitreous body of rabbits, it has damaged the visual cells, while ordinary linoleic acid was much less toxic.[a] *Lipoperoxide* formed by irradiation of retina appears to have analogous injurious effect.[b]

Linoleic hydroperoxide and **linolenic hydroperoxide,** prepared from the corresponding acids, injected into the vitreous body in rabbits has caused progressive irreversible decrease in the ERG's, eventually to extinction.[d]

a. Hiramitsu T: The effect of lipoperoxides on respiration of rabbit retina. *ACTA SOC OPHTHALMOL JPN* 73:1706–1710, 1969.

b. Kawamura Y, Miyata M: Studies on retinitis pigmentosa. *ACTA SOC OPHTHALMOL JPN* 73:1789–1800, 1969.

c. Kojima K, Ookochi Y: The opacity of rat lens caused by fatty acid peroxide. *ACTA SOC OPHTHALMOL JPN* 72:1732–1733, 1968.

d. Armstrong D, Hiramitsu T, et al: Studies on experimentally induced retina degeneration. *EXP EYE RES* 35:157–171, 1982.

Lint, consisting of cotton fibers, mainly cellulose, have many times been discovered in the anterior chamber after intraocular surgery, having come from swabs of absorbent cotton or gauze, or from drapes of cloth or paper used at operation.[a,c,f,h,i] Air, and intraocular irrigating solutions if not carefully filtered, as well as surgical instruments and sponges, are recognized vehicles for the lint fibrils. In most instances the fibrils have been tolerated in the eye indefinitely without obvious reaction, but in 3 cases Vail attributed moderately severe, but transient iritis to these particles.[i]

In rabbits introduction of pieces of cotton from 0.5 × 0.5 mm to 1 × 1 mm into the anterior chamber produced no reaction recognizable by slit-lamp biomicroscopy, but by histologic examination a cellular reaction was found, strictly limited to iris where it was in contact with the foreign particles.[e,g]

Finely chopped cotton fibers have been introduced into the anterior chamber of the eyes of rabbits to obstruct outflow of aqueous humor and they have rapidly induced elevation of ocular pressure. The pressure has been maintained at 38 to 48 mm Hg for at least a month.[b] The effect may represent a physical obstruction by small particles, not a toxic action.

a. Brockhurst RJ: Cotton fibrils in the anterior chamber after surgery. *ARCH OPHTHALMOL* 52:121–124, 1954.
b. De Carvalho CA: Histopathology of retina and optic nerve with experimental glaucoma. *ARCH OPHTHALMOL* 67:483–487, 1962.
c. Gurtler E: Cotton fibers in the anterior chamber after eye-opening operations. *WIEN KLIN WOCHENSCHR* 6:686–689, 1949. (German)
d. Mukai H: Swab fibers in the anterior chamber after cataract operation. *KLIN MONATSBL AUGENHEILKD* 76:88–90, 1926. (German)
e. Peiffer RL, Safrit HD, et al: Intraocular response to cotton, collagen and cellulose in the rabbit. *OPHTHALMIC SURG* 14:582–587, 1983.
f. Purtscher F: Cotton threads in the anterior chamber after intracapsular lens extraction. *KLIN MONATSBL AUGENHEILKD* 102:844, 1939. (German)
g. Savar DE: Intraocular effects of lint particles from disposable drapes. *ANN OPHTHALMOL* 10:1607–1609, 1978.
h. Shoemaker RE: Lint in the anterior chamber after surgery. *ARCH OPHTHALMOL* 52:807, 1954.
i. Vail D: Lint in the anterior chamber following intraocular surgery. *TRANS AM OPHTHALMOL SOC* 48:243–258, 1950.

Lipidosis, or **phospholipidosis,** is a drug-induced intralysosomal accumulation of lipids that can affect all cells of the body. Lipidosis involving the eye has been shown to have affected the cornea, conjunctiva, lens, ciliary body, and retina. Drug-induced lipidosis has been reviewed in detail by D'Amico (1981)[b], Lullmann (1975, 1978)[g,i], and Seiler (1977).[j] Examples of effects on the eye that are most familiar clinically are the deposits in the cornea from *chloroquine* and *amiodarone,* and, possibly, the retinopathy from *chloroquine*. Other types of eye involvement have been produced in experimental animals.

Drugs which have the peculiar property of inducing lipidosis are widely varied in their pharmacologic, toxicologic, and chemical properties, but have one feature in common. They all have in their molecular structure highly hydrophobic and hydrophilic portions in close proximity, and they are cationic. They are said to be "amphiphilic" or "amphipathic." They can penetrate into cells and then into the lysosomes of the cells, where they become strongly associated with intralysosomal phospholipids. The polar lipids formed by this combination are not readily digested or degraded, and therefore tend to accumulate in the lysosomes, gradually changing the lysosomes to residual cytoplasmic inclusion bodies. These bodies are of two types, multilamellated and crystalloid. They are recognizable by electron microscopic ultrastructural study, but generally not by ordinary light microscopy. However, when present in large amount in transparent structures, such as cornea and lens, they may produce grossly visible opacities. To what extent the presence of lipidosis can be correlated with other toxic phenomena is yet to be learned. For instance, in *chloroquine* retinopathy it is uncertain whether loss of rods and cones is a consequence of impairment of polar lipid catabolism, or due to some other toxic mechanism.[g]

Experimental work on retinal lipidosis has been carried out by Lullmann-Rauch (1976),[h] examining in rats the effect on the retinal pigment epithelium (RPE) from feeding several drugs that interfere with enzymatic degradation of phospholipids. This has special interest because an important function of the RPE is continuous phagocytosis and digestion of old discs of visual cell outer segments, which have high phospholipid content. Several weeks of feeding *chlorphentermine, iprindole, chloroamitriptyline, imipramine,* or *clomipramine* resulted in doubling in height of the RPE due to accumulation of crystalloid cytoplamic inclusions. Inclusions were found also in the neuroretina, mostly in the ganglion cells. These inclusion bodies were both lamellated and crystalloid. After withdrawal of the drugs, the changes were reversible. To what degree visual function might have been affected was not investigated. Further work on retinal lipidosis by Drenckhahn and Lullmann-Rauch (1978)[f] showed that different drugs produced different distributions of inclusion bodies. *Triparanol* affected only the RPE and Muller cells. *Chlorcyclizine* affected the RPE, neurons, and Muller cells equally. *Diethylaminoethoxyhexestrol* (Coralgil; Trimanyl) affected principally neurons and Muller cells. *Chloroquine,* the only one known clinically to be retinotoxic, was the only one to affect visual cells, not the outer segments, but the cytoplasm near the outer limiting membrane. However, *chloroquine* caused greater changes in ganglion cells, neurons, and Muller cells. *Amiodarone* fed to rats was found by Bockhardt and colleagues (1978)[a] to produce cytoplasmic inclusions in RPE cells, retinal ganglion cells, some Muller cell processes, and epithelial layers of ciliary body and iris, but not in photoreceptor cells. D'Amico and colleagues (1982)[d], utilizing cultured RPE and conjunctiva, showed that lipidosis could be induced in these tissues by addition of *gentamicin, tobramycin,* or *streptomycin.*

Lens opacities have been produced experimentally in rats by drug-induced lipidosis. Drenckhahn and Lullmann-Rauch (1977)[e] found that feeding *chloroquine chlorphentermine,* or *iprindole* for several weeks produced diffuse anterior and posterior subcapsular lens opacities, and also sutural opacities. The opacities were attributed to light scattering by lamellated inclusions and vacuoles in the lens epithelium. Lens cells that were growing during the period of drug feeding seemed to be most affected, presumably due to interference in the polar lipid metabolism of those cells. The most pronounced cortical opacities were visible to the naked eye; others were discernible by slit-lamp microscopy.

Fine deposits in the corneas of patients taking *chloroquine* or *amiodarone,* and some other drugs, are well known clinically, often showing a characteristic whorl-like or cat's whisker pattern when examined with a slit-lamp biomicroscope. D'Amico and colleagues (1981)[c] showed by examining corneal epithelial and conjunctival biopsies and a cataractous lens from one patient on amiodarone that typical intracytoplasmic lysosomal inclusions were present in these tissues. Bockhardt and colleagues (1978)[a] found that these cytoplasmic inclusions could be induced in all layers of the corneas of rats, especially in the epithelium, by repeated local application of *amiodarone*.

It is remarkable that such widespread ultrastructural changes in eye tissues have been found in a number of drug-induced lipidoses from drugs in clinical use, yet so far these mostly seem to have been tolerated without serious results. The corneal deposits produced by *chloroquine* and *amiodarone* have seemed innocuous, and it is not known to what degree lipidosis may play a part in the visual disturbances of chloroquine retinopathy.

For ***additional numerous examples*** and information, see *Lipidosis* and *Retinal lipidosis* in the INDEX.

a. Bockhardt H, Drenckhahn D, Lullmann-Rauch R: Amiodarone-induced lipidosis-like alterations in ocular tissues in rats. *GRAEFES ARCH OPHTHALMOL* 207:91–96, 1978.

b. D'Amico DJ, Kenyon KR: Drug-induced lipidoses of the cornea and conjunctiva. *INT OPHTHALMOL* 4:67–76, 1981.

c. D'Amico DJ, Kenyon KR, Ruskin JN: Amiodarone keratopathy. Drug-induced lipid storage disease. *ARCH OPHTHALMOL* 99:257–261, 1981.

d. D'Amico DJ, Kenyon KR, et al: Lipid inclusions in human ocular tissues *in vitro* induced by aminoglycoside antibiotics. *BIRTH DEFECTS* 18:411–420, 1982.

e. Drenckhahn D, Lullmann-Rauch R: Lens opacities associated with lipidosis-like ultrastructural alterations in rats treated with chloroquine, chlorphentermine, or iprindole. *EXP EYE RES* 24:621–632, 1977.

f. Drenckhahn D, Lullmann-Rauch R: Drug-induced retinal lipidosis: Differential susceptibilities of pigment epithelium and neuroretina toward several amphiphilic cationic drugs. *EXP MOL PATHOL* 28:360–371, 1978.

g. Lullmann H, Lullmann-Rauch R, Wassermann O: Drug-induced phospholipidoses. *CRC CRIT REV TOXICOL* 4:185–218, 1975.

h. Lullmann-Rauch R: Retinal lipidosis in albino rats treated with chlorphentermine and with tricyclic antidepressants. *ACTA NEUROPATHOL (Berlin)* 35:55–67, 1976.

i. Lullmann H, Lullmann-Rauch R, Wassermann O: Lipidosis induced by amphiphilic cationic drugs. *BIOCHEM PHARMACOL* 27:1103–1108, 1978.

j. Seiler KV, Thiel HJ, Wassermann O: Chloroquine keratopathy as an example of drug-induced phospholipidosis. *KLIN MONATSBL AUGENHEILKD* 170:64–73, 1977. (German)

Lithium hydride is a strong respiratory irritant even at very low concentrations, and it has been observed to cause irritation and inflammation in the eyes in rats, rabbits, and guinea pigs at concentrations which were very irritating to the respiratory tract.[b] (Compare *Lithium hydroxide*.)

A serious eye injury by lithium hydride has been described by Cracovaner in 1964 in a man who had massive exposure from explosion of a cylinder, heavily contaminating both eyes.[a] The immediate effects and treatment were not described, but in two and one-half weeks the corneas were extensively opacified and ulcerated. "Multiple keratoplasties" were done, ultimately successful in one eye. However, from inhalation of the dust the patient developed strictures of the larynx, trachea, bronchi, and esophagus requiring many operations.

a. Cracovaner AJ: Stenosis after explosion of lithium hydride. *ARCH OTOLARYNGNOL* 80:87–92, 1964.

b. Spiegl CJ, Scott JK, et al: Acute inhalation toxicity of lithium hydride. *ARCH IND HEALTH* 14:468–479, 1956.

Lithium hydroxide (lithium hydrate), a white, strongly alkaline powder which forms an acrid irritating dust, has been used to absorb carbon dioxide from the air in space capsules. On one occasion an unintended dispersal of the dust in the air is reported to have caused much irritation of the eyes and respiratory tract of astronauts.[a]

In tests on eyes of animals solutions of lithium hydroxide are similar to solutions of sodium hydroxide of equal pH in rate of penetration and severity of injury to the cornea.[81]

a. Space. *TIME* (*MAGAZINE*), July 29, 1966, pp 28–29.

Lithium salts have had changing uses in human nutrition and medical treatment. Lithium citrate has been used in soft drinks, but apparently in concentrations too low to be toxic. Lithium chloride was at one time used as a dietary substitute for salt in low-sodium diets. Around 1950 there were several reports of poisonings, some fatal, from excessive lithium intake in food, coupled with reduced sodium intake. Some of these reports described temporarily blurred vision, but no definitive study of the cause was made. Measurements of visual acuity, visual field, intraocular pressure and observations on the fundi were lacking.[c,g,m,o,p] Possibly the visual disturbance was of cortical origin, since it was said to be accompanied by confusion, insomnia, irritability, and abnormalities of the encephalogram.[252] An earlier report of an acute overdose gave a similar picture. A healthy person who took 4 g of lithium chloride by mouth on one occasion, and on another occasion took 2 g after each meal for three meals, both times experienced blurring vision so marked that he was able to read only the largest headlines of a newspaper. This was accompanied by tinnitus, generalized weakness, staggering, and tremor. The vision returned to normal in about a day and the other symptoms disappeared in four or five days.[b]

Now the main use of lithium salts in human beings is in treatment of manic-depressive psychosis, mainly as lithium carbonate (Lithane, Eskalith, Lithotabs, Lithonate, Lithobid). Exophthalmos with thyroid disturbance has become recognized as a significant complication, affecting 5 out of 44 patients in one prospective study during at least 6 months' treatment for psychiatric disease,[n] and documented also in a number of random cases.[e,h,i,l] Apart from exophthalmos and thyroid disturbance, a systematic ophthalmologic study of 73 patients who had been receiving lithium treatment for several years in a psychiatric clinic did not uncover any eye disease thought to be attributable to lithium.[h] Separately, two instances of papilledema have been reported,[j,k] and questions have been raised about possible maculopathy, but so far there has been no convincing evidence for this.[f,312] Severe photophobia has been reported in one case of lithium intoxication.[s]

Application of lithium chloride solutions from 0.1 to 17 M to rabbit's eyes after removal of the corneal epithelium to facilitate penetration caused no evident injury, but produced long-lasting flattening of the cornea.[d,81]

The intraocular pressure in rabbits has not been affected by administering suble-thal amounts of lithium chloride intravenously, subconjunctivally, or intravitreally.[b]

In rodents teratogenic ocular anomalies have been produced by doses of lithium chloride that were very toxic to the mother.[r]

a. Berggren L: The intraocular pressure in rabbits after lithium administration. *ACTA OPHTHALMOL* 45:229–238, 1967.

b. Cleaveland SA: A case of poisoning by lithium presenting some new features. *J AM MED ASSOC* 60:722, 1913.

c. Corcoran AC, Taylor RD, Page IH: Lithium poisoning from the use of salt substitutes. *J AM MED ASSOC* 139:685–688, 1949.

d. Cress J, Maurice DM: An attempt at a chemical treatment of myopia. *ARCH OPHTHAL-MOL* 86:692–693, 1971.

e. Dry J, Aron-Rosa D, Pradalier A: Occurrence of exophthalmos during treatment with lithium bicarbonate. *THERAPIE* (Paris) 29:701–708, 1974. (French)

f. Fraunfelder FT: Questions and answers—Lithium carbonate therapy and senile macular degeneration. *J AM MED ASSOC* 249:2389, 1983.

g. Hanlon LW, Romaine M, et al: Lithium chloride as a substitute for sodium chloride in the diet. *J AM MED ASSOC* 139:688–692, 1949.

h. Hiroz CA, Assimacopoulos T, et al: Ophthalmological side effects of lithium. *ENCEPHALE* 7:123–128, 1981. (French)

i. Leverger JC, et al: Lithium salts and endocrine glands. *SEM HOP PARIS* 52:2017–2020, 1976. (French)

j. Lobo A, Pilek E, Stokes PE: Papilledema following therapeutic dosages of lithium carbonate. *J NERV MENT DIS* 166:526–529, 1978.

k. Pesando P, Nuzzi G, Maraini G: Bilateral papilledema in long term therapy with lithium carbonate. *PHARMAKOPSYCHIATRIE/NEURO-PSYCHOPHARMAKOLOGIE* 13:235–239, 1980. (German)

l. Schoenberg M, et al: Single case study Grave's disease manifesting after maintenance lithium. *J NERV MENT DIS* 16:575–577, 1979.

m. Schou M, Juel-Nielsen N, et al: The treatment of manic psychoses by the administra-tion of lithium salts. *J NEUROL NEUROSURG PSYCHIATR* 17:250–257, 1954.

n. Segal RL, Rosenblatt S, Eliasoph I: Endocrine exophthalmos during lithium therapy of manic-depressive disease. *N ENGL J MED* 289:136–138, 1973.

o. Stern RL: Severe lithium chloride poisoning with complete recovery. *J AM MED ASSOC* 139:710–711, 1949.

p. Talbott JH: Use of lithium salts as substitute for sodium chloride. *ARCH INTERN MED* 85:1–10, 1950.

q. Todd J, Jerram TC: Thyrotoxicosis during lithium treatment. *BR J CLIN PRACT* 32:201–203, 1978.

r. Tuchmann-Duplessis H, Mercier-Parot L: Effect of lithium on pregnancy and prenatal development of the rat and mouse. *C R SOC BIOL* 167:183–186, 1973.

s. Caplan RP, Fry AH: Photophobia in lithium intoxication. *BR MED J* 285:1314–1315, 1982.

Locoweed poisoning of livestock in North America is caused by grazing on *Astragalus* and *Oxytropis* plants; a similar poisoning in Australia is caused by grazing on *Swainsona* plants. The poisoning in cattle, sheep and horses causes ataxic gait and behavior suggesting "partial blindness", which has been described in vague terms, such as sheep "obviously unaware of their surroundings", cattle with "blind staggers", "dull eyes with a staring look", and animals "that walk into obstructions."[b,c,e] A probable explanation for these abnormalities is offered by electron microscopy, which shows widespread vacuolation of the cytoplasm of cells and neurons of the central nervous system and of the ganglion cells of the retina.[e-g] The findings have the characteristics of lysosomal storage disease, quite similar to findings in mannosidosis. Experimental feeding of an extract of locoweed to animals has reproduced the disease, and additional experiments have provided evidence that this has been associated with reversible inhibition of the enzyme α-mannosidase. Normally this enzyme acts upon mannose-containing compounds to prevent their accumulation, but when the enzyme is inhibited, or genetically absent, lysosomal accumulation of mannose-containing oligosaccharides results. The disease mannosidosis in human beings is attributed to an inborn genetic deficiency of the enzyme α-mannosidase resulting in the same type of lysosomal storage disease as locoweed poisoning in livestock, and serious disturbance of the central nervous system. In the case of locoweed or Swainsona-induced mannosidosis in animals the vacuolation in the central nervous system is at least partially reversible when feeding of the toxic weeds is discontinued and active enzyme is allowed to regenerate.[b] The alkaloids *swainsonine* and *swainsonine N-oxide*, which have been isolated from *Swainsona canescens*, and have been shown to inhibit the enzyme α-mannosidase, has also been isolated from locoweed (*Astragalus lentiginosus*), offering an attractive explanation for why Australian Swainsona and American locoweed poisoning are so much alike.[e]

The loss of vision in poisoned animals, which has been deduced from their gross behavior, could be explained on the basis of histologic examinations which showed widespread vacuolation of neurons in the central nervous system, and more specifically on the basis of involvement of retinal ganglion cells, with vacuolar degeneration of their cytoplasm.[f,g] Interestingly, in human mannosidosis cataracts have been noted in several cases,[a,d] but cataracts have not yet been reported in the poisoned animals.

a. Arbisser AI, Murphree AL, et al: Ocular findings in mannosidosis. *AM J OPHTHALMOL* 82:465–471, 1976.

b. Dorling PR, Huxtable CR, Vogel P: Lysosomal storage in *Swainsona spp* toxicosis, an induced mannosidosis. *NEUROPATHOL APPL NEUROBIOL* 4:285–295, 1978.

c. James LF, Hartley WJ, Van Kampen KR: Syndromes of *Astragalus* poisoning in livestock. *J AM VET MED ASSOC* 178:146–150, 1981.

d. Letson RD, Desnick RJ: Punctate lenticular opacities in type II mannosidosis. *AM J OPHTHALMOL* 85:218–224, 1978.

e. Molyneux RJ, James LF: Loco intoxication; Indolizidine alkaloids of spotted locoweed (*Astragalus lentiginosus*). *SCIENCE* 216:190–191, 1982.

f. Van Kampen KR, James LF: Ophthalmic lesions in locoweed poisoning of cattle, sheep, and horses. *AM J VET RES* 32:1293–1295, 1971.

g. Van Kampen KR, James LF: Sequential development of the lesions in locoweed poisoning. *CLIN TOXICOL* 5:575–580, 1972.

Lomotil, a combination of *diphenoxylate hydrochloride* and a small amount of *atropine sulphate,* used orally in treatment of diarrhea, has been reported to have caused severe but nonfatal poisoning from overdosage in a two-year-old child. Pinpoint pupils were one of the noteworthy signs. The child vomited and staggered about for some hours before becoming stuporous. He then had slow shallow respiration and elevated temperature. The pinpoint pupils gave the clue to poisoning. Despite treatment with levallorphan, the patient remained unconscious for three days.[a] A 10-month old child became comatose after taking 4 tablets, and had apparent cortical blindness, presumably due to cerebral edema secondary to hypoxia.[b] Vision returned in 3 weeks. (*Diphenoxylate* has narcotic properties; treatment of overdose with an opioid antagonist such as levallorphan, nalorphine, or naloxone is appropriate.)

    a. Riley ID: Lomotil poisoning. *LANCET* 1:373, 1969.
    b. Wasserman GS: Lomotil ingestions in children. *AM FAMILY PHYSICIAN* 11:93, 1975.

Lonicera plants (honeysuckles) have berries which contain an unidentified toxin. If eaten they are said to cause severe gastrointestinal irritation, reddening of the face, particularly the eyelids, also mydriasis and photophobia.[142]

Lorazepam (Ativan), a tranquilizer, has been tested at a daily oral dose of 1 to 2 mg in patients with chronic open-angle glaucoma, and found to have no effect on intraocular pressure, nor to manifest anticholinergic effects.[a]

    a. Calixto N, De Costa Maia JA: Influence of lorazepam on intraocular pressure. *CURR THER RES* 17:156–160, 1975.

Lupin seeds when ingested are reported to cause mydriasis, but the constituent responsible is not identified.[214]

Lysergide (LSD, lysergic acid diethylamide), a psychotomimetic serotonin antagonist, is well known for inducing visual hallucinations, and this has stimulated considerable investigation of effects on the visual pathways from retina back to visual cortex in animals and man.[z]

In human beings, lysergide may produce acute intoxication resembling atropine poisoning, consisting of visual hallucinations, disorientation, elevated body temperature, increased heart rate, and dilated pupils, but most of these effects are sympathomimetic, rather than anticholinergic. In lysergide intoxication the skin characteristically shows "goose pimples." These are not seen in atropine poisoning, which produces red, dry skin.[1,26,118] Effects on the pupil and accommodation have been studied in normal human volunteers after oral administration of lysergide, substantiating the mydriatic effect and demonstrating weakening of accommodation.[za,26]

Intraocular pressure in human volunteers given LSD 1 μg/kg orally rose less than 2 mm Hg, but in rabbits given 100 μg/kg a mean rise of 3.6 mm Hg was obtained.[o,p]

The visual hallucinogenic effects of lysergide have been well reviewed by Hoffer and Osmond in their book on hallucinogens,[118] and will not be considered further here. Afterimages that may interfere with driving have been described.[zg,zh]

Cortical visually evoked potentials are influenced by lysergide in man, monkeys, cats, and rats.[j] Blocking action on the lateral geniculate synapses has been reported, particularly in monkeys.[d,e,x,zb,zf]

Modifications of the ERG and of dark adaptation in human beings have been reported in people who had hallucinations from lysergide, but totally blind subjects without a functioning retina, who had previously had sight, could experience visual hallucinations when given lysergide, indicating that the retina was not the source, or at least not the only source.[u,v] In cats, lysergide produced changes in the ERG or electric potential of the eye only when very large doses were administered, and these appeared to be nonspecific, such as might be induced by large amounts of barbiturates.[t] In severely poisoned cats, spontaneous action potentials have appeared in the ERG, with exaggerated responses to stimulation by light. Simultaneously, large spikes appeared in recordings from the occipital visual cortex, and these spikes disappeared when the optic nerves were cut, suggesting that this spontaneous visual activity originated in the retina.[c]

The ERG of *excised* human, cat, or monkey retina has not been affected by lysergide.[t]

Behavior suggesting blindness has been observed in cats, pigeons, and monkeys under the influence of lysergide.[f,i,zd,ze] In monkeys this has been interpreted as "psychic blindness" and has been associated with loss of contact with the surroundings and impairment of skilled movements involving oculomotor control.[i] In cats that acted blind after large doses of lysergide, electrical potentials have been picked up in the CNS, showing that although there might be effects on retina and optic nerve the changes were insufficient to cause blindness.[zd,ze]

There is a report, from a comparison of former users of LSD with controls, suggesting that some users may have irreversible impairment of color discrimination,[a] but no published reports were found of blindness or of persistent alteration of the eyes or of vision in human beings after intoxication by lysergide, apart from effects of sun-gazing. Some actual persistent impairment of visual acuity, and persistent tiny central scotomas, have resulted from gazing at the sun while under the influence of LSD. A series of cases have been reported in which early decrease in visual acuity from sun gazing has been associated with macula edema, changing later to mottled pigmentation of the maculas, usually with at least partial recovery of vision.[k,m,n,zc] There has been no evident difference from solar maculopathy developed in the absence of LSD. A report by Milman on an accidentally poisoned five-year-old girl has been cited by others as having featured "disorganization of visual motor functions for several months", perhaps implying disturbance of vision, but it should be noted that the original report included no actual evaluation of vision or mention of eye examination other than note of dilated pupils. The "visual motor function disorganization" was judged solely on the basis of bizarre copying of geometric figures and drawings of human figures.[y]

A teratogenic effect of lysergide on the lens has been shown to result from administration of large doses to pregnant mice, causing histologically observable abnormalities in the lens epithelium similar to effects produced by x-irradiation.[q] In human beings a series of cases of ocular malformations have been reported in infants of mothers who took LSD during pregnancy.[b,g,h,r,s,w] In some cases cataracts were noted.[b,g,h] Severe bilateral optic disc hypoplasia,[s] bilateral optic nerve colobomas,[s] and unilateral anophthalmia[w] have been reported.

a. Abraham HD: A chronic impairment of colour vision in users of LSD. *BR J PSYCHIATRY* 140:518–520, 1982.

b. Apple DJ, Bennett TO: Multiple systemic and ocular malformations associated with maternal LSD usage. *ARCH OPHTHALMOL* 92:301–303, 1974.

c. Apter JT, Pfeiffer CC: The effect of the hallucinogenic drugs LSD–25 and mescaline on the electroretinogram. *NY ACAD SCI* 66:508–514, 1957.

d. Bishop PO, Burke W, Hayhow WR: Lysergic acid diethylamide block of lateral geniculate synapses and relief by repetitive stimulation. *EXP NEUROL* 1:556–568, 1959.

e. Bishop PO, Field G, et al: Action of d-lysergic acid diethylamide on lateral geniculate synapses. *J NEUROPHYSIOL* 21:529–549, 1958.

f. Blough DS: Effect of lysergic acid diethylamide on absolute visual threshold of the pigeon. *SCIENCE* 126:304–305, 1957.

g. Bogdanoff B, Rorke LB, et al: Brain and eye abnormalities; possible sequelae to prenatal use of multiple drugs including LSD. *AM J DIS CHILD* 123:145–148, 1972.

h. Chan CC, Fishman M, Egbert PR: Multiple ocular anomalies associated with maternal LSD ingestion. *ARCH OPHTHALMOL* 96:282–284, 1978.

i. Cole J, Glees P: Behavioral effects of lysergic acid diethylamide in monkeys. *ARZNEIMITTELFORSCHUNG* 17/3:401–404, 1967.

j. Connors B, Dray A, et al: LSD's effect on neuron population in visual cortex gauged by transient responses of extracellular potassium evoked by optical stimuli. *NEUROSCI LETT* 13:147–150, 1979.

k. von Domarus D: Solar maculopathy under the influence of LSD. *KLIN MONATSBL AUGENHEILKD* 166:547–549, 1975. (German)

l. (Editor's comment.) *N ENGL J MED* 277:1209, 1967.

m. Ewald RA: Sun gazing associated with the use of LSD. *ANN OPHTHALMOL* 3:15–17, 1971.

n. Fuller DG: Severe solar maculopathy associated with the use of lysergic acid diethylamide (LSD). *AM J OPHTHALMOL* 31:413–416, 1976.

o. Green K: Ocular effects of diacetyl morphine and lysergic acid diethylamide in rabbit. *INVEST OPHTHALMOL* 14:325–329, 1975.

p. Holliday AR, Sigurdson T: The effects of lysergic acid diethylamide. *PROC WEST PHARMACOL SOC* 8:51, 1965.

q. Hanaway JK: Lysergic acid diethylamide: Effects on the developing mouse lens. *SCIENCE* 164:574–575, 1969.

r. Holmes LB: Ocular malformations associated with maternal LSD usage. *ARCH OPHTHALMOL* 93:1061, 1975.

s. Hoyt CS: Optic disc anomalies and maternal ingestion of LSD. *J PEDIATR OPHTHALMOL* 15:286–289, 1978.

t. Jacobson JH, Gestring GF: Spontaneous retinal electrical potentials. *ARCH OPHTHALMOL* 62:599–603, 1959.

u. Krill AE, Alpert HU, Ostfeld AM: Effects of a hallucinogenic agent in totally blind subjects. *ARCH OPHTHALMOL* 67:180–185, 1962.

v. Krill AE, Wieland AM, Ostfeld AM: The effect of two hallucinogenic agents on human retinal function. *ARCH OPHTHALMOL* 64:724–733, 1960.

w. Margolis S, Martin L: Anophthalmia in an infant of parents using LSD. *ANN OPHTHALMOL* 12:1378–1381, 1980.

x. McKay JM, et al: Effects of LSD on receptive fields of single cells in the lateral geniculate nucleus of the cat. *NATURE* 229:347–349, 1971.

y. Milman DH: An untoward reaction to accidental ingestion of LSD in a 5-year-old girl. *J AM MED ASSOC* 201:821–827, 1967.

z. Ostfeld AM: Symposium on effects of hallucinogenic drugs in man. *FED PROC* 20:876–883, 1961.

za. Payne JW: LSD-25 and accommodative convergence ratios. *ARCH OPHTHALMOL* 74:81–85, 1965.

zb. Rebentisch E: The influence of serotonin and LSD on light-induced activity of the visual cortex of the rat. *PSYCHOPHARMACOLOGIA* (BERLIN) 13:106–117, 1968. (German)

zc. Schatz H, Mendelblatt F: Solar retinopathy from sun-gazing under the influence of LSD. *BR J OPHTHALMOL* 57:270–273, 1973.

zd. Schwartz AS, Cheney C: Retinal effects of high doses of LSD in the cat. *EXP NEUROL* 13:273–282, 1965.

ze. Schwartz AS, Cheney C: Effect of LSD on the tonic activity of the visual pathways of the cat. *LIFE SCI* 4:771, 1965.

zf. Shagass C: Effects of LSD on somatosensory and visual evoked responses and on the EEG in man. *RECENT ADVANCES BIOL PSYCHIAT* 9:209–227, 1966.

zg. Woody GE: Visual disturbances experienced by hallucinogenic drug abusers while driving. *AM J PSYCHIATRY* 127:683–686, 1970.

zh. Woody GE: Hallucinogens and afterimages. *AM J PSYCHIATRY* 128:367, 1971.

Lysophosphatidyl choline is normally at a much lower concentration in the aqueous and vitreous humors than in the blood, but, in rabbits, when the blood-aqueous barrier is chronically broken down by experimentally induced uveitis, the concentration has been shown to rise to levels that are demonstrably damaging to the permeability of the rabbits lens, and cataracts result.[a,b] Thus there is evidence that lysophosphatidyl choline is involved in production of cataract in uveitis.

a. Cotlier E, Baskin M, et al: Lysophosphatidyl choline and cataracts in uveitis. *ARCH OPHTHALMOL* 94:1159–1162, 1976.

b. D'Ermo F, Secchi AG: Phospholipase A and lysophosphatidyl choline in the pathogenesis of "permeability-cataract". *KLIN MONATSBL AUGENHEILKD* 170:433–436, 1977. (German)

Lysosomes from peritoneal polymorphonuclear leucocytes in rabbits have been shown to be toxic to the corneal endothelium, both in vivo and in culture.[a,b]

a. Arya DV, Mannagh J, et al: Effect of lysosomes on corneal endothelium. *INVEST OPHTHALMOL* 11:655–661, 1972.

b. Arya DV, Mannagh J, Irvine AR: Effects of lysosomes on cultured rabbit corneal endothelial cells. *INVEST OPHTHALMOL* 11:662–667, 1972.

Magnesium hydroxide is a white powder which is slightly soluble in water, imparting a mildly alkaline reaction, not enough to be damaging to the surface of the eye. *Milk of magnesia* is a suspension of magnesium hydroxide in water which has been given by mouth-as- an antacid and laxative, and has been occasionally employed in treatment of acid burns of the eye.

Tests of milk of magnesia on rabbit eyes by application twice a day for three or four days caused damage to the corneal epithelium demonstrable by staining with fluorescein.[27] After the applications of milk of magnesia were discontinued, the corneas returned to normal in two or three days. It was found that injury was induced only by certain brands of milk of magnesia, and it appeared to be due to a mechanical scratching of the epithelium by sharp crystals of magnesium hydroxide known as *brucite,* which formed gradually during storage.[27]

Magnesium metal introduced experimentally into the anterior chamber of human and rabbit eyes generated hydrogen bubbles, but caused no apparent injury.[340] The intraocular pressure remained subnormal for several weeks while the metal was being absorbed.[b] In animal eyes a 2 mm splinter has been observed to disappear in about ten days either from anterior chamber or vitreous body without causing irritation. Absorption from under the conjunctiva is much slower and is said not to influence the tension of the eye.[a]

<ul style="list-style:none">
<li>a. Morax V, Chiazzaro: On the resorption of magnesium metal in the body, and especially in the globe of the eye. *BULL SOC OPHTALMOL PARIS* 6:342–345, 1930. (French)</li>
<li>b. Romer P: Experimental studies on hypotony. *BER DTSCH OPHTHALMOL GESELLSCH* 42:55–60, 1920. (German)</li>
</ul>

Magnesium salts, such as ***magnesium chloride*** and ***magnesium sulfate,*** are essentially innocuous when applied in solution to the eyes.[a] Magnesium chloride at a concentration of 1% for ten minutes, or 10% for half a minute causes no damage to the eye or alteration of the pupil, when applied to rabbit eyes after mechanical removal of the corneal epithelium to facilitate penetration.[81] Injection of 0.08 M magnesium sulfate into the rabbit cornea similarly causes no reaction.[123]

Old reports alleging corneal opacification from magnesium chloride or sulfate were concerned primarily with an artificial fertilizer named Kainit, which contained various magnesium and potassium salts.[46, 253] Guillery in 1910, investigating some of the components, found that a slurry of magnesium chloride crystals applied to rabbit eyes caused a spotty clouding of the cornea and anterior lens cortex, which soon cleared. Application of concentrated magnesium sulfate and potassium sulfate solutions to Guillery's own eye caused only a moderate burning sensation.[253]

Systemic administration of 25 mg of magnesium chloride per kg body weight intravenously to rabbits daily for seven to ten months is reported to have induced xerophthalmia demonstrable histologically.[c]

Magnesium poisoning of six patients occurred during hemodialysis because of a mistake in preparing the dialysate solution with 15 instead of 1.5 mEq of magnesium chloride per liter. Three complained of blurring of vision but none had an objective visual defect, and the cause for the symptom of blurring was undetermined. All recovered rapidly.

Magnesium chlorate (not to be confused with *magnesium chloride*) has been used as a defoliant, and has been tested for toxicity in rats. Given orally for 10 to 45 days, it caused damage to the corneas, conjunctivae, lenses, and retinas.

a. Cote G, Smith G, Rochette J: Use of magnesium in the treatment of herpetic ulcer of the cornea. *CAN J OPHTHALMOL* 5:231–238, 1970. (French)

b. Govan JR, Porter CA, et al: Acute magnesium poisoning as a complication of intermittent hemodialysis. *BR MED J* 2:278–279, 1968.

c. Ogawa G: On changes in the cornea from magnesium chloride injection. *TRANS JPN PATH SOC* 13:48, 1924.

d. Rezhabek OY, Khalnazarov KA: Morphological changes in the eyes of rats exposed to the defoliant magnesium chlorate for a prolonged time. *ZDRAVOOKHR TURKM* 16:6–10, 1972.

Makare (cherry mahogany) is an African wood employed in cabinet making. Its dust causes skin and ocular irritation with lacrimation and swelling of the eyelids.[252]

Maleic acid (toxilic acid) is injurious to the cornea of rabbits, but less injurious than *maleic anhydride.* Aged aqueous solutions of either substance exhibit equal toxicity owing to conversion of the anhydride to the acid by reaction with water.

On rabbit eyes 10% maleic acid in water at pH 1 applied for thirty seconds causes permanent opacity and vascularization.[81] A 1% solution applied for two minutes causes cloudiness of the cornea, but no injury remains the next day. A 5% solution has similar but more intense effect, with recovery delayed six to seven days.[a]

Neutral 1 M *ammonium maleate* applied for five minutes to the cornea after mechanical removal of the epithelium to facilitate penetration causes corneal edema and hyperemia of the iris, but the eye returns to normal in a few days.[81] It seems that the maleate ion is much less toxic to the cornea than is maleic acid or maleic anhydride.

a. Winter CA, Tullius EJ, (1950):—see reference under *Maleic anhydride.*

Maleic anhydride (toxilic anhydride) is a crystalline material which powders and sublimes readily, producing fumes which are powerfully irritating to the eyes and respiratory tract.[a,c,51,252] Although cases have been reported of workmen exposed to the dust or vapors developing intense burning sensation in the eyes and punctate epithelial keratitis, the eyes have recovered in a few days, more rapidly than the respiratory tract.[a,b,c,165] Pulmonary edema or pneumonitis is a threat.[b] Solid maleic anhydride is potentially extremely injurious to the eyes and is caustic to the skin. Experimentally in rabbits it produces damage as severe as that caused by strong alkalis.[b,d,27,81] Its toxicity may be attributable to a conjugated double-bond system which is highly reactive, and may cause enzyme inhibition and protein denaturation. Irrigation with water is appropriate first aid treatment.

In contact with water, maleic anhydride changes to maleic acid. The acid is less injurious to the eye than is the anhydride.[101] (See also *Maleic acid.*)

a. Ghezzi I, Scotti P: Clinical contribution to knowledge of the pathology from phthalic and maleic anhydrides. *MED LAVORO* 56:746–752, 1965.

b. Heersink ME, Duane TD: Ocular disaster plan. *AM J OPHTHALMOL* 81:242–243, 1976.

c. Kowalski Z, Slusarczyk-Zalobna A, et al: *MED PRACY* 18:238–252, 1967. (*CHEM ABSTR* 68:20575, 1968.)

d. Russo L, Zannini D: Acute mass poisoning with maleic anhydride. *FOLIA MED (NAPLES)* 42:62–76, 1959. (*CHEM ABSTR* 53:15359.)
e. Winter CA, Tullius EJ: The irritating effects of maleic acid and maleic anhydride upon the eyes of rabbits. *AM J OPHTHALMOL* 33:387–388, 1950.

Malondialdehyde, produced by autoxidation of docosahexenoic acid, has been demonstrated in the vitreous humor of rabbits after intravitreal injection of docosahexenoic acid.[a] Posterior subcapsular cataracts developed as a result of the injection. It was postulated that formation of cataracts in association with retinal and choroidal degenerative diseases might involve release of docosahexenoic acid from rod outer segments, diffusion forward in the vitreous body, and autoxidation to toxic malondialdehyde in the vicinity of the lens.

a. Goosey JD, Tuan WM, Garcia CA: A peroxidative mechanism for posterior subcapsular cataract formation in the rabbit. *INVEST OPHTHALMOL VIS SCI* 25:608–612, 1984.

Manchineel (*Hippomane mancinella,* manzanillo tree, beach apple) is a small tree of the family Euphorbiaceae which grows along the seashore of Florida, the West Indies, and Central America.[252] Contact with any part of the plant, most commonly with the leaves, causes severe vesicular or bullous dermatitis within twenty-four hours. When the eyes are involved, symptoms of tearing, conjunctival hyperemia, chemosis, and swelling of the lids begin within one to two hours.[46] In exceptional cases, severe keratoconjunctivitis with temporary loss of corneal epithelium occurs.[c] The reaction is reproducible in rabbits.[b] No specific antidotal treatment is known other than irrigation of the eyes and washing the skin to decontaminate. Topical corticosteroid might help reduce irritation and inflammation. Recovery without complications is the rule.[a]

a. Grana PC: Conjunctivitis and dermatitis due to "Beach Apple". *ARCH OPHTHALMOL* 35:421–422, 1946.
b. Harley R: Keratoconjunctivitis caused by the Manzanillo tree. *AM J OPHTHALMOL* 27:628–631, 1944.
c. Snow JS, Harley RD: Dermatitis venenata and keratoconjunctivitis caused by the manzanillo tree. *ARCH DERM SYPH* (*CHICAGO*) 49:236–239, 1944.

Manganese compounds in the form of dust or fumes may be absorbed by inhalation and cause a peculiar form of poisoning. This usually has occurred after long exposure, especially in mining of manganese ores. Characteristically there is impaired mentation, increased fatigability and sleepiness, with ataxia, difficulty in walking, and mask-like facies, resembling parkinsonism.

The most conspicuous involvement of the eyes is in decreased movement of the eyelids and eyes.[c] It is said, however, that neither paresis of the eye muscles nor nystagmus occurs, and that manganese poisoning differs from postencephalitis parkinsonism in having no accompanying oculogyric crisis or loss of Bell's phenomenon.[a, 194]

The visual fields and ocular fundi in manganese poisoning as a rule remain normal.[a, b, 33] One instance of alleged constriction of the fields has been reported, but the author of the report expressed strong suspicion that the patient had a functional neurosis and was suffering from manganophobia without actual manganese poisoning.[a] Retrobulbar neuritis may possibly have occured in one case.[129] Also in one experimentally poisoned monkey a papillomacular type of degeneration was found in the intracranial portion of the optic nerves, in association with several other lesions in the nervous system, particularly atrophy of the cerebellar cortex.[d]

Local contact of manganese compounds with the cornea does not appear to be a problem industrially, but experimentally the manganous ion is not innocuous to the corneal stroma. Exposure of the rabbit cornea to 0.1 M manganous chloride solution at pH 5 or 6 for ten minutes after mechanical removal of the epithelium appears initially to cause no serious injury, but in the course of two to three days a severe reaction develops which results in opacification and vascularization of the cornea.[81]

(The injurious effects of *Potassium permanganate* are described elsewhere under that heading.)

a. Jaksch RV: On manganese toxicosis and manganophobia. *MUNCH MED WOCHENSCHR* 54:969–972, 1907. (German)
b. Leschke E: *CLINICAL TOXICOLOGY.* Translated by C.P. Stewart and O. Dorrer. London, Churchill, 1934, p 346.
c. Penalver R: Diagnosis and treatment of manganese intoxication. *ARCH IND HEALTH* 16:64–66, 1957.
d. Van Bogaert L, Dallelmagne MJ: Experimental approachs to the neurologic problems of manganism. *MSCHR PSYCHIAT NEUROL* 111:60–89, 1945–1947.

Manganese metal has been tested for toxicity as a foreign body in the eyes of rabbits, and during one year was found to be well tolerated.[340]

Mazindol (Mazanor; Sanorex), an anorexic, is stated in one manufacturer's literature to be contraindicated in glaucoma, but no explanation is given. Also in this literature it is noted that in dogs long-term treatment with high dosage has caused reversible corneal opacities, but this effect had not been seen in human beings.

Menadione (2-methyl-1,4-naphthoquinone; vitamin K) tested in the form of a water-soluble derivative, menadione sodium bisulfite, by dropping on rabbit eyes, caused immediate discomfort and conjunctival congestion, but the eyes rapidly returned to normal.[53] Injected into the corneal stroma or dropped on the cornea after removal of the epithelium, a 0.05 M solution caused moderate reaction.[123] Subcutaneous administration to guinea pigs caused death with liver damage but no evidence of damage to the eyes.[a]

a. Simonelli M: Experimental poisoning with vitamin K and ocular effects. *G ITAL OFTALMOL* 3:183–187, 1950.

Menthol is employed as a flavoring material and as an anti-pruritic. Rubbing the eyelids with hands contaminated by menthol or peppermint oil causes a burning sensation of fifteen to thirty minutes duration, without aftereffect.[153]

In rabbit eyes, application of menthol has been reported to cause severe damage, graded 9 on a scale of 1 to 10 at twenty-four hours.[27] However, complete recovery has been observed two weeks after application of 10 mg of menthol crystals for five minutes to a rabbit's cornea.[81] Slight corneal haze appeared during exposure, and for a few days became worse, accompanied by intense hyperemia of the iris, and miosis, but this was followed by spontaneous clearing.

Oral administration of 5 to 7 g of menthol in olive oil to a rabbit has been reported to cause death with convulsions in a few minutes, with cataracts developing while the animal was dying, increasing to complete whiteness during two hours postmortem.[153]

Mephenesin (Myanesin, Tolserol, Tolyspaz) is a muscle relaxant. Several reports have described nystagmus in all directions, including rotary and vertical nystagmus, drooping of the lids, and drowsiness after intravenous injection.[c-e] Mephenesin has no adverse effect on intraocular pressure.[a,b]

  a. Avasthy P: Myanesin elixir in 150 cases of cataract extraction. *BR J OPHTHALMOL* 39:623–625, 1955.
  b. Hofmann H: On the effect of muscle relaxants on the eye. *KLIN MONATSBL AUGENHEILKD* 130:32–37, 1957. (German)
  c. Hunter AR, Waterfall JM: Myanesin in hyperkinetic states. *LANCET* 366–367, 1948.
  d. Schlesinger EB, Drew AL, Wood B: Clinical studies in the use of myanesin. *AM J MED* 4:365–372, 1948.
  e. Stephen CR, Chandy J: Clinical and experimental studies with myanesin. *CAN MED ASSOC J* 57:463–468, 1947.

Mephenytoin (Mesantoin), an anticonvulsant, has occasionally caused nystagmus.[174] It has not been found to affect the ocular pressure in glaucomatous patients.[190] In guinea pigs, prolonged administration is reported to cause exophthalmos with damage to cornea, lens, and vitreous.[a]

  a. Craviotto C: Experimental exophthalmic syndrome in guinea pigs by prolonged administration of 3-methyl-5-ethylphenyllhydantoin. *RIV ANAT PAT ONCOL* 19:473–479, 1961. (*CHEM ABSTR* 58:10605, 1963.)

Meprobamate (Equanil, Miltown), a tranquilizer, has been used by a very large number of people without causing important disturbances of the eyes or vision. Large overdoses sufficient to cause coma have had no permanent effects on the eyes.[g] The pupils during coma from excessive meprobamate have shown no uniform behavior, variously being reported dilated, constricted, reactive, fixed, or changing.[g] With ordinary dosage, complaints concerning vision have been rare. Exceptionally a reversible weakness of accommodation for near has been reported in patients under the age of natural presbyopia,[m] and in experimental investigation of the influence of 800 mg taken orally by normal young people some investigators have detected slight alterations of binocular vision, particularly in stereopsis, simultaneous perception, and amplitude of fusion on a synoptophore, with slight tendency to exophoria,[c] while other investigators have reported that this same dose causes no change in visual acuity, depth perception, or phorias, and even 1,200 to 1,600 mg orally has been reported not to disturb significantly the extra-ocular muscle balance or amplitude of fusion in normal people.[q] Specifically, 800 mg has not interfered with performance in simulated automobile driving,[l] and a study on 120 volunteers in Switzerland has shown that driving skill tested under actual driving conditions was not affected by 400 mg of meprobamate.[i]

The ERG in normal human subjects has been unaffected by 800 mg given orally.[e] Slight changes in critical flicker fusion frequency have been detected in normal subjects given 400 to 800 mg orally, apparently reflecting pharmacologic influence on the state of the central nervous system as from other sedative drugs, not a toxic effect.[a,d,n,q] Dark adaptation curves according to some investigators have shown little or no effect on light sense threshold after doses up to 1,600 mg orally in normal subjects, but a slight, 5° to 10° concentric functional contriction of visual field in most subjects.[f,h] The opposite has also been reported, enlargement of perimetric fields and lowered threshold of peripheral photoreceptors.[b]

The intraocular pressure in rabbits has been found reduced only by very large doses (400 mg per rabbit) which also produced mydriasis.[o] In patients there appears to be no adverse effect on intraocular pressure. A reduction of pressure averaging 3.7 mm Hg in normal patients and 8.6 mm Hg in glaucomatous patients has been reported during the first day after administration of 800 to 1,600 mg, but the pressure has been unaffected by 400 mg.[f,k] In treatment of glaucoma, occasional beneficial tension reduction has been reported, but in most glaucomatous patients there has been no significant or sustained reduction of pressure.[j,r]

a. Alagna G, Petrosillo O: Effect of tranquilizers on critical frequency. *ARCH OTTALMOL* 64:237–249, 1960. (Italian)

b. Coriglione G, Gorgone G, Schillaci C: Sensory modifications induced by psycho-pharmaceuticals (Meprobamate). *MINERVA OFTALMOL* 8:109–115, 1966. (Italian)

c. Coriglione G, Gorgone G, Schillaci C: On modifications of motor and sensory activity of binocular vision induced by psychopharmaceuticals (meprobamate). *MINERVA OFTALMOL* 9:15–18, 1967. (Italian)

d. Corglione G, Gorgone G, Schillaci C: Pharmacodynamic study of the F.C.F. and its physiologic significance. *MINERVA OFTALMOL* 9:167–171, 1967. (Italian)

e. Coriglione G, Gorgone G, Schillaci C: The ERG under the influence of psychodepressive drugs. *ANN OTTALMOL CLIN OCUL* 93:677–682, 1967.

f. DiMartino C: Experimental investigation of the activity of meprobamate in ophthalmology. *ARCH OTTALMOL* 62:131–144, 1958. (Italian)

g. Gitelson S: Methaqualone-Meprobamate poisoning. *J AM MED ASSOC* 201:977–979, 1967.

h. Guiffre V: Influence of meprobamate and the visual field and light sense. *G ITAL OFTALMOL* 4:324, 1957. (Italian)

i. Kielholz P, Goldberg L, Oberssteg JI, et al: Street traffic, tranquilizer and alcohol. *DTSCH MED WOCHENSCHR* 92:1525–1531, 1967. (German)

j. Leydhecker W: Meprobamate in glaucoma and in preparation for eye operations. *KLIN MONATSBL AUGENHEILKD* 132:224–233, 1958. (German)

k. Malec J: Influence of meprobamate on the retinal circulation. *SBORN LEK* 67:211–214, 1965. (*ZENTRALBL GES OPHTHALMOL* 95:257, 1965.)

l. Marquis DG, Kelly EL, Miller JG, et al: Behavioral effects of meprobamate on normal subjects. *ANN NY ACAD SCI* 67:701–710, 1957.

m. Mayer LL: (Meprobamate) Letters to the Journal. *J AM MED ASSOC* 178:966, 1961.

n. Mislak H, Zenhausern R, Salafia WR: Continuous temporal evaluation of the effect of meprobamate on critical flicker frequency in normal subjects. *PSYCHO-PHARMACOLOGIA* 9:457–461, 1966. (*CHEM ABSTR* 65:14316, 1966.)

o. Paul SD, Leopold IH: The effect of tranquilizing and ganglion blocking agents on the eyes of experimental animals. *AM J OPHTHALMOL* 42:752–759, 1956.

p. Tavolara L: Influence of meprobamate on the intraocular pressure in normal and glaucomatous subjects. *BOLL OCULIST* 38:11–24, 1959. (Italian)

q. Toselli C, Guzzinati GC: The influence of meprobamate on motor and sensory functions of binocular vision. *ANN OTTALMOL CLIN OCUL* 84:341–347, 1958. (Italian)

r. Vukov B: The role of meprobamate in treatment of glaucoma. *SRPSKI ARCH CELOK LEK* 89:1273–1279, 1961. (*ZENTRALBL GES OPHTHALMOL* 85:263, 1962.) (German abstract)

2-Mercaptobenzothiazole (2-benzothiazolethiol, Captax), a rubber vulcanization accelerator, is reported to be very irritating to the eyes and to emit highly toxic fumes when decomposed by heat or acid.[215]

a. Kowalski Z, Bassendowska E: The effects of certain vulcanization accelerators. *MED PRACY* 16:35–42, 1965. (*CHEM ABSTR* 63:18930, 1965.)

2-Mercaptoethanol applied undiluted to the rabbit eye is toxic to the conjunctiva and causes long-lasting moderately severe corneal opacity.[a]

a. White K, Bruckner JV, Guess WL: Toxicological studies of 2-mercaptoethanol. *J PHARM SCI* 62:237, 1973.

Mercurial diuretics, including *chlormerodrin, meralluride, mercaptomerin,* and *mercuderamide,* appear to have had no significant adverse effect on the eyes. Intraocular pressure in rabbits was reduced slightly by *mercaptomerin* or *mercuderamide* given intramuscularly, but not by topical administration.[a, b]

a. Auricchio G, Diotallevi M: Effect of mercurial diuretics on intraocular pressure. *ANN OTTALMOL CLIN OCUL* 89:763–766, 1963. (Italian)

b. Auricchio G, Diotallevi M: Can the recovery rate of the intraocular volume be used for measurements of the aqueous inflow. *ACTA OPHTHALMOL* 43:245–251, 1965.

Mercuric chloride is seriously toxic on absorption and is severely caustic in concentrated solution or as a solid.[171] Acute systemic poisoning appears seldom to have caused disturbance of the eye, but in three young people bilateral mydriasis, hyperemia of the optic nerveheads, and retinal venous distension with rapid decrease in visual acuity have been reported. These patients recovered, but had persistent visual disturbance, which was not explained in the available abstract.[a] Another man believed to have had normal eyes before swallowing a 0.5 g tablet of mercuric chloride, which caused diarrhea and moderate albuminuria for a few days, two years later had vision 20/60 O.D. 20/200 O.S. The media were clear, but in both fundi many discrete white areas were seen deep to the retina in the whole central area and around the disc, with patches of degeneration with glistening crystalline appearance, but no vascular abnormalities or appearances to suggest inflammation. (For more concerning systemic poisoning and its possible effect on the eye, see *Mercury, inorganic.*)

In cultured retina, mercuric chloride 5×10^{-6} M causes degeneration of rod cells.[99, 157] However, from the bloodstream it seems that mercuric chloride may not readily have access to the retina. Intracarotid injections of mercuric chloride in rabbits in doses that were lethal in one to six days have caused no ophthalmoscopically recognizable change in the retina.[b]

External contact with mercuric chloride solutions has caused severe burns in human eyes.[153,253] Dusting of the eye with powdered mercuric chloride mistakenly in place of mercurous chloride has caused devastating damage of all structures of the anterior segment of the eye.[c,f] In very rare instances vision has recovered despite severe damage and necrosis in the conjunctiva.[c,d] On rabbit eyes, tests of solutions of mercuric chloride have shown the cornea to be severely injured by 0.5% (0.018 M) solution.[e]

Treatment of rabbit eyes by irrigation with 0.03 M sodium edetate (EDTA) solution for thirty minutes after exposure to 0.1 M solution of mercuric chloride for ten minutes did not prevent severe corneal opacification and necrosis, although some recovery of circulation in conjunctival blood vessels was obtained by the treatment, in contrast to control eyes treated with sodium chloride solution in which the circulation was permanently interrupted.[81]

a. Beradze NI, Antelava DN, Sharashenidze SV: Changes occuring in the organ of vision following granizan poisoning. *VESTN OFTAL* 78:43–45, 1965. (*ZENTRALBL GES OPHTHALMOL* 95:228, 1965.)

b. D'Agostino A, Vecchione L, Tieri O: Further contribution to the study of experimental retinal degeneration. *ARCH OTTALMOL* 66:417–422, 1962. (Italian)

c. Schmelzer H: Sublimate burn of the eye. *KLIN MONATSBL AUGENHEILKD* 90:96–97, 184–190, 1933.

d. Strebel J: Sublimate burn of the eye. *KLIN MONATSBL AUGENHEILKD* 90:522–523, 1933.

e. Yamashita K: Studies of the caustic action of silver nitrate and some disinfecting agents on the eye. *JBER KURASIKI Z HOSP,* No.5:235–248, 1930. (*ZENTRALBL GES OPHTHALMOL* 26:523, 1932.)

f. Sood GC, Sofat BK, et al: Eye injury with mercuric chloride. *BR J OPHTHALMOL* 56:687–689, 1972.

Mercuric iodide resembles *mercuric chloride* in local and systemic toxicity. In contact with the eye it has been known to cause damage,[253] and injected into the anterior chamber of rabbits has caused purulent exudation and inflammation.[150]

Of possible historical interest when *potassium iodide* was administered systemically and *mercurous chloride* was applied to the conjunctival sac a local interaction took place forming *mercuric iodide,* inducing more irritation of the conjunctiva than ordinarily produced by *mercurous chloride* alone. (Compare *Mercurous chloride.*)

Mercuric oxide (yellow) has been used as an antiseptic in the form of 1% or 2% ointment, chiefly for inflammation of the eyelids and conjunctivae.[171] Frequent applications to the lids for many years has induced a bluish-gray darkening of the lids and conjunctivae.[a–e] Slight discoloration has also been seen in the cornea in the peripheral portions of Descemet's membrane, and a brownish, lusterless opacity superficially in the pupillary area of the lens, but with no interference with the transparency of the media or disturbance of visual acuity.[a] In the bulbar conjunctiva dark pigment granules may be distributed about the blood vessels near the cornea.

The discoloration of cornea and lens is similar to that which occurs in chronic systemic absorption of mercury. It appears to be harmless and causes no symptoms.

Mercuric oxide injected experimentally into the anterior chamber of rabbits has been observed regularly to cause inflammation and a purulent exudate.[150] (Compare *Mercury, inorganic.*)

a. Abramowicz I: Deposition of mercury in the eye. *BR J OPHTHALMOL* 30:696–697, 1946.
b. Kern AB: Mercurial pigmentation. *ARCH DERMATOL* 99:129–130, 1969.
c. Lamar LM, Bliss BO: Localized pigmentation of the skin due to topical mercury. *ARCH DERMATOL* 93:450–453, 1966.
d. Long JC, Danielson RW: Mercurial discoloration of the eyelids. *AM J OPHTHALMOL* 34:753–756, 1951.
e. Wheeler M: Discoloration of the eyelids from prolonged use of ointment containing mercury. *AM J OPHTHALMOL* 31:441–444, 1948.

Mercuric oxycyanide (mercury oxycyanate), a violently poisonous compound, has been used as an antiseptic, but in a series of twelve cases proved to be severely damaging to the cornea when 1:5,000 solution was introduced into the anterior chamber post-operatively. There was severe corneal edema with wrinkling of Descemet's membrane, hyperemia of the iris, thickening and opacification of the hyaloid and anterior lens capsule, and formation of posterior synechias. In three eyes the corneas cleared in three to six weeks, but in seven eyes the corneas remained permanently clouded. Secondary glaucoma developed in some, and vision was reduced to counting fingers. The injurious nature of the antiseptic was proved in rabbits by placing two drops of 1:5,000 mercuric oxycyanide solution in the anterior chamber. This caused intense edema and clouding of the cornea within twenty-four hours. The corneas cleared partially in two weeks but never cleared completely.[a]

a. Stein R: Complications in eye surgery due to introduction into the anterior chamber of solutions erroneously prepared with an antiseptic. *AM J OPHTHALMOL* 52:261–263, 1961.

Mercuric sulfide (red) (vermilion, cinnabar) has been used as a pigment, and formerly for syphilis.[171] Injected as a suspension into the anterior chamber of rabbits it induces a slight fibrinous and leukocytic reaction. In many weeks it is mostly removed by leukocytes, but some remains for a long time in the cells in the iris.[150]

Mercuric sulfide has been used medically as a pigment for tattooing corneas of rabbits and patients to hide corneal scars, and is said to have given permanent coloration without irritation.[199]

Mercurous chloride (calomel) formerly was applied as a dusting powder to the eye in treatment of corneal ulcers. Topical calomel was usually tolerated well, causing only slight transient redness and swelling,[d] but in exceptional cases induced inflammation and scarring of the conjunctiva.[a]

A severe local reaction occurred when soluble iodides were given systemically at the same time that mercurous chloride was applied to the eye.[b,c,d] In the absence of soluble iodides, mercurous chloride in the conjunctival sac normally remained white, but when applied within a day of systemic administration of soluble iodides, the material which collected in the lower conjunctival sac was characteristically discolored gray and greenish. The attendant inflammation, which was usually restricted to the lower bulbar and palpebral conjunctiva, was associated with membranous patches on the conjunctiva, edema of the lids, hyperemia of the eye, tearing, and mucoid or purulent discharge.[b] The cornea was rarely involved except in the most severe cases, in which transient erosions of the corneal epithelium and clouding of the cornea occurred.[d]

Several investigations in animals and experiments *in vitro* have substantiated that mercurous chloride and soluble iodides react to form *mercuric iodide* and *metallic mercury.* It is the formation of finely divided metallic mercury which accounts for the greenish or darkened appearance of the material in the conjunctival sac. The *mercuric iodide* which is formed is responsible for the local irritation and injury.[b,c,d] Tests of *mercuric iodide* and *mercuric bromide* on rabbit eyes have shown them to be irritating and caustic, similar to *mercuric chloride,* whereas the poorly soluble *mercurous chloride* or *mercurous iodide* induce only slight reaction in the absence of soluble iodides or bromides.

a. Dehenne A: On ocular injuries. *REC OPHTHALMOL* 7:1–28, 1885. (French)
b. Friedenwald H, Crawford AC: Calomel conjunctivitis. *AM J OPHTHALMOL* 10:239–247, 1893.
c. Schlaefke W: On the use of potassium iodide and calomel in ophthalmology. *GRAEFES ARCH OPHTHALMOL* 25:251–279, 1879. (German)
d. Schloms B: On injuries of the eye from calomel-dusting of the conjunctival sac with simultaneous systemic administration of halogen salts. *ARCH AUGENHEILKD* 73:220–241, 1913. (German)

Mercury fulminate dust causes conjunctival irritation and itching erythema and swelling of the lids, face and other exposed skin. In contact with the skin it has vesicant action.[124,129,176,252]

Mercury (inorganic) poisoning and its effects on the eyes are described here in general terms regardless of the inorganic form of mercury responsible. (Effects of organic compounds of mercury are not included here. For these, see *Organomercury compounds* in the INDEX.)

Systemic poisoning from absorption of mercury vapor or inorganic mercury compounds may occur acutely or chronically. Acute poisoning, which is most commonly caused by ingestion of soluble salts of mercury, has no characteristic effect on the eyes. Chronic poisoning more often has been caused by occupational absorption of metallic mercury through the respiratory tract and skin, or by mercury compounds administered medically, usually occurring insidiously during prolonged exposure. There are characteristic changes in personality (knows as "erethism"), muscular incoordination, inflammation of the mouth and gums, and excessive salivation.[171,252] The cranial nerves are seldom affected. Disturbances of the eyes in mercury poisoning consist of discoloration of the cornea and lens, tremor of the eyelids, and possibly, in very rare instances, disturbances of vision and extraocular muscles. The discolorations have been well documented, but neurological effects involving the eyes are open to considerable questioning.

In very young children acrodynia is a special manifestation of mercury (inorganic) poisoning. As described by Walsh and Hoyt, it is characterized by skin eruptions, weakness, irritability, and hyperesthesia, with ocular symptoms in half of the cases.[256] Photophobia is an outstanding symptom, often the earliest, usually associated with conjunctivitis, itching of the eyes, sometimes with discharge. Keratitis is said to be slight, and to occur rarely. Under treatment Walsh and Hoyt's patients recovered.

Chronic absorption of mercury by dentists, thermometer-makers, hatters, and others handling mercury, or exposed to its vapors, has led to a characteristic discoloration of the front surface of the lens. Apparently in no case has it interfered with vision. Mercurialentis has been described and studied many times.[c,d,h,i,n,p-r,t,v,x-z]

A rose-brown or pinkish homogeneous reflex is seen with the slit-lamp biomicroscope, in some cases involving the whole anterior surface of the lens, but sometimes limited to an anterior subcapsular disc. One observer has described the reflex as coffee brown.[v] At the very first, only a very thin lamina of faint gray is discernable at the anterior surface of the lens. Very fine deposits of black or dark brown pigment have been found histologically beneath the lens epithelium.[d,y] Chemical analyses showing accumulation of mercury in the lens in mercurialentis have been reported by Abrams.[a]

Mercurialentis has been reported not only in people chronically exposed to mercury vapor and mercury compounds occupationally but also it has been reported a number of times from chronic local application of medications containing mercury compounds, such as mercuric oxide (in ointment) or organic mercury preservatives (in eyedrops). (See *Mercuric oxide* and *Phenylmercuric salts.*)

In many cases, discoloration of the cornea as well as lens has been observed with few or no other indications of systemic intoxication. Discoloration of the cornea has been produced experimentally in animals by repeated systemic administration of mercury.[zd] In the cornea the discoloration is similar to that observed after many years of daily application of mercuric oxide ointment to the eye. It consists of a grayish ring in the cornea just anterior to the endothelium extending approximately 2 mm from the limbus.

A few patients chronically exposed to metallic mercury vapor are reported to have developed band keratopathy. Also in two cases fine glistening particulate opacities have been described centrally in the corneal stroma, with the periphery remaining clear.[x] (Also see *Mercury metal* for more details.)

Impairment of vision from optic neuropathy has occasionally been attributed to poisoning by mercury,[zc] but such reports have been seriously criticized. In 1931 Uhthoff and Metzger pointed out that many of the reports claiming injury of the optic nerve by mercury had been made prior to the use of the ophthalmoscope, and that more recent reports had not been convincing in establishing a direct injurious action on the optic nerve.[247] Usually the affected patients had syphilis or other diseases which could account for the disturbances of vision. In 1932 Sattler similarly reviewed the evidence and expressed doubt that any reports of injury of the optic nerve by mercury were correct, and believed that probably all were more properly attributable to pre-existing disease which was under treatment with mercury.[214]

A strong basis for this opinion was provided by a 431 page monograph published in 1861 by Kussmaul, summarizing and reviewing essentially the whole literature on mercurial poisoning to that time.[u] Special attention was given in that monograph to distinguishing between the effects of mercury and syphilis, and for that purpose a comprehensive study was made of the effects of occupational poisonings, distinct from medical poisonings induced in treatment of disease by mercury. In hundreds of cases, many of his own as well as from the literature, Kussmaul rarely found evidence of impairment of vision or hearing. Furthermore, cases of keratitis, iritis, or complete paralysis of extraocular muscles were practically never encountered, but in rare instances conjunctivitis or tremor of the eyelids was noted. In the rare instances in which complaint was made of weakness of vision, no anatomic basis or special characteristics were established.

A further survey of the literature on ocular involvement from 1865 to 1959 by Toselli also provided little basis for disagreeing with Uhthoff, Metzger, and Sattler.[zc]

Considering only reports of *inorganic* mercury poisoning, it is difficult to find any case in either the nineteenth or twentieth century in which the optic nerve has unquestionably been injured by mercury. Cases with optic neuropathy suggested, but unproven, have been published by Square (1867),[zb] Galezowski (1878),[m] Church (1887),[j] and Spillman (1904).[za]

Retinal disturbances have been reported very rarely in association with inorganic mercury poisoning. In three such cases the authors of the reports were themselves unconvinced of a relationship.[f,o]

The extraocular muscles are rarely affected in inorganic mercury poisoning. A tremor of the lids has occasionally been noted in chronic mercurialism, usually accompanying the characteristic tremor of fingers and hands, and presumably of similar central origin.[b,k] In rare instances ptosis has been reported, in one instance monolateral and associated with hemiparesis which may have come from causes other than mercury.[zc] In another instance a partial ptosis came on gradually in a middle-aged man who was exposed to mercury and had some suggestive personality changes, but no typical discoloration of the lens or other evidence of poisoning.[zc]

Single instances of paresis of lateral conjugate movement[zc] and of paresis of one lateral rectus[p] have been observed in association with chronic exposure to mercury. In the case of monocular lateral rectus palsy the patient had typical symptoms of chronic mercurialism and characteristic brown discoloration of the lenses, but also had acute recurrent episodes of vertigo, vomiting, and nystagmus, suggestive of acute labyrinthitis, which is not characteristic of mercury poisoning, and may have been coincidental.[p] Another patient who worked with mercury and had headache and tremor developed diplopia suddenly but recovered completely in two to three weeks.[f,v] Recurrent tenonitis in a single case is said to have improved when work with mercury was discontinued.[s]

No characteristic effect of mercury poisoning on the pupils has been recognized.

It seems fair to conclude from the evidence so far examined that apart from the discoloration of lens and cornea, which has been well established, if inorganic mercury poisoning does have toxic effect on the eyes, it must be extremely rare and presents no consistent pattern.[129,194]

In conflict with this opinion are the following reports. First, there is a remarkable report by Baldi and associates (1954) of high incidence of constriction of visual fields in Italian hatters chronically poisoned by vapors of inorganic mercury.[e] In twelve out of eighteen hatters the fields were found to be smaller than normal, usually by 20° to 40°. The constriction was concentric and without scotomas. Visual acuity was normal with or without glasses in all but one patient. (This patient had vision no better than 2/10 and 3/10, and fields reduced to 10°.) No significant abnormality was found in the fundi. Yearly reexaminations from 1948 to 1953 showed the fields to become more constricted in nine cases, to remain unchanged in three cases, and not to improve in any.

A claim of similar effect was made from Poland in 1969, stating that half the people working in an environment of mercury vapor had narrowing of visual fields for red, but no other changes in the eyes.[g] Also, in a report from Czechoslovakia in 1964 it was remarked that three out of 127 people working with mercury had constriction of visual fields.[t]

Against these claims is to be weighed a report by Locket and Nazroo in which no abnormality of visual fields, either central or peripheral, was found in England in a survey of forty-nine individuals chronically exposed to sufficient concentrations of mercury vapor to induce characteristic discoloration of the lens in twelve cases.[v] (In contrast, compare *Methyl mercury compounds,* which do notoriously constrict visual fields.)

Rabbits exposed to 5 mg Hg/cu m of air for two hours a day every day have become irritable, developed tremors, lost weight, and died in three to eight months. The brains showed edema about the small vessels and later a more diffuse edema involving the occipital lobes. A few hemorrhagic foci and zones of demyelinization appeared in the corpora quadrigemina, and neuroglial cells seemed to be increased in the chiasm. If similar changes occurred in human beings, they might account for constriction of visual fields.[e]

In treatment of mercury poisoning, favorable results in promoting excretion and relieving neurologic signs have been obtained by treatment with N-acetyl-D,L-penicillamine.[x,ze]

a. Abrams JD, Majzoub U: Mercury content of the human lens. *BR J OPHTHALMOL* 54:59, 1970.

b. Agate JN, Buckell M: Mercury poisoning from fingerprint photography. *LANCET* 2:451, 1949.

c. Atkinson WS: A colored reflex from the anterior capsule of the lens which occurs in mercurialism. *AM J OPHTHALMOL* 26:685–688, 1943.

d. Atkinson WS, vonSallman L: Mercury in the lens. *TRANS AM OPHTHALMOL SOC* 44:65–70, 1946.

e. Baldi G, Marenghi B, Picollo H: Eye disturbances in chronic mercurialism. Experimental clinical investigations. *MED LAV* 45:214–224, 1954. (Italian)

f. Bidstrup PL, Bonnell JA, et al: Chronic mercury poisoning in men repairing direct-current meters. *LANCET* 2:856–861, 1951.

g. Brodziak-Krzesiekowa K, Ogielska E: Field changes in persons working in the presence of mercury vapour. *KLIN OCZNA* 39:761–763, 1969.

h. Burn RA: Mercurialentis. *PROC ROY SOC MED* 55:322–326, 1962.

i. Caffi M, Straneo G: Metallic impregnation of the posterior aspect of the cornea and of the capsule of the lens in a case of mercurialism. *ANN OTTALMOL CLIN OCUL* 87:38–42, 1961. (Italian)

j. Church HM: On a case of poisoning by corrosive sublimate. *EDINBURGH MED J* 32:795–800, 1887.

k. Clinton M: Mercury. *AM PETROL INST TOXIC REV,* Sept. 1948.

l. Fischer FP: Mercuriosis of the lens. *ANN OCULIST (PARIS)* 180:508, 1947. (French)

m. Galezowski: Optic atrophy following mercurial poisoning. *REC OPHTALMOL* 5:226–230, 1878. (French)

n. Gourlay JS: Mercurialentis. *TRANS OPHTHALMOL SOC UK* 74:441–447, 1954.

o. Guilbert: Mercurial exanthems. *BULL SOC FR OPHTALMOL* 13:351–353, 1895.

p. Hunter D, Lister A: Mercurialentis. *BR J OPHTHALMOL* 37:234–235, 1953.

q. Iannaccone A, Lamphis R, Marras O: Changes in the crystalline lens of eye in chronic mercurial poisoning. *INT CONGR OCCUP HEALTH 14th, MADRID,* 1963:876–878, 1964.

r. Kipling MD: Mercury and the eye. *ANN OCCUP HYG* 8:81–83, 1965.

s. Kipp CJ: Inflammation of Tenon's capsule in mercurial poisoning. *TRANS AM OPHTHALMOL SOC* 6:415–419, 1892.

t. Kuruc F, Streicher T, Krajcovic S: Mercuria lentis. *CS OFTAL* 20:382–385, 1964.

u. Kussmaul A: *Untersuchungen uber den constitutionellen Mercurialismus.* Wurzburg, 1861.

v. Locket Z, Nazroo IA: Eye changes following exposure to metallic mercury. *LANCET* 1:528–530, 1952.

x. Parameshvara V: Mercury poisoning and its treatment with N-acetyl-D,L-penicillamine. *BR J IND MED* 24:73–76, 1967.

y. Rosen E: Mercurialentis. *AM J OPHTHALMOL* 33:1287–1288, 1950.

z. Rosen E: A newly observed ophthalmologic occupational hazard in dentistry. *ORAL SURG* 3:1041–1043, 1950.

za. Spillman L, Blum P: A case of subacute poisoning by mercuric chloride. *ANN HYG PUBLIC* 2:126–135, 1904. (French)

zb. Square W: Optic neuritis in connexion with mercurial poisoning. *OPHTHALMOL HOSP REP* 6:54, 1867.

zc. Toselli C: Clinical contribution to the study of ocular complications in chronic poisoning by mercury. *ANN OTTALMOL CLIN OCUL* 85:83–89, 1959. (Italian)

zd. Velhagen K: On argyrosis of the cornea. *KLIN MONATSBL AUGENHEILKD* 122:36–42, 1953. (German)

ze. Kark RAP, Poskanzer DC, et al: Mercury poisoning and its treatment with N-acetyl-D,L-penicillamine. *N ENGL J MED* 285:10–16, 1971.

Mercury metal (quicksilver) is a silvery, heavy liquid which is slightly volatile at ordinary temperatures. Both the vapor and the metal have caused ocular disturbances.

Band keratopathy has been reported in several individuals exposed to mercury vapor and to dusts of its inorganic salts, mostly in removing hair from rabbit pelts.[c, h] Galin and Obstbaum studied a patient who developed bilateral keratopathy without mercurialentis or other evidence of mercurialism, after 20 years in manufacture of mercury thermometers.[h] In this patient the corneal opacity was shown to be calcific, and after removal from each eye, either with edetate solution or by scraping, vision improved and tonometry indicated lower intraocular pressures. It was concluded that abnormal rigidity of the corneas with calcific deposits had earlier led to spurious indications of elevated intraocular pressure.

In two cases chronic exposure to mercury vapor has been described as producing fine glistening particulate opacities in the axial portions of the corneal stroma in addition to mercurialentis.[f]

Mercury has entered the eye, and had toxic effects, in the following various ways: (a) by injection of droplets of mercury into various parts of the eye from the outside, (b) by diffusion from the outer surface into the eye, (c) from the bloodstream reaching the eye as embolic droplets, and (d) from the bloodstream in dissolved form in systemic mercury poisoning.

When mercury metal droplets are in the epithelium, rather than the corneal stroma or anterior chamber, they are extruded rapidly with little reaction, as was reported in a patient who was sprayed forcefully with metallic mercury and was observed to have many fine silvery globules beneath the epithelium of the cornea. These globules were seen to have penetrated the corneal epithelium and stopped at Bowman's membrane. Two days after the accident the cornea was found to have become cleared of the droplets, and vision was normal.[b]

A droplet of mercury metal injected into the anterior chamber of a rabbit or into the corneal stroma causes a purulent reaction around the droplet, forming an abscess in the adjacent cornea, leading ultimately to expulsion of the foreign material. Leber originally observed this, and I have repeated the observation.[81,150] In patients in rare instances mercury has been introduced accidentally into the anterior chamber in association with a penetrating injury. To remove the droplets of mercury from the anterior chamber, Ivanov has utilized an ingenious procedure. A specially prepared and amalgamated (mercury wetted or coated) brass probe was introduced through an incision into the anterior chamber into contact with the droplets. The droplets became adherent to the probe and were withdrawn. Ivanov noted in one patient that a tiny droplet was inaccessible to the probe and remained in a crypt in the iris, but it apparently was so small that it did not cause injurious reaction, and was gradually absorbed.[d]

Mercury metal was injected by Leber also into the vitreous humor of rabbits, and a purulent reaction with shrinkage of the vitreous, detachment of the retina, and shrinkage and atrophy of the eye was observed.[150]

Diffusion and absorption of mercury into the tissues from the outer surface of the eye have been demonstrated. Mercury metal in contact with the conjunctiva has been shown in rabbits to be absorbed and ultimately to be detectable in the urine. Though in contact with the conjunctiva, metallic mercury produced no clinical signs of conjunctivitis, histologically an inflammatory reaction has been demonstrable, and histochemically mercury has been detected in conjunctival tissues. External contact with mercury vapor has repeatedly been observed to induce a characteristic discoloration of the crystalline lens (mercurialentis).[e]

Accidental injection of mercury metal into the arterial circulation through cardiac catheters has caused embolism of the central retinal artery with resultant acute blindness, according to Valloton (1964) and Buxton (1965). Globules of mercury could be seen ophthalmoscopically in the retinal arteries and were demonstrable elsewhere in the body by x-ray.[a,g]

In systemic mercury poisoning from absorption of mercury vapor through the respiratory tract, the skin, and the gastrointestinal tract, mercurialentis has many times been observed. Even when overt signs of mercury poisoning are lacking, chronic exposure to low concentrations of mercury vapor are known to induce mercurialentis, but acute exposure to high concentrations of mercury vapor can induce acute systemic mercury poisoning before any discoloration of the lens is detectable. (Systemic mercury poisoning and mercurialentis are described in more detail under the heading *Mercury (inorganic) poisoning.*)

a. Buxton JT, Hewitt JC, et al: Metallic mercury embolism. *J AM MED ASSOC* 193:103–105, 1965.

b. Fleischanderl A: Impregnation of the cornea with mercury. *KLIN MONATSBL AUGEN-HEILKD* 104:432, 1940.

c. Harrison WJ: Primary zonular opacity of the cornea. *ARCH OPHTHALMOL* 16:469–471, 1936.

d. Ivanov VV: A procedure for removing mercury from the anterior chamber of the eye. *VESTN OFTAL* 78:65–66, 1965.

e. Kulczycka B: Resorption of metallic Hg by the conjunctiva. *NATURE* 206:943, 1965.

f. Parameshvara V: Mercury poisoning and its treatment with N-acetyl D,L-penicillamine. *BR J IND MED* 24:73–76, 1967.

g. Vallotton WW, Stokes HR: Mercury embolism of the central retinal artery. *AM J OPHTHALMOL* 57:476–478, 1964.

h. Galin MA, Obstbaum SA: Band keratopathy in mercury exposure. *ANN OPHTHALMOL* 6:1257–1261, 1974.

Mesaconic acid (methyl fumaric acid) on rabbit eyes causes moderate acid-type injury. An 11% solution at pH 1.9 causes rapid white coagulation of the epithelium, but damages the stroma only if the epithelium has been removed, and even under these circumstances healing is complete in a week.[81]

Mescaline (3,4,5-trimethoxyphenethylamine) obtained from mescal buttons or peyote, the flowering heads of a cactus, causes hallucinations of vision, particularly appearance of colors and forms without loss of consciousness.[246,252] The visual effects resemble those caused by lysergic acid diethylamide. In cats within ten minutes of administration of severely poisonous doses of either of these substances there are spontaneous action potentials which appear to originate in the retina, and are detectable from the eye, the optic nerve, and the occipital visual cortex.[a] No ocular injury or permanent alteration of vision has been attributed to either substance. In rats, intraocular injection of mescaline inhibits axoplasmic transport of proteins from retinal ganglion cells up the optic nerves.[b]

a. Apter JT, Pfeiffer CC: Effect of hallucinogenic drugs on the electroretinogram. *AM J OPHTHALMOL* 42:206–210, 1956.

b. Paulson JC, McClure WO: Inhibition of axoplasmic transport by mescaline and other trimethoxyphenylalkylamines. *MOL PHARMACOL* 9:41–50, 1973.

Mesidine (2,4,6-trimethylaniline) is reported to have produced morphologic changes in the retina when given to rats and rabbits. Also workers engaged for eleven to twenty years in the manufacture of mesidine and aniline were reported to have narrowing of peripheral visual fields, increase in size of the blind spot, and decrease in "photosensitivity", for which mesidine was thought to be responsible.[a]

> a. Laryukhina GM: Toxic action of mesidine (aniline derivative) on the organ of vision. *VESTN OFTALMOL* 83:75–78, 1970. (English summary)

Mesityl oxide applied as a drop to rabbit eyes caused mild presumably reversible injury, graded 5 on a scale of 1 to 10 after twenty-four hours.[27,222] The vapor induces a sensation of irritation which is detectable to human eyes at 25 ppm in air, and definitely irritating to the nose and eyes at 200 ppm.[b,217] Mice, rabbits, and guinea pigs give evidence of considerable eye and nose irritation at concentrations which are not injurious, and only at very much higher concentrations is corneal damage produced.[a,b] It appears that the vapors have adequate warning properties to prevent damaging exposures of human beings, and that splash injury is not likely to be serious.

> a. Hart ER, Schick JA, Leake CD: The toxicity of mesityl oxide. *UNIV CALIF PUB PHARMACOL* 1:161, 1939.
> b. Smyth HF, Seaton J, Fischer L: Response of guinea pigs and rats to repeated inhalation of vapors of mesityl oxide and isophorone. *J IND HYG* 24:46–50, 1942.

Mesoridazine (Lidanar, Serentil), an antipsychotic related to thioridazine, has been evaluated for adverse eye effects by comprehensive ophthalmologic examinations of 53 schizophrenic patients who were given 150 to 250 mg per day for an average of 132 days.[a] There were no significant changes in the eyes or in vision that could be definitely attributed to the medication, except for a possible mild acquired red-green color vision defect in one patient. Also, no distinctive ocular toxicity has been reported from Fraunfelder's National Registry as of 1982.[312]

> a. Posner RE, Burhan AS, Jagerman L: Ophthalmologic studies on mesoridazine. *AM J OPHTHALMOL* 69:143–146, 1970.

Mesquite thorn, the thorn from *Prosopis Chiliensis* or *glandulosa,* a tree growing in regions of the western United States, is said on penetrating the eye to cause an intraocular inflammation greater than expected from the degree of physical injury. The irritation has been attributed to a wax present in glands in the thorn and on its surface. Experimental injection of a suspension of the wax into the anterior chamber of an animal is reported to have caused a severe intraocular inflammation with disturbance of the cornea demonstrable by diffuse staining with fluorescein. Experimental introduction of a mesquite thorn into the animal's anterior chamber caused moderate reaction around the thorn in forty-two hours, but cleared in five days, with no disturbance of the cornea. It has been speculated that cerotic acid in the wax was the principal irritant, but no evidence has been presented to support this.[a]

> a. Brunner H, Bieberdorf F: The effects of the mesquite thorn on the human eye. *TRANS AM ACAD OPHTHALMOL* 54:595–597, 1949–50.

Metaldehyde ingested by animals is very toxic, frequently causing deaths, and sometimes blindness which may be reversible in survivors. Metaldehyde is commonly used as a molluscicide, and may be accessible to animals in the form of slug-bait pellets composed of metaldehyde and bran or wheat. A metaldehyde-poisoned dog had convulsions, complete incoordination, a period of barbiturate-induced unconsciousness, and total blindness upon regaining consciousness, though ophthalmoscopy and pupillary light reflex were normal.[a] The dog's vision returned slowly to normal in 3 weeks. Poisoned cows have been described similarly as incoordinated, with muscular spasms, and blindness, but without examination of their eyes.[b]

> a. Bishop CH: Blindness associated with metaldehyde. *VET REC* 96:438, 1975.
> b. Stubbings DP, Edington AB, et al: Three cases of metaldehyde poisoning in cattle. *VET REC* 98:356–357, 1976.

Methacrylonitrile on the skin causes dermatitis after a latent period, and systemically it is poisonous somewhat like hydrogen cyanide. The vapor is said to be lacrimatory.[171] A drop of the liquid applied to a rabbit eye caused immediate blepharospasm and shaking of the head, showing much irritation, but one hour later, and twenty-four hours later, the eye was completely normal, graded 1 on a scale of 1 to 10.[a,228]

> a. McOmie WA: Comparative toxicities of methacrylonitrile and acrylonitrile. *J IND HYG* 31:113–116, 1949.

Methacycline, an antibacterial, has caused yellow-brown discoloration of exposed conjunctiva, without disturbance of ocular function, and greyish-black pigmentation of skin exposed to light. Extracellular pigment deposition has been seen microscopically. This complication was estimated to occur in only 3% of long-term treated patients with total dose of 400 to 1600 g.

> Dyster-Aas K, Hansson H, et al: Pigment deposits in eyes and light-exposed skin during long-term methacycline therapy. *ACTA DERM VENEREOL* 54:209–221, 1974.

Methadone (Adanon, Althose, Dolophine), a narcotic analgesic with effects similar to morphine, but effective in treatment of opiate addiction, has caused reversible cortical blindness, apparently secondary to anoxia, in a young child. The child had severe depression of respiration and deep unconsciousness, from which it awoke after a week, apparently unable to see, although the pupils reacted to light and the fundi appeared normal. During the next four to five weeks the EEGs returned from severe generalized abnormality to normal, and vision seemed to recover completely.[b] Even a small amount of methadone is life-threatening to children, due to respiratory depression, and many have been accidentally poisoned, but disturbance of vision as in the case just summarized must be rare.[e] The pupils in methadone-poisoned children are characteristically miotic. After a nalorphine type antidote they become less miotic, but with hypoxic brain damage they may become dilated.[e]

In mice, systemic administration of methadone has caused rapid appearance of opacities on the front of the crystalline lenses which are reversible and apparently similar to those induced by morphine, pethidine, and other drugs that suppress blinking and allow exposure and drying of the cornea with attendant dehydration of the lens.[c,d,261] Development of the opacities can be prevented by keeping the lids closed.[a,c]

a. Fraunfelder FT, Burns RP: Effects of lid closure in drug-induced experimental cataracts. *ARCH OPHTHALMOL* 76:599–601, 1966.
b. Ratcliffe SC: Methadone poisoning in a child. *BR MED J* 1:1056–1070, 1963.
c. Weinstock M, Steward HC, Butterworth KR: The action of drugs on the formation of transient lens opacities. *EXP EYE RES* 2:28–32, 1963.
d. Weinstock M, Marshall AS: Factors influencing the incidence of reversible lens opacities in solitary and aggregated mice. *J PHARMACOL EXP THER* 170:168–172, 1969.
e. Aronow R, Paul SD, Wooley PV: Childhood poisoning, an unfortunate consequence of methadone availability. *J AM MED ASSOC* 219:321–324, 1972.

Methamphetamine, a CNS stimulant, has received some attention with respect to intraocular pressure. In rabbits a very slight increase has been obtained in both intraocular and blood pressure from subcutaneous and intravenous injections.[a] In patients with "chronic simple glaucoma", or with eyes that had had filtering operations for glaucoma, only a 1 or 2 mm Hg change in intraocular pressure appears to have been induced by subcutaneous administration.[b,c]

a. Takayama H: Effect of intravenous injection of methamphetamine HCl on intraocular pressure and blood pressure. *FOLIA OPHTHALMOL JPN* 9:147–152, 1958.
b. Thiel R: On the cause of primary glaucoma. *BUECH AUGENARZT* 21:9–52, 1952. (German)
c. Thiel R, Hollwich F: Eye-midbrain reflex and intraocular pressure. *BUECH AUGENARZT* 23:166–209, 1955. (German)

Methanol (methyl alcohol) has been one of the most notorious toxic causes of loss of vision, the subject of hundreds of articles since first noted in the 1870's. Only the most noteworthy or representative of these articles can be included in the bibliography accompanying this synopsis. They are listed alphabetically by first author's name.

This synopsis will consider various aspects in the following order: (a) clinical character of intoxication of human beings, with pathological findings and treatment, (b) animal experiments and investigations of the mechanism of intoxication, (c) the effects of external contact of methanol with the eye.

Many reports have described mass poisonings and individual cases. A reasonably consistent picture is presented by most of this material (Aquilonius; Benton; Dethlefs; Durang; McLean; Roe; Sekkat). Poisoning usually results from drinking methanol. It so resembles ethanol (ethyl alcohol) in taste and smell that it has many times been substituted for the latter in alcoholic beverages without the victim being aware of its toxicity until many hours later. Susceptibility to poisoning varies greatly from one person to another, but 15 to 30 ml may lead to serious poisoning.

In very few seemingly authentic cases poisoning has been ascribed to absorption through the skin or to inhalation of high concentration of vapor (Tyson; Weill). Walsh and Hoyt described a case of acute loss of vision and subsequent recovery which was probably, but not positively, due to inhalation of methanol vapor.[256] More questionably, Perli ascribed irreversible retrobulbar neuritis in one patient to a habit of inhaling methanol vapors several times a day for two years. (Whether there is a chronic form of methanol poisoning is open to question, and if it exists it must be very rare.)

When several ounces are rapidly consumed, the first reaction may be nausea and vomiting from irritation of the gastrointestinal tract. However, the special toxic effects of methanol usually first appear after a latent period of eighteen to forty-eight hours. Methanol is metabolized very much more slowly than ethanol, and a significant amount may remain in the body for several days. Typically, within eighteen to forty-eight hours poisoned patients develop nausea, abdominal pain, vomiting, headache, and shortness of breath. This is accompanied by failing vision. The visual symptoms have ranged from spots before the eyes or mistiness of vision to markedly reduced visual acuity and complete blindness. The most severely poisoned patients become comatose and may die of respiratory failure. Those who recover from coma may be found blind on regaining consciousness.

Clinical examinations of the eyes of patients have been particularly well described by Benton and Calhoun from a study of 320 victims of a mass poisoning, and their observations are in generally good agreement with previously published descriptions. In the acute phase of poisoning, typically visual acuity is impaired by central or cecocentral scotomas. Rarely are these accompanied by constriction of peripheral fields in the early phase. Impaired visual acuity is accompanied by proportionately impaired pupillary response to light. No impairment of pupillary reaction is found unless vision has been affected. The pupils continue to react normally to accommodation.

Ophthalmoscopic examination has been rather uniformly described as showing hyperemia or reddish appearance of the optic nerveheads when vision is first impaired, then development of edema of the disc margins and adjacent retina in the course of the next twenty-four hours. The edema has been described as appearing chiefly in the nerve fiber layer and tending to follow the course of the major retinal vessels. With development of retinal edema the retinal veins usually appear engorged (Muller). In rare cases subhyaloid, flame-shaped hemorrhages have occurred (Sathiavakesan).

The subsequent course, depending on the severity of poisoning and the adequacy of treatment, ranges from complete recovery with disappearance of retinal edema and return of vision to normal, to the other extreme of persisting edema of the retina for as long as two months, with atrophy of the optic nervehead becoming visible in one to two months, and vision completely and permanently gone. Between the extremes are many cases of vision partially but permanently impaired. Vision may be temporarily impaired, then worsen (Rossazza).

In general it appears that if normal vision is to be regained, it is regained within six days after the onset, and if not regained by this time, may actually deteriorate further. Exceptionally, some recovery is possible over a longer time (Scrimgeour). Of particularly bad prognostic implication are the findings of severe initial impairment of vision, wide dilation and unresponsiveness of the pupils to light, and severe edema of the retina.

In patients whose vision does not completely recovery, the scotomas in the central field remain, and as optic atrophy develops, the peripheral fields may constrict.

The appearance of optic atrophy caused by methanol has the characteristics of so-called primary optic atrophy, showing whiteness of the nervehead with distinct margins and little or no surrounding abnormality. In a noteworthy small proportion of cases, but with numerous examples scattered through the literature, the atrophic nervehead has become cupped, and its appearance has closely resembled the cupping and atrophy of glaucoma (Friedman; Klar; Larco). With very rare exceptions, no elevation of intraocular pressure has been detected in association with methanol poisoning to account for this peculiarity.

Electroretinography in methanol poisoning of human beings has shown minor alterations, particularly reduction of the b-wave, suggesting to Ruedemann and to Salorio that there is some injurious action on sensory receptors of the retina or the outer plexiform layer. However, Durang and associates demonstrated in one case that the ERG was essentially normal though the patient remained blind after the acute stage of poisoning and acidosis had passed, at a time when optic atrophy was developing. Also, Ingemansson reported no abnormality of the ERG, early or late, in nine typical cases of poisoning (Ingemansson). This seems to be consistent with the belief that the principal injurious action of methanol is on retinal ganglion cells and optic nerve fibers.

The histologic pathology of the eyes in methanol poisoning in human beings presents in the late stages evidence of degeneration of retinal ganglion cells and optic nerve fibers as part of the picture of optic atrophy (Benton; McGregor; McLean; Muller). However, in specimens from patients who have died from very severe poisoning in the first day or two, either the retinal ganglion cells and optic nerve fibers have appeared morphologically normal, or slight abnormalities in their appearance have generally been attributed to postmortem changes (Benton; McGregor; Muller). Most recently, demyelinating retrolaminar optic neuropathy has been described as an early finding (Sharpe).

Clinically, one of the most striking features of methanol poisoning is acidosis. The severity of the acidosis appears to have great influence on the course and outcome of the poisoning. Acidosis is manifested by shortness of breath, acid urine, and by reduced carbon dioxide-combining power of the blood (Benton; Chew; Gilger; Roe).

The degree of acidosis has been found to parallel closely the severity of poisoning (Benton; Roe). With normal carbon dioxide-combining power of 26 mEq/liter or 55 vol % in the blood there is no significant poisoning or disturbance of vision. If the carbon dioxide-combining power remains more than two thirds of normal, the symptoms of poisoning are as a rule mild, and even moderate visual loss is uncommon. When the carbon dioxide-combining power is half of normal or less, the incidence of visual disturbances and severe poisoning becomes high.

It is well recognized that the acidosis itself is not responsible for the damage of the eye in methanol poisoning, since equally severe acidosis occurs in other conditions, such as diabetes, without damaging the optic nerve or retina. However, in methanol poisoning, correcting the acidosis does dramatically improve the general condition of the patient.

Acidosis in methanol poisoning appears to be caused primarily by formation and accumulation of formate in the blood, but increased lactate is also found, varying from case to case in a manner yet to be fully explained.

In addition to alkalinizing therapy to combat the acidosis, attempts to hasten the excretion of unchanged methanol from the body appear logical, since this substance, unlike ethanol, is slowly metabolized and persists in the body for several days, presumably continuing to form toxic metabolites. Ethanol interferes with the metabolism of methanol, and is beneficial in treatment of methanol poisoning. This has been indicated by comparisons of the relative amounts of ethanol and methanol consumed by various individuals and the severity of their poisoning, also by clinical and experimental investigations by Roe.

Hemodialysis, and to a lesser degree peritoneal dialysis, have been acclaimed in the treatment of acute methanol poisoning, and their effectiveness has been demonstrated. Dialysis removes methanol from the body much more rapidly than it would be excreted or metabolized naturally. Rapid removal of methanol before it can be metabolized to more toxic metabolites has proved of great importance in several cases of poisoning.

Now, as pointed out particularly by McLean, with hemodialysis, cardiopulmonary support, and improved management of acid-base balance, more of the severely poisoned patients who formerly would have died are surviving. These new survivors unfortunately may not only be permanently blind with optic atrophy, but also have serious damage to the central nervous system. This ranges from "moderate polyneuropathy" mentioned by Aquilonius, to rigidity, spasticity and hypokinesis reported by Guggenheim, and a Parkinson-like extrapyramidal syndrome with mild dementia described by McLean. Neurologic disturbances have been rarely encountered in the past. For instance, in a study of 323 cases of methanol poisoning Bennett reported in 1953 no permanent sequelae except optic atrophy. However, Guggenheim has pointed out 3 reports in earlier German literature. When disability in walking and use of the arms has occurred, it has in some cases developed and become worse during weeks and months following difficult survival from poisoning with methanol. Damage to the putamen has been a peculiarly specific part of the central nervous system damage, even in patients without obvious motor disability. Damage to the putamen has been demonstrable clinically by computerized tomography, and confirmed by autopsy (Aquilonius; McLean).

Experimental investigations in animals have been attempted repeatedly for more than sixty years, but until recently have yielded results of little relevance to poisoning of human beings. The principal difficulty has been that in all commonly employed laboratory animals, except subhuman primates, the type of poisoning induced by methanol differs significantly from that in human beings. In lower animals death can be readily and acutely produced by large doses of methanol acting apparently as a narcotic, but acidosis is not induced, and seldom have optic nerve and retina been injured in the manner in which they are injured in human beings. In all experimental work on methanol, it is most important to recognize the differences among species, and particularly to be cautious in relating results to human beings.

A similarity between methanol poisoning in rhesus monkeys and human beings has been reported by Potts, Gilger, Farkas and their associates. Some acutely poisoned monkeys developed severe acidosis, and edema of the optic nervehead and retina, similar to that in human beings. They were benefited by treatment with sodium bicarbonate, and they were at least partially protected against lethal poisoning by administration of ethanol (Gilger; Potts; Praglin). However, Cooper and Felig reported mostly an acute narcotic type of intoxication without acidosis, and only exceptionally acidosis and blindness, which was temporary.

Subsequently, a team of investigators, with ophthalmological aspects represented by Hayreh and Hayreh, carried out further experiments on monkeys, reported in a series of articles (Baumback; Hayreh; Martin-Amat; McMartin). They confirmed that when monkeys were acutely, lethally poisoned with methanol they usually died with little evidence of toxic effect on the eyes, but when monkeys were sublethally poisoned by repeated smaller doses of methanol they became blind and showed edema of the optic nervehead the same as human beings. The dosage of methanol was regulated to induce a level of acidosis like that encountered in poisoned human beings. Histologically, the optic nerve heads showed edema the same as produced by elevated cerebrospinal fluid pressure, but this pressure was found to be normal. No abnormality was found in the retinal ganglion cells. Abnormality of the optic nerve fibers was localized to the optic nerve head and the retrolaminar and intraorbital portions. It appeared that swelling of oligodendroglia compressed the optic nerve axons and interfered with axoplasmic flow, causing accumulation of material in the axons at the optic disc and providing the characteristic appearance of papilledema.

One crucial question remaining to be answered was why does papilledema from increased cerebrospinal fluid pressure not impair vision, while identical-appearing papilledema from methanol definitely was associated with loss of vision. It appeared that methanol must have an effect on nerve conduction and vital function in addition to its morphologically evident effect on axoplasmic flow.

Other crucial questions have been answered by this series of studies. It has long been thought that methanol itself is not the direct cause of toxic effects on the eye, but that one of its metabolites, either formaldehyde or formic acid, was more likely responsible, but it remained uncertain which to blame. Now in this series of monkey experiments no evidence was found to inculpate formaldehyde (McMartin), but giving formic acid or formate reproduced the characteristic blinding effects of methanol (Martin-Amat; McMartin). Interestingly, this same toxic action was obtainable even in the absence of acidosis.

Formate is found to be metabolized to carbon dioxide and water by a folate-dependent pathway, but so slowly in monkeys, and presumably in humans, that it can accumulate. Its toxic effect on the optic nerves has been postulated to involve inhibition of cytochrome oxidase and NaKATPase (Baumback; Martin-Amat). Administration of folate to monkeys has been shown to increase the rate of formate oxidation, and folate deficiency has been shown to increase the susceptibility to methanol poisoning (McMartin).

Although now the evidence strongly indicates that formate is the important toxic intermediate, there have been reasons in the past to suspect formaldehyde. In rare instances formaldehyde has been detected in the vitreous and aqueous humors and in other fluids and tissues of the body of animals poisoned by methanol. Also rarely formaldehyde has been detected during oxidation of methanol by tissues *in vitro*

(Keeser). Intravenous drip of formaldehyde in monkeys causes immediate change in the ERG (Potts). However, it has not been possible to reproduce the blindness and CNS effects of methanol poisoning by giving formaldehyde intravenously over a period of several hours (Potts). Administration of formate to monkeys in doses comparable to toxic amounts of methanol has also been found to cause a definite change in the ERG in one or two hours (Potts).

The biochemical aspects of methanol poisoning, particularly in monkeys, were examined in a series of investigations by Cooper and Kini. Kini and Cooper showed that formaldehyde is formed from methanol through the action of alcohol dehydrogenase in the retina itself, and that formaldehyde can inhibit retinal respiration, glycolysis, oxidative phosphorylation, and generation of ATP, indicating significant toxicity to the retina.

4-Methylpyrazole, an inhibitor of alcohol dehydrogenase, interferes with oxidation of methanol to formaldehyde and formate. Ingemansson has shown that administering 4-methypyrazole to monkeys can prevent toxic changes in the ERG when methanol is given.

External contact of methanol with the eye has been alleged to have caused corneal opacities,[46] but this must be far from the rule. Tests on rabbit eyes indicate that the danger is slight. In rabbits after application of a drop, a mild reversible reaction, graded 3 on a scale of 1 to 10 has been observed after twenty-four hours.[27] On excised beef corneas 30% methanol has had slight effect on adhesion of epithelium to stroma.[107] By exposure of cats to methanol vapor an attempt has been made to induce vacuoles in the corneal epithelium similar to those produced by other solvents, but this has been unsuccessful.[216] (Compare *Solvent vapors.*) No poisonous effect on the retina or optic nerve is observed after splash of a drop of methanol on the eye.

One case has been reported briefly by McDonald in which for a month after a patient splashed a mixture of chloroform and methyl alcohol in the eye the cornea had persistent staining with fluorescein.

Aquilonius SM, Askmark H, et al: Computerized tomography in severe methanol intoxication. *BR MED J* 2:929–930, 1978.

Baumback GL, Cancilla PA, et al: Methyl alcohol poisoning. *ARCH OPHTHALMOL* 95:1859–1865, 1977.

Bennett IL Jr, Cary FH, et al: Acute methyl alcohol poisoning: A review based on experiences in an outbreak of 323 cases. *MEDICINE* 32:431–463, 1953.

Benton CD Jr, Calhoun FP Jr: The ocular effects of methyl alcohol poisoning: Report of a catastrophe involving 320 persons. *TRANS AM ACAD OPHTHAL OTOL* 56:875–885, 1952; *AM J OPHTHALMOL* 36:1677–1685, 1953.

Chew WB, Berger EH, et al: Alkali treatment of methyl alcohol poisoning. *J AM MED ASSOC* 130:61–64, 1946.

Cooper JR, Felig P: The biochemistry of methanol poisoning. *TOXICOL APPL PHARMACOL* 3:202–209, 1961.

Cooper JR, Kini MM: Biochemical aspects of methanol poisoning. *BIOCHEM PHARMACOL* 11:405–416, 1962.

Dethlefs R, Naraqi S: Ocular manifestations and complications of acute methyl alcohol intoxication. *MED J AUSTRALIA* 2:483–485, 1978.

Durang L, Ravault MP, et al: Acute neuritis from poisoning with methyl alcohol. *BULL SOC OPHTALMOL FRANCE* 68:46–48, 1968. (French)

Friedman B: Deep cupping of nervehead in atrophy of optic nerve due to methyl alcohol. *ARCH OPHTHALMOL* 26:6–11, 1941.

Gilger AP, Farkas IS, Potts AM: Studies on visual toxicity of methanol. *AM J OPHTHALMOL* 48:153–160, 1959.

Gilger A, Potts A: Studies on the visual toxicity of methanol. *AM J OPHTHALMOL* 39:63–86, 1955.

Gilger AP, Potts AM, Farkas IS: Studies on the visual toxicity of methanol. *AM J OPHTHALMOL* 42:244–251, 1956.

Guggenheim MA, Couch JR, Weinberg W: Motor dysfunction as a permanent complication of methanol ingestion. *ARCH NEUROL* 24:550–554, 1971.

Hayreh MS, Hayreh SS, et al: Methyl alcohol poisoning. III. Ocular toxicity. *ARCH OPHTHALMOL* 95:1851–1858, 1977.

Hayreh MMS, Hayreh SS, et al: Ocular toxicity of methanol, an experimental study. Pages 35–53 in Merigan and Weiss (1980).[358]

Ingemansson SO: Studies of the effect of 4-methylpyrazole on retinal activity in the methanol poisoned monkey. *ACTA OPHTHALMOL* (Suppl 158):1–24, 1983.

Ingemansson SO: Clinical observations on ten cases of methanol poisoning. *ACTA OPHTHALMOL* 62:15–24, 1984.

Keeser E, Vincke E: On formation of formaldehyde by break-down of methyl alcohol. *KLIN WOCHENSCHR* 19:583–585, 1940. (German)

Kini MM, Cooper JR: Biochemistry of methanol poisoning. *BIOCHEM PHARMACOL* 8:207–215, 1961.

Klar J: How does the excavation of the papilla develop following poisoning with methyl alcohol? *ANN OCULIST* 184:959, 1951. (French)

Lasco F: Pseudoglaucoma following poisoning by methyl alcohol. *ANN OCULIST* 191:235–241, 1958. (French)

Martin-Amat G, McMartin KE, et al: The monkey as a model in methanol poisoning. *ALCOHOL ALDEHYDE METAB SYST* 2:419–428, 1977.

Martin-Amat G, Tephyl TR, et al: Methyl alcohol poisoning. III. Development of a model for ocular toxicity in methyl alcohol poisoning using the rhesus monkey. *ARCH OPHTHALMOL* 95:1847–1850, 1977.

Martin-Amat G, McMartin KE, et al: Methanol poisoning: Ocular toxicity produced by formate. *TOXICOL APPL PHARMACOL* 45:201–208, 1978.

McDonald JE: Chemical burns of the eye. *J AM MED ASSOC* 192:271, 1965.

McGregor IS: A study of the histopathological changes in the retina and late changes in the visual field in acute methyl alcohol poisoning. *BR J OPHTHALMOL* 27:523–543, 1943.

McLean DR, Jacobs H, Mielke BW: Methanol poisoning: a clinical and pathological study. *ANN NEUROL* 8:161–167, 1980.

McMartin KE, Martin-Amat G, et al: Methanol poisoning. V. Role of formate metabolism in the monkey. *J PHARMACOL EXP THER* 20:564–572, 1977.

McMartin KE, Martin-Amat G, et al: Methanol poisoning: role of formate metabolism in the monkey. *ALCOHOL ALDEHYDE METAB SYST* 2:429–440, 1977.

McMartin KE, Martin-Amat G, et al: Lack of a role for formaldehyde in methanol poisoning in the monkey. *BIOCHEM PHARMACOL* 28:645–649, 1979.

Muller H: Histologic study of an eye in acute lethal methyl alcohol poisoning. *KLIN MONATSBL AUGENHEILKD* 116:135–145, 1950. (German)

Perli R, Orioli F, Berkman S: Retrobulbar neuritis due to inhalation of methyl alcohol. *ARCH OFTALMOL B AIR* 38:430–435, 1963.

Potts AM: Studies on the visual toxicity of methanol. *AM J OPHTHALMOL* 39:86–92, 1955.

Potts AM, Praglin J, Farkas I, et al: Studies on the visual toxicity of methanol. *AM J OPHTHALMOL* 40:76–83, 1955.

Praglin J, Spurney R, Potts AM: An experimental study of electroretinography. *AM J OPHTHALMOL* 39(2, Part II):52–62, 1955.

Roe O: Methanol poisoning; its clinical course, pathogenesis and treatment. *ACTA MED SCAND* (Suppl.), 182, 1946.

Roe O: Past present and future fight against methanol blindness and death. *TRANS OPHTHALMOL SOC UK* 89:235–242, 1969.

Rossazza C, Delplace MP, et al: Significant but transitory visual improvement after poisoning by methanol. *BULL SOC OPHTALMOL FRANCE* 83:545–548, 1983. (French)

Ruedemann AD Jr: The electroretinogram in chronic methyl alcohol poisoning in human beings. *TRANS AM OPHTHALMOL SOC* 59:480–526, 1961. (*AM J OPHTHALMOL* 54:34–53, 1962.)

Salorio M: Intoxication by methyl alcohol. *OPHTHALMOLOGICA* 158:141–148, 1969. (French)

Sathiavakesan S: Unusual findings in methyl alcohol poisoning. *J ALL INDIA OPHTHALMOL SOC* 17:121–122, 1969.

Scrimgeour EM, Dethlefs RF, Kevau I: Delayed recovery of vision after blindness caused by methanol poisoning. *MED J AUST* 2:481–483, 1982.

Sekkat A, Maillard P, et al: Optic neuropathy in the course of an acute poisoning by methanol. *J FR OPHTALMOL* 5:797–804, 1982. (French)

Sharpe JA, Hostovsky M, et al: Methanol optic neuropathy: A histopathological study. *NEUROLOGY* 32:1093–1100, 1982.

Tyson HH: Amblyopia from methyl alcohol. *ARCH OPHTHALMOL* 41:459, 1912; *TRANS AM OPHTHALMOL SOC* 13:146, 1912.

Weill G: Serious ocular disturbances from inhalation of impure acetone. *BULL SOC FR OPHTALMOL* 47:412–414, 1934. (French)

Methaqualone (Quaalude), a sedative-hypnotic, has had no documented specific toxic effects on the eyes, or on the pupils after overdosage.[a,b] However, Fraunfelder indicates that some patients in "toxic states" have dilated pupils.[312] In one case after deep coma the patient developed widespread purpura with a small hemorrhage in the conjunctiva of one eye, but no hemorrhages in the fundi.[b] Another patient who developed acute purpura with thrombocytopenia had retinal hemorrhages.

a. Gitelson S: Methaqualone-meprobamate poisoning. *J AM MED ASSOC* 201:977–979, 1967.

b. MacDonald HRF, Lakshman AD: Poisoning with Mandrax. *BR MED J* 1:500–501, 1967.

c. Trese M: Retinal hemorrhage caused by overdose of methaqualone (Quaalude). *AM J OPHTHALMOL* 91:201–203, 1981.

Methazolamide (Neptazane), a carbonic anhydrase inhibitor related to acetazolamide, has adverse effects qualitatively like those of acetazolamide, but quantitatively somewhat different. Rather than repeat here much that has been said in the section on acetazolamide, the reader is referred to that section, and here will be reviewed only what has been reported specifically about adverse effects of methazolamide itself.

Nearly all that has been reported about acetazolamide has been reported about methazolamide, but in much smaller numbers.

Urinary stones were thought to be less likely to form in patients treated with methazolamide, because of less reduction of urinary citrate, but several cases of this complication have now been reported.[a,d,g]

Similarly, blood dyscrasias, particularly aplastic anemia, have relatively seldom been associated with methazolamide, but there have been a small number of cases where a connection has been strongly suspected.[f,i,j,k]

Methazolamide, like acetazolamide, has caused acidosis with unpleasant symptoms that can be partially relieved by giving sodium bicarbonate or acetate.[c,e] Both have caused respiratory failure in the presence of respiratory disease.[b] Both have caused decreased libido.[h]

No cross-sensitization with antimicrobial sulfonamides is evident, and in some patients skin rash has been associated with either acetazolamide or methazolamide, but not with both.

a. Becker B: Use of methazolamide (Neptazane) in the therapy of glaucoma. *AM J OPHTHALMOL* 49:1307–1311, 1960.

b. Coudon WL, et al: Acute respiratory failure precipitated by a carbonic anhydrase inhibitor. *CHEST* 69:112–113, 1976.

c. Dahlen K, Epstein DL, et al: A repeated dose-response study of methazolamide in glaucoma. *ARCH OPHTHALMOL* 96:2214–2218, 1978.

d. Ellis PP: Urinary calculi with methazolamide therapy. *DOC OPHTHALMOL* 34:137–142, 1973.

e. Epstein DL, Grant WM: Carbonic anhydrase inhibitor side effects. *ARCH OPHTHALMOL* 95:1378–1382, 1977.

f. Gangitano JL, Foster SH, Contro RM: Nonfatal methazolamide-induced aplastic anemia. *AM J OPHTHALMOL* 86:138–139, 1978.

g. Shields MB, Simmons RJ: Urinary calculus during methazolamide therapy. *AM J OPHTHALMOL* 81:622–624, 1976.

h. Wallace TR, Fraunfelder FT, et al: Decreased libido—a side effect of carbonic anhydrase inhibitor. *ANN OPHTHALMOL* 11:1563–1566, 1979.

i. Weblin TP, Pollack IP, Liss RA: Aplastic anemia and agranulocytosis in patients using methazolamide for glaucoma. *J AM MED ASSOC* 241:2817–2818, 1979.

j. Weblin TP, Pollack IP, Liss RA: Blood dycrasias in patients using methazolamide (Neptazane) for glaucoma. *OPHTHALMOLOGY* 87:350–354, 1980.

k. Wisch N, Fischbein FI, et al: Aplastic anemia resulting from the use of carbonic anhydrase inhibitors. *AM J OPHTHALMOL* 75:130–132, 1973.

Methicillin, an antibacterial, was found to alter transiently the corneal endothelium of rabbits when placed in the anterior chamber,[341] but to be non-toxic to the retina when used in vitreous replacement fluid at 25 μg/ml.[361]

Methixene (Trest), an anticholinergic smooth muscle relaxant administered orally, has less effect on pupils and accommodation than atropine given for the same purpose. It seldom affects pupil or accommodation[a,b] and has been reported to have no effect on intraocular pressure in chronic open-angle glaucoma or in patients subject to angle-closure glaucoma.[b]

a. Strang, RR: Clinical evaluation of chlorphenoxamine with caffeine in the treatment of Parkinson's disease, including a comparison with methixene. *J CLIN PHARMACOL* 7:214–220, 1967.

b. Marcotte D: Use of a new antispasmodic in glaucomatous patients. *ROCKY MOUNTAIN MED J* 63:66–68, 1966.

Methocarbamol (Robaxin), a skeletal relaxant, is said to have produced drowsiness, vertigo, nystagmus, blurred vision, and diplopia after intravenous, and oral administration. Apparently these have all been transitory functional disturbances, and the cause and nature of the blurred vision have not been elucidated.[4,171] To answer a question as to the effect of Robaxin intravenous solution (diluted for injection) on accidental contact with the eye, several drops were instilled in the conjunctival sac of a normal volunteer, and no irritation or injury resulted.

Methotrexate (amethopterin), an antineoplastic and antipsoriasis agent, has been tested as a potential chemotherapeutic agent in rabbit eyes. A concentration of 10 mg/ml injected into the vitreous humor has caused membranes to form,[b] but 400 μg/ml is reported non-toxic.[277] Subconjunctival injection of 6.25 mg/kg in rabbits and re-examination at 24 and 48 hours showed no remaining fluid bleb and no toxic effect on cornea or conjunctiva discernible by biomicroscopy.[d]

Systemically administered methotrexate was first noted clinically to cause eye irritation by Johnson and Burns in 1965 in a patient who developed blepharocon-junctivitis.[333] In 1983, Fraunfelder stated that at least 25% of patients develop "ocular irritation, including periorbital edema, blepharitis, conjunctival hyperemia, epiphora, and photophobia," though the anterior segments of these patients' eyes may appear normal.[313] Doroshow reported that 4 out of 13 patients who received high-dose intravenous infusions of methotrexate developed uncomfortable burning, itching and gritty sensation, but not until several days later, and then lasting only a few days.[a] This appeared to be associated with a marked temporary reduction of tear production, but otherwise normal-appearing anterior segments. A different type of reaction was reported by Lischka in a patient who experienced pain and excess tearing with defects in the corneal epithelium and wrinkling of Descemet's membrane while receiving daily intramuscular methotrexate for psoriasis.[f] There was complete recovery from the keratitis when the treatment was discontinued. A question whether systemic methotrexate treatment for psoriasis could delay healing of a herpetic corneal ulcer was posed to two ophthalmologists and a dermatologist, eliciting opinions ranging from no to yes.[c]

From intrathecal administration of methotrexate in treatment of lymphoma a case of transient bilateral ophthalmoplegia with exotropia has been reported, with evidence that demyelination was cause by a combination of the drug and irradiation.[e]

a. Doroshow JH, Locker GY, et al: Ocular irritation from high-dose methotrexate. *CANCER* 48:2158–2162, 1981.

b. Ericson L, Karlberg B, et al: Trials of intravitreal injections of chemotherapeutic agents in rabbits. *ACTA OPHTHALMOL* 42:721–726, 1964.

c. Fields LM, Kaufman HE, Levine SB, Voorhees JJ: Can methotrexate therapy delay healing of corneal ulcer? *J AM MED ASSOC* 223:1170, 1973.

d. Gudauskas G, Ostry A, Rootman J: Concentrations of tritiated methotrexate in ocular compartments, serum and urine after subconjunctival and intravenous injection. *CAN J OPHTHALMOL* 15:179–182, 1980.

e. Lepore FE, Nissenblatt MJ: Bilateral internuclear ophthalmoplegia after intrathecal chemotherapy and cranial irradiation. *AM J OPHTHALMOL* 92:851–853, 1981.

f. Lischka G: Surprisingly rapid effect of methotrexate; side effects on the eye. *HAUTARZT* 19:473, 1968. (German)

Methotrimeprazine (levomepromazine, Levoprome, Nozinan), a phenothiazine analgesic, has been said to produce pigmentation of the lens and cornea like that produced by chlorpromazine.[311] However, many people treated with this drug probably have also received chlorpromazine at some time, and at least in some cases it is possible that it was the chlorpromazine that was actually responsible.[a, b] Gerhard reported finding anterior segment pigmentation in patients who had received chlorpromazine, but never in patients who had received only methotrimeprazine, also no retinopathy or disturbance of vision.[d] However, Kassman has reported anterior segment pigmentation in four patients who were believed to have received only methotrimeprazine.[e] One case of bilateral maculopathy and central scotomas is reported in a 38 year old patient who had received methotrimeprazine for 15 years, but no other phenothiazine drug, and had no anterior segment pigmentation.[c]

a. Calluaud JL, DiBattista JC, et al: Ocular pigmentation and phenothiazine derivatives. *BULL SOC OPHTALMOL FRANCE* 77:661–664, 1977. (French)

b. Delorme R, Ballereau L, et al: Major adverse ocular effect of phenothiazines. *BULL SOC OPHTALMOL FRANCE* 73:591–593, 1973. (French)

c. Deodati F, Bec P, et al: Maculopathy and levomepromazine. *BULL SOC FR OPHTALMOL* 86:191–197, 1973. (French)

d. Gerhard JP, Franck H, et al: Incidence of ophthalmologic complications of treatment with phenothiazines. *REV OTO-NEURO-OPHTALMOL* 47:71–77, 1975. (French)

e. Kassman T: Lens opacities and prophobilinogen-like substance in urine associated with levomepromazine. *ACTA PSYCHIATR SCAND* 43:163–168, 1967.

Methoxsalen (8-methoxypsoralen, xanthotoxin, ammodoin, Meloxine, Methoxa Dome, Oxsoralen) is a psoralen found in a number of plants, including *Psoralea coryliafolia, Ammi majus,* parsley, celery, wild carrots, parsnips, figs, and limes.[m] It is one of the constitutents that may cause photosensitization reactions of the skin and eyes in animals that eat these plants, e.g. in ducklings that have eaten seeds of *Ammi majus.*[zc] Another psoralen, *trioxsalen* (Trisoralen), will be included in the discussion of methoxsalen, because of close similarity of properties and uses.

Medically, psoralens have been administered topically or orally to patients some hours prior to exposure to sunlight or long wavelength ultraviolet (UVA) in treatment of psoriasis, and to aid skin pigmentation in vitiligo. However, there has been concern that this treatment might cause patients to develop cataracts. This apprehension has been based in part on indications that environmental UVA by itself may have a role in development of senile cataracts.[w] It has been thought that this effect might be enhanced by the photosensitizing action of the psoralens. Supporting this idea, intensive exposure of animals to a combination of psoralens and UVA has produced opacities in their lenses, as well as effects on the cornea and skin, varying from species to species. However, there has so far been no proof of cataract induction in human beings by current standard treatment with psoralens and UVA, so called PUVA. Transient slight actinic-type keratitis has been reported in some patients.[b]

In 1979 in a report on patients who had been treated for vitiligo with methoxsalen and sunlight (usually without protective goggles), it was noted that this regimen had been in use for at least 28 years with no report of ocular damage.[h,i] A follow up study was performed in which patients were selected according to the following criteria: they were under 40 years of age (to avoid confusion from possible presence of senile cataracts), had taken large doses of methoxsalen, and had exposed their vitiligo lesions to the sun over a period of 5 or more years. Fifteen patients who met these criteria were given comprehensive eye examinations. The duration of their treatment had ranged from 5 to 23 years, and had terminated from one month to 20 years before the study. Dosages had ranged from 40 to 120 mg per day, with totals from 73 to 262 g. No significant ocular abnormalities were discovered, particularly no signs of cataracts.[i]

Since 1974, photochemical treatment of psoriasis (PUVA) with methoxsalen or trioxsalen has been used in thousands of patients, but special goggles to shield the eyes from UVA have been advised for at least 24 hours after administration of the photosensitizing drug.[z,ze] By 1980 a prospective trial and evaluation of this treatment had enlisted one to two thousand patients in 16 clinical centers with twice weekly treatments, but none had developed cataracts that were thought to be related to the treatment.[m,n,q] Independent observations, some on series of 42 to 96 patients, similarly were negative.[a,o,zb,zd]

In 1980 one clinical report raised a suspicion of cataracts from PUVA associated with possible inconsistent use of protective goggles in treatment of vitiligo.[g] At first eye examination, more than a year and a half after the patient started treatment with trioxsalen orally, all was normal except that by slit lamp examination in the anterior cortex of both lenses there were stellate opacities composed of multicolored speckles extending in zonular configuration to the posterior cortex. Trioxsalen was stopped on the assumption that it plus insufficient use of protective goggles might be responsible. In 1984, in a 28-month follow-up of 78 PUVA-treated patients, small lens opacities developed in three, without affecting visual acuity; failure to wear dark glasses after medication was a suspected factor in two of the patients.[s]

In 1982, although there was yet no real proof that PUVA treatment without special protection would cause cataracts in human beings, it was being advised that special protective goggles be used for two days each time that methoxsalen was taken.[j]

Experimentally in various animals lens opacities have been induced acutely, but they generally have been reversible, except in instances of the most extreme dosage and exposure. Accounts of animal studies indicating danger to the eyes from photosensitization by methoxsalen began to appear in 1960 when severe reactions were reported in guinea pigs given very large doses, 40 mg of methoxsalen by intraperitoneal injection one hour before they were exposed to UVA continuously for 24 hours.[d,f] White guinea pigs developed ulceration of the lids, edema of the corneas, congestion of iris vessels, permanently dilated pupils, and multiple anterior cortical punctate opacities in the lenses. (The retinas were not evaluated.) In black guinea pigs the lids and iris were less damaged. Guinea pigs given 80 to 100 mg of methoxsalen per kg showed no damage to the eyes unless they were also exposed to UVA.[l]

Albino mice reacted severely when given 4 mg of methoxsalen daily intraperitoneally and were exposed to UVA for 10 minutes a day for 5 months.[e] At the end of this time 45 out of 75 eyes had lens opacities, mostly anterior cortical, whereas only 6 out of 76 control eyes had opacities after exposure to UVA without the drug. During 5 months of further observation, but no more treatments, the experimental eyes showed worsening conditions, and some had mature cataracts.

In rabbits some attempts to induce lens opacities with methoxsalen and UVA have been negative.[c,za] However, assays have shown extraordinarily rapid disappearance of the drug in rabbits, and when the exposure to UVA has been scheduled at a time when methoxsalen concentration is elevated in the lens, but low in the aqueous humor and serum, lens opacities have been produced similar to those in guinea pigs and mice, presenting a gray-white flecked appearance beneath the anterior lens capsule.[m] The daily dosage of methoxsalen and UVA to produce cutaneous photosensitization in rabbits is less than required to produce cataracts.[za]

In rats, systemically administered methoxsalen has been shown to enter the lens,[t] and to bind to lens proteins under the influence of light.[r,u] Cataracts, corneal opacities, and devascularization of the iris have been produced by a combination of methoxsalen and UVA.[u] In vitro, methoxsalen plus UVA has induced unscheduled DNA synthesis in rat lens epithelial cells, and this could be part of a mechanism to produce lens opacities.[p] Severe acute damage of lens epithelial cells has been found in rat lenses after very large doses of methoxsalen (40 mg per rat) and UVA.[y] After smaller doses (1 mg per kg), tritiated methoxsalen concentrations were much lower in the lens than in other parts of the eye, and there was no suggestion of accumulation of the drug or its metabolites in the lens. Under the influence of UVA no specific binding of low-dose methoxsalen was demonstrated.[zg] In pigmented rats, autoradiography showed that the highest concentrations were in the retina, ciliary body and iris, suggesting binding to melanin.[zf]

In patients the apprehension that a chronic or cumulative action of the drug might develop as a result of photo-induced binding in the lens, particularly to DNA, has been the basis for repeated advice for patients to wear special protective goggles to exclude UVA during the period when the drug is present. In attempts to determine how long the drug may be in the lens after it is administered, volunteer patients about to undergo cataract extraction have taken the drug, and their lenses have been assayed after removal. Free drug has been reported in human lenses 12 hours after oral administration,[v] but not after 24 hours.[x]

There has been one report of transient visual disturbances in 3 patients, related to dosage of methoxsalen in PUVA therapy.[k] One had photophobia with central scotoma lasting as long as 20 minutes and occurring up to 3 times a day. A second patient had "tunnel vision" in episodes lasting up to 5 minutes. The third patient had "tunnel vision" for 8 hours. All had normal eyes. The episodes stopped when dosages were reduced.

a. Back O, Hollstrom E, Thorburn W: Absence of cataract ten years after treatment with 8-methoxypsoralen. *ACTA DERM-VENEREOL* 60:79–80, 1980.

b. Backman HA: The effects of PUVA on the eye. *AM J OPTOM PHYSIOL OPT* 59:86–89, 1982.

c. Becker SW Jr, West B: Detection of photosensitizers in tissue. *ARCH DERMATOL* 92:457–460, 1965.

d. Cloud TM, Hakim R, Griffen AC: Photosensitization of the eye with methoxsalen. *ARCH OPHTHALMOL* 64:346–351, 1960.

e. Cloud TM, Hakim R, Griffen AC: Photosensitization of the eye with methoxsalen. II. Chronic effects. *ARCH OPHTHALMOL* 66:689–693, 1961.

f. Cogan DG: Photosensitization and cataracts (Editorial). *ARCH OPHTHALMOL* 66:612–613, 1961.

g. Cyrlin MN, Pedvis Leftick A, Sugar J: Cataract formation in association with ultraviolet photosensitivity. *ANN OPHTHALMOL* 12:786–790, 1980.

h. DeWitte E, Coppens A, Missotten L: Can PUVA treatment and artificial sunlight cause ocular lesions? *BULL SOC BELGE OPTALMOL* 185:111–118, 1979. (French)

i. El-Mofty AM, El-Mofty A: Retrospective ocular study of patients receiving oral 8-methoxypsoralen for the treatment of vitiligo. *ANN OPHTHALMOL* 11:946–948, 1979.

j. Farber EM, Epstein JH, et al: Current status of oral PUVA therapy for psoriasis. Eye protection revisions. *J AM ACAD DERMATOL* 6:851–855, 1982.

k. Fenton DA, Wilkinson JD: Dose-related visual field effects in patients receiving PUVA therapy. *LANCET* 1:1106, 1983.

l. Freeman RG: Morphologic changes resulting from photosensitization of the eye with 8 methoxy psoralen a comparison with conventional ultraviolet injury. *TEX REP BIOL MED* 24:588–596, 1966.

m. Glew WB: Determination of 8-methoxypsoralen in serum, aqueous, and lens: relation to long-wave ultraviolet phototoxicity in experimental and clinical photochemotherapy. *TRANS AM OPHTHALMOL SOC* 77:464–514, 1979.

n. Glew WB, McKeever G, et al: Photochemistry and the eye: photoprotective factors. *TRANS AM OPHTHALMOL* SOC 78:243–251, 1980.

o. Hammershoy O, Jessen F: A retrospective study of cataract formation in 96 patients treated with PUVA. *ACTA DERM VENEREOL* 62:444–446, 1982.

p. Jose JG, Yielding KL: Photosensitive cataractogens, chlorpromazine and methoxypsoralen, cause DNA repair synthesis in lens epithelial cells. *INVEST OPHTHALMOL VIS SCI* 17:687–691, 1978.

q. Kearns TP: in discussion of Glew WB[n]

r. Koch HR, Beitzen R, et al: 8-Methoxypsoralen and long ultraviolet effects on the rat lens. *GRAEFES ARCH OPHTHALMOL* 218:193–199, 1982.

s. Lafond G, Roy PE, Grenier R: Lens opacities appearing during therapy with methoxsalen and long-wavelength ultraviolet radiation. *CAN J OPHTHALMOL* 19:173–175, 1984.

t. Lerman S, Borkman RF: A method for detecting 8-methoxypsoralen in the ocular lens. *SCIENCE* 197:1287–1288, 1977.

u. Lerman S, Jocoy M, Borkman RF: Photosensitization of the lens by 8-methoxypsoralen. *INVEST OPHTHALMOL VIS SCI* 16:1065–1068, 1977.

v. Lerman S, Megaw J, Willis I: Potential ocular complications from PUVA therapy and their prevention. *J INVEST DERMATOL* 74:197–199, 1980.

w. Lerman S: Editorial. UV radiation photodamage to the ocular lens: diagnosis and treatment. *ANN OPHTHALMOL* 14:411–413, 1982.

x. Marqversen J, Axelsen I, et al: 8-methoxypsoralen and the eye. *ARCH DERMATOL RES* 270:387–390, 1981.

y. Mikuni I, Fujiwara T, Obazawa H: Effect of 8-methoxypsoralen on the crystalline lens of mammals. *TOKAI J EXP CLIN MED* 2:243–253, 1977.

z. Parrish JA, Fitzpatrick TB, et al: Photochemotherapy of psoriasis with oral methoxsalen and longwave ultraviolet light. *N ENGL J MED* 291:1207–1211, 1974.

za. Parrish JA, Chylack LT Jr, et al: Dermatological and ocular examinations in rabbits chronically photosensitized with methoxsalen. *J INVEST DERMATOL* 73:250–255, 1979.

zb. Ronnerfalt L, Lydahl E, et al: Ophthalmological study of patients undergoing long-term PUVA therapy. *ACTA DERM VENEREOL* 62:501–505, 1982.

zc. Singer L, Romem M, et al: Methoxsalen-induced ocular lesions in ducks. *OPHTHALMIC RES* 8:329–334, 1976.

zd. Sterk CC, Geldof CA, Ten Jet Foei HG: The lens and PUVA therapy. *DOC OPHTHALMOL* 55:149–152, 1983.

ze. Wennersten G: Photoprotection of the eye in PUVA therapy. *BR J DERMATOL* 98:137–139, 1978.

zf. Wulf HC, Hart J: Accumulation of 8-methoxypsoralen in the rat retina. *ACTA OPHTHALMOL* 56:284–290, 1978.

zg. Wulf HC, Andreasen MP: Concentration of ^{3}H-8-methoxypsoralen and its metabolites in the rat lens and eye. *INVEST OPHTHALMOL VIS SCI* 22:32–36, 1982.

Methoxyflurane (Penthrane), an inhalation anesthetic, may lower intraocular pressure in patients, as do other general anesthetics, but less than halothane.[e,f] Three patients who had subnormal renal function and who underwent prolonged general anesthesia with this agent developed generalized oxalosis accompanied by disturbance of their ocular fundi described as "numerous yellow-white punctate lesions scattered throughout the posterior poles and midperiphery of both eyes."[a–d] Visual acuity was not reduced. Post-mortem examinations established this "flecked retina" appearance to be due to deposits of calcium oxalate in the retinal pigment epithelium; some was intracellular. The oxalate presumably came from metabolic breakdown of the methoxyflurane. Experimentally in rabbits the same changes were produced by administering dibutyl oxalate.[a] (See also *Dibutyl oxalate.*)

a. Albert DM, Bullock JD, et al: Flecked retina secondary to oxalate crystals from methoxyflurane anesthesia. *TRANS AM ACAD OTOL* 79:817–826, 1975.

b. Bullock JD, Albert DM, et al: Calcium oxalate retinopathy associated with generalized oxalosis. *INVEST OPHTHALMOL* 13:256–265, 1974.

c. Bullock JD, Albert DM: Generalized oxalosis with retinal involvement following methoxyflurane anesthesia. *ANESTHESIOLOGY* 41:296–302, 1974.

d. Bullock JD, Albert DM: Flecked retina; appearance secondary to oxalate crystals from methoxyflurane anesthesia. *ARCH OPHTHALMOL* 93:26–31, 1975.

e. Schettini A, Owre ES, Fink AI: Effect of methoxyflurane anesthesia on intraocular pressure. *CAN ANAESTH SOC J* 15:172, 1968.

f. Tammisto O, Hamalainen L, Tarkkanen L: Halothane and methoxyflurane in ophthalmic anesthesia. *ACTA ANAESTH SCAND* 9:173–177, 1965.

4-Methoxy-m-phenylenediamine, a hair-dye constituent, tested on rabbits' eyes caused only a mild conjunctival reaction.[347]

Methyl acetate, a solvent, at 10,000 ppm in air causes irritation of the eyes, nose, and throat in human beings, also in cats. This vapor induces vacuoles visible with the microscope in the corneal epithelium of cats, but no serious or irreversible injury of the cornea has been reported from it, either in cats or human beings.[188,216] Owing to the possibility of methyl acetate hydrolyzing to methanol, it has been suspected that methyl acetate might be toxic to the optic nerve.[56] One case of bilateral optic atrophy has been reported following inhalation of methyl acetate.[a] (Also see *methyl formate.*)

Testing by application to rabbit eyes caused injury to the cornea graded 5 on a scale of 1 to 10.[228] From a splash in a human eye one might expect spontaneously reversible corneal and conjunctival epithelial injury.

> a. Lund A: Toxic amblyopia after inhalation of methyl acetate. *UGESKR LAEG* 106:308–311, 1944. (*CHEM ABSTR* 39:4689.)

Methylal (formal, dimethoxymethane), a solvent, is made from the notoriously toxic substances *methanol* and *formaldehyde.* For this reason it has been investigated with special attention to possible injurious effect on the eyes. Exposures of mice and guinea pigs to much higher concentrations of methylal vapor than would be encountered industrially caused damage to the lungs, liver, heart, and kidneys, and occasional superficial irritation of the eyes, but no histologically demonstrable abnormality of the optic nerve or retina.[a] Tests for free formaldehyde and formic acid in the vitreous humor and urine were negative. (Newer knowledge of characteristics of methanol toxicity to the optic nerves suggests that testing on monkeys would be much more meaningful.) For continuous industrial exposure a vapor concentration of 1,000 ppm has been considered safe.[56]

> a. Weaver FL, Hough AR, Highman V, Fairhall LE: The toxicity of methylal. *BR J IND MED* 8:279, 1951.

1-α-Methylallylthiocarbamoyl-2-methylthiocarbamoylhydrazine (I.C.I.33,828), an experimental drug of interest because of effect on the pituitary, has been found to produce cataracts in rats, with the incidence strikingly related to the rate of administration, an incidence of 52 percent when 250 mg/kg were given every day for sixteen weeks, but zero incidence if the same dose was given daily for only five days out of each week for ten months. The drug was found to have rapid turnover and not to accumulate in the eye. It produced no diabetes. The cataractous lenses have been examined histologically, but the mechanism of cataractogenesis has not been determined. A few patients have been given the drug for as long as two years without developing abnormalities of the eyes, but the dosage and number of patients is not stated.[a]

> a. Baker SB deC, Alcock SJ: An apparent change in toxicity of a compound when dosed for seven days a week instead of five. *PROC EUROP SOC STUDY DRUG TOXICITY* 6:213–228, 1965.

Methyl amine, similar to ammonia, may irritate the eyes and respiratory tract.[171] A drop of 5% solution in water applied to animal eyes caused hemorrhages in the conjunctiva, superficial corneal opacities, and edema.[63] A higher concentration, or liquefied methyl amine presumably would be at least as severely damaging to the eye as is ammonia.

Methylamyl acetate tested in vapor form on the eyes of human volunteers causes sensation of irritation at 100 ppm in air.[217]

Methyl arsine dichloride (methyldichloroarsine) is an extremely poisonous liquid with vapor that is an extremely powerful lacrimatory irritant of the eyes and nose, also very irritating to the skin and respiratory tract. The vapor is said to cause necrosis of the corneal epithelium. It has been studied primarily as a potential war gas.[61,155]

Methylatropine nitrate (atropine methylnitrate, Eumydrin, Metropine), an anticholinergic, tested in non-glaucomatous human beings by giving 3 to 6 mg per day orally and subcutaneously for eleven days caused no significant rise of intraocular pressure.[b] (See also *Anticholinergic drugs.*)

Large overdose from ingestion of Eumydrin eye drops has caused severe poisoning in children, with the same characteristics as atropine poisoning.[a] (See *Atropine.*)

a. Meerstadt PWD: Atropine poisoning in early infancy due to Eumydrin drops. *BR MED J* 285:196, 1982.
b. Passow A: On eye symptoms with internal use of medications that act on the parasympathetic nervous system. *ARCH AUGENHEILKD* 97:432–439, 1926.

Methylazoxymethanol acetate (MAM), an antimitotic agent known to cause selective destruction of neurons in the developing brain in rats, has also been tested for effects on developing retina. Latker and associates in 1982 summarized the considerable literature on this agent, and carried out a study relating the stage of development to the vulnerability of the retina.[a] The retina was most sensitive during gestation and the early postnatal period, but could recover. Eventually the retina became refractory to the agent. Rosettes in the photoreceptor layer was the lesion most commonly seen. (Also see Cycasin, page 294.)

a. Latker CH, Eiden LE, Zatz M: The effect of methylazoxymethanol acetate (MAM) on the developing rat retina. *EXP EYE RES* 35:351–361, 1982.

Methyl bromide causes no immediate irritation of the eyes, nose, or respiratory tract, even at severely poisonous concentrations. It is readily liquefied under pressure and has been employed as a fire extinguisher, fumigant, extractant solvent, and as a methylating agent. At least sixty articles have been written concerning its poisonous properties.

Characteristically during exposure to the gas there are no warning sensations, but after a latent period of several hours the victim has headache, nausea, vomiting, vertigo, and staggering. He may then also have lacrimation from irritation of the eyes, and may experience blurring and diplopia. Transient dimming of vision and blindness for twelve hours has been reported associated with severe nausea and vomiting, but with recovery within a few days.[p] In other cases, nystagmus on lateral gaze,[a,b] diplopia,[a,n] and blurring of vision, especially when attempting to read,[a,b] have been associated with the general neurologic disturbances. In severe cases, convulsions, delirium, and sometimes mania ensue, followed by collapse and possible death. Patients who recover may have a protracted period of apathy and depression, incoordination, tremors, and bothersome visual complaints. As a rule those who recover eventually recover completely.

Visual disturbances have been noted rather prominently in many reports of poisoning, although rarely have they been studied thoroughly. Disturbance of the eyes by methyl bromide apparently was first described by Jaquet in 1901 in three cases.[i] In the first, a man had several episodes of transient blurring at his work of transferring methyl bromide from one container to another. On one occasion he had especially pronounced blurring accompanied by temporary diplopia, associated with ataxia and delirium necessitating hospitalization. Although the ocular fundi were found normal, the patient continued to complain for several weeks of slightly blurred vision, particularly while attempting to read. In a second case, after chronic and then acute exposure to methyl bromide, a man became ill and could not clearly distinguish objects of moderate size. For some hours all objects seemed doubled. After several days, vision returned to normal. The author of the original report was himself accidentally acutely exposed to methyl bromide gas, and he wrote that by evening of the same day print appeared so unclear to him that reading was impossible. However, by the next morning he was all well.

Similarly, Drawneek et al in 1964 reported on a patient in whom there was thought to be diffuse organic cerebral damage from repeated episodes of methyl bromide poisoning during fourteen years of work as a fumigator. He had an episode of diplopia for five days, blackouts, and impaired distant vision associated with protracted severe frontal headache and ataxia.[d] Ophthalmoscopy showed only a small patch of healed choroiditis which must have been old and unrelated to the visual complaints. Though no measurements of visual acuity or visual fields were reported, the clinical description seemed to imply that the visual complaints were transitory. No squint was found to account for the diplopia, but in two other patients transient convergent strabismus has been reported.[k]

In a more severe case, described in 1918, a man exposed to pure methyl bromide gas for about half an hour became weak and stupified, unable to walk, but able to crawl out of the room.[h] He saw lights doubled, and they appeared to dance in front of his eyes. He could not place his hands on things accurately. He had neither headache nor vomiting, but in the next few days ataxia increased so that he could scarcely stand, and he had marked intention tremor of the hands. The eyes appeared normal externally, and he made no complaint of ocular irritation. The optic nerveheads were described as abnormally red. The retinal arteries seemed normal, but the veins were distended and tortuous. In one eye a retinal hemorrhage slightly larger than the disc extended from the nervehead inferiorly along the course of the nerve fibers. Visual acuity varied from 3/4 to 1. There seemed to be slight paresis of abduction in each eye, but psychic disturbance made testing difficult, and the patient complained not only of doubled vision, but of seeing things four or five fold. Ataxia and psychic symptoms became more severe, with hallucinations of hearing and vision, epileptiform attacks and periods of coma. The hemorrhage in the fundus spread, and it was postulated that the patient must have small hemorrhages in various parts of the central nervous system.[h]

In a carefully studied case in 1937, a man exposed to methyl bromide while filling fire extinguishers did not develop symptoms until forty-eight hours later; then he began to have vertigo, aphasia, and ataxia.[c] At the end of a week, when speech was improving, he noted that the contour of objects appeared blurred. His amblyopia became worse, approaching almost complete blindness in a few days. At the same time, vertigo became worse, and one arm was paralyzed. Three weeks after exposure he began to discern objects better, and there was general improvement. At a month, vision in both eyes could not be improved beyond 5/10 with glasses, but the pupils and fundi were normal. There appeared to be weakness of accommodation (requiring 3.5 D for near vision), and central scotomas were found for green, but not for white. By two months, vision in each eye improved to 8/10, and only 1.5 D was required for near vision. His other neurologic disturbances had also subsided.[c]

Generalizing from observation on twelve cases of intoxication but without detailed descriptions, Gaultier has reported that edema of the papilla and punctiform hemorrhages may be found in the retina in accompaniment with headache and vertigo, and that these abnormalities may rapidly disappear. The same author claims to have observed retrobulbar neuritis in two cases; in one the visual acuity remained 1/10 for more than six months before recovery.[g]

Optic atrophy and constriction of visual fields from methyl bromide poisoning appear to have been described in only one report.[f] The report making both of these rare observations was concerned with examination of twelve individuals one year after probable chronic intoxication by methyl bromide leaking from fire extinguishers. A variety of ophthalmic abnormalities were found in all. The findings were listed in tabular form with few details. Of three patients listed as having optic atrophy, two were said to have improved in the course of a year, but one was said to have remained blind. Although only one of the twelve workers apparently had permanent visual impairment, ten were said to have had disturbances of central color vision, and all were listed as having slight to marked constriction of visual fields.[f] Eight cases of contracted visual fields have been reported from Japan.[r]

Autopsy in a case in which there had been blurring of vision and an appearance of flickering lights, double vision, and pain behind the eyes showed many minute hemorrhages throughout the brain, heart, spleen, and kidneys.[n]

Results of extensive observations on animals and the postmortem findings in human cases of fatal methyl bromide poisoning have been summarized by vonOettingen. Little, other than scattered hemorrhages, has been found to explain the visual disturbances observed clinically. As noted in some of the cases already described, small hemorrhages in the retina have also been noted occasionally clinically.

The mechanism of intoxication by methyl bromide appears unlike that of methanol, but similar to that of methyl chloride and methyl iodide. Acidosis does not appear to be a feature of the poisoning by these methyl halides nor is there much production of formate, both of which are features of poisoning by methanol. It seems probable that a methylation (alkylation) reaction which is common to the three methyl halides is the basis for their peculiar toxicity.[d,h,l] There is no sound evidence to support old ideas that bromide liberation accounted for toxicity.[d] No specific treatment for poisoning by methyl bromide has been devised as yet. (See also *Methyl chloride* and *Methyl iodide*.)

Local contact of methyl bromide with the eye either as concentrated vapor or as a splash of liquid has resulted in no more than transient irritation and conjunctivitis in the few cases in which this accident has been observed.[g,q]

Experimental exposure of a rabbit's eye to pure methyl bromide gas at room temperature for one and one-half minutes caused immediate loss of surface luster, followed in several hours by loss of corneal epithelium, and much edema of the conjunctivae and lids. A day later the corneal stroma was bluish, much swollen, and nearly opaque, but within five days the cornea started to clear.[81] This was much more severe exposure than would occur by accident.

a. Carter AB: Methyl bromide poisoning, effect on nervous system. *BR MED J* 1:43, 1945.
b. DeJong RN: Methyl bromide poisoning. *J AM MED ASSOC* 125:702–703, 1944.
c. Dixon M, Needham DM: Biochemical research on chemical warfare agents. *NATURE* 158:432–438, 1946.
d. Drawneek W, O'Brien MJ, et al: Industrial methyl bromide poisoning in fumigators. *LANCET* 2:855–856, 1964.
e. Duvoir M, Fabre R, Layani F: Poisoning by methyl bromide. *BULL SOC HOP PARIS* 34:1504–1554, 1937. (French)
f. Eross S, Szobor A: Ophthalmological and neurological signs of chronic methyl bromide poisoning. *ORV HETIL* 34:944–946, 1953. (English abstract)
g. Gaultier M: Ocular disturbances in poisoning by methyl bromide. *PROC 9th INT CONGR INDUSTR MED LONDON* 1948:523–525, 1949.
h. Grant WM: Drug intoxications and chemical injuries of the eye. In Sorsby, A. (Ed.): *SYSTEMIC OPHTHALMOLOGY.* London, Butterworth, 1951 and 1958.
i. Jaquet A: On methyl bromide poisoning. *DEUTSCH ARCH KLIN MED* 71:270–286, 1901. (German)
j. Kakizaki T: Methyl bromide poisoning. *IND HEALTH (KAWASAKI)* 5:135–143, 1967. (*CHEM ABSTR* 69:9439, 1968.)
k. Prain JH, Smith GH: A clinical-pathological report of 8 cases of methyl-bromide poisoning. *BR J IND MED* 9:44–49, 1952.
l. Rathus EM, Landy PJ: Methyl bromide poisoning. *BR J IND MED* 18:53–57, 1961.
m. Steiger O: On methyl bromide poisoning. *MUNCH MED WOCHENSCHR* 65:753–755, 1918. (German)
n. Viner N: Methyl bromide poisoning; a new industrial hazard. *CAN MED ASSOC J* 53:43–45, 1945.
o. vonOettingen WF: *The Toxicity and Potential Dangers of Methyl Bromide.* National Institutes of Health Bull 185, Washington, 1946.
p. Watrous RM: Methyl bromide, local and mild systemic toxic effects. *IND MED* 11:575–579, 1942.
q. Wyers H: Methyl bromide intoxication. *BR J IND MED* 2:34–39, 1945.
r. Araki S, Ushio K, et al: Methyl bromide poisoning; a report based on fourteen cases. *SANGYO IGAKU* 13:507–513, 1971.

Methyl bromoacetate vapors are irritating to all mucous membranes, especially to the eyes. Five ppm in air is unbearable for more than a minute.[61] Exposure for several hours to lower concentrations, is said to have caused corneal erosion.[252] The toxic properties are probably attributable to the reactivity of bromoacetate with tissue thiol groups. (Also see *Ethyl bromoacetate* and *Lacrimatory action.*)

Methyl Cellosolve (2-methoxyethanol, ethyleneglycol monomethylether), tested by applying three drops to rabbit eyes, was found to be only slightly irritating causing only temporary reddening and swelling of the conjunctiva, graded 3 on a scale of 1 to 10 after twenty-four hours.[27,151,222] One instance of contamination of a human eye with methyl Cellosolve has been recorded, and in this case recovery was complete within forty-eight hours.[165]

Methylcellulose (Methocel) forms a neutral viscous solution in cold water. Applied to the surface of the eye it is innocuous. Injected into the anterior chamber of rabbits, 0.1 ml of 0.5 to 1% methylcellulose in 0.9% sodium chloride solution causes mild·iridocyclitis, but in a balanced salt solution it causes no clinically evident reaction. Methylcellulose is detectable in the anterior chamber for three days after injection, but is gone after the fourth day.[f,j] A 1 or 2% solution has been used clinically as a lubricant aid to the insertion of intraocular lenses.[c-e,h] *Hydroxypropylmethyl cellulose* 2% in balanced salt solution has been used in the anterior chamber without complication in hundreds of operations, always irrigated out of the anterior chamber at the end of operation.[k]

When the aqueous humor is replaced by 0.5 to 2% methylcellulose in rabbits and not irrigated out the intraocular pressure may rise to 60 mm Hg or more during the next hour or two.[a,b,g,i]

a. Bonomi L, Raquetti E: On the effect of administering guanethidine on experimental hypertension in the rabbit eye. *BOLL OCULIST* 43:319–325, 1964. (Italian)
b. De Freitas F, Morin JS: The changes in the blood supply of the posterior pole of rabbits with ocular hypertension. *CAN J OPHTHALMOL* 6:139–142, 1971.
c. Fechner PU: Methyl cellulose as lubricant substance for implantation of artificial intraocular lenses. *KLIN MONATSBL AUGENHEILKD* 174:136–138, 1979. (German)
d. Fechner PU, Fechner MU: Methylcellulose and lens implantation. *BR J OPHTHALMOL* 67:259–263, 1983.
e. Fechner PU: The effect of sodium hyaluronate, chondroitin sulfate, and methylcellulose on the corneal endothelium and intraocular pressure. *AM J OPHTHALMOL* 96:256–257, 1983.
f. Fleming TC, Merrill DL, Girard LJ: Studies of the irritating action of methylcellulose. *ARCH OPHTHALMOL* 61:565–567, 1959.
g. Lorenzetti OJ, Sancilio LF: Procedure for evaluating drug effects on increased intraocular pressure. *ARCH OPHTHALMOL* 78:624–628, 1967.
h. MacRae SM, Edelhauser HF, et al: The effects of sodium hyaluronate, chondroitin sulfate, and methylcellulose on the corneal endothelium and intraocular pressure. *AM J OPHTHALMOL* 95:332–341, 1983.
i. Paul W, Vick HP: On perforation of the globe from experimental elevation of the intraocular pressure in the rabbit. *GRAEFES ARCH OPHTHALMOL* 181:207–215, 1971. (German)
j. Swan KC: Use of methyl cellulose in ophthalmology. *ARCH OPHTHALMOL* 33:378–380, 1945.
k. Fechner PU: Methylcellulose. *TRANS OPHTHALMOL SOC UK* 103:259–262, 1983.

Methyl chloride (chloromethane) formerly was widely used in refrigerators. It is still employed in chemical manufacture as a methylating agent. The vapor has no noticeable irritating effect on eyes, nose, or respiratory tract even in concentrations which are dangerously toxic.

Typically, individuals exposed to methyl chloride gas have not been discomforted during exposure, or have merely been aware of a slight sweetish odor, and have presented the first signs of poisoning after a latent period of several hours. In some cases the first symptoms have been nausea, vomiting, and diarrhea. More commonly the victims have developed somnolence, confusion, headache, ataxia, and vertigo. The most severely affected have gone into coma with or without convulsions, and some have died. Autopsy has revealed injury to kidneys and liver, and hyperemia and edema of the brain.[f]

At least forty articles have been published describing this poisoning, and disturbances of the eyes are commonly mentioned, yet there is very little exact information on this aspect of the poisoning. Marked reduction in vision was first reported in 1914 in a patient who had several episodes of poisoning but recovered.[c] In this case the poor vision persisted for two weeks after the patient was otherwise well, but the nature of the visual impairment was not determined. In 1927, sixteen out of twenty-one patients who suffered drowsiness, intoxication, nausea, anorexia, and staggering from poisoning by methyl chloride in a refrigerator factory had visual disturbances ranging from slight blurring of vision to diplopia.[a] Occasional ptosis was also mentioned.

In a survey of twenty-nine cases of poisoning, with firsthand observations on seven, by Kegel and associates in 1929, blurring of vision was a complaint in eleven cases, commonly persisting after recovery from other symptoms of poisoning.[f] Among these cases there were ten deaths, and in the most severely poisoned, the pupils were usually widely dilated and either unreactive or sluggishly reactive to light. Of the survivors, one could not recognize people five feet away a week after exposure. His pupils remained dilated for at least two weeks, and he was said to be unable to focus, but no measurements were given and no information on the effect of correcting lenses. Two other patients in the same group noted that they were able to read only large print for as long as three months. No details of ophthalmic examination were given in any of these cases.

In 1942 Jones reported on visual disturbances in four cases.[e] Misty vision principally for near objects was noted and thought to be associated with difficulty in accommodation. Intermittent diplopia was also observed. No details of ophthalmic examination were given except that in one case the fundus was noted to be normal.

In reports of individual cases of poisoning, one person was observed to be ataxic, staggering, weak, and to have twitching in his arms and legs for ten days, while his vision was said to be blurred so that he could neither read nor write, but he had no diplopia.[n] Another patient who had had drowsiness, ataxia, confusion, and psychosis for a day or two, complained of double vision and "admitted having had difficulty in focusing for several days."[j] Yet another became extremely somnolent and ataxic in a manner to suggest encephalitis; his pupils reacted normally, but he could not read two-inch type for two weeks.[m] In each of these cases recovery was spontaneous and complete. In none of the cases was the basis for the visual distur-bance investigated.

In another case development of bilateral paracentral scotomas with reduced visual acuity and slight temporal pallor of the discs was ascribed to methyl chloride, but on very little evidence.[b]

In 1964 MacDonald summarized experiences with thirty cases of methyl chloride intoxication which had occurred in a synthetic rubber plant since 1952 and noted that in cases of brief severe exposure the symptoms consisted of "visual disturbances," dizziness, nausea, and severe headache, all tending to improve in a few hours, except the headache, which tended to last for two to three days.[h] In more severely poisoned patients there were loss of coordination, nausea and vomiting, and severe headache persisting intermittently for seven to ten days. Although blurring of vision was mentioned as a feature in five cases, nothing was said as to its nature, nor were any tests of vision or eye examinations described In reports on single cases of poisoning by Gummert and by Mackie in 1961, the same mention was made of blurred vision, with no information on its basis.[d,i]

Scharnweber in 1974 reported six cases of poisoning from exposure to 200 to 400 ppm at work for 2 to 3 weeks before development of symptoms, including "blurred vision" in three, and "diplopia" in two.[k] There were no further details.

Spevac in 1976 reported on acute poisoning of four members of a family, and mentioned that all had nystagmus, optic, oculomotor and facial nerve involvement, but gave no details, and no measurements of visual acuities.[l]

We have so far progressed scarcely at all in our understanding of the nature and cause of the visual disturbances from methyl chloride.

So far there seems to have been no case in which undoubted methyl chloride poisoning has resulted in optic atrophy or any other permanent eye disturbance. Although autopsies have revealed hyperemia and edema of the brain, it remains quite uncertain in what manner to explain the transitory impairment of vision, diplopia, and ptosis which have been observed. Experiments on animals have not been concerned with effects on the eye or vision.

The chemical basis for the toxicity of methyl chloride has not been established, but it is evident that it differs from that of methanol, since acidosis is not a feature of methyl chloride poisoning. The metabolism of methyl chloride has been studied extensively. It reacts with glutathione, forming methylglutathione, which in turn is converted to other potentially toxic substances. Among the known products, *methanethiol* is particularly suspected to be an intermediary in the neurotoxic action of methyl chloride.[g] The similarity of methyl chloride to methyl bromide and methyl iodide, both in respect to chemical methylating activity and toxicity to the central nervous system, suggests that a methylation reaction may be fundamental to the poisoning by all three. (Also see *Methyl bromide* and *Methyl iodide.*)

Local effects of methyl chloride on the eye are relatively insignificant. In only one instance has a burn of the eye been reported in a human being, presumably from a spray of liquid, and healing was prompt.[165] Exposure of a rabbit's eye to pure methyl chloride gas at room temperature for ninety seconds caused only slight conjunctival hyperemia.[81] Also in an experiment in which two rabbits were exposed for five days to concentrations from 250 to 465 ppm in air, there were no changes in the corneas, nor in pupillary reactions to light.[81]

a. Baker, HM: Intoxication with commercial methyl chloride. *J AM MED ASSOC* 88:1137–1138, 1927.
b. Garde A, Etienne R: Retrobulbar optic neuritis from methyl chloride. *REV OTO-NEUROOPHTAL* 23:480–482, 1951. (French)
c. Gerbis H: Peculiar narcosis condition after industrial work with methyl chloride. *MUNCH MED WOCHENSCHR* 61:879, 1914. (German)
d. Gummert M: Wilson-Block after methyl chloride poisoning. *Z GES INN MED* 16:677–680, 1961. (German)
e. Jones AM: Methyl chloride poisoning. *QUART J MED* 11:29–43, 1942.
f. Kegel AH, McNally WD, Pope AS: Methyl chloride poisoning from domestic refrigerators. *J AM MED ASSOC* 93:353, 1929.
g. Kornbrust DJ, Bus JS: The role of glutathione and cytochrome P-450 in the metabolism of methyl chloride. *TOXICOL APPL PHARMACOL* 67:246–256, 1983.
h. MacDonald JDC: Methyl chloride intoxication. *J OCCUP MED* 6:81–84, 1964.
i. Mackie IJ: Methyl chloride intoxication. *MED J AUST* 48:203–205, 1961.
j. Macrae MM: A case of methyl chloride poisoning. *BR MED J* 1:1134, 1954.
k. Scharnweber HC, Spears GN, Cowles SR: Chronic methyl chloride intoxication in six industrial workers. *J OCCUP MED* 16:112–113, 1974.
l. Spevak L, Nadj V, Felle D: Methyl chloride poisoning in four members of a family. *BR J IND MED* 33:272–274, 1976.
m. Van der Kloot A: Methyl chloride poisoning. *ILLINOIS MED J* 65:508–509, 1934.
n. vanRaalte HGS, Thoden van Velzen HGEC: Methyl chloride intoxication. *IND MED* 14:707–709, 1945.

2S-Methyl-4-chloro-6-methyl pyrimidine is known industrially as a volatile lacrimator, and a case of severe skin reaction has been reported, but without direct involvement of the eyes.[73]

4(2-Methyl-4-chlorophenoxy) butyric acid is a weed killer which is not irritating to the skin, but the undiluted material is said to cause pain and irritation when introduced into the conjunctival sac.[70]

Methylcholanthrene injected intraocularly in rats is reported to have produced carcinomas, malignant tumors resembling melanomas and fibrosarcoma of the choroid.[a,272]

a. Patz A, Wulf LB, Rogers SW: Experimental production of ocular tumors. *AM J OPHTHALMOL* 48:98–117, 1959.

Methyl cyclohexanol, a solvent, has occasionally been noted to be irritating to the eyes and throat of workers, but so far without producing significant injury.[21] Rabbits exposed to 2.3 mg/liter of air show symptoms of irritation of the eyes.[385]

Methyl cyclohexanone has been reported to cause irritation of the eyes the same as methyl cyclohexanol at equal vapor concentrations.[385]

Methyl dichlorisone has been used like dichlorisone acetate (Diloderm) orally to stimulate the hair follicles in patients with alopecia, a treatment observed to be complicated by posterior subcapsular cataracts in six out of ten patients treated for more than eighteen months.[a]

    a. Griboff WI, Futterweit W: Effects of new 9,11-dihalogenated corticosteroids in various types of alopecia. J MOUNT SINAI HOSP 32:121–129, 1967.

Methyl-α,β-dichloropropionate appears to be nonirritating when it is first applied as a liquid to the skin or as a vapor to the eyes, but in a few hours after exposure, a painful keratitis and dermatitis with vesication develops, postulated due to gradual change to *methyl α-chloroacrylate* which is very irritating.[a]

    a. Oettel H: Danger to health from synthetic substances? *NAUNYN–SCHMIEDEBERG'S ARCH EXP PATH PHARMAK* 232:77–132, 1957. (German)

Methyldopa (Aldomet), an antihypertensive, has caused no elevation of intraocular pressure in normal or glaucomatous rabbit or human eyes. It has occasionally been thought to reduce the intraocular pressure slightly, but not enough to be practically useful in treatment of glaucoma.[a–d] One case has been published reporting reversible keratitis sicca in a patient who developed methyldopa fever,[e] and Fraunfelder's National Registry reports knowledge of a number of such cases.[312]

    a. Laibson PR, Krishna N, Leopold IH: Intraocular pressure studies with α-methyl-dopa. *ARCH OPHTHALMOL* 68:648–650, 1962.

    b. Peczon JD: Effect of methyldopa on intraocular pressure in human eyes. *AM J OPHTHALMOL* 60:82–87, 1965.

    c. Suda K, Wakae K: The hypotensive effect of aldomet on glaucomatous eyes. *J CLIN OPHTHALMOL* 18:191–194, 1964. (*ZENTRALBL GES OPHTHALMOL* 92:37, 1964.)

    d. Tuovinen E, Esila R, Liesmaa M: The effect of alpha-methyldopa on the intraocular pressure in the rabbit eye. *ACTA OPHTHALMOL* 44:669–675, 1966.

    e. Chan W: Less common side effects of methyldopa. *MED J AUST* 2:14–15, 1977.

Methylene blue (Methylthionine chloride) is a basic cationic dye. A good review of its properties and corneal staining attributes has been published by Norn, along with experiments showing that a 1% solution at pH 3.78 made isotonic with tears by sodium sulphate caused a stinging sensation in 30 out of 100 patients when applied to the conjunctival sac, producing epiphora in ten of the patients, but no damage and no persistent staining of normal or pathological cornea or conjunctiva.[d] This type of solution has been employed for vital staining of corneal nerves.[186] High concentrations or solid dye in contact with the eye have been known to have caused corneal and conjunctival injury in human beings[250,251] and in rabbits.[78,81,123] Patients who have applied methylene blue eye drops to their eyes for years have developed strong staining of bulbar and palpebral conjunctiva, the lid margins, and slight staining of the corneal epithelium.[c,e]

Intracameral (anterior chamber) injection in rabbits causes loss of cells from the anterior polar region of the lens, with temporary opacity in this region, clearing as repopulation of cells takes place from the periphery.[g–i]

Systemic administration of methylene blue to patients has in rare instances caused transient spasm of accommodation,[f] and blue coloration of the vitreous humor without injury to the eyes.[b] Walsh and Hoyt have reported a case in which methylene blue was injected into the lumbar subarachnoid space, causing paralysis in the lower half of the body and diplopia with subsequent blurring of the disc margins, hydrocephalus, and partial optic atrophy with much loss of vision.[256] In another case, injection into the cisterna magna resulted in a several-week period of papilledema, impairment of upward gaze, and impairment of accommodation.[256] Transitory blackout was reported by one patient who was given 50 ml of a 1% solution intravenously.[256]

a. Briggs RC, Wainwright N, Rothstein H: Biochemical events associated with healing of a chemical injury in the rabbit lens. *EXP EYE RES* 24:523–529, 1977.
b. Gerber A, Lambert RK: Blue appearance of the fundus caused by the prolonged ingestion of methylthionine chloride. *ARCH OPHTHALMOL* 16:443–446, 1936.
c. Morax S, Limon S, Forest A: Exogenous conjunctival pigmentation by methylene blue. *ARCH OPHTALMOL (PARIS)* 37:708A–708B, 1977. (French)
d. Norn MS: Methylene blue (methythionine) vital staining of the cornea and conjunctiva. *ACTA OPHTHALMOL* 45:347–358, 1967.
e. Pasticier-Florquin, Boski, et al: Ocular tattooing from abuse of methylene blue collyrium. *BULL SOC OPHTALMOL FRANCE* 77:147–148, 1977. (French)
f. Pilicque J: Acute spasm of accommodation. (Adverse effect of methylene blue?) *BULL SOC OPHTALMOL PARIS* 7:617–621, 1936. (French)
g. Unakar NJ, Weinsieder A, Reddan JR: Ultrastructural changes associated with the induction and removal of a chemically induced cataract. *OPHTHALMIC RES* 9:296–307, 1977.
h. Weinsieder A, Briggs R, et al: Induction of mitosis in ocular tissue by chemotoxic agents. *EXP EYE RES* 20:33–44, 1975.
i. Weinsieder A, Reddan J, Wilson D: Aqueous humor in lens repair and cell proliferation. *EXP EYE RES* 23:355–363, 1976.

Methylene chloride (dichloromethane), a volatile solvent widely used as a paint remover and degreaser, causes a burning sensation on contact with the skin. Many splash contacts with the eye must have occurred, yet little is to be found in the literature concerning the effects. First-hand observers report that typically there is an immediate burning sensation in the eye, but that when the eye is flushed with water the discomfort subsides in 15 to 20 minutes.[e] Generally there is no persisting damage to the eye, but one patient who accidentally splashed his eye with a paint-remover containing methanol and propylene dichloride in addition to methylene chloride flushed his eye with water immediately, but lost about 20% of his corneal epithelium.[b] Fortunately, the eye healed completely in two days. A more surprising observation has been reported in a boy who had methylene chloride splashed into his eyes from an exploding bubbling-type christmas-tree ornament, and had cells in the anterior chambers, which, with corticosteroid eye drops, cleared in six weeks.[g]

On rabbits' eyes a single application of 0.1 ml of methylene chloride has caused lacrimation persisting for a week, hyperemia of the conjunctivae and lid margins, small hemorrhages and marked edema of the conjunctiva, subsiding in a week.[a] The corneas lost epithelium and became swollen for a week or two in some rabbits, usually associated with signs of iritis. Exceptionally there was peripheral vascularization of the corneas. Intraocular pressure rose a few mm Hg in the first hour, and was normal again in three days. Response to a smaller drop (0.01 ml) of methylene chloride was milder and less persistent.[a] Other tests on rabbits indicate irritancy to the eye to be similar to that from chloroform or slightly less.[c] The response of rabbit eyes appears to have been more severe than what is generally experienced by human beings.

Vapor exposure of rabbits for 10 minutes to 17,500 mg/m^3 produced no obvious injury, but slight temporary increase in corneal thickness and intraocular pressure.[a] In dogs exposed to 5,000 ppm 5 days a week for 7 hours daily for 6 months no eye abnormalities were found.[d] Monkeys exposed to 5 mg/L for 6 hours per day for 13 weeks had no obvious eye abnormalities except that the outline of the nucleus of the lenses became more distinct.[f] In human beings psychological testing of visual-motor performance and critical flicker frequency showed some impairment by methylene chloride vapor.[h]

a. Ballantyne B, Gazzard MF, Swanston DW: The ophthalmic toxicology of dichloromethane. *TOXICOLOGY* 6:173–187, 1976.
b. Cook, Robin: personal communication.
c. Duprat P, Delsaut L, Gradiski D: Irritant power of the principal aliphatic chlorinated solvents on rabbit skin and ocular mucosa. *EUR J TOXICOL ENVIRON HYG* 9:171–177, 1976.
d. Heppel LA, Neal PA, et al: Toxicology of dichloromethane (methylene chloride). *J IND HYG TOXICOL* 26:8, 1944.
e. Ives, Cindy: personal communication, 1978.
f. Meltzer N, Rampy L, et al: Skin irritation inhalation toxicity studies of aerosols using methylene chloride. *DRUG COSMET IND* 120:38, 1977.
g. Pippitt, Richard: personal communication, 1973.
h. Winneke G, Kastka J, Fodor GG: Disturbance of vigilance and visual-motor performance resulting from air pollutants and drugs. *ADVERSE EFF ENVIRON CHEM PSYCHOTROPIC DRUGS* 1:193–202, 1975.

4,4'-Methylenedianiline has been considered a possible human carcinogen, and is one of the substances considered suspect in development of choroidal melanoma in chemical industry.[272]

Methylergonovine maleate (Methergine), an oxytocic, has been associated with a case of transitory cortical blindness after delivery, thought due to vasospasm.[a]

a. Creze B, Truelle JL, et al: Transitory cortical blindness after delivery using Methergin. *REV FR GYNECOL OBSTET* 71:353–356, 1976.

Methyl ethyl ketone (MEK, 2-butanone) is a widely used volatile solvent. Testing of a drop on rabbit eyes indicates moderate reversible injuriousness, graded 5 on a scale of 1 to 10.[228] The effect of a splash in human eyes should be similar to that of acetone. However, one case has been described with a most unusual course.[b] A workman splashed his eye accidentally, but the next day had only slight conjunctival hyperemia, no residual corneal injury. Despite the mildness of the injury, in the next few days the affected eye developed severe anterior uveitis, which resolved after intensive treatment. Such an extraordinary reaction might be attributable to a latent tendency to uveitis triggered by slight trauma.

MEK vapor causes a sensation of irritation to human eyes detectable at a concentration of 350 ppm in air.[183] A concentration of 3,300 ppm has a strong odor and is moderately irritating to the eyes and nose of workmen; 10,000 ppm (1%) causes almost intolerable irritation of the eyes and nose after several inhalations.[a] Guinea pigs exposed to 1% vapor in air also evidence severe irritation of the nose and eyes by rubbing the nose with the paws and closing their eyes after two to four minutes.

Injury of the eyes from contact with vapor of methyl ethyl ketone has been induced in guinea pigs only by extreme condition of exposure, such as 10% vapor for thirty minutes or more. Under these conditions the guinea pigs' corneas have become opaque, but eight days later they returned to normal.[a]

Smyth has mentioned that in one episode of industrial eye injuries associated with exposure to methyl ethyl ketone vapor he found the injuries to be caused by an unsaturated ketone impurity that was accidentally present, but he seems not to have published a description of the nature of the eye injuries or an identification of the impurity responsible.[227] Possibly this was the same episode and the same material that Cogan and Grant investigated (but did not publish) in 1943, involving fifteen workers who were exposed to vapors from a plastic which was thinned with methyl ethyl ketone for spreading on cloth to make raincoats. No symptoms were noted during the work day, but in the evening and the following day the patients had much pain in their eyes and blurring of vision, which were due to bilateral erosion and loss of corneal epithelium in the palpebral fissures, with swelling and haziness of the corneal stroma. The eyes were hyperemic, but there was no infiltration of the stroma, and there was a clear zone between the corneal lesion and the limbus. The eyes all healed.

In one quite inconclusive case a young man used methyl ethyl ketone as a paint remover for one and a half hours, then had headache, vertigo, and decrease in vision to 20/200 bilaterally. Except for the vision, and transient superior arcuate scotomas, eye examination was normal.[c] Vision returned to 20/20 in 36 hours. Methanol was found in the blood, and gradually disappeared in six days; the concentration was unstated. There was no history of drinking methanol, and no statement concerning its possible presence in the paint remover.

   a. Patty FA, Schrenk HH, Yant WP: Acute response of guinea pigs to vapors of some new commercial organic compounds. VIII. Butanone. *PUBLIC HEALTH REP* 50:1217–1228, 1935.
   b. Johnson, Trimble J: personal communication, 1980.
   c. Berg EF: Retrobulbar neuritis. *ANN OPHTHALMOL* 3:1351–1353, 1971.

Methyl ethyl ketone peroxide has been tested by applying two drops of 40% solution in dimethyl phthalate to rabbit eyes, and this has been found to cause severe damage, graded 6 on a scale of 0 to 7. (The solvent was not significantly injurious.) At 3% a moderate reaction occurred lasting for two days, followed by rapid improvement.[59] Washing the eyes with water within four seconds after application prevented injury of the eye in all cases.[59] (Also see *Peroxides, organic.*)

Methyl fluoroacetate is highly poisonous but different from *methyl bromoacetate* or *methyl iodoacetate* in that the fluorine atom is essentially unreactive, and the compound has no lacrimatory effect on rabbit eyes. Systemic poisoning with methyl fluoroacetate is similar to that of sodium fluoroacetate. Animals become apathetic for 30 to 120 minutes, then excitable and apparently unable to see. Convulsions follow for two to four minutes. Postmortem no anatomical lesions have been found. (See *Fluoroacetate* for further details.)

Methyl fluorosulfate (methyl fluorosulfonate, Magic Methyl), a methylating agent, has delayed toxic effects, like dimethyl sulfate. Exposure of human beings to the vapor can cause corneal epithelial damage with consequent severe eye irritation lasting for 24 hours.[a] Similarly, severe irritation is induced in the eyes of rabbits.[b] Sufficient can be absorbed after application to rabbits' eyes to cause systemic poisoning and death.

   a. Alder RW, Sinnott ML, et al: Methyl fluorosulfate. *CHEM ENGIN NEWS* p. 56, Sept. 11, 1978.
   b. Hite M, Rinehart W, et al: Acute toxicity of methyl fluorosulfonate (Magic Methyl). *AM IND HYG ASSOC J* 40:600–603, 1979.

Methyl formate, a very volatile solvent and fumigant, causes no eye irritation in animals at 1,500 ppm in air,[188] but does cause some irritation at 3,500 ppm.[46]

Eye disturbances have been described in a factory in which boiling methyl formate and other esters (ethyl formate, methyl acetate, and ethyl acetate) were employed.[a] Methyl formate was probably responsible for causing irritation of the eyes and tearing which affected ten out of fifteen women employees. One woman complained of difficulty with her vision for two days while at work and two days after leaving work. Another employee was said to have lost her vision temporarily, but to have regained it in about twelve days. Purportedly the ophthalmologist who took care of this patient could find no abnormality of her eyes and concluded that her optic nerves had been affected. In neither case were any details of ophthalmic examination or measurement of vision reported.

   a. Duquenois P, Revel P: Occupational poisonings by the vapors of some esters employed as solvents. *J PHARM CHIM* 19:590–600, 1935. (French)

Methylhydrazine (monomethylhydrazine) has been found to be peculiarly toxic to the cornea.[a] When applied to the skin of dogs, it is absorbed and carried by the bloodstream to the eyes where it enters the aqueous humor and injures the endothelium of the cornea, causing corneal edema in five to six hours. In excised corneas solutions as dilute as 10^{-7} M promote swelling of the cornea, presumably from injurious effect on the endothelium.

   a. Takahashi GH, Dasher CE: Effects of MMH (monomethylhydrazine) upon the cornea and studies on the blood-aqueous barrier to MMH. *AERO-SPACE MED* 40:279–283, 1969.

Methyl iodide (iodomethane), a methylating agent, causes the same type of delayed vesicular burning of the skin as does methyl bromide.[b] Methyl iodide appears to share with *methyl bromide* and *methyl chloride* a high systemic toxicity with delayed action, but slight immediate irritative or warning properties. All three methyl halides appear to have serious toxic effects on the central nervous system, with psychotic or depressive sequelae.

Exposure of mice to rapidly lethal concentrations of vapor (25 to 85 mg/liter of air) has caused immediate irritation of the eyes, but exposure to only 5 mg/liter of air for ten minutes caused no signs of irritation of the eyes in most animals, although all died within the next day.[b]

In three case reports of poisoning in human beings ocular disturbances from methyl iodide have resulted from inhalation of the vapor. One patient felt weak and dizzy, walking as though drunk. Objects appeared doubled and he stumbled over obstacles as though not seeing them. Intermittently he thought he could not see at all. He had no headache or nausea, despite a sensation of movement of the environment. Eight days later the eyes were examined clinically and found normal, and he subsequently had no further visual troubles. However, he became progressively disoriented and psychotic, and was unable to work.[d]

In the second case, poisoning was fatal. Its onset was accompanied by drowsiness and inability to walk. The patient's speech was slurred and incoherent. The only description concerning the eyes was of nystagmoid movements and slight right internal strabismus, but the fundi were said to be normal. The vision was not evaluated. The patient became comatose and died. Autopsy showed bronchopneumonia and congestion of all organs except the heart.[c]

In the third case a chemical worker developed diplopia, ataxia, and somnolence, later stiffness of the neck, vomiting and semicoma, suggesting an encephalitis. This was followed by mental disturbance which cleared only after four months.[a]

(There appears to be some confusion in the literature, particularly in toxicology texts and reviews, in ascribing constriction of visual field to methyl iodide. This type of field change has been induced by *methyl mercuric iodide*, but apparently not by methyl iodide.)

    a. Baselga-Monte M, Estadella-Botha S, et al: Occupational methyl iodide intoxication. *MED LAV* 56:592–595, 1965. (*CHEM ABSTR* 64:10295, 1966.)
    b. Buckell M: The toxicity of methyl iodide. *BR J IND MED* 7:122–124, 1950.
    c. Garland A, Camps FE: Methyl iodide poisoning. *BR J IND MED* 2:209–211, 1945.
    d. Jaquet A: On methyl bromide poisoning. *DTSCH ARCH KLIN MED* 71:370, 1901. (German)

Methyl iodoacetate, like ethyl iodoacetate, is a lacrimator and a very effective inhibitor of thiol enzymes.[160]

Methyl isobutyl ketone (MIK, isobutyl methyl ketone, hexone, isopropylacetone, 4-methyl-2-pentanone) is employed as a solvent. Its vapor is increasingly irritating to the eyes and nose of human beings from concentration of 200 to 1,000 ppm in air.[56,217] Exposure of guinea pigs to higher concentrations causes much irritation with lacrimation and salivation. The irritant effect apparently provides adequate warning against exposure to concentrations which might have systemic effects.[56] (Contrast *methyl n-butyl ketone*. See INDEX.)

Methyl isocyanate (MIC) became notorious for its toxicity in the diaster at Bhopal in India in 1984, when accidental release of a cloud of heavy vapor in a short time killed some 2000 people in the neighborhood, by injury to their lungs. The vapor also caused painful burning of the eyes and acute loss of epithelium from the corneas of the victims, either punctate or diffuse with corneal edema.[a] The eyes of survivors recovered completely, with apparently no irreversible damage.[a]

Proctor and Hughes in 1978[372] cited earlier investigations of toxicity to human beings by experimental exposure to MIC vapor, showing that 2 ppm caused lacrimation, and 21 ppm caused "unbearable irritation of eyes, nose, and throat." Rye in 1973 stated that methyl isocyanate and *ethyl isocyanate* could "cause permanent eye damage," but did not elaborate.[c] Presumably this was from liquid contact. Smyth and Carpenter (1969) rated injury of rabbit cornea 10 on a scale of 10.[228] *Methyl diisocyanate*, according to Rye, did not cause "appreciable irritant reaction in the eye."[c]

Addition of MIC to young rat lenses *in vitro* has produced reversible opacities.[b]

    a. Anderson N, Muir MK, et al: Bhopal eye; Bhopal diaster. *LANCET* 2:1481,1984; 1:761–762, 1985.
    b. Harding JJ, Rixon KC: Lens opacities induced in rat lenses by methyl isocyanate. *LANCET* 1:762, 1985.
    c. Rye WA: Human responses to isocyanate exposure. *J OCCUP MED* 15:306–307, 1973.

Methyl isothiocyanate (methyl mustard oil) is irritant and vesicant, similar to allyl and ethyl isothiocyanates, and similarly appears to be a lacrimator.[73]

Methyl mercury compounds (including dimethyl mercury, methyl mercury hydroxide, methyl mercury iodide, methyl mercury nitrate, methyl mercury phosphate, and methyl mercury thioacetamide) are notorious for their toxic effects, particularly as they have affected vision, caused ataxia and paralysis, and in many cases have caused death. (*Ethyl mercury compounds* have similar effects, but have received less attention. They are described under a separate heading. See INDEX.)

In 1940 Hunter and associates described four cases of poisoning from inhalation of *methyl mercury* in a fungicide factory. In each case there was gross constriction of the visual fields, down to small central islands in three of the cases, yet central visual acuity was little if at all affected.[j] One of these patients was followed for fifteen years, continuing to have extreme concentric narrowing of the visual fields, dysarthria, and ataxia until his death. At autopsy, atrophy of the visual cortex, greatest at the anterior ends of the calcarine fissures with relative sparing of the occipital poles, was found to explain the narrowing of the visual fields, and atrophy of the cerebellum explained the ataxia.[h] The optic chiasm and nerves were normal.

In the 1940's also were described the cases of two men who had sprayed methyl mercury wood preservative for five years, then developed numbness of the hands, incoordination, ataxia, and bilateral concentric contraction of the visual fields.[a,r] Both became completely blind, and died.

From these early isolated cases the principal features of methyl mercury poisoning had become known, but more was to be learned from epidemics of poisonings to follow, and from experimental investigations. Most notoriously, in Japan many people were poisoned by eating fish from Minamata Bay which had become contaminated by industrial wastes, and in Iraq many were poisoned by eating grain which had been treated with methyl mercury compounds to protect it for use as seed. The history and features of "Minamata Disease" have been described by Walsh and Hoyt.[256] Numerous other series of case reports also give information on ophthalmologic findings from the Japanese epidemics,[l-n, p, q, u, w, zd] the epidemic in Iraq,[b, za, zb] and from smaller epidemics[x, y] of methyl mercury poisoning. The larger epidemics involved hundreds and thousands of people.

The findings in systemic poisoning by *methyl mercury compounds* have been remarkably uniform. In all cases the symptoms and signs have been quite different from those of inorganic mercury poisoning. Instead of producing tremor, salivation, stomatitis and discoloration of the lens, poisoning by methyl mercury has involved principally the nervous system. Characteristically in poisonings from *methyl* or *dimethyl mercury,* several weeks or months after acute exposure of as little as two weeks' duration, or after chronic exposure to low concentrations for several months or years, the victims have developed numbness and tingling of fingers, lips, and tongue and have become clumsy. In some cases, symptoms have not appeared until several weeks after exposure has ceased. Typically the initial clumsiness has progressed rapidly to severe dysarthria and ataxia. Speech has been seriously affected in most cases, becoming quite indistinct or impossible, usually for several months. Hearing has usually been impaired. Several patients have become aware that they could see distinctly straight ahead, but that they had difficulty with peripheral vision. Concentric constriction of visual fields has been soundly established as a characteristic of this poisoning. Constriction has been observed to progress markedly in the course of two weeks, even after exposure to methyl mercury compounds was discontinued. Apparently spontaneous recovery of visual fields has been observed rarely, but central vision has recovered in some cases of blindness.[za] Most children who became blind remained blind.[b] In all cases in which the fundi have been examined, the optic discs and retinal nerve fibers have been found normal, despite blindness or constriction of fields to small central islands. Pupillary responses to light have remained normal, consistent with cortical type of visual loss. Electroretinograms remained normal. Visual evoked cortical responses under ordinary illumination were reduced only when fields were severely constricted, but in scotopic illumination the VER was reduced in association with only moderate constriction.[m] Arden grating tests revealed abnormalities comparable to abnormalities of VER with pattern reversal stimulus.[w]

Exceptionally, slight ptosis and irregular nystagmus on extremes of gaze have been noted. Disturbances of eye movements have been brought out more clearly by use of electro-oculography, indicating that "jerky pursuit" and abnormal saccadic movements were very common.[n, zd]

The early histopathologic findings of Hunter and associates are corroborated in findings in victims of the various epidemics, showing most characteristically involvement of occipital visual cortex and cerebellum with disappearance of neurons and proliferation of glial cells, but no histologic alterations in optic radiations, lateral geniculate body, optic chiasm or optic nerve.[m]

Experimental or accidental poisoning of animals with methyl mercury has reproduced the cerebral damage and blindness in cats,[e] swine,[d, v, y] and most extensively in monkeys.[c,g,h,o,s,t,z,zc,ze] Results in rabbits[m] and rats[f,i] have been less satisfactory. Results in monkeys appear to have been closely similar to results of poisoning in human beings, with an exception that the cerebellum characteristically is affected in human beings, but not in monkeys.[zc] In monkeys the severity of poisoning has been dose-related.[h,s] Complete blindness with cerebral cortical damage, but normal pupillary reaction to light, has been produced.[g,h] At lower dose levels, impairment of visual discrimination and flicker sensitivity have been most readily detected at reduced levels of illumination.[g,t] Visual fields have become constricted, as in human beings.[t,z] Similar results have been obtained in infant monkeys.[ze] Electro-oculography has revealed spontaneous and positional nystagmus at relatively low doses of methyl mercury.[o]

a. Ahlmar A: Poisoning by methyl mercury compounds. *BR J IND MED* 5:117–119, 1948.

b. Amin-Zaki L, Majeed MA, et al: Methylmercury poisoning in Iraqi children. *BR MED J* 1:613–616, 1978.

c. Berlin M, et al: Neurotoxicity of methylmercury in squirrel monkeys. *ARCH ENVIRON HEALTH* 30:340–348, 1975.

d. Davies TS, Nielsen SW, Kircher CH: The pathology of subacute methylmercurialism in swine. *CORNELL VET* 66:32–55, 1976.

e. Davies TS, Nielsen SW: Pathology of subacute methylmercurialism in cats. *AM J VET RES* 38:59–67, 1977.

f. Dye RS, Eccles C, Annau Z: Evoked potential alterations following prenatal methyl mercury exposure. *PHARMACOL BIOCHEM BEHAV* 8:137–141, 1978.

g. Evans HL, Garman RH: Scotopic vision as an indicator of neurotoxicity. Pages 135–147 in Merigan and Weiss (1980).[358]

h. Finocchio DV, Luschei ES, et al: Effects of methylmercury on the visual system of rhesus macaque. Pages 113–122 in Merigan and Weiss (1980).[358]

i. Gramoni R: Retinal function of rats exposed to organomercurials. Pages 101–111 in Merigan and Weiss (1980).[358]

j. Hunter D, Bomford RR, Russell DS: Poisoning by methylmercury compounds. *QUART J MED* 9:193–213, 1940.

k. Hunter D, Russell DS: Focal cerebral and cerebellar atrophy in a human subject due to organic mercury compounds. *J NEUROL NEUROSURG PSYCHIATR* 17:235–241, 1954.

l. Iwata K: Neuroophthalmological findings and their transition of organic mercury poisoning, "Minamata Disease", in Agano area of Niigata prefecture. *ACTA SOC OPHTHALMOL JPN* 77:1788–1834, 1973.

m. Iwata K: Neuroophthalmologic indices of Minamata disease in Niigata. Pages 165–185 in Merigan and Weiss (1980).[358]

n. Kairada K, Nomura Y, et al: Neuroophthalmological findings of Minamata disease, with special reference to eye movement. *ACTA SOC OPHTHALMOL JPN* 30:1366–1370, 1979.

o. Kato I, Aoyagi M, et al: Electrooculographic evaluation of methylmercury intoxication of monkeys. *EXP NEUROL* 72:51–62, 1981.

p. Kurland LT, Faro SN, Siedler H: Minamata Disease. *WORLD NEUROL* 1:370–395, 1960.

q. Li Y: An autopsy case of chronic organic mercury poisoning. *ACTA PATH JPN* 16:411–420, 1966.

r. Lundgren K, Swenson A: Occupational poisoning by alkyl mercury compounds. *J IND HYG* 31:190–200, 1949.

s. Luschei E, Mottet NK, Shaw CM: Chronic methylmercury exposure in the monkey. *ARCH ENVIRON HEALTH* 32:126–131, 1977.

t. Merigan WH: Visual fields and flicker thresholds in methylmercury-poisoned monkeys. Pages 149–163 in Merigan and Weiss (1980).[358]

u. Mikuni M, Iwata K, et al: Ocular findings of organic mercury poisoning in Agano area. *ACTA SOC OPHTHALMOL JPN* 74:1152–1163, 1970.

v. Miller E, Earl FL, et al: Chronic neurotoxic effect of methyl mercury in miniature swine. *PROC WORLD VET CONG* 3:2455–2456, 1975.

w. Mukuno K, Ishikawa S, Okamura R: Grating test of contrast sensitivity in patients with Minamata disease. *BR J OPHTHALMOL* 65:284–290, 1981.

x. Okinaka S, et al: Encephalomyelopathy due to an organic mercury compound. *NEUROLOGY* 14:69–76, 1964.

y. Pierce PE, Thompson JF, et al: Alkyl mercury poisoning in humans. *J AM MED ASSOC* 220:1439–1442, 1972.

z. Rice DC, Gilbert SG: Early chronic low-level methylmercury poisoning in monkeys impairs spatial vision. *SCIENCE* 216:759–761, 1982.

za. Rustam H, Hamdi T: Methyl mercury poisoning in Iraq. *BRAIN* 97:499–510, 1974.

zb. Sabelaish S, Hilmi G: Ocular manifestations of mercury poisoning. *BULL W H O* 53:(suppl) 83–86, 1976.

zc. Shaw C, Mottet NK, Chen WJ: Effects of methylmercury on the visual system of rhesus macaque. Pages 123–134 in Merigan and Weiss (1980).[358]

zd. Tsutsui J: Clinical and pathological studies of eye movement disorders in Minamata disease. Pages 187–202 in Merigan and Weiss (1980).[358]

ze. Willes RF, Truelove JF, Nera EA: Neurotoxic response of infant monkeys to methylmercury. *TOXICOLOGY* 9:125–135, 1978.

Methyl methacrylate is a liquid which can be polymerized to form the transparent plastics Lucite, Plexiglas, and Perspex, which have been used in hard contact lenses and intraocular lenses. Contact lenses have appeared to cause no chemical injury when polymerization is complete.[56] However, some depolymerization and re-formation of methyl methacrylate can occur under various circumstances, and this has caused some concern in the case of intraocular lenses, raising the question whether the monomer is toxic in the eye, and whether it is present clinically in significant amount. Rabbit experiments in which the polymerized plastic with monomer content of 3.7% was placed in the anterior chamber gave no evidence of toxicity during a year of observation.[b,c] A less realistic and more drastic test of intraocular toxicity in rabbits has been made by introducing a 10 μl droplet of methyl methacrylate into the anterior chamber.[d] A localized fibrin mass, damage of corneal endothelium and swelling of the cornea, with partial vascularization, developed acutely. Where the fibrin and droplets were in contact with the lens, anterior lens opacity rapidly appeared. As the reaction subsided, areas of iris atrophy were found. Smaller volumes of methyl methacrylate produced less effect. Although this chemical clearly has the potential of intraocular toxicity, it is questionable whether significantly toxic amounts are actually released from intraocular polymeric plastic with low content. No evidence has been found for involvement of an immune mechanism.[e]

Externally applied to the rabbit eye, methyl methacrylate has caused irritation requiring several days for recovery.[f]

Isolated frog retina shows a dose-related depression of the ERG at concentrations above 1 mM.[a]

a. Borchard U, Bohling HG: Investigation of the neurotoxicity of monomeric methyl-methacrylate and homologous chemicals. *ACTA PHARMACOL TOXICOL* [Suppl] 41:421, 1977.

b. Galin MA, Chowchuvech E, Turkish L: Uveitis and the intraocular lens. *TRANS OPHTHALMOL SOC UK* 96:166–167, 1976.

c. Galin MA, Turkish L, Chowchuvech E: Detection, removal and effect of unpolymerized methylmethacrylate in intraocular lenses. *AM J OPHTHALMOL* 84:153–159, 1977.

d. Holyk PR, Eifrig DE: Effects of monomeric methylmethacrylate on ocular tissues. *AM J OPHTHALMOL* 88:385–395, 1979.

e. Jennette J, Eifrig DE, et al: The inflammatory response to secondary methylmethacrylate challenge in lens-implanted rabbits. *AM INTRAOCULAR IMPLANT SOC J* 8:35–37, 1982.

f. Speakman CR, Main RJ, et al: Monomeric methyl methacrylate. Studies on toxicity. *IND MED* 14:292–298, 1945.

N-Methyl morpholine (4-methyl morpholine), has been tested by application to rabbit eyes and found to cause moderate injury, graded 5 on a scale of 1 to 10 after twenty-four hours.[224] Application of one drop to a rabbit's cornea, without subsequent irrigation and with the lids kept closed, caused corneal haze, sloughing of the epithelium, and hyperemia of the conjunctiva within five minutes.[170] Methyl morpholine is one of a series of amines that has caused transient edema of the corneal epithelium in workers chronically exposed to vapor concentrations of 40 ppm or more in air, particularly in the manufacture of polyurethane foams.[40,164,170] Typically the vapor has not caused objectionable irritation of the eyes during exposure, but at the end of the work day vision has become blurred, with blue haze or fog and haloes about lights, which have usually cleared within several hours after work. This effect has been especially objectionable in automobile driving, particularly at night. The visual disturbance has been attributed to optical irregularity produced by edema of the corneal epithelium. A volunteer who exposed his eyes to the vapor developed temporary "grey haziness" of his vision, but this effect was not produced by inhalation.[a] (See also INDEX for *Amines* for other substances with this effect.)

a. Jones WT, Kipling MD: Glaucopsia—blue-grey vision. *BR J IND MED* 29:460–461, 1972.

1-Methyl-3-nitro-1-nitrosoguanidine (NSC-9369) injected into pregnant rabbits has caused fetal ocular malformations consisting of dysgenesis of the anterior segment, hypoplasia of the iris stroma, and ectopia of the ciliary body.[a]

a. Alfieri G, Alfieri-Rolla G: Ocular alterations in the new-born rabbit after treatment of the mother during gestation with N-methyl-N[1]-nitro-N-nitrosoguanidine. *ARCH RASS ITAL OTTAL* 3:247–256, 1973. (Italian)

N-Methyl-N-nitrosourea, closely related to N-Methyl-N-nitrosourethane, a mutagen, carcinogen, and methylating agent, causes damage to the retina in Syrian hamsters. Seven days after one or two doses of 5 mg have been injected intravenously, the retinas of these animals have shown arcades in the outer nuclear layer, degeneration of the pigment epithelium, and destruction of rods and outer nuclear layer, leading to thinning of the whole retina and migration of pigment.[a] In rats, 70 mg/kg has induced retinal atrophy and cataracts.[b,356]

> a. Herrold KM: Pigmentary degeneration of the retina induced by N-methyl-N-nitrosourea. *ARCH OPHTHALMOL* 78:650–653, 1967.
> b. Murthyl AS, Vawter GF, et al: Retinal atrophy and cataract in rats following administration of N-methyl-N-nitrosourea. *PROC SOC EXP BIOL MED* 139:84–87, 1972.

Methylpentynol (meparfynol, Dormison), a sedative-hypnotic, has been reported through Fraunfelder's registry to be capable of producing nystagmus, diplopia, ptosis, and mydriasis.[312]

Methylphenidate (Ritalin, Methidate), a mild CNS stimulant and antidepressant administered orally, was claimed in 1955 to cause a rise of ocular pressure in glaucomatous patients, but without discriminating as to type of glaucoma, and with no control comparisons without medications.[a] Tablets crushed and injected intravenously have caused multiple small retinal emboli.[b,312]

> a. Thiel R, Hollwich F: Eye-midbrain reflex and intraocular pressure. *BUECH AUGEN-ARZT* 23:166–109, 1955. (German)
> b. Gunby P: Methylphenidate abuse produces retinopathy. *J AM MED ASSOC* 241:546, 1979.

1-Methyl-4-phenyl-1,2,5,6-tetrahydropyridine (MPTP), a by-product of meperidine-analog synthesis, taken intravenously by several people has caused Parkinsonism with diminution of blinking, apraxia of eyelid opening, and limitation of vertical gaze.[a] Some victims were said to be paralyzed for a time and able only to move their eyes.[b]

> a. Langston JW, Ballard P, et al: Chronic Parkinsonism in humans due to a product of meperidine-analog synthesis. *SCIENCE* 219:979–980, 1983. (*N ENGL J MED* 309:310, 1983.)
> b. Blume E: Street drugs yield primate Parkinson's model. *J AM MED ASSOC* 250:13–14, 1983.

Methyl propyl ketone (2-pentanone, ethyl acetone) is a moderately volatile solvent. Men exposed to 1,300 to 1,500 ppm in air found even brief exposure was severely irritating to the eyes and nose, but this produced no damage.[a,b] No ocular injury from the vapors has been reported from industrial use.[21] Tested in liquid form on rabbit eyes, it caused only moderate injury, graded 3 on a scale of 1 to 10 after twenty-four hours.[228]

> a. Specht H, Miller JW, et al: Acute response of guinea pigs to inhalation of ketone vapors. *U.S. PUBLIC HEALTH SERV, NAT INST HLTH, BULL* No. 176, 1940.
> b. Yant WP, Patty FA, Schrenk HH: Acute response of guinea pigs to vapors of some new

organic compounds. IX. Pentanone (methyl propyl ketone.) *U.S. PUBLIC HEALTH REP,* 51:392, 1936.

Methyl salicylate (wintergreen oil) employed for flavoring and as a counterirritant on the skin, in contact with the eye causes discomfort but only temporary irritation. Testing by application of a drop to rabbit eyes has caused slight and reversible injury, graded 3 on a scale of 1 to 10 after twenty-four hours.[27]

Ingestion of 5 to 30 ml may cause severe poisoning. More than ninety cases of poisoning have been reported, with deaths in about half. Treatment has been directed toward correcting acidosis and ketonuria by intravenous administration of sodium bicarbonate, sodium lactate, and glucose.[c]

In reviews of methyl salicylate poisoning, dimness of vision is mentioned as occurring in about 15 per cent of all cases, but the nature of the impairment has been poorly characterized, and the impression is given that it is a manifestation of disturbance of the central nervous system.[b,c] Rarely has any definitive observation been made on the visual effects.

For instance, one patient complained of dimness of vision and difficulty in hearing on first regaining consciousness after ingestion of 30 ml of methyl salicylate, after going through severe acidosis, coma, and convulsions, which were treated with intravenous amytal, sodium lactate, and calcium gluconate.[b] Vision and hearing were said to have returned to normal within two weeks, but no actual measurements of visual acuity, visual fields or examination of the fundi were reported. Another patient, who took 24 ml of methyl salicylate in the course of forty-eight hours, complained of xanthopsia and inability to read. This patient was reported to have recovered in about five days after the drug was discontinued, but the reason for the inability to read was not explained.[a]

Apparently there have been no permanent disturbances of vision from methyl salicylate. (The relationship of methyl salicylate poisoning to methanol poisoning has not been established, but acidosis is a feature of both and requires similar treatment.)

a. Baum WL: Toxic amblyopia from oil of wintergreen. *OPHTHAL REC,* 1903, p.25.
b. Cancelmo JJ: Methyl salicylate poisoning. *U.S. NAVAL MED BULL* 47:1077–1085, 1947.
c. Stevenson C: Oil of wintergreen (methyl salicylate) (Report of 3 cases, 1 with autopsy, and a review of the literature.) *AM J MED SCI* 193:772–778, 1937.

Methyl silicate (tetramethyl silicate; tetramethoxysilane) is a liquid which resembles dimethyl sulfate in both physical and toxic properties. Both liquids are severely damaging to the eyes, and both have sufficient vapor pressure to present serious hazard to the eyes of people exposed to open containers of the liquids. Both substances resemble mustard gas in having an insidious delayed action, causing slight or no immediate effect, followed after a latent period of several hours by a potentially serious reaction. On the skin, liquid methyl silicate is less injurious than dimethyl sulfate or mustard gas, but on rabbit eyes, test application of a droplet has caused severe injury, graded 9 on a scale of 1 to 10 after twenty-four hours, with permanent opacification.[27,225]

The results of exposure of human eyes to vapors or possibly to mist of methyl silicate under working conditions have not been described in detail, but it is known that in some cases the epithelium of the cornea has been injured, and that pain and swelling of the lids and conjunctivae have developed several hours after exposure. In most cases the eyes have recovered completely. In exceptional instances the deeper layers of the cornea have been involved, resulting in permanent opacification, and in one patient, causing loss of the eye.[a, b]

Trimethoxysilane apparently has toxic effects on the eye similar to those of tetramethyl silicate, judging by a report on six people who were engaged in purifying trimethoxysilane and had onset of severe irritation of the eyes eight to twelve hours after finishing work. The discomfort was like that of ultraviolet keratitis, and the same type of keratitis epithelialis was observed. It reached its maximum in twelve to twenty-four hours, but was surprisingly slow in healing, returning completely to normal only after twenty to ninety days.[c] Tests on rabbit eyes showed that trimethoxysilane applied as a solution or spray caused damage of the cornea and conjunctiva similar to that in the patients. There was loss of corneal epithelium and edema of the cornea, maximum in twelve to twenty-four hours, healing completely in twenty to twenty-five days.[c]

Hexamethoxydisiloxane, a probable hydrolysis product of trimethoxysilane, tested on rabbit eyes was not damaging.[c]

   a. Cogan HD, Setterstrom CA: Properties of ethyl silicate. *CHEM ENGIN NEWS* 24:2499, 1946.
   b. Fawcett HH: Laboratory safety. *CHEM ENGIN NEWS* 29:1302, 1951.
   c. Tamura A, Yuri H, et al: Clinical and experimental investigation of ocular damage caused by trimethoxysilane. *ACTA SOC OPHTHALMOL JPN* 72:40–47, 1968.

α-**Methylstyrene** (isopropenylbenzene) has been tested by application of a drop to rabbit eyes and has been found to cause only slight transient evidence of conjunctival irritation and no corneal damage demonstrable with fluorescein.[265]

Surprising observations from Russia on 231 workers exposed to "*α*-methylstyrol" in a synthetic rubber plant included constriction of retinal arteries, rise of ocular tension, decrease in light sensitivity, and narrowing of the visual field for red and blue, all reversible.[a] The original data should be reviewed for question of statistical significance and adequacy of controls. Possibly related, biochemical studies of retinas of rats exposed to *α*-methylstyrene for 4 months are reported by the same author to have shown accumulation of acid mucopolysaccharides and metabolic malfunctions.

   a. Vilisova LF: Changes in the retina and its vessels occurring under the effect of *α*-methylstyrol. *VESTN OFTALMOL* 82(1):44–45, 1969. (English abstract)
   b. Vilisova LF: Histochemical changes in rat retina under the action of *α*-methylstyrene. *FR KRASNOYARSK GOS MED INST* 9(1):22–23, 1969. (English abstract)

Methyl trichlorosilane has been tested by application of a small drop to rabbit eyes and has been found to cause severe damage.[211] (See also *Chlorosilanes.*)

Methyl triethoxysilane has been tested by application of 0.02 ml to rabbit eyes and found to cause immediate irritation but no corneal damage. The eyes were normal within twenty-four hours.[211]

2-Methyltryptamine (α-methyltryptamine), a monoamine oxidase inhibitor, tested by oral administration, produced a feeling of elation or intoxication and produced significant though slight enlargement of the pupils. Visual disturbances were reported by three of twelve subjects, principally blurring of vision; one noted a few flashes of light. The mechanism was not investigated.[a] Similar effects were produced by *Etryptamine* (α-ethyl tryptamine).

  a. Murphree HB, Dippy RH, et al: Effects in normal man of α-methyltryptamine and α-ethyltryptamine. *CLIN PHARMACOL THER* 2:722–726, 1961.

Methyl vinyl carbinol causes a sensation of irritation of the eyes in human beings at concentrations as low as 50 ppm in air.[217]

Methyl vinyl ketone has a powerfully irritating odor. It is a skin irritant and lacrimator.[215] In the synthetic rubber industry in Czechoslovakia it has been suspected of causing conjunctivitis and injury to the corneal epithelium. (See *Chloroprene.*)

Methylviolet (pyoktanin) is a basic cationic dye which in contact with human eyes has caused injury of the cornea and conjunctiva, sometimes very severe, either as a result of contamination with powdered dye or from indelible pencil in which it has been widely used.[a,141,153] Severe injury has also been produced experimentally in rabbits.[b,141,153,250,251] (See also *Pencils, indelible,* and *Dyes, cationic.*)

  a. Passow A: On the danger to the eyes from colored pencils. *KLIN MONATSBL AUGENHEILKD* 115:680–690, 1949. (German)
  b. Linksz A: On the question of so-called physiologic pupillary block. *ARCH AUGEN-HEILKD* 105:526–536, 1932. (German)

β-Methylxylocholine, a sympatholytic agent, as eyedrops (a 2.5% solution) caused a small reduction of intraocular pressure, but was too irritating to be useful in glaucoma.[a]

  a. Krishna A, Fajardo RV, Leopold IH: Sympatholytic agent SKF No. 6890. *ARCH OPHTHALMOL* 67:600–607, 1962.

Methysergide (Sansert), a vasoconstrictor used for migraine, has rarely had untoward effects on the eyes or on vision. In one series of eighty-seven patients one patient had eye symptoms, complaining of "spots before the eyes," and no eye examination was reported.[b] In another series a 1 per cent incidence of "disturbance of vision" is mentioned in 850 cases, but without details as to the nature of the complaint.[a]

  a. Leyton N: Methysergide in the prophylaxis of migraine. *LANCET* 1:830, 1964.
  b. Lloyd-Smith DL, McNaughton FL: Methysergide (Sansert) in the prevention of migraine. *CAN MED ASSOC J* 89:1221–1223, 1963.

Metiapine, an antipsychotic, has been tested on albino rats and beagle dogs, but no drug-induced changes in cornea, lens, or retina have been detected, although the drug is known to have affinity to melanin.[a]

    a. Gibson JP, Rohovsky MW, et al: Toxicity studies of metiapine. *TOXICOL APPL PHARMACOL* 25:220–229, 1973.

Metoclopramide (Reglan), an anti-emetic, has caused oculogyric crises and dystonic head-neck syndrome, particularly in children, sometimes with nystagmus. These episodes are acute, alarming and distressing, but cease shortly after the medication is stopped.[a,312]

    a. Berkman N, Frossard C, Moury F: Oculo-gyric crises and metoclopramide. *BULL SOC OPHTALMOL FRANCE* 81:153–155, 1981. (French)

Miconazole, an antifungal, has been tested for toxicity to the lens, vitreous body, and retina after intravitreal injections in rabbits and monkeys.[a,b] Doses of 100 to 1000 μg produced cataracts, inflammation in the vitreous body, retinal hemorrhages and necrosis. Doses of 10 to 80 μg caused some retinal necrosis in rabbits, but not in monkeys. Clinical use of as much as 40 μg was thought justifiable in desperate cases.[b] Tested externally as eye drops on rabbits, 1% miconazole did not retard closure of corneal epithelial defects.[309]

    a. Perrone S, Moschini GB, et al: Toxic effects of the intravitreous injection of miconazole. *BOLL OCULIST* 58:571–580, 1979.

    b. Tolentino FI, Foster CS, et al: Toxicity of intravitreous miconazole. *ARCH OPHTHALMOL* 100:1504–1509, 1982.

Millipore filters, have been widely used for removal of particles and microorganisms from solutions, but a warning has been issued that for preparation of solutions to be used within the eye one should be careful to avoid a type of filter that contains a wetting agent (Triton X-100) which may injure the corneal endothelium; one should use a toxin-free type.[a]

    a. Meltzer DW, Drew RC, Hajek AS: Millipore filters in ophthalmic surgery. *AM INTRAOCUL IMPLANT SOC J* 7:143–146, 1981.

Mimosine (leucenol) can be isolated from the plants *Leucaena glauca* and *Mimosa pudica.* Cataracts develop in young rats fed the seeds or leaves.[b] Feeding the crystalline compound has caused severe inflammatory changes in the anterior segments of the eyes two or three days after the start of feeding,[a] and has produced cataracts in rats.[c]

Local application of 0.5% solution twice daily for twenty-one days produced no similar effect. In the feeding experiments the vessels of the conjunctiva and iris became engorged, and bleeding occurred into the conjunctiva, anterior and posterior chambers. The corneas became cloudy and vascularized. Degenerative changes in the lens epithelium were detectable by the time corneal and iris damage was evident. It appeared that the development of cataract was a primary effect of a toxic agent on the lens.[a] No instance of injury to human eyes is known.

a. von Sallman L, Grimes P, Collins E: Mimosine cataract. *AM J OPHTHALMOL* 47:107–117, 1959.
b. Yoshida (1944), referred to by von Sallman et al.[a]
c. Tittarelli R, Catalino P, Bucci MG: Contribution to the study of experimental cataract from leucinol. *BOLL OCULIST* 40:619–634, 1961. (Italian)

Minocycline (Minocyn), an antibacterial, and tetracycline were taken orally for several years by two patients who developed pigment deposits in cysts in the palpebral conjunctivae, closely resembling those produced by epinephrine; the patients had not used epinephrine, and were asymptomatic.[a, b]

Benign intracranial hypertension, with 6th nerve palsy and papilledema, has been reported in a girl taking minocycline, gradually resolving when the drug was stopped.[c]

a. Brothers DM, Hidayat AA: Conjunctival pigmentation associated with tetracycline medication. *OPHTHALMOLOGY* 88:1212–1215, 1981.
b. Messmer E, Font RL, et al: Pigmented conjunctival cysts following tetracycline/minocycline therapy. *OPHTHALMOLOGY* 90:1462–1468, 1983.
c. Monaco F, et al: Benign intracranial hypertension after minocycline therapy. *EUROP NEUROL* 17:48–49, 1978.

Minoxidil (Loniten), an antihypertensive, had been given to a patient for six months, along with prednisone and azathioprine, after renal transplantation, when he complained of his vision, which was reduced to counting fingers at five feet in one eye, 20/100 in the other.[a] There were central scotomas with swollen, hyperemic discs, diagnosed as optic neuritis. Subsequently vision did not improve, and optic atrophy developed, with pigmented lesions at the posterior pole of both eyes, and yellowish scar in the macula of the worse affected eye.

a. Gombos GM: Bilateral optic neuritis following minoxidil administration. *ANN OPHTHALMOL* 15:259–261, 1983.

Miotics constrict the pupil, either by weakening the iris dilator muscle, or by stimulating the iris sphincter muscle. The first type (anti-alpha-adrenergic) will be described elsewhere under *Thymoxamine*. (See INDEX). The second type only will be described here. These are employed mainly in treatment of glaucoma, and to a small extent in strabismus in children. Miotics employed in treatment of glaucoma include pilocarpine, carbachol, aceclidine, and methacholine, which are parasympathomimetic or cholinergic substances acting in a manner similar to acetylcholine at the parasympathetic myoneural junctions. Other miotics used for treating glaucoma are physostigmine, neostigmine, demecarium, and alkyl phosphate esters such as isoflurophate, diisopropylfluorophosphate, echothiophate (Phospholine iodide), and paraoxon (Mintacol, Arminium), which are inhibitors of cholinesterase. The drugs in the latter category closely resemble in toxic and pharmacologic effect a large group of substances used as insecticides and nerve gases. Phosphate insecticides, such as parathion and TEPP, and nerve gases characteristically induce miosis, as well as other effects on the eyes the same as produced by the miotic drugs. (See INDEX for *Organophosphorus pesticides.*)

The literature on adverse effects of miotics on the eyes is so extensive that the bibliography is planned to be selective, rather than complete. Selection favors publications that are recent and provide numerous additional references. The effects will be summarized under the following headings: (1) *Lids*, (2) *Conjunctiva*, (3) *Cornea*, (4) *Iris*, (5) *Ciliary processes*, (6) *Ciliary muscle*, (7) *Glaucoma*, (8) *Cataract*, (9) *Retina*, and (10) *Systemic*.

1. The *lids* often respond by twitching after local contact or systemic poisoning with cholinesterase-inhibiting miotics. The muscles of the lids, most commonly the lower lid, contract spasmodically, causing a twitching which is felt by the subject and is often visible to others. This occurs commonly during use of cholinesterase inhibitors in treatment of glaucoma, and may be annoying but not harmful.

2. The *conjunctiva* under the influence of parasympathomimetic drugs regularly becomes slightly hyperemic owing to the vasodilating action of these drugs. An asymptomatic and apparently harmless hypertrophy of conjunctival follicles may result from repeated application, as in treatment of glaucoma. Contact allergy or sensitivity develops occasionally. A serious disturbance of the conjunctiva has been produced in several patients by application of *furtrethonium iodide* daily for several years. This particular miotic caused formation of a membrane on the surface of the conjunctiva, obstructing the lacrimal passages and leading to much discomfort and disability. (Also see INDEX for *Furtrethonium iodide*.)

Ocular cicatricial pseudopemphigoid was diagnosed in two patients who had been taking echothiophate iodide eye drops for glaucoma for 6 and 9 years respectively.[zc] In each case these drops had been used in only one eye of each patient, and only the treated eyes had developed the pseudopemphigoid, which seemed a strong argument for cause and effect. Pseudopemphigoid has also been seen bilaterally in patients who have used this medication in both eyes, but these have been anecdotal and rare, not very convincing in themselves. So far there has been no documented systematic study proving a significantly abnormal incidence of this possible complication.

3. The *cornea* presented a bizarre reaction in two patients who used pilocarpine drops several times a day for many years in treatment of glaucoma, and gradually developed burning discomfort in the eyes with much tearing and blurring of vision, but no itching or disturbance of the skin suggestive of allergy.[31] The corneal epithelium in both patients became gray. Superficial vascularization extended onto the cornea for 3 or 4 mm, in the whole circumference. The conjunctiva appeared beefy red, but exhibited no membrane or follicular hypertrophy. When the pilocarpine drops were discontinued, the patients began to feel better within a day or two, and in a few weeks the corneal epithelium cleared so that the vision was much improved. In the course of a few years the vessels practically disappeared. It is not certain that the apparent idiosyncratic reaction in these patients was due to the pilocarpine, rather than some associated preservative. A series of patients have been described with a different type of corneal disturbance, an atypical band keratopathy, following chronic use of pilocarpine eye drops containing *phenylmercuric salts* as preservative. (See INDEX for *Phenylmercuric salts*.)

4. The *iris* is peculiarly affected by miotic drugs repeatedly applied to the eye. Cysts or nodules of the pigment epithelium develop at the pupillary margin both in

young and old patients, most frequently from use of the cholinesterase inhibitor miotics which tend to make the pupil smaller than do the direct-acting cholinergic or muscarinic miotics. Pupillary cysts often have been observed in children treated with miotics for accommodative strabismus. The cysts may grow to 2 mm in diameter, and sometimes interfere with vision when the pupil is small. They were described in 1920 by Vogt and have been observed many times since. Simultaneous use of phenylephrine has been found helpful in preventing formation of these pupillary cysts.[h]

Other side effects on the iris are dilation of the vessels, release of fine pigment particles into the aqueous humor on initial vigorous miosis, and rarely iritis. One of the commonest complaints of patients who must use miotic eyedrops is a darkening or dimming of the environment, particularly at night or indoors in artificial illumination, because the contracted pupil greatly reduces the amount of light that can enter the eye. It is a serious handicap to automobile driving at night.[86] Use of a mydriatic, such as phenylephrine, and brighter lights indoors help to compensate.

5. The *ciliary processes* have also in rare instances been thought to form cysts analogous to those at the pupil under the influence of strong miotics.[u]

6. The *ciliary muscle* under the influence of miotics contracts, with spasm of accommodation, blurring of vision for distance, and aching of the eye if the cyclotonia is severe. These side effects are familiar to ophthalmologists and patients who use potent miotics, particularly the cholinesterase inhibitors, but are disturbing and disabling to normal individuals poisoned by miotic insecticides or nerve gases.[zi] Spasm of accommodation and blurring of vision are particularly dangerous to airplane pilots employed in crop dusting with miotic insecticides. Unequal spasm of accommodation in the two eyes may cause disastrous inability to judge distances.[zi]

7. *Glaucoma* may result when the lens accommodates for near as a result of the action of the miotic drugs that cause contraction of the circular or sphincter-like fibers of the ciliary muscle. The zonules that suspend the lens become relaxed and allow the lens to change from a flattened to a thicker or more globular form. The loosening of the zonules and change in shape of the lens can significantly affect the depth of the anterior chamber, and can precipitate angle-closure glaucoma in certain eyes. In an eye with unusually small anterior segment and disproportionately large lens, if the front of the lens moves forward, pushing against the pupillary portion of the iris, this can cause an increase in resistance to the normal flow of aqueous humor from the posterior chamber, where it is formed, forward through the pupil to the anterior chamber, from which it normally leaves the eye. Resulting increase in pressure in the posterior chamber can cause the periphery of the iris to balloon or bulge forward and to close the drainage angle of the anterior chamber. This is followed by a rapid rise in intraocular pressure, constituting an acute attack of angle-closure glaucoma.[291] Strong miotics that contract the ciliary muscle are more likely to precipitate this kind of an attack than are relatively weak or dilute miotics that have less effect on the ciliary muscle, yet still constrict the pupil, and, in fact, tend to prevent angle-closure glaucoma by pulling the periphery of the iris toward the pupil, away from the angle wall. A related, but more complicated type of glaucoma, can also be precipitated by miotics after intraocular operation for angle-closure glaucoma. This type of glaucoma seems to involve pressure from the vitre-

ous body which pushes lens, ciliary body and iris forward when the lens zonules are relaxed. It has been known as malignant glaucoma or ciliary-block glaucoma.[291]

8. *Cataract* from miotic eye drops has received a great deal of attention. A unique instance of transient clouding of the lenses associated with use of DFP (diisopropyl fluorophosphate, isofluorophate) locally in treatment of strabismus was reported in 1960 by Harrison.[p] The patient was thirteen years old and had normal eyes except for esotropia. After daily application of 0.025% DFP to both eyes for three months, a delicate rosette of silvery gray lines in petal pattern became visible by slit-lamp biomicroscope in the anterior subcapsular region of both lenses. At four months, cysts developed at the pupillary margins, and treatment was stopped. Within the next three weeks the lenses cleared completely. The patient's vision was at all times unaffected.

Intensive clinical surveys particularly by Axelsson and by Shaffer showed that many patients who had been under treatment with the strongest miotics for glaucoma had abnormalities in their lenses that appeared to have been caused by the treatment.[d,zf] and these observations have been corroborated by others.[i,v,ze,zg]

However, not all reports have agreed. Both Morton[zb] and Thoft[zh] reported prospective studies in which the miotic eyedrops were administered monocularly. No deterioration of vision was observed by Morton in eyes treated with 4% pilocarpine or 0.03% echothiophate. Thoft similarly found very little indication of lens changes at the lowest concentrations of echothiophate. In children no cataracts were discovered in 205 eyes of patients between two and fourteen years of age treated for accommodative esotropia by means of echothiophate or DFP eyedrops daily for three to forty months.[e]

From the weighing of evidence so far, it appears that chronic use of all of the long-acting cholinesterase inhibitor miotics, including iso-flurophate, echothiophate, paraoxon, and demecarium, can produce anterior subcapsular vacuoles in the lenses of patients, best seen with a slit-lamp microscope. Subsequently posterior subcapsular and nuclear changes develop, which in some cases may have led to complete opacification of the lens within less than a year, although usually visual impairment has not been obvious during the first two years of treatment. In some cases, discontinuing medication appears to have prevented progression of clouding of the lens, but in other cases, when clouding has already progressed, it has continued after the medication was withdrawn. Most observers have agreed with Axelsson that clouding of the lenses tends to be more rapid in patients over sixty years of age than in younger patients. Axelsson found no greater tendency to induction of cataract by cholinesterase inhibitor miotics in patients with pseudoexfoliation than in others. Much remains to be determined regarding the relationship of type of miotic, concentration and type of eye that is prone to development of lens changes. Axelsson has estimated that at least 50 percent of glaucomatous eyes treated with echothiophate iodide during three years will suffer some visual impairment owing to changes in the lenses induced by the drug.

Clinically, as a consequence of these findings, there has been a tendency to use pilocarpine eye drops as usual, because of no proof so far of cataractogenic effect, but to reserve the strong cholinesterase-inhibitor miotics for aphakic eyes or desperate cases of glaucoma. Considering that glaucoma can produce irreversible loss of vision if not treated, whereas cataracts can usually be removed with complete restoration of vision if they do advance to a stage requiring operation, it seems that even the threat of induction of cataract is insufficient reason for witholding cholinesterase inhibitors if they are needed for control of the glaucoma. Fortunately, other means of treatment have been multiplying, and a decision on use of cholinesterase inhibitors has become less often necessary.

In monkeys, cataracts have been induced by chronic topical administration of cholinesterase inhibitor miotics,[a,r-t,za] though not in subprimates.[d] Vacuoles and opacities have appeared quite similar to those seen in human beings. Simultaneous administration of atropine has had an inhibiting effect.[s] However, reducing accommodation by detachment of the ciliary muscle has not prevented development of characteristic lens changes in monkeys.[a,t]

Experimental studies on animal lenses endeavoring to elucidate the toxic mechanism have included a number of biochemical investigations. Most interesting so far have been studies on rabbit lenses surviving in tissue culture, in which both demecarium bromide and echothiophate iodide have been shown to induce subcapsular vacuoles and to cause decrease of the potassium content of the lens and increase of sodium and water, which are fundamental derangements that have been observed in lenses which have been subjected to other cataractogenic influences.[y,z] In rabbits, echothiophate eye drops increase glyolysis and reduce the activity of pentose phosphate and sorbitol pathways in the lens, according to measurements of metabolite levels.[o]

9. The *retina* has become detached in several cases after use of strong miotics, and the circumstances have suggested that the miotic was in some way responsible, but the mechanism has not been established. Comprehensive reviews of the evidence have been provided by Alpar,[c] Beasley,[f] and Freilich,[k] giving references to published cases. In essence, when administration of miotic eye drops is started, the sooner that symptoms and signs of retinal detachment develop, the stronger the circumstantial evidence of a cause and effect. A majority of ophthalmologists appear to believe that it is likely that miotic eye drops can precipitate retinal detachment, and that the stronger the miotic the more the risk. Furthermore, myopic eyes and eyes with pre-existing retinal lesions are probably at special risk. However, most agree that so far there has been no proof. Hypotheses have mostly blamed mechanical effects of contraction of the ciliary muscle. An instance of macular hole developing after starting pilocarpine has been reported, but is an extraordinary rarity, compared to retinal detachment in association with miotics.[m]

10. *Systemic toxic effects of miotic eye drops* are encountered occasionally, and are similar for the direct acting drugs, such as pilocarpine, and the cholinesterase inhibitors, though the pilocarpine type usually is involved in acute overdoses, and the cholinesterase inhibitors more likely to cause chronic intoxication. A comprehensive review and bibliography has been published by Hermans.[q]

Instances of acute poisoning by pilocarpine have developed in treatment of acute angle-closure glaucoma when drops were applied repeatedly every few minutes, causing profuse sweating, salivation, nausea and retching, tremor and decreased blood pressure, but essentially normal temperature.[j,n] Fortunately, spontaneous recovery is usual when pilocarpine is discontinued.

Chronic intoxication from absorption of anticholinesterase eye drops tends particularly to cause diarrhea. Severe chronic diarrhea may be accompanied by fatigue, muscle weakness, and chronic sweating.[b,x,za,zj] Stopping the medication can bring about remarkable improvement within a couple of days.

The cholinesterase inhibitor miotic eyedrops when administered chronically have been repeatedly shown to depress the activity of cholinesterases in the blood, particularly serum pseudocholinesterase, and also erythrocyte cholinesterase. However, in many patients it has been shown that the cholinesterase activity can be very much depressed without producing symptoms. In the absence of symptoms, the main concern is the possible danger to patients who might need surgery and might be given suxamethonium (succinylcholine) in conjunction with their general anesthetic. There is the possibility of prolonged apnea because of persistence of suxamethonium when this is not broken down at a normal rate because of lack of the specific active enzyme. (See also *Suxamethonium.*)

Pancreatitis has been reported from cholinergic stimulation in human beings, but a systematic study of 44 patients regularly taking echothiophate iodide for glaucoma has fortunately shown no significant elevation of serum lipase or serum amylase.[1]

In pregnancy, use of miotic eye drops to treat glaucoma has raised concern for the welfare of the unborn infant, but so far there appear to be no suspicions of congenital abnormalities. However, it is not known how many patients have been treated during pregnancy with miotics without difficulty. A case report by Birks recorded 0.125% echothiophate iodide twice a day having been used until the last 2 months of pregnancy with no abnormality except a possible temporary depression of serum pseudocholinesterase.[g]

Counteraction or treatment of the effects of excessive miotics is not often called for, but cholinergic effects can be counteracted by intramuscular injection of atropine sulfate, usually 1 mg per injection. (Findings suggesting need for atropine, and intravenous fluids to compensate for dehydration, are sweating, salivation, nausea, tremor, slowing of the pulse, and decrease of blood pressure.) In the case of poisoning from miotics of the phosphate ester cholinesterase inhibitor types such as DFP, echothiophate, and paraoxon, administration of cholinesterase reactivators may be indicated in addition to the administration of atropine.[za] (See *Pralidoxime.*)

In patients who have not been acutely intoxicated, but who have depressed erythrocyte cholinesterase as a result of chronic use of echothiophate eyedrops, it has been shown that a gradual partial reactivation can be accomplished by repeated oral administration of pralidoxime chloride during several weeks.[w]

a. Albrecht M, Barany E: Early lens changes in Macaca fascicularis monkeys under topical treatment with echothiophate or carbachol studied by slit-image photography. *INVEST OPHTHALMOL VIS SCI* 18:179–187, 1979.

b. Alexander WD: Systemic side effects with eye drops. *BR MED J* 282:1359, 1981.

c. Alpar JJ: Miotics and retinal detachment. *ANN OPHTHALMOL* 11:395–401, 1979.

d. Axelsson U: Cataracts following the use of long-acting cholinesterase inhibitors in glaucoma patients. *PROC EUR SOC DRUG TOXICITY* 12:199–203, 1971.

e. Baldone JA, Clark WB: Absence of lenticular changes from cholinesterase inhibitors in 205 eyes of children. *J PEDIATR OPHTHALMOL* 6:81–83, 1969.

f. Beasley H, Fraunfelder FT: Retinal detachments and topical ocular miotics. *OPHTHALMOLOGY* 86:95–98, 1979.

g. Birks DA, Prior VJ, et al: Echothiophate iodide treatment of glaucoma in pregnancy. *ARCH OPHTHALMOL* 79:283–285, 1968.

h. Chin NB, Gold AA, Breinin GM: Iris cysts and miotics. *ARCH OPHTHALMOL* 71:611–616, 1964.

i. de Roetth A Jr: Lens opacities in glaucoma patients on Phospholine iodide therapy. *AM J OPHTHALMOL* 62:619–628, 1966.

j. Epstein E, Kaufman I: Systemic pilocarpine toxicity from overdosage. *AM J OPHTHALMOL* 59:109–110, 1965.

k. Freilich DB, et al: Miotic drugs, glaucoma, and retinal detachment. *MOD PROBL OPHTHALMOL* 15:318–322, 1975.

l. Friberg TR, Thomas JV, et al: Serum cholinesterase, serum lipase, and serum amylase levels during long-term echothiophate iodide therapy. *AM J OPHTHALMOL* 91:530–533, 1981.

m. Garlikov RS, Chenoweth RG: Macular hole following topical pilocarpine. *ANN OPHTHALMOL* 7:1313–1316, 1975.

n. Greco JJ, Kelman CD: Systemic pilocarpine toxicity in the treatment of angle closure glaucoma. *ANN OPHTHALMOL* 5:57–59, 1973.

o. Harkonen M, Tarkkanen A: Effects of Phospholine iodide on the metabolites of the glycolytic pentose phosphate and sorbitol pathways in the rabbit lens. *ACTA OPHTHALMOL* 54:445–455, 1976.

p. Harrison R: Bilateral lens opacities associated with use of diisopropyl fluorophosphate. *AM J OPHTHALMOL* 50:153–154, 1960.

q. Hermans G: Systemic effects associated with use of miotic eye drops. *BULL SOC BELGE OPHTALMOL* 186:9–19, 1979. (French)

r. Kaufman PL, Axelsson U, Barany EH: Induction of subcapsular cataracts in cynomolgus monkeys by echothiophate. *ARCH OPHTHALMOL* 95:499–504, 1977.

s. Kaufman PL, Axelsson U, Barany EH: Atropine inhibition of echothiophate cataractogenesis in monkeys. *ARCH OPHTHALMOL* 95:1262–1268, 1977.

t. Kaufman PL, Erickson KA, Neider MW: Echothiophate iodide cataracts in monkeys. *ARCH OPHTHALMOL* 101:125–128, 1983.

u. Kraft H: Development of cystic changes in the ciliary processes with long-term use of cholinesterase-inhibitors. *KLIN MONATSBL AUGENHEILKD* 104:584, 1962. (German)

v. Levene RZ: Echothiophate iodide and lens changes. *Symposium on Ocular Therapy*, Vol. 4, pp. 45–52, St. Louis, CV Mosby Co, Ed. by Leopold IH, 1969.

w. Lipson ML, Holmes JH, Ellis PP: Oral administration of pralidoxime chloride in echothiophate iodide therapy. *ARCH OPHTHALMOL* 82:830–835, 1969.

x. Markman HD, Rosenberg P, Dettbarn WD: Diarrhea as the first symptom of echothiophate iodide toxicity. *N ENGL J MED* 27:197–198, 1964.

y. Michon J Jr, Kinoshita JH: Experimental miotic cataract. I. *ARCH OPHTHALMOL* 79:79–86, 1968.

z. Michon J Jr, Kinoshita JH: Experimental miotic cataract. II. *ARCH OPHTHALMOL* 79:611–616, 1968.

za. Moore WKS: Two cases of poisoning with di-isopropyl fluorophosphonate (DFP). *BR J IND MED* 13:214–216, 1957.

zb. Morton WR, Drance SM, Fairclough M: Effect of echothiophate iodide on the lens. *AM J OPHTHALMOL* 68:1003–1010, 1969.

zc. Patten JT, Cavanagh HD, Allansmith MR: Induced ocular pseudopemphigoid. *AM J OPHTHALMOL* 82:272–276, 1976.

zd. Philipson B, Kaufman PL, et al: Echothiophate cataracts in monkeys. *ARCH OPHTHALMOL* 97:340–346, 1979.

ze. Pietsch RI, Bobo CB, et al: Lens opacities and organophosphate cholinesterase inhibiting agents. *AM J OPHTHALMOL* 73:236–242, 1972.

zf. Shaffer RN, Hetherington J Jr: Anticholinesterase drugs and cataracts. *TRANS AM OPHTHALMOL SOC* 64:204–216, 1966. (*AM J OPHTHALMOL* 62:613–618, 1966.)

zq. Tarkkanen A, Karjalainen K: Cataract formation during miotic treatment for chronic open-angle glaucoma. *ACTA OPHTHALMOL* 44:932–939, 1966.

zh. Thoft RA: Incidence of lens changes in patients treated with echothiophate iodide. *ARCH OPHTHALMOL* 80:317–320, 1968.

zi. Upholt WM, Quinby GE, et al: Visual effects accompanying TEPP-induced miosis. *ARCH OPHTHALMOL* 56:128–134, 1956.

zj. Wood JR, Anderson RL, Edwards JJ: Phospholine iodide toxicity and Jones' tubes. *OPHTHALMOLOGY* 87:346–349, 1980.

Mirex, an insecticide, has been shown to produce cataracts in suckling rats when fed to the mother.[a] The mother's milk is the main vehicle.

a. Gaines TB, Kimbrough RD: Oral toxicity of mirex in adult and suckling rats. *ARCH ENVIRON HEALTH* 21:7–14, 1970.

Misonidazole desmethyl derivative (Ro-9963), a radiosensitizer, has been tested for ocular toxicity by subconjunctival injection. In rabbits, 140 mg caused loss of corneal epithelium, damage to endothelium, and swelling of corneal stroma for a week. There was hemorrhage and inflammatory-cell infiltration of the ciliary processes. Injection of half that amount caused transient iritis, localized corneal edema, and no denuding of corneal epithelium. After the lower dose the eyes were essentially back to normal in a week.[a]

a. Rootman J, Josephy PD, et al: Ocular absorption and toxicity of a radiosensitizer and its effect on hypoxic cells. *ARCH OPHTHALMOL* 100:468–471, 1982.

Mitomycin C, an antineoplastic, has been used in eyedrops after operation for pterygium in an attempt to prevent recurrence. When a 0.04% solution has been used three to six times a day for only a week, no serious side effects have been noted, just occasional reversible blepharo-conjunctivitis. However, after more extensive use, later iridocyclitis, degeneration of the sclera, and secondary glaucoma have been reported in six cases.[a,c,d]

Injection of mitomycin C into the vitreous humor of rabbits has caused severe destruction of most of the cells of the retina, particularly the nuclei and outer segments of the visual cells, and has extinguished the ERG.[b] However, a dose no greater than 2 μg (or 0.8 μg/ml) is reported not to be significantly toxic to the rabbit retina.[277,369]

a. Mori S, Murakami N, Kunitomo N: Postoperative treatment of pterygium with mitomycin C. *JPN J OPHTHALMOL* 12:30–36, 1968.

b. Yamamoto K, Tokunga S, et al: Experimental degeneration of the retina. *FOLIA OPHTHALMOL JPN* 18:52–60, 1967.

c. Yamanouchi U, Mishima K: Eye lesions due to mitomycin C instillation after pterygium operation. *FOLIA OPHTHALMOL JPN* 18:854–861, 1967.

d. Yamanouchi U: A case of scleral calcification due to mitomycin C instillation after pterygium operation. *FOLIA OPHTHALMOL JPN* 29:1221, 1978.

Mitotane (o,p -DDD, Lysodren), an antineoplastic, has, according to Fraunfelder[313] been reported to have caused blurred vision, lens opacities, and retinopathy with hemorrhages and papilledema.[a]

a. Hoffman DL, Mattox VR: Treatment of adrenocortical carcinoma with o,p -DDD. *MED CLIN NORTH AM* 56:999–1012, 1972.

Molybdenum metal implanted in rabbits' eyes has been found inert.[340] Gilded molybdenum wire placed in the sclera or episclera has not caused inflammation, though in some cases the wire gradually penetrated the sclera and choroid.[a]

a. Zehetbauer G, Prammer G: Clinical observations on gilded molybdenum wire remaining in eye tissues. *KLIN MONATSBL AUGENHEILKD* 171:779–781, 1977.

Monoamine oxidase inhibitor drugs have been extensively reviewed by Levy and Michel-Ber,[a] and by Hermans[328] with respect to toxicology and adverse effects from medical use.

Drugs for which there is information on ocular side effects are the following:

Etryptamine (Monase)
Iproniazid (Marsalid)
Isocarboxazid (Marplan)
Isoniazid
Methyltryptamine
Modaline

Nialamide (Niamid)
Octamoxin (Nimaol, Xymaol)
Pargyline (Eutonyl)
Phenelzine (Nardil, Nardelzine)
Pheniprazine (Catron)
Tranylcypromine (Parnate)

Optic neuritis and retrobulbar neuritis have been reported in numerous cases from *Pheniprazine* and *Octamoxin*, and in a few cases from *Isoniazid*, but there appears to have been no proven optic neuritis from the other MAO inhibitor drugs listed above, nor from *Mebanazine* (Actomol).

(*Ethyl pyridine*, used in manufacture of *isoniazid*, has been suspected of producing central scotomas in one patient.) *Tranylcypromine* in two cases may have caused temporary decrease in visual acuity and alteration of ERG.

Vague episodes of blurring of vision, without definite explanation of the cause, has been reported from *Etryptamine, Iproniazid, Isocarboxazid, Methyltryptamine, Modaline,* and *Nialamid*, but none of these has been shown to produce optic neuritis.

Mydriasis, which may have been partially responsible for some of the complaints of blurred vision, has been noted from *Etryptamine, Methyltryptamine, Modaline, Pargyline, Phenelzine,* and *Tranylcypromine.* Several of these drugs produced mydriasis only when overdosage was taken.

(See INDEX for details of ocular effects of each of the drugs.)

a. Levy J, Michel-Ber E: Difficulties and complications caused in man by monoamine oxidase (MAO) inhibitors, with special reference to their specific and secondary pharmacological effects. *PROC EUROP SOC STUDY DRUG TOXICITY* 9:189–222, 223–245, 1968.

Monobenzone (monobenzyl ether of hydroquinone, Alba, Benoquin), a depigmentor used topically in vitiligo, has caused lysosomal storage abnormalities in cornea and conjunctiva of patients, but no known intraocular abnormality.[a] One patient who had applied monobenzone for a year to much of her body, including her face and probably her eye lids, developed asymptomatic fine wavy brownish lines in the corneal epithelium just below the vertex. Vision was undisturbed, and eye examination was otherwise normal. Two other patients developed diffuse pigmentation of the bulbar conjunctiva after several months. Biopsies of the corneal epithelium and conjunctiva showed lipid-like inclusions in lysosomal residual bodies. Unlike the parent chemical, hydroquinone, which can be seriously damaging to the eyes, monobenzone has not been known to affect vision. (See INDEX for *Lipidosis*.)

> a. Hedges TR, Kenyon KR, et al: Corneal and conjunctival effects of monobenzone in patients with vitiligo. *ARCH OPHTHALMOL* 101:64–68, 1983.

Monochloroacetic acid (chloroacetic acid) vapors appear in one instance to have caused corneal epithelial injury.[a] Chloroacetate appears to be less toxic than *bromoacetate* or *iodoacetate*, having none of their injurious effect on the retina of rabbits.[231]

> a. Knapp P: On the question of traumatic keratitis from the action of gases. *SCHWEIZ MED WOCHENSCHR* 4:702, 1923. (German)

Moon flower has caused temporary mydriasis in a child who ate the bark, a reaction such as produced by stramonium and other anticholinergic plant alkaloids.[a]

> a. Hornsby P: A case of accidental mydriasis due to the bark of the moon flower. *EAST AFR MED J* 46:527, 1969.

Morel is an edible fungus which during industrial preservation has been associated with punctate stippling of the corneal epithelium with scratchy discomfort, photophobia, and blurring of vision. The substance responsible has not been identified, but *helvellic acid* might be split off during water rinsing,[a] or *amines*, which might be released on contact with water in cooking, have been considered.[61]

> a. Pick L: Eye and mucous membrane disturbances from morel vapors (occupational mass illness). *ZENTRALBL AUGENHEILKD* 61:325–332, 1927. (German)

Morning glory seed (*Ipomoea tricolor*), caused an acute psychiatric disturbance in a young woman who ate 250 seeds, with pupils dilated for at least forty-eight hours.[a]

> a. Ingram AL: Morning glory seed reaction. *J AM MED ASSOC* 190:1133–1134, 1964.

Morphine toxic effects on the eyes are very rare. Case reports of serious disturbances of vision from morphine seem all to date from the nineteenth century. The older literature was summarized in 1913 by Lewin and Guillery.[153] They expressed doubt about the validity of some of the reports and suggested that some visual disturbances had been caused by other poisonous substances, such as lead.

Miosis is regularly induced by ordinary systemic doses of morphine supposedly reflecting a release of the pupilloconstrictor center in the central nervous system.[214]

In fatal poisoning from large overdosage of morphine the pupils are said to dilate just before death,[196] but miosis may persist.[g] Occasional transient weakness of convergence has been noted after large doses.[e] Rarely transient myopia has been observed, causing slight blurring of vision for distant objects.[d] Also a reduction of visual field has been claimed.[159]

In morphine addicts, among the effects of withdrawal are said to be excessive tearing, irregularity of the pupils, paresis of accommodation, and occasionally diplopia.[e, 252, 255]

Morphine applied in eyedrops is said to have weak miotic effect on normal human beings, a concentration of 5% morphine sulfate producing only 0.4 to 0.7 mm miosis, compared to 1.4 mm miosis obtained from 15 mg intramuscularly.[i] This miosis can be antagonized by locally applied nalorphine,[h,i] or naloxone.[b]

Studies have been made on reversible lens opacities developed in mice, rats, and guinea pigs in less than an hour after administration of morphine and other narcotics, which has been explained by a reduction in blinking, a resultant exposure of the cornea, increased evaporation, and dehydration of the anterior segment of the eye, causing temporary loss of transparency.[c,l,m,n,261]

The distribution of tritiated morphine in various parts of the rabbit eye has been determined after intravenous injection.[a] Although considerable was found in the cornea, it did not interfere with corneal grafting, nor did it affect cell division or protein synthesis by corneal cells *in vitro* unless more morphine was added.

In rats, morphine has been reported to interfere with protein synthesis and axonal transport in the retina.[k]

a. Basu PK, Kapur BM, et al: Distribution of morphine in the eye tissues and fluids of rabbits after systemic administration. *CAN J OPHTHALMOL* 18:241–245, 1983.

b. Franciullacci M, Boccuni M, et al: The naloxone conjunctival test in morphine addiction. *EUR J PHARMACOL* 61:319–320, 1980.

c. Fraunfelder FT, Burns RP: Effects of lid closure in drug induced experimental cataracts. *ARCH OPHTHALMOL* 76:599–601, 1966.

d. V. Graefe A: On muscular asthenopia. *GRAEFES ARCH OPHTHALMOL* 8:314–367, 1861. (German)

e. Guillery: On the influence of poisons on the eye movement apparatus. *PFLUG ARCH* 77:321–404, 1899. (German)

g. Kaczander P: Fatal, suicidal morphine poisoning. *SAMML VERGIFTUNGSF* 2:177–180, 1931. (German)

h. Leopold IH, Comroe JH Jr: Effect of intramuscular administration of morphine, atropine, scopolamine and neostigmine on the human eye. *ARCH OPHTHALMOL* 40:285–290, 1948.

i. Nomof N, Elliott HW, Parker KD: The local effect of morphine, nalorphine and codeine on the diameter of the pupil of the eye. *CLIN PHARMACOL THER* 9:358–364, 1968.

k. Tuluany FC, Takemori AE: The effect of morphine on the incorporation of ^{3}H-leucine into retinal proteins and subsequent axonal transport. *LIFE SCI* 16:551–560, 1975.

l. Weinstock M: Similarity between receptors responsible for the production of analgesia and lenticular opacity. *BR J PHARMACOL* 17:433–441, 1961.

m. Weinstock M, Stewart HC: Occurrence in rodents of reversible drug-induced opacities in the lens. *BR J OPHTHALMOL* 45:408–414, 1961.

n. Weinstock M, Scott JD: Effect of various agents on drug induced opacities of the lens. *EXP EYE RES* 6:368–374, 1967.

Morpholine is widely employed as a solvent. High vapor concentrations have caused respiratory irritation and lacrimation.[a] At low concentrations in air, morpholine has been listed, along with its N-ethyl and N-methyl derivatives, among the amines which have caused transient edema of the cornea and temporary foggy blue-grey vision with haloes around lights in workers exposed to the vapors for many hours, the symptoms usually coming on after work and clearing spontaneously by the next day.[b,c] (See also *Amines.*)

Liquid morpholine is a strong base and is corrosive to human skin. Tested by application of a drop to rabbit eyes, morpholine has caused moderate injury with ulceration of the conjunctiva and clouding of the cornea, graded 7 on a scale of 1 to 10 after twenty-four hours.[27,222]

a. Clinton M: Morpholine. *AM PETROL INST TOXIC REV,* Sept. 1948.
b. Jones WT, Kipling MD: Glaucopsia-blue-grey vision. *BR J IND MED* 29:460–461, 1972.
c. Mastromatteo E: Heterocyclic amine exposure with urethane foams. *J OCCUP MED* 7:507, 1965.

Mortar is composed of lime (calcium hydroxide), cement, sand, and water. Injury to the eyes from a splash of mortar is attributable mainly to the strongly alkaline calcium hydroxide which it contains. Corneal and conjunctival injury has the same character as that described under *Calcium hydroxide* and should be treated in the same manner. The eyes should be irrigated with water as promptly as possible, and special efforts should be made to remove particles from the recesses of the conjunctival sac. Decontamination is facilitated by use of a solution of sodium EDTA (see *Calcium hydroxide*).

Moths of genus *Hylesia* have been reported to cause discomfort from irritation of the eyes, with dermatitis developing later.[a] No actual injuries of the eyes are reported.

a. Zaias, Ioannides G, Taplin D: Dermatitis from contact with moths (genus *Hylesia*). *J AM MED ASSOC* 207:525–527, 1969.

Moxalactam disodium (Moxam), an anti-infective, has been tested by intravitreal injection in rabbits, evaluating toxicity by ophthalmoscopy, ERG, and light and electron microscopy.[a] A dose 1.25 mg did not cause damage to the retina, but 2.5 mg caused some degeneration of photoreceptors, and 5 to 10 mg caused severe functional and morphologic changes. The anterior segment of the eyes appeared undamaged.

a. Fett DR, Silverman CA, Yoshizumi MO: Moxalactam retinal toxicity. *ARCH OPHTHALMOL* 102:435–438, 1984.

Mucuna pruriens is a Central American plant which has seed pods equipped with fine spicules. In contact with the eyes the spicules cause burning and conjunctivitis, and on the skin induce unbearable itching and dermatitis. A proteolytic enzyme, *mucunain*, is said to be responsible for the irritation.[252]

Mushrooms of certain types are very toxic, but ocular effects are rare.[153] Uhthoff in 1931, reviewing reports of ocular effects of mushrooms, concluded that they caused no organic changes in the optic nerve or retina.[247] Good reviews and surveys of mushroom poisoning have been published by Buck[b] and Tyler,[c] incidentally mentioning effects on vision.

Mushrooms of unidentified type were held responsible in one case for reduction of vision to light perception for several days, in association with transitory elevated systemic and retinal blood pressure, albuminuria and hematuria, but only slight abnormalities were seen in the fundi, and the cerebrospinal fluid and intraocular pressures remained normal.[a]

(The effects of specific types of mushrooms and of substances that are found in mushrooms are described under the following headings: *Amanita muscaria, Amanita phalloides, Bufotenine, Morel, Muscarine, Muscimol, Psilocybin*—see INDEX.)

a. Cattaneo D: Transitory blindness from retinal arterial hypertension. *ANN OTTALMOL CLIN OCUL* 65:81–92, 1937. (Italian)
b. Buck RW: Mushroom toxins—A brief review of the literature. *N ENGL J MED* 265:681–686, 1961.
c. Tyler VE Jr: *Progress in Chemical Toxicology.* New York, Academic, 1963.

Mustard gas (bis(2-chloroethyl) sulfide; β,β'dichloroethyl sulfide; Yperite; Gelbkreuz; Senfgas; Lost) has low but significant vapor pressure at ordinary temperatures. Mustard gas is of scientific historic interest as the first substance recognized to cause severe injury of the eyes and other tissues through *alkylation* reaction.

Studies of the mechanisms of the toxic actions of mustard gas have been numerous, and these have several times been reviewed.[e,h,n] In essence, mustard gas in an aqueous medium rearranges into a cyclic sulfonium form which is highly reactive with sulfhydryl, carboxyl, amino, and other groups of proteins, and with hydroxyl ions of water. In most of its reactions with tissues or with water, mustard gas loses one or two molecules of hydrogen chloride, but formation of acid is, contrary to old ideas, insignificant toxicologically. Most important is the alkylation reaction by which mustard gas minus its chlorides becomes firmly attached through one or both of its β-carbon atoms to tissue components, altering their functional and physico-chemical properties. Cytotoxic effects of mustard gas have most specifically been related to a double alkylation reaction in which the two reactive ends of the mustard gas molecule attach to adjacent strands of DNA, forming cross-links that prevent replication of cells.[d,h,l]

Many therapeutic attempts have been made to remove the mustard gas residue from its combination with tissue components, but any means which have been successful have been themselves excessively drastic and injurious. The reaction has so far proved practically irreversible under physiological conditions.

First observations of injurious effect of mustard gas on the eye were made in 1891 by Leber, who found that a tiny drop applied to the eye of a rabbit caused a very severe reaction. Also he determined that a tiny amount introduced into the anterior chamber of a rabbit's eye caused severe inflammation, necrosis, purulent reaction, and breakdown of the cornea.[150]

During World War I, mustard gas was used as a vesicant and poisonous war gas, inflicting upon the eye many transient injuries and a smaller number of permanent, relapsing injuries. During World War II, the chemical and biochemical aspects of injury by mustard gas were intensively investigated. A thorough review of the literature on mustard gas injuries of the eyes up to 1942 was provided by Hughes.[j] Collections of information on investigations of mustard gas toxicity to the eye during World War II were published in 1948 by Friedenwald and his associates, and by Mann and her associates.[f,m,161] A good review of the whole subject was provided in 1954 by Duke-Elder.[46]

Mustard gas in contact with the eye or other tissues promptly reacts chemically and is fixed to the tissue by very stable bonds in a matter of seconds or minutes, but no discomfort or injury appears at that time, although definite abnormalities are demonstrable chemically, physically, and metabolically.[k] Mustard gas denatures proteins and inactivates enzymes just as rapidly as it reacts with them, but it is characteristic in highly organized tissues such as cornea, conjunctiva, and skin that no clinical indication of injury becomes evident until after a latent period usually of several hours. (A delayed reaction is a characteristic also of other alkylating agents, such as dimethyl sulfate.)

After several hours the gross biological evidences of injury begin to appear as edema, hyperemia, and irritation. In the eye the corneal epithelium becomes edematous, the lids and conjunctiva become red and swollen, and the patient experiences burning discomfort and photophobia, inducing tearing and blepharospasm.[g] Simultaneously, areas of contaminated skin become blistered and inflamed. This delay in reaction is similar to that associated with injury by ultraviolet radiation in ultraviolet keratitis or in sunburn of the skin.

Exposure to vapor of mustard gas has induced uncomfortable and temporarily disabling reactions of the eyes and respiratory tract in many cases, but the victims have in most instances recovered completely. In mild vapor burns the damage is usually superficial, and the injured epithelium is spontaneously replaced by normal cells during healing.

More severe injuries with lasting effects have been produced by contact of liquid droplets with the eye, or by exposure to unusually high concentrations of vapor for extraordinarily long periods. In the more severe cases, the injury has involved not only the epithelium but also the deeper layers. The corneas have become cloudy and infiltrated and in the most severe cases have become totally opaque. Associated injury to blood vessels has caused local thrombosis, and has led after several days to a hemorrhagic phase, characterized by leakage of blood from blood vessels peripheral to the ischemic areas, followed by proliferation of the blood vessels. These new vessels have in some cases extended beyond the limbus and extensively invaded the cornea.

Peculiar to severe mustard gas burns is a development and persistence of porcelain white areas in the episcleral tissues adjacent to the cornea and a formation of large sausage-shaped or varicose vessels in these areas. These abnormal vessels are tortuous and show striking variation in diameter. Grossly enlarged segments join abruptly at either end to vessels of normal diameter and appearance. Similar abnormal vessels may be seen in burned skin. Characteristically, the areas of white abnormal tissue have been subject to repeated ulceration over many years.

Numerous case reports in the ophthalmic literature are concerned primarily with these late recurrences of mustard gas keratitis.[a,b,i,m,o] Typically, patients discharged from the Army after having had mustard gas burns of the eyes in World War I were asymptomatic at the time of discharge, and may even have had normal vision despite porcelain-white ischemic areas and dilated veins adjacent to the limbus. Subsequently, sometimes during more than forty years, the corneas have repeatedly ulcerated and gradually deteriorated.

During the recurrences of ulceration, the patients have had photophobia, pain, and lacrimation. Conjunctival graft of the ulcerated area has been recommended for relief of discomfort.[p] The ulcers have healed intermittently, but have left the corneas progressively more irregular and scarred. Fat, calcium, and cholesterol have infiltrated the corneas, contributing to impairment of vision.[c]

In patients having poor vision primarily from corneal irregularity without excessive opacity, considerable improvement in vision has been obtained, at least temporarily, by use of contact lenses.[m] In more severe cases, lamellar or penetrating keratoplasty has provided relief from recurring discomfort, and has provided worthwhile improvement in visual acuity.[i,c]

a. Amalric P, Bessou P, Farenc M: Late recurrences of mustard gas keratitis. *BULL SOC OPHTALMOL FRANCE* 65:101–106, 1965. (French)

b. Atkinson WS: Delayed keratitis due to mustard gas (dichlorodiethylsulfide burns); Report of two cases. *ARCH OPHTHALMOL* 40:291–301, 1948.

c. Blodi FC: Mustard gas keratopathy. *INT OPHTHALMOL CLIN* 11:1–13, 1971.

d. Crathorn AR, Roberts JJ: Mechanism of the cytotoxic action of alkylating agents in mammalian cells and evidence for the removal of alkylated groups from DNA. *NATURE* 211:150–153, 1966.

e. Dixon M, Needham DM: Biochemical research on chemical warfare agents. *NATURE* 158:432–438, 1946.

f. Friedenwald JS, et al: Collection of studies on mustard gas. *BULL JOHNS HOPKINS HOSP* 82:1948.

g. Geeraets WJ, Abedi S, Blanke RV: Acute corneal injury by mustard gas. *SOUTH MED J* 70:348–350, 1977.

h. Gilman A, Phillips FS: The biological actions and therapeutic applications of the β-chloroethyl amines and sulfides. *SCIENCE* 103:409–415, 436, 1946.

i. Hertzberg R: Delayed mustard gas keratitis. *MED J AUST* 1:529–530, 1959.

j. Hughes, WF: Mustard gas injuries to the eyes. *ARCH OPHTHALMOL* 27:582–601, 1942.

k. Kinsey VE, Grant WM: Determination of the rate of disappearance of mustard gas and mustard intermediates in the corneal tissue. *J CLIN INVEST* 25:776–779, 1946.

l. Lawley PD, Brookes P: Molecular mechanism of the cytotoxic action of difunctional alkylating agents and of resistance to this action. *NATURE* 206:480–483, 1965.

m. Mann I: A study of 84 cases of delayed mustard gas keratitis fitted with contact lenses. *BR J OPHTHALMOL* 28:441, 1944.

n. Peters RA: Biochemical research at Oxford upon mustard gas. *NATURE* 159:149–151, 1947.

o. Scholtyssek H: Late keratitis after mustard gas injury and the importance of early diagnosis for treatment and appraisal. *KLIN MONATSBL AUGENHEILKD* 136:243–254, 1960. (German)

p. Sourdille GP: Keratitis from mustard gas; treatment by conjunctival graft. *OPHTHAL-MOLOGICA* 118:893–908, 1949. (French)

Mustard oil from mustard seed has been known for more than a century to cause burning, redness, and vesication of the skin and to be dangerous to the eyes. Experiments have been performed on the role of the axon reflex in the relationship of conjunctival chemosis to pain from application of mustard oil to the eyes of rabbits, cats, and rats off and on since 1910, with conflicting reports on inhibition of the chemosis by local anethetics and denervations.[c]

The vapor released by grinding mustard seed has been known to cause extensive corneal epithelial irregularity in the palpebral fissure, composed of numerous fine dots, which under magnification appear like tiny lusterless droplets or vacuoles in the epithelium.[a, 153, 253] This heals spontaneously on discontinuing exposure. While present, it causes photophobia, pain, lacrimation, and blurring of vision.

In one unusual case, a splash of the liquid in the face of a pharmacist caused the lids and conjunctivae to become red, swollen, and painful. The corneas of this patient appeared to remain normal for six hours, but then vision became foggy and for two days the cornea was so cloudy that the ophthalmoscopic view of the fundus was much blurred. However, the eyes returned to normal in six to seven days.[153]

A drop on rabbit eyes similarly causes intense transitory conjunctivitis, keratitis, and iritis. The reaction is said to be strikingly reduced by large doses of phenylbutazone.[b]

In rats, mustard oil applied as a saturated aqueous solution causes pain and blepharospasm, and if Evans blue is injected intravenously, the conjunctivae and lids become abnormally blue, but the amount of dye in these tissues is the same whether or not pain was prevented by a local anesthetic.[130] (Also see *Allyl isothiocyanate.*)

a. Bischler: Changes in the cornea from mustard oil. *OPHTHALMOLOGICA* 114:56, 1947. (French)

b. Kurus E, Bach B: On the effectiveness of Butazolidine in inflammatory disturbances of the anterior segment of the eye. *KLIN MONATSBL AUGENHEILKD* 137:198–210, 1960. (German)

c. Bruce AN: Vaso-dilator axon-reflexes. *QUART J EXP PHYSIOL* 6:339–354, 1913.

Mycotoxins from several fungi have been shown to be toxic to the cornea, as follows:

Diacetoxyscripenol, from *Fusarium equiseti,* has produced corneal opacities when applied to the eyes of rabbits.[a]

Patulin, a mycotoxin, has produced corneal opacities when applied to eyes of rabbits.[b]

Sporidesmin, from *Pithomyces chartarum,* has caused corneal opacity when applied to eyes of rabbits.[c]

A mycotoxin from *Aspergillus ochraceus* when fed to rats produced interstitial keratitis and edema, with iridocyclitis and hypopyon.[e] *Ochratoxin A* interfered with the carbohydrate metabolism of the lenses.[f]

A mycotoxin from *Penicillium viridicatum* produced similar effects in rat's eyes when fed the killed fungus.[d]

a. Brian PW, Dawkins AW, et al: Phytotoxic compounds produced by *Fusarium equiseti. J EXP BOT* 12:1, 1961.

b. Brown WA, Bulbring E, et al: The pharmacology of patulin. *BR J EXP PATHOL* 25:195, 1944.

c. Done J, Mortimer PH, et al: The production of sporidesmolides by *Pithomyces chartarum. J GEN MICROBIOL* 26:207, 1961.

d. McCracken MD, Carlton WW, Tuite J: *Penicillium viridicatum* mycotoxicosis in the rat. *FOOD COSMET TOXICOL* 12:79–88, 1974.

e. Zimmerman JL, Carlton WW, Tuite J: Mycotoxicosis produced in rats by cultural products of an isolate of *Aspergillus ochraceus. FOOD COSMET TOXICOL* 16:449–461, 1978.

f. Rankov BG, Tosmova S: Studies on the influence of ochratoxin A on rat lenses. *GRAEFES ARCH OPHTHALMOL* 205:135–139, 1978.

Mydriatics dilate the pupil either by blocking the normal parasympathetic innervation of the pupillary sphincter muscle, or by sympathomimetic action. The side effect of parasympatholytic mydriatics on accommodation and on ocular hydrodynamics are discussed under the heading of *Anticholinergic drugs* and *Parasympatholytic agents.* The relationship of pupillary size to precipitation of angle-closure glaucoma is discussed under that heading.

The parasympatholytic agents characteristically induce cycloplegia in addition to mydriasis, but sympathomimetic drugs only slightly impair accommodation for near, and actually slightly enhance it for distance. The effect of the sympathomimetic agents on accommodation is ordinarily too small to be noticed by patients. Aside from the slight effect on accommodation, sympathomimetic mydriatics may slightly and temporarily impair visual acuity simply from enlarging the pupil, because the optical quality of the refractive system is usually not as good with a large pupil as with a small pupil.

Toxic effects of mydriatics on the eye are slight, and seldom encountered. Conjunctivitis and blepharitis occur in hypersensitized individuals. Blanching of the vessels of the anterior segment by sympathomimetic mydriatics may be followed by a somewhat unsightly stage of reactive hyperemia, but this appears to have no serious implications.

An insignificant formation of discrete small brown deposits in the conjunctiva has been noted occasionally following prolonged daily application of *epinephrine.*

A trivial side effect of sympathomimetic mydriatics, such as *phenylephrine,* and also of *cocaine,* is a slight appearance of staring, produced by elevation of the upper lid, caused by contraction of the sympathetically innervated portion of the levator muscle.

Dilating the pupils with adrenergic eyedrops sometimes causes a shower of pigment particles to appear in the aqueous humor. This pigment is released from the posterior pigment layer of the iris. Adrenergic mydriatic eyedrops may cause a considerable transitory rise of intraocular pressure, though the angle of the anterior chamber stays open at all times.[a,c] This pressure rise may be prevented by miotic eyedrops.[a]

In occasional patients, eyedrops containing 1% to 2% *epinephrine* cause considerable aching discomfort in the eyes, without evident relation to the size of the pupil or the intraocular pressure. The basis for this is not known.

Except in very small infants, systemic intoxication is rarely produced by adrenergic mydriatic eyedrops in ordinary amounts, but administration of 10% *phenylephrine hydrochloride* has occasionally caused a rise of systemic blood pressure in both infants and adults. (See INDEX for *Phenylephrine*.)

a. Lee P-F: The influence of epinephrine and phenylephrine on intraocular pressure. *ARCH OPHTHALMOL* 60:863–867, 1958.

b. McReynolds WU, Havener WH, Henderson JW: Hazards of the use of sympathomimetic drugs in ophthalmology. *ARCH OPHTHALMOL* 56:176–179, 1956.

c. Epstein DL, Boger WP III, Grant, WM: Phenylephrine provocative testing in the pigmentary dispersion syndrome. *AM J OPHTHALMOL* 85:43–50, 1978.

Nafoxidine hydrochloride, an anti-estrogen, structurally related to clomiphene and chlorotrianisene, is said to have caused cataracts in dogs and cats, but not in hamsters.[a, 301] (Clomiphene has produced cataracts in rats.) A 46 year old woman developed cataracts in both eyes after having taken nafoxidine for three years, but cause and effect was unproven.[a] The fact that the drug causes photosensitivity of the skin in some people provided grounds for suggesting that patients wear sunglasses while taking it.[a]

a. Bloom HJG, Boesen E: Antioestrogens in treatment of breast cancer. *BR MED J* 2:7–10, 1974.

Nail hardener, a liquid preparation probably containing aldehydes for hardening and preventing fingernails from breaking, has caused conjunctivitis. This is presumably due to contact allergic reaction when the eyelids have been touched or rubbed with the fingers. One patient had conjunctivitis for a year, and this did not respond to ordinary topical treatments, but was cured when use of the nail hardener was stopped.

a. Gundersen T: Personal communication, 1966.

Nail polishes (enamels, lacquers, finishes) are composed of a plastic or resin, dissolved in a volatile solvent, plus plasticizers and dyes or pigments. Splash of a drop of a typical nail polish in the eye can cause uncomfortable temporary solvent burns such as those produced by plastic cement or acetone.

Repeated contact with the nonvolatile components carried by the fingers to the skin about the eyes has been reported in numerous hypersensitive individuals to have caused dermatitis venenata characterized by swelling and vesiculation of the lids, and itching.[a, b]

a. Ormsby O: Dermatologic lesions about the eyes. *AM J OPHTHALMOL* 26:850–855, 1943.

b. Osborne ED, Jordon JS, Campbell PS: Dermatitis venenata due to nail polish, 100 cases. *ARCH DERMATOL SYPH* 44:604–615, 1941.

Nail polish removers are composed principally of acetone, alcohol, ethyl acetate, butyl acetate, amyl acetate, and benzene to dissolve the plastic or resinous coating from the nails. Splash in the eye may be expected to cause immediate pain and damage of the corneal and conjunctival epithelium, but prompt recovery in twenty-four to forty-eight hours.

Nalidixic acid (Cybis, NegGram, Wintomylon), an antibacterial, has had numerous side effects on the eyes or vision. Davidson's reporting system for ocular adverse effects in 1973 called attention to the fact that 288 involved nalidixic acid.[298] Fraunfelder's registry has also received numerous reports.[312] Among the cases summarized by Davidson were 208 in which the main feature was a brightly colored appearance of objects which appeared soon after the drug was taken. Also there were 20 cases of severe loss of vision which lasted from a half hour to 72 hours. Blurring, photophobia, and disturbance of color vision, have also been reported.[i,298] Four cases of disturbance of color vision have been reported separately by Haut, all transient and characterized by rapid onset of a violet or rose-colored appearance of objects.[h] Scintillating scotomas as from ophthalmic migraine have been described by Dralands in a review of the subject.[301] Apparently all the visual disturbances of rapid onset have been reversible, either spontaneously, or when nalidixic acid was discontinued or dosage was reduced.

Pseudotumor cerebri has been induced by nalidixic acid in several cases, much less commonly than the acute visual disturbances.[a,b,d-g,j,k] The characteristics, have been reviewed by Van Dyk.[386] Principally infants and children have been affected. Elevated intracranial pressure has produced papilledema and sixth nerve palsies. Stopping the medication has brought relief.

Nalidixic acid has been tested for adverse effect on the cornea and sclera in rabbits, because of discovery of disturbances in articular cartilages, but no adverse effect was found.[c]

a. Anderson EE, Anderson B Jr, Nashold BS: Childhood complications of nalidixic acid. *J AM MED ASSOC* 216:1023–1024, 1971.

b. Boreus LO, Sundstrom B: Intracranial hypertension in a child during treatment with nalidixic acid. *BR MED J* 2:744–745, 1967.

c. Bouissou H, Caujolle D, et al: Resistance of ocular conjunctival tissues of the rabbit to nalidixic acid. *J FR OPHTALMOL* 3:607–608, 1980. (French)

d. Cohen DN: Intracranial hypertension and papilledema associated with nalidixic acid therapy. *AM J OPHTHALMOL* 76:680–682, 1973.

e. Comelli A, et al: A case of pseudotumor cerebri during treatment with nalidixic acid. *MINERVA PEDIATR* 25:969–971, 1973. (Italian)

f. Deonna T, et al: Acute intracranial hypertension after nalidixic acid administration. *ARCH DIS CHILD* 49:743, 1974.

g. Guran P, et al: Acute and transitory intracranial hypertension in a 9-year-old child treated with nalidixic acid. *ARCH FR PEDIATR* 29:1107–1111, 1972. (French)

h. Haut J, Haye C, et al: Disturbances of color perception after taking nalidixic acid. *BULL SOC OPHTALMOL FRANCE* 72:147–149, 1972.

i. Marshall BY: Visual side-effects of nalidixic acid. *THE PRACTITIONER* 19:222–224, 1967.

j. Rao KG: Pseudotumor cerebri associated with nalidixic acid. *UROLOGY* 4:204–207, 1974.

k. Walker SH, Salanio I, Standiford WE: Nalidixic acid in childhood urinary tract infections. *CLIN PEDIATR* 5:718, 1966.

Nalorphine (N-allylnormorphine, Nalline), a narcotic antagonist, is not toxic to the eye, but constricts the pupils when given systemically to normal people, and causes the pupil to dilate in people who already have miosis associated with dependence on opioid drugs, such as heroin and morphine.[a, c, 163] Applied as eyedrops to normal human volunteers, a 5% solution causes miosis, and it antagonizes miosis induced by morphine.[b]

    a. Eckenhoff JE, Elder JD, King BD: N-Allylnormorphine in treatment of morphine or demerol narcosis. *AM J MED SCI* 223:191, 1952.
    b. Nomof N, Elliott HW, Parker KD: The local effect of morphine, nalorphine, and codeine on the diameter of the pupil of the eye. *CLIN PHARMACOL THER* 9:358–364, 1968.
    c. Way EL, Mo BPN, et al: Evaluation of the nalorphine pupil diagnostic test for narcotic usage in long-term heroin and opium addicts. *CLIN PHARMACOL THER* 7:300–311, 1966.

Naloxone (N-allylnoroxymorphone, Narcan), a narcotic antagonist, like nalorphine, has no effect on the pupil when administered systemically to normal people, but in people who are dependent on opioid drugs such as morphine and heroin, it causes the pupils to dilate.[a, 163] Topically the effect is similar.[b]

    a. Jasinski DR, Martin WR, Haertzen CA: The human pharmacology and abuse potential of N-allylnoroxymorphone (naloxone). *J PHARMACOL EXP THER* 157:420–426, 1967.
    b. Fanciullacci M, Boccuni M, et al: The naloxone conjunctival test in morphine addiction. *EUR J PHARMACOL* 61:319–320, 1980.

Naphazoline (Privine), a sympathomimetic nasal and ocular vasoconstrictor used topically, has been said to cause moderate mydriasis when applied at 0.1% concentration in eyedrops, but this did not raise the intraocular pressure in normal or glaucomatous patients in whom it was tested.[a]

    a. Gandolfi C: Therapeutic ocular application of sympathomimetic substances. *BOLL OCULIST* 26:397–400, 1947.

Naphthalene (naphthaline, naphthene) has caused little trouble from direct external contact with the eye, but has been of great interest because of severe intraocular effects which can be produced by systemic administration. Formerly it was administered internally as an antiseptic and anthelmintic.

External contact of naphthalene with the eyes is irritating but not injurious unless actual particles are allowed to remain in contact with the cornea.[c] Experimentally when crystals of naphthalene were applied to rabbit eyes and allowed to remain for an unspecified period, local epithelial injury and slight turbidity of the underlying stroma resulted, but in two weeks the cornea cleared and healed completely.[35] In human beings, probably no corneal damage has been produced by the vapors of naphthalene. However, a sensation of eye irritation from the vapor is said to start at a concentration of 15 ppm in air.

Systemic poisoning from ingestion, inhalation, or absorption through the skin causes nausea and vomiting, hematuria from acute hemolysis, hemolytic anemia, injury of the liver, convulsions, and coma.[i, 171] Serious toxic effects on the eye have been well established in poisoned animals, but injury of human eyes from systemic poisoning is uncertain, and rather scantily documented.[g,n,q]

Probably the first instance in which naphthalene was blamed for producing cataract in a human being occurred in 1900.[q] A thirty-six-year-old pharmacist was given 5 g of unpurified naphthalene in an emulsion of castor oil in divided doses in the course of thirteen hours. On awakening eight to nine hours later he had severe pain in the bladder, and found that he was nearly blind, although previously he had had good vision. At examination, almost a year later, according to the published dates, the vision was found to be reduced to finger-counting at 1.5 meters, unimproved by glasses, and the visual fields were constricted to 30° to 50°. In both lenses were seen countless fine whitish opacities arranged as a zonular cataract about the nucleus with a narrow clear zone at the equator. Ophthalmoscopically, the fundi could not be seen clearly because of the changes in the lenses, but the retinas appeared pale and turbid, the vessels were narrowed, and the temporal portions of the papillas seemed pale. A small bright red dot with irregular margins was seen near the macula in the retina of one eye. The clouding of the lenses did not progress.

Around 1900, at the time this case was observed, naphthalene was apparently in common medical use at doses of 3 to 5 g a day, and pain in the urinary tract was a common side effect. No disturbance of vision had been noted previously, and it was pointed out that in the case of the unfortunate pharmacist the naphthalene which was administered had not been purified, whereas other patients received only the purest material.[q]

In 1906 suspicion was expressed that naphthalene had caused cataract and chorioretinitis in other patients.[n] A forty-four-year-old man who worked with naphthalene was found to have vision of 5/8 with spokes of beginning cataract in both lenses and a streak of blood in the retina of one eye. A co-worker, after working with naphthalene powder for three years, had decrease of visual acuity to 5/30 in one eye, and in this eye was found to have chorioretinitis, both recent and old. This patient's other eye was completely normal. In neither case was there other evidence of naphthalene poisoning, nor was there definite evidence to establish that the eye diseases of these patients were related to their contact with naphthalene.[n]

Similarly, a patient briefly mentioned by Koelsch in 1926 was described as having bilateral optic neuritis and a history of having worked with naphthalene for a long time.[77] No evidence of naphthalene poisoning was mentioned. The patient recovered completely in four to five weeks.

In 1956 examination of workers in a plant producing a dye-intermediate from naphthalene was reported to have revealed pinpoint and diffuse opacities in the lenses of eight out of twenty-one employees who ranged in age from twenty to sixty years.[g] However, other industrial surveys have revealed no abnormalities of the eyes in men exposed for years to naphthalene.[d,z]

Among the cases in which naphthalene has been suspected of causing disturbances of the eye, it is noteworthy that only one (the first) involved acute or definite poisoning. On the other hand, several cases of severe acute poisoning from ingestion, inhalation, and probably from skin contact have been reported, with no observed injury to the retina or lens.[a,r]

In rabbits, cataracts from naphthalene added to the diet were observed in 1886, many years before it was suspected in any human case, and since that time it has been studied very extensively in animals.[46] In essence, it has been established that feeding a dose of 1 g/kg induces a variety of changes in the eyes, beginning within a few hours. Nearly all parts of the eyes are affected, but in varying degrees and differing from animal to animal. Early there is usually miosis and hyperemia of the iris and ciliary body. Vitreous opacities appear, and the retina and choroid may develop edema, exudates, crystals, hemorrhages, separation, abnormal pigmentation, and atrophy. Necrosis in the retina has been ascribed to thrombosis of small arteriole branches.[zm] Hemorrhages have been described, principally in the ciliary body. Lens changes in rabbits have been described as appearing as early as the first day, sometimes developing into mature cataract in two weeks.[b,o,44,46,247] On the basis of extensive experience, van Heyningen has stated, "the appearance of cataract was very variable; in some animals there were severe changes after a few days and in others there were no changes after 1–2 weeks of daily dosage. Sometimes only the lens was damaged and sometimes only the retina. Sometimes both tissues were affected and sometimes neither. But the variable response was not related to the pigmentation of the animal."[zl]

Cataracts also develop in rats, but appear to differ from those in rabbits.[h,p,zl] In particular, pigmented rats are much more prone to develop naphthalene cataracts than are albinos.[p,zl] Van Heyningen has provided evidence that in rats an enzyme associated with pigmented tissues, polyphenol oxidase, plays a crucial role, whereas in rabbits an enzyme in the lens, catechol reductase, plays the crucial role and is unrelated to tissue pigments.[zl] Otherwise, the metabolism of naphthalene and formation of cataractogenic intermediates appears to be the same in rabbits and rats.

Many factors which might conceivably be involved in the experimental production of cataract by naphthalene have been explored by a long list of investigators. It was long ago ascertained that naphthalene was ineffectual in inducing cataracts when introduced directly into the eye.[j] Changes in the composition of the lens and aqueous humor, such as decrease of ascorbate and glutathione, have particularly been noted, and much attention has been given to changes in permeability of the blood-aqueous barrier.[v,zg] There is a loss of potassium and gain of sodium and chloride in the lens,[x] and a loss of amino acids and glutathione from the lens, giving a transient elevation in the aqueous humor while opacities are developing.[o,12] Several studies on enzyme activities in naphthalene cataractous lenses have been made.[y,zf,zh] Additive injurious influences have also been demonstrated by Hockwin and associates showing in rabbits that development of naphthalene cataracts can be enhanced by subjecting the eyes to x-irradiation, paracentesis, or subconjunctival injection of pilocarpine.[l]

The morphology of changes in the lens has been examined by light and electron microscopy, showing characteristic changes in the epithelium of the lens, and aggregates of insoluble proteins, but normal capsule.[s,t] Abnormalities have also been seen in the epithelium of the ciliary body and in the retinal pigment epithelium.[t,zb] Severe damage of the retina in naphthalene-fed rabbits has been studied in flat preparations. Spotty circular patches of abnormality of pigment epithelium and overlying retina are visible both ophthalmoscopically and in flat preparation. Damage of the retinal pigment epithelium may precede damage of the retina itself.[zb] The metabolism of naphthalene and the toxicity of its metabolites to the lens have been studied extensively by Pirie and van Heyningen, who have shown that in rabbits 1,2-dihydroxynaphthalene and 1,2-naphthoquinone (β-naphthoquinone) are produced enzymatically and by autoxidation, and that they are the metabolic intermediates responsible for naphthalene cataractogenesis.[za-zc,ze,zi-zk] Naphthalene poisoning and cataract production can be imitated by administering 1,2-naphthoquinone to animals.[zn-zq] (Also see INDEX for *1,2-naphthoquinone.*)

Van Heyningen in a resume published in 1979 considered that it was then "generally accepted, that one or more metabolic products of naphthalene reaches the eye by way of the bloodstream, reacts with the constituents of the lens and thus disrupts its integrity and transparency.[zl]" Three metabolites in the blood of poisoned rabbits that could be enzymatically converted to the toxic intermediate 1,2-dihydroxynaphthalene were naphthalene diol, naphthalenediol glucuronide, and 1,2-dihydroxynaphthalene sulfate. (Naphthalene diol caused cataracts when dropped on the rabbit's eye, and produced retinal lesions when injected systemically.[zi-zl])

Naphthoquinone, which is produced in the eye by autoxidation of 1,2-dihydroxynaphthalene, reacts with several constituents of the lens and causes degenerative changes. Also naphthoquinone catalyzes oxidation of ascorbic acid in the aqueous and vitreous humors, ultimately producing oxalic acid, which precipitates as calcium oxalate, forming the vitreous opacities that are seen in rabbits poisoned with naphthalene.[za-zc,zl]

Besides, 1,2-naphthoquinone, certain other compounds related to naphthalene have toxic effects on the eyes similar to those of naphthalene. Naphthol has been suspected of producing cataract in human beings. In animals, cataracts have been induced by means of decahydronaphthalene, tetrahydronaphthalene, and 2-methoxy-1,2,3,4-tetrahydronaphthalene.[307] Retinal degeneration has been induced by naphthol.

Among the means of detoxication of naphthalene in rabbits is conjugation with glucuronic acid, which may have a protective influence against development of naphthalene cataract.[u,w] An inhibitory effect on development of naphthalene cataracts in the rabbit by means of Catalin has been demonstrated, presumably by interference with toxic reaction of quinones with lens sulfhydryl groups.[m]

(For further information on various compounds mentioned above related to Naphthalene, see the INDEX.)

a. Abelson SM, Henderson AI: Moth ball poisoning. *U.S. ARMED FORCE MED J* 2:491–493, 1951.

b. Adams DR: The nature of the ocular lesions produced experimentally by naphthalene. *BR J OPHTHALMOL* 14:49–60, 397–401, 545–576, 1930.

c. Anonymous: Naphthalene. *AM PETROL INST TOXIC REV,* 1959.

d. Axenfeld: Is naphthalene protection against lice-nuisance and are naphthalene vapors of concern for the eye? *KLIN MONATSBL AUGENHEILKD* 54:517, 1915. (German)

f. Fujiwara T: Studies on the total glutathione of aqueous humor in cataract. *ACTA SOC OPHTHALMOL JPN* 72:1744–1752, 1968.

g. Ghetti G, Mariani L: Eye changes due to naphthalene. *MED LAVORO* 47:533–538, 1956. (Italian)

h. Goldmann H: Experimental supranuclear cataract and nuclear sclerosis. *KLIN MONATSBL AUGENHEILKD* 83:433–438, 1929. (German)

i. Grigor WG, Robin H, Harley JD: An Australian variant on "full-moon disease." *MED J AUST* 2:1229–1230, 1966.

j. Hess C: On the naphthalene-induced changes in massage cataract of the rabbit eye. *BER DTSCH OPHTHALMOL GESELLSCH* 19:54, 1887. (German)

l. Hockwin O, Okamoto T, et al: Genesis of cataracts: Cumulative effects of subliminal noxious influences. *ANN OPHTHALMOL* 1:321–325, 1969.

m. Hockwin O, Weigelin E, et al: The effect of Catalin on experimentally induced lens opacities in the rabbit. *BER DTSCH OPHTHALMOL GESELLSCH* 69:452–457, 1969. (German)

n. van der Hoeve J: Chorioretinitis in human beings from the action of naphthalene. *ARCH AUGENHEILKD* 56:259–262, 1906. (German)

o. Igersheimer J, Ruben L: On the morphology and pathogenesis of naphthalene-induced changes in the eye. *GRAEFES ARCH OPHTHALMOL* 74:456, 1910. (German)

p. Koch HR, Doldi K, Hockwin O: Naphthalene cataracts in rats. *DOC OPHTHALMOL PROC SER* 8:293–303, 1976.

q. Lezenius A: A case of naphthalene cataract in a human being. *KLIN MONATSBL AUGENHEILKD* 40:129–140, 1902. (German)

r. MacGregor RR: Naphthalene poisoning from ingestion of mothballs. *CAN MED ASSOC J* 70:313–314, 1954.

s. Matsuto T: Scanning electron microscopic studies on the lens of rabbits with experimental naphthalin cataract. *FOLIA OPHTHALMOL JPN* 27:885, 1976. (English summary)

t. Matsuura H: Electron microscopic studies of lens and ciliary body of rabbits with experimental naphthalene cataract. *ACTA SOC OPHTHALMOL JPN* 72:1708–1732, 1968.

u. Mizukawa T, Takagi Y, Hama H: The inhibitive action of glucuronic acid upon the development of naphthalene cataract. *JPN J OPHTHALMOL* 2:30–35, 1958.

v. Mizukawa T, Takagi Y, et al: Studies on the cause of naphthalene cataract of rabbit. *ACTA SOC OPHTHALMOL JPN* 62B:1401–1409, 1958.

w. Okamura H: Relation between the development of naphthalene cataract and the fluctuation of conjugated glucuronic acid in serum. *ACTA SOC OPHTHALMOL JPN* 66:290–303, 1962.

x. Oshima T: Studies on the electrolytes and water of the various experimental cataracts. *ACTA SOC OPHTHALMOL JPN* 72:1753–1758, 1968.

y. Ozawa H: Histochemical studies on the transparent ocular tissue. *ACTA SOC OPHTHALMOL JPN* 73:1155–1164, 1969.

z. Pike MH: Ocular pathology due to organic compounds. *J MICHIGAN MED SOC* 43:581–584, 1944.

za. Pirie A, van Heyningen R: Reactions of 1,2-dihydroxynaphthalene and of 1,2-naphthoquinone with eye constituents. *BIOCHEM J* 100:70P–71P, 1966.

zb. Pirie A: Pathology in the eye of the naphthalene-fed rabbit. *EXP EYE RES* 7:354–357, 1968.

zc. Pirie A, van Heyningen R: Naphthalene cataract (2). In Dardenne M, Nordmann J. (Eds.): BIOCHEMISTRY OF THE EYE. Base/New York, Karger, 1968, pp. 410–412.

zd. Ponte F: Action of naphthalene and some of its derivatives on anaerobic glycolysis. *BOLL SOC ITAL BIOL SPER* 33:1792–1794, 1957.

ze. Rees JR, Pirie A: Possible reactions of 1,2-naphthoquinone in the eye. *BIOCHEM J* 102:853–863, 1967.

zf. Salmony D: Some biochemical changes in naphthalene cataract. *BR J OPHTHALMOL* 44:29–34, 1960.

zg. Sapuppo C: Histamine and experimental cataract from naphthalene. *G ITAL OTTAL-MOL* 11:193–198, 1958. (Italian)

zh. Srivastava SK, Nath RL: Metabolic alterations in experimental cataract. *INDIAN J MED RES* 57:225–227, 1969. (*CHEM ABSTR* 7:37203, 1969.)

zi. van Heyningen R, Pirie A: The metabolism of naphthalene by the rabbit eye. *BIOCHEM J* 100:70P, 1966.

zj. van Heyningen R, Pirie A: Naphthalene cataract (1). In Dardenne M, Nordmann J, (Eds.): BIOCHEMISTRY OF THE EYE. Basel/New York, Karger, 1968, pp. 407–409.

zk. van Heyningen R, Pirie A: The metabolism of naphthalene and its toxic effect on the eye. *BIOCHEM J* 102:842–852, 1967.

zl. van Heyningen R: Naphthalene cataract in rats and rabbits; a resume. *EXP EYE RES* 28:435–439, 1979.

zm. Verdi GP: Histologic and pathogenetic study of experimental retinal lesions after naphthaline intoxication. *BOLL OCULIST* 37:50–66, 1958. (*AM J OPHTHALMOL* 46:765, 1958.)

zn. Yuge T: Cataract and hexose monophosphate shunt of lens. Mechanism of cataract caused by β-naphthoquinone. *ACTA SOC OPHTHALMOL JPN* 66:1135–1144, 1962.

zo. Yuge T, Ueda K, Nose Y: Biochemical studies on naphthalene cataract *JPN J OPHTHALMOL* 7:36–47, 1963.

zp. Yuge T: Additional biochemical studies on naphthalene cataract. *ACTA OPHTHALMOL SOC JPN* 70:533–536, 1966.

zq. Yuge T: Na-K-ATPase of the lens and its role on the lens swelling. *JPN J OPHTHALMOL* 10:142–148, 1966.

Naphthalenebutylsulfonate, sodium (Nekal) is a textile-wetting agent. As a dust in the air it has caused severe irritation of the eyes and respiratory tract of human beings and animals.[a]

a. Scaglioni C, Brina A: Experimental study of the pathology of sodium naphthalenebutyl-sulfonate or nekal. *MED LAVORO* 37:140–146, 1946.

Naphthaphenanthridine is said to have caused a rise in intraocular pressure in the monkey, but this is still to be confirmed.[149]

1-Naphthol (α-naphthol), in rabbits produced fine yellow spots in the retina according to van der Hoeve in 1910 and Takamura in 1911, after repeated intravenous injection.[a, 153] (See also *2-Naphthol*.)

1-Naphthol on the surface of rabbit eyes is irritating,[b] causing damage, graded 9 on a scale of 1 to 10,[228] and scarring of cornea and conjunctiva.[c]

a. van der Hoeve J: Effect of naphthol on the eye of human beings and animals, and on fetal eyes. *GRAEFES ARCH OPHTHALMOL* 85:305–317, 1913. (German)

b. Lloyd GK, Liggett MP, et al: Assessment of the acute toxicity and potential irritancy of hair dye constituents. *FOOD COSMET TOXICOL* 15:607–610, 1977.

c. Nemtsev GI, Piatnitskaya LV: Action of alpha- and beta-naphthol and intermediates on the cornea and conjunctiva. *OFTALMOL ZH* 28:471–472, 1973. (English summary)

2-Naphthol (β-naphthol) has had medical uses as a counterirritant in alopecia, also as an anthelmintic, and as an antiseptic in treatment of scabies.[171] Toxic effects on the eyes have been described by van der Hoeve in patients and in rabbits.[a,b]

A forty-year-old man treated with 3% 2-naphthol salve for eczema of the neck and face developed irritation of the eyes, and about a half year later was found to have opacities of the posterior cortex of both lenses. An eleven-year-old girl treated for loss of hair by application of 10% 2-naphthol ointment to the scalp for several months developed white spots and edema in the ocular fundus, with reduction of vision. She eventually developed hundreds of small slightly pigmented spots in the fundi, but no cataracts. A twenty-one-year-old patient developed transitory streaks in the posterior portion of one lens after application of 10% ointment to the head, and this was accompanied by some reduction of vision. A twenty-eight-year-old patient taking 4 g of *benzonaphthol* a day for sixteen weeks for intestinal complaints had normal vision but many yellow-white spots in both fundi.[a]

Twenty patients who were treated for scabies by rubbing 50 g of a salve containing 7.5% 2-naphthol over the whole body morning and evening for two days were reported to have developed hyperemia of the fundus and many had very small white and pigmented spots in the retina. Vitreous opacities were noticed in two cases. Only in one case was abnormality of the lens observed, and this was only a dot in the posterior cortex. Visual acuity was reported to be impaired in two cases, but neither of these had normal eyes before the treatment.[b]

Experimentally in rabbits the most consistent ocular change induced by administering 2-naphthol either by stomach or by application to the skin was a development in the retina of small white shiny flecks which soon became pigmented.[b] These became more numerous and increased in size as daily administration of the chemical continued. The retinal vessels and the iris commonly became hyperemic. The aqueous was sometimes slightly turbid, and the vitreous commonly became turbid early, but then cleared despite continuing administration of naphthol. The cornea and conjunctiva were never involved.

Changes in the lenses were observed by van der Hoeve in many rabbits, but other investigators failed to find them.[a,b] They were described as a change in refractile properties, or as glass-clear spokes, with later development of small opacities at the equator, at the posterior suture, or at the posterior pole of the lens, but never developing to complete cataracts. These changes in the lenses did not appear regularly. They appeared to have no relationship to the incidence of the more constant retinal changes, and were sometimes completely absent in spite of marked retinal abnormality. When 2-naphthol was administered to pregnant rabbits, the offspring had congenital cataracts, degeneration of the neuroepithelium, and hypertrophy of the retinal pigment cells.[b] In the retinas of poisoned adult rabbits spotty degeneration of the rods and cones and irregular variation in the amount of pigment in the pigment epithelium were observed. Vacuoles were present in the nuclear and nerve fiber layer and the ciliary epithelium.[b]

In rabbit lenses surviving in culture, very little disturbance of either cation transport or glycolysis has been produced by 2-naphthol.[126]

In rats, Fitzhugh and Buschke produced perinuclear cataracts in the form of a shell by feeding *naphthalene,* and also by feeding 2-naphthol.[307] Similar cataracts were produced by the following series of naphthol derivatives: *2-naphthylethyl ether;*

2-naphthylmethyl ether; 2-naphthylsalicylate; 1,2,3,4-tetrahydro-2-naphthol (β-tetralol); 1,2,3,4-tetrahydro-2-naphthylpropionate.[307] Cataracts in rats were also produced by repeated parenteral injections of *2-naphthoxyacetic acid* and *2-naphthylsalicylate.*[362]

(For information on other compounds related to 2-naphthol, see INDEX for *Naphthalene; 1-Naphthol; 1,2-Naphthoquinone; 2-Naphthyl benzoate;* and *2-(2-Naphthyloxy) ethanol.*)

a. van der Hoeve J: On the injurious action of β-naphthol in therapeutic doses on the human eye. *GRAEFES ARCH OPHTHALMOL* 53:74–78, 1901. (German)
b. van der Hoeve J: Action of naphthol on human and animal eyes and on fetal eyes. *GRAEFES ARCH OPHTHALMOL* 85:305–317, 1913. (German)

1,2-Naphthoquinone (β-naphthoquinone) appears to be the metabolite in naphthalene poisoning that reacts with ocular tissues and is responsible for production of cataract and damage to the retina. This quinone is probably formed by autoxidation of 1,2-dihydroxynaphthalene, another metabolite of naphthalene, but it reacts so readily with lens constituents that only the characteristic products, oxalate in the case of ascorbic acid, and discolored proteins in the lens, are evidences of its formation and reaction.[e,f] Reactions have also been demonstrated with various amino acids, glutathione, and proteins in the lens.[c,e] In cultured lenses 1,2-naphthoquinone inhibits the NaK–ATPase of the epithelium, reducing the uptake of potassium and increasing sodium uptake, leading to formation of vacuoles beneath the capsule and swelling of the lens as in naphthalene poisoning. Cation transport, glycolysis, and passage of lactate out of the lens are interfered with.[b,c,e–j] Acid production by embryonic chick lens in culture is inhibited.[a] The morphology of cultured lens epithelium with addition of naphthoquinone has been studied by electron microscopy.[d] (Also see *Naphthalene.*)

a. Edwards A, Marsh J, et al: Use of embryonic chick lens for screening potentially toxic chemicals. *EXP EYE RES* 10:288–292, 1970.
b. Friedburg D, Mayer U: Effect of β-naphthoquinone on glycolytic enzymes of lens epithelium. *GRAEFES ARCH OPHTHALMOL* 183:152–157, 1971. (German)
c. Ikemoto F, Iwata S, Narita F: Biochemical studies on the enucleated lens. *YAKUGAKU ZASSHI* 99:945–949, 1968.
d. Koniszewski G, Mayer U: Electron-microscopic changes in surviving eye tissue after addition of naphthoquinone. *BER DTSCH OPHTHALMOL GESELLSCH* 74:676–681, 1977.
e. Rees JR, Pirie A (1967):—see *Naphthalene* bibliography.
f. Van Heyningen R, Pirie A (1967):—see *Naphthalene* bibliography.
g. Yuge T (1962,1966):—see *Naphthalene* bibliography.
h. Yuge T: The effect of β-naphthoquinone upon Na and K levels and Na-K–ATPase of calf lens. *ACTA SOC OPHTHALMOL JPN* 70:2176–2178, 1966.
i. Yuge T, Takeda H: An autoradiographic study on naphthalene cataract. *FOLIA OPHTHALMOL JPN* 24:187–189, 1973. (English summary)
j. Yuge T, Takeda H, Tani M: Studies on naphthalene cataract and ion transport of rabbit lens. *NIPPON GANKA GAKKAI ZASSHI* 81:1437–1441, 1977. (English summary)

2-Naphthyl benzoate (betanaphthol benzoate, benzonaphthol) apparently has toxic effects similar to those of 2-naphthol to which it is supposed to be hydrolyzed in the body. One patient is known to have taken 4 g a day for sixteen weeks, after which the optic papillas were hyperemic and many yellowish white dots were seen in the fundi. The vision however was 6/6 and 6/8.[153] (Compare *2-Naphthol.*)

2-(2-Naphthyloxy) ethanol (β-naphthoxyethanol, Anavenol), an intravenous anesthetic in animals, has been reported to have produced retinal hemorrhages and infarcts of retinal vessels in horses.[64]

Naproxen, a non-steroidal anti-inflammatory, as of 1982 had no proven adverse ocular effects, and the instances of possible "decreased vision", "subcapsular cataracts", or "optic neuritis" reported to Fraunfelder's National Registry were too few to raise serious suspicions.[312]

Natrin (sodium 2,4,5-trichlorophenoxyethyl sulfate; 2,4,5-TES), a weed killer, according to information from a manufacturer, is said to cause "moderate skin irritation and severe damage to the eyes," but more specific information has not been given.[70]

Neoarsphenamine (Neosalvarsan, Novarsenobenzol) differs chemically and in toxic effects from the various derivatives of arsanilic acid which cause optic neuritis and atrophy. Neoarsphenamine has no recognized tendency to injure the optic nerve or retina when given systemically, though it has been shown to cause selective degeneration of the rod cells when added at a concentration of 5×10^{-6}M to animal retina surviving in tissue culture.[99]

Cases of blindness attributed to neoarsphenamine have been rare, and possibly caused by syphilis or other disease. One woman receiving neoarsphenamine became suddenly and permanently blind, and when examined on the second day had constricted, ensheathed retinal arteries and pale optic nerveheads.[c] In three other cases, loss of vision has been associated with intraocular inflammation with exudates into the vitreous, more likely caused by disease than by the drug.[a,b]

Transient myopia, similar to that which has been noted with arsphenamine, has been observed as a rare side effect.[d] Typically the pupils have not been disturbed, but myopia has increased to a maximum in about eighteen hours after injection and subsided in the course of two days.

Applied to the eyes of animals, 1% neoarsphenamine has caused temporary corneal opacification and edema.[e] (See also *Arsenicals, organic.*)

a. Gregorio S: Changes in the ocular fundus during treatment with Neosalvarsan. *BOLL OCULIST* 3:351–358, 1924. (Italian)
b. Gouin J, Bienvenue A, LeBigot: Blindness after Novarsenobenzol. *BULL SOC FRANC DERM* 42:317–318, 1935. (French)
c. Juler F: A case of blindness after NAB. *BR MED J* 3852:809–810, 1934.
d. Redslob E, Levy G: Spasmodic myopia from Novarsenobenzol. *REV OTOL* 6:801–804, 1928. (French)
e. Ross EL, Lederer LG: Influence of some toxic substances on the inner ear. *TRANS AM OTOL SOC* 27:327–344, 1937.

Neodymium chloride, one of the rare-earth salts, tested as a 50% solution by application of 0.1 ml to rabbit eyes, caused ulceration of the conjunctiva, but no opacity of the cornea,[a] and as a 25% solution at approximately pH 5 applied repeatedly during ten minutes it also did not produce corneal opacity. However, when applied in the same manner after mechanical removal of the epithelium from the cornea to permit penetration, it produced severe damage to the stroma of the cornea, much as other rare-earth or lanthanide salts do. Within one day after the denuded cornea was exposed, it developed dense gray opacities. These persisted, the cornea becoming hard and dense within four weeks.[90] (See also, *Rare-earth salts.*)

a. Haley TJ, Komesu N, et al: Pharmacology and toxicology of praseodymium and neodymium chlorides. *TOXICOL APPL PHARMACOL* 6:614–620, 1964.

Neomycin, an antimicrobial, has a tendency to cause allergic reaction of the eye and skin upon prolonged repeated use.[a,c,d,f] Characteristic lesions of the corneal epithelium in the form of tiny snowflakes, usually associated with sensation of irritation, may develop and may persist for weeks after application of neomycin to the eye is discontinued.[a] Kaufman has noted blepharitis apparently caused by inspissation of meibomian gland secretion by neomycin.[336] Studies on corneal wound healing have shown topical neomycin not to interfere at low concentrations that are effectively antibacterial.[354,368,382] However, at high concentrations of 1 to 10% applied to rabbit eyes for 30 days degeneration of corneal nerves has been reported.[g] A single instance of temporary difficulty in swallowing, speaking, and breathing has been attributed to disturbance of neuromuscular transmission by absorption of eye drops containing both neomycin and polymyxin B.[b]

Cotlier has described in detail damage of the lens and formation of cataract in rabbits from intravitreal injection of polymyxin B sulfate, and has said that "similar effects" were obtained with neomycin sulfate.[297]

No toxic reaction was observed clinically in 250 human eyes after post-operative irrigation of the anterior chamber with 0.25 to 0.5 ml of a solution containing 0.5% neomycin plus 0.1% polymyxin B, and in rabbits no evidence of injury was found histologically after similar treatment.[e]

a. Dohlman CH: (Reply to Query). *ARCH OPHTHALMOL* 76:902, 1966.
b. Koenig A, Ohrloff C: Influence on neuromuscular transmission from local application of Isoptomax eye drops. *KLIN MONATSBL AUGENHEILKD* 179:109–112, 1981. (German)
c. Kruyswijk MRJ, Van Driel LMJ, Go-Sennema AA: Contact allergy following administration of eyedrops and eye ointments. *DOC OPHTHALMOL* 48:251–253, 1980.
d. Maucher OM: Periorbital eczema as iatrogenic disturbance. *KLIN MONATSBL AUGENHEILKD* 164:350–356, 1974. (German)
e. McCoy DA, McIntyre MW, Turnbull DC: Irrigation of anterior chamber with neomycin-polymyxin solution in intraocular surgery. *ARCH OPHTHALMOL* 79:506, 1968.
f. Schubert H: Contact eczema in the region of the eye. *KLIN MONATSBL AUGENHEILKD* 151:457–464, 1967. (German)
g. Verzin AA, Mirzayants MG: Local use of neomycin. Histomorphological changes in the neuroreceptor apparatus of rabbit cornea. *ANTIBIOTIKI (MOSCOW)* 21:79–81, 1976. (English abstract)

Neurine (trimethylvinyl ammonium hydroxide) in 5% aqueous solution damages rabbit eyes in the same manner as 5% trimethylamine, causing hemorrhagic conjunctivitis and corneal edema with superficial opacities.[63] Neutral *Neurine chloride* is not known to be injurious to the cornea.[80]

Niacin (Nicotinic acid), a vitamin, has been used as a systemic vasodilator. Adverse ocular effects have rarely been reported with adequate documentation. In rare instances in which rise of intraocular pressure in glaucoma has been attributed to nicotinic acid the evidence has been vague and questionable.[a,f] Systematic, controlled studies have shown no significant tendency for nicotinic acid to raise the intraocular pressure in open-angle glaucomatous eyes.[c,193]

Concerning possible effects of nicotinic acid on vision, Parsons and Flinn in 1957 noted that one patient taking 3 to 6 g per day complained of medication-related blurring of vision, but no ocular abnormalities were found after the high dosage was discontinued.[d] Toxic amblyopia was suspected in another patient as a result of taking 4 to 6 g per day for a year, but this diagnosis was based only on a complaint of slight blur, with a change in vision with glasses from 20/20 in both eyes to 20/30 in one eye and 20/25 in the other, associated with paracentral relative scotomas. The suspicion seemed to be supported by relief of the patient's complaint within three days after stopping nicotinic acid, and by return of visual acuity to 20/20.[b] Another patient was said to have developed proptosis and ocular edema on similar dosage.[b] Gass in 1973 reported three patients who lost central vision from an atypical form of cystoid macular edema, without fluorescein leakage, while being given 3 to 5 g of nicotinic acid per day for hypercholesterolemia. When the medication was stopped, the vision and maculas improved. One of the patients had two recurrences when he resumed taking large doses of nicotinic acid.[f]

No injuries of the eye appear to have been reported from direct contact with nicotinic acid.

a. Gallois J: Nicotinic acid and the principle of elective minimal vasodilatation in ophthalmology. *ARCH OPHTALMOL (PARIS)* 5:197–208, 1945. (French)
b. Harris JL: Toxic amblyopia associated with administration of nicotinic acid. *AM J OPHTHALMOL* 55:133, 1963.
c. Miura M: A new functional test for aqueous outflow with vasodilators. *FOLIA OPHTHALMOL JPN* 18:396–409, 1967.
d. Parsons WB Jr, Flinn JH: Reduction in elevated blood cholesterol levels by large doses of nicotinic acid. *J AM MED ASSOC* 165:234, 1957.
e. Zaverucha FM: Nicotinic acid in glaucoma. *VESTN OFTALMOL* 31:31–35, 1952. (English summary)
f. Gass JDM: Nicotinic acid maculopathy. *AM J OPHTHALMOL* 76:500–510, 1973.

Nialamide, an antidepressant, has been held in some suspicion as a possible cause of optic neuritis because it is a monoamine oxidase inhibitor, but there has been no proof. Vague visual symptoms have occasionally been mentioned without elucidation. In one case the question was raised whether the damage caused to the optic nerve by *pheniprazine,* a definitely toxic MAO inhibitor, could have been aggravated by subsequent administration of nialamide, but this was inconclusive.[b] In another case retrobulbar neuritis developed in a patient receiving nialamide, but the evidence was not clear that this was the only drug involved; another definitely toxic MAO inhibitor, *octamoxin,* may also have been involved.[a]

Intraocular pressure in rabbits has been acutely reduced by intravenous injection of nialamide, and the MAO in the ciliary body was shown to be inhibited.[c] In patients no effect on intraocular pressure has been reported. (See also *Monoamine oxidase inhibitors.*)

a. Sourdille MJ: Optic neuritis from inhibitors of monoamine oxidase. *BULL SOC OPHTALMOL FRANCE* 64:981–990, 1964. (French)
b. Stenkula S, Wranne I: Can optic atrophy caused by pheniprazine treatment become aggravated by subsequent nialamid treatment? *ACTA OPHTHALMOL* 44:387–389, 1966.
c. Tarkkanen A, Mustakallio A: Inhibition of monoamine oxidase in the rabbit cillary epithelium. *ACTA OPHTHALMOL* 44:558–563, 1966.

Nibufin (dibutyl-p-nitrophenyl phosphate), a cholinesterase inhibitor, is reported to have caused not only increased tear production but transient change in the b-wave of the ERG, when applied as 0.33% solution to the conjunctival sac of dogs and rats.[a]

a. Lapina IA, Sukhinin VP: Action of Nibufin on the electric activity in the eye and on the function and morphology of the lacrimal gland. *FARMIKOL TOXIK* 1:18–22, 1968. (*RUSSIAN PHARMACOL TOXIC* 31:12, 1968.)

Nickel is a well-known cause of contact dermatitis in sensitized individuals. In the region of the eyes it has resulted from contact with nickel spectacle frames, but the eye itself has not been involved.[e,46] Workers employed in nickel plating have developed conjunctivitis and epiphora when ventilation was poor.[b]

Nickel carbonyl has induced ocular anomalies, including anophthalmia and microphthalmia, in the offspring of rats when inhaled early in pregnancy.[d]

Nickel metal implanted as a foreign particle in the vitreous body of rabbits has caused an inflammatory reaction with damage to ciliary body and lens, cyclitic membrane, and detachment of the retina.[340] Clinically, intraocular foreign bodies of nickel are severely damaging.

Nickel subsulfide injected into the vitreous body of rats has induced malignant tumors in 14 out of 15 eyes.[a]

Nickel salts added to the feed of sheep is said to cause blindness.[c]

a. Albert DM, Gonder JR, et al: Induction of ocular neoplasms by intraocular injection of nickel subsulfide. *INVEST OPHTHALMOL VIS SCI* 22:768–782, 1982.
b. Nechipurenko NP: Eye lesions in workers in nickel industry and their prevention. *VESTN OFTAL* 78:42, 1965.
c. Roslyakov AK, Baiturin MA, Izbasarov ZU: Prevention of nickel blindness of sheep in the Aktyubinsk Region. *TR ALMA-AT ZOOVET INST* 24:142–144, 1972. (English abstract)

d. Sunderman FW Jr, Allpass PR, et al: Eye malformations in rats; induction by prenatal exposure to nickel carbonyl. *SCIENCE* 203:550–553, 1979.

e. Taylor W, Fergusson A: Dermatitis from wearing Army spectacles. *BR MED J* July 1945, p.40.

Nifedipine (Adalat; Procardia), a coronary vasodilator, administered sublingually, has had no adverse effect on intraocular pressure of normal or glaucomatous people.[a]

a. Schnell D: Responses of intraocular pressure in normal subjects and glaucoma patients to single and repeated doses of the coronary drug Adalat. In: Lochner W, et al, ed. NEW THERAPY IN ISCHEMIC HEART DISEASE. Berlin, Springer, 1975, pp.290–302.

Nigericin, a carboxylic ionophore, when added to the medium in which mouse lenses are cultured, causes change in the lens sodium to potassium ratio, leading to irreversible opacification of the periphery of the lens after several hours of incubation.[a]

a. Iwata S, Horiuchi M: Studies on experimental cataracts induced by ionophores. *EXP EYE RES* 31:543–551, 1980.

Niobium pentachloride (columbium pentachloride) has been tested on rabbit eyes by applying 1 mg, which caused blinking and redness of the conjunctivae during the first hour, but in twenty-four hours the eyes were entirely normal.[a]

a. Haley TJ, Monesu N, Raymond K: Pharmacology and toxicology of niobium chloride. *TOXICOL APPL PHARMACOL* 4:385–392, 1962.

Nitric acid in contact with the eye causes immediate opacification of the corneal and conjunctival epithelium, imparting a yellow color when the acid is concentrated. In general the burns resemble those of other strong acids, such as hydrochloric acid.

In the most serious cases, as in accidental application of nitric acid to the eyes of newborn children in place of dilute silver nitrate solution, several eyes have been lost as a result of corneal opacification, symblepharon, and shrinkage of the globe.[a] In milder cases, involving a very small quantity, a low concentration, or rapid decontamination with water, the epithelium which is initially opacified may slough off in a day or two revealing clear underlying cornea. In such cases the eye may return completely to normal as the epithelium regenerates.[153] Good visual results have been obtained even in occasional instances in which it was felt necessary to perform a transplant of buccal mucosa because of the degree of conjunctival necrosis.[b,c]

Experimentally, nitric acid changes the physical properties of excised pieces of corneal stroma so that they do not swell in water in a normal manner. The effect of nitric acid is not notably different from that of other common acids, such as hydrochloric or sulfuric acid.[79] Nitric acid has no exceptional tendency to penetrate through the cornea.[79]

a. Ask F: Four cases of severe injury of the eye from interchanging Credé solution with nitric acid. *SVENSK LAKARTIDNINGEN* 22:449–453, 1953.

b. Catsourakis N: A case of corneal and conjunctival burn by nitric acid. *BULL SOC HELLEN OPHTALMOL* 17:165, 1950.

c. Veasey CA: Nitric acid burn of eye-ball. *OPHTHAL REC* 14:238, 1905.

m-Nitroaniline in test application of 10 to 20 mg of powder to an unanesthetized rabbit's eye caused no evident discomfort and no injury.[81]

Nitrobenzene (nitrobenzol) can be absorbed through the skin as well as by breathing the vapor, and can induce methemoglobinemia. The most reliably established ocular effects are secondary to discoloration of the blood from methemoglobinemia, and consist of brown discoloration of the vessels of the fundus and the conjunctiva.[a, 153]

Information on possible effects on vision is much less reliable, because most exposures to nitrobenzene have occurred industrially and have usually involved a mixture of substances, such as dinitrobenzene, nitrochlorobenzene, chlorodinitrobenzene, and aniline. It has been claimed that both nitrobenzene and dinitrobenzene have caused diminution of central visual acuity, contraction of visual fields, and rarely central scotoma.[b, 41, 247] The effects of dinitrobenzene on vision are better documented than those attributed to nitrobenzene

  a. Yoshida K: A case of nitrobenzene poisoning with ophthalmoscopic changes. ACTA SOC OPHTHALMOL JPN 39:862–864, 1935.
  b. Yoshida K: A case of nitrobenzene poisoning with ophthalmoscopic changes. JPN J MED SCI X OPHTHALMOL 2:559, 1940.

o-Nitrobenzylchloride is a significantly stronger lacrimogenic eye irritant than simple benzylchloride, and it has been noted to cause irritation of the eyes in people working with it in the pharmaceutical industry.[155, 176]

2-Nitro-1-butene has been examined for irritant effects in relation to smog, and found at 0.1 to 0.5 ppm of air to cause sensation of eye irritation in normal people in about three minutes.[143]

Nitrocellulose paint or **lacquer,** now less used than formerly, was composed of nitrocellulose dissolved in volatile solvents, mixed with plasticizers and colored pigments, dyes, or lakes. Ocular disturbances ranging from keratitis to optic neuritis have been ascribed to various of the components, but in most cases the relationship has been indefinite; rarely has there been satisfactory identification of a specific component responsible for the alleged toxic effects.

In a report from the Soviet Union, which is difficult to evaluate, it has been claimed that the *nitrocellulose* itself has caused special type of cataract in paintsprayers.[a] A peculiar peripheral opacity was said typically to develop in the form of a ring, concentric with the lens equator.

  a. Glezerov CY: Cataract caused by nitro-paint. *VESTN OFTAL* 5:46–49, 1956.

Nitrofurantoin (Furadantin, Furantoin, Macrodantin), a urinary antibacterial administered orally, is reported in some patients to have produced severe itching and burning of the eyes, with excess tearing. The symptoms are said to have persisted in some cases for weeks after the medication was stopped.[d] Other adverse effects on the eyes apparently have been very rare. Only one instance of retrobulbar neuritis seems to have been published[a] during the time that 137 cases of sensorimotor peripheral neuropathy, mostly affecting the legs were reported in the world literature.[f] In notifications to registries of adverse drug reactions, in Sweden with 921 reports, effects on eyes or vision were unlisted,[b] in the United Kingdom, with 92 reports of either polyneuropathy or CNS reaction, only 2 cases of "abnormal vision" (undefined) were included,[c] and in the United States Fraunfelder has noted a few cases of paralysis of extraocular muscles, and called attention to two published cases of papilledema from pseudotumor.[312] Walsh and Hoyt described one case of unilateral paralysis of the third cranial nerve, with recovery when administration of nitrofurantoin was discontinued.[256] Vertical diplopia and ataxic gait, both reversible, developed in one out of fourteen volunteers after taking 400 mg a day for 10 days.[e]

   a. Hakamies L: Nitrofurantoin polyneuropathy. *SCHWEIZ MED WOCHENSCHR* 100: 2212–2215, 1970. (German)
   b. Holmberg L, Boman G, et al: Adverse reactions to nitrofurantoin. *AM J MED* 69:733–738, 1980.
   c. Penn RG, Griffin JP: Adverse reactions to nitrofurantoin in the United Kingdom, Sweden, and Holland. *BR MED J* 284:1440–1442, 1982.
   d. Perritt RA: Eye complications resulting from systemic medications. *MED SCI* Feb. 10, 1960, pp.179–181.
   e. Toole JF, Gergen JA, et al: Neural effects of nitrofurantoin. *ARCH NEUROL* 18:680–687, 1968.
   f. Toole JF, Parrish ML: Nitrofurantoin polyneuropathy. *NEUROLOGY* 23:554–559, 1973.

Nitrofurazone (Amifur, Eldezol, Furacin, Nitrofural), a topical anti-infective, has been reported to cause an increase in oxygen utilization *in vitro* by rabbit and pig retina, to cause clumping of retinal pigment in rabbits when injected subcutaneously daily for 20 days, to reduce the a and b waves of the ERG, and to slow the recovery of the ERG from pressure ischemia.[a]

   a. Weiss H, Kosmath B: Furacin retinopathy in rabbits. *GRAEFES ARCH OPHTHALMOL* 181:130–139, 228–233, 1971.

1-(5-Nitro-2-furfurylideneamino)guanidine (Furaguanidine, Guanofuracin), an antibacterial used for treatment of conjunctivitis, caused the eyelashes to turn white and the skin of the eyelids to become depigmented in 10 to 20 per cent of chronic users in Japan. The whitening of the cilia was permanent.[a] The possibility of confusion with vitiligo has been pointed out.[b]

   a. Moutou Y, Boo-Chai K: Transplantation of hair for eyelash replacement. *PLAS RECONSTR SURG* 29:573–580, 1962.
   b. Stegmaier OC: Cosmetic management of nevi and pigmentary disturbances. *J AM MED ASSOC* 172:559–561, 1960.

Nitrogen in liquefied form is used in cryotherapy of skin lesions, but there seems to have been no report of accidental injury from splash contact with the eye, and experiments on rabbits indicate that danger from splash is very slight. Liquid nitrogen poured onto the eyes of rabbits for one or two seconds with the lids held apart produced no discernible injury. When the exposure was extended to five seconds, the corneal epithelium showed a trace of staining when tested with fluorescein, but by the next day all eyes were entirely normal.[a]

Nitrogen gas at room temperature injected into the anterior chamber of rabbits, replacing part of the aqueous humor, is non-toxic and is absorbed in two or three days.[81]

Awake guinea pigs in a pressure chamber with nitrogen pressure raised to 16 atmospheres have been found to have 15% reduction of the potentials of the ERG and optic chiasm, and 32% reduction of visual cortex potentials.[b]

  a. Grant WM: Low temperature liquids and eye injuries. *J AM MED ASSOC* 188:769, 1964.
  b. Hempel FG, Burns SP, Kaufmann PG: Responses of retinal and visual pathway potentials of the guinea pig to nitrogen and helium at high pressure. *AVIAT SPACE ENVIRON MED* 50:792–798, 1979.

Nitrogen dioxide has been examined for toxicity to the eye in relation to its use in rocket propellants and in relation to smog. The liquid form, known as *nitrogen tetroxide,* can be expected to cause severe burns on even brief contact with the skin or eyes.[a] The gas at 70 ppm of air causes irritation of the eyes and nose, and has been lethal to most animals exposed for eight hours. The corneas of rabbits that survived such exposures developed persisting opacities.[b] However, up to 20 ppm in air and exposure of four hours has produced no significant damage to the corneas of rabbits.[114,172,173]

  a. Boysen JE: Health hazards of selected rocket propellents. *ARCH ENVIRON HEALTH* 7:71–75, 1963.
  b. Steadman BL, Jones RA, et al: Effects on experimental animals of long-term continuous inhalation of nitrogen dioxide. *TOXICOL APPL PHARMACOL* 9:160–170, 1966.

Nitrogen mustards (particularly Chlormethine; Mechlorethamine; Mustine, HN2; N-methyl-2,2'-dichlorodiethylamine, and Chlormethine oxide) have been used medically as antineoplastic alkylating drugs. Comprehensive clinical and pharmacological reviews have been provided by Dralands and by Francois.[g,i] These compounds, as well as diethyl-2-chloroethyl amine, dimethyl-2-chloroethylamine, and trichlorotriethylamine, were originally developed as war gases.[f,o] The nitrogen mustard gases in contact with the eye are severely damaging, acting similar to the sulfur mustard gas, but with more immediate effect and greater tendency to injure deeper ocular structures, particularly the iris and lens. Accidental burns of human eyes have been observed,[p,161] and irritation of the eyes, nose, skin and respiratory tract have been reported following industrial exposure to vapors of *diethyl-2-chloroethylamine* and *dimethyl-2-chlorethylamine.*[q]

In patients treated for intracranial cancer by carotid perfusion with nitrogen mustard, severe necrotizing uveitis has been induced.[a]

Extensive animal experiments have been carried out with these substances.[b,j–n,p,161] In rabbits, small amounts have increased permeability of the blood-aqueous barrier[e] and caused transient increase in intraocular pressure.[d] Nitrogen mustard injected into the vitreous body in rabbit eyes is very damaging.[h] In mice, nitrogen mustard has induced cataracts similar to radiation cataracts.[c]

A series of studies have been carried out using *mechlorethamine* in particular as a substance that is irritative and injurious to the eye, lending itself well to experiments aimed at analyzing the mechanisms of response of the eye.[b,j-l,n] Application to the eye of a rabbit causes miosis and transient rise of intraocular pressure to peak in 40 minutes, dependent upon a sensory neural axon type reflex that can be blocked by prior denervation or induction of local anesthesia in various ways, or by prior treatment with capsaicin to deplete stores of substance P. A second rise of pressure peaks in 6 to 12 hours with increased permeability of the blood aqueous barrier, involving a prostaglandin mechanism, which can be blocked by indomethacin.

a. Anderson B, Anderson B Jr: Necrotizing uveitis incident to perfusion of intracranial malignancies with nitrogen mustard or related compounds. *TRANS AM OPHTHALMOL SOC* 58:95–104, 1960.

b. Camras CB, Bito LZ: The pathophysiological effects of nitrogen mustard on the rabbit eye. I. *EXP EYE RES* 30:41–52, 1980; II. *INVEST OPHTHALMOL VIS SCI* 19:423–428, 1980.

c. Conklin JW, Upton AC, et al: Comparative late somatic effects of some radiomimetic agents and X-rays. *RADIAT RES* 19:156, 1963.

d. Davson H, Huber A: Effects of nitrogen mustard on the intraocular pressure. *BR MED J* 1:939–940, 1950.

e. Davson H, Quilliam JP: The effects of nitrogen mustard on the permeability of the blood aqueous humor barrier to Evans blue. *BR J OPHTHALMOL* 31:717–721, 1947.

f. DeVincentiis M, DeGennaro G: Investigations of the effect of methyl-bis-(β-chloroethyl) amine hydrochloride on the metabolism of the retina. *OPHTHALMOLOGICA* 137:384–389, 1959. (German)

g. Dralands L: Cytostatics. Chapter 18 in Michiels report (1972).[359] (French)

h. Ericson L, Karlberg B, Rosengren BHO: Trials of intravitreal injections of chemotherapeutic agents in rabbits. *ACTA OPHTHALMOL* 42:721–726, 1964.

i. Francois J. Van Oye R: Immunodepressors in ophthalmology. *ANN OCULIST* 210:89–110, 1977. (French)

j. Jampol LM, Neufeld AH, Sears ML: Pathways for the response of the eye to injury. *INVEST OPHTHALMOL* 14:184–189, 1975.

k. Jampol LM, Axelrod A, Tessler H: Pathways of the eye's response to topical nitrogen mustard. *INVEST OPHTHALMOL* 15:486–489, 1976.

l. Jampol LM, Noth J: Further studies of the ipsilateral and contralateral responses to topical nitrogen mustard. *EXP EYE RES* 28:591–600, 1979.

m. LaMotte WO Jr, Leopold IH: The pathologic changes in rabbit eyes resulting from exposure to liquid nitrogen mustards. *AM J OPHTHALMOL* 29:1553–1562, 1946.

n. Maul E, Sears ML: Objective evaluation of experimental ocular irritation. *INVEST OPHTHALMOL VIS SCI* 15:308–312, 1976.

o. Ross WCJ: Aryl-2-haloalkylamines. *J CHEM* SOC 183–191, 1949.

p. Uhde GI: Burns from nitrogen mustard (β-chlorethylamine) gas (1149); clinical study. *ARCH OTOLARYNGOL* 44:701–709, 1946.

q. Watrous RM, Martins J, Schulz HN: Two chlorinated tertiary amines (diethyl-2-chlorethylamine and dimethyl-2-chlorethylamine): Toxicity in industrial use. *IND MED* 17:237–241, 1948.

Nitrogen trichloride (nitrogen chloride, Agene) vapor is pungent and irritating to the nose and eyes.[61,129,171] In swimming pools it is said that chlorine added for sanitation may react with ammonia (formed by decomposition of urea) and may produce nitrogen trichloride when the pH is less than 7.8, and that nitrogen chloride is one of the substances responsible for chemical irritation of the eyes. (For additional information, see *Hypochlorite and ammonia mixtures* and *Swimming pool water.*)

Nitroglycerin (glyceryl trinitrate) is used in explosives, and medically as a vasodilator. Ocular toxic effects have not been well documented, but observations made more than fifty years ago are commonly quoted.

It was said that when workers exposed to nitroglycerin were about to develop an acute toxic reaction, one premonitory sign was a transient loss of vision, either in one or both eyes. Then, extremely severe headache developed, but not until sight was completely restored.[b] Lewin and Guillery in 1913 accepted without doubt that nitroglycerin given experimentally or medicinally could cause decreased visual acuity and foggy vision, assuming this to be related to some vascular effect.[153] One patient with normal intraocular pressure of 15 mm Hg has been observed to have this pressure fall to 6 mm Hg within ten minutes after taking 0.6 mg sublingually, and this was associated with transient partial blackout of vision, presumably due to fall of blood pressure as in fainting. The symptom was relieved promptly by inhalation of spirits of ammonia.[c]

Tests for an adverse influence on the intraocular pressure have been made in rabbits and in normal and glaucomatous patients, some with very narrow anterior chamber angles, but no significant elevation of intraocular pressure has been observed after oral or intravenous administration.[a,c,d,e,266] Some patients had transient decrease of intraocular pressure.[c] There appears to be no specific report of precipitation or aggravation of glaucoma by nitroglycerin. (See also *Vasodilators.*)

    a. Brodehl D, Steinback PD: How does nitroglycerin act on intraocular pressure? *KLIN MONATSBL AUGENHEILKD* 166:784–791, 1975.
    b. Laws CE: Nitroglycerine head. *J AM MED ASSOC* 54:793, 1910.
    c. Whitworth CG, Grant WM: Use of nitrate and nitrite vasodilators by glaucomatous patients. *ARCH OPHTHALMOL* 71:492–499, 1964.
    d. Wizemann AJS, Wizemann V: Organic nitrate therapy in glaucoma. *AM J OPHTHALMOL* 90:106–109, 1980.
    e. Zahn K: The effect of nitroglycerine on the retinal circulation. *CS OFTAL* 13:146–149, 1957. (*ZENTRALBL GES OPHTHALMOL* 72:235, 1957.)

Nitronaphthalene vapors have been thought to cause a special type of keratitis. However, it is not entirely certain that nitronaphthalene is responsible, since the industrial atmospheres causing the keratitis have contained a mixture of substances, and attempts to induce keratitis with the pure compound in animals have been unsuccessful.[a,b,c,d,153] Other compounds reported to be present along with nitronaphthalene when keratitis has occurred industrially were *naphthalene, dinitronaphthalene,* and in one instance *dinitrotoluene.*

Typically, exposure of workers for several months in munitions manufacture induced a fine punctate disturbance of the corneal epithelium limited to the palpebral fissure, and stopping on either side 1 mm from the limbus.[153] The epithelium appeared to have innumerable tiny transparent vacuoles visible with magnification against the dark background of the pupil. Visual acuity was reduced. In bright light, objects appeared to be in a fog, but in dim light they might appear normal. Haloes could be observed about lights, but the tensions remained normal. Typically there was no pain, inflammation, or vascularization. When exposure was discontinued, the corneal epithelium cleared and vision returned to normal.[a,b,d] Exceptionally, chalky deposits formed in the corneas, and in rare cases the stroma of the cornea was reported to have become infiltrated or to have developed grayish striations.[a,33]

One worker is reported to have developed a disturbance of the corneal epithelium four or five months after having several times sprayed a benzene solution of nitronaphthalene in his eyes; this cleared spontaneously after many months.[d]

In only one instance has an opacity of the lens been reported, and this is said to have cleared after exposure was discontinued.[a]

a. Caspar L: Toward knowledge of occupational eye injuries from naphthalene. KLIN MONATSBL AUGENHEILKD 59:142–147, 1917. (German)
b. Frank W: Corneal changes from the action of nitronaphthalene. BEITR AUGEN-HEILKD 4:93–99, 1898. (German)
c. Hanke V: Nitronaphthalene-clouding of the cornea. WIEN KLIN WOCHENSCHR 12:725–726, 1899. (German)
d. Silex P: On nitronaphthale-clouding of the cornea. Z AUGENHEILKD 5:178–181, 1901. (German)

Nitro-olefins (nitro derivatives of unsaturated aliphatic hydrocarbons) as a group yield vapors which are very irritating to the eyes, of interest particularly in connection with smog. Nitroethylene has been noted at a concentration of 0.1 ppm in air to have especially strongly lacrimogenic vapor, causing symptoms such as encountered in smog.[d] Normal people detect eye irritation from 2-nitro-2-butene and from 2-nitro-2-hexene at 0.1 to 0.5 ppm in about three minutes, and from 2-nitro-2-nonene at concentration just above 1 ppm.[b,c]

Exposure of rat, chick, and rabbit eyes to vapors of compounds ranging from 2-nitro-2-pentene to 3-nitro-3-nonene at concentrations from 10 to 1,400 ppm in air caused conspicuous eye irritation.[a]

Nitro-olefins tested by application of drops to rabbit eyes, all caused dilation of the superficial blood vessels, lacrimation, and whitening of the corneal epithelium, which sloughed in about twenty-four hours.[a,b] The end results are not reported, but presumably the eyes recovered, since only the epithelium was described as being injured. Approximately the same effects were produced by the following compounds:

2-nitro-2-butene	2-nitro-2-octene
2-nitro-2-pentene	3-nitro-2-octene
3-nitro-2-pentene	3-nitro-3-octene
3-nitro-3-pentene	4-nitro-3-octene
2-nitro-2-hexene	4-nitro-4-octene
3-nitro-2-hexene	2-nitro-2-nonene
3-nitro-3-hexene	3-nitro-2-nonene
2-nitro-2-heptene	3-nitro-3-nonene

3-nitro-2-heptene	4-nitro-3-nonene
3-nitro-3-heptene	4-nitro-4-nonene
4-nitro-3-heptene	5-nitro-4-nonene

a. Deichman WB, Keplinger ML, Lanier GE: Acute effects of nitro-olefins upon experimental animals. *ARCH IND HEALTH* 18:312–319, 1958.
b. Deichman WB, MacDonald WE, et al: Nitro-olefins as potential carcinogens in air pollution. *IND MED SURG* 34:800–807, 1965.
c. Lampe KF, Mende TJ, et al: Evaluation of conjugated nitro-olefins as eye irritants in air pollution. *IND MED SURG* 27:375–377, 1958.
d. McCabe LC: Atmospheric pollution. *IND ENG CHEM* 43:89A, 1951.

Nitroparaffins, nitroderivatives of saturated aliphatic hydrocarbons, including *nitromethane, nitroethane, nitropropane, nitrobutane,* and *nitropentane,* yield vapors which are irritating to the eyes.[46,61,171] Human volunteers noted eye irritation from *nitropropane* at a concentration of 150 ppm in air.[217]

Nitrophenide (bis (m-nitrophenyl) disulfide), an anticoccidial veterinary medication, in dogs has caused temporary ataxia, vertigo, nystagmus, mydriasis, and opisthotonus.[70]

Nitrophenol (o- or p-nitrophenol) has been tested by feeding to chicks and found not to produce cataract.[a]

a. Dietrich WC, Beutner R: Failure of o- and p-mononitrophenol to produce cataract. *FED PROC* 5:174, 1946.

Nitroprusside (sodium nitroprusside, Nipride, Nitropress), an antihypertensive, when given intravenously to rabbits has caused decrease in blood pressure and a parallel, but much smaller decrease in intraocular pressure.[b] Applied externally to the eyes of rabbits it has caused a rise in intraocular pressure, indicated by tonographic measurements to be attributable to increase in rate of aqueous formation.[a] The elevation is prevented by alpha-adrenergic blocking, but not by antiprostaglandin drugs.

a. Krupin T, Weiss A, et al: Increased intraocular pressure following topical azide or nitroprusside. *INVEST OPHTHALMOL* 16:1002–1007, 1977.
b. Pinto G, Giraldi JP, et al: Action of sodium nitroprusside on the intraocular pressure. *BOLL OCULIST* 59:665–671, 1980. (Italian)

Nitroquinolones and a series of related *4-hydroxy-quinoline derivatives* have been examined for toxic effects on the eyes. Most notably, 1,3-dimethyl-6-nitro-4-quinolone was found to cause opacity of the lens in guinea pigs, observable in a few hours after administration of 150 mg/kg.[a] The substituent in the 3-position of 1,3-dimethyl-6-nitro-4-quinolone could be varied considerably without affecting the fundamental toxicity of the compound. Other related but not specifically identified 6-nitro-4-quinolone derivatives also produced cataract in guinea pigs, but derivatives of 4-quinolone that had a chloro, amino, or hydroxyl in the 6-position instead of 6-nitro did not produce cataract.[a]

Speaking in generalities about nitroquinolones, Paget has mentioned that some of these compounds produced irreversible structural changes in the lenses and corneas of guinea pigs after oral administration for a few days, demonstrated in histologic sections of the eyes.[b,c] These compounds produced minimal changes in lenses of rabbits and monkeys, but rats, mice, and dogs were immune to this toxic action.[b,c] The compounds apparently have not been tested on human beings. (See also *Quinoline derivatives.*)

    a. Duncan WAN: The importance of metabolism studies in relation to drug toxicity. *PROC EUR SOC STUDY DRUG TOXICITY* 2:67–77, 1963.

    b. Paget GE: Symposium on clinical drug evaluation and human pharmacology. *CLIN PHARMACOL THER* 3:381–384, 1962.

    c. Paget GE, Lemon P: Toxicological aspects. In Herxheimer A. (Ed.): DRUGS AND SENSORY FUNCTIONS. Boston, Little, 1968, pp.5–11.

Nitrosamines have been examined as potential war gases, and are said to have effects somewhat like a combination of sulfur mustard gas and nitrogen mustards.[161] After a latent period there is both corneal damage and uveitis, leading to permanent injury and depigmentation of the iris.

Nitrosomethyl urethane is used in preparation of *diazomethane.* Both substances have similar toxic effect. Since 1895 they have been known to be vesicant on the skin, and in the form of vapor to cause painful irritation of the eyes and severe respiratory irritation following an asymptomatic latent period after exposure.[b,153,258] Blurring of vision is associated with inflammation of the eyes and is presumably attributable to edema of the corneal epithelium.

In 1965 a chemist exposed presumably only to the vapors felt burning and scratching pain in the eyes after about two and one-half hours. Examination showed hyperemia, blepharospasm, chemosis, and keratitis epithelialis. This was followed by partial loss of corneal epithelium. Discomfort was greatest in the early stages. The eyes were entirely normal five months later.[a]

Nitrosomethyl urea, from which diazomethane may also be prepared, appears not to have the same type of toxicity.[258] (See also *Diazomethane.*)

    a. Neu HJ, Eistert B: Toxic effects of the action of a nitroso-compound on the eye and the whole organism. *KLIN MONATSBL AUGENHEILKD* 147:254–258, 1965. (German)

    b. Wrigley R: Toxic effects of nitroso-methyl urethane. *BR J IND MED* 5:26–27, 1948.

Nitrosyl chloride (NOCl) is a very corrosive reddish yellow gas, which is said to be intensely irritating to the eyes and skin, and to be severely injurious to the lungs.[171]

Nitrous oxide (dinitrogen monoxide, laughing gas) is a nonirritating slightly sweetish gas, not to be confused with the poisonous and irritating oxides of nitrogen. Nitrous oxide employed as an inhalation anesthetic may induce anoxia and damage to the central nervous system when high concentrations are employed without adequate accompanying oxygen. Walsh has pointed out that prolonged unconsciousness after anesthesia suggests brain damage, and that there is distinct tendency to involvement of the visual system.[255] He has observed that with loss of vision on regaining consciousness the chance of vision returning to normal is less than even.

Several cases of permanent cortical visual impairment and blindness have been reported.[255]

After vitrectomy, loss of air which is injected into the vitreous cavity is reported to be undesirably hastened by nitrous oxide used in general anesthesia.[a]

a. Boucher MC, Meyers E: Effects of nitrous oxide anesthesia on intraocular air volume. *CAN J OPHTHALMOL* 18:246–247, 1983.

Norepinephrine (levarterenol, noradrenalin), an adrenergic vaso-constrictor, has many times been reported to reduce ocular pressure, particularly in glaucoma, when administered topically or systemically, and has rarely raised the pressure. In patients a rise of as much as 6.8 mm Hg in intraocular pressure has been observed in association with 15 to 20 mm Hg rise of blood pressure from 5μg intravenously.[a] In rats a similar rise of intraocular pressure associated with induced systemic hypertension has been observed, but in an unexplained manner continuing to increase after blood pressure became steady.[b]

a. Komor K, Medgyaszay A, Polgar E: Change of intraocular pressure after intravenous administration of norepinephrine. *GRAEFES ARCH OPHTHALMOL* 168:577–580, 1965. (German)
b. Ohnesorge FK, Soyka H, et al: On the influence of systemically administered catecholamine on the intraocular pressure of rats. *GRAEFES ARCH OPHTHALMOL* 173:241–249, 1967. (German)

Norethindrone (Norethisterone), a progestin, is reported to have caused an increase of 5 mm Hg in intraocular pressure on two occasions in one postmenopausal female patient with "simple glaucoma" when 10 mg was administered orally.[a]

a. Paterson GD, Miller SJH: Hormonal influence in simple glaucoma. *BR J OPHTHALMOL* 47:129–137, 1963.

Novobiocin an antibacterial, has been known to cause skin rashes with conjunctivitis,[4] but forty-two children treated with large amounts of novobiocin had no adverse ocular effects.[a]

a. Keith CG, DeHaller J, Young WF: Side effects to antibiotic administration and to severity of pulmonary involvement. *ARCH DIS CHILD* 41:262–266, 1966.

Nutmeg (Myristica, *nux moschata*) is the aromatic seed of a tropical tree, *Myristica fragrans*, much used as a spice. Taken in excess, nutmeg has caused poisoning in a number of cases.[153] The signs and symptoms of nutmeg poisoning resemble those of atropine poisoning, including visual hallucinations. Because of the possibility of confusing the two conditions, some authors have proposed that the size of the pupils might serve as a diagnostic differentiating feature, knowing the pupils to be dilated in atropine poisoning, and supposing them not to be dilated by nutmeg.[c,e] However, Ahmad and Thompson reviewed all cases of nutmeg poisoning in which the pupils had been described, finding some were normal, some constricted, and some dilated.[a–d,f] They concluded that pupillary signs should not be depended upon in the diagnosis.[a] Accommodation is not known to be affected.[a,d,f]

Apart from visual hallucinations, little has been said about vision, but vision was affected in a woman who ate four or five nutmegs, and within six hours became extremely weak and had a fast, weak pulse. Her pupils were semidilated and unresponsive to light or accommodation. Objects seemed to her to be far off and in the left half of the visual field appeared to be a chocolate brown, but in the right half appeared normal. Sitting up caused blackout of vision, suggesting impairment of circulation.[c]

Nutmeg oil administered to cats intraperitoneally or externally to the eye did not affect the pupil, and when injected into the vitreous body caused miosis and severe uveitis.[a]

a. Ahmad A, Thompson HS: Nutmeg mydriasis. *J AM MED ASSOC* 234:274, 1975.
b. Green RC Jr: Nutmeg poisoning. *J AM MED ASSOC* 171:1342–1344, 1959.
c. Hinman EE: A case of nutmeg poisoning. *ALBANY MED ANN* 22:669–670, 1901.
d. Payne RB: Nutmeg intoxication. *N ENGL J MED* 269:36–38, 1963.
e. Shafran I: Nutmeg toxicology. *N ENGL J MED* 294:849, 1976.
f. Truitt EG Jr, Callaway E III, et al: Pharmacology of myristicin-psychopharmacology of nutmeg. *J NEUROPSYCHIAT* 2:205–210, 1961.

Octamoxin ([1-methylheptyl] hydrazine), a monoamine oxidase inhibitor, has caused optic neuritis in several patients.[a-f] In most cases central visual acuity was reduced and color vision disturbed by retrobulbar neuritis with cecocentral scotomas. There was no abnormality in appearance of the optic nerveheads at first. Generally the visual disturbances developed during several months when a total of 2 to 5 g had been taken, though less often decrease in vision was noted in one to two months after start of medication.[b] Reduction of visual acuity to 1/10 was common. In some cases after octamoxin was discontinued, the vision gradually recovered,[c,d] but in other cases recovery was incomplete, and partial optic atrophy developed.[a,b,e] (See also *Monoamine oxidase inhibitors* for other drugs of this category which have produced optic neuritis.)

a. Ardouin M, Urvoy M, et al: Electroretinographic study of a case of intoxication by monoamine oxidase inhibitors. *BULL SOC OPHTALMOL FRANCE* 67:920–924, 1967. (French)
b. Delay J, Deniker P, et al: Preliminary trials of a new monoamine oxidase inhibitor, 2-hydrazinooctane (D-1514) as antidepressant. *ENCEPHALE* 51:517–530, 1962. (French)
c. Joseph E, Berkman N: Ocular complications due to monoamine oxidase inhibitors. *PRESSE MED* 73:1627–1629, 1965. (French)
d. Kalt M: Bilateral optic neuritis of acute onset in an atherosclerotic patient, heavy smoker, intoxicated by a monoamine oxidase inhibitor. *BULL SOC OPHTALMOL FRANCE* 65:194–199, 1965. (French)
e. Paufique L, Charleux J, et al: Warning on the monoamine oxidase inhibitors. *BULL SOC OPHTALMOL FRANCE* 66:560–562, 1966. (French)
f. Sourdille MJ: Optic neuritides from monoamine oxidase inhibitors. *BULL SOC OPHTALMOL FRANCE* 64:981–990, 1964. (French)

Octanol (octyl alcohol, caprylic alcohol) has caused transient injury of the corneal epithelium, with recovery in forty-eight hours.[165]

Octatropine (anisotropine methyl bromide, Valpin), an anticholinergic, used orally in 10 mg doses four times a day did not dilate the pupils and did not cause clinically significant increase in intraocular pressure in nonglaucomatous or glaucomatous patients under anti-glaucoma treatment.[a]

a. Pilger IS, Holzhauer A: Effect of a new antispasmodic drug, anisotropine methylbromide, on intraocular pressure. *EYE EAR NOSE THROAT MONTHLY* 43:58–59, 62, 64, 1964.

tert-Octylamine vapor was observed by Munn (1967)[363] to have caused temporary mistiness of vision in industrial workers from corneal epithelial edema the same as produced by vapors of a number of other amines. (See INDEX for *Amines.*)

Octyl trimethylammonium bromide in 0.1 M solution dropped on rabbit eyes for ten minutes caused transient irregularity of the corneal epithelial surface, with return to normal in two or three days. Exposure after removal of the epithelium caused swelling of the corneal stroma and permanent opacification and vascularization.[80,81]

Ointment bases fall into the following four classes: *hydrocarbon bases* mainly of petrolatum; *absorption bases* in which there is an emulsion of water, petrolatum, and lanolin; *water-removable bases* composed of an oil-in-water emulsion; and *water-soluble or greaseless ointment bases* composed of water-soluble constituents such as polyethylene glycol. For ophthalmic ointments any of the four classes may be used.

Ointment applied to the skin of the lids has been shown to spread into the conjunctival sac, mainly via the canthal regions. This has been demonstrated with dye-colored ointments,[n] and has been evident in cases of glaucoma caused by corticosteroid ointments applied to the lids. (See *Corticosteroids.*) Also this mechanism has been involved in episodes of keratitis from water-soluble or greaseless ointments which were applied to the face. (See *Vick's Vapo-Rub.*)

Ointments applied to the eyes themselves have had the following adverse effects:

(1) *Interference with corneal wound healing.* This has been reported in rabbits, but inconsistently, and not from commercial ointment bases consisting mainly of petrolatum and mineral oil. Taniwaki in 1965 and 1966 reported experimental corneal epithelial wounds to heal most slowly in the presence of water-soluble ointments.[u,v] Similar earlier experiments by Berens (1943), Smelser (1944,1946), Leopold (1945), Friedenwald (1944), and Heerema (1950) were reviewed by Hanna and Fraunfelder in 1973, pointing out their varied results, and the fact that commercial ophthalmic ointments had become different from those in the earlier tests.[j] Hanna et al in their own tests on rats, rabbits, and monkeys found that the rate of healing of corneal abrasions or of non-penetrating keratectomies was not influenced by the currently used commercial ophthalmic ointments based on soft petrolatum, mineral oil and sometimes a small amount of purified lanolin.[j] This agreed with clinical impressions in use of ointments after operation or injury.

(2) *Entrapment of ointment in the cornea.* This has been a very rare complication of application of ointments to injured corneas. Fraunfelder and Hanna found in experimental animals that they could not cause the common mixture of petrola-

tum and mineral oil to become entrapped in the cornea unless they purposely injected it, or placed it in a pouch of cornea allowing stroma to envelop and heal around the ointment. Essentially no inflammatory reaction resulted, and localized vascularization occurred only if the foreign material was close to the limbus.[f,g] The same investigators pointed out that ointment droplets could become temporarily lodged in a depression in the cornea in a firmly bandaged eye, without actually being entrapped, a "pseudoentrapment."[h]

(3) *Ointment in the anterior chamber.* This is a complication that occurs after trauma or after operation when ointment is used while a penetrating, somewhat gaping wound is present. Leber in 1897 is credited by Flament[e] as having first reported the problem. Many cases have been reported since then,[a,b,d,e,i,k-m,o-t,243] and experiments in animals have been performed.[p,q,s] In some clinical cases a small amount of ointment has been seen floating in the anterior chamber for weeks or months without serious reaction,[a,k,p,q] but in most cases there has been an inflammatory reaction, leading to surgery to remove the foreign material in a few cases.[b,c,e,i,o] The composition of the ointments involved is varied, and the course is varied, but it seems that in an average case one might see a globule or droplet of melted ointment floating free in the uppermost part of the anterior chamber, with signs of iritis or iridocyclitis, and that in time the globule might come to rest on the surface of the iris, with dulling of its surface and formation of an enveloping veil holding it partly in the interstices of the iris. At this stage, if there is enough inflammatory reaction to indicate it, iridectomy can remove the attached ointment, and quiet the eye.[e] In most cases, surgical removal of the ointment has not been necessary, and eventually the foreign material has disappeared. Clinical opinion is that, if wounds of the anterior segment are well sutured, ointments can be used with very little risk of entering the anterior chamber.[c]

  In experiments in rabbits by Scheie, only slight reaction was induced by 0.05 ml of petrolatum, mineral oil or peanut oil in the anterior chamber, but a devastating reaction was produced by crude lanolin.[p] Three commercial atropine ointments similarly injected by Sugar caused some localized corneal clouding and vascularization, but no secondary glaucoma or destruction of the globe.[q] A mixture of petrolatum and wool fat similarly injected by Sykowski caused severe reaction only when a large amount (5 mm in diameter) was injected.[s]

(4) *Keratitis from water-soluble or greaseless ointment bases.* This has been described by Popp and by Dahl and Grant. In both reports there was a characteristic lack of discomfort during exposure of the eyes to the ointment bases, possibly due to partial anesthesia induced by surfactant materials,[162] until onset of blurring and discomfort from keratitis after a latent period of many hours. Popp's observations are described in more detail elsewhere under *Polyethyleneglycol ethers,* and Dahl and Grant's observations are described under *Vick's Vapo-Rub.* In the latter report an experimental greaseless preparation was applied to the face and unintentionally contaminated the eyes.

  a. Benitez Del Castillo JM: Foreign body (ointment) in anterior chamber. *ARCH SOC OFTAL HISP-AMER* 24:520–523, 1964. (Spanish)

b. Binder DK: Ointment absorbed through corneal wound. *ARCH OPHTHALMOL* 38:830–832, 1947.

c. Castroviejo R: Ointment bases in the anterior chamber. *ARCH OPHTHALMOL* 74:143, 1965.

d. Colombi C: On a possible contingency in the use of ointment in ophthalmic surgery; penetration into the anterior chamber. *RASS ITAL OTTALMOL* 29:91–100, 1957. (Italian)

e. Flament J, Payeur G, Bronner A: On the trouble with applying ointment after perforating ocular injury. *BULL SOC OPHTALMOL FRANCE* 71:463–467, 1971. (French)

f. Fraunfelder FT, Hanna C, et al: Entrapment of ophthalmic ointment in the cornea. *AM J OPHTHALMOL* 76:475–484, 1973.

g. Fraunfelder FT, Hanna C: Ophthalmic ointment. *TRANS AM ACAD OPHTHALMOL OTOL* 77:467–475, 1973.

h. Fraunfelder FT, Hanna C, Woods AH: Pseudentrapment of ointment in the cornea. *ARCH OPHTHALMOL* 93:331–334, 1975.

i. Gandolfi C: Mobile formation of traumatic origin free in the anterior chamber. *BOLL OCULIST* 16:1076–1083, 1937. (Italian)

j. Hanna C, Fraunfelder FT, et al: The effect of ophthalmic ointments on corneal wound healing. *AM J OPHTHALMOL* 76:193–200, 1973.

k. Hermann MP: Concerning a drop of oil in the anterior chamber. *BULL SOC OPHTAL-MOL FRANCE* 64:678–679, 1964. (French)

l. Hill D: personal communication, 1976.

m. Metzger E: Fat droplets in the upper part of the anterior chamber after perforating injury. *KLIN MONATSBL AUGENHEILKD* 77:515, 1926. (German)

n. Norn MS: Eyelid ointment penetrating into conjunctival sac. *ACTA OPHTHALMOL* 50:206–209, 1972.

o. Salvi GL: Contribution to the knowledge of the nature of free pseudocysts of the anterior chamber. *BOLL OCULIST* 29:578–584, 1950. (Italian)

p. Scheie HG, Rubenstein RA, Katowitz JA: Ophthalmic ointment bases in the anterior chamber. *ARCH OPHTHALMOL* 73:36–42, 1965.

q. Sugar HS, Airala MA: Introduction of some ophthalmic atropine ointments into the anterior chamber. *ANN OPHTHALMOL* 4:367–374, 1972.

r. Sykowski P: Ointment in the anterior chamber. *AM J OPHTHALMOL* 33:800–801, 1950.

s. Sykowski P: Experiments with ointment base in the anterior chamber. *AM J OPHTHAL-MOL* 35:1030–1031, 1952.

t. Tietze HM: Unusual retrocorneal phenomenon. Globule of prontosil in anterior chamber. *BR MED J* 1:665, 1943.

u. Taniwaki T: Experimental studies on corneal damage due to ophthalmic ointments and oils. *ACTA SOC OPHTHALMOL JPN* 69:809–831, 1965.

v. Taniwaki T: Experimental studies on corneal damage by ophthalmic ointment and oil. *JPN J OPHTHALMOL* 10:9–10, 1966.

Oleander (Nerium oleander) is a plant with toxic properties resembling those of squill and digitalis. In poisoning by oleander, mydriasis characteristically accompanies vertigo, convulsions, coma, and bradycardia.[171]

Oleic acid has been important in studies by Cogan and Kuwabara on aberrant lipogenesis.[a] They observed that oleic acid or neutralized sodium oleate injected into the corneas of rabbits caused the eyes to become inflamed within a few hours, to develop corneal abscess within a few days, and to become extensively scarred and vascularized. There was necrosis in the immediate region of the injection, and formation of fat droplets in surviving surrounding corneal cells.

Calcium oleate, Methyl oleate, and *Polysorbate 80,* an oleic acid ester, when injected into the rabbit cornea also induced intense necrosis and lipogenesis in adjacent surviving cells.

Compared to several other fatty acids tested in the same manner, oleic acid was not exceptionally necrotizing or pyogenic, but oleic acid and the oleates were unique in causing the cells to produce sudanophilic neutral fat.

a. Kuwabara T, Cogan DG: Experimental aberrant lipogenesis. *ARCH PATHOL* 63:496–501, 1957.

Olive oil applied to the surface of the eye is well tolerated and nonirritating. However, if injected into the anterior chamber of rabbits, it produces an inflammatory reaction, attracting leukocytes and causing endothelial proliferation. Fibrinous white sheets develop, and the cornea becomes turbid and vascularized.[a, 150] Injection of olive oil into the vitreous humor of rabbit eyes also has caused an inflammatory reaction with uveitis and cataract.[a]

a. Moro F: Research on the effect of benzopyrene injected into the vitreous chamber of the rat's eye. *ATTI 37 CONGR SOC OTTAL ITAL* 10:173–189, 1948. (Italian)

Onion vapors cause smarting of the eyes and lacrimation. The principal substances responsible have been said to be *allyl propyl disulfide,*[a] *diallyl disulfide,*[b] and *propenylsulfinic acid.*[b, c] In working with onions the maximum concentration of allyl disulfides which people can tolerate appears to be 2 to 3 ppm.[a] The precursor of the lacrimogenic substance *propenyl-sulfinic acid* in onions is said to be *S-(1-propenyl) -cysteine sulfoxide.*[c]

There seems to have been no study of the mechanism of action of these substances on the eye.

a. Feiner B, Burke WJ, Baliff J: An industrial hygiene survey of an onion dehydrating plant. *J IND HYG* 28:278, 1946.
b. Strong FM: Naturally occurring toxic factors in plants and animals used as food. *CAN MED ASSOC J* 94:568–573, 1966.
c. Virtanen AI: *Organic sulfur compounds in vegetables and their importance in human nutrition.* Address before the Am Chem Soc Northeastern Sect Oct 12, 1961.

Opiates, opioids, and **opioid antagonists** are outlined here concerning general properties, but specific details and bibliography are to be found elsewhere, under the names of the individual drugs. For the opiates or opioids, there are descriptions elsewhere under *Codeine, Cyclazocine, Heroin, Levorphanol, Methadone, Morphine, Opium, Pentazocine,* and *Pethidine.* For the opioid antagonists there are descriptions under *Levallorphan, Nalorphine,* and *Naloxone.*

In general, miosis is produced in human beings by systemic administration of opioids, and also by the opioid antagonists, levallorphan and nalorphine. However, when miosis has been induced by one of the opioids, the pupils can be made to dilate by administering one of the antagonists, and this is the basis for a screening test for narcotic use or addiction.[b]

In poisoning, miosis is characteristic; but if the patient is deeply unconscious and apneic, the pupils may be large and unreactive, becoming constricted only after correction of the anoxia, as exemplified by a case of poisoning by a combination of an opiate drug, dipipanone, with methaqualone and diphenhydramine.[d] In such cases treatment with adequate amounts of the antagonist nalorphine is helpful in relieving the poisoning, and the miosis is counteracted.

Nystagmus is not characteristic of opiate or opioid poisoning and suggests that also a sedative drug is present, especially a barbiturate.[c]

Opacities of the lens in mice and rats have been produced experimentally by a series of drugs, including several opiates, the principal mechanism apparently being suppression of blinking, in some cases with lid retraction, exposing the small rodent eye to evaporation and dehydration, resulting in reversible changes in transparency of the front of the lens. (This is described in more detail separately in connection with the individual drugs involved.) In human beings, when natural blinking is suppressed, there is measurable dehydration and reduction of intraocular pressure, but no known effect on lens transparency.[a] (There is a much larger volume of fluid between cornea and lens in the human than in small rodents.)

a. Grant WM, English FP: An explanation for so-called consensual pressure drop during tonography. *ARCH OPHTHALMOL* 69:314–316, 1965.
b. Martin WR: Opioid antagonists. *PHARMACOL REV* 19:463–506, 1967.
c. Sapira JD: The narcotic addict as a medical patient. *AM J MED* 45:555–588, 1968.
d. Wright N, Syme CW: Nalorphine in opiate poisoning. BR MED J 2:360, 1969.

Opium given systemically induces miosis and accommodation for near, and may also induce ptosis transiently. In opium addicts pallor of the optic nerveheads has been described,[a,41] but an injurious effect on retina or optic nerve has not been proven. Occasional instances of blurring of vision have been explained on the basis of miosis and altered accommodation.[246] Instances of amblyopia may be related to malnutrition and vitamin deficiency. (See also *Morphine* and *Opiates*.)

a. Motegi A, Saigan S: Ophthalmologic observations in 101 cases of chronic opium intoxication. *KLIN MONATSBL AUGENHEILKD* 93:367–371, 1934. (German)

Orange oil from orange peel has been claimed to have caused elevation of intraocular pressure in rabbits when it, or a hydrochloric acid extract, was given orally or subcutaneously, or was injected into the anterior chamber of the rabbit.[b,c] Also, it has been claimed that feeding orange peels to monkeys raised the intraocular pressure measurably, and further that *citral* was the component responsible for the pressure rise in both rabbits and monkeys.[b] A rise of a few millimeters of mercury from giving $2\mu g$ to $5\mu g$ per day orally, was said to be accompanied by histologic changes in Schlemm's canal.[a]

These claims need to be investigated further. They appear to have been neither corroborated nor challenged.

a. Leach EH: Ocular changes in monkeys fed with sanguinarine and other substances. *TRANS OPHTHALMOL SOC UK* 75:425–430, 1955.
b. Leach EH, Lloyd JFP: Experimental ocular hypertension in animals. *TRANS OPHTHAL-MOL SOC UK* 76:453–459, 1956.
c. Lloyd JFP: Argemone oil and sanguinarine poisoning in monkeys. *TRANS OPHTHAL-MOL SOC UK* 75:431–433, 1955. ·

Organophosphorus pesticides have, in widely varying degrees, two well recognized toxic actions. The first is inhibition of cholinesterase enzymes. The second is production of "delayed distal axonopathy." Numerous other toxic actions have been ascribed to these compounds, but with much less certainty.

Inhibition of ocular cholinesterases can result from contact of organophosphorous compounds with the surface of the eye or from systemic poisoning. Some organophosphorus cholinesterase inhibitors have been used in eye drops in treatment of glaucoma. Compounds used in this way have included *echothiophate iodide, isoflurophate (DFP), tetraethylpyrophosphate,* and *paraoxon.* A detailed description of the effects of cholinesterase inhibition on the eyes (including lids, conjunctiva, cornea, iris, ciliary processes, ciliary muscle, lens and retina) is given in the section of this book titled "*Miotics*". (See INDEX). In essence, contact of the eye with a strong cholinesterase inhibitor causes hyperemia of the conjunctiva, constriction of the pupil, and spasm of accommodation (focusing), with aching pain in and about the eye, and temporary blurring of vision.[j] Atropine, and other anticholinergic eye drops, give relief. Systemic poisoning, by ingestion or absorption through the skin, usually causes, in addition to the ocular effects, abdominal cramps, diarrhea, muscular weakness, and confusion.[e,o] Relief can be obtained with systemic pralidoxime and anticholinergic eye drops. Upbeat nystagmus has been noted in systemic poisoning.[i] As described in the section on "Miotics", in very rare cases acute angle-closure glaucoma can be provoked by topical or by systemic poisoning with a cholinesterase inhibitor.[f] This can occur only in an individual with a very special anatomic predisposition to angle-closure glaucoma, with abnormally shallow anterior chamber and narrow angle of the anterior chamber.

"Delayed distal axonopathy," the second well-recognized toxic effect induced by some organophosphorus pesticides, appears to have no particular relationship to anticholinesterase activity or to the eyes. This special poisoning is attributed to action on a "neurotoxic esterase" causing paralytic effects on legs and arms. After acute exposure to the poison there is characteristically a delay of weeks before paresthesias and paralyses of the limbs develop. It is most readily demonstrable in animals, and rarely has been produced in human beings by organophosphorus pesticides.[c] (Many cases of delayed distal axonopathy in human beings have resulted from acute poisoning with another type of organophosphorus compound, *tricresyl phosphate.* See INDEX.) An unusual series of ten human cases has been reported in which characteristic acute signs and symptoms of anticholinesterase poisoning developed and subsided as the first phase of organophosphorus pesticide poisoning, then, after a two to four week delay, paralytic neuropathy developed in the limbs.[m]

Tests on hens are used to detect a propensity to produce "delayed distal axonopathy" in organophosphorus compounds that are being considered for pesticidal use. This type of toxic action is considered quite undesirable for safety reasons. It is interesting to note that *isoflurophate* (DFP) has produced distal axonopathy in test animals, but has not been known to produce this type of poisoning in human beings who have been treated for glaucoma with eye drops or ointment containing this compound.[a,c]

A comprehensive review by Plestina and Piukovic-Plestina in 1978 of effects of anticholinesterase pesticides on the eye and on vision describes a third group of alleged toxic effects which they regard as controversial, because they are inconsistent with their own findings and with the findings of other investigators outside of Japan.[l,o] They give a bibliography of 179 references, many from Japan, but only a few key references will be quoted here. Most conveniently the controversial observations from Japan have been reviewed in a chapter by Ishikawa, the leading proponent, published in 1980.[h]

Ishikawa and associates published numerous reports primarily claiming that the incidence of myopia in local school children was related to the amounts of *parathion, malathion* and other pesticides sprayed in the Saku district of Japan.[q] In addition, reduced vision from corneal astigmatism, narrowing of peripheral visual fields, with or without central scotoma, congestion or atrophy of optic nerves, difficulty with ocular pursuit movements, and abnormality of ERG's, they also ascribed to chronic environmental pesticide exposure.[h] This became known as Saku disease. Miosis was seldom noted. Recovery after prolonged treatment with pralidoxime was taken as supporting evidence that pesticides were responsible.[l] Experimentally, they said that in Beagle dogs daily administration of *ethylthiometon* or *fenitrothion* for two years resulted in a mean of 1.25 diopter myopia more than in controls, and that "destructive changes" were found in the ciliary muscle cells.[n] The optic nerves showed a reduced number of nerve fibers and proliferation of glial cells. The retinas showed partial necrosis of retinal pigment epithelial cells and Muller cells, but the retinal ganglion cells remained intact.[r]

Separate tests in rats have shown change in the ERG and retinal pigmentary degeneration from *fenthion*,[g] changes in the ERG in mice from *parathion*,[289] *mevinphos* and *malathion*.[b] In cats, both ERG and VER have been affected by *chlorfenvinphos*.[p]

The comprehensive review by Plestina and Piukovic-Plestina in 1978 provides an extensive tabulation of reports on clinical observations on eyes and vision in relation to organophosphorus pesticides, while the reviewers indicate the unsatisfactory nature of the evidence, concluding that any cause and effect connection in most cases is purely speculative.[l]

The following observations were not included in the Plestina review. Several cases of cranial palsies (3rd, 6th, or 7th bilaterally) have been reported after suicidal attempts, mostly with *diazinon*, regularly with a period of miosis, but no optic nerve involvement.[s] Macular degeneration was suspected to be associated with prolonged exposure to pesticides. Fourteen sprayers out of a total of 64 employed in spraying *Baytex, Temophos,* and *Paris Green* for an average 7 years had decreased visual acuity and ophthalmoscopic appearance of pigmentary maculopathy.[k] One patient developed bilateral iridocyclitis 15 days after a possible air-borne exposure to *Bromophos,* but, with no history of miosis and in view of the length of time after exposure, a relationship seems hardly credible.[d]

A follow-up study of 232 people three years after a history of organophosphorus pesticide poisoning disclosed only one person with slight residual blurring of vision that might have been related to the earlier poisoning, though at the time of poisoning over one third of the people had blurring, which lasted only a day or two after exposure was discontinued.[o] The possible exceptional case had findings suggestive of basilar artery insufficiency, rather than effects of poisoning.

a. Bouldin TW, Cavanagh JB: Organophosphorus neuropathy. *AM J PATHOL* 94:241–248, 253–262, 1979.

b. Carricaburu P, Lacroix R, Lacroix J: Electroretinographic study of the white mouse intoxicated by organo-phosphorus. *TOXICOL EUR RES* 3:87–91, 1981.

c. Davies CS, Richardson RJ: Organophosphorus compounds. Pages 527–544 in Spencer and Schaumburg (1980).[378]

d. Deodati F, Bechac G, et al: Bilateral uveitis from organo-phosphorus insecticide. *BULL SOC OPHTALMOL FRANCE* 77:857–859, 1977. (French)

e. Ecobichon DJ, Ozere RL, et al: Acute fenitrothion poisoning. *CAN MED ASSOC J* 116:377–379, 1977.

f. Francois J, Verbraeken H: Acute glaucoma after poisoning with an organo-phosphate ester. *BULL SOC BELGE OPHTALMOL* 176:19–22, 1977; *J FR OPHTALMOL* 1:39–40, 1978. (French)

g. Imai H, Miyata M, et al: Retinal degeneration in rats exposed to an organophosphorus pesticide (Fenthion). *ENVIRON RES* 30:453–465, 1983.

h. Ishikawa S, Miyata M: Development of myopia following chronic organophosphate pesticide intoxication. Pages 233–254 in Merigan and Weiss (1980).[358]

i. Jay WM, Marcus RW, Jay MS: Primary position upbeat nystagmus with organophosphate poisoning. *J PEDIATR OPHTHAL STRABISMUS* 19:318–319, 1982.

j. LeHunsec J: Ocular disturbances provoked by use of organo-phosphoric insecticides. *BULL SOC OPHTALMOL FRANCE* 67:929–931, 1969. (French)

k. Misra UK, Nag D, et al: Macular degeneration associated with chronic pesticide exposure. *LANCET* 1:288, 1982.

l. Plestina R, Piukovic-Plestina M: Effect of anticholinesterase pesticides on the eye and on vision. *CRC CRIT REV TOXICOL* 6:1–23, 1978.

m. Senanayake N, Johnson MK: Acute polyneuropathy after poisoning by a new organophosphate insecticide. *N ENGL J MED* 306:155–157, 1982.

n. Suzuki H, Ishikawa S: Ultrastructure of the ciliary muscle treated by organophosphate pesticide in Beagle dogs. *BR J OPHTHALMOL* 58:931–940, 1974.

o. Tabershaw IR, Cooper WC: Sequelae of acute organic phosphate poisoning. *J OCCUP MED* 8:5–20, 1966.

p. Taked Y, Tsukahara I, Takaori S: Effects of chlorfenvinphos, an organophosphate insecticide, on afferent transmission in the central visual system. *JPN J OPHTHALMOL* 20:195–203, 1976.

q. Tamura O: Organophosphorous pesticides as a cause of myopia in school children. *EXCERPTA MEDICA ICS* 1:202–206, 1979.

r. Uga S, Ishikawa S, Mukuno K: Histopathological study of canine optic nerve and retina treated by organophosphate pesticide. *INVEST OPHTHALMOL* 16:877–881, 1977.

s. Wadia RS, Sadagopan C, et al: Neurological manifestations of organophosphorous insecticide poisoning. *J NEUROL NEUROSURG PSCHIATRY* 37:841–847, 1974.

Ornithine, an amino acid, has been injected into the vitreous body in rats' eyes and monkeys' eyes, and has been shown to cause striking swelling of the retinal pigment epithelial cells, maximal in 4 hours.[b] Although the swelling disappeared in 24 hours, some of the cells degenerated in areas. In these areas the photoreceptor cells also disappeared. There was no inflammatory reaction. *Arginine,* a metabolic precursor of ornithine, injected intravitreally did not damage the retinal pigment epithelium.[b]

The particular importance of these observations is in their probable relevance to the human eye disease, gyrate atrophy, in which the ornithine concentration in blood and tissues is 10 to 20 times higher than normal, due to an inherited inborn defect in the enzyme ornithine ketoacid transaminase. The disease is characterized by myopia and failing vision in childhood, with night blindness and progressive constriction of visual fields associated with equatorial chorioretinal atrophy of striking appearance.[c] Cataracts form in early adult life. Ornithine has been shown to be toxic not only to the retina, but also to muscle fibers of patients with the disease.[a] Withholding of the precursor arginine in one young patient reduced the blood ornithine level and improved vision.[c] A low protein diet has also been helpful.[d] Evidence that ornithine inhibits the enzyme arginine-glycine amidinotransferase and interferes with endogenous formation of creatine has been presented, and there has been evidence of slowing of the disease progress by feeding creatine.[e]

a. Kaiser-Kupfer MI, Kuwabara T, et al: Systemic manifestations of gyrate atrophy of the choroid and retina. *OPHTHALMOLOGY* 88:302–306, 1981.

b. Kuwabara T, Ishikawa Y, Kaiser-Kupfer MI: Experimental model of gyrate atrophy in animals. *OPHTHALMOLOGY* 88:331–334, 1981.

c. McInnes RR, Arshinoff SA, et al: Hyperornithinaemia and gyrate atrophy of the retina. *LANCET* 1:513–517, 1981.

d. Rinaldi E, Andria G, et al: Long-term follow-up of some early-treated aminoacidophathies associated with ocular abnormalities. *OPHTHALMIC PAEDIATR GENET* 2:135–138, 1983.

e. Sipila I, Rapola J, et al: Supplementary creatine as a treatment for gyrate atrophy of the choroid and retina. *N ENGL J MED* 304:867–870, 1981.

Orphenadrine (Mephenamine, Norflex, Banflex, Disipal), a skeletal-muscle relaxant and antihistaminic, can cause dryness of the mouth, dilation of the pupils, and blurred vision, the last presumably from interference with accommodation.[298,312] One patient with extremely narrow anterior chamber angles and no previous symptoms of glaucoma was observed to develop acute angle-closure glaucoma in one eye soon after starting to take orphenadrine for arthritis.[b] As with other anticholinergic drugs, this possibility has to be considered in anatomically predisposed eyes. Overdosage, as might be expected, produces widely dilated unreactive pupils.[a,c] (See also *Anticholinergic drugs.*)

a. Bosche J, Mallach HJ: On anatomic and chemical-toxicologic findings in a fatal poisoning by orphenadrine. *ARCH TOXIK* 25:76–82, 1969. (German)

b. Chandler PA: Personal communication, June 1964.

c. Heinonen J, Heikkila J, et al: Orphenadrine poisoning. *ARCH TOXIK* 23:264, 1968.

Orsudan (sodium 3-methyl-4-acetylaminophenylarsonate) in one case caused contraction of the visual fields with optic neuritis and optic atrophy similar to other derivatives of arsanilic acid.[a,214]

a. Clarke E: Optic atrophy following use of arylarsonate in treatment of syphillis. *TRANS OPHTHALMOL SOC UK* 30:240–251, 1910.

Osmium tetroxide (osmic acid) is a crystalline solid which sublimes readily, forming a poisonous vapor. Aqueous solutions also yield osmium-containing vapors. For more than one hundred years it has been known that the eyes are peculiarly susceptible to injury by vapors of osmium tetroxide. With sufficient concentrations a sensation of irritation with lacrimation and sensation of foreign body is induced immediately. This may be accompanied by irritation of the nose and throat. Respiratory irritation may accompany the eye disturbance, and with repeated exposure asthma may develop. The maximum concentrations which are said to be tolerated without aftereffects are 0.1 ppm in air for one-half hour, or 0.0001 ppm for six hours.[61]

Concentrations of vapor which do not cause immediate sensation of irritation have an insidious cumulative action with a latent period before the onset of smarting and lacrimation, which may be delayed from one to several hours after start of exposure. In either case the symptoms and signs are those of keratitis epithelialis with corneal epithelial edema. The victim sees haloes or colored rings around lights, and suffers blurring of vision and a painful scratchy sensation in the eyes. The signs and symptoms resemble those of ultraviolet keratitis, increasing in intensity for several hours after the onset, but recovery is spontaneous and usually complete in twenty-four to forty-eight hours.[a,c] No permanent effect has been noted, even when several episodes of keratitis epithelialis have been experienced.

As an example, a laboratory worker who heated osmium in a crucible under conditions in which osmium tetroxide would be formed developed pain in his eyes, blepharospasm, photophobia, epiphora, and hyperemia of the eyes. Visual acuity was reduced, but pupils, accommodation, and visual fields remained normal. The patient recovered after a day. All signs and symptoms pointed to the cornea as the site of the disturbance; there was no evidence to support a suspicion of poisoning of the retina.[c] Early case reports in which a poisonous influence on the retina was postulated, are not to be relied upon.[c] In all instances blurring of vision is explicable on the basis of alterations of the corneal epithelium discernible with the slit-lamp biomicroscope.

In no patient has injury of the retina or optic nerve been observed, and in no instance has blindness resulted from exposure to osmium tetroxide vapor.

Application of a drop of 1% solution of osmic acid to rabbit eyes causes severe corneal damage.[a,188] Brown staining of the cornea and conjunctiva appears rapidly, ultimately resulting in moderate permanent opacity and superficial vascularization.

a. Brunot FR: The toxicity of osmium tetroxide. *J IND HYG* 15:136–143, 1933.
b. McLaughlin AIG, Milton R, Perry KMA: Toxic manifestations of osmium tetroxide. *BR J IND MED* 3:183–186, 1946.
c. Noyes HD: Amblyopia produced by osmic acid. *N.Y. MED J* July, 1866. (*TRANS AM OPHTHALMOL SOC* 1:34–35, 1866.)

Ouabain, a cardiotonic drug, has been of great interest for investigative purposes as an inhibitor of the enzyme system NaK–ATPase, particularly in study of transport mechanisms involving sodium in the cornea, lens, ciliary body epithelium, and retina. Toxic effects in these structures have almost all been induced experimentally, and there have been very few instances of eye injury or intoxication occuring clinically in human beings.

The corneas of experimental animals have been exposed to ouabain at various concentrations, *in vitro* and *in vivo*.[m] Studies have been made on effects on electrical properties, permeability, and swelling of the cornea, indicating that in the corneal endothelium and probably also in the epithelium there is a sodium pump that can be inhibited by ouabain at concentrations which do not alter endothelial permeability.[f,p,r,v,w,za,zf] On the human eye, eyedrops containing 0.25 mg ouabain per ml have been applied experimentally with no notable effect on the cornea.[ze]

Lenses in tissue culture exposed to ouabain have shown evidences of interference with active transport of cations,[j,o] but there seems to be no report of cataractogenesis from poisoning of animals or human beings. Cataract has been induced in cultured lenses.[h,i,n]

Retinal activity measured by electroretinography in animals and in isolated retinas has been shown to be rapidly reduced by exposure to ouabain.[s,x,z] This has not been observed in low-sodium media.[l] Intravitreal injection in rabbits has caused rapid loss of vision, without gross inflammation, but with extensive loss of cells from the retina evident histologically in two months, while pigment epithelium, ciliary processes, lens, and cornea remained morphologically normal.[s] In fish, degeneration of retinal cell bodies and nerves have been reported.[zi] Apparently there have been no clinical observations of toxicity to the retina in use of ouabain for digitalization of patients, but a variety of visual disturbances of unknown origin have been reported as side effects of several digitalis-type drugs. (See also *Digitalis glycosides.*)

Investigations have been carried out on the effects of ouabain on the epithelium of the ciliary body, on formation of aqueous humor and on intraocular pressure.[b,zd,zh] Ouabain reduces activity of NaK–ATPase in the ciliary body and reduces aqueous formation and intraocular pressure in animals when injected into the vitreous body,[b] probably less effectively when injected into the anterior chamber, and only at very high doses when given systemically.[zd,zh] Not all investigators have been able to confirm an inhibitory effect on formation of aqueous humor by ouabain injected into the vitreous body or the posterior chamber.[q,y] Related observations have been made on other enzyme activity, electrical activity, secretory pumping of sodium, and on electron microscopic morphology in the ciliary epithelium after exposure to ouabain.[a,c-g,k,zb,zc]

Extraocular topical administration of ouabain as eyedrops in patients has caused no reduction of intraocular pressure,[ze] but repeated subconjunctival injection in rabbits is said to have reduced the pressure.[zg]

In cats the circumferential artery of the iris is reported to be constricted by ouabain.[t,u]

a. Akita K: Electron microscopic studies on the ciliary epithelium after administration of ocular tension depressants. *ACTA SOC OPHTHALMOL JPN* 70:1405–1423, 1966.

b. Becker B: Ouabain and aqueous humor dynamics in the rabbit eye. *INVEST OPHTHALMOL* 2:325–331, 1963.

c. Berggren L: Effect of composition of medium and metabolic inhibitors on secretion in vitro by ciliary processes of the rabbit eye. *INVEST OPHTHALMOL* 4:83–90, 1965.

d. Bonting SL, Becker B: Studies on sodium-potassium activated adenosine-triphosphatase. *INVEST OPHTHALMOL* 3:523–533, 1964.

e. Bonting SL: Physiological chemistry of the eye. *ARCH OPHTHALMOL* 74:561–578, 1965.

f. Brown HD, Jackson RT, Waitzman MB: Ciliary process ATPase; aza steroid and erythrophleum alkaloid inhibition. *LIFE SCI* 6:1519–1527, 1967.

g. Cole DF: Location of ouabain-sensitive adenosine triphosphatase in ciliary epithelium. *EXP EYE RES* 3:72–75, 1964.

h. Duncan G, Marcantonio JM: Changes in lens amino acid transport and protein metabolism during osmotic cataract produced by ouabain. *TRANS OPHTHALMOL SOC UK* 102:314–317, 1982.

i. Gupta JD, Edwards A, et al: Toxicity of ouabain to embryonic chick lens. *AUST J EXP BIOL MED SCI* 49:305–308, 1971.

j. Harris JE: The temperature-reversible cation shift of the lens. *TRANS AM OPHTHALMOL SOC* 64:675–699, 1966.

k. Holland M: *In vitro* studies of ciliary body ion transport. *AM J OPHTHALMOL* 62:1128–1135, 1966.

l. Honda Y: Some observations of the mode of action of ouabain upon the electrical activity of mammalian retinas. *INVEST OPHTHALMOL* 11:706–710, 1972.

m. Kaye GI, Donn A: Studies on the cornea. *INVEST OPHTHALMOL* 4:844–852, 1965.

n. Kinoshita JH: Mechanisms initiating cataract formation. *INVEST OPHTHALMOL* 13:713–724, 1974.

o. Korte I, Hockwin O, et al: On the influence of ouabain on the metabolism of bovine and calf lenses. *GRAEFES ARCH OPHTHALMOL* 175:242–245, 1968.

p. Lambert B, Donn A: Effect of ouabain on active transport of sodium in the cornea. *ARCH OPHTHALMOL* 72:525–527, 1964.

q. Langham ME, Eakins KE: Influence of the cardiac glycoside ouabain on the intraocular pressure and dynamics of the rabbit and the cat. *J PHARMACOL EXP THER* 144:421–428, 1964.

r. Langham ME, Kostelnik M: The effect of ouabain on the hydration and the adenosine triphosphatase activity of the cornea. *J PHARMACOL EXP THER* 150:398–405, 1965.

s. Langham ME, Ryan SJ, Kestelnik M: The Na, K ion dependent adenosinetriphosphatase of the retina and the mechanism of visual loss caused by cardiac glycosides. *LIFE SCI* 6:2037–2047, 1967.

t. Macri FJ: The constrictor action of antiglaucoma drugs on the iris artery of the cat. *INT J NEUROPHARMACOL* 3:205–212, 1964.

u. Macri FJ, Dixon R, Rall DP: Aqueous humor turnover rates in the cat. *INVEST OPHTHALMOL* 5:386–390, 1966.

v. Mishima S, Trenberth SM: Permeability of the corneal endothelium to non-electrolytes. *INVEST OPHTHALMOL* 7:34–43, 1968.

w. Muneoka A: The inhibition of the active transport of Na^+ of the cornea by ouabain. *ACTA SOC OPHTHALMOL JPN* 72:962–968, 1968.

x. Nasu K: Retinal degeneration induced by medical agents. *FOLIA OPHTHALMOL JPN* 19:87–88, 1968.

y. Oppelt WW, White ED Jr: Effect of ouabain on aqueous humor formation rate in cats. *INVEST OPHTHALMOL* 7:328–333, 1968.

z. Ostrovskii MA, Dettman P: The effect of ouabain on electroretinogram of isolated washed frog retina. *BIOFIZIKA* 11:724–726, 1966. (*CHEM ABSTR* 65:14289, 1966.)

za. Peyman GA, Sanders DR, Ligara TH: Dextran 40—containing infusion fluids and corneal swelling. *ARCH OPHTHALMOL* 97:152–155, 1979.

zb. Reddy DV: Intraocular transport of taurine. *BIOCHEM BIOPHYS ACTA* 158:246–254, 1968.

zc. Riley MV: The sodium-potassium-stimulated adenosine triphosphatase of rabbit ciliary epithelium. *EXP EYE RES* 3:76, 1964.

zd. Simon KA, Bonting SL, Hawkins NM: Studies on sodium-potassium-activated adenosine triphosphatase. *EXP EYE RES* 1:253–261, 1962.

ze. Smith JL, Mickatavage RC: The ocular effects of topical digitalis. *AM J OPHTHALMOL* 56:889–894, 1963.

zf. Trenberth SM, Mishima S: The effect of ouabain on the rabbit corneal endothelium. *INVEST OPHTHALMOL* 7:44–52, 1968.

zg. Waitzman MB, Jackson RT: Effects of topically administered ouabain on aqueous humor dynamics. *EXP EYE RES* 4:135–145, 1965.

zh. Warner DM, Drance SM: Effect of intravenous cardiac glycosides on the aqueous humor dynamics of the cat. *BR J OPHTHALMOL* 50:701–704, 1966.

zi. Wolburg H: Time- and dose-dependent influence of ouabain on the ultrastructure of optic neurones. *CELL TISSUE RES* 164:503–517, 1975.

Oven cleaners, designed to aid in the cleaning of household ovens, commonly have consisted of strongly alkaline pastes, often containing 7% to 8% sodium hydroxide, applied with a stiff brush or as a pressurized spray. The higher the content of caustic sodium hydroxide, the greater the hazard to the eyes. There have been many injuries of the corneal epithelium and conjunctiva of housewives from accidental spatter or from accidental spraying in the eye. In cases of slight contamination the eye felt irritated, with foreign-body sensation, and showed fine stippling of the corneal epithelium, which stained with fluorescein. More severe spatters have caused more diffuse damage and loss of corneal epithelium. Fortunately the amount of caustic material spattered or sprayed on the surface of the eye in this type of accident has ordinarily been so small that the injury has remained superficial, without significant damage to the corneal stroma. Generally the eyes have healed completely within one to a few days.

Efforts have been made by manufacturers to provide less caustic preparations, with lower content of sodium hydroxide, by adding sodium silicate, glycols, detergents, and ammonia.

Oxalic acid has caused burns of the human eye in a few instances when solutions accidentally came in contact with the eye. The injury has been epithelial and recovery has been prompt, the epithelium regenerating usually within two days.[a, 165]

In rabbits the response is similar. Application of a 5% solution for thirty seconds caused coagulation of the epithelium, but the cornea recovered within six days.[81] Guillery in 1910 applied a saturated solution of oxalic acid to eyes of rabbits and found that application for several minutes induced turbidity of the corneal epithelium, but that this was practically clear again the next day. With more intensive and prolonged exposure the deeper layers of the cornea became clouded and showed histologic evidence of damage.[96]

Severe systemic poisoning by oxalic acid has been reported in one case to have been associated with loss of vision, but no details were provided on the nature of the loss or on the degree of recovery.[153]

Oxalate ions from exogenous sources, from metabolism of oxalate precursors, or from inborn errors of metabolism, react with calcium ions in blood or tissues to form calcium oxalate. Calcium oxalate has low solubility and precipitates in various parts of the body, including the eyes. This condition, known as "oxalosis" is discussed in following paragraphs.

    a. Suker GF: Injury to cornea from oxalic acid. OPHTHAL REC 23:40, 1913.

Oxalosis, a condition in which there is an abnormal amount of oxalate in the blood or tissues, leading to precipitation of *calcium oxalate,* has been produced in human beings by prolonged inhalation of *methoxyflurane,* and has been characterized by an appearance of "flecked retina" with yellow-white punctate lesions in the fundi composed of deposits of calcium oxalate in the retinal pigment epithelium. In rabbits, the same changes have been produced by administering *dibutyl oxalate.* In poisoning by *ethylene glycol,* calcium oxalate deposits are found in the kidneys and other tissues, but none have been described in the eyes. In poisoning by *naphthalene* and related compounds in animals, oxalate is formed by conversion of ascorbic acid and the resulting calcium oxalate forms vitreous opacities. There is also a primary hereditary oxalosis which produces the flecked-type retinopathy, as well as deposition of myriads of yellow crystals throughout the retina,[f] and has been fatal for some infants.[a-f]

(See INDEX for further information on each substance mentioned above.)

    a. Besio R, Meerhoff E, et al: Oxalosis. *AM J OPHTHALMOL* 95:397–398, 1983.
    b. Fielder AR, Garner A, Chambers TL: Ophthalmic manifestations of primary oxalosis. *BR J OPHTHALMOL* 64:782–788, 1980.
    c. Richard G, Promesberger H: Fundus albipunctatus in primary oxalosis. *OPHTHAL-MOLOGICA* 185:32–36, 1982. (German)
    d. Toussaint D, Vereerstraeten P, et al: Primary hyperoxaluria. *ARCH OPHTALMOL (PARIS)* 36:97–112, 1976. (French)
    e. Zak TA, Buncic R: Primary hereditary oxalosis retinopathy. *ARCH OPHTHALMOL* 101:78–80, 1983.
    f. Meredith TA, Wright JD, et al: Ocular involvement in primary hyperoxaluria. *ARCH OPHTHALMOL* 102:584–587, 1984.

Oxalyl chloride is a poisonous fuming liquid causing irritation of the eyes and respiratory distress. One man, after having worked with oxalyl chloride and having experienced respiratory disturbances observed in the evening colored rings about all lights.[a] This patient was found to have no cataract, and it is most likely that the appearance of the colored rings were induced by edema of the corneal epithelium, which is the most common cause of this optical phenomenon.

    a. Gerbis H: Occupational poisoning with oxalyl chloride. *ZENTRALBL GEWER-BEHYGIENE* 6:293–294, 1929. (German)

Oxazepam (Adumbran, Serax), a tranquilizer, has been tested for effects on vision with oral doses of 30 mg, but caused no change in visual acuity, accommodation, or eye movement, except possibly an enhancement of existing heterophorias.[a] Visually induced EEG potentials have been little influenced.[b] Readaptation after a flash of light may be delayed.[c]

a. Aust W: Ophthalmological investigations of the compatibility of 7-chloro-1,3-dihydro-3-hydroxy-5-phenyl-2H-1,4-benzodiazepin-2-one. *ARZNEIMITTELFORSCHUNG* 15: 379–382, 1965.
b. Dolce G, Kaemmerer E: Effect of benzodiazepine, Adumbran, on the resting and sleeping EEG and the visual reaction potentials in the adult man. *MED WELT* 9:510–514, 1967.
c. Bergman H, Borg S, et al: The effect of oxazepam on ocular readaptation time. *ACTA OPHTHALMOL* 57:145–150, 1979.

Oxprenolol (Trasicor), coronary vasodilator, beta-adrenergic blocker, is recorded by Fraunfelder's National Registry as having been the subject of a number of informal reports associating it with "sudden onset keratoconjunctivitis sicca with marked conjunctival hyperemia."[312] In published case reports, one patient noted red eyes only after 15 months of treatment, and 3 months later, still without discomfort or change in visual acuity, developed punctate corneal epithelial opacities.[b] On discontinuing oxprenolol, the eyes looked much better in a week. Another patient had psoriasiform eruption of the skin and dryness of the eyes with reduced tear production after 6 months of treatment.[a] After stopping oxprenolol she was improved in a week, but had return of symptoms on retrial of the drug. One other patient developed dry eye discomfort and hyperemia after 2 months of treatment, and largely recovered in 2 weeks off treatment. On re-trial of the drug, symptoms worsened in 72 hours. A patient who had received both practolol and oxprenolol suffered a corneal perforation.[d]

a. Holt PJA, Waddington E: Oculocutaneous reaction to oxprenolol. *BR MED J* 2:539–540, 1975.
b. Knapp MS, Galloway NR: Ocular reaction to beta-blockers. *BR MED J* 2:557, 1975.
c. Lewis BS, Setzen M, Kokoris N: Ocular reaction to oxprenolol. *S AFR MED J* 50:482–483, 1976.
d. Lall JRW: Ocular reactions to beta-blockers. *BR MED J* 2:247, 1975.

Oxygen effects involving the eyes or vision are outlined below.

(1) *The effects of hyperbaric oxygen on the eyes of men* has received great attention in relation to aerospace and underwater living as well as use of hyperbaric oxygen in treatment of disease. The primary response of the adult retina to hyperoxia is retinal vasoconstriction (Anderson). In hypoxia the retinal arterioles and venules dilate (Dollery; Frayser; Ramalho; Ring; Saltzmann; Touraids). Young healthy men can breathe pure oxygen at 3 atm pressure for three hours without distressing symptoms. However, in the fourth hour they have been reported to have progressive contraction of the visual fields, impaired central vision, and mydriasis, all of which are reversible if exposure is discontinued.[188,252] The pressure of oxygen is an important factor. At atmospheric pressure, breathing oxygen for four and one half hours caused no change in visual fields or visual acuity (Miller).

A case has been reported in which acute decrease in vision in one eye occurred in a young man during exposure to oxygen at high pressure (Nichols). The patient had been well except for a history of two episodes of unilateral retrobulbar neuritis. During exposure the vision in that eye gradually decreased to light perception. After the exposure was discontinued, the peripheral visual field returned to normal but a central scotoma persisted. Systemic corticosteroid treatment was started and in a week vision had recovered fully.

Profound permanent loss of vision in both eyes in an adult human being has resulted from being kept for months in an 80% oxygen atmosphere on account of myasthenia gravis (Kawasaki; Kobayashi). Ophthalmoscopic and electroretinographic findings indicated both arrest of retinal circulation and deterioration of visual cells.

(2) *Experiments on adult animals* have turned up interesting effects in various species. In adult dogs observations have been made on toxic effects of oxygen on retina and choroid (Beehler). Dogs exposed to pure oxygen for forty-eight hours were found to develop retinal and choroidal detachments, protein in the aqueous humor, and sometimes hemorrhages in the retinas, but no holes in the retinas. The intraocular pressure was usually below normal. When exposure was prolonged, the retinas showed degenerative changes and cysts developed in the ciliary bodies. Dogs which had been given promazine as a tranquilizer prior to exposure were particularly prone to these exudative retinal detachments. When this tranquilizer was omitted, the oxygen alone produced only "focal retinal elevations" in about 20% of the dogs and caused no complete detachments. Toxicity of oxygen to the dog eyes could be enhanced by other phenothiazine drugs and by chloroquine. Lesions in the medicated and oxygen-poisoned dogs' eyes appeared first in the tapetum, at first focal and scattered, but then became enlarged and coalesced to give exudative retinal detachments, and later produced pigmentary changes and degeneration in the retina (Beehler). Dogs which received no medications but were exposed to 100% oxygen showed much less reaction than medicated dogs, but developed retinal detachments as though from leakage of fluid from the choroid into the subretinal space (Yanoff). In comparison with the central nervous system, it appeared that danger to the eyes might be a limiting factor to the extent of use of hyperbaric oxygen (Margolis).

In adult rabbits oxygen toxicity studies have been concerned with relating effects on the ERG to the duration and pressure of oxygen exposure (Bridges; Criswick; Perdriel; Watanabe). Generally, after preliminary increase in size of the a- and b-waves, if oxygen is given at sufficient pressure and for sufficient time the ERG can be abolished. By suitable choice of conditions the extinction can be reversible or irreversible. Degeneration of the visual cells in rabbits after exposure to high concentrations of oxygen has been demonstrated morphologically by electron microscopy (Bresnick). Several days exposure of albino rabbits to abnormally high concentrations of oxygen has been found to produce irreversible degeneration of the rods, changes in the ERG, and edema of the ciliary body and iris, with increased permeability of the blood-aqueous barrier (Noell). The higher the oxygen pressure, the more rapidly these changes appeared.

In rats, lens mitoses are increased by hyperoxia at elevated pressure, but not at atmospheric pressure (Scullica). In mice, cataracts have been produced by repeated exposure to hyperbaric oxygen (Schocket). In guinea pigs, irreversible changes in the epithelium of the lens, and thinning of the corneal endothelium have been seen after exposure to 3 to 5 atmospheres of 100% oxygen (Nichols).

(3) *Effects of oxygen on the eyes of the newborn* has received the greatest attention, because of the hundreds of children each year who have severe permanent loss of vision from oxygen inhalation that they require because of premature birth, and inability to survive without it. Retinopathy of prematurity, or retrolental fibroplasia, was first recognized as a clinical entity in the early 1940's. The role of oxygen-supplementation in incubators for the premature was not appreciated until several years later, from clinical evidence and from study of an oxygen-induced model of the disease in kittens (Ashton; Kinsey; Patz). Later study of the effect of hyperoxia in developing rabbit retinas added to the picture (Ashton; Tripathi). A detailed history of early developments in this disease is available (James).

When the role of oxygen was recognized, an effort was made to reduce the amount of oxygen used in incubators, but a satisfactory compromise between life-saving and vision-saving levels has proven extremely difficult to achieve, and re-ports of clinical experiences during the 1960's and 1970's emphasize this problem (Ashton 1980; Campbell 1983; Kalina 1982; Patz 1979; Weiter 1981). From the clini-cal experience gained over those years, the clinical and histopathologic character-istics of the disease have become well known (Flynn; Kushner). In essence, both clinical and animal studies have shown that prematurely-born, underweight individuals respond to oxygen breathing by retinal vascular obliteration, then upon returning to breathing air they respond by vascular proliferation in periph-eral portions of the retina, sometimes with cicatrization and retinal detachment.

In addition to clinical studies carried on in the hopes of finding a solution to the dilemma, research continues in animals and in cultured retina to learn more about the biochemical aspect. However, one report argues that the long-honored kitten model presents some important differences from the human disease (Gole). Biochemically for a long time there has been suspicion, and some evidence, of an important role for a free radical mechanism (Feeney; Slater). Inactivation of retinal sodium-potassium ATPase is found in experimental oxygen poisoning (Ubels). Lipid peroxides experimentally cause retinal degeneration.[274]

Vitamin E, as an antioxidant and free radical scavenger has been tested as a preventive measure in kittens and premature infants with some promise (Hittner; Phelps).

Retinal disease closely resembling that caused by oxygen in premature new-borns has been recognized as occurring occasionally in full-term infants who were never given oxygen treatment. Collections of such cases, and their differen-tial diagnoses, have been published (Schulman; Stefani).

(4) *Myopia from oxygen* has been described in premature infants, with the degree related to severity of cicatricial retinopathy of prematurity (Nissenkorn). However, adults too have been found to have a slow increase in myopia from change in the

refractive properties of the lens during several months of repeated exposure to hyperbaric oxygen (Anderson; Lyne). This tends to affect older people and tends to disappear gradually, but nuclear cataracts which were persistent have been produced in a series of patients by hyperbaric oxygen treatments, total 200 to 850 hours (Palmquist).

Anderson B Jr: Retinal responses to ischemia and hyperoxia. *N CAROLINA MED J* 26:446–449, 1965.

Anderson B Jr, Saltzman HA, Gebel E: Duration of hyperbaric oxygenation related to delay in ischemic visual blackout. *SOUTHERN MED J* 58:1047–1049, 1965.

Anderson B Jr, Saltzman HA, Frayser R: Changes in arterial pCO_2 retinal vessel size with oxygen breathing. *INVEST OPHTHALMOL* 6:416–419, 1967.

Anderson B Jr: Ocular effects of changes in oxygen and carbon dioxide tension. *TRANS AM OPHTHALMOL SOC* 66:423–474, 1968.

Anderson B Jr, Farmer JC Jr: Hyperoxic myopia. *TRANS AM OPHTHALMOL SOC* 76:116–124, 1978.

Ashton N: Retrolental fibroplasia. *AM J OPHTHALMOL* 39:153–159, 1955.

Ashton N: Oxygen and the growth and development of retinal vessels. *In vivo* and *in vitro* studies. *AM J OPHTHALMOL* 62:412–435, 1966.

Ashton N: Ocular hazards in oxygen therapy. *TRANS OPHTHALMOL SOC UK* 88:707, 1968.

Ashton N: Some aspects of the comparative pathology of oxygen toxicity in the retina. Donders Lecture, 1967. *BR J OPHTHALMOL* 52:505–531, 1968.

Ashton N, Tripathi B, Knight G: Effect of oxygen on the developing retinal vessels of the rabbit. *EXP EYE RES* 14:221–232, 1972.

Ashton N: Oxygen and the retinal blood vessels. *TRANS OPHTHALMOL SOC UK* 100:359–362, 1980.

Beehler CC, Newton NL, et al: Ocular hyperoxia. *AEROSPACE MED* 34:1017–1020, 1963.

Beehler CC, Newton NL, et al: Retinal detachment in adult dogs resulting from oxygen toxicity. *ARCH OPHTHALMOL* 71:665–670, 1964.

Beehler CC: Oxygen and the eye. *SURVEY OPHTHALMOL* 9:549–560, 1964.

Beehler CC, Roberts W: Experimental retinal detachments induced by oxygen and phenothiazines. *ARCH OPHTHALMOL* 79:759–762, 1968.

Bresnick GH: Oxygen-induced visual cell degeneration in the rabbit. *INVEST OPHTHALMOL* 9:372–387, 1970.

Bridges WZ: Electroretinographic manifestations of hyperbaric oxygen. *ARCH OPHTHALMOL* 75:812–817, 1966.

Campbell PB, Bull MJ, et al: Incidence of retinopathy of prematurity in a tertiary newborn intensive care unit. *ARCH OPHTHALMOL* 101:1686–1688, 1983.

Criswick VG, Harris GS: Effect of hyperbaric oxygen on adult rabbit retina. *ARCH OPHTHALMOL* 78:788–793, 1967.

Dollery CT, Hill DW, et al: High oxygen pressure and the retinal blood vessels. *LANCET* 2:291–292, 1964.

Dollery CT, Bulpitt CJ, Kohner EM: Oxygen supply to the retina from the retinal and choroidal criculations at normal and increased arterial oxygen tensions. *INVEST OPHTHALMOL* 8:588–594, 1969.

Feeney L, Berman ER: Oxygen toxicity; membrane damage by free radicals. *INVEST OPHTHALMOL* 15:789–792, 1976.

Flynn JT, O'Grady GE, et al: Retrolental fibroplasia. *ARCH OPHTHALMOL* 95:217–223, 1977.

Frayser R, Saltzman HA, et al: The effect of hyperbaric oxygenation on retinal circulation. *ARCH OPHTHALMOL* 77:265–269, 1967.

Gole GA, Gannon BJ, Goodger AM: Oxygen induced retinopathy; the kitten model re-examined. *AUST J OPHTHALMOL* 10:223–232, 1982.

Hittner HM, Godio LB, et al: Retrolental fibroplasia; efficacy of vitamin E. *N ENGL J MED* 305:1365–1371, 1981.

James SL, Lanman JT (eds.): History of oxygen therapy and retrolental fibroplasia. *PEDIATRICS (SUPPL)* 57:591–642, 1976.

Kalina RE, Karr DJ: Retrolental fibroplasia. *OPHTHALMOLOGY* 89:91–95, 1982.

Kawasaki K, Okumura T, et al: Oxygen induced ocular syndrome in an adult. *JPN J CLIN OPHTHALMOL* 27:137–140, 1973.

Kinsey VE: Retrolental fibroplasia. *ARCH OPHTHALMOL* 56:481–529, 1956.

Kobayashi T, Murukami S: Blindness of an adult caused by oxygen. *J AM MED ASSOC* 219:741–742, 1972.

Kushner BJ, Essner D, et al: Retrolental fibroplasia. *ARCH OPHTHALMOL* 95:29–38, 1977.

Lyne AJ: Ocular effects of hyperbaric oxygen. *TRANS OPHTHALMOL SOC UK* 98:66–68, 1978.

Margolis G, Brown IW: Hyperbaric oxygenation: The eye as a limiting factor. *SCIENCE* 151:466–468, 1966.

Miller EF: Effect of breathing 100% oxygen upon visual field and visual acuity. *J AVIATION MED* 29:598–602, 1958.

Nichols CW, Lambertsen CJ, Clark JM: Transient unilateral loss of vision associated with oxygen at high pressure. *ARCH OPHTHALMOL* 81:548–552, 1969.

Nichols CW, Lambertsen CJ: Effects of high oxygen pressures on the eye. *N ENGL J MED* 281:25–30, 1969.

Nichols CW, Yanoff M, et al: Histologic alterations produced in the eye by oxygen at high pressure. *ARCH OPHTHALMOL* 87:417–421, 1972.

Nissenkorn I, Yassur Y, et al: Myopia in premature babies with and without retinopathy of prematurity. *BR J OPHTHALMOL* 67:170–173, 1983.

Noell WK: Metabolic injuries of the visual cell. *AM J OPHTHALMOL* 40:60–70, 1955.

Palmquist BM, Philipson B, Barr PO: Nuclear cataract and myopia during hyperbaric oxygen therapy. *BR J OPHTHALMOL* 68:113–117, 1984.

Patz A, Eastham AB: Oxygen studies in retrolental fibroplasia. *AM J OPHTHALMOL* 44:110–117, 1957.

Patz A: The effect of oxygen on immature retinal vessels. *INVEST OPHTHALMOL* 4:988–999, 1965.

Patz A: Present status of retrolental fibroplasia. *SIGHT SAV REV* 36:67–69, 1966.

Patz A: Oxygen administration to the premature infant. *AM J OPHTHALMOL* 63:351–353, 1967.

Patz A: New role of the ophthalmologist in prevention of retrolental fibroplasia. *ARCH OPHTHALMOL* 78:565–568, 1967.

Patz A: The role of oxygen in retrolental fibroplasia. *TRANS AM OPHTHALMOL SOC* 66:940–985, 1968.

Patz A: Retrolental fibroplasia. *SURVEY OPHTHALMOL* 14:1–29, 1969.

Patz A: Symposium on retrolental fibroplasia; introduction. *OPHTHALMOLOGY* 86:1685–1689, 1979.

Perdriel G, Desbordes P, et al: Note concerning the effect of hyperoxia on the electroretinogram of the rabbit. *BULL SOC OPHTALMOL FRANCE* 65:25–29, 1965. (French)

Phelps DL, Rosenbaum AL: Observations of vitamin E in experimental oxygen-induced retinopathy. *OPHTHALMOLOGY* 86:1741–1748, 1979.

Phelps DL, Rosenbaum AL: Vitamin E in kitten oxygen-induced retinopathy. *ARCH OPHTHALMOL* 97:1522–1526, 1979.

Ramalho PS, Dollery CT: The effects of oxygen on retinal circulation. *OPHTHALMOLOGICA ADDIT AD* 158:506–512, 1969.

Ring HG, Fujino T: Observations on the anatomy and pathology of the choroidal vasculature. *ARCH OPHTHALMOL* 78:431–444, 1967.

Saltzman HA, Hart L, et al: Retinal vascular response to hyperbaric oxygenation. *J AM MED ASSOC* 191:290–292, 1965.

Schocket SS, Esterson J, et al: Induction of cataracts in mice by exposure to oxygen. *ISRAEL J MED SCI* 8:1596–1601, 1972.

Schulman J, Jampol LM, Schwartz H: Peripheral proliferative retinopathy without oxygen therapy in a full-term infant. *AM J OPHTHALMOL* 90:509–514, 1980.

Scullica L, Bisantis C: Changes induced in the lens epithelium by hyperoxia. *BOLL OCULIST* 47:281–299, 1968. (Italian).

Slater TF, Riley PA: Free radical damage in retrolental fibroplasia. *LANCET* 2:467, 1970.

Stefani FH, Ehalt H: Non-oxygen induced retinitis proliferans and retinal detachment in full-term infants. *BR J OPHTHALMOL* 58:490–513, 1974.

Touraids T, Coburn KR: Retinal vascular response to oxygen at increased partial pressures. *AEROSPACE MED* 38:611–612, 1967.

Tripathi B, Knight G, Ashton N: Effect of oxygen on the developing retinal vessels of the rabbit. *EXP EYE RES* 19:449–475, 1974.

Ubels JL, Hoffert JR: Ocular oxygen toxicity. *EXP EYE RES* 32:77–84, 1981.

Watanabe I, Miyake Y, Ando F: The effect of hyperbaric oxygen on ERG. *ACTA SOC OPHTHALMOL JPN* 73:1920–1933, 1969.

Weiter JJ: Retrolental fibroplasia; an unsolved problem. *N ENGL J MED* 305:1404–1406, 1981.

Yanoff M, Miller WW, Waldhausen JA: Oxygen poisoning of the eyes. *ARCH OPHTHALMOL* 84:627–629, 1970.

Oxymetazoline hydrochloride, an adrenergic vasoconstrictor, tested as 0.025% eye drops, had no adverse effect on the eyes of rabbits or human volunteers.[a, b]

   a. Duzman E, Anderson J, et al: Topically applied oxymetazoline. *ARCH OPHTHALMOL* 101:1122–1126, 1983.
   b. Samson CR, Danzig MR, et al: Safety and toleration of oxymetazoline ophthalmic solution. *PHARMATHERAPEUTICA* 2:347–352, 1980.

Oxypertine, an antidepressant, when administered for several months to beagle dogs caused a gradual, reversible decrease in a- and b-waves of the ERG, slight impairment of dark adaptation, decrease in brilliance of the tapetum lucidum viewed ophthalmoscopically, but no histologic abnormality.[a]

   a. Legros J, Rosner I, Berger C: Ocular effects of chlorpromazine and oxypertine in beagle dogs. *BR J OPHTHALMOL* 55:407–415, 1971.

Oxyphenbutazone (Oxalid; Tandearil), anti-inflammatory, has been used topically and systemically for ocular inflammations. In one series of 326 patients treated chronically with 10% ophthalmic ointment there were no notable adverse effects.[c] However, a patient treated for uveitis by oral administration developed fatal epidermal bullous necrolysis with evidence of severe immunosuppression and thrombocytopenia.[b]

No cataractogenic tendency was detected in experiments in which oxyphenbutazone 10% ointment was applied to eyes of rabbits which were developing naphthalene cataracts, or eyes of rats developing galactose cataracts.[a]

a. Koch HR, Hockwin O, et al: Investigations into the possibility of additive cataractogenic side-effects with oxyphenbutazone. OPHTHALMIC RES 5:272–274, 1973.
b. Neetens A, Zelencova L: Toxic epidermal necrolysis. BULL SOC BELGE OPHTALMOL 178:77–85, 1977.
c. Nemetz U: Treatment of diseases of the outer eye with Tanderil eye ointment. KLIN MONATSBL AUGENHEILKD 160:618–623, 1972.

Oxytocin, an oxytocic hormone, came under suspicion when a woman who had been given oxytocin intravenously in combination with methylergonovine developed blurred vision and exudative retinal retachment in both eyes. The patient had no toxemia or hypertension. There was complete recovery in two weeks. The cause of the detachment was not established nor is it certain that either of the drugs was directly responsible.[a]

Another woman developed acute water retention as a result of 6 hours of intravenous infusion producing a vasopressin-like effect.[b] She had marked edema of face and hands, diplopia and blurring of vision, and conjunctival hemorrhages, which gradually cleared. Intraocular pressure was not reported, and the cause of diplopia or blurring not explained.

a. Gombos GM, Howitt D, Chen S: Bilateral retinal detachment occurring in the immediate postpartum period after methylergonovine and oxytocin administration. EYE EAR NOSE THOAT MONTHLY 48:680–682, 1969.
b. Storch AS: Acute water retention with continuous slow infusion of oxytocin. OBSTET GYNECOL 37:109–111, 1977.

Ozone is a strongly oxidizing gas produced by action of the ultraviolet in sunlight on the oxygen of the air. It is formed also by artificial ultraviolet sources and by electrical discharges in air. It is commercially available in refrigerated concentrated form for chemical use and water purification. At concentrations greater than 1 ppm in air, ozone has been found irritating to the eyes and nose and injurious to the respiratory tract.[61,171] Concentrations of 2 to 3.7 ppm caused sensation of irritation to normal human eyes within six minutes.[a]

Ozone has been among the substances suspected of causing ocular irritation in smog, because it is characteristically found in higher concentration in smog than under smogless conditions. It is doubtful, however, that ozone is directly responsible.

At concentrations that are irritating to human eyes, ozone appears not to be demonstrably injurious to corneas of experimental animals. Exposure of rabbits to 2 to 2.8 ppm for four hours daily for one to twenty-five days caused no injury to the corneas detectable by ordinary clinical means, by measurement of rate of repair of artificial epithelial wounds, by histology, or by measurement of the activity of several enzymes in the epithelium.[a,e,f] Exposure of dogs for six hours daily for one year to concentrations of ozone higher than attained in urban atmospheres induced no symptoms of irritation, and all parts of the eyes remained normal, according to complete clinical examination.[h]

Mechanisms of systemic toxicity of ozone have been extensively reviewed and discussed by Stokinger and Jaffe.[b,c,g] They have quoted without criticism a report of experiments on human subjects exposed for periods of three and six hours to concentrations of 0.2 to 0.5 ppm of ozone in air estimated to be in the range that might be found in airplanes flying at high altitudes in the lower layers of the ozonosphere, showing no definite effect on ordinary visual acuity, on color vision, stereopsis, or vertical phorias, but describing frequent change in horizontal phoria measurements, also an odd increase in pheripheral vision and a slight reduction in visual acuity during dark adaptation tests.[d] It seems double-masked reexamination is needed to establish whether these effects are to be attributed to the ozone or to other factors in the conditions of the experiment.

Systemically absorbed ozone has been shown to affect electrical signals from the visual cortex of the brain of rats induced visually by flashes of light, believed to represent an effect on the CNS rather than on the eyes.[i]

a. Hine CH, Hogan MJ, et al: Eye irritation from air pollution. *J AIR POLLUT CONTROL ASSOC* 10:17–20, 1960.
b. Jaffe LS: Biological effects of photochemical air pollutants on man and animals. *AM J PUBLIC HEALTH* 57:1269–1277, 1967.
c. Jaffe LS: The biological effects of ozone on man and animals. *AM IND HYG ASSOC J* 28:267–277, 1967.
d. Lagerwerff JM: Prolonged ozone inhalation and its effects on visual parameters. *AEROSPACE MED* 34:479–486, 1963.
e. Mettier SR Jr, Boyer HK, et al: Study of the effects of air pollutants on the eye. *ARCH IND HEALTH* 21:1–6, 1960.
f. Mettier SR Jr, Boyer HK, et al: Effects of air pollutant mixtures on the eye. *ARCH ENVIRON HEALTH* 4:103–107, 1062.
g. Stokinger HF: Ozone toxicology. A review of research and industrial experience: 1954–1964. *ARCH ENVIRON HEALTH* 719–731, 1965.
h. Stokinger HE, Wagner WD, Dobrogorski OJ: Ozone toxicity studies. *ARCH IND HEALTH* 16:514–522, 1957.
i. Xintaras C, Johnson BL, et al: Application of the evoked response technique in air pollution toxicology. *TOXICOL APPL PHARMACOL* 8:77–87, 1966.

Palladium chloride can be used without toxic effect for cosmetic tatooing of leukomas of the cornea. A 2% solution applied to the cornea after removal of the epithelium followed by application of 5% ascorbic acid solution to reduce the salt to a black deposit has given better results than platinum chloride.[a,b,c] (See also *Tatooing.*)

a. Tota, G.: Tatoo of the cornea with palladium chloride. *BOLL OCULIST* 44:45–54, 1965. (Italian)
b. Valu L, Sallai S: Tatooing of the cornea. *DEUTSCH GES WOCHENSCHR* 21:1409–1411, 1966. (German)
c. Fodor F: Tatooing of the cornea with palladium chloride. *BER DTSCH OPHTHALMOL GESELLSCH* 71:236–237, 1971.

Pamaquine (plasmochin, aminoquin) is a derivative of 8-aminoquinoline, employed, usually as the naphthoate salt, in treatment of malaria.[171] It has toxic effects on the blood. In one case of fatal reaction a patient had diminution of vision and disturbance of speech, and was found at autopsy to have degenerative changes in the ocular motor nuclei.[a,194]

In dogs pamaquine has caused an apparent enophthalmos and pupillary constriction, as from sympathetic paralysis, and it has been reported to cause divergent strabismus. Histologically in these animals no damage was found in the sympathetic pathways in the spinal cord, but moderate damage was evident in the motor nuclei of the third, fourth, and sixth cranial nerves.[b] Similar injuries to the extraocular motor nuclei have been caused by closely related compounds, *Pentaquine, Isopentaquine* and *Plasmocid.*

Pamaquine apparently has not been suspected of causing impairment of vision except possibly in the fatal case already mentioned. In this respect it differs from a closely related substance, *Plasmocid,* which has damaged vision in many cases. (Compare *Pentaquine, Isopentaquine, Plasmocid,* and *Quinoline derivatives.*)

 a. Loken AD, Haymaker W: Pamaquine poisoning in man with a clinico-pathologic study in one case. *AM J TROP MED* 29:341, 1949.
 b. Schmidt IG, Schmidt LH: Neurotoxicity of the 8-aminoquinolines. *J NEUROPATH EXP NEUROL* 7:368–398, 1948.

Papain, a vegetable pepsin, has been used to tenderize meat, clean contact lenses, and to treat wounds. Subconjunctival injection of 2 mg in rabbits and patients is said to have caused no unfavorable aftereffects, but rather to be helpful in treatment of vitreous hemorrhages and posterior synechias in uveitis.[a,b]

 a. Starkov GL, Savinykh VI: Papain as a measure for the struggle with organization processes in the eye. *OFTAL Z* (Keiv) 24:89–94, 1969.
 b. Starkow GL, Sawinych WI: Papain treatment of eye diseases. (English summary) *KLIN MONATSBL AUGENHEILKD* 159:755–769, 1971. (German)

Papaverine, a smooth muscle relaxant and vasodilator, apparently does not raise intraocular pressure, at least for a dose of 50 mg orally in patients with systemic hypertension.[266]

Parabens (Parasepts; esters of p-hydroxybenzoic acid), widely used as antimicrobials in preservation of pharmaceutical preparations, may be used in the region of the eyes, and occasionally cause redness and swelling of the eyelids from allergic contact dermatitis.[b,c]

Methyl paraben and propyl paraben as saturated aqueous solutions have been noted to be moderately irritating to the eye, but at lower concentrations are useful in eyedrops as antimicrobial preservatives.[d] Eyedrops containing 0.02% propyl paraben and 0.04% methyl paraben in 0.9% sodium chloride solution are said to have caused smarting of the eyes in about three fourths of patients on whom comparative tests were made, but no persistent irritation or toxicity was noted.[7] In a methylcellulose gel (2.5%, 4,000 cps) methyl paraben 0.023% and propyl paraben 0.01% have been well tolerated by patients' eyes when this has been used in contact with the cornea for several minutes under gonioscopy contact lenses.[a]

Ethyl paraben (0.6%) applied to eyes of rabbits for 30 minutes caused only loss of the most superficial corneal epithelial cells.[300]

   a. Miller D, Aquino MV, Fiore AS: Gonioscopy ointment. *AM J OPHTHALMOL* 67:419–421, 1969.
   b. Schorr WF: Paraben allergy. *J AM MED ASSOC* 204:859–862, 1968.
   c. Schubert H: Contact eczema in the region of the eye. *KLIN MONATSBL AUGENHEILKD* 151:457–464, 1967. (German)
   d. Vaughan DG, Riegelman S: Management of corneal ulcers. In Kimura SJ, Goodner EK (Eds.): *Ocular Pharmacology and Therapeutics and the Problems of Medical Management.* Philadelphia, F.A. Davis, 1963, pp. 129–135.

Paraffin used in ointment bases is innocuous in contact with the eye. Formerly employed in cosmetic surgery by melting and injection into tissues, it caused much tissue reaction, and instances of loss of vision from emboli reaching the retinal arteries.[a, 153] Severe reactions in orbital tissues, thrombosis of orbital veins, and reactions in the lids have been reported.[153] In the anterior chamber of rabbits, paraffin has caused slight inflammatory reaction accompanied by clouding of the cornea.[153]

   a. Mintz: Amaurosis from paraffin injections into the nose. *OPHTHALMIC YEAR BOOK* 3:179, 1905.

Paraldehyde a hypnotic and sedative, causes miosis as in sleep,[247] but in overdosage causes mydriasis.[153] Paraldehyde appears to have no direct injurious action on the optic nerve or retina,[247] but visual hallucinations have been experienced by paraldehyde addicts during withdrawal.[255] In one instance a cerebrovascular accident with left homonymous hemianopsia and loss of corneal reflex followed a paroxysm of violent coughing after intravenous injection of 0.5 cc of the drug.[255]

Paraldehyde has been tested for influence on intraocular pressure when administered systemically to dogs and to normal and glaucomatous rabbits, and was found to cause no elevation, possibly a slight reduction of pressure.[a, b]

   a. Schmerl E, Steinberg B: The role of diencephalon in regulating ocular tension. *AM J OPHTHALMOL* 31:155–158, 1948.
   b. Stone HH, Prijot EL: The effect of a barbiturate and paraldehyde on aqueous humor dynamics in rabbits. *ARCH OPHTHALMOL* 54:834–840, 1955.

Paraphenylenediamine (p-phenylenediamine; p-diaminobenzene), a hair dye constituent, is usually encountered as the hydrochloride. In aqueous solution it rapidly absorbs oxygen, and passing through quinone intermediates, forms dark products which are the basis for the hair dyeing action. Paraphenylenediamine and its oxidation products appear not to be caustic or injurious unless there is hypersensitivity to them. Apparently hypersensitivity is spontaneously present in some individuals, and is readily developed by many others.

On normal rabbit eyes, 2.5% solution causes only mild conjunctival reaction.[347] On eyes from which the corneal epithelium had been removed, application of 0.02M solution at pH 4 or 8 continuously for ten minutes caused transient slight conjunctival edema and stromal grayness, but the eyes returned to normal promptly. The same type of exposure after allowing the solutions to age and darken in contact with air produced essentially the same results with only slightly slower healing.[81] Application of dry powdered paraphenylenediamine hydrochloride to rabbit eyes caused some discomfort, but no persistent injury of cornea or conjunctiva.[53]

N, N-dimethyl and *N, N-diethyl* derivatives of paraphenylenediamine tested as 1% aqueous solutions of unstated pH, but presumably as free bases, have been reported to cause conjunctivitis and corneal opacities in rabbits.[o]

In human beings many instances of inflammation and damage of periocular and ocular tissues have been reported from contact with hair dyes containing paraphenylenediamine, presumably in hypersensitized individuals. Reactions which have followed application of dyes containing paraphenylenediamine to the hair of the head characteristically have consisted of dermatitis of the head, forehead, and neck, associated with edema of the lids and conjunctiva, with tearing and exophthalmos. In at least two cases there has been limitation of eye movements associated with proptosis.[w] Involvement of the cornea with loss of epithelium and infiltration has occurred infrequently, and in most such cases the cornea has recovered rapidly.[k, m, x, zb, 153, 214]

More severe ocular reactions have followed application of paraphenylenediamine hair dyes to the eye lashes. Characteristically the reaction in these cases has been of rapid onset, with pain and burning of the eyes, redness and swelling of the lids, and edema and hyperemia of the conjunctiva. In numerous cases the corneal epithelium has become eroded, and iritis and iridocyclitis have developed. In several cases vision has been lost or permanently impaired by severe corneal ulceration.[b, c, j, l, p, r, t, u, v, za]

In the 1930's a cosmetic preparation known as Lashlure became notorious as a cause of serious ocular injuries of this type. Cosmetic use of paraphenylenediamine in the region of the eyes is no longer permitted in the United States.

A second and quite different type of ocular toxicity in human beings has been ascribed to both p-phenylenediamine and m-phenylenediamine. This second type of intoxication has also been attributed to contact with hair-coloring materials, but the supposed victims have had no notable dermatitis. Instead they have been described as having retrobulbar neuritis with central scotoma, or more rarely an optic neuritis with papilledema.[a, d, e, f, s]

The evidence to inculpate the phenylenediamines has been purely circumstantial and not very convincing. All patients improved when contact was discontinued, but this does not establish that poisoning was responsible for visual disturbance in these cases, because spontaneous recovery is common in retrobulbar neuritis such as is associated with multiple sclerosis. This is a disease which may present few other symptoms for some years, and which principally affects women in an age group most likely to use hair dyes.

Experimentally, systemic poisoning of rabbits, cats, and dogs by oral or parenteral administration of paraphenylenediamine has not been found to induce optic neuritis, but has caused a peculiar selective edema of the head and neck, in some instances producing temporary protrusion of the eyes, owing to edema of orbital tissues and conjunctiva.[g,i,m,o,y,z] Chemosis, exophthalmos, edema of face and larynx have also been observed in human beings poisoned by absorption through the skin or by ingestion.[h,n]

Yet a fourth type of ocular toxicity in human beings has been ascribed to hair dyes or paraphenylenediamine. In India a clinical suspicion that users of hair dyes developed cataracts more often than non-users led to comparison of slit-lamp examinations and refractions in those who would give a history of hair dye use and in a "matched" non-user group, apparently in an open, unmasked manner.[q] Lenticular changes were described in 89% of the first group and 23% of the second, but in most cases visual acuity was not affected, despite slit-lamp finding of lens changes. In the same study, albino rats and rabbits were treated with paraphenylenediamine in various ways. In rats, 5 to 15% solution applied daily for up to 3 months caused corneal opacities. Lenticular opacities were observed after 4% solution was applied to the head for a year. In rabbits, intravitreal 0.25 mg or more, or 4 mg per week subconjunctivally for 11 months, resulted in changes in lens transparency.[q] A number of questions have been left unanswered.

a. Berger E: Visual disturbance as a result of use of an aniline-containing hair dye. *ARCH AUGENHEILKD* 38:397, 1909. (German)

b. Bourbon OP: Severe eye symptoms due to dyeing the eyelashes. *J AM MED ASSOC* 101:1559–1560, 1933.

c. Brav A: Toxic ocular manifestations resulting from the use of eyelash dye. *AM J OPHTHALMOL* 19:894–895, 1936.

d. Busacca A: Neuroretinitis from use of hair dye, with a macular star. *FOLIA CLIN BIOL S PAULO* 6:45–49, 1934. (Italian)

e. Chiari C: Concerning a derivative of aniline (paraphenylenediamine). *ANN OTTAL-MOL CLIN OCUL* 38:882, 1909. (Italian)

f. Chiari C: Visual trouble from cosmetic use of anilin derivatives. *ARCH OPHTHALMOL* 30:706, 1911. (*OPHTHAL YEAR BOOK* 8:211, 1911.)

g. Dubois, Vignon: C R ACAD 107:533–535, 1888.

h. El-Ansary EH, Ahmed MEK, Clague HW: Systemic toxicity of para-phenylenediamine. *LANCET* 1:1341, 1983.

i. Erdmann E, Vahlen E: On the effects of p-phenylenediamine and quinonediimine. *NAUNYN-SCHMIEDEBERG'S ARCH EXP PATH PHARMAK* 53:401, 1905. (German)

j. Forbes SB, Blake WC: Fatality resulting from the use of Lashlure, on the eyebrows and eyelashes. *J AM MED ASSOC* 103:1441–1442, 1934.

k. Fuchs: Poisoning by a hair dye (paraphenylenediamine). *DTSCH MED WOCHENSCHR* p.2098, 1906. (German)

l. Greenbaum SS: Dermatoconjunctivitis due to Lashlure, an eyelash and eyebrow dye. *J AM MED ASSOC* 101:362–364, 1933.

m. Grunert: Eye symptoms in poisoning. *WIEN KLIN WOCHENSCHR* 31:712, 1900. (German)

n. Grunert K: Eye symptoms from poisoning by paraphenylenediamine. *BER OPHTHAL-MOL GESELLSCH HEIDELBERG* 208–217, 1904. (German)

o. Hanzlik PJ: The pharmacology of some phenylenediamines. *J IND HYG* 4:386–409, 448–462, 1922.

p. Harner CE: Dermato-ophthalmitis due to the eyelash dye Lashlure. *J AM MED ASSOC* 101:1558–1559, 1933.

q. Jain IS, Jain GC, et al: Cataractogenous effect of hair dyes. *ANN OPHTHALMOL* 11:1681–1686, 1979.

r. Jamieson RC: Eyelash dye (Lash-lure) dermatitis with conjunctivitis. *J AM MED ASSOC* 101:1560, 1933.

s. Keschner M, Rosen VH: Optic neuritis caused by coal tar hair dye. *ARCH OPHTHALMOL* 25:1020–1024, 1941.

t. Machlin IM: Injuries of the eyes from dyeing of the eyebrows and eyelashes. *VESTN OFTALMOL* 13:271–275, 1938.

u. McCally AW, Farmer AG, Loomis EC: Corneal ulceration following use of Lashlure. *J AM MED ASSOC* 101:1560–1561, 1933.

v. Moran CT: Bilateral necrosis of the cornea following the use of hair dye on the eyebrows and lashes. *J AM MED ASSOC* 102:286–287, 1934.

w. Naffziger HC: Our present knowledge of exophthalmos and its surgical treatment. *ANN WESTERN MED SURG* 2:397–401, 1948.

x. Neuschuler L: Allergic blepharo-conjunctivitis from cosmetic. *BOLL OCULIST* 13:1098–1111, 1934. (Italian)

y. Pollak: A case of paraphenylenediamine poisoning. *WIEN KLIN WOCHENSCHR* 31:712, 1900. (German)

z. Puppe: Concerning paraphenylenediamine poisoning. *VJSCHR GERICHTL MED* 116:1896. (German)

za. Sallman Lv: Four cases of eye injury from dyeing the eyelashes. *Z AUGENHEILKD* 93:99–100, 1937. (German)

zb. Sgrosso S: On some rare eye afflications from hair dye. *ARCH OTTALMOL* 32:545–555, 1925. (Italian)

Paraquat (methyl viologen), a dipyridylium or bipyridyl herbicide commonly employed in combination with a related compound, diquat, in commercial preparations known as Preeglone Extra, Weedol, and Gramoxone, has been involved in several serious splash injuries of the eye. Though in tests on rabbit eyes pure paraquat at 50% concentration caused only mild superficial inflammation, developing in twelve hours and clearing in two to four days with no damage to the cornea,[c] and pure diquat proved even less irritating,[a] splashes of the commercial preparations which contain surfactants have been serious. Presumably the surfactants rather than the paraquat or the diquat has been responsible for the severity of these injuries. In several patients after a splash there have been increasing signs and symptoms of irritation of the eye, with loss of corneal and conjunctival epithelium, and with mild iritis in some cases. Some eyes have gradually recovered within a week or two, but in at least four cases there has been residual corneal scarring.[b,d,e] One eye has required corneal transplantation.[d] The slow development of signs and symptoms after contamination and the slow recovery seem to have been characteristic, and these are consistent with injury from a surfactant. (See also *Diquat.*)

Tests of a commercial "concentrate" of paraquat containing 242 mg/ml on rabbits' eyes showed severe corneal opacification when a 50% dilution was applied.[g] A 12.5% dilution caused relatively slight corneal damage, but much reaction of the conjunctiva and lids. (Testing of the vehicle minus the paraquat was not reported.)

Several human deaths from ingestion or subcutaneous injection of paraquat have been reported, characterized by few symptoms at first, but gradually developing lung damage becoming lethal usually in three weeks, but with no associated effects on the eyes or vision noted so far.

a. Akhavein AA, Linscott DL: The dipyridylium herbicides, paraquat and diquat. *RESIDUE REV* 23:97–145, 1968.
b. Cant JS, Lewis DRH: Ocular damage due to paraquat and diquat. *BR MED J* 1:224, 1968; 2:59, 1968.
c. Clark DG, McElligott TF, Hurst E: The toxicity of paraquat. *BR J IND MED* 23:126–132, 1966.
d. Joyce M: Ocular damage caused by paraquat. *BR J OPHTHALMOL* 53:688–690, 1969.
e. Swan AAB: Ocular damage due to paraquat and diquat. *BR MED J* 1:624, 1968; 2:187, 1968.
f. Peyresblanques J: Eye burn by Gramoxone. *BULL SOC OPHTALMOL FRANCE* 69:928, 1969. (French)
g. Sinow J, Wei E: Ocular toxicity of paraquat. *BULL ENVIRON CONTAM TOXICOL* 9:163–168, 1973.

Parathion (Thiophos; E605; diethyl-p-nitrophenylthiophosphate) is an anti-cholinesterase insecticide with general properties as described under the heading "Organophosphorus pesticides." (See INDEX). Absorption from contact with eyes, through the skin, or by inhalation, causes miosis and spasm of accommodation for near, which may be accompanied by aching pain about the eyes and blurred vision for distant objects. In systemic poisoning the pupils have generally been pinpoint and vision blurred,[f,i] but the pupils are not always constricted. In a number of cases of severe poisoning, the pupils have appeared widely dilated.[a,b,d,e] In some cases the wide and unreactive pupils have been associated with deep unconsciousness.[a,b,d] In one patient the pupils changed dramatically from wide and unreactive to pinpoint when the general conditions improved slightly.[a]

Suspicions of disturbances of vision from slight and possibly repeated intoxications with parathion have been raised, but without strong evidence. One agricultural worker, without real evidence of poisoning by parathion, developed optic neuritis; the relationship to parathion appeared extremely tenuous.[c] One young man with a history suggesting previous intoxications by parathion was found to have constricted visual fields and a scotoma extending from the blind spot, but visual acuity and fundi were normal.[h] Evidence to rule out other disease or to inculpate parathion seemed very weak in these cases.

a. Barckow D, Neuhaus G, Erdmann WD: On treatment of severe parathion-(E605)-poisoning with the cholinesterase-reactivator obidoxim (Toxogonin). *ARCH TOXIKOL* 24:133–146, 1969. (German)
b. Bogolepov NK, Kaplan SL, Luzhetskaia TA: Apoplectiform and epileptiform syndrome in thiophos poisoning. *SOV MED* 31:132–133, 1968.
c. Brihaye M, Graff E, Smulders J: Retrobulbar optic neuritis; anatomo-clinical study (Poisoning by parathion?). *BULL SOC BELGE OPHTALMOL* 126:1083–1099, 1960. (French)
d. DiComite A, DiComite P: Paradoxical behavior of the pupil (Mydriasis in the course of poisoning by organophosphorus compounds). *MINERVA OFTALMOL* 9:114–115, 1967. (Italian)

e. Eitzman DV, Wolfson SL: Acute parathion poisoning in children. *AM J DIS CHILD* 114:397–400, 1967.
f. Ganelin RS, Mail GA, Cueto C Jr: Hazards of equipment contaminated with parathion. *ARCH ENVIRON HEALTH* 8:826–828, 1964.
g. Gilsenan LD: A fatal case of parathion poisoning. *MED J AUST* 2:251, 1957.
h. Pejouan H, Moulin J, et al: Visual field defects and poisoning by parathion. *BULL SOC OPHTALMOL FRANCE* 64:138–139, 1964. (French)
i. Simon RD: Parathion poisoning. A case report. *AM J DIS CHILD* 105:527, 1963.

Pargyline (Eutonyl), a monoamine oxidase inhibitor and antihypertensive, seems to have produced no disturbances of the optic nerve or vision such as produced by certain other monoamine oxidase inhibitors. In one case of poisoning in a child the pupils were dilated and sluggishly reactive to light, and there were conspicuous wandering movements of the eyes, but within a day the poisoning was relieved by peritoneal dialysis and the pupils returned to normal size and reactivity.[a]

No adverse effect on intraocular pressure has been reported. On the contrary, a slight reduction of pressure has been induced in rabbits[b] and glaucomatous patients[312] by topical application, which produces mydriasis in rabbits.[c]

a. Lipkin D, Kushnick T: Pargyline hydrochloride poisoning in a child. *J AM MED ASSOC* 201:135–136, 1967.
b. Zeller EA, Shock D, et al: Enzymology of the refractory media of the eye. *INVEST OPHTHALMOL* 6:618–623, 1967.
c. Balacco-Gabrieli C: Effects of the monamine oxidase inhibitor, pargyline, on the motility of the iris. *BOLL SOC ITAL BIOL SPER* 47:33–35, 1971. (Italian)

Paris quadrifolia (in German, *Einbeere*) is said to be a type of berry eaten mostly by children and causing acute gastroenteritis and constriction of the pupils.[177]

Peat dust may cause irritation of the eyes when accidentally introduced into the conjunctival sac.[a] The irritation is said to be caused by acid salts and silica spicules, and is mechanically aggravated by rubbing. Treatment consists of irrigation and cleansing of the conjunctival sac.

a. Powell BJ: Uniocular conjunctivitis from peat dust. *AM J OPHTHALMOL* 17:206–208, 1934.

Pelargonic acid morpholide (pelargonic morpholide) is a potent lacrimator of short duration. It is highly irritating to the eyes of animals and human beings and has been considered as a potential tear gas for civilian use.[155, 204, 205] *Pelargonic acid* (nonanoic acid) itself is also a strong irritant,[171] but no description of its eye effects was found.

Pelletierine, an alkaloid from *Cortex granati,* the root bark of the pomegranate tree, has been employed in the treatment of tapeworm infections and has caused decrease in visual acuity, diplopia, and ptosis.[153] (See also *Cortex granati.*)

Pempidine, a ganglion blocking agent, is said to have caused blurring of vision,[171] presumably from interference with accommodation, but tests by systemic administration to glaucomatous patients have shown no adverse effect on intraocular pressure.[a]

a. Ernyei S: KLIN MONATSBL AUGENHEILKD 148:523–527, 1966.

Pencils, indelible or colored (aniline pencils, copying pencils) have caused a great number of ocular injuries. At least seventy articles have been published on this subject, and an extensive bibliography has been furnished by Duke-Elder.[46] The injuriousness of these pencils to the eye is attributable to the cationic or basic dyes, usually methyl violet or closely related phenylmethane dyes, used in them. (The general subject of injury of the eye by dyes is to be found discussed separately under the headings of *Dyes,* and *Dyes, cationic.*)

Fortunately, reports of serious eye injury from colored pencils have become increasingly rare, owing presumably to a recognition of the toxic properties of basic dyes, and a shift to the relatively nontoxic acidic or anionic dyes. Many of the colored pencils in use at present are not injurious when tested on rabbit eyes.[81]

However, as late as 1963 in Poland, indelible pencils containing crystal violet were available and a series of cases (42 eyes) of very severe self-induced damage of the eyes was reported from placing ground-up violet indelible pencil in the conjunctival sac for hours or days.[i] In seven eyes in this series very severe refractory glaucoma associated with iridocyclitis developed six to eight weeks after injury. A granuloma of the lid was reported from a benzidine yellow pencil in Japan in 1972,[g] and an orbital reaction from a violet pencil in France in 1970.[h]

Most of the reports of serious eye injuries come from an earlier period, the first forty years of this century, when indelible pencils containing basic or cationic dyes were common. The injuries generally resulted from accidentally striking the eye with an indelible pencil, causing the tip of the pencil to break off and remain in the tissues. The nature and severity of the resulting reaction was dependent on the location of the foreign material and its content of cationic dye.

In many instances permanent corneal opacification resulted from direct implantation of the pencil tip in the cornea or in the conjunctival sac in a position to be in intimate contact with the cornea. Pain, inflammation, much swelling of the lids, and purple discharge have been the usual reactions. In some instances there was panophthalmitis.[d] Tissues close to the foreign material typically became necrotic, but infection was rare. The necrotizing action was sometimes limited to ulceration of the conjunctiva in the fornix.[e]

Indelible pencil particles embedded in the orbit became surrounded by inflammation and necrosis, but as a rule a fistula remained, discharging colored material, usually purple. If the fistula opened into the conjunctival sac, the eye could be severely damaged and scarred by the discharge.[i] Discharge through the lid, not involving the conjunctival sac was less dangerous, but caused scarring and deformity of the lid.[a] Exceptionally the foreign material formed a cyst in the orbit, accompanied by much swelling of lids and orbital contents, with proptosis of the globe,[b,c] potentially with brain abscess if the dura was penetrated.[f,i]

Experiments in which violet indelible pencil grindings have been placed on rabbit corneas demonstrated clear relationships between amount of material applied, length of time allowed to remain before washing off, and effects produced.[i] Irrigation of the eye was helpful as late as thirty minutes after application of the grindings if the amount was not excessive. The purple dye took more than an hour to penetrate into the aqueous humor.

From many reports it is quite evident that surgical removal of every trace of particulate pencil material from the ocular or orbital tissues is the most essential and most effective part of the treatment. Of secondary importance are various chemical treatments which are discussed under *Dyes, cationic.*

a. Curdy RJ: Anilin injuries of the eye. *ARCH OPHTHALMOL* 45:243–246, 1916.
b. Drews LC: Aniline pencil in the orbit. *AM J OPHTHALMOL* 23:89–90, 1940.
c. Drews LC: Aniline pencil cyst of the orbit. *AM J OPHTHALMOL* 25:72–74, 1942.
d. Dunn J: Two cases of enucleation necessitated by getting into the conjunctival sac the point of an aniline pencil. *ARCH OPHTHALMOL* 39:120, 1910.
e. Elmer WH: Caustic burn of the eye from indelible ink or lead. *J AM MED ASSOC* 74:246–247, 1920.
f. Foy P, Sharr M: Cerebral abscesses in children after pencil-tip injuries. *LANCET* 2:662–663, 1980.
g. Matsuo N, Okabe S, Yamamoto K: A case of lid granuloma induced by a yellow pencil. *JPN J CLIN OPHTHALMOL* 26:113–121, 1972. (English summary)
h. Michail S, Nuta M, Niculescu A: Anatomic-pathologic study of a case of ocular injury caused by a chemical pencil. *ARCH OPHTALMOL (PARIS)* 30:227–230, 1970.
i. Segal P, Mrzygold S, et al: Self-inflicted eye injuries. *AM J OPHTHALMOL* 55:349–362, 1963.
j. Van Den Heuvel JEA: Clinical demonstrations. II. Aniline necrosis in orbital roof, dura mater and cerebrum. *OPHTHALMOLOGICA* 152:537–539, 1966.

Penicillamine (Cuprimine, Depen, Metalcaptase), a chelating agent for copper and heavy metals, has been used in treatment of Wilson's hepatolenticular degeneration, rheumatoid arthritis, and cystinuria. Originally DL-penicillamine was used, but this has been replaced by D-penicillamine, which is less toxic. Most toxic effects on the eye have been rare, consisting of isolated cases of optic neuritis, retinopathy, myopia, and superficial irritations, but there have been a number of cases of ocular myasthenia. Details on these side effects follow.

Two cases of axial optic neuritis have been associated with use of DL-penicillamine in treatment of Wilson's disease.[f,p] The first patient had reduction of vision to 20/70 and 20/200, with slight papilledema, tortuosity of the retinal veins, and development of new vessels at the margin of the left disc; but when the dosage was reduced and pyridoxine was administered, the centrocecal scotomas gradually disappeared and vision returned to normal.[p] In the second patient, vision became 20/40 in both eyes, in association with slight papilledema, a small hemorrhage near one disc, and obliteration of some small vessels. This patient was already receiving multiple vitamins when the optic neuritis developed. After the dosage of DL-penicillamine was reduced, the vision gradually returned to normal and the optic nerveheads improved with only slight residual evidence of the previous disturbance.[f] In neither patient was DL-penicillamine the only drug being given when optic neuritis appeared; in the first case primidone was also being given; in the second case, carbacrylamine resin.

In a third case of optic neuritis, D-penicillamine, rather DL, was used in treatment of Wilson's disease in a young patient who had partial optic atrophy already present from meningitis in infancy.[c] While receiving the drug the visual acuity became worse, the fields contracted, and the optic nerves looked more atrophic. These improved when pyridoxine was given.

Another patient, a seven-year-old child receiving D-penicillamine for cystinuria, was observed to have two small flame-shaped hemorrhages near the optic nervehead in one eye, but the nervehead itself continued to appear normal. The hemorrhages disappeared without change in the treatment, but later two other hemorrhages developed in the same eye. Vision was not appreciably affected.[b]

Retinopathy has been described in two patients. In one, defects in the retinal pigment epithelium were seen to develop during the 7th to 10th years of medication, appearing as numerous drusen-like lesions in dense white clusters throughout the posterior poles, but with normal visual acuity.[d] The other case was quite different, consisting of rapidly developed drug-induced thrombocytopenia with bilateral serous detachments of the maculas, and rapid decrease of visual acuity, but rapid recovery when penicillamine was discontinued. An underlying choroidal hemorrhage in the macular region of each eye was noted.[h] Fraunfelder's National Registry reports having received information on cases of retinopathy resembling retinitis pigmentosa.[312]

Change in refraction, gradually increasing myopia, has been noted in two patients. To explain this, a change in curvature of the lens, possibly from some influence on cystein metabolism of the lens, has been postulated.[k] Cataracts have been mentioned in a patient receiving penicillamine for Wilson's disease,[l] but it was not stated explicitly whether this referred to the deposits that may be seen beneath the lens capsules in patients with this disease and which can disappear, as do the Kayser-Fleischer rings from the cornea, during penicillamine treatment,[f,n] or whether the patient had some ordinary type of cataract.

Skin reactions to penicillamine treatment have been observed, and conjunctival inflammation with photophobia and lacrimation have been mentioned as side effects.[j,n] Chalazion in the eyelids of both eyes in two patients with blepharo-conjunctivitis may have been caused by penicillamine.[i]

Ocular myasthenia gravis was recognized as a definite complication of penicillamine treatment in the mid-1970's. Within a few years more than 20 articles have been published describing typical cases, some articles recording collections of several cases. In most instances symptoms of ocular myasthenia have occurred in patients with rheumatoid arthritis who had been receiving penicillamine for several months.[a,e,g,m] It has also been encountered in the presence of scleroderma.[o] Patients with Wilson's disease apparently are not subject to this complication. Presumably an immunologic mechanism is involved. Ptosis of the upper lids, often asymmetrical, and diplopia from weakness of extraocular muscles are characteristically the first indications of this complication. Tensilon testing as a rule has been dramatically positive. Treatment with cholinesterase inhibitors has been helpful. In most cases the eyes have slowly returned to normal after penicillamine has been discontinued. References to 20 publications on ocular myasthenia from penicillamine, in addition to those in the following bibliography, are to be found in the bibliographies of the articles by Francois (1978),[e] Kimbrough (1981),[g] and Schmidt (1976),[m] in which there is surprisingly little duplication.

a. Atcheson SG, Ward JR: Ptosis and weakness after start of D-penicillamine therapy. *ANN INTERN MED* 89:939–940, 1978.

b. Bigger JF: Retinal hemorrhages during penicillamine therapy of cystinuria. *AM J OPHTHALMOL* 66:954–955, 1968.

c. Damaske E, Althoff W: Optic neuritis in a child with Wilson's disease. *KLIN MONATSBL AUGENHEILKD* 160:168–175, 1972. (German)

d. Dingle J, Havener WH: Ophthalmoscopic changes in a patient with Wilson's disease during long-term penicillamine therapy. *ANN OPHTHALMOL* 10:1227–1230, 1978.

e. Francois J, Verbraeken H, et al: Myasthenia syndrome after peroral treatment with penicillamine. *BULL SOC BELGE OPHTALMOL* 182:126–130, 1978. (French)

f. Goldstein NP, Hollenhorst RW, et al: Possible relationship of optic neuritis, Wilson's disease, and DL-penicillamine therapy. *J AM MED ASSOC* 196:734–735, 1966.

g. Kimbrough RL, Mewis L, Stewart RH: D-penicillamine and the ocular myasthenic syndrome. *ANN OPHTHALMOL* 13:1171–1172, 1981.

h. Klepach GL, Wray SH: Bilateral serous retinal detachment with thrombocytopenia during penicillamine therapy. *ANN OPHTHALMOL* 13:201–203, 1981.

i. Loffredo A, Sammartino A, et al: Hepatolenticular degeneration. *ACTA OPHTHALMOL* 61:943–946, 1983.

j. McDonald JE, Henneman PH: Stone dissolution in vivo and control of cystinuria with D-penicillamine. *N ENGL J MED* 273:578, 1965.

k. Michiels J, Saterre C, Dumoulin D: Ocular manifestations of Wilson's disease treated with penicillamine. *BULL SOC BELGE OPHTALMOL* 132:552–561, 1962. (French)

l. Scheinberg IH: D-Penicillamine with particular relation to Wilson's disease. (Editorial) *J CHRON DIS* 17:293–298, 1964.

m. Schmidt D, Kommerell G: Ocular myasthenia through D-penicillamine treatment. *KLIN MONATSBL AUGENHEILKD* 168:409–413, 1976. (German)

n. Sternlieb I, Scheinberg IH: Penicillamine therapy for hepatolenticular degeneration. *J AM MED ASSOC* 189:748–754, 1964.

o. Torres CF, et al: Penicillamine-induced myasthenia gravis in progressive systemic sclerosis. *ARTH RHEUM* 23:505–508, 1980.

p. Tu J, Blackwell RQ, Lee PF: DL-Penicillamine as a cause of optic axial neuritis. *J AM MED ASSOC* 185:83–86, 1963.

Pentaborane, a rocket propellant, causes constriction of the pupils as an early sign of poisoning in dogs exposed to sublethal vapor concentrations.[b] The miosis disappears in three days after exposure is terminated. The mechanism has not been elucidated. In human beings, mention has been made of difficulty in focusing the eyes and of visual disturbances after inhalation of low concentrations, but these effects seem not to have been given detailed study.[a, 215]

a. Boysen JE: Health hazards of selected rocket propellants. *ARCH ENVIRON HEALTH* 7:71–75, 1963.

b. Weir FW, Seabaugh VM, et al: Short exposure inhalation toxicity of pentaborane in animals. *TOXICOL APPL PHARMACOL* 6:121–131, 1964.

Pentachlorophenol (Penta, Santophen 20) employed for preservation of wood, and for slime and algae control, is also used for the same purposes in the form of a water-soluble salt, sodium pentachlorophenate (Santobrite, Dowicide G). Dust and vapor of pentachlorophenol are irritating to the eyes, causing lacrimation.[a]

In 1952 monocular retrobulbar neuritis was reported in three patients who were exposed to a mixture containing pentachlorophenol, o- and p-dichlorobenzene, and DDT, but the specific substance responsible was not identified.[d]

From then until 1968 the only additional instance in which pentachlorophenol may have been implicated as a possible cause of retrobulbar neuritis appears in a report of a man who regularly sprayed wood with a proprietary mixture (not named) containing pentachlorophenol, dieldrin, and possibly unknown substances in a petroleum distillate solvent. The patient's vision became impaired, owing to dense 20° central scotomas in both eyes. The optic nerveheads were said to be slightly congested but not swollen. Bilateral retrobulbar neuritis was diagnosed. No associated neurologic symptoms were noted, and medical and neurologic studies were negative.[e] In both of the case reports in which instances of retrobulbar neuritis occurred in people exposed to pentachlorophenol, there appears to have been none of the characteristics of systemic poisoning by pentachlorophenol, and the relationship of the optic nerve disturbance to this chemical is entirely unproven.

People who have had severe acute poisoning by pentachlorophenol have characteristically had fever, sweating, weakness, and weight loss.[b,h] When death has occurred, it has been associated with high temperature, dehydration, or heart failure.[b] Pentachlorophenol interferes with the coupling of phosphorylation to oxidation, similar to the action of 2,4-dinitrophenol, and in addition pentachlorophenol inhibits mitochondrial adenosine triphosphatase.[b,g]

It seems particularly noteworthy that in instances of severe poisoning there has been no mention of disturbance of the eyes or of vision.[b,h] Also, large numbers of workmen have been chronically exposed industrially without disturbance of vision. For example, a report by Bidstrup and associates in 1969 notes that during a ten-year period among 1,853 men working full time on application of wood preservation fluids containing pentachlorophenol, no case of peripheral neuritis had occurred, and effects on vision or optic neuritis were not even mentioned.[c]

It is of further interest that despite the similarity in toxic properties to 2,4-dinitrophenol, there appear to have been no reports of induction of cataract by pentachlorophenol, either in experimental animals or in human beings. In rabbits it has been shown capable of penetrating through the cornea to the lens.[i] In a single case a fifty-year-old patient developed cataracts in both eyes peripherally in the anterior cortex in the course of work with a pentachlorophenol wood preservative, but there was no evidence to indicate poisoning, or to establish that the pentachlorophenol was responsible.[f] (Compare *2,4-Dinitrophenol.*)

a. Baader EW, Bauer HJ: Industrial intoxication due to pentachlorophenol. *IND MED SURG* 20:286, 1951.
b. Bergner H, Constantinidis P, Martin JH: Industrial pentachlorophenol poisoning in Winnipeg. *CAN MED ASSOC J* 92:448–451, 1965.
c. Bidstrup PL, Gauvain S, et al: Toxic chemicals and peripheral neuropathy. *PROC ROY SOC MED* 62:208–210, 1969.
d. Campbell AMG: Neurological complications associated with insecticides and fungicides. *BR MED J* 2:415–417, 1952.

e. Jindal HR: Bilateral retrobulbar neuritis due to insecticides. *POSTGRAD MED J* 44:341–342, 1968.

f. Nelson JH: Personal communication, Feb. 1969.

g. Weinbach, EC: Biochemical basis for the toxicity of pentachlorophenol. *SCIENCE* 124:940, 1956.

h. Toxicity of pentachlorophenol. *LANCET* 1:647–648, 1966.

i. Ismail RM, Salminen L, Korte F: Distribution of topically applied environmental chemicals in the rabbit eye. *CHEMOSPHERE* 6:797–802, 1977.

Pentaerythrityl tetranitrate (pentaerythritol tetranitrate, PETN, Equanitrate, Peritrate), a coronary vasodilator, in tests on patients with open-angle glaucoma and with eyes subject to angle-closure glaucoma produced no elevation of intraocular pressure when an ordinary amount of drug was given by mouth as in the treatment of angina pectoris. (See also *Vasodilators*.)

a. Whitworth CG, Grant WM: Use of nitrate and nitrite vasodilators by glaucomatous patients. *ARCH OPHTHALMOL* 71:492–496, 1964.

Pentamethylenediamine (cadaverine) is a poisonous, strongly basic, fuming liquid.[171] Tested in dilute aqueous solution on rabbit eyes, it has caused no significant injury.[123] A 12% solution applied six times a day for six days caused temporary mucoid discharge, but the eyes rapidly returned to normal when exposure was discontinued.[63] Test of the full-strength chemical on the eye seems not to have been reported.

Pentaquine is a derivative of *8-aminoquinoline*, related to *isopentaquine, pamaquine,* and *plasmocid*. Pentaquine is employed in prevention and treatment of malaria. Experimentally all four substances have been found to cause injury to the nuclei of the third, fourth, and sixth cranial nerves in dogs and monkeys,[a] but in human beings the principal toxic effect of pentaquine is on the blood.[171] (Compare *Isopentaquine, Pamaquine, Plasmocid,* and *Quinoline derivatives*.)

a. Moe GK, Peralta B, Seevers MH: Central impairment of sympathetic reflexes by 8-aminoquinolines. *J PHARMACOL EXP THER* 95:407–413, 1949.

Pentazocine (Talwin), an analgesic, constricts the pupil in normal people when administered systemically.[163] Pentazocine has produced visual hallucinations and disorientation in many people after intramuscular injection of as little as 30 mg.[a, 298, 312]

a. Gould WM: Central nervous disturbance with pentazocine. *BR MED J* 313–314, 1972.

Pentolinium tartrate (Ansolysen) a ganglion blocking antihypertensive, has frequently caused mydriasis and impairment of accommodation for near.[255] However, the intraocular pressure has not been raised in normal eyes or chronic (presumably open-angle) glaucoma.[a]

a. Tarkkanen A, Becker B: Aqueous humor dynamics. *AM J OPHTHALMOL* 46:499–508, 1958.

Pentylenetetrazol (Metrazol, Cardiazol), is a CNS stimulant employed in shock therapy for psychoses.[171] Walsh has described scintillating scotoma, chromatopsia, and xanthopsia accompanying petit mal type of convulsive attacks induced by intravenous administration of this drug.[255]

Peplomycin sulfate (pepleomycin sulfate), antineoplastic, tested on rabbit eyes by application of 10mg in 0.1 ml caused only moderate dilation of conjunctival vessels.[a]

> a. Abe F, Koyu A, et al: Safety evaluation of pepleomycin. *JPN J ANTIBIOT* 31:859–871, 1978.

Pepper is the dried unripe fruit of *Piper nigrum,* a tropical plant.[171] It is used chiefly as a spice. Contact with powdered pepper can cause redness of the eyes and swelling of the lids. This has been attributed to the *piperine* which it contains.[129]

Peppermint oil contains not less than 50% menthol plus numerous other substances.[171] In one instance splash of peppermint oil in the eye caused a loss of corneal epithelium, corneal infiltration, release of pigment into the anterior chamber with deposits on the back of the cornea, but in the course of sixteen days the irritation subsided and vision improved to 5/4.[a] (See also *Menthol.*)

> a. Becker: Peppermint oil injury of the eye. *KLIN MONATSBL AUGENHEILKD* 81:386–387, 1928. (German)

Peracetic acid at a concentration of 0.1% in water has been found to be an effective disinfectant for Schiotz tonometers,[b] and not to be irritating to rabbit's eyes.[a,b] However, 10% solution causes ulceration and perforation of the cornea and formation of symblepharon, despite prompt irrigation with water after application to the rabbits' eye.[a]

> a. Duprat P, Gradiski D, et al: Irritant action of various concentrations of Javelle water and peracetic acid on rabbit skin and eye. *REV MED VET (TOULOUSE)* 125:879–895, 1974. (French)
> b. Pambor R, Kiessig R: On the use of peracetic acid for disinfection of tonometers. *KLIN MONATSBL AUGENHEILKD* 169:270–271, 1976. (German)

Perchlorate salts, tested intravenously and compared with *iodate* salts, have been shown to increase permeation of ^{131}I from blood to aqueous humor by acting on the ciliary body, rather than acting on the retinal pigment epithelium like *iodate.*[a]

> a. Davson H, Hollingsworth JR: The effects of iodate on the blood-vitreous barrier. *EXP EYE RES* 14:21–28, 1972.

Perfluorocarbon gases are the equivalent of saturated hydrocarbons in which all of the hydrogen atoms have been replaced by fluorine atoms. In ophthalmology they have been of interest as gas bubbles to inject into the aqueous or vitreous chambers, particularly for their physical effect in helping hold detached retinas in desired positions for a longer time than can be accomplished by means of bubbles of air. Those that have been examined for this purpose include:

perfluoromethane,[d,e,f,h,i] *perfluoroethane,*[e,f,h,i] *perfluoropropane,*[e,f,h,i] *perfluoro-n-butane,*[g,h,i] *octafluorocyclobutane,*[a,c,d,j,k,l] and *perfluoropentane.*[b]

Their physical properties have been of prime interest, i.e. their low solubility in water, their slow disappearance from the eye, and their increase in volume due to absorption of normal gases from tissue fluids. Intraocular pressure can be elevated by enlargement of the gas bubble. Toxicity to the eye has been minor in most cases, usually consisting of temporary clouding of portions of cornea in direct contact with bubbles in the anterior chamber, and persistent clouding of the lens when in broad contact with bubbles.

Octafluorocyclobutane has been tested for toxicity in rabbits, monkeys, and human beings, in both the anterior and the vitreous chambers. In rabbits, 0.15 ml in the anterior chamber caused corneal edema, iritis, cataracts, peripheral anterior synechias, elevated intraocular pressure, iris atrophy, and buphthalmos.[a] If less than 0.1 ml was injected, the formation of synechias and lens opacities were less, and the corneal edema was reversible.[a]

In rabbits, 0.1 ml in the vitreous chamber caused no inflammatory reaction or histologic disturbance,[l] while 0.2 ml caused transient flare and cellular invasion.[d]

In monkeys, 1 ml of 70% octafluorocyclobutane with air in the vitreous chamber caused no persistent lens changes, or retinal damage,[c] but 1.5 ml undiluted caused posterior subcapsular cataracts in 8 to 14 days, but no histologically evident damage to the retina.[j] There was a temporary increased vascular permeability to blood proteins.[c] In monkeys' anterior chambers 0.2 to 0.3 ml of gas caused anterior subcapsular cataract in ten days, maturing in 2 to 3 months.[j] Smaller volumes or dilution with air limited the disturbances to clinically acceptable levels.

In human beings, a 40% mixture of octafluorocyclobutane with 60% air injected into the vitreous cavity during operations for detached retina in volumes less than 4 ml was reported to have no pathologic effect on lens or retina.[k]

a. Brubaker S, Peyman GA, Vygantas C: Toxicity of octafluorocyclobutane after intracameral injection. *ARCH OPHTHALMOL* 92:324–328, 1974.

b. Constable IJ: Perfluoropentane in experimental ocular surgery. *INVEST OPHTHALMOL* 13:627–629, 1974.

c. Constable IJ, Swann DA: Vitreous substitution with gases. *ARCH OPHTHALMOL* 93:416–419, 1975.

d. Lincoff H, Kreissig I: Posterior lip traction caused by intravitreal gas. *ARCH OPHTHALMOL* 99:1367–1370, 1981.

e. Lincoff H, Madirossian J, et al: Intravitreal longevity of three perfluorocarbon gases. *ARCH OPHTHALMOL* 98:1610–1611, 1980.

f. Lincoff A, Haft D, et al: Intravitreal expansion of perfluorocarbon bubbles. *ARCH OPHTHALMOL* 98:1646, 1980.

g. Lincoff A, Lincoff H, et al: Perfluoro-n-butane. *ARCH OPHTHALMOL* 101:460–462, 1983.

h. Lincoff H, Coleman J, et al: The perfluorocarbon gases in the treatment of retinal detachment. *OPHTHALMOLOGY* 90:546–551, 1983.

i. Lincoff H, Maisel JM, Lincoff A: Intravitreal disappearance rates of four perfluorocarbon gases. *ARCH OPHTHALMOL* 102:928–929, 1984.

j. Peyman GA, Vygantas CM, et al: Octafluorocyclobutane in vitreous and aqueous humor replacement. *ARCH OPHTHALMOL* 93:514–517, 1975.

k. Peyman GA, Namperumalsamy P, Vygantas C: Clinical trial of intravitreal C_4F_8 in retinal detachment surgery. *CAN J OPHTHALMOL* 10:218–221, 1975.

l. Vygantas CM, Peyman GA, et al: Octafluorocyclobutane and other gases for vitreous replacement. *ARCH OPHTHALMOL* 90:235–236, 1973.

Perfume in accidental contact with the eye, particularly by spraying, occasionally causes mild superficial transient injury of the corneal epithelium with immediate burning sensation and foreign-body-type discomfort, with gray dots observable by slit-lamp biomicroscope in the corneal epithelium, stainable, better the next day without special treatment.

Perhexiline maleate (Pexid), coronary vasodilator, has adverse side effects of peripheral polyneuropathy and papilledema.[a-h] The peripheral neuropathy involves segmental demyelination.[273] It produces muscle pain, and weakness of distal muscle groups. The mechanism of the optic nerve disturbance is yet to be established. Papilledema has been estimated to occur in about half of the cases of peripheral perhexiline neuropathy in which ophthalmoscopic examination has been done,[g] but it may occur independently[e] or in advance of the peripheral neuropathy.[h] Papilledema, usually accompanied by headache and enlargement of the blind spot, occurs after perhexiline has been taken for several months. Some observers have presumed that the intracranial pressure is elevated, without having measured it,[f] while in a few cases in which it has been measured it was normal.[d,h] Visual acuity in most cases has not been reduced, but in a few cases there has been moderate reduction, which has persisted after perhexiline was discontinued and the papilledema disappeared.[h] Peripapillary vascular engorgement and flame-shaped hemorrhages have been described associated with the papilledema.[b,g] Keratitis sicca was reported in one case, relieved when perhexiline was discontinued.[g]

Gibson and associates in 1984 described a man who had definite elevation of cerebrospinal fluid pressure (320 mm) and papilledema with decrease in visual acuity.[c] The patient had taken 200 mg perhexilene maleate daily for 8 to 9 months when his vision became reduced to 6/18 right, 6/24 left. After withdrawal of the drug, the cerebrospinal fluid pressure dropped, the papilledema subsided, and vision improved to 6/9 right, 6/12 left at 6 weeks and 6 months, with residual temporal pallor of the discs.

This same patient is also noteworthy for the fact that he had lipidosis of his corneal epithelium, with the same clinical biopsy appearance as corneal deposits from amiodarone or chloroquine. This is the first report of this condition from perhexiline. Lullmann and Lullmann-Rauch had shown in 1978 that perhexiline could produce generalized lipidosis in rats. (For further information, see INDEX for *Lipidosis.*)

a. Bouche P, Bousser MG, et al: Perhexiline maleate and peripheral neuropathy. *NEUROLOGY (Minneap)* 29:739–743, 1979.

b. Detilleux JM, Rausin G: Papilledema and perhexiline maleate. *BULL SOC BELGE OPHTALMOL* 180:27–32, 1978. (French)

c. Gibson JM, Fielder AR, et al: Severe ocular side effects of perhexilene maleate. *BR J OPHTHALMOL* 68:553–560, 1984.

   d. Hutchinson WM, Williams J, Gawler J: Papilloedema in patients taking perhexiline maleate. *BR MED J* 1:305, 1978.

   e. Mandelcorn M, Murphy J, Colman J: Papilledema without peripheral neuropathy in a patient taking perhexiline maleate. *CAN J OPHTHALMOL* 17:173–175, 1982.

   f. Stephens WP, Eddy JD: Raised intracranial pressure due to perhexiline maleate. *BR MED J* 1:21–22; 509, 1978.

   g. Turut P, Hache JC, et al: Ophthalmologic complications of Pexid. *BULL SOC OPHTALMOL FRANCE* 77:1003–1007, 1977. (French)

   h. Van Effenterre R, Poisson M, et al: Edematous optic neuropathy from perhexiline maleate associated with peripheral polyneuropathy. *ARCH OPHTALMOL* (PARIS) 37:709–714, 1977. (French)

Periciazine (propericiazine), a phenothiazine derivative anti-psychotic, evaluated in groups of 45 and 43 patients under treatment for a year or longer, revealed no ocular side-effects except in five patients a stellar deposit under the anterior capsule of the lens, such as is known to be produced by chlorpromazine.[a,b] Because of use of multiple drugs, it could not be proven that periciazine alone was responsible.

   a. Oniki S: Periodic observation of ocular changes associated with propericiazine therapy. *JPN J OPHTHALMOL* 23:132–139, 1979. (English summary)

   b. Tamai A, Setogawa T, et al: Temporal aspects of ophthalmological findings on neuropsychiatric patients during psychopharmacotherapy. *FOLIA OPHTHALMOL JPN* 29:577, 1978. (English summary)

Peroxides, organic, have been tested on rabbit eyes, giving reactions ranging from insignificant to devastating.[a,b] Organic peroxides for which there is information on eye effects are *Arachidonic hydroperoxide, Benzoyl peroxide, t-Butyl hydroperoxide, t-Butyl peracetate, t-Butyl perbenzoate, Cumene hydroperoxide, Cyclohexanone peroxide, Diacetyl peroxide, Di-t-butyl peroxide, Docosahexenoic hydroperoxide, Lauryl peroxide, Linoleic acid peroxide, Linoleic hydroperoxide, Linolenic hydroperoxide, Methylethyl ketone peroxide, Peroxyacetyl nitrate, Peroxybenzoyl nitrate.* (See INDEX).

Of these, the *benzoyl peroxide,* the *di-t-butyl peroxide,* and *lauryl peroxide* were practically nonirritating and noninjurious to the eye when applied externally, whereas severe injury was caused by *cumene hydroperoxide, methyl-ethyl ketone peroxide, cyclohexanone peroxide,* and *diacetyl peroxide.*

In the most severe injuries induced in rabbit eyes there has been great chemosis and formation of gas bubbles in the conjunctiva, cornea, and anterior chamber. The conjunctiva has become necrotic and the cornea opaque.

Treatment of contaminated eyes by irrigation with water within four seconds prevented injury in all instances, but if irrigation was delayed for sixty seconds after contact with the most toxic compounds, devastating injury was not prevented. Washing within thirty seconds did not consistently prevent damage, but did reduce the severity of the reactions. Experimental comparison of 2% sodium bicarbonate and 10% ascorbic acid solution as irrigating solutions showed slight advantage over plain water, but tannin solution offered no advantage, and definite worsening of the injuries resulted when olive oil was used.

Cataract formation and retinal damage from oxygen free radicals and hydrogen peroxide are believed to involve peroxidation of lipid cellular membranes, and to involve breakdown of lipid peroxides to form *malondialdehyde.*

Intravitreal injection of *docosahexenoic acid* has produced posterior subcapsular cataracts in rabbits, evidently through autoxidation through a peroxide form, and breakdown to malondialdehyde.

Irreversible retinal degeneration and severe reduction of the a-, b-, and c- waves of the ERG has been produced in rabbits by intravitreal injection of *arachidonic hydroperoxide, docosahexenoic hydroperoxide, linoleic hydroperoxide,* and *linolenic hydroperoxide. Malondialdehyde* also was shown to be toxic to the retina.

   a. Armstrong D, Hiramitso T, et al: Studies on experimentally induced retinal degeneration. *EXP EYE RES* 35:157–171, 1982.
   b. Bhuyan KC, Bhuyan DK, et al: Increased lipid peroxidation and altered membrane functions in Emory mouse cataract. *CURR EYE RES* 2:597–606, 1983.
   c. Floyd EP, Stokinger HE: Toxicity studies of certain organic peroxides and hydroperoxides. *AM IND HYG ASSOC J* 19:205–212, 1958.
   d. Goosey JD, Tuan WM, et al: A lipid peroxidative mechanism for posterior subcapsular cataract formation in the rabbit. *INVEST OPHTHALMOL VIS SCI* 25:608–612, 1984.
   e. Kuchle HJ: Investigations of the eye injuring action of organic peroxides. *ZENTRALBL ARBEITSMED* 8:25–31, 1958.

Peroxyacetyl nitrate (PAN) is one of the components of smog thought to be responsible for discomfort of the eyes. Tests of 0.05 to 1 ppm in air caused significant sensation of eye irritation in human volunteers in ten to fifteen minutes.[a,365] (Also see *Smog.*)

   a. Jaffe LS: Biological effects of photochemical air pollutants on man and animals. *AM J PUBLIC HEALTH* 57:1269–1277, 1967.

Peroxybenzoyl nitrate has been suspected to be one of the components of smog particularly responsible for sensation of eye irritation, producing definite sensation in human volunteers at concentrations as low as 0.01 to 0.02 ppm in air.[110,365] (Also see *Smog.*)

Perphenazine (Trilafon, Fentazin), an antipsychotic and anti-emetic derivative of chlorophenothiazine, has caused transient blurring of vision and a temporary Parkinson-like syndrome, as have other phenothiazine derivatives.[70,171] Young people appear particularly prone to develop oculogyric crises,[d,f,g] as well described in the case of an eight-year-old girl who received 1 mg at bedtime because of restlessness following a severe respiratory infection.[f] During the following day she was apathetic and complained that her eyes hurt. Twenty-four hours after the single dose she had a seizure lasting thirty minutes, during which both eyes turned up and to the right. Her neck was held in a painfully opisthotonic position and she was unable to close her lids or control the muscles of her eyes and neck. She remained alert and able to walk about during this seizure but complained of pain in the eyes and neck. Without further treatment she slept or was apathetic until forty-one hours after the single dose, when she had another oculgyric crisis the same as the first, but lasting two hours. Subsequently the patient recovered completely. A family history of epilepsy may possibly have provided a hereditary basis for exceptional susceptibility to the drug in this case. A 13-year-old girl has written an even more dramatic first-hand account of her painful experience.[d] She obtained relief from diazepam.

Unilateral internuclear ophthalmoplegia was present temporarily in a man who was comatose from an overdose of perphenazine, but recovered completely.[c]

Toxic amblyopia and transient blindness was alleged to have been caused by perphenazine in one instance, but the only evidence was suggestive behavior by the patient, who before receiving the drug was mentally deficient, irrational, and hallucinating.[e]

Mydriasis of less than 2 mm and cycloplegia of 1 to 1.5 D, but no change in intraocular pressure was observed in 7 normal young subjects given 16 mg orally.[b] Two patients developed acute angle-closure glaucoma while receiving the drug, raising the question whether the mydriatic effect might be involved.[b, 298]

Deposits in the corneal stroma of dogs similar to those from chlorpromazine have been induced by administering perphenazine,[278] and in rats the ERG has been altered,[h] but it is not clear whether pigment deposits or any form of retinopathy has been produced by perphenazine in patients.

b. Bonomi L, Levi-Minzi S: Disturbances of pupils, accommodation and tensions in patients treated with perphenazine. *BOLL OCULIST* 50:115–123, 1971. (Italian)
c. Cook FF, Davis RG, Russo LS Jr: Internuclear ophthalmoplegia caused by phenothiazine intoxication. *ARCH NEUROL* 38:465–466, 1981.
d. Forrester RM: Side-effects of perphenazine. *LANCET* 1:1383–1384, 1975.
e. Johnson W: Toxic amblyopia from perphenazine. *J MENT SCI* 106:352–354, 1960.
f. Kozinn PJ, Wiener H: Oculogyric crisis after a small dose of perphenazine. *J AM MED ASSOC* 17:304–305, 1960.
g. Paton A: *BR MED J* 3:344, 1974.
h. Uematsu I, Supachai C, et al: Change in oscillatory potential by perphenazine. *JPN J CLIN OPHTHALMOL* 34:897–902, 1980.

Pethidine (meperidine, Demerol, Mepadin), a narcotic analgesic, usually does not affect the pupils or vision in ordinary dosage. Miosis, if any, is very slight, usually less than 0.5 mm.[b] However, overdosage has been known to cause miosis in some patients and mydriasis in others.[255] The intraocular pressure in normal patients is not elevated by 100 mg intramuscularly, but may be reduced about 2 mm Hg.[a]

In mice a reversible opacity of the front of the lens has been observed to develop acutely after systemic administration of pethidine, because of reduced blinking, exposing the eye to evaporation and causing dehydration of the lens. The effect could be completely prevented by keeping the lids of the mice closed. Artificial exposure of the eyes to drying without use of drugs produced the same type of reversible opacities.[c]

In manufacture of pethidine its dust is said to cause blepharitis and conjunctivitis.[176]

a. Burn RA, Hopkin AB, et al: Sedation for ophthalmic surgery. *BR J OPHTHALMOL* 39:333–342, 1955.
b. Carlson VR: Individual pupillary reactions to certain centrally acting drugs in man. *J PHARMACOL EXP THER* 121:501–506, 1957.

c. Fraunfelder FT, Burns RP: Effect of lid closure in drug-induced experimental cataracts. *ARCH OPHTHALMOL* 76:599–601, 1966.

Petroleum products to be considered here include *Benzine, Gasoline, n-Hexane, Kerosene, Naphtha, Paraffin oil, Petroleum benzine, Petroleum ether, Petroleum hydrocarbons, Liquid petrolatum, Stoddard solvent, Deo-Base.* (Other petroleum products such as *petroleum asphalt* and *cyclic aromatic hydrocarbons* are discussed separately under the headings *Asphalt,* and *Benzene.*)

The various liquid hydrocarbons of petroleum cause little or no injury on direct external contact with the eye. In particular, kerosene, Deo-Base, Stoddard solvent, and petroleum oil on rabbit and human corneas are essentially innocuous.[27,81] Liquid petrolatum and purified, deodorized kerosene such as used for insecticide solvent can be applied to human eyes without causing discomfort or signs of irritation.

More volatile derivatives, high-test gasoline in particular, cause smarting and pain on splash contact with the eye, but only slight transient corneal epithelial disturbance.

Experimental exposure of rabbit eyes to gasoline with and without tetraethyl lead have been carried out, and the effects have been evaluated by biomicroscope and by testing with fluorescein.[81] A single drop applied without local anesthetic caused obvious discomfort and immediate blepharospasm which lasted several minutes. The conjunctiva became mildly hyperemic and the corneal epithelium stained faintly, but all returned rapidly to normal. Ten drops applied during five minutes after induction of local anesthesia by means of topical proparacaine hydrochloride caused blepharospasm lasting fifteen minutes. The conjunctiva became moderately edematous and hyperemic. The cornea stained definitely with fluorescein, but the injury was superficial and transient. Recovery was prompt and complete. Gasoline containing tetraethyl lead caused no more injury than plain gasoline.

Experimental exposure of human volunteers to vapors of gasoline indicates essentially no ocular irritation at a concentration of 140 ppm in air, but a detectable sensation of irritation of eyes and throat at 270 to 900 ppm.[h] This sensation is perceived by the subject before signs of irritation, such as conjunctival hyperemia, are visible.[c] The vapor of Stoddard solvent is perceptibly irritating to human eyes at 400 ppm.[183]

Repeated exposure of albino rabbits' eyes to gasoline vapor (3 mg/liter of air daily for ten months) has been reported to cause disturbances of the corneal and conjunctival epithelium recognizable histologically.[f] In workers chronically exposed in the Russian petroleum industry, there is said to be a related irreversible gradual loss of corneal and conjunctival sensibility.[f]

In experiments on rats in Russia, chronically inhaling gasoline vapor (1 g per cu m) is reported to have caused damage to cornea, retina and ciliary body in 6 to 9 months, with reversible damage to blood vessels of the eye being particularly noted.[g]

In human beings, inhaling gasoline vapor may cause inebriation and may lead to unconsciousness.[c,d,188] During inebriation, miosis has been noted, and in comatose individuals, mydriasis and nystagmus.[247]

Inhaling *n-hexane,* a constituent of petroleum benzine and petroleum ether, is a notorious cause of peripheral neuropathy, and in several cases "blurred vision" has been mentioned. However, the possible effects on vision need much more thorough study. This is discussed in more detail under *n-Hexane.* (See INDEX).

Visual and CNS disturbances from chronic inhalation of hydrocarbon vapors have been of particular interest in Russia, and a report of examinations of 865 workers in the petroleum industry has indicated disturbances of color vision and of peripheral visual fields to be not uncommon.[f]

Cataracts have been induced in 70 per cent of rats exposed to a C_9-C_{10} fraction of high octane motor fuel for two months, and were confirmed histologically.[180] Many other systemic toxic effects were noted in the rats, but the mechanism of cataract induction was not examined. The petroleum fraction was composed mainly of alkyl benzenes, not more specifically identified, but contained no naphthalene. Rats exposed to n-decane vapor under similar conditions have also been examined for lens opacities, but no cataracts were found.[180]

Accidental subconjunctival injection of petroleum benzine in a patient who had been under treatment for chorioretinitis caused immediate pain, rapid development of chemosis, corneal clouding, exophthalmos, and limitation of motion. These reactions resolved in fifteen days, but degenerative changes were seen in the retina. It was not clear whether these were caused by the accident or the previous eye disease.[j]

Injection of *mineral oil* or *liquid paraffin* into the anterior chamber of rabbits, replacing the aqueous humor, has been used to obstruct aqueous outflow and to induce glaucoma experimentally.[b,e] This presumably is a mechanical effect rather than a toxic reaction.

Injection of liquid petrolatum into the lacrimal system of patients with chronic epiphora produced a mass in the lower lid with inflammation in one, and infiltration of the orbit with interference in motion of the eye in another, both requiring surgery for relief.[a]

a. Crehange JR, Arouete J, et al: Palpebral vaselinomas after injection of medications into the lacrimal ducts. *BULL SOC OPHTALMOL FRANCE* 70:1202–1206, 1970. (French)
b. Cole DF: Effects of some metabolic inhibitors upon the formation of the aqueous humor in rabbits. *BR J OPHTHALMOL* 44:739–750, 1960.
c. Davis A, Schafer LJ, Bell ZG: Effects on human volunteers of exposing to air containing gasoline vapor. *ARCH ENVIRON HEALTH* 1:548–554, 1960.
d. Drinker P, Yaglou CP, Warren MF: The threshold toxicity of gasoline vapor. *J IND HYG* 25:225–232, 1943.
e. Garg KN, Sangha SS: Experimental glaucoma and ocular hypotensive effects of urea and mannitol. *ORIENT ARCH OPHTHALMOL* 2:121–127, 1964.
f. Giniyatullina AK: The effect of petroleum products on the organ of vision in the crude oil and petroleum processing industries. *VESTN OFTAL* 78:36–43, 1965.
g. Sunargulov TS, Giniyatullina AK, Ivanova TS: Histomorphochemical changes of eye tissues in experimental poisoning of animals with gasoline. *OFTALMOL ZH* 31:20–24, 1976. (English summary)
i. Speert H: Noxious vapors in aircraft cabins. *OCCUP MED* 2:101–115, 1946.
j. Takaku I: A case with subconjunctival injection of petroleum benzine by mistake. *JPN J CLIN OPHTHALMOL* 18:1113–1114, 1964.

Phenacetin (acetophenetidin), an analgesic, was under suspicion in the case of a man who had yellow vision for two days after taking 2 g, while the headache for which the medication had been taken disappeared.[a,153,214] The visual acuity and fundi remained normal. In another nebulous case, an elderly man who was addicted for years to a mixture of phenacetin and aminopyrine had poor central vision for several years, associated with large central scotomas, many scattered drusen of both fundi, and slightly pale discs. Autopsy after a cerebrovascular accident showed essentially normal optic nerves, but marked demyelination of the central core of both optic tracts.

a. Hilbert: On subjective pathologic color appreciation as a result of poisoning. *KLIN MONATSBL AUGENHEILKD* 45:518–523, 1907. (German)
b. Neetens A, Martin J, et al: Possible iatrogenic action of phenacetin at the levels of the visual pathway. *BULL SOC BELGE OPHTALMOL* 178:65–76, 1977.

1,10-Phenanthroline, a metal chelator, injected daily intraperitoneally for 30 days in rats produced unusual osmiophilic inclusion bodies in the retinal pigment epithelium, with the same appearance as those produced by dithizone.[a] It is postulated that this may represent sequestration of zinc in the retina by these chelators.

a. Leurre-du Pree AE: Electron-opaque inclusions in the rat retinal pigment epithelium after treatment with chelators of zinc. *INVEST OPHTHALMOL VIS SCI* 21:1–9, 1981.

Phenarsazine chloride (diphenylaminechloroarsine, phenazarsine, adamsite, DM), a very poisonous and irritating substance, has been used as a war gas dispersed in the air in the form of minute particles.[171] Maximum effects on the eyes is reached four to six hours after exposure, with necrosis of corneal epithelium associated with lacrimation and severe symptoms of eye irritation.[155]

Phenazone (antipyrine), an analgesic, has frequently induced sensitivity reactions, with swelling of the lids, dermatitis, and conjunctivitis. In exceptionally severe cases keratitis has occurred, characterized by gray stippling and fine defects of the corneal epithelium with infiltrate in the corneal stroma near the limbus.[153,214]

Transitory amblyopia or amaurosis has been recorded in four or five cases following overdosage.[a,2,42,74] Blindness has lasted from a few minutes to as long as eight days, but most patients have recovered completely.[157,246] Chronic use of antipyrine for sixteen years was thought in one case to have been responsible for development of optic atrophy.[24]

a. Hotz FC: A case of antipyrin amaurosis induced by 130 grains taken in 48 hours. *ARCH OPHTHALMOL* 35:160–163, 1906.

Phenazopyridine hydrochloride (Pyridium), a urinary tract analgesic, administered therapeutically or experimentally to dogs has caused keratoconjunctivitis sicca with reduced tear flow in 7 to 10 days.[a,b] The drug has been found to accumulate in the tear glands of dogs and to cause degeneration of the secretory cells. In severe cases the dogs have had purulent conjunctivitis and ulceration of the corneas. So far, human beings and cats have not shown this adverse effect.

a. Bryan GM, Slatter DH: Keratoconjunctivitis sicca in by phenazopyridine in dogs. *ARCH OPHTHALMOL* 90:310–311, 1973.
b. Slatter DH, Davis WC: Toxicity of phenazopyridine. *ARCH OPHTHALMOL* 91:484–486, 1974.

Phencyclidine (Sernyl, "Angel Dust"), formerly an intravenous anesthetic, now a psychotogenic, illicit street drug, produces miosis, nystagmus, and visual hallucinations.[312]

Phenelzine (phenethylhydrazine, Nardil), a monoamine oxidase inhibitor antidepressant, in large overdosage in one case has caused the pupils to be widely dilated and unresponsive to light, with signs of excess epinephrine and norepinephrine in the blood, although the patient was not unconscious. The ocular fundi were normal and the pupils became normal within two days.[a]

In rats that were given phenelzine subcutaneously, no changes in the lenses have been observed, but when serotonin was injected four hours after the phenelzine a reversible anterior capsular opacification developed in the lenses in one to three hours, and began to disappear after an hour.[b] This combination suppressed blinking, presumably exposing the eyes to dehydration from evaporation and leading to reversible lens opacification.

a. Solberg CA: Phenelzine intoxication. *J AM MED ASSOC* 177:572–573, 1961.
b. Tilgner S, Kusch T: Studies on the reversible lens clouding in rats and mice after combined administration of phenelzine and serotonin. *OPHTHALMOLOGICA* 159:211–222, 1969. (German)

Phenformin (phenethylbiguanide, DBI, Debinyl), an antidiabetic agent taken orally, is reported to have caused acute transitory myopia in a diabetic patient.[a] A few hours after the patient took the drug, the refraction of one eye, which was phakic, went from its normal of +0.50 D to −1.25 D, while the other eye, which was aphakic, underwent no change in refraction. The attack lasted approximately one day. The mechanism was not known, except that it apparently involved the crystalline lens, but whether it was related to change in blood sugar or was on some other basis, like the acute myopias induced by many other drugs that do not influence blood sugar, is not known. (Also see *Myopia, acute transient.*)

Phenformin has been withdrawn from use in some countries, including the United States, because of danger of producing fatal lactic acidosis. Two instances of severe reduction of vision related to severe acidosis have been reported. Both patients were diabetic and had been under chronic treatment with phenformin. One had taken a considerable amount of alcohol, and on awakening had widely dilated pupils, and could not distinguish light from dark. Ophthalmoscopy was essentially normal. There was severe lactic acidosis, and no methanol. Vision returned to normal during treatment with bicarbonate, insulin, and glucose. It was presumed that inhibition of oxidative mechanisms in the retina had temporarily interfered with retinal function. In the second case there was no mention of alcohol, but the patient had been vomiting, and vision rapidly decreased from hazy vision to light perception before fatal coma developed. There was marked edema of the nerve heads and retinas, and narrowing of arteries and veins, with a few fresh hemorrhages.

a. Scialdone D, Artifoni E: Transitory myopia in the course of treatment with Debinyl. *G ITAL OFTAL* 16:92–101, 1963. (Italian)
b. Sorensen PN: Transitory blindness during ethanol and phenethylbiguanide induced lactic acidosis in a subject with diabetes mellitus. *ACTA OPHTHALMOL* 55:177–182, 1977.
c. Roggenkamper P, Hirsch E: Eye symptoms in biguanide-induced lactic acidosis. *KLIN MONATSBL AUGENHEILKD* 172:115–117, 1978. (German)

Pheniprazine (Catron, 1-phenyl-2-hydrazinopropane) is a monoamine oxidase inhibitor which formerly was employed in depressive states and in treatment of hypertension, but is no longer used in most countries because of visual disturbances which it induced in probably less than 1 per cent of patients taking it. Usually the visual symptoms were not associated with other notable neurologic defects. The disturbance of vision was reversible in most instances, but occasionally was not. Most characteristically there was gradual development of red-green blindness within weeks or months on oral dosage in the range of 18 to 50 mg a day. Often the loss of ability to discriminate between red and green was accompanied by a complaint of blurring of vision. The blurring, which was not due to any effect on accommodation,[b,c] was often but not always associated with reduction of visual acuity. More than twenty cases of this general type, mostly completely reversible within a few weeks after discontinuing treatment, have been reported.[a–c,f,g,i,k–o]

In occasional patients with reduced visual acuity a definite central scotoma for white has been demonstrated. In rare cases this persisted indefinitely after treatment was discontinued, and partial optic atrophy developed.[a,f,j] In two special cases there is a possibility that administering nialamide, another monoamine oxidase inhibitor, after administration of pheniprazine was discontinued, may have contributed to the development of partial optic atrophy.[l] Exceptionally, constriction of the fields has been reported.[n,o]

Apart from one case in which loss of myelin cylinders in both optic nerves and tracts were detectable histologically at autopsy,[f] there has been no localization of the initial site of the toxic action of pheniprazine affecting vision in patients.

In pigeons, chronic feeding of pheniprazine has caused reversible alteration of discrimination of different colors.[d] In dogs poisoned with pheniprazine and seeming to have impairment of vision, lesions in the central nervous system have been detected histologically but not in locations to explain loss of vision.[e] In rabbits, systemic administration of pheniprazine has been reported to cause slight degeneration of the outer segments of the rods and proliferation of the pigment in the retina, giving an appearance similar to retinitis pigmentosa.[h] Injection of pheniprazine into the vitreous body in rabbits has caused more drastic damage to the retina, causing loss of visual cells and the outer nuclear layer with migration of pigment into all layers of the retina.[h] The findings in rabbits seem most suggestive and point to a possible primary site of toxic action in the retina.

The fact that disturbance of red-green color vision has been the outstanding feature of the effect in human beings has been urged by Jaeger (1977)[p] as evidence in favor of optic neuropathy such as found in postmortem examination by Jones (1961).[f]

a. Frandsen E: Toxic amblyopia during antidepressant treatment with pheniprazine (Catran). *ACTA PSYCHIATR SCAND* 38:1–14, 1962.

b. Gillespie L, Terry LL, Sjoerdsma A: The application of a monoamine oxidase inhibitor, 1-phenyl-2-hydrazinopropane (JB 516), to the treatment of primary hypertension. *AM HEART J* 58:1–12, 1959.

c. Gillespie L (Discussion) *ANN NY ACAD SCI* 80(Art. 3): 954–959, 1959.

d. Hanson HM, Witoslawski JJ, Campbell EH: Reversible disruption of a wavelength discrimination in pigeons following administration of pheniprazine. TOXICOL APPL PHARMACOL 6:690–695, 1964.

e. Highman B, Maling HM: Neuropathologic lesions in dogs after prolonged administration of phenylisopropylhydrazine (JB 516) and phenylisobutylhydrazine (JB 835) *J PHARMACOL EXP THER* 137:344–355, 1962.

f. Jones OW III: Toxic amblyopia caused by pheniprazine. ARCH OPHTHALMOL 66:29–36, 1961.

g. Kinross-Wright VJ: (Discussion) *ANN NY ACAD SCI* 80(Art. 3):840–842, 1959.

h. Mizuno K: Etiology and treatment of retinitis pigmentosa. *ACTA OPHTHALMOL JPN* 64:2186–2195, 1960.

i. Palmer CAL: Toxic amblyopia due to pheniprazine. *BR MED J* 1:38, 1963.

j. Simpson JA, Evans JI, Sanderson ID: Amblyopia due to pheniprazine. *BR MED J* 1:331, 1963.

k. Stenbeck A: Ocular damage during Catran medication. *ACTA OPHTHALMOL* 44:381–385, 1966.

l. Stenkula S, Wranne I: Can optic atrophy caused by pheniprazine treatment become aggravated by subsequent nialamid treatment? *ACTA OPHTHALMOL* 44:387–389, 1966.

m. Westerholm B: Adverse reactions induced by monoamine oxidase inhibitors: Swedish experiences. *PROC EUROP SOC STUDY DRUG TOXICITY* 6:157–162, 1965.

n. Wranne I: Pheniprazine amblyopia. *ACTA OPHTHALMOL* 42:236–242, 1964.

o. Ytteborg J: Optic neuropathy during treatment with Catron. *ACTA OPHTHALMOL* 44:377–379, 1966.

p. Jaeger W: Acquired color-vision defects caused by side effects of drugs. *KLIN MONATSBL AUGENHEILKD* 170:453–460, 1977. (German)

Phenmetrazine (Preludin), an anorexic, in overdosage has caused mydriasis with impaired pupillary response to light and accommodation-convergence, associated with general physical overactivity, cardiac stimulation and palpitation, abnormalities of mood, hallucinations, and disorientation, all reversible.[a, 229] Ordinary oral dosage of 12.5 to 50 mg of phenmetrazine appears to have little influence on the pupils.

A CNS stimulatory effect seems to be reflected in a significant increase in critical flicker frequency in normal people three to six hours after an ordinary dose.[219]

Phenmetrazine was suspected in the development of posterior subcapsular cataracts in two women under thirty-nine years of age who without supervision of their dosage attempted intense weight reduction and succeeded in losing 8 to 12 kg in two or three months after starting the medication. No other cause for the cataracts was known. The cataracts developed rapidly, reducing vision significantly. Vision returned to normal after the cataracts were removed surgically.[b] (Compare *Phentermine.*)

Phenmetrazine was suspected in 4 out of 6 cases of monocular central or branch

retinal vein occlusions in young adults while taking anorexics in greater than
advised dosage.[c]

   a. Bartholomew AA, Marley E: Toxic response of 2-phenyl-3-methyltetrahydro-1,4-oxazine
       hydrochloride (Preludin) in humans. *PSYCHOPHARMACOLOGIA* 1:124–139, 1959.
   b. LeGrand J, Chevannes H: Opacifications of the lens in treatments for obesity. *BULL
       SOC OPHTALMOL FRANCE* 65:943–945, 1965. (*ANN OCULIST (PARIS)* 199:714, 1966.)
       (French)
   c. Rouher F, Cantat MA: Anorexic medications and retinal venous thromboses. *BULL
       SOC OPHTALMOL FRANCE* 62:65–71, 1962. (French)

Phenol (carbolic acid) is poisonous and caustic, causing second or third degree
burns of the skin unless very promptly removed. Alcohol commonly is used for
decontaminating the skin in case of accidental contact with concentrated phenol. For
immediate irrigation of contaminated eyes, water is recommended, since nothing
has been proven to be simpler, more effective, or as easily available. A claim has
been made that immediate irrigation with 1% aqueous diethylenetriamine neutralized to pH 7.5 to 8.5 has been effective first aid for phenol contaminated eyes, but
carefully controlled animal experiments would be needed to compare with the
standard irrigation with water.[d] Lang has reported clinical experiences in treatment
of fifteen patients with phenol burns of the eye by irrigation as quickly as possible
with a 30% to 50% solution of polyethyleneglycol 400, which he believed to be
superior to either alcohol or water for first aid irrigation of the phenol-contaminated
eye.[k]

On rabbit eyes, crystalline or concentrated aqueous phenol causes almost instanta-
neous white opacification of the corneal epithelium[35,96] Eight hours after application the cornea is anesthetic, the surface ulcerated, and the stroma opaque. In five
weeks there is entropion, scarring of the conjunctiva, and opacity of the cornea. On
human eyes, concentrated phenol has had severe effects characteristically rendering
the conjunctiva chemotic, and the cornea white and hypesthetic. The lids have
become edematous, and in some cases, have been so severely damaged that they
required plastic surgery.[a,h] Severe iritis has accompanied the corneal injury in at
least one case.[j] The final visual results have varied from complete recovery,[a] to
partial recovery,[j] to blindness and loss of the eye.[h] In one instance a spray of 12.5%
phenol dissolved in 25% glycerol in water struck both eyes of a patient, and induced
faint haze in the corneal epithelium, associated with fine gray stippling visible by
slit-lamp biomicroscope, causing temporary impairment of vision to 6/12 and 6/18.
The corneas cleared within 4 days, and vision returned to normal.[g]

Chronic systemic absorption of phenol has caused gray coloration of the sclera
with brown spots near the insertion of rectus muscle tendons, associated with blue or
brown discoloration of the tendons over the knuckles of the hands. This is a form of
ochronosis, known as *carbolochronosis*, of which twenty cases were collected from the
literature up to 1942 by Smith.[i]

Glaucoma has been induced experimentally in rabbits by injecting 5% phenol in
almond oil subconjunctivally in all four quadrants. According to initial reports, this
caused flattening of the tonographic curve, gradual elevation of intraocular pressure
to 30 to 60 mm Hg, persisting for weeks.[e,f] However, some investigators have not

succeeded in producing glaucoma by this means.[c] A related substance, cresol, has been found to induce glaucoma in the eyes of monkeys when injected into the anterior chamber. (See *Cresol.*)

a. Carter JC: Instillation of pure carbolic acid into the eye. *J AM MED ASSOC* 47:37, 1906.

c. Hessburg PC, Kraus X: Experimental glaucoma in the rabbit. *AM J OPHTHALMOL* 67:767–768, 1969.

d. Krejci L, Jansa J: Diethylenetriamine as first aid in eye burns due to phenol and aldehydes. *CS OFTAL* 24:132–134, 1968.

e. Luntz MH: Experimental glaucoma in rabbits. *TRANS OPHTHALMOL SOC UK* 82:271–282, 1962.

f. Luntz MH: Experimental glaucoma in the rabbit. *AM J OPHTHALMOL* 61:665–680, 1966.

g. Pollock WBI: Burn of the cornea from carbolic acid seen with the slit-lamp. *TRANS OPHTHALMOL SOC UK* 45:723–724, 1925.

h. Sheehan JF: Phenol burns of the left eyelids, eyeball, upper face and temporal area. *LARYNGOSCOPE* 35:55, 1925.

i. Smith JW: Ochronosis of the sclera and cornea complicating alkaptonuria. *J AM MED ASSOC* 120:1282–1288, 1942.

j. Winkler A: Phenol burn of both eyes and general consequences, with some comments on the treatment of eye burns. *KLIN MONATSBL AUGENHEILKD* 102:810–815, 1939. (German)

k. Lang K (1969)—reference under *Polyethyleneglycol.*

Phenolphthalein, a cathartic, has caused edema of the eyelids and conjunctival ecchymoses accompanying widespread reactions of the skin, which may be severe.[252]

Phenothiazine (thiodiphenylamine, dibenzothiazine, Nemazine) an anthelmintic in animals and human beings,[171] causes a photosensitized keratitis with corneal edema in pigs and cattle after oral administration. The keratitis develops only in bright sunlight, and if one eye is shielded from light, does not develop in that eye. The same effect is obtained when the compound is injected into the anterior chamber as when given systemically.[a]

The effects on the eyes of pigs and cattle are particularly well known in New Zealand. The corneal edema or clouding and the interference with vision usually come on in 12 to 36 hours, but clear within a few days or a week. The keratitis has been observed also in sheep and birds, but sheep are said to be less susceptible because in sheep the photosensitizing agent, identified as *phenothiazine sulfoxide,* is more rapidly converted to an inactive derivative than in the other animals.[64]

In human beings, photosensitization of the skin has been noted,[171] but keratitis has been reported only among workers handling the compound,[176] and in this instance the nature of the keratitis has not been described, and it is not clear whether it is due to mechanical irritation by crystals of the substance or from hydrogen sulfide liberated in its manufacture.

Psychotropic derivatives of phenothiazine, such as chlorpromazine, have been shown by Potts to have a high affinity for the pigmented uveal tissues and to become stored in the pigment granules,[201,202] but phenothiazine itself does not behave in this way, and has not been known to affect retinal function or morphology. (Compare *Phenothiazine-derivative drugs*.)

a. Whitten LK, Clare NT, Filmer DB: A photosensitized keratitis in cattle dosed with phenothiazine. *NATURE* 157:232, 1946.

Phenothiazine-derivative drugs that have antipsychotic or major tranquilizing actions have been widely used in treatment of schizophrenia and other psychoses. Some also have been used as antiemetics. Specific toxic effects involving the eyes have been reported and confirmed for *Chlorpromazine, Piperidylchlorophenothiazine,* and *Thioridazine*. Only *chlorpromazine* has been shown undoubtedly to produce deposits in the crystalline lens, the cornea, the conjunctiva, and the skin, but very likely *levomepromazine* and *periciazine* have similar effect, since they have been reported to have produced deposits in the lenses in four or five patients who had not used any other phenothiazine derivatives. Only *piperidylchlorophenothiazine* and *thioridazine* have been proven to induce pigmentary retinopathy that can impair vision. (*Thioridazine* appears to be safe within specific dosage limits. *Piperidylchlorophenothiazine* is no longer used.) All other psychotropic phenothiazine derivative drugs continue under clinical scrutiny for possible similar actions, since some may eventually be found to have similar effects.

There are a number of other influences on the eyes that are common to a larger number of phenothiazine drugs and are relatively nonspecific. These include occasional slight blurring of vision, assumed to be an anticholinergic interference with accommodation, occasional oculogyric crises associated with dystonic or dyskinetic reactions, and idiosyncratic acute transitory myopia in rare cases.

Anticholinergic symptoms of slight blurring of vision and dryness of the mouth have been reported from *acetophenazine, chlorprothixene, pecazine, thiopropazate, trifluoperazine,* and *triflupromazine*.

Oculogyric crises have been reported from *fluphenazine, perphenazine, prochlorperazine,* and *trifluoperazine*.

Meier-Ruge in an authoritative review and commentary in 1977[357] pointed out an important observation, first recorded by Boet in 1970, that all sorts of chronically administered phenothiazine-derivative drugs eventually produce a brown discoloration of the macula due to lipofuscin deposition in retinal ganglion cells, increasing gradually with age and duration of treatment. Meier-Ruge emphasized that this macula pigmentation is a harmless side effect, unrelated to toxic retinal damage such as produced by piperidylchlorophenothiazine or thioridazine.

Further details on the ocular side effects of the individual phenothiazine derivative drugs are given elsewhere in this book under their individual names. Also several reviews discussing these side effects are available.[b,c,f–h,i]

(It is unfortunate that some otherwise well done and potentially valuable clinical studies describing pigmentary retinopathy, changes in vision, and electro-oculographic measurements have failed to identify the specific phenothiazine drugs involved.)[a,d,e]

a. Alkemade PPH: Phenothiazine-retinopathy. *OPHTHALMOLOGICA* 155:70–76, 1968.
b. Apt L: Tranquilizing agents. Chapter 11, 102–108, 1067. In Leopold, IH (Ed.): *Ocular Therapy, Complications and Management.* St. Louis, Mosby, vol.2, 1966.

c. Ayd FJ: A survey of drug-induced extrapyramidal reactions. J AM MED ASSOC 175:1054–1060, 1961.

d. Boet DJ: Phenothiazine retinopathy. *OPHTHALMOLOGICA ADDIT AD* 158:574–582, 1969.

e. Henkes HE: Electro-oculography as a diagnostic aid in phenothiazin retinopathy. *TRANS OPHTHALMOL SOC UK* 87:285–287, 1967.

f. Hollister LE: Current concepts in therapy. Complications from psychotherapeutic drugs. *N ENGL J MED* 264:291–293, 1961.

g. Nelson NM: Toxic hazards. Severe neurologic reactions to antemetics. *N ENGL J MED* 260:1296–1298, 1959.

h. Siddall JR: Phenothiazines in ophthalmology. *INT OPHTHALMOL CLIN* 7:207–216, 1967.

i. Garner LL, Wang RIH, Hieb E: Eye changes following phenothiazine administration. *WIS MED J* 73:119–121, 1974.

Phenoxybenzamine (dibenzyline), an adrenergic blocking agent used as an anti-hypertensive, may produce slight conjunctival hyperemia associated with nasal stuffiness and slight ptosis. It has had no adverse effect in glaucoma, but rather has occasionally been suspected to reduce the intraocular pressure slightly.

Phenprocoumon (Liquamar), an anticoagulant, taken daily by 30 patients for 3 to 15 years was associated with petechial retinal hemorrhages in 20 cases, more extensive retinal hemorrhages in 10, and subconjunctival hemorrhages in 6.[a]

a. Neumann L: Conjunctival, retinal, and vitreal hemorrhages in the course of long-term anticoagulant treatment. *BULL SOC FR OFTALMOL* 86:164–166, 1973. (French)

Phentermine (Ionamin, Linyl), an anorexic, has in overdosage produced dilated pupils associated with tachycardia and extreme restlessness,[b] but the only suggested possible serious adverse ocular effect has been in one woman under thirty-nine years of age who took this drug along with Dipleil and Diteriam in unsupervised dosage to obtain 8 to 12 kg loss of weight in two to three months, and developed posterior subcapsular cataracts with reduction of vision several months later.[a] No relationship to phentermine has actually been proven. (Compare *Phenmetrazine.*)

In studies on drug-induced lipidosis, Drenckhahn and Lullmann-Rauch pointed out that phentermine lacks the lipidosis-inducing effect of *chlorphentermine*, and, unlike the latter, did not produce lens opacities in rats during prolonged feeding experiments.[303]

a. Le Grand J, Chevannes H: Lens opacities in treatments for obesity. *BULL SOC OPHTALMOL FRANCE* 65:943–945, 1965. (French)

b. Rubin RT: Acute psychotic reaction following ingestion of phentermine. *AM J PSYCHIATR* 120:1124–1125, 1964.

L-Phenylalanine, an aminoacid present in excess in children suffering from phenyketonuria, has been shown to cause pyknosis and necrosis of cells in the retinal bipolar and ganglion layers when administered to newborn rats parenterally from the first to seventh postnatal day.[a] When administered to older rats, phenylalanine has not caused abnormalities of the corneas such as are produced by tyrosine.[b]

>   a. Colmant G: Investigation of the problem of phenylketonuria in the retina of newborn rats. *GRAEFES ARCH OPHTHALMOL* 202:259–273, 1977. (German)
>
>   Landolfo A, Albini L, Savastano S: Toxicity of tyrosine and phenylalanine for the eye of the albino rat. *ANN OTTALMOL CLIN OCUL* 102:135–144, 1976. (Italian)

Phenylarsine oxide (Arzene) has caused devastating injury when tested in 0.01 M solution on rabbit eyes by injection into the corneal stroma or by dropping on the surface after removal of the corneal epithelium.[123]

Phenylbutazone (Butazolidin), an antirheumatic, has caused numerous toxic side effects, including agranulocytosis and a variety of eye disturbances.

In several instances phenylbutazone has been associated with development of Stevens-Johnson syndrome or epidermal necrolysis with involvement of the eyes, characterized by severe keratitis with involvement of the conjunctivae, corneas, and tear glands, which may result in scarring of the corneas with opacification, vascularization, and symblepharon.[a,b,g]

Rare ocular complications possibly related to use of phenylbutazone, but not proved, include a case of a woman who developed diplopia from paralysis of the right abducens muscle within three weeks of starting daily dosage of 100 mg.[c] Also one patient receiving both phenylbutazone and sulfinpyrazone for severe gout developed optic neuritis with dense central scotoma in one eye.[i] These anecdotal cases without further substantiation carry little weight. In reports to registries toxic amblyopia has rarely been reported.[298,312]

One patient has been described in whom after four weeks of systemic treatment with phenylbutazone for rheumatic pains, blood vessels were noted deep in the cornea of one eye which two years earlier has had an ulcerative keratitis. This vascular reaction in the cornea subsided in the course of a month after the medication was discontinued. Walsh and Hoyt observed an instance of "peripheral stromal corneal vascularization and conjunctival injection" similar to this in association with use of phenylbutazone but gave no further details.[256]

In experimental animals phenylbutazone has been found to inhibit the incorporation of sulfate into the sulfomucopolysaccharides of the cornea,[e] but apart from the cases mentioned above there have been very little clinical indications of toxicity to the cornea. In rabbits a 20% solution has been found too irritating to administer subconjunctivally as a potential therapeutic agent, but a 5% ointment has been tolerated on the surface of the eye without notable effect.[j]

In experimental studies phenylbutazone appears to have no specially noteworthy influence on metabolism of the lens[f] or retina.[d]

>   a. Anderes W: On a case of "Toxic Epidermal Necrolysis" (Lyell) with severe eye complications. *OPHTHALMOLOGICA* 145:291–296, 1963. (German)
>   b. Bruna F: A fatal case of Stevens-Johnson syndrome from phenylbutazone. *BOLL OCULIST* 37:3–16, 1958. (Italian)

   c. Crismer R, Pirot G, et al: A case of diplopia caused by phenylbutazone intoxication affecting the abducens nerve. *REV MED LIEGE* 20:549–550, 1965. (French)

   d. de Conciliis V: Effect of Butazolidin on the metabolism of retina and lens. *ARCH OTTALMOL* 62:209–214, 1958. (Italian)

   e. Greiling H, Stuhlsatz HW: Biochemical study of mechanism of action of phenylbutazone and some of its derivatives. *Z RHEUMAFORSCH* 24:491–426, 1965. (German)

   f. Kleifeld O, Hockwin O: The effect of dinitrophenol, ethylenediaminetetraacetate, Diamox and Butazolidin on metabolism of the lens. *GRAEFES ARCH OPHTHALMOL* 158:54–63, 1956. (German)

   g. Oppel O: Eye involvement in toxicoderma. *BER DTSCH OPHTHALMOL GESELLSCH* 65:52–59, 1963. (German)

   h. Raymond LF: Neovascularization of the cornea due to Butazolidin toxicity. *AM J OPHTHALMOL* 43:287–288, 1957.

   i. Scott AW: Personal communication, 1965.

   j. Yourish N, Paton B, et al: Effect of phenylbutazone on experimentally induced ocular inflammation. *ARCH OPHTHALMOL* 53:264–266, 1955.

Phenylcarbylamine chloride, used as a military poison gas, is a potent lacrimator, but requires concentrations several times as high as chloroacetophenone for comparable effect.[155]

Phenylethyl alcohol (2-phenylethanol, benzyl carbinol) has been used in 0.5% concentration as an antibacterial agent in ophthalmic solutions. Tests on rabbit eyes indicate that higher concentrations should not be used for this purpose; irritation of the conjunctiva and transient clouding of corneal epithelium were induced by application of 1% solution.[a,b] Drying of the corneal tear film in rabbits is hastened by 0.3% solution.[305]

   a. Nakano M: Effect of various antifungal preparations on the conjunctiva and cornea of rabbits. *YAKUZAIGKU* 18:94–99, 1958. (*CHEM ABSTR* 53:8420e, 1959.)

   b. Soehring K, Klingmuller O, Neuwald F: *ARZNEIMITTELFORSCHUNG* 9:349–351, 1959. (*CHEM ABSTR* 53:17432c, 1959.)

Phenylephrine (Neo-synephrine), an adrenergic mydriatic and vasoconstrictor, has adverse side effects principally on intraocular pressure, systemic blood pressure, and the cornea, conjunctiva and lids. In normal human eyes it has little or no effect on the pressure or on accommodation. In open-angle glaucomatous eyes, it has little effect on the pressure in most case, but occasionally reduces the pressure temporarily in some eyes, while in other eyes it may cause an elevation of 6 to 23 mm Hg, with the angle of the anterior chamber remaining open.[g,k,o] It is likely that the transient elevation of pressure in open-angle glaucomatous eyes is, at least in some cases, attributable to release of pigment from posterior surface of the iris into the aqueous humor, causing temporary obstruction of the aqueous outflow channels while pigment is escaping from the eye. However, this effect does not relate to degree of iris transillumination and is not useful for identifying latent glaucoma in patients with pigmentary dispersion syndrome.[g]

In human eyes with abnormally shallow anterior chambers and abnormally narrow anterior chamber angles, phenylephrine has precipitated angle-closure glaucoma in a few published and many unpublished cases.[w,zb,zc] Angle-closure glaucoma is more likely to occur at a stage of moderate dilation than when the pupil is widely dilated.[31] Eyedrops containing 0.12% phenylephrine hydrochloride have caused sufficient mydriasis to cause angle-closure glaucoma,[zc] and in cases in which 10% solution has rapidly produced wide mydriasis, the onset of acute angle-closure glaucoma has usually occurred later, during the time the pupil was becoming smaller. Limitation of the degree of mydriasis by simultaneous use of pilocarpine may enhance the risk of angle closure.[m,w] After peripheral iridectomy has been performed, the risk of again inducing angle-closure glaucoma by applying phenylephrine is very greatly reduced.

Systemic reactions to 10% phenylephrine hydrochloride eyedrops have been reported, consisting of temporary increase in blood pressure, with headache, trembling, and perspiration. These systemic hypertensive side effects from 10% phenylephrine hydrochloride have occurred in such a small proportion of people in fair or normal health that series of a considerable number of routinely treated cases have been reported with no dangerous elevations of blood pressure.[a,d,h] Despite the low incidence, phenylephrine has been so widely used that it has been easy to gather reports on many adult individuals with hypertensive reactions.[i,l,n,t,u,x,zd,ze,346] Also, there have been series of tests of the responses of infants which have shown infants to be at significantly greater risk than adults.[b,c,p,s,y] From the incidents reported it has been learned that in adults phenylephrine is safer used in lower than 10% concentration, such as 5% or 2.5%, in elderly people with cardiovascular disease;[i] insulin-dependent diabetics;[t] hypertensive patients taking reserpine or guanethidine;[t] patients taking monamine oxidase inhibitors, tricyclic antidepressants, or beta-adrenergic blockers;[l] patients with aneurysms, and patients with idiopathic systemic hypertension.[x] Use of conjunctival packs or conjunctival injection appears to increase the hazard.[u] It has been urged that some of the reactions during angiography that have been blamed on fluorescein should be attributed to the phenylephrine used to obtain mydriasis.[ze]

In infants, routine blood pressure measurements have made a good case in neonates for reducing the concentration of phenylephrine, or for using alternative mydriatics such as tropicamide or cyclopentolate.[b,c,zd] Studies on premature or low-weight infants have shown significant rise of blood pressure even from 2.5% phenylephrine eyedrops.[p,s,y]

Toxicity of phenylephrine to corneal endothelial cells has been shown in rabbits, cattle, cats, and human beings. When the epithelium is present, it affords the endothelium protection from even 10% phenylephrine eyedrops, but when the epithelium is removed, the function and morphology of the endothelium are disturbed, and the cornea swells.[e,f] When introduced into the anterior chamber of human eyes at operation, especially if in conjunction with air or Miochol, 10% phenylephrine causes as much as a 30% decrease in endothelial cell density, though the cornea may remain grossly clear.[zf] Cytotoxicity is demonstrable also in bovine corneal endothelium in culture.[za]

Pseudopemphigus[z] and epidermalization of the conjunctiva, with occlusion of the lacrimal puncta[q] have been reported clinically from chronic topical use of phenylephrine in conjunction with other eye medications. Instances of allergic dermatoconjunctivitis have also been recorded.[j,r]

Acute reversible lens opacities from evaporation and temporary dehydration have been studied in hamsters after application of phenylephrine.[v]

a. Brown MM, Brown GC, Spaeth GL: Lack of side effects from topically administered 10% phenylephrine eyedrops. *ARCH OPHTHALMOL* 98:487–489, 1980.

b. Borromeo-McGrail V, Bordiuk JM, Keitel H: Systemic hypertension following ocular administration of 10% phenylephrine in the neonate. *PEDIATRICS* 51:1032–1036, 1973.

c. Caputo AR, Schnitzer RE: Systemic response to mydriatic eyedrops in neonates. *J PEDIATR OPHTHALMOL* 15:109–122, 1978.

d. Coffman MR, Klein JW, Tredici TJ: The effect of topical Mydriacyl and phenyleph-rine on cardiac rate and rhythm. *ANN OPHTHALMOL* 12:286–290, 1980.

e. Cohen KL, Van Horn DL, et al: Effect of phenylephrine on normal and regenerated endothelial cells in cat cornea. *INVEST OPHTHALMOL VIS SCI* 18:242–249, 1979.

f. Edelhauser HF, Hine JE, et al: The effect of phenylephrine on the cornea. *ARCH OPHTHALMOL* 97:937–947, 1979.

g. Epstein DL, Boger WP III, Grant WM: Phenylephrine provocative testing in the pigmentary dipersion syndrome. *AM J OPHTHALMOL* 85:43–50, 1978.

h. Epstein DL, Murphy E: Effect of combined 1% cyclopentolate — 10% phenylephrine eye drops on systemic blood pressure of glaucoma patients. *ANN OPHTHALMOL* 13:735–736, 1981.

i. Fraunfelder FT, Scafidi AF: Possible adverse effects from topical ocular 10% phenyl-ephrine. *AM J OPHTHALMOL* 85:447–453, 1978.

j. Hanna C, Brainard J, et al: Allergic dermatoconjunctivitis caused by phenylephrine. *AM J OPHTHALMOL* 95:703–704, 1983.

k. Hill K: What's the angle on mydriasis? *ARCH OPHTHALMOL* 79:804, 1968.

l. Kim JM, Stevenson CE, et al: Hypertensive reactions to phenylephrine eyedrops in patients with sympathetic denervation. *AM J OPHTHALMOL* 85:862–868, 1978.

m. Kirsch RE: A study of provocative tests for angle-closure glaucoma. *ARCH OPHTHAL-MOL* 74:771–776, 1965.

n. Lansche RK: Systemic reactions to topical epinephrine and phenylephrine. *AM J OPHTHALMOL* 61:95–98, 1966.

o. Lee PF: The influence of epinephrine and phenylephrine on intraocular pressure. *ARCH OPHTHALMOL* 60:863–867, 1958.

p. Lees BJ, Cabal LA: Increased blood pressure following pupillary dilation with 2.5% phenylephrine hydrochloride in preterm infants. *PEDIATRICS* 68:231–234, 1981.

q. Lisch K: Conjunctival disturbances by sympathomimetics. *KLIN MONATSBL AUGEN-HEILKD* 173:404–406, 1978. (German)

r. Mathias CGT, Maibach HI, et al: Allergic contact dermatitis to echothiophate iodide and phenylephrine. *ARCH OPHTHALMOL* 97:286–287, 1979.

s. Merritt JC, Kraybill EN: Effect of mydriatics on blood pressure in premature infants. *J PEDIATR OPHTHALMOL* 18:42–46, 1981.

t. Meyer SM, Fraunfelder FT: Phenylephrine hydrochloride. *OPHTHALMOLOGY* 87:1177–1180, 1980.

u. Miller SA, Mieler WF: Systemic reaction to subconjunctival phenylephrine. *CAN J OPHTHALMOL* 13:291–293, 1978.

v. Peterson LH: Cation changes in the lens and aqueous during the induction of acute reversible lens opacity in the hamster. *INVEST OPHTHALMOL* 10:147–150, 1971.

w. Renard P: On the danger of treatment of certain glaucomas by means of eye drops combining pilocarpine and phenylephrine. *BULL SOC OPHTALMOL FRANCE* 68:344–350, 1968. (French)

x. Robertson D: Contraindication to the use of phenylephrine in idiopathic orthostatic hypotension. *AM J OPHTHALMOL* 87:819–822, 1979.

y. Rosales T, Isenberg S, et al: Systemic effects of mydriatics in low weight infants. *J PEDIATR OPHTHALMOL* 18:42–44, 1981.

z. Saraux H, Offret H, DeRancourt E: Ocular pseudopemphigus induced by eye drops. *BULL SOC OPHTALMOL FRANCE* 80:41–42, 1980. (French)

za. Staatz WD, Van Horn DL, et al: Effects of phenylephrine on bovine corneal endothelium in culture. *OPHTHALMIC RES* 12:244–251, 1980.

zb. Tapie R: Acute bilateral glaucoma after instillation of 5% phenylephrine eye drop. *BULL SOC OPHTALMOL FRANCE* 57:691–693, 1957. (French)

zc. Weiss DI, Shaffer RN: Mydriatic effects of one-eighth percent phenylephrine. *ARCH OPHTHALMOL* 68:727–729, 1962.

zd. Wellwood M, Goresky GV: Systemic hypertension associated with topical administration of 2.5% phenylephrine HCl. *AM J OPHTHALMOL* 93:369–370, 1982.

ze. Wesley RE: Phenylephrine eyedrops and cardiovascular accidents after fluorescein angiography. *J OCULAR THER SURG* 2:212–214, 1983.

zf. Lang RM, Hassard DTR: Effects on the corneal endothelium of anterior chamber reconstituents instilled during intracapsular extraction. *CAN J OPHTHALMOL* 16:70–72, 1981.

Phenylhydrazine hydrochloride has been injected into the vitreous humor in rabbit eyes in a study of mechanism of absorption of vitreous hemorrhages. Injection of 0.56 mg caused inflammation, chorioretinitis, and degeneration of the retina, but 0.023 mg seemed to be innocuous.[14]

Phenylmercuric salts to be described here include *phenylmercuric acetate, chloride, nitrate, oleate,* and also the *hydroxide.* They have been employed as antimicrobial agents, often in eyedrops. Concentrated solutions are irritating to the skin and injurious to the cornea. A severe reaction is induced by 0.1 M *phenylmercuric chloride* or *hydroxide.*[123] *Phenylmercuric acetate* and *oleate* at sufficient concentration are vesicants (and would also be expected to be injurious to the eye externally.)[73] However, *phenylmercuric acetate* diluted to 0.005 M (0.167%) can be applied daily as a microdrop to the eyes of guinea pigs and rats for a month without causing corneal opacities.[6]

(Phenylmercuric dinaphthylmethane disulfonate is described elsewhere under the name *Hydrargaphen.* (See INDEX))

When phenylmercuric salts are used as antimicrobial agents in eyedrops, very low concentrations are employed, so that they do not cause injury to the eye, and generally they are well tolerated.[326] For instance, *phenylmercuric nitrate* in eyedrops at a concentration of 0.001% has been shown to cause no discomfort.[7] Also, at this concentration it does not interfere with the "temperature reversal" phenomenon in corneas of excised rabbits' eyes.[383]

Phenylmercuric acetate used as a preservative in eyedrops at a concentration of 0.002% can produce a microscopic discoloration and change in transparency of the front of the lens in patients after long chronic use, as in treatment of glaucoma. This so-called mercurialentis apparently is due to direct penetration from the surface of the eye to the front of the lens in the pupil.[b] This is illustrated by an example of an ophthalmologist who applied 1% epinephryl borate (*Eppy*) eyedrops containing *phenylmercuric acetate* 0.002% to one eye twice a day for more than five years, while keeping the pupil small with pilocarpine. There was no disturbance of vision, but by slit-lamp biomicroscope the treated eye developed in the front surface of the lens a fine gray lamina with faint brown hue composed of an extremely fine mosaic pattern. This developed only in the eye under treatment and was limited to a small diffuse axial disc corresponding to the size of the pupil. When the pupil was dilated with mydriatic drops, the peripheral portions of the anterior surface were entirely clear and normal.

Mercurialentis, discoloration of the front of the lens by mercury, is well known from absorption of inorganic or metallic mercury, as discussed elsewhere under "Mercury". (See INDEX). Mercurialentis has been observed in series of patients . who have been treated for years with eyedrops containing *phenylmercuric nitrate*, as in the case described above. Abrams (1963, 1970)[a,b] and Garron (1977)[d] have reported numerous cases in which pilocarpine eyedrops containing this antimicrobial have produced mercurialentis after having been applied in treatment of glaucoma 3 or 4 times a day for an average of 10 years, but exceptionally for as little as 3 years. Characteristically the discoloration of the anterior surface of the lens gradually advanced from lusterless gray to yellowish brown to reddish brown. When the pupils were dilated, the discoloration was obviously limited to correspond to the size of the miotic pupil. This differed from the involvement of the whole front surface of the lens reported in some patients exposed to mercury vapor, suggesting that the mercurial compound from eyedrops might reach the lens by passage through cornea and anterior chamber only to the area not covered by the iris, while in some cases of mercury vapor exposure there might be in addition a systemic absorption and entry into the aqueous humor, having access to the whole front surface of the lens. Microscopy of lenses from patients who had mercurialentis from eyedrops showed electron-dense particles in the affected areas of the lens at all levels in the lens capsule, as well as in lens epithelial cells. Assays for mercury have shown that a very small amount can produce striking changes in appearance by microscopy. There has been no evidence that mercurialentis interferes with vision or causes cataract.

Corneal involvement was rarely seen in the series of cases reported by Abrams and by Garron, while Kennedy (1974) reported on 48 cases in which the circumstances of exposure were the same, but their most notable feature was atypical band keratopathy.[f] In Kennedy's cases after an average of 10 years use of pilocarpine eyedrops containing *phenylmercuric nitrate* a veil of opacification developed in and under the corneal epithelium, near the corneal vertex and spreading peripherally. This appeared to be same as band keratopathy, or corneal calcification, which is associated with systemic hypercalcemia, except that the latter tends to start more peripherally and spread to the vertex. When in the pupillary area, band keratopathy of both sorts interferes with vision, but can be easily and satisfactorily treated by scraping the corneal epithelium and dissolving the calcific deposit by means of a solution of sodium edetate.

Using *thimerosal* in place of *phenylmercuric salts* in eyedrops seems to avoid the production of mercurialentis and band keratopathy. (See INDEX for *Thimerosal.*)

In rats, analyses for mercury have shown both *phenylmercuric nitrate* and *acetate* applied in eyedrops to penetrate not only to the lens but also to iris, ciliary body, and retina.[c] However, no toxic effects on the retina have been noted in patients. *Phenylmercuric acetate* added to cultures of retina has caused degeneration of the rod cells at 5×10^{-6} M,[99] but daily subcutaneous *phenylmercuric borate* 1 mg kg for 7 weeks in rats has not affected the E.R.G.[e]

a. Abrams JD: Iatrogenic mercurialentis. *TRANS OPHTHALMOL SOC UK* 83:263–269, 1963.
b. Abrams JD, Majzoub U: Mercury content of the human lens. *BR J OPHTHALMOL* 54:59–61, 1970.
c. Ancill RJ, Richens ER, Norton DA: Aspects of the penetration and distribution of organic mercurials within the eye. In Pigott PV (Ed.): *Evaluation of Drug Effects on the Eye.* London, F.J. Parsons, 1968.
d. Garron LK, Wood IS, et al: A clinical pathological study of mercurialentis medicamentosus. *TRANS AM OPHTHALMOL SOC* 74:295–320, 1977.
e. Gramoni R: Retinal function of rats exposed to organomercurials. Pages 101–111 in Merigan and Weiss (1980).[358]
f. Kennedy RE, Roca PD, Platt DS: Further observations on atypical band keratopathy in glaucoma patients. *TRANS AM OPHTHALMOL SOC* 72:107–122, 1974.

1-Phenylpiperazine (N-Phenylpiperazine) applied to the surface of rabbit eyes is severely injurious to the cornea.[228] When administered systemically to dogs, it did not produce cataracts. (For reference, see next entry.)

2-(4-Phenyl-1-piperazinylmethyl) cyclohexanone when chronically administered systemically to dogs has caused mucopurulent discharge and lens opacities. Related compounds have similar effect, but the simpler compound *phenylpiperazine* did not cause cataract.[a]

a. Phillips BM, Hong E et al: Biological disposition of 2-(4-Phenyl-1-piperazinylmethyl) cyclohexanone-1-[14]C(MA1050-^{14}C). *J PHARM SCI* 54:899–902, 1965.

Phenylpropanolamine (Norephedrine, Propadrine), an adrenergic vasoconstrictor, appears to have little or no effect on the pupils in normal people when given in ordinary doses of 25 to 50 mg of the hydrochloride salt. In one person with active pupils a dose of 150 mg, which induced dryness of the mouth, had no effect on the pupils.

Phenytoin (diphenylhydantoin, Dilantin, Diphenine, Diphentoin, Epanutin), an anticonvulsant antiepileptic drug, when given in excessive dosage causes nystagmus and ataxia, and less commonly diplopia, weakness of accommodation, and convergence.[1] Nystagmus, ataxia, and dulled or stuporous mental state may also occur occasionally in individuals who have a deficiency in the enzyme system required for metabolism of the drug.[b,d,f] Evidences of intoxication tend to appear in the order: nystagmus, ataxia, and mental disturbance, usually at blood concentrations of $20\mu g$, $30\mu g$, and

$40\mu g$ per ml.[j,m] Many instances have been reported in which disturbances of the eyes were reversible when the dosage of phenytoin was reduced.[c,d,h,j-m,o] In exceptional cases, nystagmus and ataxia has persisted for twenty months or more after phenytoin has been discontinued.[h] Degenerative changes in the cerebellum which could explain these persistent toxic effects have been induced in rats and cats with large doses of phenytoin,[h] and disappearance of Purkinje's cells from the cerebellum has been described at postmortem examination after intensive treatment with phenytoin.[f] When no nystagmus is detectable by ordinary observation, a very fine periodic dancing of the eyes vertically or horizontally, termed oscillopsia, has been described as a reversible effect of treatment with phenytoin. It is best seen when looking at details of the ocular fundus with an ophthalmoscope.[c] The patient who has oscillopsia may complain that his vision is jumbled.

In two cases described by Orth, overdosage caused rapid onset of nearly complete external ophthalmoplegia lasting about a day, followed by several days of nystagmus.[l] Five other patients who received large doses had their eyes temporarily fixed in mid-position, with no response to flexion or rotation of the head, or to irrigation of the ear with ice-water, yet the effect was not particularly related to the level of consciousness, being present not only in coma but also persisting for a while when not in coma.[n] Phenytoin apparently can interfere with the vestibulo-ocular reflex arc.

Apart from neurologic side effects, phenytoin has caused dermatitis and conjunctivitis, and rarely Stevens-Johnson syndrome.[e] Phenytoin is believed to stimulate formation of collagen, but has not interfered with healing of penetrating wounds of the cornea in rabbits.[i]

No adverse effect on intraocular pressure in open-angle glaucoma was detected in twelve patients given 100 mg three times a day for one to five days.[190]

One article has raised a question whether phenytoin might hasten cataract formation, on the clinical basis of two patients aged 43 and 40 who had been under treatment with this drug and phenobarbital for 7 years, with one patient having mature cataract in one eye incipient cataract in the other, and with the second patient having only subcapsular opacities with vision 6/12, 6/10.[b] These isolated instances seem hardly worth considering as evidence, but the same article has reported that rats given comparable dosage for 3 months developed slight subcapsular lens clouding in significantly larger number than did control rats. None developed any more definite opacification.

Malformations involving the eyes of infants born to epileptic mothers who have taken phenytoin during pregnancy has become known as the "fetal hydantoin syndrome", but it is not yet proven whether the epilepsy or the drug is primarily responsible.[a] The eye malformations, usually associated with a number of non-ocular malformations, have included hypertelorism, ptosis, strabismus, epicanthal folds, abnormality of the lacrimal apparatus,[q] optic nerve hypoplasia,[g,r] retinoschisis,[g] and congenital glaucoma.[k,p]

a. Apt L, Gaffney WL: Is there a "fetal hydantoin syndrome?" *AM J OPHTHALMOL* 84:439–440, 1977.

b. Bar S, Feller N, Savir H: Presenile cataracts in phenytoin-treated epileptic patients. *ARCH OPHTHALMOL* 101:442–425, 1983.

c. Bender MB: Oscillopsia. *ARCH NEUROL* 13:204–213, 1965.

d. Frantzen E, Hansen JM, et al: Phenytoin (Dilantin) intoxication. *ACTA NEUROL SCAND* 43:440–446, 1967.

e. Greenberg LM, Mauriello DA, et al: Erythema multiforme exudativum (Stevens-Johnson syndrome) following sodium diphenylydantoin therapy. *ANN OPHTHALMOL* 3:137–139, 1971.

f. Hofmann WW: Cerebellar lesions after parenteral Dilantin administration. *NEUROLOGY* 8:210–214, 1958.

g. Hoty CS, Billson FA: Maternal anticonvulsants and optic nerve hypoplasia. *BR J OPHTHALMOL* 62:3–6, 1978.

h. Kokenge R, Kutt H, McDowell F: Neurological sequelae following Dilantin overdose in a patient and in experimental animals. *NEUROLOGY* 15:823–829, 1965.

i. Kolbert GS: Oral diphenylhydantoin in corneal wound healing in the rabbit. *AM J OPHTHALMOL* 66:736–738, 1968.

j. Kutt H, Wolk M, et al: Insufficient parahydroxylation as cause of diphenylhydantoin toxicity. *NEUROLOGY* 14:542–548, 1964.

k. Meadow SR: Glaucoma, maternal epsilepsy, and anticonvulsant drugs. J PEDIATR 90:499, 1977.

l. Orth DN, Almeida H, et al: Ophthalmoplegia resulting from diphenylhydantoin and primidone intoxication. *J AM MED ASSOC* 201:485–487, 1967.

m. Patel H, Crichton JU: Neurological hazards of diphenylhydantoin in childhood. *J PEDIATR* 73:676–684, 1968.

n. Spector RH, Davidoff RA, Schwartzman RJ: Phenytoin induced ophthalmoplegia. *NEUROLOGY (Minneap)* 26:1031–1034, 1976.

o. Tenckhoff H, et al: Acute diphenylhydantoin intoxication. *AM J DIS CHILD* 116:442–425, 1968.

p. Tunnessen WW Jr, Lowenstein EH: Glaucoma associated with the fetal hydantoin syndrome. *J PEDIATR* 89:154–155, 1976.

q. Wallar PH, Genstler DE, George CC: Multiple systemic and periocular malformations associated with the fetal hydantoin syndrome. *ANN OPHTHALMOL* 10:1568–1572, 1978.

r. Wilson RS, Smead W, Char F: Diphenylhydantoin teratogenicity. *J PEDIATR OPHTHAL-MOL STRABISMUS* 15:137–140, 1978.

pHisoHex is a germicidal soap employed in preparatin for surgery. It contains *hexachlorophene* and a *detergent.* In contact with the human eye for several minutes, it has caused severe corneal edema in two cases.[a] The endothelium appeared to be injured, but the eyes gradually recovered in several weeks. Experimentally in rabbits and dogs the injury was reproduced by exposures of two to four minutes, and when the individual components were tested, it was determined that hexachlorophene in the concentration present (3%) did not cause significant corneal damage, but that the detergent, 80% *sodium octylphenoxyethyl ether sulfonate,* also known as Entsufon or Triton, did damage the cornea in the same manner as did the original mixture. (*Hexachlorophene* systemically absorbed has serious neurotoxic effects. See INDEX for *Hexachlorophene.*)

a. Browning C, Lippas J: pHisoHex keratitis. *ARCH OPHTHALMOL* 53:817–824, 1955.

Phlorizine (phloridzin) has been employed experimentally to produce glycosuria in animals.[171] In rabbits, it is said to have caused convulsions and exudate between retina and pigment epithelium.[153]

Phloxine B is an anionic, acid dye. Anionic dyes as a rule are not significantly toxic to the cornea and conjunctiva, but phloxine B appears to be an exception. It has induced moderate injury and opacification when applied to rabbit eyes as 0.02 M solution at pH 7 to 7.8 for ten minutes after mechanical removal of the corneal epithelium.[81] Both chromatographically purified dye and commercial dye had this toxicity.

Phoradendron flavescens (American mistletoe) is said to contain toxic substances, possibly sympathomimetic, which when ingested cause mydriasis, delirium, hallucinations, and vascular collapse.[142]

Phosgene (carbonyl chloride) is a colorless, highly toxic gas. At 4 to 10 ppm in air it causes irritation of the respiratory tract and of the eyes.[d,61,171,252] Exposure to the gas may cause conjunctival hyperemia, but at irritating concentrations there is automatic protection through blepharospasm, and by far the greatest danger is to the lungs.[b]

Liquid phosgene splashed in the eyes has, however, caused complete opacification of both corneas in one patient, leading ultimately to perforation and formation of symblepharon.[a] Experimentally in cats it has been possible to cause corneal opacification by high concentrations of gas.[c]

a. D'Osvaldo E: Clinical contribution concerning the action of a war gas (phosgene). *ANN OTTALMOL CLIN OCUL* 56:154, 1928. (Italian)
b. Everett ED, Overholt EL: Phosgene poisoning. *J AM MED ASSOC* 205:243–245, 1968.
c. Laquer E, Magnus R: On war-gas poisoning. *Z GES EXP MED* 13:200, 1921. (German)
d. Kuzelova M, Kos J, et al: Industrial mass poisoning by phosgene in 52 workers at a chemical plant. *PRAC LEK* 27:115–117, 1975. (English abstract)

Phosphine (hydrogen phosphide) gas poisoning of human beings and experimental animals has been reported, but no characteristic ocular or visual effects are known. In acute poisoning, the pupils are said to be usually widely dilated.[155]

Phosphonoacetate disodium, in a petrolatum ointment base at 5% concentration, pH 7, tested on rabbits' eyes by repeated application for 42 days caused no abnormality detectible by clinical or histological examination.[a]

a. Gordon YJ, Lahav M, et al: Effect of phosphonoacetic acid in the treatment of experimental herpes simplex keratitis. *BR J OPHTHALMOL* 61:506–509, 1977.

Phosphoric acid (orthophosphoric acid, metaphosphoric acid) topically may irritate and injure the eyes, owing to its acidity, but systemically phosphate has no poisonous action on the eye. Tested on human eyes, 0.16 M *orthophosphoric acid* buffered to pH 2.5 caused moderate brief stinging sensation but no injury when applied as a single drop. A drop of the same solution adjusted to pH 3.4 caused no discomfort. Irrigation of a rabbit's eye for five minutes with *orthophosphoric acid* diluted to pH 3.8 caused slight transient epithelial edema and conjunctival hyperemia, but the eye was completely normal by the next day.[81] On the other hand when injected into the rabbit corneal stroma or applied to the cornea after removal of the epithelium, *metaphosphoric acid* caused detectable injury below pH 5.5.[123] Phosphoric acid has been held responsible for burns of the eye from *superphosphate fertilizers.*

Phosphorus, the element, has two forms, *red phosphorus* and *white phosphorus,* that are entirely different in external contact toxic effects, as well as in physical and chemical properties.

Red phosphorus is a red to violet powder which is much less reactive and toxic than white phosphorus. In contrast to white phosphorus, it is not caustic to the skin or eyes and does not burn spontaneously in air unless heated. The relatively slight local toxicity of red phosphorus is exemplified by a case in which a mixture of powdered red phosphorus with an oxidizing agent exploded in a boy's face and drove many fine red particles deep into the corneas, as well as into conjunctivae and skin. All wounds healed promptly, and the red particles were watched by slit-lamp biomicroscope for many months thereafter, causing no signs or symptoms of irritation or reaction in the surrounding corneas. Vision was normal. The particles in the corneas had the same characteristic size, color, and shape as an authentic sample of pure red phosphorus.[81] However, an entirely different course has since been described from Czechoslovakia, in a boy who was reported to have burns of both eyes with red phosphorus, and to have suffered for more than two years from inflamed conjunctiva and photophobia.[c] It is surprising that the effect of red phosphorus seems to have been so different in these two cases.

Experimentally, a small amount of an aqueous suspension of red phosphorus has been injected into the corneas of both eyes of a rabbit, and into the anterior chamber in one eye. During the next two weeks the particles in the corneal stroma appeared to induce no infiltration or other reaction in the cornea, as though the particles were inert and innocuous foreign bodies. However, while the cornea seemed unreactive, the iris developed numerous fine abnormal vessels. Furthermore, in the eye in which the red phosphorus had been injected into the anterior chamber, a gross hypopyon developed and the vessels of the iris in that eye became conspicuously dilated.

The difference in severity of reaction of the two patients may be explainable by a difference in the amount of red phosphorus that entered the eyes. The rabbit experiment shows that when enough of this substance is present it can produce considerable inflammation in the eye, even while appearing inert in the cornea. Apparently the amount that can be tolerated without inflammation is very small, as in the first patient, in whom the particles were so fine that they could be seen only with a slit-lamp biomicroscope.

White (or yellow) phosphorus, in contrast to red phosphorus, is a highly reactive solid which sublimes and gives off white fumes in air, igniting spontaneously at 30° in moist air. Both the fumes and the solid are poisonous. White phosphorus fumes are irritating to the respiratory tract and cause severe ocular irritation with blepharospasm, photophobia, and lacrimation.[b] Particles of white phosphorus are caustic and seriously damaging in contact with tissues.

In one instance of burn of the eye only small areas of cornea were rendered opaque, but interstitial vascularization and episcleritis developed. Episodes of inflammation recurred for many years, but good vision was maintained.[a]

In another case of burn of the eye, particles of white phosphorus were spattered into both eyes and became embedded in the bulbar and tarsal conjunctivae.[b] Smoke was seen to be emanating from these particles until the eyes were irrigated and several drops of 3% copper sulfate solution were applied. (In emergency treatment of skin contamination by white phosphorus, copper solutions have long been employed to form a relatively unreactive coating on the phosphorous particle.) The copper sulfate solution was applied to the eyes several times within fifteen minutes, and the embedded particles were removed mechanically. Areas of gray necrosis were evident at the burned sites in the conjunctivae, but the eyes otherwise returned to normal within two days. The corneas were not involved.

In chronic systemic phosphorus poisoning in human beings, isolated instances of retinal edema, retinal hemorrhages, neuritic and edematous changes in the optic nerveheads have been reported, but none in recent times.[77,153,214,247] Teleky in his toxicology text describes chronic phosphorus poisoning, and says that it can lead to loss of one or both eyes from a necrotic and destructive process in the maxilla extending into the orbit, causing destruction of the orbit and the globe. He presents a photograph of such a case.[239]

Experimental chronic poisoning of dogs and cats for two to three weeks is reported to have caused retinal hemorrhages, degenerative changes in all layers of the retina, leukocytic infiltration, papilledema and fatty and hyalin degeneration of the blood vessels.[7,153,214,247]

a. Lyle TK, Cross AG: Sclero-keratitis following phosphorus injury of the eye. *BR J OPHTHALMOL* 26:301–303, 1942.
b. Scherling SS, Blondis RR: The effect of chemical warfare agents on the human eye. *MIL SURG* 96:70–78, 1945.
c. Sedlacek J: Eye burns with phosphorus. *CS OFTAL* 25:36–38, 1969.

Phosphorus pentoxide (phosphoric anhydride) as powder or fumes in air are irritating to the eyes and respiratory tract. Particles of solid phosphorous pentoxide in contact with the eye react vigorously, and even small amounts may cause burns of the lids, conjunctivae, and corneas, producing blue-white opacities, which may be permanent.[a,171]

a. Augstein R: On blinding in work with artificial fertilizer through accidental sprinkling in the eye. *KLIN MONATSBL AUGENHEILKD* 45:563–566, 1907. (German)

Phosphorus oxychloride (phosphorylchloride) is a strongly fuming liquid with vapor and fumes that are strongly irritating to the eyes and respiratory tract.[a] Burns of the human cornea by phosphorus oxychloride have been noted in two cases to be slow in healing, but no details have been reported.[165]

a. Sassi C: Occupational poisoning by phosphorus oxychloride. *MED LAVORO* 45:171–177, 1954. (Italian)

Phosphorus pentachloride vapor and fumes are irritating to the eyes and respiratory tract.[171,252]

Phosphorus sesquisulfide (tetraphosphorus trisulfide) dust is irritating to the eyes and respiratory tract, and it has caused contact dermatitis in numerous instances.[129,188,242] In several cases contact dermatitis caused by matches containing this compound has been accompanied by blepharitis and conjunctivitis.[129]

Phosphorus trichloride is toxic, irritating and corrosive to skin and mucous membranes.[171,252] The vapors are irritating to the respiratory tract and eyes. Experimentally in cats 2 to 4 ppm in air in the course of six hours has caused respiratory difficulty and conjunctivitis. At 23 to 90 ppm in air in the course of six hours the corneas became clouded and the systemic effects were severe.[61]

Phthalic anhydride dust, vapor, or fumes are irritating to the eyes and respiratory tract, causing persistent conjunctivitis, but no permanent injury.[a,56,129,165,252]

a. Ghezzi I, Scotti P: Clinical contribution on the pathology induced by phthalic and maleic anhydrides. *MED LAVORO* 56:746–752, 1965.

Phthalofyne (Whipcide; phthalic acid 1-ethyl-1-methyl-2-propynyl ester) has been employed as an anthelmintic in dogs and human beings. Ocular complications have developed in about one out of ten patients receiving a dose of 100 to 200 mg/kg, and in all patients receiving more than 200 mg/kg. In twelve hours after oral medication there has been onset of burning sensation in the eyes and redness of the conjunctivae, usually progressing to a "generalized filmy keratitis" with considerable pain and photophobia. In the most severe cases a moderately dense corneal opacity 1.5 to 2.0 mm in diameter has developed near the vertex within twenty-four hours, and in one instance, after a dose of 385 mg/kg, a patient developed almost complete opacity of both corneas within twenty-four hours. In two cases there was deafness. All eye lesions and deafness cleared completely, usually within seven to eight days, and in the most severe case within three weeks. Similar ocular effects have been noted in chimpanzees but not in monkeys or dogs.[a]

The corneal lesions have not been described in sufficient detail to reveal which layer of the cornea was first affected or whether the opacities were caused by edema, cellular infiltrates, or other material.

a. Hoekenga MT: Ocular toxicity of Whipcide (3-methyl-1-pentyn-3-yl acid phthalate) in humans. *J AM MED ASSOC* 161:1252, 1956.

Physostigmine (eserine), an alkaloid from Calabar beans, is an anticholinesterase agent used in eyedrops and ointment as a miotic medication in glaucoma. It produces miosis and enhances accommodation for near, reducing intraocular pressure by facilitating aqueous outflow. Its local side effects include conjunctival hyperemia from dilation of superficial vessels, twitching of the lids, variable discomfort from contraction of ciliary muscle, and frequent development of contact allergic blepharoconjunctivitis during chronic use. (For more relating to glaucoma, see INDEX for *Miotics.*)

Systemic poisoning from drinking small amounts of physostigmine eyedrops may cause perspiration, gastrointestinal hyperactivity, slowing of the heart, and faintness, also miosis and blurring of vision from spasm of accommodation.

Massive overdosage, such as a gram of the alkaloid taken with suicidal intent, has produced very severe poisoning characterized by nausea and severe abdominal pain, frightening visual hallucinations, sweating and salivation, and development of semicoma. In such severe poisoning the pupils rather than being constricted have been found dilated and sluggishly reactive to light, apparently analogous to the paradoxical mydriasis observed in severe poisoning by pesticidal phosphate ester anticholinesterases. As an antidote, it is logical to give atropine systemically, but in very severe poisoning this has caused ventricular tachycardia. This dangerous complication can be prevented by giving propranolol (5 mg) slowly intravenously, permitting use of atropine to aid in keeping respiratory passages dry.[a, b]

In cases of systemic poisoning by atropine-like anticholinergic agents, physostigmine has been administered therapeutically for its antagonistic effect. (See also *Anticholinergic agents.*)

a. Cumming G, Harding LK, Prowse K: Treatment and recovery after massive overdose of physostigmine. *LANCET* 2:147–149, 1968.
b. Valero A: Treatment of severe physostigmine poisoning. *LANCET* 2:459–460, 1968.

α-Picoline (2-methyl pyridine) on rabbit eyes has caused moderate injury, graded 8 on a scale of 1 to 10 after twenty-four hours, but the final result is not reported.[225] It has been alleged that workmen exposed to picoline vapors may develop diplopia as a result of disturbance of the eye muscles.[a] This belief appears to have existed for a hundred years, but no firsthand reliable observation of such an effect seems to have been published.

a. Ludwig H: On the toxicology of pyridine and its homologs. *ARCH GEWERBEPATH GEWERBEHYG* 5:564–664, 1934. (German)

Picric acid (trinitrophenol) dust or fumes cause irritation of the eyes of men and animals,[61, 176] and this may be aggravated by sensitization. Corneal injury is said to have resulted from accidental squirt of picric acid solution in the eye.[153] Experimentally, a solution of picric acid injected into the corneal stroma of rabbit eyes has been found to be injurious even when the solution is neutralized to the range of pH 7 to 9.[123]

Experimental ingestion of 0.3 g has been reported to cause objects to have a yellowish appearance, but not significantly to disturb the perception of other colors. The effect has been described as beginning in two minutes, reaching a maximum at thirty minutes, and lasting not more than two hours.[a] Although this dose has been thought to be too small to color the transparent media of the eye,[247] doses of picric acid large enough to cause severe systemic poisoning are said to color all tissues yellow, including the conjunctiva and aqueous humor, and yellow vision appearing under these circumstances seems to be explainable on a simple optical basis.[171,252]

a. Hilbert R: On subjective pathologic color perception as a result of poisonings. *KLIN MONATSBL AUGENHEILKD* 45:518–523, 1907. (German)

Picrotoxin (cocculin), a stimulant of the central nervous system, has caused severe poisoning of human beings.[171,252] There appears to be difference of opinion as to whether the pupils are constricted or dilated.[196,214,252]

An unusual case of poisoning with eye involvement occurred in a young woman who ate fish that had been killed by picrotoxin.[d] She developed headache, chills, salivation, and loss of vision, with the pupils dilated and unreactive. Both retinas were observed to be edematous. Despite these severe effects, the patient recovered completely.

Experiments in cats and rabbits have shown both reduction and enhancement of electrical activity of optic nerve neurons and visual evoked cortical responses, depending on the dosage of picrotoxin.[a,c,e] Inhibitory effect on frog retina activity has been shown.[b]

a. Barnes CD, Moolenaar GM: Effects of diazepam and picrotoxin on the visual system. *NEUROPHARMACOLOGY* 10:193–201, 1971.
b. Burchardt DA: Effects of picrotoxin and strychnine upon electrical activity of the proximal retina. *BRAIN RES* 43:246–249, 1972.
c. Heiss WD: The protracted activity of retinal neurons under the influence of strychnine and picrotoxin. *VISION RES* 7:583–598, 1967.
d. Lauterstein M: On a case of bilateral retinal edema and internal ophthalmoplegia after partaking of poisoned fish (picrotoxin poisoning.) *ZENTRALBL GES AUGENHEILKD* 80:58–63, 1933. (German)
e. Tsuchida Y: Effects of intravitreous injection of several chemicals on the ERG and light-induced optic nerve potential in the albino rabbit. *ACTA SOC OPHTHALMOL JPN* 72:2151–2161, 1968.

Pig weed, a plant of the family *Chenopodiaceae,* is said to have caused keratitis in agricultural workers, possibly on an allergic basis.[176] (See also *Chenopodium oil.*)

Pilocarpine, a parasympathomimetic natural alkaloid is used topically, mostly in eyedrops, in treatment of glaucoma. The adverse side effects are much like those of other drugs described together under the heading "Miotics". (See INDEX). Pilocarpine's adverse effects from use on the eye commonly consist of a sensation of dimness of surroundings owing to constriction of the pupil and reduction of amount of light entering the eye, also enforced accommodation for near, causing pseudomyopia and improper focusing of distant objects by people below the age of presbyopia.[e] Aching discomfort in the eye from contraction of the ciliary muscle occurs occasionally at the start of treatment with strong pilocarpine eyedrops.

Retinal detachment occurs occasionally in patients using pilocarpine or other miotic eyedrops, sometimes shortly after starting the medication, which particularly suggests a cause and effect relationship. In one case in which pilocarpine was suspected of having caused a retinal tear, ultrasonography showed that in this case the posterior surface of the lens moved forward under the influence of pilocarpine, suggesting a physical mechanism for vitreoretinal traction as a cause of the retinal tear.[a] Whether the interpretation is valid remains to be determined.

Cataracts occur occasionally in patients using pilocarpine or other miotic eyedrops, but cataracts also occur commonly in patients using no medication. There has been clinical evidence of increased incidence of lens changes in patients using anticholinesterase eyedrops, but no conclusive clinical evidence to link pilocarpine and cataracts. Experimental studies since 1956 have focused mainly on biochemical, metabolic, and morphologic changes in lenses *in vivo* and *in vitro*.[f-h,j] It was found that 10^{-3}M pilocarpine *in vitro* caused at least 50% inhibition of the respiration of the lens, and that application of 2% pilocarpine to rabbit eyes also inhibited respiration of the lens. However, pilocarpine produced no cataracts in animals. Hockwin and associates showed that pilocarpine administered in addition to naphthalene or x-irradiation favored induction of cataracts in rabbits at levels of naphthalene or irradiation that were not cataractogenic by themselves.[f,g] Several invesigators measured the concentration of pilocarpine in the aqueous humor after the drug was applied as eyedrops, but with considerable differences in results. Review of the data by Klauber indicates that during ordinary topical medication the concentration in the aqueous humor approximates 5×10^{-4}M, but to definitely suppress oxygen consumption by the lens may require as much as 10^{-2}M.[h] This suggests that under clinical circumstances the glycolytic activity of the lens may not be affected.

The cornea is seldom affected by pilocarpine in a clinically notable way, but two cases of pemphigoid or pseudo-pemphigus have been reported in association with use of a combination of pilocarpine and phenylephrine.[k] Haziness of the corneal epithelium and superficial corneal vascularization with redness of the conjunctiva have been observed by Chandler in two patients after long-continued use of pilocarpine eyedrops.[31] The ordinary signs of contact allergy were absent. There was much improvement when the drops were discontinued. It was not established whether the pilocarpine itself or some other constituent of the eyedrops was responsible. Allergic conjunctival reactions to pilocarpine do occur, but are rare.

On rabbit corneas, a 2 minute exposure to 2% pilocarpine hydrochloride has caused no increase in permeability to fluorescein.[320] Tests on the endothelium of rabbit corneas with longer exposures to concentrations above 0.25% produce changes measurable by increase in corneal thickness and by electron microscopy, with the rate of onset and severity related to concentration.[b]

Systemic intoxication from absorption of pilocarpine eyedrops is rare, but occasional patients are peculiarly sensitive and develop sweating and gastrointestinal overactivity with ordinary amounts. Overdosage (e.g. thirty drops of 2%,[a] or sixty drops of 3%,[e]) can produce sweating, salivation, nausea, and tremor, with slowing of the pulse and decrease in blood pressure. In moderate poisoning, spontaneous recovery is to be expected, and is aided by intravenous fluids to compensate for dehydration.[d] For severe poisoning, atropine would be a natural pharmacologic antagonist to pilocarpine. Also, Curti has extrapolated from experiments on mice that pulmonary effects might be antagonized by intravenous ambroxol.[c] Apparently one can survive very large overdoses, as illustrated by two cases reported by Lisch (1976).[346] Accidentally in retrobulbar injections pilocarpine hydrochloride was substituted in place of a local anesthetic, and two patients each received 4.5 ml of 4% solution. They became agitated, with profuse perspiration, and colic. However, they recovered gradually in a few hours under treatment with pentylenetetrazol and oxygen inhalation. Chlorpromazine, which they had been given prior to the injections, may have helped.

a. Abramson DH, Mackay C, Coleman DJ: Pilocarpine-induced retinal tear. *GLAUCOMA* 3:9–12, 1981.
b. Coles WH: Pilocarpine toxicity. *ARCH OPHTHALMOL* 93:36–41, 1975.
c. Curti PC, Renovantz HD: The effect of accidental overdosage with pilocarpine on the pulmonary surfactant of the mouse. *KLIN MONATSBL AUGENHEILKD* 179:113–115, 1981. (German)
d. Epstein E, Kaufman I: Systemic pilocarpine toxicity from overdosage. *AM J OPHTHAL-MOL* 59:109–110, 1965.
e. Greco JJ, Kelman CD: Systemic pilocarpine toxicity in the treatment of angle closure glaucoma. *ANN OPHTHALMOL* 5:57–59, 1973.
f. Hockwin O, Okamoto T, et al: Genesis of cataracts; cumulative effects of subliminal noxious influences. *ANN OPHTHALMOL* 1:321–325, 1969.
g. Hockwin O, Okamoto T, et al: Effect of pilocarpine on lens metabolism. *OPHTHAL-MOLOGICA* 152:46–56, 1966.
h. Klauber A: In vitro investigations on the effect of pilocarpine on the metabolism in pig lenses. *ACTA OPHTHALMOL* 55:597–604, 1977.
i. Lindstrom EE, Tredici TJ, et al: Effects of topical ophthalmic 2% pilocarpine on visual performance of normal subjects. *AEROSPACE MED* 39:1236–1240, 1968.
j. Muller HK, Kleifeld O, et al: The influence of pilocarpine and Mintacol on the metabolism of the lens. *BER DEUTSCH OPHTHALMOL GESELLSCH* 60:115–120, 1956. (German)
k. Saraux H, Offret H, De Rancourt E: Ocular pseudopemphigus induced by eyedrops. *BULL SOC OPHTALMOL FRANCE* 80:41–42, 1980. (French)

Pimaricin, an antimicrobial used medically and to prevent food spoilage, has been tested externally on rabbit eyes and found to be essentially non-irritating.[a] However, 0.25 to 2.5 mg injected into the anterior chamber showed increasingly severe reactions in the anterior segment, yet eventual recovery. In eyes infected with *Aspergillus fumigatus,* injection of any more than 0.25 mg into the aqueous caused unacceptably damaging reactions. In rabbit eyes with *Aspergillus fumigatus* endophthalmitis, 0.025 mg injected into the vitreous body was tolerated, but was therapeutically ineffective. Higher doses in either infected or normal eyes caused loss of retinal function, vitreous retraction, and detachment of the retina.

a. Levinskas GJ, Ribelin WA, Shaffer CB: Acute and chronic toxicity of pimaricin. *TOXICOL APPL PHARMACOL* 8:97–109, 1966.
b. Ellison AC, Newmark E: Intraocular effects of pimaricin. *ANN OPHTHALMOL* 8;987–995, 1976.
c. Ellison AC: Intravitreal effects of pimaricin in experimental fungal endophthalmitis. *AM J OPHTHALMOL* 81:157–161, 1976.

Pimelic acid (1,7-heptanedioic acid), applied to rabbit eyes caused moderate irritation of the conjunctivae and swelling of the lids, plus "a trace of diffuse corneal opacity," all of which gradually cleared in seven days.[37]

Pine-flower pollen (pine pollen), which is scattered from pine trees in the spring, can cause irritation of the eyes from direct contact, the severity depending upon the amount of pollen.[a] Kinnas has described nine cases, ranging from severe irritation lasting more than a week after being struck in the face by pollen sacs or by the flowers themselves, to slight transient irritation by pollen blown one to three yards from the tree. The reaction was interpreted as a toxic or allergic effect, although in the first case the discomfort was intense and immediate, and after violent rubbing of the lids there were epithelial erosions of corneas and lids, edema of conjunctiva and lids, ecchymoses, and many papillae.

a. Kinnas JS: Ophthalmic lesions due to pine-flower pollen. *BR J OPHTHALMOL* 55:714–715, 1971.

Pine oil consists mainly of terpene alcohols obtained by steam distillation or solvent extraction from pine woods. It is irritating to the eyes and mucous membranes but appears to have produced no injuries.[70]

Piperazine (diethylenediamine) is a strong organic base. Tested full strength by application of a drop to rabbit eyes, it has caused severe injury, graded 9 on a scale of 1 to 10 after twenty-four hours.[27] However, no injury was caused by a 0.2 M aqueous solution at pH 7.5 dropped continuously on rabbit eyes for ten minutes after mechanical removal of the corneal epithelium to permit penetration.[81]

Medicinally, *piperazine citrate* (Antepar) has been employed as an anthelmintic. Toxic effects occur mostly from overdosage, which may produce diarrhea, urticaria, weakness, tremor, and disturbance of coordination and equilibrium. Miosis appears occasionally to be induced by interference with the sympathetic supply to the eye, and slight disturbances of accommodation may have the same basis.[a, b, 171, 252] Descriptions of the visual effects are vague, variously characterized as difficulty in vision, difficulty in focusing, disturbance of color vision, or occurrence of flashes on closing the eyes at night, usually associated with giddiness, lack of coordination, and a sense of detachment. In any case the visual disturbances appear to be rare and inconsequential.[a–c]

Lateral rectus muscle paralysis on one side has in one child seemed related to treatment with piperazine.[d]

a. Brown HW, Chan KF, Hussey KL: Treatment of enterobiasis and ascariasis with piperazine. *J AM MED ASSOC* 161:515–520, 1956.
b. Mossmer A: On the effectiveness, dosage, and toxic effects of piperazine preparations. *MED MSCHR* 10:517–526, 1956. (German)
c. Neff L: Another severe psychological reaction to side effects of medication in an adolescent. *J AM MED ASSOC* 197:218–219, 1966.
d. Rouher F, Cantat MA: Instructive observation of an ocular paralysis after taking piperazine. *BULL SOC FRANC OPHTALMOL* 75:460–465, 1962. (French)

Piperidine (hexahydropyridine) is a strongly basic organic liquid miscible with water. In testing on rabbit eyes without control of pH, it caused severe injury of the cornea, graded 9 on a scale of 1 to 10 at twenty-four hours.[228] Tested in aqueous solution at 0.023 M concentration by continuous application for ten minutes after mechanical removal of the corneal epithelium to permit penetration, at pH 11 the solution caused slight reversible graying of the cornea, and at pH 10 caused no significant injury.[81, 89]

Piperidylchlorophenothiazine (NP 207) was introduced into clinical use in 1954 as a major tranquilizer for psychoses, but it was soon found to cause retinal degeneration.[a, c, d, f–h.] Individuals were found to differ in their susceptibility to injury by this drug, but dosage had an important influence on incidence of ocular complications.

A daily dose of 0.3 to 0.4 g for two to three months did not appear to have toxic effects on the retina,[c] but most patients receiving 0.4 to 0.8 g per day for two or three months developed visual disturbances.[h] Visual disturbances appeared only after four to eight weeks. In some cases, effects on the eyes did not appear until after the drug had been discontinued.[g, h]

An initial symptom typically was impairment of vision in dim light. In more severe cases, visual acuity was reduced, and visual fields became moderately contracted. At the onset, the optic discs in some cases appeared more red than normal, the retinal vessels appeared dilated, and the retina seemed to have edema.[a, c] However, these changes were not seen by all observers.[g]

Abnormal retinal pigmentation developed, at first very fine, giving a pepper-and-salt appearance, distributed sometimes peripherally and sometimes in the macular region, better visible with reflected light than with direct light.[g] As pigmentation progressed, black patches appeared, of uniform size in a given individual, but variable from one patient to another. The pigment appeared to be in the deepest portions of the retina or behind it and did not necessarily follow the course of the retinal vessels.[g]

The pigmentary retinopathy had superficial similarity to that of retinitis pigmentosa but was recognizably different. The main difference was lack of change in the vessels and nervehead when the pigment was fully developed. Also, ring scotoma was rarely found. In most severe cases pigment dots coalesced to form larger clumps, and in the most severe there were sheets of pigment with spoke-like or scalloped edges toward the periphery.[a, c]

Detailed functional examination of vision in two patients gave evidence of severe damage to both cones and rods. Dark adaptation was delayed and final thresholds high. The poisoned patients differed from patients having retinitis pigmentosa, in that the ERG was not completely extinguished in the patients affected by piperidylchlorophenothiazine. Also, the function of their rod system was less affected than in patients having retinitis pigmentosa.[a]

After discontinuance of medication, most patients showed considerable functional improvement, sometimes continuing for many months. Some recovered normal visual acuity and had much improvement in dark adaptation and visual fields. In the most severely affected patients, recovery was incomplete, and a small number remained practically blind.

The mechanism of injury of the retina by piperidylchlorophenothiazine was studied mainly by Meier-Ruge, Cerletti, Werthemann, and Kalberer, who produced a series of publications from 1966 to 1969 on the subject.[b, e, 166-169] They succeeded in inducing retinopathy in cats, evident as grayish black pigmentation in the retina, visible ophthalmoscopically four to five weeks after beginning of administration. They found that the drug accumulated selectively in the melanin of the choroid, forming a reservoir which had direct access to the visual receptors of the retina. These investigators pointed out that there was close similarity between cats and human beings in features of their retinal circulation and metabolism, and particularly in the relationship of the choriocapillaris, pigmented epithelium, and visual cells. They believed that this accounted for the success in producing the retinopathy in this species (cats), and accounted for failures to produce it in rabbits, rats, guinea pigs, and dogs,[c, g, h] whose eyes appeared to be less like the human eye in these important respects.

Histochemical studies and assays of enzyme activities *in vitro* led to a concept that the toxic effect was mainly on the ellipsoids of the rods, and that accompanying inhibition of ATPase and lactic dehydrogenase, the outer rod segments disintegrated. The pigment epithelium was disturbed by excessive shedding of disintegrated outer rod segments and resorption by the pigment epithelium. Storage of light-absorbing products of disintegrated rods in the pigment epithelium produced the appearance of pigment retinopathy. The Muller cells of the retina early showed a supposedly partly compensatory activation of lactic dehydrogenase associated with inhibition of metabolism in the visual cells. Cerletti and Meier-Ruge have further postulated that a fundamental factor in this toxic mechanism may be inhibition of oxidative phosphorylation secondary to blocking of flavine nucleotides by the drug.

Electrophysiologic studies on acutely and chronically poisoned cats by Bornschein and associates, including ERG *in situ* and in isolated retina, single nerve fiber activity of the optic nerve, and VER, showed in essence effects on the c-wave of the ERG and optic nerve single fiber activity that indicated a primary effect of the drug on the receptors, consistent with reported histologic findings.[i]

a. Burian HM, Fletcher MC: Visual functions in patients with retinal pigmentary degeneration following the use of NP 207. *ARCH OPHTHALMOL* 60:612–629, 1958.

b. Cerletti A, Meier-Ruge W: Toxicological studies on phenothiazine induced retinopathy. *PROC EUROP SOC STUDY DRUG TOXICITY* 9:170–188, 1968.

c. Goar EF, Fletcher MC: Toxic chorioretinopathy following the use of NP 207. *TRANS AM OPHTHALMOL SOC* 54:129–140, 1956. (*AM J OPHTHALMOL* 44:603–608, 1957.)

d. Kinross-Wright V: Clinical trial of a new phenothiazine compound NP 207. *PSYCHIATR RES REP AM PSYCHIATR ASSOC* 4:89–94, 1956.

e. Meier-Ruge W, Cerletti A: On the experimental pathology of phenothiazine retinopathy. *OPHTHALMOLOGICA* 151:512–533, 1966. (German)

f. Rintelen F, Hotz G, Wagner P: On the clinical and experimental pathology of the pigment epithelial disturbance after medication with a piperidine-phenothiazine. *OPHTHALMOLOGICA* 133:277–283, 1957. (German)

g. Verrey F: Pigmentary degeneration of the retina of drug origin. *OPHTHALMOLOGICA* 131:296–303, 1956.

h. Wagner P: Investigations of the effects of phenothiazine-derivatives on the ocular fundus of animals. *KLIN MONATSBL AUGENHEILKD* 129:772–781, 1956. (German)

i. Bornschein H, Hoyer J, et al: Animal experimental study with a substance harmful to the visual system (NP 207). *GRAEFES ARCH OPHTHALMOL* 190:13–25, 1974. (German)

Piperonyl butoxide is a liquid of slight volatility used as an ingredient of insecticides. Tests on eyes and skin of rabbits, rats, cats, and dogs showed that it was not damaging, although it may be irritating.[56,171]

Piperoxan (Benodaine, Benzodioxane), an adrenergic blocking agent, has been tested intravenously in glaucomatous patients and had neither adverse nor beneficial effect on the intraocular pressure.[a]

a. Muller CR, Leopold IH: Adrenergic blocking agents in treatment of glaucoma. *ARCH OPHTHALMOL* 46:549–552, 1951.

Pitch is the black residue from distilling tar. In contact with the eyes of workmen it has been known to cause irritation, and if long in contact has caused chemosis of the conjunctiva, ulceration and infiltration of the cornea, hypopyon, and adherent leukoma.[b] Chronic exposure to pitch dust has been found to cause deep staining of the cornea in the palpebral fissure, conjunctival discoloration and irritation, and deformities of the lower lid.[b,129] In one case a peripheral, brownish annular discoloration of the cornea was found to be associated with fine subepithelial pigmented granules.[a]

Tests on rabbit eyes confirm the irritating and injurious effects of pitch.[35] It appears that pitch from *coal tar* is more injurious than pitch from *petroleum*.[129]

A study of roofers occupationally exposed to vapors from hot coal-tar pitch disclosed that they suffered from burning sensation in their eyes that was aggravated by sunlight.[c] This led to experiments in rabbits in which $10\mu l$ of coal-tar pitch distillate was applied to the eyes, some exposed to ultraviolet irradiation, and some not.[c] (The irradiation alone was insufficient to cause injury.) Without ultraviolet, the pitch distillate caused slight, transient irritation and corneal epithelial edema, but with ultraviolet the eyes developed much greater reaction, with severe corneal edema and loss of corneal epithelium, taking 3 or 4 days to heal completely. Phototoxic damage to the cornea and conjunctiva was thus well demonstrated.

a. Bischler: Pigmentation of the corneal limbus in pitch injury. *OPHTHALMOLOGICA* 11:456, 1947. (French)
b. Moret: Ocular lesions produced by pitch. *OPHTHALMOLOGY* 8:381, 1912.
c. Emmett EA, Stetzer L, Taphorn B: Phototoxic keratoconjunctivitis from coal-tar pitch volatiles. *SCIENCE* 198:841–842, 1977.

Pivalic acid has been tested for toxicity to the cornea because it is a part of the ophthalmic pro-drugs *dipivefrin* and *pivalylphenylephrine*, from which it is released by ocular esterases. On rabbit eyes, topical 1.4% pivalic acid (pH unstated) did not alter corneal thickness, whether the epithelium was present or had been removed by scraping. The morphology of cultures of bovine corneal endothelial cells was unaffected by 0.1% pivalic acid, but changes started to appear with 1.0%.

Staatz WD, Edelhauser HF, et al: Cytotoxicity of pivalylphenylephrine and pivalic acid to corneal endothelium. *ARCH OPHTHALMOL* 98:1279–1282, 1980.

Placebo is a pharmacologically inactive medication made to resemble a medicine that is believed to be active, in order to conceal from the patient, and sometimes from the tester, which one is being administered. The intention is to help in distinguishing imagined from real effects. A great many reports of eye symptoms attributed to drugs and chemicals have been inconclusive when they have lacked such controls. A good survey by Schindel in 1968 has called attention to several reports in which placebos have been blamed for effects on the eye, including instances of loss of vision, miosis, and in one study blurred vision in 18.3 per cent of patients receiving a placebo.[a]

a. Schindel L: Placebo-induced side-effects. In Meyler L, Peck HM (Eds.): *Drug Induced Diseases*. Amsterdam, Excerpta Med Foundation, 1968, vol. 3, pp. 323–330.

Plasmocid (8-[3-diethylaminopropylamino]-6-methoxyquinoline, and the related compounds, pamaquine, pentaquine, and isopentaquine) are derivatives of 8-aminoquinoline employed as antimalarials. Plasmocid has, like the related compounds, caused selective injury to the third, fourth, and sixth cranial nerve nuclei in monkeys, and also to the vestibular and cochlear nuclei, inducing nystagmus, ataxia, and internal and external ophthalmoplegia.[e, 194] The nystagmus observed in patients after taking plasmocid is said generally to have been nonpersistent after the drug was discontinued, but in one young woman the nystagmus persisted for many years.[f]

Plasmocid appears to be more toxic to the optic nerve than the related compounds, in that it has been reported to have caused optic neuritis and impaired vision in numerous patients, whereas pamaquine and the others have rarely done so. Almost all reports on visual effects of plasmocid are in the Russian literature in the period 1935 to 1940. An analysis of the literature, also in Russian, in 1968 is a potential source of further information on the incidence and nature of eye complications from plasmocid.[f]

At least ninety cases of optic atrophy have been reported, apparently always from overdosage, sometimes from a single large dose.[a, 194] Typically, vision has been acutely reduced, with central scotoma. The pupils become dilated and react poorly to light, but the visual fields are not as a rule constricted. Weakness of convergence, ataxia, and polyneuritis may also be present. Improvement of vision is uncommon and optic atrophy usually results. Toxic effects on the optic nerve and retina have been demonstrated in cats, rabbits, and dogs.[a, c] In rats severe lesions have been observed in the extraocular muscles.[b]

Experimental poisoning of monkeys with plasmocid has provided a clear histopathologic basis for disturbances observed in eye movements. Light and electron microscopy have shown neuronal vacuolar lesions selectively affecting the nuclei of cranial nerves III, IV, VI, and VIII, while the cerebral and cerebellar cortices remained normal.[d, g] Ultrastructural findings have suggested that the primary effect of the drug is on neuronal mitochondria.[g] Typical functional disturbances in poisoned monkeys have included nystagmus, disturbance of equilibrium, paresis of extraocular muscles (even complete ophthalmoplegia), and abnormality of pupillary light reflex.

(Also, see INDEX for *Pamaquine, Pentaquine, Isopentaquine,* and *Quinoline derivatives.*)

a. Askalonowa T: *VESTN OFTAL* 10:91–94, 1937; 13:26–37, 1938.
b. Hicks SP: Brain metabolism in vivo. *ARCH PATH* 50:545–561, 1950.
c. Krassnow M, Lewkojewa E, Dorsovzewa P: The effect of plasmocid on the organ of vision in the light of clinical experimental and pathologic anatomic findings. *VESTN OFTAL* 10:73–78, 1937.
d. Lyle DJ, Schmidt IG: The selective effect of drugs upon nuclei of the oculogyric system. *AM J OPHTHALMOL* 54:706–716, 1962.
e. Schmidt IG, Schmidt LH: Neurotoxicity of the 8-aminoquinolines. *J NEUROPATH EXP NEUROL* 7:368–398, 1948.
f. Smirnov AA: Protracted nystagmus due to plasmocid poisoning. *VESTN OFTAL* 81:84–85, 1968.
g. Sipe JC, Vick NA, et al: Plasmocid encephalopathy in the rhesus monkey. *J NEUROPATHOL EXP NEUROL* 32:446–457, 1973.

Plaster employed for plastering walls and ceilings has variable composition. The most important component from the standpoint of ocular injury is *calcium hydroxide,* which may produce the so-called limeburn of the eye. Other components, such as *plaster of Paris,* or *calcium sulfate,* are relatively innocuous. Plaster is most injurious as a powder before mixing with water, and as a paste when freshly mixed with water. The older and drier the plaster becomes, the more completely the calcium hydroxide is converted to calcium carbonate by absorption of carbon dioxide from the air. As the calcium hydroxide content decreases, the alkalinity and possibility of injurious action on the eye decreases. Old dried plaster acts principally as a chemically inert foreign body in the conjunctival sac.

Freshly prepared plaster may adhere to the eye and become lodged in the conjunctival fornices, requiring not only copious irrigation but mechanical removal with firm swabs. Removal is facilitated by use of sodium edetate (EDTA) solution. (See also *Calcium hydroxide,* and *Edetate.*)

Plastics in solid forms, and their toxic effects on the eye, come into consideration mainly in connection with contact lenses, intraocular lenses, keratoprostheses, ocular protheses, scleral buckling materials, aqueous humor drainage devices, lacrimal drainage tubes, and sutures.

Evaluation of toxicity has often been based on clinical observation and histopathology in experimental animals and patients, or has involved use of cell cultures in which to test for cellular toxicity.[e] Interpretation of results in experimental animals and patients can be complicated There have been many examples of mechanical and physical difficulties with plastics in relation to the eye.[b,j,l,o] *Silastic sponges* and *Silicone* implants of nearly insignificant toxicity have caused pressure atrophy.[b,o] Also inert *polytetrafluoroethylene (Teflon)* membranes implanted in the cornea have had adverse effects by interfering with diffusion within the cornea, rather than by toxic action.[l]

One test for ocular toxicity that has been commonly used has been based on placing the material to be tested in the anterior chamber of rabbits, and observing the reaction of eye tissues in subsequent months. The sample to be tested is made small and smooth to try to minimize physical trauma to eye tissues. This procedure presumably would be most suitable for testing intraocular lens materials. A comprehensive review (111 references) of development and testing of intraocular lenses has been provided by Ehrich.[c]

Rohen has pointed out that different ocular tissues (e.g. cornea, conjunctiva, sclera, iris) react in different ways to plastics or suture materials. It seems therefore that testing for ocular toxicity in animal eyes should be carried out in the same type of eye tissue in which there may be interest in using a plastic or suture material clinically.

Plastics made by polymerization may contain small amounts of original monomer, but also small amounts of a number of other substances necessary in the manufacture. *Polymethylmethacrylate* (PMM), on occasion has been suspected of some toxic effect in rabbit eyes,[c] or of causing intraocular inflammation after implantation as an intraocular lens,[m] yet in standard manufacture has been found not to contain, or to release, sufficient of the monomeric methylmethacrylate to be considered a toxic threat.[e-h, n]

Polytetrafluoroethylene in an expanded form tested in rabbits as an intrascleral implant was tolerated without evidence of toxicity, permitting a presumably desirable infiltration of connective tissue into the plastic.[i]

Polyurethane in the rabbit anterior chamber gave some evidence of a toxic effect.[e]

Polyvinyl and *silicone* drains in the anterior chamber of rabbits' eyes showed no irritation or other evidence of toxicity.[b]

Proplast, a vitreous, carbon-Teflon fluorocarbon polymer was tolerated without toxic reaction after implantation in corneas of rabbits.[a]

a. Barber JC, Feaster F, Priour D: The acceptance of a vitreous carbon alloplastic material, Proplast, in the rabbit eye. *INVEST OPHTHALMOL VIS SCI* 19:182–191, 1980.
b. Egerer I: The behavior of tubes of synthetic materials in the anterior segment of the rabbit's eye. *KLIN MONATSBL AUGENHEILKD* 169:746–749, 1976. (German)
c. Ehrich W: Plexiglass (PMMA) in the anterior chamber. *KLIN MONATSBL AUGEN-HEILKD* 168:493–501, 1976. (German)
d. Ehrich W: On biological tolerance of purified polyurethane (PUR). *GRAEFES ARCH OPHTHALMOL* 205:237–243, 1978. (German)
e. Galin MA, Chowchuvech E, Galin A: Tissue culture methods for testing the toxicity of ocular plastic materials. *AM J OPHTHALMOL* 79:665–669, 1975.
f. Galin MA, Chowchuvech E, Turkish L: Uveitis and intraocular lenses. *TRANS OPHTHALMOL SOC UK* 96:166–167, 1976.
g. Galin MA, Turkish L, Chowchuvech E: Detection, removal, and effect of unpolymerized methylmethacrylate in intraocular lenses. *AM J OPHTHALMOL* 84:153–159, 1977.
h. Galin MA, Salamone JC, et al: Chemical effects of alkali on polymethylmethacrylate intraocular lenses. *INVEST OPHTHALMOL VIS SCI* 21:354–357, 1981.
i. Lobes LA Jr, Grand MG, et al: Polyletrafluoroethylene in experimental retinal detachment surgery. *ANN OPHTHALMOL* 13:921–923, 1981.
j. Refojo MF: Current status of biomaterials in ophthalmology. *SURVEY OPHTHALMOL* 26:257–265, 1982.
k. Rohen JW, Futa R: Tissue reaction to synthetic material implants from the histologic aspect. *BER DTSCH OPHTHALMOL GESELLSCH* 75:51–59, 1977. (German)

l. Schmitt H: Corneal changes after Teflon implantation. *KLIN MONATSBL AUGEN-HEILKD* 168:518–526, 1976. (German)

m. Shepard DD: The "toxic lens" syndrome. *CONTACT LENS* 6:156–161, 1980.

n. Turkish L, Galin MA: Methylmethacrylate monomer in intraocular lenses of poly-methylmethacrylate. *ARCH OPHTHALMOL* 98:120–121, 1980.

o. Witschel H, Fanlborn J: Tissue reaction to buckling and encircling material polyamide-silicone-polyester. *GRAEFES ARCH OPHTHALMOL* 206:217–226, 1978. (German)

Platinum salts such as *ammonium* or *sodium chloroplatinate* or *platinic chloride* may cause severe contact dermatitis, mainly on the basis of acquired hypersensitivity. (For *diammindichloroplatinum*, see *Cisplatin* in the INDEX.) The dusts of soluble platinum salts cause a burning sensation in the eyes, lacrimation, and conjunctival hyperemia, sometimes associated with photophobia, which suggests that the corneal epithelium may be involved. This is accompanied by severe irritation of the respiratory tract.[171,252]

Flooding the surface of the eye of normal albino rabbits with 2% to 5% solutions of *platinum chloride* for ten minutes causes only slight temporary irritation and no discoloration, but if the epithelium is first removed to permit penetration, the cornea stains light brown. Within ten days the stain disappears and the epithelium regenerates.[199] Attempts to use platinum salts in tatooing the cornea have been unsuccessful in patients, because the dark color does not persist.[a,b,199]

Experimental comparison of tattooing of rabbit corneas after removal of the epithelium has shown 10% platinum chloride reduced with 2% hydrazine to be inferior to 2% *palladium chloride* reduced with 5% ascorbic acid.[c]

Metallic platinum is inert. In the anterior chamber of rabbit eyes finely divided platinum or platinum black is tolerated as well as metallic gold.[150] In the vitreous body platinum metal causes some changes in amino acid composition.[d]

a. Duggan JN, Narravala BP: Tattooing of corneal opacity with gold and platinum chloride. *BR J OPHTHALMOL* 20:419–425, 1941.

b. Pischel DK: Corneal tattooing with gold chloride and platinum chloride. *ARCH OPHTHALMOL* 3:176, 1930.

c. Tota G: Tattooing the cornea with palladium chloride. *BOLL OCULIST* 44:45–54, 1965. (Italian)

d. Welge-Luessen L, Domeier A: Amino acids in the vitreous humor after intravitreal platinum splinter implantation. *BER DTSCH OPHTHALMOL GESELLSCH* 71:411–416, 1972. (German)

Pleomycin is an antibiotic substance produced by *Streptomyces pleofaciens*, which is effective *in vitro* against many microorganisms, but highly toxic to mammals.[171] Topical application of a 0.1% solution to rabbit eyes is reported to have induced corneal opacity.[a]

a. Machlowitz RA, Charney J, et al: *Antibiotics Annual*, 1954–55. New York, Medical Encyclopedia, p.806.

Podophyllum (May apple, mandrake root) has been used in preparation of *Podophyllum resin* or *Podophyllin*.[171] Podophyllum and its products have been used as a purgative and in treatment of warts and cutaneous carcinoma. The dust formed in grinding the roots of the plant is notorious for its severely irritant effect on the eyes.[253]

Carried to the eyes by the air or fingers, it produces a very painful keratitis and conjunctivitis. The conjunctivitis is delayed in its onset for four to six hours after exposure. Both conditions last several days.[33,46,153] There is burning discomfort, epiphora, and conjunctival hyperemia.[a-d] After slight exposures the reaction subsides spontaneously, but greater exposure may involve loss of corneal epithelium, severe iritis, and deposits on the back of the cornea. Descemet's membrane may become wrinkled from edema of the cornea, and vision may temporarily be blurred. In one case a faint nebulous scar remained after healing of an unusually severe keratitis which was induced by contact with podophyllum oleoresin.[b] Severe edema of the cornea without fluorescein staining of the epithelium has been described, suggesting that the endothelium is the prime site of attack.[c]

Application of dry powdered podophyllum to rabbit eyes has been reported to cause immediate discomfort and blepharospasm, with a rapidly progressive inflammatory reaction.[53] However, rabbit corneas are reported to be much less affected than human corneas.[c]

Treatment includes irrigation of the surface of the eye to remove residual podophyllum, administration of mydriatic-cycloplegic drops, and in severe cases topical application of corticosteroids.

The mechanism of toxic action of podophyllum on the cornea has not been explained, but it may be relevant that podophyllum and colchicine, which also causes severe keratitis after a latent period, appear to have in common an unusual inhibitory effect on mitotic processes of cells.[a]

a. King LS, Sullivan M: Effects of podophyllum and colchicine on normal skin, on condyloma acuminatum and on verruca vulgaris. Pathological observations. *ARCH PATHOL* 43:374–386, 1947.

b. Rosner RS: Corneal insult from podophyllin. *AM J OPHTHALMOL* 29:1448–1450, 1946.

c. Calogero R: On a case of corneal injury from podophyllum. *ANN OTTALMOL CLIN OCUL* 95:554–560, 1969. (Italian)

d. Pedersen B, Bramsen T: Accidental injury to the cornea by podophyllin. *UGESKR LAEG* 142:452–453, 1980. (English summary)

Poison ivy (*Rhus radicans*) and *Poison oak* (*Rhus toxicodendron*) are North American climbing plants and shrubs which have on their surface powerfully allergenic substances, derivatives of 3-pentadecylcatechol.[171] Contact causes dermatitis after a latent period of several hours. Contact with the eye, usually occurring secondary to contamination of the hands or face, causes redness and swelling of the lids and conjunctivae. The cornea may be involved, causing pain, photophobia, and blepharospasm. Small limbal infiltrates have been observed.[a,46] The symptoms of severe ocular involvement may be relieved by topical use of atropine and steroids. Microhemangiomas of the pupillary border have been considered possibly related to a poison ivy reaction,[b] but these can occur spontaneously.

a. Scherer JW: Conjunctivitis and keratitis from poison ivy. *OPHTHALMOL REC* 25:191–193, 1916.

b. Awan KJ: Microhyphema. *CAN J OPHTHALMOL* 12:153–154, 1977.

Polyacrylamide, made by polymerization of *acrylamide,* has been experimentally used as a substitute for vitreous humor in rabbits.[a] If the polyacrylamide gel was not freed of residual toxic *acrylamide* before it was used to replace vitreous humor, it caused iridocyclitis with cells and flare visible for 4 months, elevation of intraocular pressure in some rabbits, and vitreal abscess in one. If purified first by dialysis to remove toxic constituents, a 1% polyacrylamide gel injected into the vitreous cavity caused iritis for two weeks, but then was well tolerated for at least 14 months, as judged by clinical and histologic examinations.

a. Mueller-Jensen K: Polyacrylamide as an alloplastic vitreous implant. *GRAEFES ARCH OPHTHALMOL* 189:147–158, 1974.

Polychlorinated biphenyls (PCB; Arochlor, Inerteen, Kanechlor, Pyranol) have accidentally become widely distributed in food, especially in Japan where contaminated cooking oil consumed by 1000 people in 1968 caused a condition known as Yushu, and later in Taiwan where a similar epidemic occurred.[c] The clinical characteristics were chloracne, brown pigmentation of skin, nails, and palpebral and bulbar conjunctiva, swelling and pigmentation of the eyelids, and eye discharge, particularly from hypersecretion from the Meibomian glands.[a,c] Babies born to mothers with this type of poisoning likewise showed palpebral and conjunctival pigmentation, cheesy secretion in the conjunctival sac, and also exophthalmus.[h]

In poisoned patients, the optic nerve heads, fundi, and visual fields were normal, and the only disturbance of vision appeared to be due to hypersecretion of the Meibomian glands, which produced a creamy discharge on the surface of the cornea.[c]

In experimental poisoning of rats[b] and monkeys[d,g] the lid abnormalities have been reproduced and studied, but rather than hypersecretion from the Meibomian glands, keratinization of the ducts was found, accounting for a peculiar stickiness of the discharge.[g] The retina and choroid of the monkeys remained normal. Toxic effects of polychlorinated biphenyls on cultured rabbit conjunctival cells also have been demonstrated and studied.[e,f]

a. Allen JR, Norback DH: Polychlorinated biphenyl- and triphenyl-induced gastric mucosal hyperplasia in primates. *SCIENCE* 179:498, 1973.

b. Aoki A: Ocular findings of chlorobiphenyls initoxication and histological changes of the palpebral conjunctiva in rats fed with Kaneclor 500. *FUKUOKA ACTA MED* 66:96–97, 1975.

c. Fu YA: Ocular manifestations of polychlorinated biphenyl (PCB) intoxication. *ARCH OPHTHALMOL* 101:379–381, 1983.

d. McNulty WP, Griffin DA: Possible polychlorinated biphenyl poisoning in rhesus monkeys. *J MED PRIMATOL* 5:237, 1976.

e. Ohnishi Y: Influences of polychlorinated biphenyls (PCB) on conjunctival cells in tissue culture. *ACTA SOC OPHTHALMOL JPN* 80:842–850, 1976.

f. Ohnishi Y, Noda S: Effects of polychlorinated biphenyls (PCB) on dissociated conjunctival cells *in vitro. JPN J OPHTHALMOL* 21:496–506, 1977.

g. Ohnishi Y, Kohno T: Polychlorinated biphenyls poisoning in monkey eye. *INVEST OPHTHALMOL VIS SCI* 18:981–984, 1979.

h. Yamashita F: Clinical features of polychlorobiphenyls (PCB)-induced fetopathy. *PAEDIA-TRICIAN* 6:20–27, 1977.

Polyethyleneglycol (Carbowaxes), manufactured in various molecular weights, are unctuous wax-like solids which dissolve in water to form transparent neutral solutions. Tested by application to rabbit eyes in molecular weights from approximately 200 to 4,000, they were found to cause no injury perceptible after twenty-four hours.[27]

Polyethyleneglycol-400 has been used on human eyes in an aqueous solution for decontamination after accidents with phenol. A 1:1 solution in water causes only slight burning sensation and no injury, and a 1:2 or 1:4 solution in completely nonirritating when used to flush the surface of the eye.[a, 338] (Compare *Polyethyleneglycolethers,* which have more toxic actions on the eye.)

a. Lang K: Treatment of phenol burns of the eye with polyethyleneglycol-400. *Z AERZTL FORTBILD (JENA)* 63:705–708, 1969. (German)

Polyethyleneglycolethers of unspecified chain length and composition are reported to have caused corneal hypesthesia, keratitis epithelialis, almost complete loss of epithelium, and corneal edema with wrinkling of Descemet's membrane in seventeen patients who had been treated with Aristamid eye salve to which was added 2% of these compounds. Without this addition the ointment was well tolerated. When the suspected material was dropped repeatedly on rabbit eyes, it caused inflammation of the conjunctiva and long-lasting ulceration and vascularization of the cornea.[a, b] (Also see INDEX for *Ointments* and *Surfactants.*)

a. Popp C: Corneal erosions from polyethyleneglycols. *KLIN MONATSBL AUGENHEILKD* 126:76–77, 1955. (German)

b. Popp C: Corneal erosions from polyethyleneglycol ether. *KLIN MONATSBL AUGEN-HEILKD* 126:176–180, 1955. (German)

Polyethylene sulfonic acid, examined first as an agent for inducing experimental retinal detachments in animals, is found to induce a variety of toxic effects when injected into the vitreous body.[a-c, 44] It induces uveitis. The vitreous humor develops opacities, partial liquefaction, and formation of strands which contract and cause detachment of the retina in rabbits and dogs. The ERG becomes abnormal. The lens develops cataract and may become dislocated. Band keratopathy, i.e., superficial calcification of the cornea, develops in relation to amount of vitamin D in the diet. With high vitamin D intake, all rabbits that receive intravitreal polyethylene sulfonic acid injections develop band keratopathy. This is thought to be a manifestation of calciphylaxis, the combined effect of alteration of the tissues by uveitis and mobilization of calcium by vitamin D.

a. Doughman DJ, Olson GA, et al: Experimental band keratopathy. *ARCH OPHTHALMOL* 81:264–271, 1969.

b. Doughman DJ, Watzke RC, Burian HM: The ocular effects of intravitreal injection of polyethylene sulfonic acid. *AM J OPHTHALMOL* 67:571–580, 1969.

c. Watzke RC: Experimental retinal detachment. *TRANS AM OPHTHALMOL SOC* 66:1022–1059, 1968.

Polygeline (Haemaccel), a plasma volume expander prepared from gelatin, has been tested by injection into rabbit eyes and has been used as a substitute for the vitreous humor in patients in treatment of retinal detachment.[a-c] In the anterior chamber of rabbits a 3.5% solution appeared to be nontoxic. The same concentration injected into the vitreous body was also nontoxic in rabbits and patients, but appeared to cause slight swelling of the vitreous and forward movement of the lens-iris diaphragm with a 5 to 10 mg Hg rise of intraocular pressure in rabbits, maximum at about twelve hours. Signs of inflammation with clouding of the vitreous after intravitreal injection in rabbits was noted with concentrations of 7% or greater. One case of persistent glaucoma in a patient developed after treatment of retinal detachment with polygeline, but this glaucoma was believed not attributable to a toxic action.

a. van Haeringen NJ, Oosterhuis JA, et al: Experiments with Haemaccel as a vitreous substitute. *EXP EYE RES* 5:235–241, 1966.

b. Oosterhuis JA, van Haeringen NJ, et al: Polygeline as a vitreous substitute. *ARCH OPHTHALMOL* 76:258–265, 1966.

c. Oosterhuis JA: Polygeline as a vitreous substitute. *ARCH OPHTHALMOL* 76:374–377, 1966.

Polyinosinic acid-polycytidilic acid polymer (Poly I-Poly C), an anti-viral interferon inducer, has been tested on rabbit eyes by repeated application to intact and scratched cornea, giving no signs of toxicity at therapeutically effective concentrations.[b,d,e] However, very intensive topical administration produced a transient conjunctival discharge.[b] Injection into the anterior chamber in rabbits produced iritis which developed several hours after the injection and was dose related.[a,b,f] Intravenous injection also produced iritis, with flare and cells or particles in the aqueous humor. One study reported posterior subcapsular lens opacities and opacities anteriorly in the vitreous body,[c] while another study showed slight clouding and pitting of the anterior capsule of the lens, but no opacities of lens or vitreous humor.[b]

a. Leonard BJ, Eccleston E, Jones D: Toxicity of interferon inducers of the double stranded RNA type. *NATURE* 224:1023, 1969.

b. McDonald TO, et al: Polyinosinic acid—polycytidylic acid in ophthalmology. *ANN OPHTHALMOL* 3:371–376; 1135–1139; 1146–1151, 1971.

c. Ostter HB, Jang OO, et al: Toxicity of poly I—poly C for rabbit eyes. *NATURE* 228:362–364, 1970.

d. Park JH, Baron S: Herpetic keratoconjunctivitis. *SCIENCE* 162:811–813, 1968.

e. Park JH, et al: Prophylaxis of herpetic keratoconjunctivitis with interferon inducers. *ARCH OPHTHALMOL* 81:840–842, 1969.

f. Pollikoff R, DiPuppo A, Cannuvale P: Vesicular stomatitis virus (VSV) infection in rabbit eye. *INVEST OPHTHALMOL* 8:488–496, 1969.

Polymyxin B as 0.1% solution plus 0.5% neomycin was reported to have been used for postoperative irrigation of the anterior chamber without causing clinically evident reaction in human eyes or histologic abnormalities in eyes of rabbits killed within thirty minutes after injection.[d] However, Fraunfelder's report from the national registry indicates that, though rare, permanent and clinically important changes in cornea and lens have resulted from intracameral injections.[b,312]

In rabbits, injection of 1 mg of polymyxin B sulfate into the vitreous body has caused total opacification of the lens.[a] Injection of 0.1mg caused no more than vacuoles and radiating posterior water clefts, while 10 mg caused congestion of iris vessels, mydriasis, and retinal detachment. It was mentioned, without specific documentation, that similar effects on the rabbit lens have been produced by *cetylpyridinium chloride, cetyltrimethylammonium bromide, neomycin sulfate,* and *polylysine,* which resemble polymyxin B in being polycations which may react with anionic sites of lens fiber membranes.

Rarely, systemically and topically administered polymyxin B, usually with neomycin, has caused temporary myasthenia.[c,312]

a. Cotlier E, Apple D: Cataracts induced by the polypeptide antibiotic polymyxin B sulfate. *EXP EYE RES* 16:69–77, 1973.

b. Francois J, Mortiers P: The injurious effects of locally and generally applied antibiotics on the eye. *T GENEESKD* 32:139, 1976.

c. Koenig A, Ohrloff C: Influence of local application of Isoptomax eye drops on neuromuscular transmission. *KLIN MONATSBL AUGENHEILKD* 179:109–112, 1981. (German)

d. McCoy DA, McIntyre MW, Turnbull DC: Irrigation of anterior chamber with neomycin-polymyxin solution in intraocular surgery. *ARCH OPHTHALMOL* 79:506, 1968.

Polyoxyethylene dodecanol (Laurithyl) is a water-soluble wetting agent which has been used in an aerosol in treatment of respiratory diseases. Tested by drop application to rabbit eyes, the pure chemical causes moderately severe damage to the cornea, improving after one week. A 10% solution causes relatively slight damage, and 1% solution causes very transient irritation.

a. Grubb TC, Dick LC, Oser M: Studies on the toxicity of polyoxyethylene dodecanol. *TOXICOL APPL PHARMACOL* 2:133–143, 1960.

Polysorbate 80 (polyoxyethylene sorbitan mono-oleate, Tween 80) is used as an emulsifying and dispersing agent in pharmaceuticals.[171] Standard tests by application to rabbit eyes have indicated polysorbate 80 to be nonirritating.[e] In U.S.P. grade it is well tolerated when dropped on the human eye in aqueous solutions in concentrations up to 20%. In combination with castor oil in a ratio of 9 to 1 it is nonirritating even after prolonged daily application to the eye.[a]

Crystalline lenses from rabbits maintained in culture medium have shown no significant increase of permeability to cations from addition of polysorbate 80 to a concentration of 0.01%.[c]

However, injection of 0.1 ml of 25% to 100% polysorbate 80 into the anterior chamber of rabbits has been reported to destroy the corneal endothelial cells, to cause much edematous swelling of the cornea and to provoke a perilimbal inflammatory reaction with increase in the permeability of the blood vessels.[d] Injected into corneas of rabbits it has provoked necrosis, with lipogenesis in adjacent surviving cells, similar to the effects of sodium oleate.[b] (See also *Oleic acid.*)

    a. Hagiwara H, Sugiwia S: The use of castor-oil and Tween 80 as an ophthalmic base. *ACTA SOC OPHTHALMOL JPN* 57:1–5, 1953.

    b. Kuwabara T, Cogan DG: Experimental aberrant lipogenesis. *ARCH PATHOL* 63:496–501, 1957.

    c. Lambert BW: The effects of progestins and estrogens on the permeability of the lens. *ARCH OPHTHALMOL* 80:230–234, 1968.

    d. Quiroga R, Klintworth GK: The pathogenesis of corneal edema induced by Tween 80. *AM J PATHOL* 51:977–999, 1967.

    e. Treon JF: Physiological properties of selected non-ionic surfactants. *SOAP PERFUM COSMET* 38:47–54, 1965. (*CHEM ABSTR* 66:93456, 1966.)

Polytetrafluoroethylene (Teflon, KelF) is a plastic which is extremely resistant to chemical attack, but when heated to 500° to 800° it gives off fumes which are irritating to the mucous membranes of animals, causing lacrimation and dyspnea. Under severe conditions the fumes have been noted to cause etching of the cornea of experimental animals. Men, however, apparently can be exposed to concentrations which are systemically toxic without noticeable irritation of the eyes. Typically, symptoms of intoxication appear after a latent period of a few hours and consist of discomfort in the chest, fever, shivering, and sweating, but recovery is rapid.[a]

    a. Pattison FLM: *Toxic Aliphatic Fluorine Compounds.* Amsterdam, Elsevier, 1959.

Polythiazide (Renese), a diuretic antihypertensive, has caused acute transitory myopia in a woman who took the drug and the next day had blurred vision, due to a 5.50 D increase in myopia, not relieved by cycloplegia, but with vision correctable to normal with glasses. Intraocular pressure was subnormal, 6 mm Hg by applanation. The anterior chamber was of normal depth, but the aqueous contained many fine cells. All returned gradually to normal by the fourth day, with tension rising to approximately normal 14 mm Hg.[a] Many other and unrelated drugs have produced myopia similar to this, although cells, flare, and hypotony, have been unusual. (See INDEX for *Myopia, acute transient.*)

    a. Gastaldi GM: Thoughts on the transitory myopia after administration of saluretic diuretics. *RASS ITAL OTTALMOL* 34:178–185, 1965–1966.

Polyurethane foams are manufactured by polymerization of diisocyanates catalyzed by amines. (Particularly, see INDEX for *Toluene diisocyanate.*) Several of the chemicals used in the process have toxic effects on the eyes. These include irritation and sensitization to *toluene diisocyanate,* episodes of hazy blue vision due to corneal epithelial edema from the amines *N-ethylmorpholine, N-methylmorpholine,* and *triethylenediamine,* and transient interference with accommodation from *tetramethylbutanediamine.*[b] The ocular effects of each of these chemicals are described further elsewhere under their individual names, and under *Amines* (see INDEX). Polyurethane foam or sponge, when free of the chemicals from which it is made, appears to have low toxicity and to be tolerated as a plastic implant in ocular surgery.[ad]

a. Bernardczykowa A, Zawilski J, Majewski C: Investigations on the tissue reaction of rabbit eye on Polish made polyurethan and vinyl sponge. *KLIN OCZNA* 37:481–486, 1967.
b. Dernehl CU: Health hazards associated with polyurethane foams. *J OCCUP MED* 8:59–62, 1966.

Polyvinyl alcohol (PVA, Polyviol), a polymer, varying in water solubility according to composition and manner of preparation, has been used in eyedrops to increase viscosity, and as a plastic sponge implant in relatively insoluble form. In eyedrops a 1.4% neutral solution of polyvinyl alcohol with molecular weight over 100,000 tested on rabbit eyes has been shown to be noninjurious and not to interfere with healing of experimental epithelial wounds.[c,d,g,h] The same concentration has been used in eyedrops on human eyes without difficulty.[g] Concentrations as high as 10% also have not been irritating.[e] Subconjunctival injection in rabbits has caused no appreciable tissue reaction, and injections into the anterior chamber and vitreous body also caused no inflammatory reaction and is said to have caused no rise of intraocular pressure.[b,d,f,i]

Polyvinyl alcohol sponge implants in rabbit corneas are infiltrated by fibroblastic vascular tissue and become opaque and vascularized in about five weeks.[j] Polyvinyl alcohol sponge implants in extraocular tissues also have not been inert histologically.[a] A foreign-body type of reaction to an orbital sponge implant of formalinized polyvinyl alcohol resin known as Ivalon has been described histologically in one patient. (See *Ivalon.*)

a. Anderson DL, Shea M: Tissue response to polyvinyl alcohol implants. *AM J OPHTHALMOL* 51:1200–1202, 1961.
b. Hara Y, Nishiioka K, Kamiya S: Replacement of vitreous by PVA hydrogel for albino rabbit. *FOLIA OPHTHALMOL JPN* 28:576, 1977. (English summary)
c. Krishna N, Brow F: Polyvinyl alcohol as an ophthalmic vehicle, effect on regeneration of corneal epithelium. *AM J OPHTHALMOL* 57:99–106, 1964.
d. Krishna N, Mitchell B: Polyvinylalcohol as an ophthalmic vehicle. *AM J OPHTHALMOL* 59:860–864, 1965.
e. Maitchuk YR: Polyvinyl alcohol medical basis of antibiotics for ophthalmological practice. *OFTAL ZH* 19:350–354, 1964.
f. Olson RJ, Kolodner H, et al: Polyvinyl alcohol as a protective coating on intraocular lenses. *ARCH OPHTHALMOL* 98:1840–1842, 1980.
g. Swanson AA, Jeter DJ, Gregor CR: The influence of ophthalmic vehicles on ^{3}H thymidine in normal rabbit corneas. *OPHTHALMOLOGICA* 156:425–436, 1968.
h. Trautmann I: Poly(vinyl alcohol) as vehicle for eyedrops. *DTSCH GES WOCHENSCHR* 22:317–320, 1967.
i. Yamaichi A, Matsuzawa Y, et al: Behavior of polyvinyl alcohol hydrogel in the vitreous body of albino rabbits. *FOLIA OPHTHALMOL JPN* 29:1922, 1978. (English summary)
j. Zigman S, Carlsson B, Stone W Jr: The response of the cornea to implantation of polyvinyl alcohol sponge. *INVEST OPHTHALMOL* 3:68–76, 1964.

Polyvinyl chloride (PVC) plastics, such as Saran, may give off irritant fumes containing hydrochloric acid when exposed to high temperatures. These fumes have irritated the eyes of personnel exposed to them, but no permanent injury has resulted.[a]

a. Fernandez RHP, Watkins JT: Portable eye irrigation unit. *BR J OPHTHALMOL* 41:626–628, 1957.

Potassium carbonate (potash) in water has a maximum pH of 11.6 at room temperature.[171] Potassium carbonate has been mentioned as a cause of eye injury,[253] but it is more likely that injury was produced by potassium hydroxide, which is significantly more alkaline. Irrigation of the surface of the eyes of rabbits with a 10% solution of potassium carbonate at pH 11.6 for thirty seconds caused pain and very slight transient optical irregularity of the epithelium. However, one to two hours later the corneas and conjunctivae appeared normal on examination with the biomicroscope, and they did not stain with fluorescein.[81] Hot solution would probably be more injurious.

Potassium chlorate ($KClO_3$) long ago was used in treatment of conjunctivitis, as a 3 to 5% eyedrop or eye bath. This was reported to be well tolerated.[a] Also, powdered potassium chlorate applied to the human conjunctiva and to the rabbit cornea appeared to cause no injury.

a. Koster W: Potassium chlorate in ophthalmology. *ZEITSCHR AUGENHEILKD* 15:524–527, 1906. (German)

Potassium hydroxide (caustic potash) is one of the strongest alkalies. It is extremely corrosive, and many reports have been made of devastating damage of the eye from contact with either the solid or solutions of potassium hydroxide.[46, 153] The type of injury is essentially the same as that produced by sodium hydroxide and other strong alkalies. (See *Alkalies* and *Sodium hydroxide.*)

Potassium hypochlorite resembles sodium hypochlorite. It is stable only in alkaline solution. It is encountered principally in the form of Javelle (or Javel) Water containing approximately 2.5% active chlorine.[171] This solution has been known to cause severe conjunctival reaction, with hemorrhages in the conjunctiva and loss of corneal epithelium in several patients.[249] In most cases the cornea cleared subsequently, but in one case there was iritis and residual leukoma.[249] The strong alkalinity of the solution is partially responsible for its injurious effect on the eye. (Compare *Sodium hypochlorite.*)

Potassium metal in contact with water reacts violently, producing potassium hydroxide and liberating heat. In rare instances particles of metallic potassium have caused severe ocular injuries. (See *Potassium hydroxide.*)

Potassium oleate 12% aqueous solution tested on rabbit eyes caused irritation comparable to 70% isopropyl alcohol.[352]

Potassium permanganate is a dark purple crystalline compound readily soluble in water. Dilute solutions generally have not been injurious to the eye, but strong solutions and crystals have caused damage.[a-c, e, f, i, j]

Characteristically in the area of contact a hardened eroded lesion has developed, colored dark brown by the manganese oxide formed from permanganate by reducing substances in the tissues.[b, 46, 153, 249, 253] This has commonly been accompanied by swelling of the lids and conjunctivae, and by subconjunctival hemorrhages. With prolonged contact, turbidity and brown discoloration of the cornea also have developed. Clinical and experimental observations have shown that the cornea is much more likely to be involved if its epithelium has been injured mechanically.

Recovery usually has been spontaneous and complete, but in one instance total leukoma is reported following application of a strong solution of potassium permanganate.[c]

Treatments, apart from first aid irrigation with water, have been aimed at reducing residual permanganate and solubilizing and removing reduced manganese compounds from the tissues. Various agents have been used and recommended for these purposes, such as solutions of ascorbic acid,[j] sodium thiosulfate,[b] hydrogen peroxide, and sodium edetate. Ascorbic acid solution has been found to hasten the reduction of permanganate,[a, i, j] and the edetate solution is said to help in removing the reduced manganese compounds.[i] Seven eyes treated in this way are said to have done well.[b] However, in one typical case of injury by permanganate crystals in which both eyes (corneas and conjunctivae) were equally affected, treatment of one eye with edetate solution proved of no apparent advantage.[f] Both eyes recovered completely. An experimental comparison of various treatments in animal eyes would be helpful in choosing the best.

Experimentally in rabbits, irrigation of the cornea with 0.003 M solution of potassium permanganate has been found to cause no injury, but injection of 0.08 M solution into the cornea caused moderately severe reaction, graded 60 on a scale of 0 to 100.[123] In a study of corneal calcification, it has been found that repeated perfusion of the anterior chamber of rabbits with 0.1% solution of potassium permanganate, and oral administration of dihydrotachysterol, results in calcification of the most anterior layers of the cornea. The permanganate causes corneal edema and decrease in corneal content of mucopolysaccharides.

a. Bostelmann I: Potassium permanganate burns of the eye. *DTSCH GES WOCHENSCHR* 17:1210–1211, 1962. (*ZENTRALBL GES OPHTHALMOL* 88:220, 1963). (German)
b. Gassler H: Therapy of eye lesions caused by potassium permanganate. *Z GESAMTE HYG* 12:931–934, 1966. (German)
c. Hempel E: On burn of the cornea by Lysol and potassium permanganate. *KLIN MONATSBL AUGENHEILKD* 49:758–763, 1911. (German)
d. Khudovekova EA: On the possible use of sodium thiosulfate in eye burns caused by potassium permanganate. *VESTN OFTALMOL* 80:86, 1967. (English summary)
e. Meitinger A: A case of eye injury from potassium permanganate crystals. *KLIN MONATSBL AUGENHEILKD* 123:493–494, 1953. (German)
f. Michaels DD, Zugsmith GS: Potassium permanganate burn of the eye. *EYE EAR NOSE THR MONTHLY* 52:97–98, 1973.
g. Obenberger J, et al: Experimental corneal calcification. *OPHTHALMIC RES* 1:175–192, 1970.
h. Obenberger J, Cejkova J, Babicky A: Experimental calcification of the cornea. *CESK OFTALMOL* 27:198–204, 1971. (English abstract)

i. Pitter J, Vyhnamek J: The treatment of eye injuries from potassium permanganate crystals. *KLIN MONATSBL AUGENHEILKD* 133:265–267, 1958. (German)
j. Tobia S: The management of potassium permanganate ocular burn. *BULL OPHTHAL-MOL SOC EGYPT* 69:645–646, 1976.

Potassium thiocyanate, a hypotensive, may cause severe poisoning in excessive doses. Several cases of poisoning have been reported in which there was delirium, swelling of the eyelids, blurred vision, and visual hallucinations.[255]

On the eye a 2% to 5% solution of potassium thiocyanate applied repeatedly has appeared nontoxic clinically, although cattle corneas exposed to 9.7% solution for an hour have had some loosening of the epithelium.[107]

Povidone (polyvinylpyrrolidone, PVP, Plasdone, Vinisil), a water-soluble polymer, has been used as a plasma expander and as an agent to increase viscosity of solutions to be used on and in the eye. A saline solution containing 25% PVP, molecular weight 160,000, produced no inflammation or tissue damage when placed in the anterior chamber of rabbits, and this solution has been used in a considerable series of patients to replace the aqueous humor after extraction of cataracts, corneal transplantation, and antiglaucoma operations. It is said to have caused no irritation, damage, or persistent glaucoma.[a] Also a 25% to 30% solution of PVP of molecular weight 12,600 to 30,000 has been used to replace the aqueous humor after cataract extractions and was said to be "non-toxic", but postoperative measurements of intraocular pressure were not specifically reported.[b] However, 0.1 ml of 40% solution in the rabbit anterior chamber did not raise the pressure.[d]

More recently, coating of intraocular lenses with povidone has been reported to be associated with cystic macular edema.[c]

Povidone has been used in hair sprays and lacquer and has been among the substances accidentally contaminating the eyes from these sprays, but it can be considered an innocuous component.

a. King JH Jr, McTigue JW: The reformation of the anterior chamber with polyvinyl-pyrrolidone. *SOUTHERN MED J* 57:1369–1372, 1964.
b. Sarda RP, Makhija JM, Sharma RG: Polyvinyl pyrrolidone (PVP) in cataract surgery. *BR J OPHTHALMOL* 53:477–480, 1969.
c. Junge J: Cystoid macular edema associated with PVP coating of an intraocular lens. *AM INTRA-OCUL IMPLANT SOC J* 6:28–29, 1980.
d. Katz J, Kaufman HE, et al: Prevention of endothelial damage from intraocular lens insertion. *TRANS AM ACAD OPHTHALMOL OTOL* 83:204–212, 1977.

Povidone-Iodine (Pharmidine; PVP-Iodine; Betadine solution), a topical anti-infective, has been evaluated for toxicity to the cornea in patients undergoing cataract extraction.[a] Eyes in which 10–20 drops of the preparation were instilled in the conjunctival sac and not washed out pre-operatively, compared with untreated controls 5 to 7 months post-operation, showed no significant difference in amount of endothelial cell loss or in corneal thickness. Even a 10% solution has "minimal corneal toxicity."[354]

Quite different from simple *solutions* are commercial skin *scrubs* (E-Z Scrub; Betadine Scrub) which contain, in addition to povidone-iodine, a detergent or surfactant which has been seen to take the corneal epithelium off a patient's eye, and when tested on rabbit eyes caused corneal epithelial edema, and loss of epithelial cells, but the eyes recovered in a week.[354]

It is obviously important to distinguish the injurious "scrubs" from the relatively harmless "solutions".

a. Wille H: Assessment of possible toxic effects of polyvinylpyrrolidone-iodine upon the human eye in conjunction with cataract extraction. *ACTA OPHTHALMOL* 60:955–960, 1983.

Practolol (Eraldin, Dalzic), a cardio-selective beta-adrenergic receptor blocking drug, was introduced into clinical use in 1969. By 1974 and 1975 it became notorious as a cause of a unique oculomucocutaneous syndrome, and in 1975 was withdrawn from general clinical use. The adverse ocular effects of chronic oral administration of practolol are believed to represent a new, and still incompletely understood, toxic mechanism peculiar to the practolol molecule, not shared by the other beta-adrenergic blocker drugs in clinical use.

Comprehensive and authoritative synopsis-reviews of the adverse side effects of practolol have been provided by Wright and Fraunfelder.[e,f,312] What is presented here has mainly been abstracted from their publications, and from a small number of other selected publications. Case reports which present similar clinical experiences with eye involvement in one or a small number of patients, and reports of adverse effects of practolol on other parts of the body, have not been included in the present bibliography.

An incidence of eye involvement of 0.2% has been estimated among patients treated with practolol. Onset ranged from 5 months to 5 years after starting treatment with practolol. In a majority of cases skin rash accompanied ocular involvement. Initial symptoms were gritty foreign-body, burning sensation, and photophobia, characteristic of keratoconjunctivitis sicca. Tear flow was much reduced, and tenacious mucus was common in the conjunctival sac. The conjunctiva typically became hyperemic and irregularly vascularized. The upper and lower fornices, and the canthi were most involved, with keratinization, shrinkage, scarring and symblepharon. The bulbar conjunctiva was involved in the most serious cases, with an elevated roll of tissue close to the limbus.

The cornea was affected slightly in most patients, with superficial punctate lesions or small erosions, but severely in other patients, with central stromal opacification, ulceration, and more rarely perforation.

Recovery after stopping practolol was rapid for the most fortunate, with improvement in tear production, and free movement of the conjunctiva over persistent subconjunctival fibrous tissue, and lessening density of symblepharon. Those who had severe involvement of the corneas were the most unfortunate, with opacities and perforations not responding well to surgery.

The histopathology in 6 cases of adverse effects of practolol on the eye featured "destruction of lacrimal gland tissue, epidermalization of the conjunctival epithelium, with epitheliolysis and stromal ulceration of the cornea."[d] Loss of goblet cells from the conjunctiva and fibrosis of the underlying stroma also appeared to be characteristic.

Study of tears from patients with ocular involvement has shown reduction of tear lysozyme and secretory IgA to low levels, consistent with atrophy of lacrimal glands.[b,c]

Serologic studies have shown a high incidence of antinuclear antibodies,[b] and an "antibody which sticks to the intercellular region of squamous epithelial tissue" associated only with the distinct type of damage to the conjunctiva induced by practolol.[a]

An animal model has been lacking, because test animals have tolerated practolol without showing changes in lacrimal gland tissue.[d]

a. Amos HE, Brigden WD, McKerron RA: Untoward effects associated with practolol. *BR MED J* 1:598–600, 1975.
b. Garner A, Rahi AHS: Practolol and ocular toxicity. *BR J OPHTHALMOL* 60:684–686, 1976.
c. Mackie IA, Seal DV, Pescod JM: Beta-adrenergic receptor blocking drugs; tear lysozyme and immunological screening for adverse reaction. *BR J OPHTHALMOL* 61:354–359, 1977.
d. Rahi AHS, Chapman CM, et al: Pathology of practolol-induced ocular toxicity. *BR J OPHTHALMOL* 60:312–323, 1976.
e. Wright P: Untoward effects associated with practolol administration; oculomucocutaneous syndrome. *BR MED J* 1:595–598, 1975.
f. Wright P, Fraunfelder FT: Practolol-induced oculomucocutaneous syndrome. Chapter 9, Leopold IH and Burns RP, editors, *Symposium on Ocular Therapy*, Vol 9, New York, John Wiley and Sons, 1976, pp. 97–110.

Pralidoxime (2-PAM, Protopam, 2-pyridine aldoxime), used as chloride, iodide, or mesylate salts, is a cholinesterase reactivator useful in the treatment or prevention of poisoning by organic phosphorous cholinesterase inhibitors, such as pesticides, nerve gases, and miotic drugs. A dose of 1 g pralidoxime mesylate by mouth in addition to atropine (2 mg) and metaraminol (10 mg), which might be used prophylactically against poisoning, has caused no appreciable systemic adverse effects nor disturbance of vision or accommodation.[k]

However, when pralidoxime iodide was given intravenously in doses of 15 to 30 mg/kg to eighteen normal human beings, it uniformly induced dizziness, and in thirteen out of eighteen subjects caused blurred vision lasting two to thirty-five minutes.[g] Eight of those so affected also experienced diplopia, which lasted almost as long. Accommodation was tested in three individuals and was found to be impaired for thirty minutes following the injection. No alteration of the pupils, nystagmus, or gross eye muscle imbalance was observed to account for the diplopia. In this study neither visual acuity nor an examination of the fundi was reported.

In treatment of people poisoned by organic phosphorous anticholinesterase agents, these unimportant side effects have been scarcely noted and presented no significant problem.[i,j]

Investigation of use of pralidoxime topically on the eye to counteract the miosis and cyclotonia induced by cholinesterase inhibitors has shown that the expected antagonistic effect is demonstrable, but takes some hours to develop. Little effect is obtained from eyedrops containing 5% pralidoxime salts. Subconjunctival injection is required, and the concentration that can be injected is limited by irritation of the ocular tissues.[h]

In patients subconjunctival injection of 0.2 ml of 4% pralidoxime iodide has been tolerated. This had no effect on the pupil in normal eyes, but antagonized the effect of 0.25% echothiophate eyedrops on pupil and facility of aqueous outflow.[c]

In rabbits, intramuscular injection of 40 to 100 mg/kg has caused the intraocular pressure to rise a few mm Hg for 4 or more hours. The mechanism was undertermined. There was no cumulative effect from repeated injections.[a,b,276]

Additional mydriasis has been obtained when phenylephrine and atropine eyedrops have been added to the pralidoxime treatment, counteracting echothiophate or DFP miosis.[d] Miosis in the human eye from application of a standard dose of paraoxon has been utilized as a basis for comparing the effectiveness of systemically administered pralidoxime and other cholinesterase reactivators.[f]

Preoperatively in human eyes to counteract strong miosis from treatment with paraoxon, an irrigation of the anterior chamber with 1% pralidoxime iodide is said not to be injurious and to permit dilation of the pupil in a few seconds.[e]

a. Ballantyne B, Gazzard MF, et al: *TOXICOL APPL PHARMACOL* 33:559–567, 1975.
b. Ballantyne B, Swanston DW: Aqueous humor pralidoxime mesylate (P2S) concentrations and intraocular tension following intramuscular P2S. *DRUG CHEM TOXICOL* 3:259–275, 1980.
c. Becker B, Pyle GC, Drews RC: The tonographic effects of echothiophate (Phospholine) iodide. Reversal by pyridine-2-aldoxime methiodide (P₂AM). AM J OPHTHALMOL 47:635–640, 1959.
d. Byron H, Posner H: Clinical evaluation of protopam. *AM J OPHTHALMOL* 57:409–418, 1964.
e. Dekking HM: Stopping the action of strong miotics. *OPHTHALMOLOGICA* 148:428–430, 1964.
f. Graupner K, Wiezorek WD, Schmautz K: Suitability of paraoxon miosis of the human eye for testing cholinesterase reactivators. *ACTA BIOL MED GERMAN* 16:232–233, 1966. (*EXCERPTA MED* (Sect. 2C), 20:2505, 1967.)
g. Jagar BV, Stagg GN: Toxicity of biacetyl monoxime and of pyridine-2-aldoxime methiodide in man. *BULL JOHNS HOPKINS HOSP* 102:203–211, 1958.
h. Krishna N, Leopold IH: Effect of Protopam on the rabbit pupil. *AM J OPHTHALMOL* 52:566–567, 1961.
i. Quinby GE: Further therapeutic experience with pralidoximes in organic phosphorous poisoning. *J AM MED ASSOC* 187:202–206, 1964.
j. Quinby GE, Loomis TA, Brown HW: Oral occupational parathion poisoning treated with 2-PAM iodide (2-pyridine aldoxime methiodide). *N ENGL J MED* 268:639–643, 1963.
k. Taylor WJR, Llewellyn-Thomas E, et al: Effects of a combination of atropine, metaraminol and pyridine aldoxime methanesulfonate (AMP therapy) on normal human subjects. *CAN MED ASSOC J* 93:957–961, 1965.

Praseodymium chloride tested by application to rabbit eyes, had the same type of effect as several other rare-earth salts. A 0.1 M aqueous solution at pH 5.3 applied for ten minutes to the eye after the corneal epithelium had been removed to facilitate penetration caused no immediate change in appearance, but a gradually increasing haze in the course of several hours, developing into dense opacities within a week, and ultimately causing complete leukoma with vascularization. By contrast, when the corneal epithelium was left intact before application of the test solution, injury of the cornea was completely prevented.[81,90] When a 50% solution of praseodymium chloride was applied to intact rabbit eyes, 0.1 ml caused immediate blinking and hyperemia of the conjunctiva that persisted for a week, but no injury of the cornea or iris was observed during observations for three weeks.[a]

> a. Haley TJ, Komesu N, et al: Pharmacology and toxicology of praseodymium and neodymium chlorides. *TOXICOL APPL PHARMACOL* 6:614–620, 1964.

Prazosin (Minipress), an antihypertensive, in a prospective clinical evaluation of 203 patients showed no adverse effects detectible by slit-lamp examination after 6 months to two years.[a]

> a. Pitts NE: Clinical evaluation of prazosin. *POSTGRAD MED* (Special Issue):117–127, 1975.

Preservatives used in eyedrops and contact lens solutions are mainly antimicrobial or antifungal agents, but an anti-oxidant (sodium bisulfite) may be used in addition to help preserve a drug such as epinephrine that is subject to oxidation. The following preservatives have been used in eyedrops: *benzalkonium chloride, benzethonium chloride, cetylpyridinium chloride, chlorhexidine, chlorobutanol, edetate, paraben esters, phenylmercuric salts,* and *thimerosal.* All are potentially toxic to the corneal epithelium and endothelium if critical concentrations or duration of exposure are exceeded. As a result of efforts to select optimal ratios of antimicrobial effectiveness to corneal toxicity, and taking into consideration also the comfort of the patient, at present the preservatives principally used are *benzalkonium, benzalkonium with edetate, chlorobutanol,* and *thimerosal.* Comparisons of the types and degrees of discomfort caused by various preservatives have been reported by Hanna.[326]

Even at concentrations that are tolerated and used clinically there are evidences of toxicity of preservatives to the corneal epithelium, which are revealed by sensitive methods of detection, such as measurement of the electrical resistance of the cornea (an index of permeability),[285] and scanning electron microscopy.[285,300] Loss of epithelial microvilli and desquamation of superficial cells are seen.[b,300] Also, abnormal permeability to fluorescein is demonstrable with use of customary concentrations of benzalkonium.[320]

At concentrations of preservatives that are customarily used in eyedrops, and with ordinary frequency of application to the eye, the endothelium of the cornea usually remains normal, as judged by endothelial microscopy.[314] However, excessively high concentrations of a preservative such as benzalkonium applied externally can severely damage the endothelium.[314]

Eyedrops, or other solutions containing preservatives, present a greater threat to the corneal endothelium if they are introduced directly into the anterior chamber, either during intraocular surgery or by injection.[a] Eyedrops or other solutions containing preservatives should be tested in animal eyes before introduction into the anterior or vitreous chambers of human beings. As an example of the consequences of failure to make such a test, when saline solution with *benzyl alcohol* preservative was used in irrigation of the anterior chamber in patients, on the assumption that it was safe because *benzyl alcohol* is commonly used in solutions for injection elsewhere in the body, severe endothelial damage and corneal opacification resulted. (See the INDEX for more specific information on the preservatives discussed in general above.)

a. Lang RM, Hassard DTR: Effects on the corneal endothelium of anterior chamber reconstituents instilled during intracapsular cataract extraction. *CAN J OPHTHALMOL* 16:70–72, 1981.

b. Maudgal PC, Cornelis H, Missotten L: Effects of commercial ophthalmic drugs on rabbit corneal epithelium. *GRAEFES ARCH OPHTHALMOL* 216:191–203, 1981.

Primidone (Primaclone, Mylepsin, Mysoline), an anticonvulsant, causes drowsiness, ataxia, mental dullness, and drooping of the eyelids.[d] One patient is said to have had blurred and narrowed vision with diplopia, but no further details were furnished.[e]

One patient developed optic neuritis while under treatment for Wilson's disease with both DL-penicillamine and primidone, but it is thought the penicillamine was more likely responsible.[f]

In glaucomatous patients, primidone has had no adverse effect on intraocular pressure in two subjects given 250 mg orally.[190]

A child with congenital glaucoma was born to an epileptic mother who took primidone and phenytoin throughout her pregnancy.[b] (See INDEX for *Phenytoin*.)

Primidone has been involved in association with phenytoin in rare instances of external ophthalmoplegia from excessive dosage.[c] Also this combination was involved in one case of ataxia and nystagmus which persisted many months after discontuance of medication, but the phenytoin was believed to be mainly responsible.[a]

a. Kokenge R, Kutt H, McDowell F: Neurological sequelae following Dilantin overdose in a patient and in experimental animals. *NEUROLOGY* 15:823–829, 1965.

b. Meadow SR: Glaucoma, maternal epilepsy, and anticonvulsant drugs. *J PEDIATR* 90:499, 1977.

c. Orth DN, Almeida H, et al: Ophthalmoplegia resulting from diphenylhydantoin and primidone intoxication. *J AM MED ASSOC* 201:485–487, 1967.

d. Sciarra D, Carter S, et al: Clinical evaluation of primidone (Mysoline), new anticonvulsant drug. *J AM MED ASSOC* 154:827–829, 1954.

e. Timberlake WH, Abbott JA, Schwab RS: Mysoline. *N ENGL J MED* 252:304–307, 1955.

f. Tu J, Blackwell RQ, Lee PF: DL-Penicillamine as a cause of optic axial neuritis. *J AM MED ASSOC* 185:83–86, 1963.

Primula (primrose, *Primula sinensis*) is a flowering herb which causes allergic contact dermatitis. Hypersensitive individuals may develop urticarial burning and itching of the face, edema of the lids, and conjunctival hyperemia. Photophobia and lacrimation suggestive of keratitis epithelialis have been known to accompany the lid and conjunctival reaction.[153] In rare instances bilateral iritis with deposits of inflammatory cells on the posterior surface of the corneas has been observed.[253] The same ocular reactions have been ascribed to *Primula obconica.*[253] The specific allergen,

2-methoxy-6-pentyl-p-benzoquinone, also known as *primin,* has been identified, and can be used for patch testing on the skin for specific sensitivity.[a]

> a. Fregert S, Hjorth N, Schulz KH: Patch testing with synthetic primin in persons sensitive to *Primula obconica. ARCH DERMATOL* 98:144–147, 1968.

Procarbazine (Matulane), an antineoplastic, was used in treatment of a patient with multiple myeloma and plasma cell leukemia in combination treatment with carmustine and cyclophosphamide for 8 days before severe bilateral optic neuritis developed. Both procarbazine and carmustine came under suspicion, because they were known to cross the blood-brain barrier.[a]

> a. Lennan RMc, Taylor HR: Optic neuroretinitis in association with BCNU and procarbazine therapy. *AUST MED PEDIATR ONCOL* 4:43–48, 1978.

Prochlorperazine (Compazine), an antiemetic, has produced head-neck spasms such as induced by other phenothiazine derivatives, particularly in children. In one case of overdosage a young child was noted to have constricted pupils and conjugate deviation of the eyes, with periods of trismus and rigidity and arching of the neck, alternating with periods of general relaxation, all transitory.[a] A young woman who received 5 mg twice a day for 3 days had her eyes uncontrollably rolled upward, not voluntarily moveable.[323] This was relieved in 3 minutes by 25 mg of diphenhydramine given slowly intravenously.

Acute transitory myopia has also occurred in rare instances in response to prochlorperazine medication.[b] This is an odd effect produced by many drugs in very low incidence, apparently an idiosyncratic type of reaction. (For further description, see INDEX for *Myopia, acute transitory.*)

> a. Epps RP, Scott RB: Tranquilizers as a source of intoxication in children. *MED ANN DC* 30:317, 1961.
> b. Yasuna E: Acute myopia associated with prochlorperazine (Compazine) therapy. *AM J OPHTHALMOL* 54:793–796, 1962.

Proflavin, under experimental evaluation for photodynamic inactivation of corneal herpes, was applied as 0.1% solution to the eyes of normal volunteers, along with irradiation with a fluorescent light. This caused ultraviolet keratitis.[a] The same report mentions production of "anterior uveitis" in animals.

> a. O'Day DM, Jones BR, et al: Proflavin photodynamic viral inactivation in herpes simplex keratitis. *AM J OPHTHALMOL* 79:941–948, 1975.

Prolonium iodide (Entodon, Intrajod) caused in ten patients a paralysis of accommodation without disturbing the pupils, the visual acuity (corrected), or the visual fields. The effect was dose related and reached its maximum in one-half hour, disappearing in three hours.[a]

> a. Kincses E, Balazs G: Accommodation paralysis after large doses of Intrajod. *KLIN MONATSBL AUGENHEILKD* 150:252–255, 1967.

Promazine (Sparine), a phenothiazine derivative tranquilizer and anticholinergic, has produced reversible opacity of the front of the lens in mice,[261] presumably due to suppression of blinking and loss of water from the front of the eye by evaporation. Rabbit lenses in culture show reduced oxygen uptake when promazine is added, but this is probably unrelated.[a] Roberts has shown that photopolymerization of lens proteins *in vitro* by ultraviolet is increased by addition of promazine, but the significance is uncertain.[b]

Promazine has been tested in dogs to determine whether it produced accumulation of granules in the corneal stroma upon prolonged oral administration, like chlorpromazine. It did not.[278]

a. Hamdy H, El-Bagoury IM, Makarem A: The effect of psychotropic drugs on the oxygen consumption of the lens. *BULL OPHTHALMOL SOC EGYPT* 66:141–157, 1973.
b. Roberts JE: The photodynamic effect of chlorpromazine, promazine, and hematoporphyrin on lens protein. *INVEST OPHTHALMOL VIS SCI* 25:746–750, 1984.

Promethazine (Anergan, Phenergan) a phenothiazine-derivative, antiemetic and antihistaminic, has in one well-studied case produced acute transitory myopia, such as produced by many other unrelated drugs, apparently as an idiosyncratic type of reaction.[a]

The intraocular pressure in patients with normal or glaucomatous eyes has not been significantly affected by promethazine.[b]

An abnormally long latent period has been observed for the appearance of occipital EEG signals after light stimulus to the eyes in four schizophrenic patients taking both promethazine and chlorpromazine.[c] No retinopathy has been reported from promethazine.

a. Bard LA: Transient myopia associated with promethazine (Phenergan) therapy. *AM J OPHTHALMOL* 58:682–685, 1964.
b. D'Ermo F, Pirodda A: Antihistamines and the eye. *BOLL OCULIST* 39:715–721, 1960. (Italian)
c. Muller W: Visual evoked cortical response in long-term treatment with high doses of Propaphenin/Prothazin. *GRAEFES ARCH OPHTHALMOL* 172:164–169, 1967. (German)

Pronase, a proteolytic enzyme, has been tested in rabbit, bovine, and human eyes as a substitute for α-chymotrypsin as an aid in cataract extraction. It is zonulolytic and has been tolerated in 1:80,000 solution in the anterior chamber of human eyes, but at higher concentration was found to be damaging when tested in the anterior chamber of rabbits.[a]

a. Kishimoto M, Mishima K, Takano T: Experimental and clinical studies on zonulolysis by the proteolytic enzyme pronase in cataract extraction. *J CLIN OPHTHALMOL (TOKYO)* 19:165–174, 1965. (English abstract)

Propanethiol (propyl mercaptan) exposure of animals to high concentrations of vapor has induced rubbing and closure of the eyes in about 15 minutes. Application of a drop to rabbit eyes caused moderate immediate irritation. Hyperemia of the conjunctiva, chemosis, and discharge increased for 1 or 2 days, but the eyes returned to normal in 8 days.[55]

Propantheline bromide (Pro-Banthine), an anticholinergic, has weak effect on pupil and accommodation when given systemically. In one series of patients oral doses of 75 mg per day caused subjective difficulty with vision in only four out of sixty-nine, presumably from interference with accommodation.[a] In another series 120 mg given orally to sixteen normal people of ages twenty to thirty-five years had no effect on near point of accommodation.[178] Salivation has been reduced and heart rate raised by oral and intramuscular doses that have had no effect on accommodation.[178] Comparison with atropine when both drugs were given by subcutaneous injection to thirteen normal men showed the potency of propantheline bromide is only 0.08 for mydriatic effect and 0.22 for cycloplegic effect compared to atropine taken as 1.0.[109]

The only tests relating to glaucoma apparently have consisted of administering doses of 15 mg propantheline bromide orally to twenty normal patients and to twenty patients with various kinds of glaucoma, and evaluating the intraocular pressure by tonometry performed hourly for three hours.[b] This was done without gonioscopy and without comparison with measurements of spontaneous diurnal variations without medication. In the experiment, the tension did not change in the normal eyes, but during the test period it rose in three chronic simple open-angle glaucomatous eyes, in one with "chronic congestive," and in one with "secondary" glaucoma.[b] Without information from gonioscopy and without comparison mentioned above without medication, it is uncertain whether the drug was responsible for these tension elevations. As with many other anticholinergic drugs, there is theoretically the possibility of precipitating angle-closure glaucoma by inducing mydriasis in eyes anatomically predisposed because of abnormally shallow anterior chambers, and the possibility of making primary open-angle glaucoma worse by inducing cycloplegia, as discussed in more detail under *Anticholinergic Drugs*, but the comparative data on propantheline bromide suggests that its effects on pupil and accommodation are sufficiently weak that it should present little actual danger, particularly in glaucoma patients who are already receiving antiglaucoma medications.

Applied as 1% eyedrops, propantheline bromide produced mydriasis lasting 6 to 7 days, but relatively slight cycloplegia.[c]

a. Freeling P: A trial of oxyphencyclimine. *PRACTITIONER* 192:797–801, 1964.
b. Mody MV, Keeney AH: Propantheline (Pro-Banthine) bromide in relation to normal and glaucomatous eyes. *J AM MED ASSOC* 159:1113–1114, 1955.
c. Gokhale AM, Gokhale SA: Ocular effect of Pro-Banthine. *BR J OPHTHALMOL* 54:683–686, 1970.

Propiolactone has been employed in the vapor phase and in freshly prepared aqueous solution as a disinfectant. The vapor is unbearable to human beings at concentrations greater than 0.1 mg/liter of air. The immediate irritation appears to be great enough to prevent people from working in the presence of vapor concentrations which might be injurious.[a]

A drop of propiolactone applied to a rabbit's eye caused immediate pain, graying of the cornea, and miosis. The next day the lids were extremely swollen and the cornea densely gray. Opacification was permanent. Application of 2% aqueous solution of propiolactone to a rabbit's eye for one minute, followed by irrigation with water, caused moderate edema of the conjunctiva to develop in a few minutes. The cornea immediately after exposure was clear, but by the next day was moderately hazy. The haze gradually cleared, and the cornea returned to normal within two weeks.[81]

a. Beears WL, Roha M: Propiolactone as a sterilant. *US GOVT RES REP* 32:22, 1959. (*CHEM ABSTR* 54:17791, 1960.)

Propionic acid tested on rabbit eyes caused severe injury, graded 9 on a scale of 10 after twenty-four hours, with particular regard to effect on the cornea.[228] Comparing rate of penetration through whole corneas *in vitro,* propionic acid was found to penetrate at pH 2 more readily than stronger acids, but at pH 1 to penetrate at the same rate as most common acids.[79] Study of the denaturing effect on pieces of cornea, by measuring swelling capacity in running water after exposure for two minutes to 0.1 M solutions adjusted to pH 2, has shown propionic acid to have greater persistent inhibitory effect than sixteen other common acids tested in the same manner.[79] These properties evaluated *in vitro* seem consistent with the report of severe damaging effect on the cornea in rabbits. No report of human eye accident was found.

Propoxur, a carbamate anticholinesterase pesticide, used in flea collars for dogs, caused miosis during the first week the collars were worn.

Fisch H, Augerhofer R, Nelson JH: Evaluation of a carbamate-impregnated flea and tick collar for dogs. *J AM VET MED ASSOC* 171:269–270, 1977.

2-Propoxyethanol (ethyleneglycol-n-propylether) has been tested by application of three drops to a rabbit's eye and was found to cause strong irritation, reddening and swelling of the conjunctivae and lids, purulent discharge, and long-lasting corneal clouding. The final result is not reported.[151]

Propoxyphene (Darvon, Darvocet, Dolene, Doloxene, Proxagesic), an analgesic, has been taken in large overdosage in a number of suicides. Optic atrophy and permanent blindness resulted in one case in which a large amount of propoxyphene was ingested in combination with aspirin and phenacetin, as "Darvon Compound 65." The patient developed respiratory and temporary cardiac arrest, with acidosis and coma, requiring maintenance in a respirator. The pupils became dilated and unreactive to light. The discs became edematous, although cerebrospinal fluid pressure was normal. In eight weeks, when the patient became responsive to stimuli, vision was found to be severely impaired, and the pupils continued widely dilated. Subsequently the discs were described as "white, flat, and sharply demarcated." Otherwise the fundi were normal except for narrowing of retinal arteries.[a]

a. Weiss IS: Optic atrophy after propoxyphene overdose. *ANN OPHTHALMOL* 14:586–587, 1982.

Propranolol (Inderal), a beta-adrenergic receptor blocking agent, has caused visual hallucinations in rare instances,[d] but no serious toxic effect on the eyes. Because of pharmacologic relationship to *practolol*, which has caused serious degeneration of tear glands, with dry eyes, and scarring of conjunctiva and cornea in some cases, this complication has been watched for when propranol has been used. There have been no comparable serious effects, though some patients have complained of gritty, dry eye sensations,[b,e] particularly when questionned.[c] Fraunfelder's national registry has reported instances to raise suspicion, but not proof, of cause and effect.[312]

Propranolol systemically, and topically as eyedrops, reduces intraocular pressure in normal and glaucomatous eyes usually without adverse side effect.[f] Topically propranolol is said to have slight corneal anesthetic effect in some eyes, but this seems to have caused no adverse effects. Most patients have tolerated 1% eyedrops used in treatment of glaucoma, only occasionally experiencing burning sensation or conjunctival hyperemia.

The ERG in rabbits has been unaffected by propranolol.[a]

a. Akita J, Shigematsu T: Effect of adrenergic blocking agents on ERG in rabbits. *ACTA SOC OPHTHALMOL JPN* 72:2190–2209, 1968.
b. Cubey RB, Taylor SH: Ocular reaction to propranolol and resolution on continued treatment with a different beta-blocking drug. *BR MED J* 4:327, 1975.
c. Dollery CT, Bulpitt CJ, et al: Eye symptoms in patients taking propranolol and other hypertensive agents. *BR J CLIN PATHOL* 4:295–297, 1977.
d. Fleminger R: Visual hallucinations and illusions with propranolol. *BR MED J* 1:1182, 1978.
e. Halloran TJ: Propranolol and eye symptoms. *J AM MED ASSOC* 241:2784–2785, 1979.
f. Ohrstrom A: Clinical experience with propranolol in the treatment of glaucoma. *ACTA OPHTHALMOL* 51:639–644, 1973.

n-Propyl alcohol (1-propanol, Optal) in aqueous solution at 1.2 to 5 M concentration has been found to have a loosening effect on the epithelium of beef corneas, resembling n-butyl alcohol, but less effective.[107] Tested on rabbit eyes, it has had moderately injurious effect on the cornea, graded 5 on a scale of 1 to 10 after twenty-four hours, but the ultimate result was not reported.[226]

n-Propylamine (1-aminopropane), a strongly irritant, volatile alkaline liquid has caused clouding of the cornea in rats during lethal exposure to 800 ppm in air.[a] Test by application to rabbit eyes caused severe injury, graded 9 on a scale of 1 to 10 after twenty-four hours.[228]

a. Hine DH, Kodama JK, et al: The toxicity of allylamines. *ARCH ENVIRON HEALTH* 1:343–352, 1960.

S-Propyl butylethylthiocarbamate (n-propyl ethyl-n-butylthiocarbamate, Tillam), a herbicide, has been tested on rabbit eyes and reported to have produced mild irritation which subsided in forty-eight hours.[70]

Propylene glycol (1,2-propanediol), unlike ethylene glycol, is considered to have low toxicity and has been employed as a solvent for various medicaments.[171] When tested by application to rabbit eyes, it has caused no more than transient slight conjunctiva hyperemia.[27,45,123,222,275,295] Tests on rabbit eyes from which the corneal epithelium had been removed have shown no injury from irrigation with a 50% solution in water for five minutes, but a moderate reaction to application of undiluted propylene glycol for five minutes.[123] Propylene glycol has been employed as an essentially noninjurious solvent for other chemicals to be tested on rabbit eyes.[222]

Although noninjurious, a drop applied to the human eye causes immediate stinging, blepharospasm, and lacrimation, the same as induced by glycerin. The discomfort lasts for several seconds until the tears wash the foreign substance away. This is followed by mild transient conjunctival hyperemia, but no residual discomfort or injury.[81] An ointment containing approximately 70% propylene glycol has been used as an osmotic agent with good results in treatment of edema of the cornea.[a]

Injection into the vortex vein of animal eyes (0.25 ml in 10 seconds) has sporadically caused slight serous detachment of the retina, and separation of the nonpigmented from the pigmented epithelium of the ciliary body, but no degeneration of the retina and no cystoid changes in the pars plana of the ciliary body.[b]

a. Bietti GB, Pecori Giraldi J: Topical osmotherapy of corneal edema. *ANN OPHTHALMOL* 1:40–49, 1969.
b. Collier RH: Experimental embolic ischemia of the choroid. *ARCH OPHTHALMOL* 77:683–692, 1967.

Propylene glycol dinitrate, a component of a torpedo propellant, caused no corneal injury when 0.1 ml was applied to a rabbit eye,[a] but exposure of human beings to propylene glycol dinitrate vapor caused headache, disturbance of equilibrium, and eye irritation.[b] Systematic investigation of the effects of low vapor concentrations in human volunteers, to determine a tolerable level for work exposure 8 hours a day, showed headache and alteration of the visual evoked cortical response (VER) to be outstanding features of exposures in the range 0.2 to 1.5 ppm, the severity of the effects increasing strikingly in this range. No change in visual acuity was reported. Eye irritation symptoms developed consistently at 1.5 ppm, and could not serve as a warning of exposure to lower levels which produced headache and loss of equilibrium. The alterations in the VER were thought to represent a general effect of central nervous system depression. All experimentally-induced effects appeared to be reversible on discontinuing exposure.

a. Jones RA, Strickland JA, Siegel J: Toxicity of propylene glycol 1,2-dinitrate. *TOXICOL APPL PHARMACOL* 22:128–137, 1972.
b. Stewart RD, Peterson JE, et al: Experimental human exposure to propylene glycol dinitrate. *TOXICOL APPL PHARMACOL* 30:377–395, 1974.

Propylene glycol dipropionate tested by applying 0.1 ml to a rabbit's eye caused doubtful to slight irritation.[a]

a. Ambrose AM: Toxicological studies of compounds investigated for use as inhibitors of biological processes. *ARCH IND HYG* 3:48–51, 1951.

Propylene glycol butyl ether applied by drop to rabbit eyes daily for five days is said to have caused much irritation and clouding of the cornea, but healing within a week.[21]

Propylene glycol ethyl ether tested by drop application to rabbit eyes is said to have had similar effect to propylene glycol butyl ether.[21]

Propylene imine (like ethylenimine) has caused severe damage when applied to rabbit eyes, similar in severity to 28% ammonium hydroxide, graded 9 on a scale of 1 to 10 after twenty-four hours.[27,223] It is also said to have caused injury to human eyes, but details have not been provided.[27]

Propylene oxide (propene oxide) resembles ethylene oxide in chemical properties, but is appreciably less toxic.[b] Liquid propylene oxide dropped on rabbit eyes has caused reversible injury similar to that caused by acetone, graded 5 on a scale of 1 to 10 after twenty-four hours.[27,223]

Exposure of monkeys and rabbits to 457 ppm vapor in air for seven hours daily had no adverse effect, but in rats and guinea pigs it irritated the eyes and induced lung edema.[a] In guinea pigs and rabbits no disturbance of the corneas is detectable by slit-lamp biomicroscope after exposure to vapor concentrations high enough to cause death of guinea pigs and rabbits from respiratory embarrassment in the course of several days, except possibly an increase in the normal punctate staining of the corneal epithelium with fluorescein.[81]

A person who had near-lethal vapor exposure, estimated 1500 mg/l for 10–15 minutes, felt eye irritation soon thereafter, but recovered.[c]

a. Rowe VK: Toxicity of propylene oxide determined on experimental animals. *ARCH IND HEALTH* 13:228–236, 1956.
b. Schrenk HH: Safe working concentrations of ethylene oxide and propylene oxide. *IND ENG CHEM* 48:101A–102A, 1956.
c. Beliaev VA, et al: Acute poisoning with propylene oxide. *GIGIENA TRUDA I PROF ZABOLEVANIYA* 15(2):48–49, 1971. (English abstract)

Prostaglandins (PG's) are a group of oxygenated fatty acids of very special structure formed in animal tissues from certain unsaturated fatty acids, particularly *arachidonic acid,* that may be released, probably from cell membranes, in response to very slight injury or irritation.[b,p] Prostaglandins induce numerous local tissue reactions. In the eye, a prostaglandin from the iris, known as *irin,* was identified by Ambache as the local mediator of a reaction of rabbit eyes to irritation that is characterized by vasodilation in the iris, leakage of protein from blood to aqueous humor, miosis, and a rise of intraocular pressure lasting an hour or two.[a] Similar responses have been induced by administering natural and synthetic prostaglandins to animal eyes.[b,c,d,n] However, Bito and associates have pointed out that injection into the anterior chamber in rabbits gives a reaction that is complicated by the trauma of injection itself, and that intravitreal injection gives clearer results, consisting of elevation of intraocular pressure, hyperemia of the iris, and protein flare in the aqueous humor, but only slight miosis, and no cellular response.[284] Similar effects are induced by administering prostaglandins in eyedrops. Different prostaglandins produce one or more signs of intraocular inflammation, but none produces all of the signs. Particularly they generally do not cause entry of polymorphonuclear cells.[c,f] Intravitreally injected prostaglandins have adverse effects on retinal function in rabbits, as evaluated by electro-retinography.[m,q] Large doses (greater than 200 μg) cause retinal vascular damage and retinal detachment.[g,j] Injection into the sclera affects the underlying choroid, causing serous detachment of pigment epithelium and retina.[r]

The prostaglandin mechanism appears to have an important role in the reactive hypertension of rabbit eyes which can be induced by a variety of irritants (e.g. topical hypertonic sodium chloride, chloroform, formaldehyde, and carrageenin) and trauma. In the chicken eye, prostaglandins and arachidonic acid cause breakdown of the blood-aqueous barrier and increase in protein in the aqueous humor similar to the effect on rabbit eyes.[o] Cats and monkeys show less reactive hypertensive response to irritants, and they appear to respond less than rabbits to prostaglandins injected into the eye. However, in monkey eyes subconjunctival injection of a prostaglandin has caused a prompt transitory rise in intraocular pressure, with increase in protein in the aqueous humor, and microscopically visible damage to the ciliary epithelium and the endothelium of the inner wall of Schlemm's canal.[i]

In human beings the influence of prostaglandins on intraocular pressure is still being investigated. Intraocular surgery (cataract extraction) in human beings has been shown to be followed by an increase of prostaglandin in the aqueous humor, which can be inhibited by indomethacin, and less postoperative pressure rise has been reported when indomethacin was given.[e,l] Conflicting reports have appeared concerning influence on human intraocular pressure from prostaglandins used for abortion. From Germany, intrauterine injection of PGF2α (*Dinoprost, Prostin F2 Alpha*) in 5 patients and PGE2 intravenously in 12 patients produced no change in the intraocular pressure in 16 out of the 17, but one patient who received intrauterine PGF2α had a rise in blood pressure, and her intraocular pressure went from 14 to 26 or 28 mm Hg in 7 minutes, dropping below 20 in 25 minutes; two days later the eyes were normal with normal open angles.[h] In Hungary, the same PGF2α given intrauterine or intravenously was noted to cause a small rise in intraocular pressure, maximum in 15 minutes.[s] When given to glaucomatous patients intravenously a rise of 1 to 12.5 mm Hg was observed in most cases.[t]

No cataracts have been attributed to prostaglandins, but in rat lenses in culture added prostaglandin suppresses mitotic activity of the epithelial cells.[k]

a. Ambache N: Properties of irin. *J PHYSIOL* 135:114–132, 1957.
b. Demailly P: Prostaglandins in ophthalmology. *ARCH OPHTALMOL (PARIS)* 31:53–62, 1971.
c. Hall DWR, Jaitly KD: Inflammatory responses of the rabbit eye to prostaglandins. *AGENT ACTIONS SUPPL* 2:123–133, 1977.
d. Kelly RGM, Starr MS: Effects of prostaglandins and prostaglandin antagonist on intraocular pressure and protein in the monkey eye. *CAN J OPHTHALMOL* 6:205–211, 1971.
e. Kremer M, Baikoff G, Charbounel B: The release of prostaglandin in human aqueous humor following intraocular surgery. *PROSTAGLANDINS* 23:695–702, 1982.
f. Kulkarni PS, Srinivasan BD: The effect of intravitreal and topical prostaglandins on intraocular inflammation. *INVEST OPHTHALMOL VIS SCI* 23:383–392, 1982.

g. Masunaga J: Effects of prostaglandin on the blood-ocular barriers. *ACTA SOC OPHTHAL-MOL JPN* 84:427–437, 1980.

h. Ober M, Scharrer A: Change in intraocular pressure during prostaglandin-induced abortion. *KLIN MONATSBL AUGENHEILKD* 180:230–231, 1982.

i. Okisaka S: The effects of prostaglanding E, on the ciliary epithelium and the drainage angle of cynomolgus monkeys. *EXP EYE RES* 22:141–154, 1976.

j. Peyman GA, Bennett TO, Vlchek J: Effects of intravitreal prostaglandins on retinal vasculature. *ANN OPHTHALMOL* 7:279–288, 1975.

k. von Sallmann L, Grimes P: Inhibition of cell division in rat lenses by prostaglandin E_1. *INVEST OPHTHALMOL* 15:27–29, 1976.

l. Rich WJCC: Prevention of postoperative ocular hypertension by prostaglandin inhibitors. *TRANS OPHTHALMOL SOC UK* 97:268–271, 1977.

m. Siminoff R, Bito LZ: The effects of prostaglalndins and arachidonic acid on the electroretinogram. *CURR EYE RES* 1:635–642, 1981–1982.

n. Starr MS: Further studies on the effect of prostaglandin on intraocular pressure in the rabbit. *EXP EYE RES* 11:170–177, 1971.

o. Stetz DE, Bito LZ: The insensitivity of the chicken eye to the inflammatory effects of x-rays in contrast to its sensitivity to other inflammatory agents. *INVEST OPHTHALMOL VIS SCI* 17:412–419, 1978.

p. Waitzman MB: Possible new concepts relating prostaglandins to various ocular functions. *SURVEY OPHTHALMOL* 14:301–326, 1970.

q. Wallenstein MC, Bito LZ: The effects of intravitreally injected prostaglandin E_1 on retinal function. *INVEST OPHTHALMOL VIS SCI* 17:795–799, 1978.

r. Watanabe S, Ohtsuki K: Experimental serous choroidopathy. *ACTA SOC OPHTHALMOL JPN* 83:808–817, 1979.

s. Zajacz M, Torok M, Mocsary P: Effect on human eye of prostaglandin and a prostaglandin analog used to induce abortion. *IRCS MED SCI LIBR COMPEND* 4:316, 1976.

t. Zajacz M, Torok M: Glaucoma tolerance test with prostaglandins. *SZEMESZET* 114:220–224, 1977.

Protamine, a simple protein containing predominantly basic amino acids and capable of inactivating heparin, has a remarkable effect when injected into the cornea of rabbits, causing no inflammation but apparently precipitating acid mucopolysaccharides, producing immediate chalk-white opacity. Despite this, the cornea regains normal appearance and transparency within two to three weeks.[b,c] Repeated application of 5% protamine eyedrops for 9 days to alkali-burned rabbit corneas did not influence the outcome.[a]

a. Ameye C, Maudgal PC, et al: Inefficacy of topical protamine as angiogenesis inhibitor in alkali-burned corneas. *BULL SOC BELGE OPHTALMOL* 207:109–115, 1983.

b. Obenberger J, Cejkova J: Experimental leucoma after injection of protamine. *CESK OFTALMOL* 23:192–197, 1967.

c. Vrabec F: Histological changes in the rabbit cornea following the intracorneal injection of protamine sulfate. *CESK OFTALMOL* 26:1–4, 1970.

Protease enzymes from bacteria are capable of damaging the cornea,[b,c,e] causing endophthalmitis,[d] and liquefying the cortex of the lens *in vitro*.[a] (Compare *Bacterial endotoxins, exotoxin,* and also *Collagenase.*)

a. Bonnet M, Tronche P: Enzymatic phaco-maturation. *BULL SOC OPHTALMOL FRANCE* 69:596–612, 1969. (French)

b. Brown SI, Bloomfield SE, Tam WI: The cornea-destroying enzyme of *Pseudomonas aeruginosa*. *INVEST OPHTHALMOL* 13:174–180, 1974.

c. Kreger AS, Griffin OK: Cornea damaging proteases of *Serratia marcescens*. *INVEST OPHTHALMOL* 14:190–198, 1975.

d. Salceda SR, Lapuz J, Vizconde R: *Serratia marcescens* endophthalmitis. *ARCH OPHTHALMOL* 89:163–166, 1973.

e. Kessler E, Mondini BJ, Brown SI: The corneal response to *Pseudomonas aeruginosa*. *INVEST OPHTHALMOL* 16:116–125, 1977.

Protriptyline (Vivactil, Triptil, Concordin), a tricyclic antidepressant, has anticholinergic side effects like those of several other drugs in this category (listed under *Tricyclic antidepressants*), and for this reason, is customarily accompanied by a warning against use in patients with glaucoma or in patients with narrow angles. (The general basis is discussed under *Anticholinergic drugs*.) The anticholinergic side effects usually are manifested as dryness of the mouth and occasional blurring of vision from impairment of accommodation for near.[a,b] Also the pupils become slightly dilated (average 0.8 mm) reaching a maximum by the twentieth day of treatment.[244]

a. Protriptyline (Vivactil)—another antidepressant. *MED LET* 10:17–18, 1968.

b. Council on Drugs: Evaluation of a new antidepressant agent. Protriptyline Hydrochloride (Vivactil). *J AM MED ASSOC* 206:364–365, 1968.

Pseudoephedrine (Novaphed, Sudafed), an adrenergic vasoconstrictor and bronchodilator, appears to have weak mydriatic action. Five drops of a 10% solution of the hydrochloride applied to the eye has caused only occasional slight mydriasis.[a] Oral administration of 120 mg caused not more than 0.75 mm mydriasis in one normal human subject with reactive pupils. Pseudoephedrine probably presents very little danger of inducing angle-closure glaucoma, and no danger of aggravating open-angle glaucoma.

a. Howard HJ, Lee TP: Effect on the eye of instillations of a ten percent solutions of pseudoephedrine. *PROC SOC EXP BIOL MED* 23:672, 1926.

Psilocybin, a derivative of dimethyltryptamine occuring in a hallucinogenic Mexican fungus, produces mydriasis, which is antagonized by chlorpromazine.[d,f,118] In human beings 1 to $1.5\mu g/kg$ causes visual distortion and visual hallucinations.[118] These effects have been the subject of electrophysiologic and psychologic investigations with mechanism of action yet to be clearly delineated.[b,c,e] In baboons an injection of 3 mg intravenously has had no effect on behavior, or on visually evoked potentials.[a]

a. Bert J, Ayats H, Bermond F: Effects of psilocybin upon the visual pathways of baboons. In *Use Nonhuman Primates Drug Eval Symp, 1967,* 1968, pp.442–448.

b. Bermond F, Bert J, Ayats J: Effect of psilocybin on evoked visual responses in *Papio papio*. *CR SOC BIOL* 160:2405–2409, 1966.

c. Hill RM, Fischer R, Warshay D: Effects of excitatory and tranquilizing drugs on visual perception. *EXPERIENTIA* 25:171–172, 1969.

d. Martin HK: Chlorpromazine antagonism of psilocybin effect. *INT J NEUROPSYCHIATR* 3:66–71, 1967.
e. Rynearson RR, Wilson MR Jr, Bickford RG: Psilocybin-induced changes in psychological function, electroencephalogram, and light-evoked potentials in human subjects. *MAYO CLIN PROC* 43:191–204, 1968.
f. Waser PG: The pharmacology of *Amanita Muscaria*. *US PUBLIC HEALTH SERV PUBL* 1645:419–439, 1967.

Putrescine (1,4-butanediamine; tetramethylenediamine) tested on rabbit eyes by dropping a 12% aqueous solution on the eye six times a day for six days induced a mucoid discharge which cleared promptly.[63] Intracorneal injection caused slight reaction.[123]

Pyracanthus extract in rabbit and guinea pig eyes caused no damage to the cornea, but a severe inflammatory reaction in conjunctiva and iris, without necrosis. The reaction has been compared in detail to that induced by acacia. (See INDEX for *Acacia*.)

Pyrazinamide, an antituberculosis agent, is said to cause some patients to complain of brightness of both daylight and artificial light. Photosensitivity reactions of the skin have also been reported.

a. Todays drugs. Drugs for tuberculosis. *BR MED J* 1:1593–1594, 1963.

Pyrazole prolongs the time required for dark adaptation. (Also see INDEX for *4-Methylpyrazole*.)

Raskin NH, Sligar KP, Steinberg RH: Dark adaptation slowed by inhibitors of alcohol dehydrogenase in the albino rat. *BRAIN RES* 50:496–500, 1973.

Pyrethrum (pyrethrum flowers) is an insecticide powder which may cause transient contact conjunctival edema and hyperemia.[46] The constituents *pyrethrin I* and *II* in pure form are said to be irritating to the eyes and mucous membranes.[171] No persistent ocular disturbance appears to have been reported.

Pyridine is a weak base, but its vapor is irritating to the eyes and lids, as well as to the respiratory tract.[61] Pure pyridine applied to rabbit eyes has caused moderate injury graded 7 on a scale of 1 to 10 after twenty-four hours.[225] Commercial pyridine (90%) applied to rabbit eyes has caused severe reaction with clouding of the cornea and scarring of the conjunctiva. Permanent mild stromal opalescence and subepithelial vascularization resulted.[35]

Experimental poisoning of rabbits with pyridine, and histologic examination of the eyes has shown no damaging effect on retina or lens.[131]

Chronic industrial exposure to the dust of a crude mixture of *pyridine, picoline, lutidine,* and *collidine* has been associated with severe central nervous disturbances in two men.[a] One had transitory losses of consciousness, transient facial paralysis, anisocoria, and ataxia. The other had headache, rapid onset of right-sided facial paralysis, and ptosis on the left side, anisocoria, and left-sided abducens paresis.

There was also horizontal nystagmus to the left and conjugate deviation of the eyes to the left, with cerebellar ataxia. Visual fields were not abnormal. Both patients recovered gradually after discontinuing exposure.

a. Ludwig H: On toxicology of pyridine and its homologs. *GEWERBEPATH GEWERBEHYG* 5:654–664, 1934. (German)

(4'-Pyridyl)-1-piperazine derivatives in which there is an alkylaryl side chain on the N-4 position induce cataracts in rats.[a]

a. Lapalus P, Luyckx J: *TOXICOL EUR PHARMACOL RES* 2:99–102, 1979.

Pyrimethamine (Daraprim), an antimalarial, taken in large overdose (450 mg) by a 14-month old child caused serious poisoning with coma and convulsions.[a] When partially recovered on the fourth day the child was blind and deaf, with moderately dilated pupils, absent cortical visual evoked response, but normal fundi and discs. By four weeks he could follow objects with his eyes, and by two years after the poisoning had "perfect vision and hearing."

a. Akinyanju O, Goddell JC, Ahmed I: Pyrimethamine poisoning. *BR MED J* 140–148, 20 October, 1973.

Pyrithione (2-pyridinethiol-1-oxide, hydroxypyridinethione, Omadine), an antifungal and antibacterial agent, and a chelating agent particularly for zinc, has caused severe ocular reaction when administered systemically to dogs, producing blindness in approximately a week, apparently through action on the zinc-containing tapetum.[a-c] During the first day or two, the dogs began to lacrimate and the superficial vessels of their eyes appeared dilated. In four to eight days the pupils became widely dilated and protein appeared in the aqueous humor. The vitreous humor became progressively clouded. Cataract developed later in some of the dogs. Most constantly they developed retinal edema, hemorrhages, and exudative detachment. Histology showed the tapetum to be necrotic, and both tapetum and choroid to be edematous and infiltrated. Since similar reactions were obtained with *dithizone,* another chelating agent, given intravenously to dogs, it was supposed that chelation of the zinc in the tapetum was responsible. However, similar toxic effects have been produced by administration of *zinc pyrithione,* which presumably would not take up zinc from the tapetum. (See INDEX for *Zinc pyrithione.*)

In rats, rabbits, and monkeys no effect has been produced like that in dogs.[a-c] In rats systemic administration of sodium pyrithione has caused only hyperemia of the superficial vessels of the eye, lacrimation, and signs of photophobia.

a. Delahunt DS, Stebbins RB et al: The cause of blindness in dogs given hydroxy-pyridinethione. *TOXICOL APPL PHARMACOL* 4:286–294, 1962.
b. Moe RA, Kirpan J, Linegar CR: Toxicology of hydroxypyridinethione. *TOXICOL APPL PHARMACOL* 2:156–170, 1960.
c. Snyder FH, Buehler EF, Winek CL: Safety evaluation of zinc 2-pyridinethiol 1-oxide in a shampoo formulation. *TOXICOL APPL PHARMACOL* 7:425–437, 1965.

Pyrogallol (1,2,3-benzenetriol) has been employed in an ointment for skin diseases, but if taken by mouth it is severely poisonous.[171] Tests of 0.008 to 0.08 M aqueous solutions on rabbit eyes by application to the corneal stroma after removal of the epithelium or by injection into the stroma has caused slight reaction, graded 7 to 10 on a scale of 0 to 100.[123]

Pyruvaldehyde (pyruvic aldehyde, methyl glyoxal) on rabbit eyes has caused slight transient injury when applied to the intact eye, graded 2 on a scale of 1 to 10 after twenty-four hours.[27] A somewhat greater reaction was induced after removal of corneal epithelium, or by injection into the stroma; 0.25% and 1% solutions caused reactions graded 10 to 60 respectively on a scale of 0 to 100.[123]

Quercetin caused cataract in 50 per cent of the rats to which it was administered in impure commercial form, but only one eye of each rat was affected, and purified quercetin did not produce cataracts.[a] An explanation was not found.

a. Nakagawa Y, Shetlar MR, Wender SH: Cataract development in rats fed commercial quercetin. *PROC SOC EXP BIOL MED* 108:401–402, 1961. (*SURV OPHTHALMOL* 7:232, 1962.)

Quinacrine (mepacrine, Atabrine, Atebrin, Acriquine, Akrichin, Italchin) has been employed in treatment of malaria and as an anthelmintic. Direct contact of quinacrine with human eyes was described when soldiers inflicted injuries on their own eyes by applying quinacrine powder. This caused yellow staining of the bulbar conjunctiva, limited sharply to the palpebral fissure, and a yellow-green staining of the whole cornea. In mild cases the cornea was slightly hazy. In more severe reactions wrinkling of the posterior surface of the cornea developed, due to edema. The original report implies gradual recovery and mentions no permanent damage.[m]

Systemically absorbed quinacrine commonly colors the skin yellow, and may induce blue-gray pigmentation in the basal layer of the conjunctival epithelium, plica semilunaris and caruncle, and in the nail beds.[l] In event of hypersensitivity, quinacrine can cause a general dermatitis with involvement of the lids.

Reports of yellow discoloration of the cornea and sclera, and complaint of seeing yellow, green, and blue or violet, presumably owing to changes in the cornea, have been noted several times.[b,c,f,g,k] These visual symptoms resemble those associated with epithelial edema, but have not been associated with discomfort, inflammation, or fluorescein stainability.[k]

In some cases the visual symptoms have been induced by systemic administration. In other cases people exposed to quinacrine dust in its manufacture have complained of seeing blue haloes or multicolored rings about lights.[h] This has been attributed to brown particles 5 to 10μ in diameter deposited in the corneal epithelium.[h] Discontinuation of exposure to quinacrine resulted in return of the corneas to normal, and relief of the associated symptoms in all cases.[h,46]

In experiments on rabbit eyes, by testing concentrations of dust higher than those encountered industrially, it has been shown that quinacrine is capable of causing moderate transient injury to all layers of the cornea.[h]

Experimental administration to normal human beings at the rate of 0.1 g per day has revealed no influence on visual accuity,[a,d] but minor temporary enlargement of the blind spot and occasional small evanescent scotomas.[d] In two patients quinacrine is alleged to have caused optic neuritis, but this does not seem positively established.[e,i,j] In one of these cases, a child having malaria, possibly pulmonary tuberculosis, and iridocyclitis in one eye, developed transient optic neuritis in the other eye after receiving several doses of quinacrine plus pamaquine.[e] In the second case the patient was taking quinine as well as quinacrine for malaria. This patient had xanthopsia for ten days before gradually becoming blind. Papilledema was the only abnormality observed in the fundus.[i] In the course of a month after quinacrine was discontinued, vision recovered completely, although quinine was still being given.

Experimental administration of 0.375 to 0.5 g of quinacrine a day to dogs for five to fifteen days produced disturbances in the histology of the optic nerves, sufficient, it was thought, to account for the transient amaurosis observed in the second patient.[j] These doses were, however, lethal for most of the animals.

a. Abbey EA, Lawrence EA: The effect of atabrine suppressive therapy on eyesight in pilots. *J AM MED ASSOC* 130:786, 1946.

b. Blumenfeld NE: Staining of the conjunctiva and cornea. *VESTN OFTALMOL* 25:39, 1946.

c. Chamberlain WP, Boles DJ: Edema of the cornea precipitated by quinacrine. *ARCH OPHTHALMOL* 35:120–134, 1946.

d. Dame LR: Effects of atabrine on the visual system. *AM J OPHTHALMOL* 29:1432–1434, 1946.

e. Ferrera A: Optic neuritis from high doses of atebrin. *RASS ITAL OTTALMOL* 12:123, 1943. (Italian)

f. Kaplan JD: On the effect of Akrichin. *VESTN OFTALMOL* 8:73–78, 1936.

g. Lapidus A: Green vision from Akrichin intoxication. *VESTN OFTALMOL* 8:79–80, 1936.

h. Mann I: "Blue haloes" in atebrin workers. *BR J OPHTHALMOL* 31:40–46, 1947.

i. Panzardi D: On a case of amaurosis from an antimalarial. *BOLL OCULIST* 24:204–214, 1945. (Italian)

j. Panzardi D, Gastaldi A: Experimental investigations concerning the action on the optic nerve of acridinic antimalaria drugs. *BOLL OCULIST* 27:246–255, 1948. (Italian)

k. Reese FM: Edema of corneal epithelium caused by atabrine. *BULL JOHNS HOPKINS HOSP* 78:325, 1946.

l. Sugar HS, Waddell WW: Ochronosis-like pigmentation associated with use of Atabrine (Quinacrine). *ILLINOIS MED J* 89:234, 1946.

m. Somerville-Large LB: Mepacrin and the eye. *BR J OPHTHALMOL* 31:191–192, 1947.

Quinidine is a stereoisomer of quinine, occuring naturally in cinchona bark, but manufactured mostly from *quinine*. Medically it is employed for cardiac arrhythmias and has been used as an antimalarial. Although *quinine* has caused profound decrease in vision in many cases, there appears to be no convincingly documented evidence that quinidine can do so. Vague statements about quinidine are encountered such as "a few patients cannot tolerate the drug because of vertigo, blurring of vision, disturbance in gait, or lightheadedness."[d] One anonymous editorial went so far as to say that large doses of quinidine caused "disturbed vision, and amaurosis," but without indicating where one might find evidence of this.[a]

The following specific instances where disturbance of eyes or vision have been suspected are worth looking at. One patient taking both quinidine and digitalis complained of blurred vision after he had taken quinidine for seventeen days; vision was then 20/50 in both eyes and the visual fields were found to be constricted.[e] In six weeks after the quinidine was stopped, vision returned to normal. Whether the digitalis played a role is unknown. In another case in which quinidine was suspected of causing decrease in vision, a young man was known to have vision reduced to 0.01 and 0.5 for some years, and this allegedly was after an attempt at suicide with overdosage of quinidine, but when a well-documented family history of Leber's hereditary optic atrophy was obtained, and studies were done on visual fields, ERG's and VER's, it appeared that the second diagnosis was more likely correct.[g]

Two rare instances have been described in which patients who developed skin rashes within weeks of starting quinidine also had bilateral mild anterior uveitis, with fine keratic precipitates and pupillary Koeppe nodules, which cleared completely with topical corticosteroid treatment.[f]

One instance of widespread small hemorrhages in the fundus was noted as a manifestation of nonthrombocytopenic purpura, in a glaucomatous patient, after 2 years of treatment with quinidine for myocardial infarct and fibrillation. The hemorrhages disappeared in three months after the quinidine was stopped.[b]

Intravenously administered quinidine has been without effect on the ERG of rabbits.[c]

Fine gray deposits in the corneal epithelium, resembling those associated with chloroquine, were seen in one patient taking metoprolol, quinidine, furosemide, isosorbide, and digoxin (with no mention of amiodarone). In two months after the quinidine was discontinued, the corneas became clear, and vision improved from 20/40 right, 20/30 left, to 20/20. Performance in central visual field testing improved, though no scotomas had been identified.[h]

a. Anonymous editorial: Is quinidine outdated? *BR MED J* 1:331–332, 1969.
b. Cernea P, Constantin F: Hemorrhagic retinopathy as a consequence of treatment with quinidine. *ANN OTTALMOL CLIN OCUL* 102:31–36, 1976. (Italian)
c. Junnemann G, Schulze J: Electroretinographic investigations of the development of quinine or chloroquine retinopathy. *KLIN MONATSBL AUGENHEILKD* 152:562–566, 1968. (German)
d. Luchi RJ: Intoxication with quinidine. *CHEST* 73:129–131, 1978.
e. Monninger R, Platt D: Toxic amblyopia due to quinidine. *AM J OPHTHALMOL* 43:107–108, 1957.
f. Spitzberg DH: Acute anterior uveitis secondary to quinidine sensitivity. *ARCH OPHTHALMOL* 97:1993, 1979.
g. Van Lith GHM: Difficulties in diagnosing Leber's optic atrophy. *DOC OPHTHALMOL* 48:255–259, 1980.
h. Zaidman GW: Quinidine keratopathy. *AM J OPHTHALMOL* 97:247–249, 1984.

Quinine, an antimalarial and medication for muscle cramps, has been known for well over a century to disturb vision and hearing. This occurs in a very small proportion of people taking average medical dosage, but has occurred in a great many who have taken overdosage for suicide or abortion. Since its first recognition, at least 300 articles must have been published concerning toxic effects of quinine on vision, many of them highly repetitious. Additional cases of quinine poisoning, with acute loss of vision, and recovery of varying degree, continue to be reported; the latest tend to supply new knowledge of the condition (Bankes 1972; Banerji 1974; Brinton 1980; Floyd 1974; Francois 1972; Friedman 1980; Gangitano 1980; Murray 1983; Oliveau 1980; Ravault 1973).

The clinical findings during the acute phase are that the pupils are dilated and unresponsive to light in proportion to the degree of blindness. The ophthalmoscopic appearances have varied considerably from case to case, and this has occasioned much dispute concerning the mechanism by which vision is affected. In some instances the retinal vessels have appeared narrowed early. In another group of cases the retina has appeared edematous and the papilla hyperemic. Occasionally a red spot in the macula has been noted with edema. In yet other cases the fundi have appeared normal at an early stage while the patient was already profoundly blind. It has been reported very frequently that at a later stage, after some days or weeks, the retinal arterioles have become strikingly narrowed, often at a time when central vision had returned, or was returning, and this has been recognized as an obviously paradoxical situation. Pallor of the optic nerve heads has often been noted developing gradually, generally proportional to the amount of permanent loss of visual field.

Therapeutic dosage is less than one gram a day, and even this has proved toxic to some patients, but more commonly a single overdose of 2 to 5 grams has been taken, in some cases much more. After a moderate overdose some patients become nauseated and vomit, and in a few hours note rapidly decreasing visual acuity and increasing deafness. Some people have loss of vision to no light perception, with dilated pupils unresponsive to light, but remain conscious. In the most severe poisonings there has been deep coma with circulatory collapse, and the patient has become aware of complete blindness only upon recovery of consciousness. In nearly all cases, central vision has recovered at least partially, sometimes in a matter of days, but quite characteristically a constriction of the peripheral fields has remained permanently. In an example of a particularly mild case, described by Lincoff, the patient took 0.8 g in 2 days, then had sudden complete bilateral blindness, tinnitus, partial deafness, and dilated pupils. By the next day visual acuity returned to normal, but the fields were permanently constricted; within 10 days the retinal vessels had become abnormally small, and the discs appeared waxy. In an example of a serious case of quinine poisoning, described by Frisius and Beyer, the patient took 7.7 g, and in 20 minutes was going into coma, with widely dilated pupils, tonic-clonic spasms, cyanosis, and heart and respiratory arrest requiring emergency assistance. During the first week there was retinal edema and progressive narrowing of retinal vessels, but vision did return in small central fields.

In some cases central vision is left significantly impaired. Children are said to be particularly susceptible, as exemplified by a case published by Bonamour and

Bonnet with a fundus photograph showing a white disc with white lines where retinal vessels had narrowed almost to the point of disappearance.

An especially instructive case has been reported by Brinton and colleagues, documented by retinal angiography, ERG and VER. Their young patient had no light perception 14 hours after taking approximately 4 g of quinine, and, although the retinas appeared slightly hazy, with mild venous distention, fluorescein angiography confirmed that the retinal artery caliber was normal. In 35 hours, visual acuity returned to normal in small central fields, with no change in the retinal angiogram, but from the fifth to ninth days, there was increasingly notable arterial narrowing, development of background fluorescence, and disc pallor. These changes were progressive during 6 months of observation, but visual acuity remained normal, and peripheral fields remained constricted. Although the reason for the arterial narrowing in quinine poisoning remains unknown, this report provides strong objective evidence supporting the many observers who have concluded that the arterial narrowing occurs too late to be blamed for the initial acute blindness.

Since the mid-1950's there have been many reports of electroretinograms from patients and from experimental animals poisoned with quinine, but they have been controversial, some reporting no significant abnormality at the time of greatest blindness, and others reporting small but significant abnormalities at a very early stage, indicating disturbance of photoreceptors and retinal pigment epithelium. In the case documented by Brinton and colleagues the ERG measurements provided evidence for early effects on the photoreceptor cell layer and inner nuclear layer, while the EOG pointed to probable disturbance of the retinal pigment epithelium.

Earlier clinical observers who found ERG evidence of acute effects on the retina included Hommer, who described three cases in which the ERG showed significant decrease in potentials in a few hours after massive overdoses of quinine, at a time when retinal vessels and papillas were normal. The potentials returned to normal in 18 to 48 hours. A second decrease in the b-wave occurred during the subsequent week in association with narrowing of the retinal vessels. Hommer postulated that those who found no change in the ERG in acute quinine poisoning made their measurements too late, after the early reversible phase was passed. Early depression of the ERG has been noted also by Auvert and Vancea.

Among those who apparently missed the very early transient change in the ERG, several have found definite change, particularly decrease or disappearance of the b-wave, when vision was returning (Auvert; Behrman; Busti). In some cases at this stage the ERG has been essentially abolished (Ricci).

Months or years after acute poisoning, with attenuated retinal vessels and permanent visual field constriction, marked changes have been described in the ERG, like those after occlusion to the central retinal artery (Chabot; Francois; Oliveau).

The EOG has received less attention in quinine poisoning than the ERG. Changes in the EOG are said to parallel changes in the visual acuity, showing no "light rise" during the initial acute loss of vision, but subsequently gradually returning to normal as vision improves (Behrman; Francois). In the later phase, when visual fields may remain constricted and red-green discrimination may be subnormal and the ERG distinctly abnormal, the EOG may be back to normal.

Abnormal VER potentials have been reported by Brinton and Gangitano.

In experimental animals ERG studies have shown the following acute effects from quinine. Junemann and Schulze reported that in rabbits given quinine dihydrochloride, 5 to 10 mg/kg intravenously, a rapid selective inversion of the c-wave developed and lasted one to two hours. They interpreted this as evidence of a direct toxic effect on the retinal pigment epithelium. They obtained the same change in the rabbit ERG by intravitreal injection of quinine. They explained the findings of an acute change in ERG in the rabbit, but not in the human victims of poisoning, as probably due to the c-wave normally being relatively inconspicuous in the human. Hommer found a disappearance of the c-wave in cats when quinine was given by intracarotid injection. In excised surviving pieces of rabbit retina, Hommer was unable to detect a c-wave, but with concentrations of quinine which would be severely toxic to animals, found the b-wave could be reversibly deleted. In rabbits, Cibis showed a rapid effect of quinine on the a- and b-waves, and showed that this abnormality was not associated with any alteration of retinal vasculature or blood supply. In sheep, Calissendorff showed acute changes in a-, b-, and c-waves, with an effect on the pigment epithelial cells especially notable at low dose.

In anatomic experiments on dogs by de Schweinitz in 1891, subcutaneous injection of 135 to 500 mg of quinine bisulfate per kg regularly caused blindness, with widely dilated pupils, in 3 to 14 hours. The ophthalmoscopic appearance resembled the appearance in poisoned human beings, with marked narrowing of the retinal arteries. One dog examined histologically two months after poisoning showed definite atrophy of the optic nerves. These severely poisoned dogs appeared to have little tendency to recover vision, in contrast to human beings. Similar experiments by Holden in 1898 and Druault in 1902, indicated early degeneration of the ganglion cell layer of the retina, but provided little clarification of the significance of retinal vascular narrowing. In beagle dogs, Heywood has confirmed that quinine causes attenuation of retinal vessels as in other dogs, but has reported also retinal detachment, without retinal atrophy. A comprehensive review by Casini in 1939 summarizes results of a number of other experiments on dogs, which mainly described production of changes in retinal ganglion cells, and will not be reiterated here.

Morphologic studies on other animals have shown vacuolization of the retinal ganglion cells, and some evidence of endarteritis and periarteritis. Controversial points in the results of experimental investigation were well reviewed and summarized by Casini up to 1939. The weight of the evidence to that time appeared to favor a direct injurious effect on retinal ganglion cells. Later experimental work has been particularly well reviewed by Hommer in 1968.

In more recent times rabbits given 20 to 100 mg quinine hydrochloride per kg intravenously or intramuscularly three times a week for ten weeks have been reported by Applemans and Grillet to show no ophthalmoscopic or histologic abnormalities in the fundus or optic nerve, and Caffi and Ripizzi similarly found no abnormality in most rabbits injected intraperitoneally with 10 mg/kg per day for twenty-one to forty days, but a small number of rabbits killed at twenty-one to twenty-seven days showed degeneration of rods and cones and vacuoles in the retinal ganglion cells.

Potts has shown that quinine, like chloroquine and phenothiazine derivatives, tends to bind to uveal pigment *in vitro,* but a relationship to toxic action remains to be demonstrated.

In human eyes, histological examination of the aftereffects of quinine poisoning has been rare, despite the great number of instances of poisoning. This is partially accounted for by the fact that fatal human poisoning has been rare. In three cases in which the eyes have been examined histologically, the retinal ganglion cells and the nerve fibers were found degenerated, and the rods and cones atrophic (Casini).

In isolated animal retinas, direct addition of quinine was shown by Casini, Hommer, and Wolff to interfere with respiration. When retinas from poisoned animals were tested they showed depression of respiration comparable to the degree of histologic degeneration which has been produced, but generally no change in oxygen or glucose consumption at the acute early stage of vision loss.

In both patients and experimental animals, dilated pupils have often been described in association with loss of vision from quinine poisoning, and this generally has been assumed to be due simply to the loss of vision, but closer attention to the irides has produced evidence that not only reduced vision but actual atrophy of the irides may be responsible. Knox, Palmer, and English have described two patients in whom the pupils were partially nonreactive. Their irides had abnormal appearing stroma, and transillumination showed a thinning of the posterior pigment layer. It was postulated that quinine had injured the arteries of the iris as well as those of the retina. Similar findings have been reported by Ravault, but with numerous synechias to the dilated irides.

Acute poisoning by quinine *in utero* has been reported by McKinna to have caused congenital hypoplasia of the optic nerves in babies in four cases in which the mothers ingested large amounts of quinine early in pregnancy, but were unsuccessful in producing abortion.

The pathogenesis of acute quinine damage to the eyes according to the evidence so far available seems to involve not only a very early effect on the outer layers of the retina and pigment epithelium, but also probably a direct toxic effect on retinal ganglion cells and optic nerve fibers, as indicated by the typical pallor of some degree of optic atrophy, and finally the characteristic paradoxical retinal artery narrowing while vision is improving. Since the natural course is for some spontaneous recovery of vision, sometimes dramatically within hours, it has been difficult to evaluate the effectiveness of various treatments. Favorable results have been reported from many different treatments, for example stellate ganglion block intended to dilate ocular blood vessels (Bankes; Murray), from exchange transfusion (Burrows), and from hemodialysis (Floyd). Vasodilating drugs were for a long time in vogue, though there was no real proof of there efficacy. It appears at present that attention to the general condition of the patient is foremost, and, as in Brinton's case, no special eye treatment is required.

Chronic exposure to quinine occurs in those who take it medically, and in heroin addicts who use quinine-adulterated drug (Brust). Although not reported in patients medicinally chronically exposed, a toxic maculopathy has been described by Maltzman and Pruzon in addicts, detectable by Amsler grid testing, but not by fluorescein retinal angiography or ERG, and not affecting visual acuity. These are patients with no evidence of acute quinine poisoning.

Segal considered quinine to be responsible in one case for "acute transitory myopia" with shallowing of the anterior chamber sufficient to cause angle-closure glaucoma. None of the characteristic signs of quinine poisoning were present in this case. (Also see INDEX for "Acute Transitory Myopia.")

Applemans M, Grillet G: Tolerance of the rabbit toward quinine hydrochloride and chloroquine diphosphate. *BULL SOC BELGE OPHTALMOL* 143:658–676, 1966. (French)

Auvert B, Samson-Dollfus D, Moncade J: Electroretinogram and poisoning by quinine. *BULL SOC OPHTALMOL FRANCE* 65:559–565, 1965. (French)

Bankes JLK, Hayward JA, Jones MBS: Quinine amblyopia treated with stellate ganglion block. *BR MED J* 4:85–86, 1972.

Banerji NK, Martin VAF: Myelo-opticoneuropathy following quinine poisoning. *J IR MED ASSOC* 67:46–47, 1974.

Behrman J, Mushin A: Electrodiagnostic findings in quinine amblyopia. *BR J OPHTHALMOL* 52:925–928, 1968.

Bonamour G, Bonnet M: Optic papilla without vessels. *ARCH OPHTALMOL* (*Paris*) 28:467–476, 1968. (French)

Brinton GS, Norton EWD, et al: Ocular quinine toxicity. *AM J OPHTHALMOL* 90:403–410, 1980.

Brust JCM, Richter RW: Quinine amblyopia related to heroin addiction. *ANN INTERN MED* 74:84–86, 1971.

Burrows AW, Hambleton G, et al: Quinine intoxication in a child treated by exchange transfusion. *ARCH DIS CHILD* 47:304–305, 1972.

Busti A, Pissani C: Electroretinographic findings in toxic amblyopia from quinine. *RASS ITAL OTTALMOL* 30:218–233, 1961. (Italian)

Caffi M, Ripizzi A: On experimental poisoning with quinine. *MINERVA OFTALMOL* 8:65–68, 1966. (Italian)

Calissendorff B: Melanotropic drugs and retinal functions. *ACTA OPHTHALMOL* 54:109–117, 1976.

Casini F: The respiratory metabolism of the retina in experimental poisoning with quinine. ARCH OTTALMOL 46:263–279, 1939. (Italian)

Chabot J, Verin P, Bouchard J: The electroretinogram in poisoning by quinine. *BULL SOC OPHTALMOL FRANCE* 63:351–357, 1963. (French)

Cibis GW, Buriam HM, Blodi FC: Electroretinogram changes in acute quinine poisoning. *KLIN MONATSBL AUGENHEILKD* 164:789–794, 1974. (German)

De Schweinitz GE: Additional experiments to determine the lesion in quinine blindness. *TRANS AM OPHTHALMOL SOC* 6:23–30, 1891.

Druault A: Research on the pathogenesis of quinine amaurosis. *ARCH OPHTALMOL* (*FRANCE*) 22:19–32, 1902. (French)

Floyd M, Hill AVL, et al: Quinine amblyopia treated by hemodialysis. *CLIN NEPHROL* 2:44–46, 1974.

Francois J, Verriest G, DeRouch A: Study of the visual functions in two cases of poisoning by quinine. *OPHTHALMOLOGICA* 153:324–335, 1967. (French)

Francois J, DeRouck A, Cambie E: Retinal and optic evaluation in quinine poisoning. *ANN OPHTHALMOL* 4:177–185, 1972.

Friedman L, Rothkoff L, Zaks U: Clinical observations on quinine toxicity. *ANN OPHTHALMOL* 12:640–642, 1980.

Frisius H, Beyer KH: Clinical aspects, toxicology and treatment of a severe quinine poisoning. *ARCH TOXIKOL* 24:201–213, 1969. (German)

Gangitano JL, Keltner JL: Abnormalities of the pupil and visual-evoked potential in quinine amblyopia. *AM J OPHTHALMOL* 89:425–430, 1980.

Heywood R: Drug-induced retinopathies in the beagle dog. *BR VET J* 130:564–569, 1974.

Holden WA: The pathology of experimental quinine blindness. *ARCH OPHTHALMOL* 27:583–592, 1898.

Hommer K: On quinine poisoning of the retina. *KLIN MONATSBL AUGENHEILKD* 125:785–805, 1968. (German)

Hommer K: The effects of quinine, chloroquine, iodoacetate and chlordiazepoxide on the ERG of the isolated rabbit retina. *GRAEFES ARCH OPHTHALMOL* 175:111–120, 1968. (German)

Hommer K, Ulrich WD, Wundsch L: The effects of antimalarial compounds on the ERG recorded in situ. *GRAEFES ARCH OPHTHALMOL* 175:121–130, 1968. (German)

Junemann G, Schulze J: Electroretinographic studies of the development of quinine and chloroquine retinopathy. *KLIN MONATSBL AUGENHEILKD* 152:562–566, 1968. (German)

Knox DL, Palmer CAL, English F: Iris atrophy after quinine amblyopia. *ARCH OPHTHALMOL* 76:359–362, 1966.

Lincoff MH: Quinine amblyopia. *ARCH OPHTHALMOL* 53:382–384, 1955.

Maltzman B, Sutula F, Cinotti AA: Toxic maculopathy. *ANN OPHTHALMOL* 7:1321–1326, 1975.

McKinna AJ: Quinine induced hypoplasia of the optic nerve. *CAN J OPHTHALMOL* 1:261–266, 1966.

Murray SB, Jay JL: Loss of sight after self poisoning with quinine. *BR MED J* 287:1700, 1983.

Oliveau GL, Audoueineix E: ERG, clinical findings, and poisoning by quinine. *BULL SOC OPHTALMOL FRANCE* 80:431–433, 1980. (French)

Potts AM: The reaction of uveal pigment *in vitro* with polycyclic compounds. *INVEST OPHTHALMOL* 3:405–416, 1964.

Pruzon H, Kiebel G, Maltzman B: Toxic maculopathy. *ANN OPHTHALMOL* 7:1475–1481, 1975.

Ravault MP, Paquet M, Ploton MM: Atrophy of the iris and poisoning by quinine. *BULL SOC OPHTALMOL FRANCE* 73:675–677, 1973. (French)

Ricci A, Mayer R, Younessian S: Importance of the ERG for interpretation of the pathogenesis of disturbances of vision in quinine poisoning. *REV OTONEUROOPHTALMOL* 36:230, 1964. (French)

Segal A, Aisemberg A, Ducasse A: Quinine transitory myopia, and angle-closure glaucoma. *BULL SOC OPHTALMOL FRANCE* 83:247–249, 1983. (French)

Vancea P, Tacorian D: The value of the ERG in interpretation and prognosis of quinine poisoning. *OPHTHALMOLOGICA ADDIT AD* 158:653–660, 1969. (French)

Wolff E: Effect of quinine on the oxygen consumption of the dog's retina. *TRANS OPHTHALMOL SOC UK* 56:162–166, 1936.

Quinoline (1-benzazine), tested by application of a drop to rabbit eyes, caused moderately severe injury, graded 8 on a scale of 1 to 10 after twenty-four hours.[225] The final result, however, is not reported. *Isoquinoline* (2-benzazine), similar to quinoline but more basic, proved slightly more injurious on rabbit eyes, graded 9 on a scale of 1 to 10 after twenty-four hours.[225]

The systemic toxicity of quinoline to the eye was first investigated in 1910 by Jess, who administered to rabbits many compounds more or less related to naphthalene with the hopes of learning more about toxicity to retina and lens.[a] One dose of quinoline tartrate (0.2 g/kg) caused in three to twenty-four hours the appearance of distinct round white flecks with small reddish rims in the retina. Repeated administration caused degeneration of all layers of the retina.[a,131,214] Crystals were found in the tissues similar to those after naphthalene poisoning, but even in animals with the most severe retinal involvement, Jess never saw cataracts develop, quite unlike the effect of nephthalene. (For effects of related compounds, see the following section on *Quinoline derivatives.*)

    a. Jess, A: The story of a forgotten retinotoxic substance (Quinoline retinopathy). *KLIN MONATSBL AUGENHEILKD* 152:649–654, 1968.

Quinoline derivatives are composed of quinoline with various groups attached to it. Many of the derivatives, as well as quinoline itself, have been reported to be toxic to the retina or optic nerve in man or animals. Certain of these substances have induced toxic effects acutely. Others have caused disturbances which developed gradually after administration for many months.

    Quinoline derivatives have usually affected the retina or optic nerve of only a small proportion of individuals receiving these substances, as though the toxic action may be partially dependent upon some idiosyncracy or individual peculiarity of metabolism.

    The quinoline derivatives which have been reported occasionally toxic to retina or optic nerves in human beings or experimental animals are listed in the following Table with the principal effects that have been attributed to each compound.

TOXIC EFFECTS OF QUINOLINE DERIVATIVES

Derivatives	Effects
Amodiaquine	Possible depression of human EOG
Amopyroquin	Retinal degeneration in rats and dogs
Broxyquinoline	Optic atrophy in 2 or 3 patients
Chloroquine	Pigmentary retinopathy
Cinchonidine	Visual disturbance (in old reports)
Cinchonine	Retinal damage in dogs
Clioquinol	Optic atrophy in rare cases
Ethylhydrocupreine	Retinopathy and optic atrophy in patients and animals
Eucupine	Visual disturbance as from quinine in three patients
Halquinols	Optic atrophy in two patients, blindness in calves
Hydroxychloroquine	Retinopathy in human beings
Iodoquinol	Pigmentary retinopathy in one patient
Plasmocid	Central scotoma, optic atrophy in patients; retinopathy in animals
Quinine	Optic atrophy in patients; retinopathy in animals
Quinoline	Retinopathy in rabbits

Quinones may be formed by oxidation of dihydric phenols or aromatic amino compounds. Quinones commonly inhibit mitotic processes, inactivate enzymes, and denature proteins. Certain quinones cause irritation or injury upon contact with the eye (e.g., *benzoquinone, chloranil, 2-methyl-1,4-naphthoquinone*). Also, the quinones which are formed through oxidation of *hydroquinone; catechol; aniline; 2,4-diaminophenol,* and *paraphenylenediamine* are probably at least partially responsible for injuries of the eyes which have been associated with the latter compounds.

Quinones were early suspected and shown to be responsible for a brown discoloration of the cornea and exposed bulbar conjunctiva which gradually developed in workers who were long exposed to vapors associated with manufacture and use of synthetic aniline dyes.[l,n]

Benzoquinone, the simplest of the quinones, also known as paraquinone or merely as quinone, is a yellow crystalline substance which has a penetrating, unpleasant, irritating odor. The vapors of benzoquinone at 0.5ppm in air are irritating to the eyes, and at 3.0 ppm they are very irritating. Benzoquinone is an intermediate in the manufacture of hydroquinone from aniline.

Hydroquinone, a reduced form of benzoquinone, is used mostly as a photographic developer. Hydroquinone is spontaneously oxidizable by air to form benzoquinone, most readily in alkaline solutions. A series of reports have described very serious changes in the corneas of people employed in manufacture of hydroquinone and exposed to both hydroquinone dust and benzoquinone vapor. (These effects and related experimental works are described under *Hydroquinone;* see INDEX.)

Other quinones have been implicated in production of cataracts and damage of the retina in animals, particularly 1,2-naphthoquinone, which is one of the metabolic intermediates of naphthalene responsible for naphthalene cataracts in animals. (More details are to be found elsewhere under *Naphthalene* and *1,2-Naphthoquinone;* see INDEX.)

a. Bachstez E: Anilin injuries of the cornea. *KLIN MBL AUGENHEILKD* 63:240, 1919.
b. Bruckner R von: Scarring and shrinkage of the conjunctiva as a result of an occupational injury in the dyeing industry. *OPHTHALMOLOGICA* 102:221–225, 1941.
c. Mackinlay JG: Intense pigmentation of corneas and conjunctiva. *TRANS OPHTHALMOL SOC UK* 6:144, 1886.
d. Senn A: Corneal injury from anilin dyes. *KORRES BL SCHWEIZ ARTZ* 27:161–164, 1897.

Radiopaque x-ray media have caused a large number of ocular complications when injected for angiography of the arteries of the neck and head. A small number of complications have come from other uses, such as orbitography and myelography. These ocular complications have been comprehensively reviewed, notably by Walsh and Hoyt.[256] The subject has not been completely reviewed again here. Only representative observations are to be presented, under the headings *Arteriography, Orbitography, Myelography,* and *Corneal Sensitivity Reaction.*

The principal radiopaque x-ray media encountered in studies of ocular complications are the following:

Acetrizoate sodium (Thixokon), Diatrizoate meglumine (Gastrografin), Diatrizoate sodium (component of Hypaque), Iodipamide meglumine (adipiodone meglumine), Iodized oil (Lipiodol), Iodopyracet (Diodrast), Iophendylate, Metrizamide, Thorium dioxide (Thorotrast).

Arteriography. After intracarotid injection of several of the radiopaque media, retinal artery obliteration or embolism has been observed,[d,k] and after intravertebral artery injection a series of cases of temporary cortical blindness.[o,x] According to a survey by Cogan, Kuwabara, and Moser, "loss of vision in one eye following carotid angiography had been documented in approximately twenty-five patients.[f]" In reporting on a case in which a shower of retinal emboli was observed ophthalmoscopically and a month later histologic examination of the eye demonstrated the emboli to consist of globules of fat, Cogan and associates concluded that the manipulation of the injection, involving inserting a needle in the carotid artery, probably has been responsible for the release of showers of emboli from the atheromatous walls in such cases. So far there has been little evidence to establish a toxic mechanism for most of the ocular complications from radiopaque angiographic media.

Experimental testing of radiopaque x-ray contrast media, as reported by Abe, has demonstrated that they are potentially irritative and toxic to ocular tissues, but there has been no clear evidence that toxicity has been a factor in the more serious ocular complications that have been observed clinically and have usually been explicable on the basis of embolism.[a]

Iodopyracet injected rapidly into a common carotid artery often has caused immediate burning pain in the face and about the eye on that side, occasionally accompanied by a sensation of a flash of light. Flushing and mydriasis have been seen on the same side.[i,z] A high incidence of petechial hemorrhages in the conjunctiva and occasionally in the retina was reported by Falls,[i] but *Thorotrast,* which was used in the same study, may have been responsible. Walsh and others noted only occasional transient petechial hemorrhages of conjunctivae.[z] Rare instances of partial or complete loss of vision, usually transient, but sometimes leaving central scotoma, have been reported after intracarotid or intravertebral arterial injection by several authors. In some cases there has been retinal edema or appearance of spasm or obstruction of retinal arteries. In other cases the fundus has appeared normal.[g,p,v,z]

Diatrizoate meglumine has also been associated with ocular complications. In comprehensive reviews by Bynke[c] and Libal,[r] homonymous hemianopia was usually associated with hemiplegia or hemiparesis and was interpreted as probably an embolic obstruction of cerebral vessels rather than a toxic effect or vascular spasm.[c] Infarcts of the retina and embolism of retinal arteries have also been reported after intracarotid injection of both *diatrizoate meglumine* and *acetrizoate sodium.*[e,f,q,r]

Orbitography. Orbital injection has been shown dramatically in one case to present possibilities of intracranial extension.[w] Retrobulbar injection of a mixture of *sodium diatrizoate* and *lidocaine* not only rapidly reduced vision and caused the pupil to dilate in that eye but also produced weakness of abduction of the other eye and produced nystagmus. X-rays demonstrated that the material had passed up the sheaths of the optic nerve and into the intracranial subdural space. The effect on vision, which was transient, may have been produced by the *lidocaine.* (See *Anesthetics, retrobulbar.*) In another case, an unidentified radiopaque medium, presumably lipid type, produced pain, edema, diplopia, and severe granulomatous reaction when injected along the floor of the orbit.[h] Orbital injections of *iodopyracet* were reported in seventeen cases to have produced edema of the lids, headaches, and in one patient a transient loss of vision.[s]

Testing in cats with surgical lesions of the optic nerves has indicated that *metrizamide* at concentration less than 300 mg/ml should be safe in the optic nerve sheath.[n]

Myelography. Injection of *iodized oil* (Lipiodol) has been reported to have caused a severe late reaction causing papilledema and partial optic atrophy. The material did not disturb vision when it was first injected and spread in the basilar subarachnoid space, though it temporarily caused papilledema, but ten years later it produced severe extensive arachnoiditis with recurrence of papilledema, retinal hemorrhages, and severe impairment of vision.[l]

Iophendylate used in myelography was associated in one patient with loss of vision 35 days later attributed to residual contrast material along the optic nerves, and with recovery after corticosteroid treatment.[y] In three other patients bilateral temporary sixth nerve palsy developed 6 days to 8 weeks after myelography.[t]

Corneal Sensitivity Reactions. Sensitivity reactions which caused rapid appearance of multiple, superficial, fluffy-appearing corneal infiltrates near the limbus developed in one patient after intravenous *diatrizoate meglumine,*[b] and in another after intravenous *iodipamide meglumine.*[u] Under corticosteroid treatment they disappeared in 2 or 3 days.

a. Abe T: Experimental studies on the effect of the contrast medium to ocular tissues. *ACTA SOC OPHTHALMOL JPN* 68:1763–1780, 1964.
b. Baum JL, Bierstock SR: Peripheral corneal infiltrates following intravenous injection of diatrizoate meglumine. *AM J OPHTHALMOL* 85:613–614, 1978.
c. Bynke HG, Stigmar G: Homonymous hemianopia following cerebral angiography. *ACTA OPHTHALMOL* 44:204–211, 1966.
d. Carlson MR, Pilger IS, Rosenbaum AL: Central retinal artery occlusion after carotid angiography. *AM J OPHTHALMOL* 81:104–104, 1976.
e. Catros A, Stabert C, et al: The syndrome of obliteration of the retinal arteries, a rare complication of carotid arteriography. *BULL SOC OPHTALMOL FRANCE* 59:576–586, 1959. (French)
f. Cogan DG, Kuwabara T, Moser H: Fat emboli in the retina following angiography. *ARCH OPHTHALMOL* 71:308–313, 1964.
g. Curtis JB: Cerebral angiography. *BR J SURG* 38:295–331, 1951.
h. Eifrig DE: Lipid granuloma of the orbit. *ARCH OPHTHALMOL* 79:163–165, 1968.
i. Falls HF, Bassett RC, Lamberts AE: Ocular complications encountered in intracranial arteriography. *ARCH OPHTHALMOL* 45:623–626, 1951.
k. Francois J, Goes F, Stockmans L: Embolus of the central retinal artery after carotid angiography. *ANN OCULIST* (Paris) 205:993–1004, 1972. (French)
l. Giroire, Charbronnel, Colas: A severe case of optochiasmatic arachnoiditis with hydrocephalus following lipiodal myelography. *REV OTONEUROOPHTALMOL* 34:239–246, 1962. (French)
m. Hauge T: Catheter vertebral angiography. *ACTA RADIOLOGICA* (Suppl 109), 1954.
n. Haughton VM, Davis JP, et al: Metrizamide optic nerve sheath opacification. *INVEST RADIOL* 15:343–345, 1980.
o. Horwitz NH, Wener L: Temporary cortical blindness following angiography. *J NEUROSURG* 40:583–586, 1974.
p. Joy HH, Ecker A, Reimenschneider PA: The role of cerebral angiography in ophthalmology. *AM J OPHTHALMOL* 37:55–68, 1954.

q. Levine RA, Henry MD: Ischemic infarction of the retina. *AM J OPHTHALMOL* 55:365–367, 1963.

r. Libal B, Schrader KE: Ocular complications after carotid angiography. *KLIN MONATSBL AUGENHEILKD* 147:39–43, 1965. (German)

s. Manchester PT Jr, Bonmati J: Iodopyracet (Diodrast) injection for orbital tumors. *ARCH OPHTHALMOL* 54:591–595, 1955.

t. Miller Ea, Savino PJ, Schatz NJ: A rare complication of water soluble contrast myelography. *ARCH OPHTHALMOL* 100:603–604, 1982.

u. Neetens A, Buroenich H: Anaphylactic marginal keratitis. *BULL SOC BELGE OPHTALMOL* 186:69–72, 1979.

v. Otenasek FJ, Markham J: Transient loss of vision following cerebral arteriography. *J NEUROSURG* 9:547–551, 1952.

w. Reed JW, MacMillan AS Jr, Lazenby GW: Transient neurologic complications of positive contrast orbitography. *ARCH OPHTHALMOL* 81:508–511, 1969.

x. Ritter G, Busse K, Rittmeier K: Cortical blindness following arteria vertebralis angiography. *RADIOLOGE* 16:424–426, 1976. (German)

y. Tabaddor K: Unusual complication of iophendylate injection myelography. *ARCH NEUROL* 29:435–436, 1973.

z. Walsh FB, Smith GW: Ocular complications of carotid angiography. J *NEUROSURG* 9:517–537, 1952.

Rafoxanide (Ranide), a veterinary anthelmintic, administered orally to dogs for 3 to 11 days has produced equatorial cataracts and papilledema, with vacuolation of the optic nerves and chiasm.[a] Increased intracranial pressure has been associated with swelling of the brain and inflammation of the meninges around the optic nerves and chiasm. This has been likened to the "status spongiosus" produced by *hexachlorophene*,[b] and the brain edema caused by *triethyltin*.[d] *Clioxanide* (Tremerad) similarly has produced vacuolation of the white matter in rats.[c]

a. Brown WR, Rubin L, et al: Experimental papilledema in the dog induced by a salicylanilide. *TOXICOL APPL PHARMACOL* 21:532–541, 1972.

b. Kimbrough RD: Review of recent evidence of toxic effects of hexachlorophene. *PEDIATRICS* 51:391–394, 1973.

c. Kurtz SM, Schardein JL, et al: Toxicologic studies with a halogenated salicylamide. *TOXICOL APPL PHARMACOL* 14:652, 1969.

d. Lock EA, Aldridge WN: Binding of triethytin to rat brain myelin. *J NEUROCHEM* 25:871–876, 1979.

Ranitidine (Zantac), an antagonist to histamine H_2 receptors, used medically for purposes similar to *cimetidine*, was suspected in one patient to have caused rise of intraocular pressure and discomfort similar to when *cimetidine* was used, associated with pressure "up to 24 mm Hg."[a]

a. Dobrilla G, Felder M, et al: Exacerbation of glaucoma associated with both cimetidine and ranitidine. *LANCET* 1:1078, 1982.

Rare-earth salts, or lanthanide salts, that have been tested for injurious effect in contact with the eye include the chlorides of *lanthanum, cerium, praseodymium, neodymium, samarium, gadolinium, dysprosium, holmium,* and *erbium.* Also the chlorides of *scandium* and *yttrium* have been tested. Specific results for each of these salts are described elsewhere under the name of each substance, but some general findings will be described here.[88, 90]

Most notably, when rare-earth salts are given good access to the stroma of the rabbit cornea they have a special severe toxic effect, causing opacification and degeneration of the cornea, but when rabbit eyes have been exposed to the same rare-earth salts with the corneal epithelium intact, they have generally caused damage only to the conjunctiva, with little or no disturbance in the cornea.

In human beings no ocular injuries by these substances have been reported so far, and no toxic effect on the cornea would be expected from accidental splash in the eye, unless at the same time the corneal epithelium was injured, either mechanically, such as by flying glass, or chemically, such as by acid mixed with the rare-earth elements. No disturbance of the eye has been reported from experimental systemic administration of these elements.

In rabbits when rare-earth salts were given access to the stroma of the cornea by removing the epithelium before bathing the eye for ten minutes with 0.1 M solutions of the salts adjusted to between pH 5.0 and 7.0, the corneas remained clear during the exposure and for at least one-half hour thereafter, but after a latent period of several hours they gradually developed diffuse gray opacities. Subsequently, during two or three weeks these opacities changed to yellow-white plaques accompanied by extensive vascularization. In the most severely affected eyes the axial portion of the cornea became necrotic and sloughed, resulting in spontaneous perforation.

Trivalent rare-earth-metal salts react with the mucoproteins and collagen of the cornea with much higher affinity than do the monovalent or divalent alkali or alkaline earth metals of groups I and II of the periodic table, tested under the same conditions of concentration and pH.[88, 90] These trivalent elements tested on excised pieces of cornea have been found to act as fixatives, greatly reducing the normal capacity of the cornea to swell in water. Furthermore, rare-earth cations render the mucoproteins of the cornea insoluble in water and prevent their extraction by water or sodium chloride solutions from the cornea. The capacity of pieces of cornea to react with and bind rare-earth cations from solution is reduced by previous extraction of mucoprotein or by blocking anionic groups of the cornea by methylation.

Chemical analyses of the corneas of live rabbits which have been exposed to neutral 0.1 M solutions of chlorides of *yttrium* and *lanthanum* show that these elements persist in the cornea, decreasing slowly in concentration in the course of several weeks, whereas innocuous cations, such as *calcium* from calcium chloride solution, disappear rapidly from the cornea, approaching the physiologic concentration within two to three hours.

Opacification of the cornea in rabbits constitutes a biological reaction to the strong binding of the trivalent cations to the mucoproteins and collagen. Excised cornea or corneas of dead rabbits exposed to 0.1 M *lanthanum chloride* did not become opaque during four days after exposure, while the corneas of live rabbits similarly exposed regularly developed definite gray opacity.

Treatment with 0.1 M neutral sodium edetate (EDTA) has been found beneficial both *in vitro* and *in vivo*. Removal of *yttrium* and *lanthanum* from combination with the tissue by treatment with edetate restores the capacity of excised pieces of cornea to absorb water. Also, irrigation of eyes of live rabbits with edetate solution immediately after ten-minute applications of near-neutral 0.1 M solutions of *yttrium* chloride or *lanthanum* chloride to the de-epithelized cornea extracts most of the toxic element and prevents most of the biological reaction and opacification. Irrigation with sodium chloride does not have this effect.[88, 90]

In case of accidental contamination of human eyes it would be appropriate to irrigate for fifteen to twenty minutes with 0.05 M solution of sodium edetate at pH 8, which has been found to be well tolerated by human eyes.

Reserpine, an antihypertensive, commonly causes the eyes of patients to appear slightly flushed, owing to dilation of conjunctival blood vessels. This may be accompanied by lacrimation and stuffiness of the nose. Reserpine also induces slight miosis.[c]

Ocular palsies have been ascribed to reserpine, but apparently these have been observed only in patients with previous brain damage.[h] Ocular spasms, presumably a form of oculogyric crisis, have been reported in a schizophrenic woman receiving reserpine intermittently for more than a year.[d] The spasms ceased promptly when the drug was discontinued.

One report has alleged serious ocular effect from reserpine in two cases, but the relationship to reserpine seems extremely questionable. In this report, involving two patients with anterior uveitis and secondary glaucoma, in one patient the author believed exacerbations and remissions were associated with giving and withholding reserpine, while in the second the reserpine was not discontinued and there was no evidence to establish a relationship to the patient's ocular disease.[k] In contrast to this alleged adverse effect on glaucoma are several reports of controlled studies in which systemically administered reserpine either had no influence or reduced the intraocular pressure in normal and glaucomatous eyes of patients and of rabbits.[g, 190, 266] From all this evidence it seems highly unlikely that reserpine has either caused glaucoma or has had an adverse influence on intraocular pressure.

Reserpine in eyedrops has been tested on rabbit eyes and found to reduce intraocular pressure and to cause hyperemia of the conjunctiva.[b, i]

Ptosis, or drooping of the upper lids, noted occasionally as a side effect of the sympatholytic action of systemic reserpine, has also been examined in animals.[a, l] It represents a complicated combination of central and peripheral actions.

Systemic reserpine suppresses the b-wave of the ERG in cats and rabbits.[e, f]

a. Aceto ME, Harris LS: Effect of various agents on reserpine-induced blepharoptosis. *TOXICOL APPL PHARMACOL* 7:329–336, 1965.

b. Bonomi L: Effects of local instillation of reserpine on the intraocular pressure of the rabbit. *ATTI 47, CONGR SOC OFTAL ITAL* 21:361–366, 1964. (Italian)

c. Freedman DX, Benton AJ: Persisting effects of reserpine in man. *N ENGL J MED* 264:529–533, 1961.

d. Fuldauer ML: Ocular spasms caused by reserpine. *NED TIJDSCHR GENEESKD* 103:110, 1959.

e. Gutierrez CO, Spiguel RD: Electroretinographic study of the effect of reserpine on the cat retina. *VISION RES SUPPL* 3:161–170, 1972.

f. Hempel FG: Modification of the rabbit electroretinogram by reserpine. *OPHTHALMIC RES* 4:65–75, 1972/73.

g. Kaplan MR, Pilger IS: The effect of *Rauwolfia serpentina* derivatives on intraocular pressure. *AM J OPHTHALMOL* 43:550–574, 1957.

h. Kline NS, Barsa J, Goline E: Management of side effects of reserpine and combined reserpine-chlorpromazine treatment. *DIS NERV SYST* 17:352–358, 1955.

i. Krnjevic H, Tomljanovic D: The local effect of reserpine on the eye bulb of the rabbit. *ARCH INT PHARMACODYN* 155:63–68, 1965.

j. Paul SD, Leopold IH: The effect of tranquilizing and ganglion-blocking agents on the eyes of experimental animals. *AM J OPHTHALMOL* 42:752–759, 1956.

k. Raymond LF: Ocular pathology in reserpine sensitivity. *J MED SOC NEW JERSEY* 60:417–419, 1963.

l. Schmidt B, et al: Effect of reserpine on sympathetic motor innervation of the eye. *NAUNYN SCHMIEDEBERG ARCH PHARM EXP PATH* 261:75–88, 1968.

Resorcinol, a keratolytic, tested as a 10% solution on rabbit eyes caused pain, conjunctival inflammation, and vascularization of the cornea.[53] Dry, powdered resorcinol applied to rabbit eyes induced necrosis sufficient to cause extensive vascularization, or perforation of the cornea.[53]

Resorcinol is readily oxidized to darker colored compounds, but unlike hydroquinone, resorcinol appears not to have induced discoloration of cornea or conjunctiva.

Rhenium trichloride has been tested on rabbit eyes by applying 3 mg of crystals, which caused immediate superficial damage to the cornea, hyperemia of the iris, and lacrimation, but the eyes recovered within twenty-four hours with no permanent damage.[a]

a. Haley TJ, Cartwright FD: Pharmacology and toxicology of potassium perrhenate and rhenium trichloride. *J PHARM SCI* 57:231–323, 1968.

Rhizoma galanga (galangal, Chinese ginger), an aromatic spice, was accidentally splashed into the eyes of a druggist, causing deep keratitis with iritis, from which he eventually recovered.[a]

a. Hartmann K: Corneal damage with Rhizoma galange. *KLIN MONATSBL AUGEN-HEILKD* 127:97–99, 1955. (*AM J OPHTHALMOL* 40:944, 1955.)

Rhodarsan, an organic arsenical of unidentified composition, is reported to have caused sudden but partially reversible blindness from severe optic neuritis in one case.[a] (See also *Arsenicals, organic.*)

a. Gerard G, Breton A: Very severe optic neuritis developed late after treatment with rhodarsan. *CLIN OPHTAL* 15:189–193, 1926. (French)

Rhodium chloride has been tested on a rabbit's eye and was found to give a peculiar delayed injurious reaction.[81,90] A 0.1 M solution adjusted to pH 7.2 with ammonium hydroxide was applied for ten minutes to the eye after the corneal epithelium had been removed by scraping. This caused orange coloration of the cornea, fading to faint yellow in two months. During the first two weeks the cornea was not opaque, but slightly hazy. In the third week, however, irregular white opacities gradually developed. Ultimately, the cornea became extensively opacified and vascularized.

Rhodomyrtus macrocarpa (Finger cherries) have caused severe loss of vision in patients who have eaten them. Some patients have retained only light projection in one or both eyes and have had optic atrophy. The literature on this type of poisoning was reviewed in 1944.[a] No cases have been reported from 1915 to 1980. The toxic factor has not been identified.[a, 255]

> a. Flecker H: Sudden blindness after eating "finger cherries" (Rhodomyrtus macrocarpa). *MED J AUST* 2:183–185, 1944.

Ricin is a highly toxic albumin present in castor oil seeds, but not in castor oil. A severely irritating effect of ricin powder on the eye was first described by Paul Ehrlich in 1891.[153] Crushed castor oil seeds have the same effect on the eye. Severe inflammation and pseudomembraneous conjunctivitis are induced in rabbits by application of the solids or a solution. Some animals react to 1:10,000 solution with strong mucopurulent discharge, others only to 1:1,000 solution.

Rifamide, an antibacterial, has been tested on rabbit eyes by applying 5% aqueous solution daily for fifteen days, causing no injury but closure of the lids for ten or fifteen minutes as though from discomfort.[a]

> a. Dezulian V, Serralunga MG, Maffii G: Pharmacology and toxicology of rifamide. *TOXICOL APPL PHARMACOL* 8:126–137, 1966.

Rifampin (rifampicin; Rifadin; Rimactane), an antibacterial, has been known to color the tears and stain soft contact lenses orange after oral administration.[h, 312] One patient on two occasions developed red painful eyes with thick white secretions within days after starting oral medication, clearing in 2 to 3 days after stopping.[d] In Chinese patients it has been reported not uncommon to have flushing, irritation, sometimes rash of face and scalp, sometimes with redness and watering of the eyes.[f] Fraunfelder's National Registry has recorded that conjunctival hyperemia or mild blepharoconjunctivitis are not uncommon.[312] Stevens-Johnson syndrome, with anterior uveitis and blepharoconjunctivitis, though rare, seems also to have been circumstantially well linked to rifampin.[i]

There have been no clinical evidences of disturbance of vision, though concern has been expressed on the basis of animal experiments. Evidence has been obtained of affinity of rifampin for uveal melanin of mice, rats, and the pigment epithelium of a human fetal eye.[a, b] Evidence of a selective effect on the retinal pigment epithelial cells in sheep has been obtained by electroretinography after intravenous injection, showing acute selective effects on the c-wave. No detrimental effect on the optic nerves of rats have been found in feeding experiments.[j]

Topical testing of rifampin on rabbit eyes as 1% solution in polyethylene glycol, every 15 minutes for 6 hours, produced no damage observable by biomicroscopy,[e] though Fraunfelder reports a 1% ointment produces symptoms of irritation of the eye.[312]

a. Boman G: Melanin affinity of a new antituberculous drug, rifampicin, investigated by whole body autoradiography. *ACTA OPHTHALMOL* 51:367–370, 1973.

b. Boman G: Tissue distribution of ^{14}C-rifampicin. *ACTA PHARMACOL TOXICOL* 36:267–283, 1975.

c. Calissendorff B: Melanotropic drugs and retinal functions. *ACTA OPHTHALMOL* 54:118–128, 1976.

d. Cayley FE, Majumdar SK: Ocular toxicity due to rifampicin. *BR MED J* 1:199–200, 1976.

e. Feldman MF, Moses RA: Corneal penetration of rifampin. *AM J OPHTHALMOL* 83:862–865, 1977.

f. Girling DJ: Ocular toxicity due to rifampicin. *BR MED J* 1:585, 1976.

g. Knave B, Persson HE, et al: Selective effect of a new antituberculous drug, rifampicin, on the c-wave of the sheep electroretinogram. *ACTA OPHTHALMOL* 51:371–374, 1973.

h. Lyon RW: Orange contact lenses from rifampin. *N ENGL J MED* 300:372–373, 1979.

i. Nyirenda R, Gill GV: Stevens-Johnson syndrome due to rifampicin. *BR MED J* 2:1189, 1977.

j. Satoyoshi E: Effect of rifampicin on optic nerve. *JPN J ANTIBIOT* 23:403–410, 1970.

Rociverine, a myolytic and parasympatholytic antipasmodic, tested on normal people by intravenous injection (20 mg) or orally (20 mg three times a day for 4 days), caused no significant changes in pupil size, intraocular pressure or iridocorneal angle.

Pardini M: *CLIN THER* 4:48–55, 1981. (Italian)

Rolitetracycline is an antibacterial used parenterally. When 0.1% to 1% solutions are injected into the anterior chamber, it is toxic to the cornea and causes intense inflammation.

a. Malik SRK, Sood GC, Aurora AL: Experiences with intracameral injection of synermycin and reverine. *ORIENT ARCH OPHTHALMOL* (Bombay), 4:21–23, 1966.

Rose bengal conforms to the general rule that anionic acidic dyes have little or no toxicity to the cornea and conjunctiva. It has been employed clinically in vital staining of the epithelium of cornea and conjunctiva in concentrations up to 5%.

a. Kronning E: Conjunctival and corneal stainability with Bengal Rose. *AM J OPHTHALMOL* 38:351–361, 1954.

Rosoxacin, an antibacterial, under study for ocular penetration in rabbits was found when injected subconjunctivally in rabbits (0.5 ml of 0.5% or 2% solution) to make the eyes red and chemotic for at least 6 hours.[a]

a. Hulem CD, Old SE, et al: *ARCH OPHTHALMOL* 100:646–649, 1982.

Rubber foreign bodies in the anterior chamber of patients after operation were described by Brockhurst in 1952, with reference to two earlier reports.[a] He described 7 cases in which tiny red particles came from the inner surface of red rubber irrigating bulbs, and lodged in crypts of the iris, or attached to hyaloid membrane or cornea. Although some of the eyes had a period of postoperative inflammation, this did not seem to involve the particles, and the particles did not seem to disturb the tissues with which they were in contact. The same particles introduced into the anterior chamber of rabbit eyes produced no inflammation or fibrosis.

   a. Brockhurst RJ: Intraocular rubber foreign bodies after surgery. *ARCH OPHTHALMOL* 47:465–469, 1952.

Rubidium chloride has been tested on a rabbit's eye and was found to cause no appreciable injury.[90] A 0.1 M solution, pH 6, was applied for ten minutes after the corneal epithelium had been removed by scraping to facilitate penetration of the solution into the cornea. The cornea remained clear and the epithelium healed without delay.

Radioactive rubidium chloride has been given intraveneously in rabbits, and uptakes by various parts of the eye have been measured as a basis for comparison in poisoned or injured eyes.[a]

   a. Obenberger J, Babicky A: Distribution of intravenously injected [^{86}Rb] Cl in different tissues of the rabbit eye. *EXP EYE RES* 25:195–197, 1977.

Ruthenium is a metal belonging to the platinum group and chemically resembling osmium. When heated, it oxidizes readily in air, and the fumes are said to have irritant effects on the eyes and respiratory passages similar to the fumes from osmium.[a]

   a. Cooper RA: Ruthenium. *J CHEM MET MINING SOC S AFRICA* 22:152, 1922.

Saccharin, a non-caloric sweetener, was reported by Lederer et al to produce ocular anomalies in offspring when fed to pregnant rats.[a,b] However, a review of the experience of other testers revealed no comparable finding.[c] Testing using saccharin meeting German standards of purity showed no abnormalities in any portion of the eyes of rat offspring.[c] Clarification was offered when Lederer et al compared pure (Maumee process) and less pure (Remsen-Fahlberg process) samples of saccharin, finding no ocular anomalies from feeding the purer material, but reaffirming that anomalies were produced by Remsen-Fahlberg saccharin, containing manufacturing by-products. Tests on the known impurities showed ocular anomalies to be produced especially by *o-sulfobenzoic acid,* less by *o-sulfamoylbenzoic acid,* and least by *o-toluene-sulfonamide.*[b]

   a. Lederer J, Pottier-Arnould AM: Influence of saccharin on development of the embryo in pregnant rats. *DIABETE* 21:13–16, 1973. (French)
   b. Lederer J: Saccharin, its pollutants and their teratogenic effect. *LOVAIN MED* 96:459–501, 1977. (French)
   c. Luckhaus G, Machemer L: Histological examination of perinatal eye development in the rat after ingestion of sodium cyclamate and sodium saccharin during pregnancy. *FOOD COSMET TOXICOL* 16:7–11, 1978.

Salicylate poisoning and salicylism are terms that have been employed inclusively for systemic poisonings by acetylsalicylic acid (aspirin), salicylic acid, and sodium salicylate. Poisoning by methyl salicylate is to be discussed elsewhere under the heading *Methyl salicylate.* Also topical contact effects on the eye are described elsewhere under the headings *Aspirin* and *Salicylic acid.*

When sodium salicylate was in common use, it was reported to have caused temporary complete or partial blindness in numerous cases.[a,d,41,153,214,247] Typically, visual disturbances were reported after ingestion of 8 to 20 g of sodium salicylate in the course of one to several days. Vision usually faded to complete blindness in the course of several hours. Commonly, but not always, visual disturbances were accompanied by tinnitus or deafness, and sometimes by headache, stupor, or coma. Blindness usually lasted from three to twenty-four hours. Then normal vision gradually returned. Slight functional disturbances occasionally persisted for a week or more.[153]

The cause of the loss of vision has not been established. Occasionally, either narrowing or widening of the retinal vessels has been described, but more often the ocular fundi appeared normal. The pupils appeared dilated in most cases, but usually continued to react to light. A functional disturbance of the optic nerve has been suspected, but the behavior of the pupils suggests that the disturbance might be in the occipital visual cortex. No characteristic change of visual field has been recognized, but narrowing of the visual fields has been observed infrequently, and in one instance hemianopsia was reported. Defective color perception was found in three cases. Nystagmus has rarely been reported.[153]

In two rare cases, low prothrombin levels after taking 4 to 6 g sodium salicylate per day for one to two months caused petechial hemorrhages in the skin and retinas, with decreased visual acuity, but recovery when medication was stopped.[c]

Since aspirin has largely replaced sodium salicylate, overdosage has caused many severe and sometimes fatal poisonings, especially in children, but descriptions of effects on the eyes or on vision have been very rare. These are described elsewhere under the heading *Aspirin.* (See INDEX)

Teratogenic effects of sodium salicylate have been reported in rats, including anophthalmia, microphthalmia, and exophthalmia in the offspring, apparently governed somewhat by the degree of acidosis induced.[b]

a. de Schweinitz GE; Experimental salicylic acid amblyopia. *TRANS AM OPHTHALMOL SOC* 7:405–408, 1895.

b. Goldman AS, Yakovac WC: Salicylate intoxication and congenital anomalies. *ARCH ENVIRON HEALTH* 8:648–656, 1964.

c. Mortada A, Abbound I: Retinal haemorrhages after prolonged use of salicylates. *BR J OPHTHALMOL* 57:199–200, 1973.

d. Snell S: A case of blindness resulting from the administration of salicylate of sodium. *TRANS OPHTHALMOL SOC UK* 21:306–308, 1901.

Salicylic acid, a keratolytic, has a pH of 2.4 in saturated aqueous solution.[171] A splash of 3% solution in collodion and a splash of 3% in a mixture of alcohol and glycerin in the eye have caused much irritation and moderate injury to the conjunctiva. No serious damage was done to the cornea, and the eyes recovered completely.[249] (For ocular effects associated with systemic poisoning by salicylates see INDEX for *Salicylates, Aspirin,* and *Methyl salicylate.*)

Samarium chloride effects on the cornea are similar to those of other rare-earth-metal salts. Irrigation of an intact rabbit's eye with 0.1 M solution at approximately pH 5 for ten minutes causes no injury. Haley has reported 1 mg in the conjunctival sac caused only transitory irritation.[a] On the other hand, when corneal epithelium has been removed before exposure, permitting penetration of the chemical into the cornea, severe injury resulted. During or shortly after the exposure there was no change in appearance of the cornea, but within a day the cornea became bluish gray and eventually became opaque and vascularized. In the course of two weeks following exposure the calcium content of the rabbit cornea increased greatly.[81,90] (See also *Rare-earth salts.*)

a. Haley TJ, Raymond K, et al: Toxicological and pharmacological effects of gadolinium and samarium chlorides. *BR J PHARMACOL CHEMOTHER* 17:526–532, 1961.

Sanguinarine (pseudochelerythrine) is obtainable from the root of *Sanguinaria canadensis,* which is also known as bloodroot or red root, and from other *Papaveraceae.* Sanguinarine is obtainable from the oil of seeds of *Argemone mexicana*[c] and from *Chelidonium majus.* It has also been synthesized. Free sanguinarine base is colorless, but quaternary salts are reddish.

In 1913 *Sanguinaria canadensis* was very briefly mentioned by Lewin and Guillery as having caused a reduction of vision when given in doses of 0.6 to 1.2 g, and this disturbance was attributed to its content of chelerythrine, but no details were furnished.[153]

In 1954 Hakim considered the possible relationship of argemone oil and sanguinarine to epidemic dropsy and a peculiar type of glaucoma.[b] He reviewed the suspicions that epidemics of dropsy in India might be related to low-protein diet and consumption of *argemone oil.* Glaucoma was described as occurring in 10 to 12 per cent of patients having this type of dropsy. This glaucoma is said to be characterized by increased protein in the aqueous humor and high intraocular pressure, which declines after several weeks. This type of glaucoma is not associated with ordinary clinical signs of ocular inflammation, and no changes in the outflow paths for aqueous humor are recognized histologically, although the capillaries of the uveal tract may be dilated and occasionally retinal hemorrhages occur.[c,46] It is said to be an acute transitory open-angle type of glaucoma.

Attempts to induce glaucoma in rabbits by systemic administration of sanguinarine or argemone oil have been unsuccessful, except in isolated instances in which lethal or near-lethal doses gave transient elevations of intraocular pressure.[c] Whether the changes of intraocular pressure in these instances were secondary to acute changes of blood pressure is unknown. Systemic administration of sanguinarine to monkeys is said to have raised the intraocular pressure.[d,h,i]

In cats, acute elevations of intraocular pressure have been reported from injections of sanguinarine chloride into the ventricles of the brain, reaching a peak between sixty and ninety minutes after the injection at a time the cats were showing many signs of systemic distress and illness.[d] This was not antagonized by decamethonium to block autonomic innervation, but whether contraction of extraocular muscles was responsible for the pressure rise apparently was not established. Numerous other isoquinoline alkaloids from poppy-fumaria plants are said to have caused acute rise of tension when injected into the cat's brain. Lists of these have been published.[d]

Increase in intraocular pressure has also been induced by injecting various substances directly into and about the eye, including argemone oil, sanguinarine, chelerythrine, quinidine, berberine, and various papaver extracts and seed oils.[c] These substances are irritative and inflammatory, and the temporary elevation of pressure induced by local administration to rabbit eyes is produced by many other locally irritating materials[a] and does not constitute a specific type of action by sanguinarine or related alkaloids. The local congestive effects are commonly antagonized by topically applied epinephrine, as also noted in the case of sanguinarine alkaloids. Injections of sanguinarine and related substances into the eyes of rabbits has been observed to cause hyperemia of the conjunctiva, constriction of the pupil, exudates into the anterior chamber, posterior synechias, and opacity of the cornea from scarring and vascularization.

In excised ox eyes, addition of sanguinarine to fluid perfusing the anterior chamber is reported to have caused a transient increase in resistance to outflow of the perfusion fluid during the first fifteen minutes after injection. However, commercial sanguinarine sometimes contains particles detectable by filtration, and the reported impediment to outflow may have been caused by such particles. No increase in resistance to aqueous outflow was found in freshly enucleated rabbit eyes perfused with a filtered solution of sanguinarine, nor in one human eye.[81]

In 1961 Dobbie and Langham provided a good review of the literature and experimentally demonstrated a lack of specific influence of sanguinarine on the intraocular pressure. In a careful reevaluation of the effects of administering sanguinarine orally, intravenously, or intraventricularly, both acutely and chronically to rabbits, cats, and hens, they showed that sanguinarine may induce transitory elevations of blood pressure, and these may transiently be reflected in rises of intraocular pressure, but that the elevations of intraocular pressure are not sustained, and the eyes are histologically unaffected. They concluded that in the literature there is good evidence that *argemone oil* may cause dropsy, but whether glaucoma is actually a specific feature is open to question, since the evidence is very incomplete.[b] Considerable speculation has been offered on the possibility of poppy-fumaria plants related to argemone in the diet as a cause of glaucoma, even without overt evidences of edema or dropsy, but these speculations are almost entirely theoretical[e,f,g] A review, without references, by Dyke in 1978 reiterates these speculations.[j]

Retinal and optic nerve degeneration have been noted in old rats fed sanguinarine or argemone oil, but this was not considered related to intraocular pressure.[d]

Investigations in the early 1970's indicated that pure sanguinarine did not produce dropsy in experimental animals, but when mixed with other substances in argemone oil it did.[k]

a. Ascher KW: The intraocular pressure. *TABULAE BIOLOGICAE (OCULUS I)* 22, 1947.
b. Dobbie GC, Langham ME: Reaction of animal eyes to sanguinarine and argemone oil. *BR J OPHTHALMOL* 45:81–95, 1961.

c. Hakim SAE: Argemone oil, sanguinarine, and epidemic dropsy glaucoma. *BR J OPHTHALMOL* 38:193–216, 1954.

d. Hakim SAE: Sanguinarine and hypothalamic glaucoma. *J ALL INDIA OPHTHALMOL SOC* 10:83–102, 1962.

e. Hakim SAE, Mijovic V, Walker J: Distribution of certain poppy-fumaria alkaloids and a possible link with the incidence of glaucoma. *NATURE* 189:198–201, 1961.

f. Hakim SAE, Mijovic V, Walker J: Experimental transmission of sanguinarine in milk. *NATURE* 189:201–204, 1961.

g. Kabelik J: Sanguinarin and glaucoma. *CESK OFTALMOL* 22(1):49–52, 1966. (*EXCERPTA MED (OPHTHAL)* 20(9):2256, 1966.)

h. Leach EH, Lloyd JPF: Experimental ocular hypertension in animals. *TRANS OPHTHAL-MOL SOC UK* 76:453–459, 1956.

i. Lloyd JPF: Argemone oil and sanguinarine poisoning in monkeys. *TRANS OPHTHAL-MOL SOC UK* 75:431–433, 1955.

j. Dyke S: Poppies and glaucoma. *NEW SCI* 1119:679–680, 1978.

k. Shenolikar IS, Rukmini C, et al: Sanguinarine in the blood and urine of cases of epidemic dropsy. *FOOD COSMET TOXICOL* 12:699–702, 1974.

Santonin has been used as an anthelminitic for more than one hundred years. Disturbances of vision commonly have followed overdosage. This was first noted in 1846. In 1913 Lewin and Guillery devoted fourteen pages to reviewing the visual disturbances from santonin which had been reported up to that time, and presented observations on changes in their own vision from taking the drug experimentally.[153] Since the review by Lewin and Guillery relatively little has been added to the literature, and most of the following description has been summarized from their treatise.

Santonin in excessive doses frequently has caused objects to be seen in other than their natural colors, most commonly as though viewed through a yellow or yellow-green filter.[c, 153] Bright objects characteristically have appeared greenish-yellow, but dark surfaces sometimes have had a violet appearance. Violet color has been observed even with the lids closed.

The degree to which different people are affected varies considerably, but generally a dose of 0.2 to 0.5 g causes some changes in color vision beginning within an hour. A dose of 0.6 to 1.25 g begins to affect color vision in ten or fifteen minutes, and the disturbance may last for twenty hours.

In 1927 and 1928 Marshall reported observations made by a single subject who took santonin by mouth (1 g) or was given it intravenously (10 mg). Violet vision was observed within a minute after intravenous administration and was most notable in dim illumination. With greater illumination, yellow vision or greenish-yellow veiling was evident, but in bright light discoloration of vision was scarcely noticeable.[e]

In one patient a differential effect of santonin poisoning on visual fields for colored test objects has been described, consisting of constriction of blue and violet more than for red and green, and no constriction for yellow.[f] Experiments on human subjects given 0.4 to 1.25 g of santonin have shown a lowered color sensitivity, particularly near the violet end of the spectrum.[g] Studies of color perception in human subjects have led to complex hypotheses, but have not established the mode of action.[c, e]

Dark adaptation appears not to be altered, but very persistent after-images have been noted. In one case the after-image of a window is said to have been observed for four days.[153]

Rarely, visual acuity has been affected in severe santonin poisoning, and in a few instances complete blindness has occurred, but has been transitory. A six-month-old child is reported to have been blind for two and one-half months after having received 0.3 g.[153] A sixty-year-old woman had great reduction of visual acuity for twenty-four hours after taking 0.12 g, but her visual acuity rapidly returned to normal although she saw green for a week.[153]

Possibly the only instance of permanent disturbance of vision was reported from Africa in 1911 by Baxler, who reported that a three-year-old child was rendered blind by santonin.[a] Ocular examination was not described.

The site of action of santonin affecting vision has been thought to be peripheral on the light-sensitive portions of the eye rather than on the central nervous system. However, as a rule the visual fields have remained normal, and the ocular media and fundi have appeared normal by ophthalmoscope. No morphologic changes have been found in the eyes of animals poisoned with santonin.[153] In frogs the amplitude and steepness of the b-wave of the ERG is reported to be increased, and this is notable on illumination with blue light only.[d]

a. Baxler EJ: Dangers of administration of santonin to children. *CLIN OPHTALMOL* 17:324–325, 1911. (French)
b. Jacobowsky B: Studies on the effect of santonin on the sense of sight. *UPSALA LAK FORH* 22:471, 1917. (*JAHRESB OPHTHALMOL* 45:322, 1916–1917.)
c. Marshall W: Color vision after intravenous injection of santonin. *J PHARMACOL* 32:189–203, 1928.
d. Muller HW: The action of strychnine, urethan and santonin on the electroretinogram of frogs after radiation with equal energy light bands of various wave-lengths. *PFLUGER ARCH GES PHYSIOL* 254:155–170, 1951. (*CHEM ABSTR* 47:11513.)
e. Schulz H: Influence of santonin and digitalis on the color sensitivity of the human eye. *DTSCH MED WOCHENSCHR* 40:996–998, 1914. (German)
f. Tamura S: On santonin xanthopsia. *ACTA SOC OPHTHALMOL JPN* 39:1876–1890, 1935.
g. Gyurdzhian AA: New data on physiology of light and color-sensitivity of the eye in experiments on the action of santonin. *DOKL ADAD NAUK SSSR* 137:472–475, 1961. (*CHEM ABSTR* 55:17897, 1961.)

Saponins (sapogenin glycosides) are widely distributed in plants. Certain saponins, such as *githagin* from Agrostemma seeds, have an injurious effect when in direct contact with the eyes.[b,c] Small amounts cause reversible superficial keratitis and conjunctivitis with tearing and pain, but large amounts may cause corneal ulceration and leukoma.

Splash of a solution of *quillaja saponin* (from *Quillaja saponica,* soap root) into the eye of a chemist, although followed quickly by washing with water, caused much irritation, beginning within a few minutes and developing within a few hours to pain, chemosis, hyperemia, photophobia, and defects in the corneal epithelium, all of which returned to normal in the course of several days.[a]

Experimentally, the same saponin applied to rabbit eyes caused similar effect, but with greater exposure led to corneal opacity and vascularization. A purified complex of cholesterol and saponin was found to cause no reaction when applied to rabbit eyes.[a] (See also *Agrostemma seeds, Chestnut shell,* and *Digitonin.*)

a. Bakker A: Clinical and experimental investigations of eye injuries from saponin. *OPHTHALMOLOGICA* 99:356–366, 1940.

b. Kobert ER: LEHRBUCH DER INTOXIKATIONEN. Stuttgart, Enke. 1902–1906, vol. 2, p. 749.

c. Krautschneider K: On self-inflicted injuries of the eyes in war. *WIEN KLIN WOCHEN-SCHR* 31:1146, 1918.

Sarin (methylfluorophosphonic acid isopropyl ester), an anticholinesterase nerve gas, produces miosis and enhancement of accommodation for near. The miosis is generally not long lasting. Impairment of visual performance in dim illumination appears to be related primarily to reduction of the amount of light entering the eye through the reduced area of the pupillary aperture.[f] No significant difference has been found in effect on visual threshold between sarin vapor and physostigmine eyedrops.[a] However, studies on dark adaptation by one group of investigators resulted in findings that could not be explained by degree of miosis, and led to suggestions of disturbance of some mechanism in the central nervous system.[c,d,e]

Volunteers who were exposed to sarin vapor and then treated with cyclopentolate eyedrops generally did not have well balanced counteraction of their miosis and cyclotonia.[b]

In the manufacture of sarin one of the intermediate compounds, *difluoro,* is very irritating and potentially damaging to the eyes. (See INDEX for *Difluoro.*)

a. Gazzard MF, Thomas DP: A comparative study of central visual field changes induced by sarin vapour and physostigmine eye drops. *EXP EYE RES* 20:15–21, 1975.

b. Moylan-Jones RJ, Thomas DP: Cyclopentolate in treatment of sarin miosis. *BR J PHARMACOL* 48:309–313, 1973.

c. Rubin LS, Goldberg MN: Effect of sarin on dark adaptation in man. *J APPL PHYSIOL* 11:439, 1957.

d. Rubin LS, Krop S, Goldberg MN: Effect of dark adaptation in man. *J APPL PHYSIOL* 11:445, 1957.

e. Rubin LS, Goldberg MN: Effect of tertiary and quaternary atropine salts on absolute scotopic threshold changes produced by an anticholinesterase (sarin). *J APPL PHYSIOL* 12:305, 1958.

f. Stewart WC, Madill HD, Dyer AM: Night vision in the miotic eye. *CAN MED ASSOC J* 99:1145–1148, 1968.

Scandium chloride, a salt of the rare-earth-metal series, when applied to rabbit eyes with the corneal epithelium intact, 0.1 ml of 1:1 solution caused slight translucent haze of the cornea which cleared completely in two days, also considerable redness and edema of the conjunctiva with small ulcerations, but all cleared in four days.[a] When tested on a rabbit's eye from which the corneal epithelium had been removed it caused severe injury of the same type as other rare-earth-metal salts. A 0.1 M solution at pH 4.5 applied for ten minutes caused no immediate change in appearance, but within the following day the cornea became moderately opaque, and within two weeks became completely opaque and vascularized.[81,90]

a. Haley T, Komesu N, et al: Pharmacology and toxicology of scandium chloride. *J PHARM SCI* 51:1043–1045, 1962.

Sclerosing injection of an aqueous solution of *undecanol* and *benzyl alcohol,* known as "Obliterol," into a cutaneous angioma of the forehead in one instance caused thrombosis of orbital vessels, blindness and phthisis on one side.[a]

a. Chamot L, Lografos L, Micheli JL: Ocular and orbital complications after sclerosing injections in a case of a frontal cutaneous angioma. *OPHTHALMOLOGICA* 182:193–198, 1981.

Scopolamine (hyoscine), employed usually as the hydrobromide salt, is an anticholinergic mydriatic, cycloplegic, and sedative, used for prevention of motion sickness and to enhance the analgesic action of narcotics.[171]

Systemic poisoning from scopolamine resembles atropine poisoning, except that in contrast to the central exciting effect of atropine, scopolamine has a narcotic effect.[177] Overdosage is accompanied by wide mydriasis and dryness of the mouth. Some of the central effects of scopolamine can be antagonized by physostigmine salicylate, 0.25 to 4 mg given intramuscularly or subcutaneously.[e,q,s]

Systemic poisonings have been reported from application of scopolamine ophthalmic ointment and from eyedrops containing 1% scopolamine hydrobromide.[h] In children, eyedrops containing only 0.2% administered 2 or 3 times have caused acute psychotic reactions, with visual hallucinations and restlessness, although the total dose (0.6 to 1.8 mg) was not enough to cause peripheral signs of dryness of the mouth, redness of the skin, or elevated temperature.[i]

The intraocular pressure in normal people is not affected by scopolamine 0.3 mg parenterally injected once or twice a day[187], and 0.7 mg orally is reported to have no effect on accommodation in normal people.[a] Intramuscular injection of 0.4 to 0.6 mg scopolamine hydrobromide has caused an average of 1 mm mydriasis in seven out of eight patients, and a measurable impairment of accommodation in thirteen out of fifteen eyes.[h] Others have reported mydriasis and paresis of accommodation in less than half the patients receiving 0.5 mg subcutaneously or 3 mg orally.[d,p]

Scopolamine eyedrops, like atropine and other anticholinergic eyedrops, have been found not to raise the intraocular pressure in normal eyes[l] and to raise the intraocular pressure in less than half of those who have open-angle glaucoma,[k,m] but there is no doubt that angle-closure glaucoma can be induced in eyes anatomically predisposed because of abnormally shallow anterior chamber and narrow angle. (The principles are further described under *Anticholinergic drugs.*)

"Transderm-V," a device that contains scopolamine, and is to be stuck to the skin behind the ear to provide a prolonged, gradual transdermal dosage for sea-sickness or dizziness, has been the source of a series of accidentally induced mydriasis and cycloplegia, sometimes unilateral, sometimes bilateral.[b,c,f,o,r] Secondarily, some patients have developed acute angle-closure glaucoma.[j,g] It seems as though transfer of scopolamine on the fingers from the device to the eye would be the most likely mechanism in such accidents.

a. Brand JJ, Colquhoun WP, Perry WLM: Side effects of 1-hyoscine and cyclizine studied by objective tests. *AEROSPACE MED* 39:999–1002, 1968.
b. Carlston JA: Correspondence. *J AM MED ASSOC* 248:31, 1982.
c. Chiaramonte JS: Correspondence. *N ENGL J MED* 306:174, 1982.
d. Christiansen P: Studies on the effects of scopolamine in man on peroral and subcutaneous administration. *ACTA PHARMACOL TOXIC* 1:336, 1946.
e. Crowell EB Jr., Ketchum JS: The treatment of scopolamine induced delirium with physotigmine. *CLIN PHARMACOL THER* 8:409–414, 1967.
f. Flora PG: Correspondence. *CAN J OPHTHALMOL* 17:135, 1982.
g. Fraunfelder FT: Correspondence. *N ENGL J MED* 307:1079, 1982.
h. Freund M, Merin S: Toxic effects of scopolamine eye drops. *AM J OPHTHALMOL* 70:637–639, 1970.
i. Hamborg-Petersen B, Nielsen MM, Thordal C: Toxic effect of scopolamine eye drops in children. *ACTA OPHTHALMOL* 62:485–488, 1984.
j. Hamil MB, Suelflow JA, Smith JA: Transdermal scopolamine delivery system and acute angle-closure glaucoma. *ANN OPHTHALMOL* 15:1011–1012, 1983.
k. Harris LS: Cycloplegic-induced intraocular pressure elevations. *ARCH OPHTHALMOL* 79:242–246, 1968.
l. Hoorn W. van: Studies of the influence of drugs on the intraocular pressure. Dissertation. Amsterdam, 1916. (*JBR OPHTHAL* 45:277, 1916–1917.) (German)
m. Kollner H: On the influence of the pupil width on the intraocular pressure in glaucoma simplex. *ARCH AUGENHEILKD* 88:58–74, 1921. (German)
n. Leopold IH, Comroe JH Jr.: Effect of intramuscular administration of morphine, atropine, scopolamine and neostigmine on the human eye. *ARCH OPHTHALMOL* 40:285–290, 1948.
o. Lepore FE: Correspondence. *N ENGL J MED* 306:824, 1982.
p. Mehra KS, Chandra P, Khare BB: Ocular manifestations of parenteral administration of scopolamine (Hyoscine.) *BR J OPHTHALMOL* 49:557–558, 1965.
q. Ullman KC, Groh RH, Wolff FW: Treatment of scopolamine-induced delirium. *LANCET* 1:252, 1970.
r. Verdier DD: Correspondence. *AM J OPHTHALMOL* 93:803–804, 1982.
s. Young SE, Ruiz RS, Falletta J: Reversal of systemic toxic effects of scopolamine with physostigmine salicylate. *AM J OPHTHALMOL* 72:1136–1138, 1971.

Scopolamine N-oxide (scopolamine aminoxide, genoscopolamine, Scopodex, Sominex), a derivative of scopolamine used as a sleeping medicine and to prevent travel sickness, appears to have effects on the eyes similar to those of scopolamine, though in reduced degree. There seem to be no systematic studies of the effects on the eyes, but I have found that taking within six hours six Scopodex pellets, each containing 0.5 mg scopolamine aminoxide hydrobromide, caused no appreciable change in pupillary size or accommodation.

Three reports of overdosage with Sominex tablets describe ocular side effects,[a–c] but two of these reports erroneously identify the alkaloid as scopolamine hydrobromide instead of the actual scopolamine aminoxide hydrobromide.[a,b] Amounts of the order of ten to thirty-six Sominex tablets equivalent to 2.5 to 9 mg of scopolamine aminoxide hydrobromide were taken. The reactions strongly resembled atropine poisoning, with disorientation, mydriasis, and blurred vision presumably from cycloplegia. There were no permanent ocular effects. According to one of these reports, physostigmine salicylate (1 mg) injected subcutaneously twice in fifteen minutes cleared the sensorium rapidly but did not reduce the size of the dilated pupils.[c]

Effects on intraocular pressure in glaucoma have not been studied, but if the recommended oral dosage has no appreciable effect on the pupil or on accommodation, it should not be a danger in any type of glaucoma. Overdosage producing dilation of the pupil could presumably induce angle-closure glaucome in anatomically predisposed eyes. (The principles are described under *Anticholinergic drugs.*)

a. Beach GO, Fitzgerald RP, et al: Scopolamine poisoning. *N ENGL J MED* 270:1354–1355, 1964.

b. Bernstein S, Leff R: Toxic psychosis from sleeping medicine containing scopolamine. *N ENGL J MED* 277:638–639, 1967.

c. Ullman KC, Groh RH, Wolff FW: Treatment of scopolamine-induced delirium. *LANCET* 1:252, 1970.

Scorpion venom from different types of scorpions varies greatly in its toxicity. Mainly the scorpions found in Mexico have been responsible for disturbances of the eye and severe systemic reactions.[b] During twelve to twenty-four hours after the sting of Mexican scorpions there may occur severe generalized pain with paresthesias and hyperesthesias, spasms of smooth and skeletal muscle, and salivation, followed by a period of depression for a day or two. During the acute phase, ocular symptoms consisting of discomfort in the eyes and tearing are present, but of slight importance compared to the severe general disturbance. Miosis is a constant finding. Strabismus, usually convergent, may occur during convulsive seizures and may cause diplopia. Transient clouding of vision of uncertain cause has been noted during the acute phase. Usually the ocular disturbances clear up promptly, but in exceptional cases paresis of extraocular muscles has lasted from several days to several weeks.

In one case, a sting on the hand by a scorpion of species *Centruroides* in the area of Lake Havesu in Arizona was followed by acute bilateral macular chorioretinitis in a 32 year old man.[c] For 24 hours after the sting the stung hand was numb, but blurring of vision was not noted until later, within 72 hours. Examination after 2 weeks of blurred vision showed bilateral macular retinal pigment epithelial disturbance, and retinal edema, with vision 20/20 right, 5/200 left. No treatment was given. Four weeks later, the edema was gone, but there were bilateral pigmented macular scars, with vision 20/20 right, 20/200 left. The time course, especially the short time for subsidence of the chorioretinitis, seemed to point to the scorpion sting as the cause. This case appears to be unique.

Two cases have been reported in which complete blindness accompanied by dilation of the pupils and loss of reaction to light occurred during the acute phase of poisoning. No other ocular abnormalities were found except slightly edematous optic nerveheads in one case and red optic papillae in the other. Recovery was complete in seven to ten days.[b]

A sting on the right eyebrow by a small gray African scorpion is reported to have caused pain and swelling about the eye of a young woman for a month. She was unable to open the eye, and when examined three months later was found to have complete ptosis with external and internal ophthalmoplegia on that side, but normal distant vision. The contralateral eye was completely normal and the patient was otherwise healthy.[d]

In one report casual mention has been made that the sting of the Brazilian scorpion may cause profuse tearing with nausea and vomiting, and in some cases may cause decreased vision and even blindness. It has been suggested that the blindness is due to lesions of cortical centers. Apparently this has been found to be the case in poisoned fowl. The report tells us nothing of the nature of the eye disturbance in human beings, nor whether it is reversible, and furnishes no bibliography.[a]

a. DeMagalhaes O: Scorpionism. *J TROP MED HYG* 41:393–399, 1938.
b. Gonzales J de J: Ocular symptoms from envenomation by a scorpion sting. *INT CONGR OPHTHALMOL* Washington, 1922, p. 81.
c. Heckenlively JR, Pearlman JT: Acute macular chorioretinitis associated with scorpion sting. *TOXICON* 16:88–91, 1978.
d. Sarkies JWR: Ophthalmoplegia following a scorpion bite. *BR J OPHTHALMOL* 35:502–504, 1951.

Sea cucumber (*Actinopya agassizi,* Holothurioidea) is said to produce a toxic agent, *holothurin,* which can produce intensely painful inflammation of the skin and is alleged to have caused loss of sight.[a] No description of the nature of the loss of sight nor case reports substantiating the purported visual disturbance were found.

a. Halstead BW: Animal phyla known to contain poisonous marine animals. In Buckley; Porges (Eds.): VENOMS. Am. Assoc. for Advancement of Science, Pub. 44, Washington, D.C., 1956.

Seeds from plants are occasionally encountered in the conjunctival sac or within the eye after penetrating injury. Most commonly the reactions provoked seem to be attributable to irritating physical properties, or to accompanying infection, rather than to toxic properties.

Abel reported from South Africa a seed in the anterior chamber which entered, along with a cilium, in a penetrating injury, and was removed without serious consequence 10 weeks later when it sprouted.

Bettman described a boy who lost an eye due to bacterial endophthalmitis after a seed of "Russian Olive," *Elaeagnus angustifolia,* was shot from an air gun and entered the vitreous humor.

Humphrey reviewed the use of *flaxseed* in folk medicine, and recounted three cases in which patients had placed the seeds in the conjunctional sac, adding mechanical irritation and possibly bacterial contamination to the eye diseases which they were trying to treat, but with no evident toxic effect.

Wild rice seed was found by Peterson to have remained in the superior conjunctional fornix of one patient for 14 months, causing only slight irritation. *Grass* seeds imbedded in the conjunctiva have caused foreign body granulomas in two children, but no indication of toxicity.

Abel S: Germinating seed in anterior chamber. *ARCH OPHTHALMOL* 97:1651, 1979.

Bettman JW Jr, Packer S, Albert DM: Penetrating ocular injury by a plant seed. *ARCH OPHTHALMOL* 85:695–698, 1971.

Humphrey WT: Flaxseeds in ophthalmic folk medicine. *AM J OPHTHALMOL* 70:287–290, 1970.

Peterson NP, Wolter JR: A wild rice seed retained under the upper eyelid for 14 months. *J PEDIATR OPHTHALMOL* 10:285–287, 1973.

Roy FH, Hanna C: Foreign body granuloma of the conjunctiva. *ANN OPHTHALMOL* 10:1361–1362, 1978.

Selenite, sodium has been tested on rabbit eyes at concentrations of 0.003 to 0.05 M by application to the cornea after removal of the epithelium, or by injection into the corneal stroma. These solutions have caused very severe injury.[123] (See also *Selenium* and *Selenium dioxide.*)

Selenium absorbed systemically is toxic to human beings in a manner similar to arsenic and tellurium. Acute poisoning causes gastrointestinal distress, convulsions, collapse, and death. Chronic poisoning causes garlic odor of the breath, debility, dermatitis, and irritation of the nose and throat. No special involvement of the eyes appears to have been reported in human poisoning. However, important ocular effects of selenium poisoning have been recognized in lower animals, and burns of the eyes have been produced by selenium dioxide and selenious acid. (See separate sections for *Selenium dioxide, Selenious acid,* and *Selenite, sodium.*)

Poisoning of cattle has occurred in Wyoming and other areas in which selenium in the soil is absorbed by plants and transported to the leaves, which are eaten by the cattle. A condition is produced known as "alkali disease." When chronic, the skin and hooves are principally affected, but if the poisoning is severe, the animals are restless, tending to wander aimlessly in circles in a condition known as "blind staggers" before onset of paralysis. It is difficult to determine from the literature whether the vision is actually affected at this stage as implied by the term "blind staggers." It appears that in most instances the aimless wandering in circles is not attributable to impairment of vision.[c,g,p] However, in severe acute poisoning, animals may have swelling of the lids, discharge from the nose and eyes, and purportedly the cornea may be involved and become opaque.[n,129] Blindness and blind staggers have been described in both cattle and sheep.[64]

In rats, the influence of dietary selenium on the lens has been of great interest. It is known that deficiency of selenium in mother and young offspring can cause cataract, yet administration of excess selenium to rats a few days old can also induce cataracts.[a,b,e,f,h-m] Nuclear cataracts develop in days, following microscopic changes in the lens cortex.[l,m,o] Excess selenium has depressed lens glutathione, as well as catalase, superoxide dismutase, and GSH peroxidase, suggesting that cataracts may have resulted from impairment of protection against toxic metabolites of oxygen.[e,f,h] Administration of other trace substances along with selenium has shown protection against cataract formation in decreasing order of effectiveness by: mercury, silver, cyanide, arsenic, cadmium, copper, and tellurium.[n] No protection was provided by: iron, zinc, lead, chromium, molybdenum, tungsten, or vanadium. (It is noteworthy that none of these trace elements produced cataracts themselves.[n]) Selenium appears to stand alone as a trace-element promoter of cataracts in young rodents, particularly in rats, but also in rabbits and guinea pigs.

The effects of several inorganic selenium compounds have been examined in the frog retina by direct injection of micro-quantities, demonstrating reversible changes in the ERG.[d]

For description of local effects of selenium compounds on the eye, see separate sections on *Selenium dioxide, Selenium sulfide,* and *Selenite, sodium.*

a. Babichy A, Ostadalova I, et al: Peculiar response of Brattleboro rats to selenite. *EXPERIENTIA* 38:839, 1982.

b. Babicky A, Ostadalova I: Protective effect of premature weaning against the appearance of selenium induced cataract in young rats. *IRCS MED SCI* 10:464, 1982.

c. Beath OA, et al: Poisonous plants of Wyoming activated by selenium. *J AM PHARMACOL ASSOC* 23:94–97, 1934.

d. Berger H: The effect of different inorganic selenium compounds on the bioelectric behavior of the frog retina. *ACTA BIOL MED GERMAN* 19:405–403, 1967.

e. Bhuyan KC, Bhuyan DK, Podos SM: Cataract produced by selenium in rat. *IRCS MED SCI* 9:195–196, 1981.

f. Bunce GE, Hess JL: Biochemical changes associated with selenite-induced cataract in the rat. *EXP EYE RES* 33:504–514, 1981.

g. Draize JH, Beath OA: Observations on the pathology of blind staggers and alkali disease. *J AM VET MED ASSOC* 86:753–763, 1935.

h. Lawrence RA, Sunde RA, et al: Glutathione peroxidase activity in rat lens and other tissues in relation to dietary selenium intake. *EXP EYE RES* 18:563–569, 1974.

i. Ostadalova I, Babicky A, Obenberger J: Cataract induced by administration of a single dose of sodium selenite to suckling rats. *EXPERIENTIA* 34:222–223, 1978.

j. Ostadalova I, Babicky A, Obenberger J: Cataractogenic effect of sodium selenite administered in a single dose to suckling male rats. *CESK OFTALMOL* 34:373–377, 1978.

k. Ostadalova I, Babicky A, Obenberger J: Cataractogenic and lethal effects of selenite in rats during postnatal ontogenesis. *PHYSIOL BOHEMOSLOV* 28:393–397, 1979.

l. Russell NJ, Royland JE, et al: Ultrastructural study of selenite-induced nuclear cataracts. *INVEST OPHTHALMOL VIS SCI* 25:751–757, 1984.

m. Shearer TR, McCormack DW, et al: Histological evaluation of selenium induced cataracts. *EXP EYE RES* 31:327–333, 1980.

n. Shearer TR, Anderson RS, Britton JL: Influence of selenite and fourteen trace elements on cataractogenisis in the rat. *INVEST OPHTHALMOL VIS SCI* 24:417–423, 1983.

o. Shearer TR, Anderson RS, et al: Early development of selenium-induced cataract. *EXP EYE RES* 36:781–788, 1983.

p. Stenn F: "Alkali Disease"—Selenium poisoning. *ARCH PATHOL* 22:398–412, 1936.

Selenium dioxide and **selenious acid** cause contact burns, although it has been said that they are not serious if promptly irrigated with water.[a] In one instance a spray of selenium dioxide, in unspecified form and concentration, into the eyes of a chemist has been described as causing superficial burns of the skin and immediate irritation of the eyes. Injury appeared slight and the corneas did not stain with fluorescein immediately after the exposure. In the course of six hours, although vision remained clear, photophobia and pain developed, and the lower portions of both corneas became stainable with fluorescein. Within sixteen hours vision was blurred and the lower three-fourths of both corneas appeared dulled, and the bulbar conjunctivae whitened. From the third to fifth days the corneas cleared from above downward, and by the sixteenth day the corneas were essentially normal.[b]

In another accident a workman received a spray of selenious acid in one eye, affecting the lower two-thirds of the cornea, extending from 4 to 8 o'clock at the limbus.[c] Eipthelization was progressing after 10 days, but was irregular, and precipitates on Descemet's membrane persisted for 15 days. Finally a superficial 1.5 mm scar remained along the limbus with a small pterygium, but vision was normal.

A third patient had a history of exposure of one eye to gaseous selenium dioxide from explosion of a selenium rectifier.[d] A year later a fibrous growth was present inferiorly on the periphery of the cornea, with a small white scar on a corresponding area of the inner surface of the lower lid. During the next 17 years, despite repeated operations, a pterygium formed, threatened the optical axis, and led to total inferior symblepharon requiring mucous membrane grafts to separate.

   a. Cerwnka EA Jr, Cooper WC: Toxicology of selenium and tellurium and their compounds. *ARCH ENVIRON HEALTH* 3:189–199, 1961.
   b. Middleton JM: Selenium burn of the eye. *ARCH OPHTHALMOL* 38:806–811, 1947.
   c. Peyresblanques J: Eye burns by selenious acid. *BULL SOC OPHTALMOL FRANCE* 76:1179–1180, 1976. (French)
   d. Wesley RE, Collins JW: Pseudopterygium from exposure to selenium dioxide. *ANN OPHTHALMOL* 14:588–589, 1982.

Selenium sulfide (Selsun, Exsel), an antifungal, antiseborrheic, is used in combination with a detergent as a shampoo for treatment of dandruff, and as an ointment for application to the lid margins in treatment of seborrheic blepharitis. The suspension employed in a shampoo for treating dandruff when tested on rabbit eyes was found to cause superficial keratitis,[b,e] but ointments containing 0.5% of selenium sulfide caused no damage to rabbit eyes,[e] and only occasional irritation or transient keratitis in human eyes.[a,b,d–g]

   a. Bahn GC: The treatment of seborrheic blepharitis. *SOUTHERN MED J* 47:749–753, 1954.
   b. Cohen LB: Use of Selsun in blepharitis marginalis. *AM J OPHTHALMOL* 38:560–562, 1954.
   c. Lavyel A: Selsunef ointment to treat squamous blepharitis. *AM J OPHTHALMOL* 49:820–821, 1960.
   d. Post CF, Juhlin E: Demodex folliculorum and blepharitis. *ARCH DERM* 88:298–302, 1963.
   e. Rosenthal JW, Adler H: Effect of selenium disulfide on rabbit eyes. *SOUTHERN MED J* 55:318, 1962.
   f. Welsh AL, Ede M: Observations on the use of selenium sulfide and hydrocortisone ointment. *ARCH DERM* 75:130–131, 1957.
   g. Wong AS, Fasanella RM, Haley LD, Marshall CL, Krehl W: Selenium (Selsun) in treatment of marginal blepharitis. *ARCH OPHTHALMOL* 55:246–254, 1956.

Serotonin (5-hydroxytryptamine) tests on the pupil and intraocular pressure in animals, generally show slight miosis and slight reduction of intraocular pressure. No elevations of intraocular pressure have been reported. The retinal vessels in rats have been observed to become attenuated after intravenous injection of serotonin, and protrusion of the eyeballs has been induced.[c] Electric potentials in the optic tract of cats, induced by exposing the eye to flashes of light, have been strongly depressed by intra-arterial injections of serotonin.[b] Electrical potentials from the cortex of rats, evoked by exposure of the eyes to flashes of light, have also been altered and this may have involved a blocking action in the lateral geniculate body.[a]

Reversible anterior capsular opacities in the lenses of rats have been produced when both serotonin and phenelzine have been injected subcutaneously to produce a near-lethal condition. The opacities developed within one to three hours while the animals lay apathetic and unblinking. The opacities gradually disappeared in another hour. Neither the serotonin nor the phenelzine separately induced this condition. The opacities were produced by suppressing blinking and allow dehydration of the anterior segment of the small rodent eye, and were prevented when the lids were kept closed.[d]

a. Rebentische E: The influence of serotonin and LSD on visual evoked cortical activity of the rat. *PSYCHOPHARMACOLOGIA* 13:106–117, 1968. (German)
b. Straschill M, Perwin J: Inhibition of retinal ganglion cells by catechol amines and gamma-aminobutyric acid. *PFLUGERS ARCH* 312:45–54, 1969.
c. Tammisto T: The effect of 5-hydroxytryptamine (serotonin) on retinal vessels of the rat. *ACTA OPHTHALMOL* 43:430–433, 1965.
d. Dietz V, Tilgner S, Schroder KD: Influence of lid closure on the development of reversible serotonin-cataract of the rat. *OPHTHALMOLOGICA* 168:230–237, 1974. (German)

Silica (quartz, silicon dioxide) has been observed to cause fibrotic nodules in the eye analogous to pulmonary silicosis.[a,c] Particles of silica predominantly in the range of 2μ to 3μ introduced into the corneal stroma of rabbit eyes cause very little reaction.[c] The same particles introduced into the anterior chamber sink to the bottom of the chamber and in the course of three to five weeks cause an inflammatory reaction with formation of fibrotic nodules in the iridocorneal angle.[f] The reaction is quite different and more severe than that induced by *brickdust, glass,* or *magnesium silicate. Silica gel* placed in the anterior chamber of rabbits has been observed to cause local corneal swelling and clouding, with accumulation of leukocytes in the anterior chamber and in the swollen part of the cornea, leading eventually to corneal vascularization.[150] However, apparently silica gel has not induced a fibrotic nodular reaction like that caused by silica dust.

Finely divided *silica* injected into the vitreous body of rabbit eyes has caused necrosis of the retina and atrophy of the choroid.[b]

An apparently unique report of involvement of the cornea in foundry workers who developed pulmonary silicosis has described gradual decrease in visual acuity due to corneal opacities in the pupillary area and has reported spectroscopic analytical evidence of an abnormally high silicon content in the cornea.[b]

Silica granulomas of the eyelids, presumably from trauma, have been described in several cases.[d,e] Birefringent crystals, best seen with polarized light, associated with foreign-body-type giant cells, and scarring, are characteristic findings. Scanning electron microscopy and x-ray analysis have proven most effective in determining the composition of the crystals.

a. Eggenschwyler H: Experimental investigations into the effect of quartz and glass dust in the anterior chamber of rabbits. *Z UNFALLMED BERUFSKR* 42:287–303, 1949. (German)

b. Hanische J, Orban T, Szakacz O: Analysis of the emissionspectrum in cases of silicosis of the cornea. *SZEMESZET* 103:88–90, 1966. (*ZENTRALBL GESAMTE OPHTHALMOL* 97:419, 1967.) (German)

c. Krummel H: Silicotic tissue reactions in animal eyes. *BEITR SILIKOSEFORSCH* 57:1–127, 1958. (*CHEM ABSTR* 53:7399, 1959.)

d. Riddle PJ, Font RL, et al: Silica granuloma of eyelid and ocular adnexa. *ARCH OPHTHALMOL* 99:683–687, 1981.

e. Teslnsky P, Fakan F, Safanda J: Silicotic granuloma of the eyelids. *CESK OFTALMOL* 33:263–268, 1977. (English summary.)

f. Vyskocil J: An experimental study of the pathogenesis of silicotic granuloma in the anterior eye chamber in rabbits. *BR J IND MED* 14:30–38, 1956.

Silicones are organo-silicon-oxide polymers which have high thermal and chemical stability. They may be fluids of varied viscosity or rubbery compounds.[171] They will be discussed under the separate headings, "Silicone oils" and "Silicone rubbers."

Silicone oils (polydimethylsiloxanes, DC 200, Dimethicone) are available in a wide range of viscosities. The lower viscosity oils cause slight transient sensation of irritation when applied to rabbit or human eyes, but no injury of the cornea.[211] However, they delay healing of experimental corneal erosions.[e] Many observations have been made on the effects of injecting silicone oils into various parts of the eye. Injection into the stroma of the cornea in rabbits and dogs appears to produce no toxic effect during several months, but the stroma anterior to the deposit of oil has become atrophied, forming a crater-like defect.[l]

Injection into the anterior chamber has produced varied results, possibly related to the purity of the silicone oil used. Some reports indicate injections of Dow Corning 200 of viscosities from 100 to 13,000 centistokes into the anterior chamber of cats, rabbits, and monkeys caused no damage,[a,b] and similarly Dow Corning 703 of 20 or 30 centistoke viscosity in the anterior chamber of rabbits has been reported to be well tolerated except for occasionally causing glaucoma.[r] However, other reports do record injurious effects from silicone oils ranging from 20 to 60,000 centistokes in the anterior chambers of rabbits.[k,m,q,w,z]

Though the fluid usually appeared to be tolerated for two or three months, it later caused edema, vascularization, and scarring of the cornea, and sometimes cataracts. In the anterior chamber of the monkey, silicone liquid has caused only a transitory elevation of intraocular pressure.[g] Limited trials of silicone oil of 100 centistoke viscosity in the anterior chamber of patients have been made in treatment of bullous keratopathy, but injurious effect on the endothelium may prove excessive.[z]

Intravitreal injections of silicone oil experimentally in animals or in patients to replace cloudy vitreous or as an aid in treatment of retinal detachment have generally given first impressions of being well tolerated.[a,d,h,s,v,y,za,zc] However, cataracts have developed in both rabbits and patients.[o,t,w]

Clinical use of silicone oil injected into the vitreous cavity as a tamponade to push detached retinas back in place met with considerable early success, but then recurrences of detachments, development of cataracts, glaucoma, and corneal edema caused many surgeons to abandon this use. However, some have said that changes in technique, particularly improvement in management of proliferating vitreoretinal membranes, improve the results and reduce the complications. It also appears that removal of the oil after the retina has reattached may reduce late complications.

Differences in opinion have been held as to whether adverse side-effects from silicone oil injected into the vitreous cavity are toxic effects or physical-mechanical effects.

Favoring the concept of toxic effects have been animal experiments which showed early post-operative formation of a silicone-vitreous emulsion, probably aided by formation of a silicone-lipid complex involving phospholipids from the retina.[u] Histology in monkey retinas showed clear spaces which apparently had been occupied by silicone oil that had passed through the internal limiting membrane.[j,u] At a late stage, degeneration of small ganglion cells and Muller's fibers was described. Human eyes examined histologically years after intravitreal silicone oil injection also showed many cavities, presumably occupied by silicone oil, in most of the tissues of the eye.[c,p,zb] Phagocytic cells were seen to have taken up the oil,[i,x] but without inflammatory reaction or necrosis such as would suggest a toxic process.[p] It appeared that a portion of the injected oil became emulsified and phagocytosed in various parts of the eye.

Those who considered that there was no evidence to prove toxicity, noted that cataract and corneal edema were usually the result of a large oil globule coming in contact with the back of the lens or back of the cornea in a manner that could physically interfere with their metabolism.[f]

Development of secondary open-angle glaucoma in a moderate proportion of patients after intravitreal silicone oil has been explained as due to oil-containing macrophages blocking the intertrabecular spaces of the trabecular meshwork.[i,x] In two well-studied eyes with glaucoma, histology showed phagocytes with oil vacuoles in the trabecular meshwork, in a situation to block aqueous outflow.[i,x]

Clinical descriptions point out that most of the eyes that develop glaucoma are aphakic, that gonioscopy in some shows fine silicone globules floating superiorly in the angle, and in some shows peripheral synechias, with or without rubeosis iridis. Occasionally the angle has appeared clinically normal.

a. Armaly MF: Ocular tolerance to silicones. *ARCH OPHTHALMOL* 68:390–395, 1962.
b. Armaly MF: The organo-silicones and the eye. *EYE EAR NOSE THROAT DIGEST* 51–65, 1964.
c. Blodi FC: Injection and impregnation of liquid silicone into ocular tissues. *AM J OPHTHALMOL* 71:1044–1051, 1971.
d. Cibis PA: The use of liquid silicone in retinal detachment surgery. *ARCH OPHTHALMOL* 68:590–599, 1962.

e. Ehrich W: Delays in healing of corneal epithelium from silicon oil. *GRAEFES ARCH OPHTHALMOL* 191:109–120, 1974. (German)

f. Haut J, Ullern M, et al: Complications of intraocular injections of silicone combined with vitrechtomy. *OPHTHALMOLOGICA* 180:29–35, 1980.

g. Kalvin NH, Hamasaki DI, Gass JDM: Experimental glaucoma in monkeys. *ARCH OPHTHALMOL* 76:94–103, 1966.

h. Labelle P, Okun E: Ocular tolerance to liquid silicone. *CAN J OPHTHALMOL* 7:199–204, 1972.

i. Leaver PK, Grey RHB, Garner A: Silicone oil injection in the treatment of massive preretinal retraction. *BR J OPHTHALMOL* 63:361–367, 1979.

j. Lee P, Donovan RH, et al: Intravitreous injection of silicones. *ANN OPHTHALMOL* 1:15–25, 1969.

k. Lepri G, Tota G: Changes in the intraocular pressure caused by introduction of silicone liquid into the anterior chamber. *ANN OTTALMOL CLIN OCUL* 93:188–200, 1967. (Italian)

l. Levenson DS, Stocker FW, Georgiade NG: Intracorneal silicone fluid. *ARCH OPHTHALMOL* 73:90–93, 1965.

m. Liesenhoff H, Schmitt J: Complications from liquid silicone in the interior chamber. *BER DTSCH OPHTHALMOL GESELLSCH* 68:643–644, 1969. (German)

n. Liesenhoff H, Rentsch FJ, et al: Observations after injection of silicone oil in vitreous cavity of rabbits and electron microscopic studies of the retina. *MOD PROBL OPHTHALMOL* 10:55–59, 1972. (German)

o. Lund OE: Silicone oil as viterous substitute. *BER DTSCH OPHTHALMOL GESELLSCH* 68:166–169, 1968. (German)

p. Manschot WA: Intravitreal silicone injections. *ADV OPHTHALMOL* 36:197–207, 1978.

q. Martola EL, Dohlman CH: Silicone oil in the anterior chamber of the eye. *ACTA OPHTHALMOL* 41:75–79, 1963.

r. Maurice DM, Zauberman H, Michaelson IC: The stimulus to neovascularization in the cornea. *EXP EYE RES* 5:168–184, 1966.

s. Moreau PG: Intraocular silicones in desperate detachments of the retina. *ANN OCULIST (Paris)* 200:257–265, 1967. (French)

t. Mori S: Development of cataract in rabbit eyes following implantation of liquid silicone into the vitreous chambers. *FOLIA OPHTHALMOL JPN* 16:827, 1965.

u. Mukai N, Lee PF, et al: A long-term evaluation of silicone retinopathy in monkeys. *CAN J OPHTHALMOL* 10:391–402, 1975.

v. Ober RR, Blanks JC, et al: Experimental retinal tolerance to liquid silicones. *RETINA* 3:77–85, 1983.

w. Ojima M: Reaction of ocular tissue against implanted liquid plastic materials. *JPN J CLIN OPHTHALMOL* 20:1427–1432, 1966.

x. Rentsch FJ, Atzler P, Liesenhoff H: Histologic and electronmicroscopic studies of a human eye several years after intravitreal silicone implantation. *BER DTSCH OPHTHALMOL GESELLSCH* 75:70–74, 1977. (German)

y. Rosengren G: Silicone injection into the vitreous in hopeless cases of retinal detachment. *ACTA OPHTHALMOL* 47:757–760, 1969.

z. Strampelli B, Restivo Manfridi ML: Experimental and clinical contribution on the intraocular use of liquid silicone. *ANN OTTALMOL CLIN OCUL* 92:415–428, 1966. (Italian)

za. Tahara H: Experimental studies on effects of intravitreous injections of silicon oil in normal rabbits. *ACTA SOC OPHTHALMOL JPN* 71:363–379, 1967.

zb. Watzke RC: Silicone retinopoiesis for retinal detachment. *SURVEY OPHTHALMOL* 12:333–337, 1967.

zc. Zakharov VD, Fedorov SN, Bedilo VY: Replacement of the vitreous body with silicon fluid. *VESTN OFTAL* 78:83–86, 1965.

Silicone rubber of various textures, including Silastic sponge, have been tested as intrascleral implants. In the cornea, preformed silicone or Silastic rubber membranes have been inserted into the stroma without toxic effects.[a,b,h] Liquid silicone rubber mixed with a catalyst has been injected into the corneal stroma in rabbits and allowed to polymerize to a rubbery material without immediate evidence of toxicity, but the mass gradually induced vascularization and was extruded.[d] Room-temperature-vulcanizing (RTV) silicone rubber has been tolerated well in orbital reconstruction.[i] Implants of silicone rubber in the sclera have been the subject mainly of clinical reports concerned with surgical technique,[f,g] but experiments with rabbits have shown granulation tissue reaction, degeneration of sclera, and changes in the choroid from deeply implanted silicone rubber.[e]

In the anterior chamber of rabbits, tests of various hydrophobic and hydrophilic silicone rubbers for toxicity have identified a number of parameters to be considered.[c]

a. Brown SI, Mishima S: The effect of intralammelar water-impermeable membranes on corneal hydration. *ARCH OPHTHALMOL* 76:702–708, 1966.

b. Dohlman CH, Dube I: The artificial corneal endothelium. *ARCH OPHTHALMOL* 79:150–158, 1968.

c. Ehrich W: Biological compatibility of silicone rubber. *CONTACTOLOGIA* 1:9–20, 1979.

d. Hanna C, Shibley S: Tissue reaction to intracorneal silicone rubber. *AM J OPHTHALMOL* 60:323–328, 1965.

e. Manuelli GF, Caffi M: Experimental study of histologic changes in the sclera secondary to implantation of silicone and of homonymic sclera. *ANN OTTALMOL CLIN OCUL* 92:451–459, 1966. (Italian)

f. Regan CDJ: The scleral buckling procedures. *ARCH OPHTHALMOL* 68:313–330, 1962.

g. Schepens CL: Scleral buckling procedures. *ACTA OPHTHALMOL* 64:868–881, 1960.

h. Steinbach PD, Sprengel G: Tissue reactions to silicone and HEMA implants in the cornea. *BER DTSCH OPHTHALMOL GESELLSCH* 75:77–80, 1977. (German)

i. Vistnes LM, Paris GL: Uses of RTV silicone in orbital reconstruction. *AM J OPHTHALMOL* 83:577–581, 1977.

Silver in the form of its salts can be locally injurious in contact with the eye. Injurious effects are described elsewhere under the names of the compounds responsible. (See *Silver ammonium compounds, Silver nitrate,* and *Silver oxide.*)

Discoloration of the eye, without injury, can be caused by silver metal, or by silver compounds, either in contact with the eye, or via systemic absorption. Discoloration by silver, known as argyrosis or argyria, is discussed here.

At least eighty original articles have been published describing argyrosis of the eye either from local contact with silver compounds or from systemic absorption of silver or its compounds. An extensive review of the literature on ocular argyrosis both from local and systemic routes was prepared in 1953 by Velhagen.[v]

In ocular argyrosis, the conjunctiva has grayish discoloration which is apparent without use of magnification. In the cornea, discoloration is observable with a slit-lamp biomicroscope, consisting most commonly of light gray or gray-blue mottled appearance in Descement's membrane, sometimes forming a peripheral ring diminishing in intensity toward the corneal axis. Typically, a thin clear rim is left outside the ring of discoloration in Descemet's membrane.[d] Gonioscopy in several patients with ocular argyrosis has shown no abnormal pigmentation in the corneoscleral trabecular meshwork.[d, 81]

With argyrosis of great intensity, a mottled blue-gray discoloration may be seen involving all layers of the corneal stroma, and from the posterior surface a bluish-green reflex or shagreen may be evident in reflected light. A good picture of ocular argyrosis in colors has been published as part of a report on thirty-one new cases occurring industrially from handling silver bromide and silver nitrate in manufacture of photographic film.[q]

In rare instances greenish iridescent discoloration under the anterior lens capsule has been observed with the slit-lamp biomicroscope in argyrosis.[c,i,l,r] In one instance linear opacites were described in both lenses of a man who had argyrosis of the cornea and skin. The opacities had an iridescent appearance with golden tint. They were located axially in the adult nucleus but did not impair visual acuity.[a]

Very rarely, the vitreous humor has been described as containing fine light-green glistening dots, and superficial layers of the retina have been reported to show a delicate blue-green veiling, but without disturbance of visual acuity, and the nature of the discoloration is uncertain.[i,l]

In a single instance, ocular argyrosis has been considered a possible cause of glaucoma,[g] but glaucoma has not been present in other cases, and no good reason has been presented for supposing it to cause glaucoma.

Diffuse ocular argyrosis has resulted from habitual application of silver-containing medications such as *silver proteinates* (Argyrol, Protargol) to the conjunctival sac during many years, and involves cornea, conjunctiva, tear sac, and eyelids.[e,j,x] Ocular argyrosis apparently has also been produced by accidental contamination with silver compounds on the fingers from habitual rubbing of the eyes.[h] Prolonged use of eyelash dyes containing silver compounds, such as *silver lactate,* can produce argyrosis of the cornea.[w] The same kind of argyrosis is produced by chronic systemic absorption of silver, except that in the latter the skin and mucous membranes of the whole body show blue-gray discoloration.

Generalized argyrosis from industrial absorption of dusts of silver compounds and of silver metal has been reported in numerous cases.[b,d,m,p,q,s,153,176]

Discoloration of Descemet's membrane by silver has been said to be the most sensitive indicator of chronic exposure to silver,[i,p] and the suggestion has been made that silver workers be examined routinely with a slitlamp biomicroscope for early detection of argyrosis before other manifestations become evident.[d] However, others have reported that the initial signs of occupational argyrosis were more likely to appear in the conjunctiva than in the cornea.[m,q]

Since no disturbance of ocular functions has been reliably attributable to argyrosis, it appears that early detection would be of concern primarily to avoid the cosmetically unattractive effects of excessive deposition of silver in eyes and skin.

Several histologic studies on eyes from patients with ocular argyrosis have been published. In a patient who had ingested silver proteinate for years, Spencer reported the highest concentration of silver deposit to be in Bruch's membrane, in Descemet's membrane, and in the basement membrane of conjunctival epithelium.[t] None was found in the trabecular meshwork, probably due to the fact that the trabecular meshwork does not have a component analogous to Bruch's or Descemet's membranes. No signs of cellular injury were found around even the densest deposits. A high concentration of sulfur was found associated with deposited silver, which could be explained by deposition as silver sulfide. A study of Hanna of eyes with deposits from prolonged topical administration showed extracellular deposition in the cornea, limited to Descemet's membrane, but in the conjunctiva silver was located intracellularly in connective tissue.[f] Light microscopy had shown silver associated with elastic fibers.[r] In the conjunctiva it had been found in phagocytes, and between the endothelial and perivascular cells of capillaries.[k,r]

Ocular argyrosis has been reproduced experimentally in the eyes of rats by chronic oral administration of silver. Attempts to relieve the argyrosis by treatment with dimercaprol have been unsuccessful.[n,o]

The most successful treatment for argyrosis of the skin, described in 1929 by Stillians and Lawless, is also effective in treatment of cosmetically objectionable argyrosis of the conjunctiva.[u] A sterile solution containing 6% sodium thiosulfate and 0.25% potassium ferricyanide, prepared within half an hour of use, can be injected into the skin to solubilize and remove the dark deposits of silver. (Solutions of 12% sodium thiosulfate and 0.5% potassium ferricyanide prepared separately are more stable, and can be mixed in equal quantities just before use to provide the appropriate solution.) The same solution has been injected subconjunctivally and has been observed to remove the gray discoloration of argyrosis without causing inflammation or injury. The solution may also be dropped in the conjunctival sac without causing irritation, but applied in this way it acts much more slowly than when injected. I have applied the solution to a denuded human cornea for seven minutes and found it not to be injurious.

On the cornea the solution has been used to remove discoloration from the anterior layers of the stroma caused by localized contact with strong silver nitrate, and has been very effective for this purpose, as described under the heading *Silver nitrate.* The treatment has not been observed to alter the discoloration present in the deepest layers of the cornea. There is, of course, no need to treat the argyrosis of the deeper layers of the cornea, since it is harmless and does not interfere with vision.

a. Bartlett RE: Generalized argyrosis with lens involvement. *AM J OPHTHALMOL* 38:402–403, 1954.
b. Bischler V: Thoughts on metallic impregnations of the cornea in relation to a case of occupational argyrosis. *OPHTHALMOLOGICA* 103:281–295, 1942. (French)
c. Bryk E: Generalized argyrosis with involvement of lenses. *KLIN OCZNA* 26:217–219, 1956.
d. Buttner-Wobst W, Opitz H: Corneal changes in the eyes of workers in the silver industry. *ARCH GEWERBEPATHOL* 13:374–381, 1954. (German)
e. Gutman FA, Crosswell HH, Jr: Argyrosis of the cornea without clinical conjunctival involvement. *AM J OPHTHALMOL* 65:183–187, 1968.

f. Hanna C, Fraunfelder FT, Sanchez J: Ultrastructural study of argyrosis of the cornea and conjunctiva. *ARCH OPHTHALMOL* 92:18–22, 1974.

g. Hua LP: Silver impregnation of the cornea and glaucoma in occupational argyrosis. *ARCH AUGENHEILKD* 102:334–338, 1930. (German)

h. Jensen SF: Argyrosis of conjunctiva in studio photographer. *ACTA OPHTHALMOL* 40:544–547, 1962.

i. Larsen B: On argyrosis of the cornea in silver nitrate workers. *GRAEFES ARCH OPHTHALMOL* 118:145–166, 1927. (German)

j. Lo Cascio G Jr: Findings with the corneal microscope in some cases of conjunctival argyrosis. *ARCH OTTALMOL* 64:229–236, 1960. (Italian)

k. McKee SH: Severe argyrosis of the conjunctiva. *CAN MED ASSOC J* 39:474, 1938.

l. Metzger: Occupational argyrosis of the eye. *KLIN MONATSBL AUGENHEILKD* 77:210, 1926. (German)

m. Moss AP, Sugar A et al: The ocular manifestations and functional effects of occupational argyrosis. *ARCH OPHTHALMOL* 97:906–908, 1979.

n. Olcott CT, Ricker WF: Experimental argyrosis. *SCIENCE* 105:67, 1947.

o. Olcott CT: Experimental argyrosis. *AM J PATHOL* 23:783–792, 1947.

p. Perrone S, Sarto F, Cardin P: Further observations on eight cases of occupational argyrosis with ocular involvement. *BOLL OCULIST* 59:621–630, 1980. (Italian)

q. Remler O: On occupational argyrosis in the photochemical industry. *KLIN MONATSBL AUGENHEILKD* 133:695–705, 1958. (German)

r. Rosen E: Argyrolentis. *AM J OPHTHALMOL* 33:787–800, 1950.

s. Schlappi V: A case of occupational argyrosis of the eye. *OPHTHALMOLOGICA* 137:214–217, 1959.

t. Spencer WH, Garron LK, et al: Endogenous and exogenous ocular and systemic silver deposition. *TRANS OPHTHALMOL SOC UK* 100:171–178, 1980.

u. Stillians AW, Lawless TK: The intradermal treatment of argyria. *J AM MED ASSOC* 92:20–21, 1929.

v. Velhagen K: On argyrosis of the cornea. *KLIN MONATSBL AUGENHEILKD* 122:36–42, 1953. (German)

w. Weiler HH, Lemp MA, et al: Argyria of the cornea due to self-administration of eyelash dye. *ANN OPHTHALMOL* 14:822–823, 1982.

x. Yanoff M, Scheic HG: Argyrosis of the conjunctiva and lacrimal sac. *ARCH OPHTHALMOL* 72:57–58, 1964.

Silver ammonium compounds are complex salts formed by reaction of soluble silver salts such as the nitrate, sulfate, or lactate, with ammonium hydroxide. They are employed in chemical processes such as silvering of mirrors. These solutions are more injurious to the eye than solutions of simple silver salts, presumably owing to the action of the strongly alkaline ammonium hydroxide.[a]

A detailed report has been made of two newborn babies who accidentally in place of regular 1% silver nitrate eyedrops had received drops of 25% to 35% ammoniacal silver nitrate solution, a dental caustic.[b] The damage was severe, the corneas were permanently opacified and the lids deformed by scarring.

a. Calvery HO, Lightbody HD, Rones B: Effects of some silver salts on the eyes. *ARCH OPHTHALMOL* 25:839–847, 1941.

b. Giffin RB Jr: Eye damage in newborns from use of strong silver nitrate solutions. *CALIF MED* 107:178–181, 1967.

Silver metal in the rabbit anterior chamber causes little reaction, and in the vitreous body induces no clinically evident inflammation, but atrophic changes in the retina have been found by microscopic examination.[150] In the cornea, silver particles become ensheathed in a connective tissue coating, and the surface is discolored by gray-white material assumed to be silver chloride, and also by black material assumed to be silver sulfide.[a]

> a. Heubner W: On the conversion of silver in the cornea. *SCI FARMACOL* (SUPPL 6):555–560, 1937. (Italian)

Silver nitrate danger to the eye depends greatly upon its concentration. At one extreme, a 1% solution has been applied almost routinely to newborn infants' eyes for prophylaxis of ophthalmia neonatorum. At the other extreme, solid silver nitrate, known as *lunar caustic,* can be very injurious to the eye.

In prophylaxis of ophthalmia neonatorum, single application of 1% silver nitrate eyedrops to the eyes of the newborn has periodically been discussed and reviewed. Critical examination of earlier literature in which 1% silver nitrate had been alleged in rare instances to have caused damage to the eyes has shown that these allegations were inadequately documented and provided no conclusive evidence that the solutions that were blamed were actually 1% concentration of silver nitrate. There seems to be no case in which permanent damage to the eye was actually proved to have been caused by a single application of 1% silver nitrate. A critical review by Barsam in 1966 is particularly noteworthy, and several other reviews and extensive clinical studies support the same conclusion.[a,b,k,n,s]

A few instances in which damage to the eyes has occurred in newborn babies from application of what was intended to be 1% silver nitrate have had explanations on the basis of use of more concentrated materials by mistake. (e.g. see *Silver ammonium compounds.*)

One infant received severe burns from use of a silver nitrate stick in place of the 1% solution.[j]

Concentrations of silver nitrate from 5% to 50% applied by mistake or accidentally splashed in the eye have caused severe injury, with permanent corneal opacification in some cases. Several references to injuries of this sort have been collected by Duke-Elder,[46] and several others have been reported.[j,q,t,34,153,249,253]

Characteristically, solutions of high concentration cause rapid appearance of edema of the conjunctivae and lids, with bloody purulent discharge from the conjunctival sac. Opacification of the cornea may result and may be permanent, but in eyes which have been contaminated with very small amounts of solution the results have been less disastrous. In cases of moderate injury, despite initial ground-glass or blue-gray appearance of the cornea, sufficient to obscure the pupil, the corneas have occasionally cleared spontaneously.[34,46,153]

Particles of solid silver nitrate in the conjunctival sac have been known to cause severe inflammation with deep injury to surrounding tissues, scarring, and symblepharon.[153] In a most unusual case of severe injury from solid nitrate described in 1891 by vonHipple, the cornea became dark brown, and the lens became cataractous.[153]

In a less dramatic but effectively treated case, a young man had been treated for corneal ulcer, probably caused by herpes simplex, by cauterization with solid silver nitrate. As a result, he had a solid white plaque in the treated area on the surface of the cornea for three to four days, but this gradually changed to dark brown, and three to four weeks later was accompanied by a blue-green discoloration of Descemet's membrane. This discoloration was most intense nearest to the plaque at the corneal vertex, diminishing in intensity peripherally. The anterior plaque of brown discoloration was removed completely by applying to it a cotton swab soaked in a mixture of potassium ferricyanide and sodium thiosulfate. The anterior discoloration was gone in seven minutes, but the coloration of Descemet's membrane was unchanged.[81] (See *Silver* for details of treatment solutions.)

Several patients have been seen in whom severe corneal injury has been produced when solid silver nitrate was used to cauterize a chalazion or conjunctival lesion. In one of the cases I have known of, a residue of the chemical in a cauterized chalazion in contact with the cornea caused loss of epithelium and two white opaque areas in the cornea. Without specific treatment the patient's cornea cleared sufficiently to restore normal vision in two months, and at that time only a green sheen persisted in the posterior layers of the cornea.[81]

In another patient, two days after the conjunctival surface of the upper lid of one eye was treated with a solid silver nitrate bead for questionable vernal conjunctivitis, much of the corneal epithelium was missing and the lower two-thirds of the cornea showed wrinkling of Descemet's membrane, fine punctate infiltration of stroma, and a dense gray opacification near the lower limbus, but no recognizable color in the cornea. It was not until about four days after the exposure that the characteristic blue discoloration of silver became recognizable in the deepest portions of the corneal strome. Healing was very slow, with wrinkling of the posterior surface and corneal edema gradually becoming less, and the epithelium healing very poorly. Even after two months there was reported still to be a defect in the epithelium in the palpebral fissure, and persistent blue discoloration deep in the stroma.

The most severe case of corneal injury from cauterization of a chalazion with solid silver nitrate has been reported by Grayson and Pieroni. Their patient had dense opacification and cataract, requiring corneal transplantation and lens extraction. Histologic examination showed silver still present in the tissue five years after the injury.[g]

The effects of applying solid silver nitrate to rabbit eyes has been extensively investigated. In one series of studies by Grawitz, involving 1,500 experiments and over 230 experimental modifications, special attention was given to corneal damage occurring in six to twenty-four hours following application of solid silver nitrate for ten seconds to the vertex of the cornea, with particular interest in the histologic changes and the inflammatory reaction at the limbus.[f]

Cauterization of the cornea of animals with concentrated solution or solid beads of silver nitrate has been used many times as a means for injuring the cornea for study of mechanisms of inflammatory reaction, vascularization, permeability, and healing processes since Hoffmann's studies on hypopyon in 1885.[c,d,e,i,o,r]

In attempts to induce glaucoma in rabbits, Luntz has injected 0.175% silver nitrate solution subconjunctivally, but found that it caused excessive local reaction to be of use for this purpose.[1]

Dose-response studies on the effect of various concentrations of silver nitrate have been reported after topical ocular applications to rabbits[322,324] and to monkeys.[322] Effects on the dog eye have been described.[p]

After chronic oral administration to rats, electronmicroscopy showed silver deposits in Bruch's membrane and in the basement membranes of the choriocapillaris and cilliary processes.[m]

Ingestion of silver nitrate repeatedly in small quantities over long periods has caused diffuse argyrosis involving the eyes and other tissues, but there appears to have been no well-established case of disturbance of vision from systemically absorbed silver.

Experimentally, a light gray cat which was poisoned by administration of 3 g of silver nitrate by stomach tube is said two days later to have had transient blindness with swelling of the optic nerveheads and dilation of retinal vessels.[h,153] The pigmentation of the fundus then resembled that of a black cat.

a. Allen JH, Barrere L: Prophylaxis of gonorrheal ophthalmia of the newborn. *J AM MED ASSOC* 162–177, 1949.

b. Barsam PC: Current concepts: Specific prophylaxis of gonorrheal ophthalmic neonatorum. *N ENGL J MED* 274(13):731–734, 1966.

c. Brown J, Soderstrom CW, Winkelmann RK: Langerhans' cells in guinea pig cornea: Response to chemical injury. *INVEST OPHTHALMOL* 7:668–671, 1968.

d. Faure JP, Graf B, et al: Microscopic study of an inflammatory reaction of the rabbit cornea. *ARCH OPHTALMOL (PARIS)* 30:39–56; 149–160; 575–588, 1970. (French)

e. Goren SB, Eisenstein R, Choromokos E: The inhibition of corneal vascularization in rabbits. *AM J OPHTHALMOL* 84:305–309, 1977.

f. Grawitz PB: Further contribution on the physiology of keratitis. *GRAEFES ARCH OPHTHALMOL* 159:459–485, 1958. (German)

g. Grayson M, Pieroni D: Severe silver nitrate injury to the eye. *AM J OPHTHALMOL* 70:227–229, 1970.

h. Harnack E: Toxicologic observations. *BER KLIN WOCHENSCHR* 47:1137–1140, 1893. (German)

i. Hoffmann FW: On keratitis and the development of hypopyon. *BER OPHTHALMOL GES HEIDELBERG* 17:67–80, 1885. (German)

j. Hornblass A: Severe silver nitrate ocular damage in newborn nursery. *NY STATE J MED* 76:1875–1878, 1976.

k. Kaivonen M: Prophylaxis of ophthalmia neonatorum. *ACTA OPHTHALMOLOGICA SUPPL* 79, 1965.

l. Luntz MH: Experimental glaucoma in the rabbit. *AM J OPHTHALMOL* 61:665–680, 1966.

m. Matuk Y, Ghosh M, McCullock C: Distribution of silver in the eyes and plasma proteins of the albino rat. *CAN J OPHTHALMOL* 16:145–150, 1981.

n. Mellin GW: Ophthalmia neonatorum, yesterday, today and tomorrow. *SIGHT SAVING REV* 31:102–113, 1961.

o. Reed JW, Fromer C, Klintworth GK: Induced corneal vascularization remission with argon laser therapy. *ARCH OPHTHALMOL* 93:1017–1019, 1975.

p. Rubin LF, et al: Silver nitrate burn of the dog cornea. *J AM VET MED ASSOC* 155:134–135, 1969.

q. Seggern V: Corneal burns with perchloric acid and silver nitrate. *KLIN MONATSBL AUGENHEILKD* 74:778, 1925. (German)

r. Szalay J, Pappas GD: Fine structure of rat corneal vessels in advanced stages of wound healing. *INVEST OPHTHALMOL* 9:354–365, 1970.

s. Thygeson P: Ophthalmia neonatorum. *J AM MED ASSOC* 201:902, 1967.

t. Vergne J: Severe ocular lesions from instillation of a solution of silver nitrate. *BULL SOC FR OPHTALMOL* 38:330–333, 1925. (French)

Silver (II) oxide (AgO) is a charcoal gray powder, having very strong oxidizing properties and said to be highly irritating to the skin, eyes, and respiratory tract.[171]

Sisomicin, an antibacterial related to gentamicin, has been found well tolerated by rabbit eyes when administered as eyedrops or by subconjunctival injection.[a]

a. Mester U, Krasemann C, Stein HJ: Experimental studies on local use of sisomicin on the eye. *KLIN MONATSBL ANGENHEILKD* 173:359–363, 1978. (German).

Skunk (*Mammalia mephitis*) is a common mammal of North America which can eject from its perineal glands a secretion having a characteristic and highly offensive odor. No recorded description of the effects of this secretion in contact with the eyes was found, but several owners of dogs have told of observing a severely irritating and damaging reaction in the eyes of their dogs. Veterinarians who have been questioned about this have corroborated the observation from their own experience, but have been unaware of descriptions in veterinary or canine literature. It appears that skunk scent sprayed into the eyes of dogs induces conjunctivitis, and in more severe cases causes the corneas to become opaque and vascularized. Purportedly irritation may be so persistent and distressing that it is necessary to kill the animal.

A man who said he was sprayed by a skunk from a distance of about five feet and felt droplets hit his face and his eyes experienced such smarting sensation in his eyes that he found it difficult to open them for five or ten minutes, but he then drove to the hospital unaided. When seen within an hour or two of the incident, he was still having discomfort consisting of burning sensation, but not pain as from a foreign body. In his corneas a very faint haze and only very slight diffuse staining of the epithelium by fluorescein was detectable. By the next day the eyes had returned entirely to normal without special treatment.[a]

The substances in skunk scent which may be responsible for irritation and injury of the eye have not been determined, but the odor is accounted for by alkyl mercaptans and disulfides (*crotyl mercaptan, isopentyl mercaptan, methyl crotyl disulfide*) known to be present.[b,c] In general, alkyl mercaptans are not especially damaging to the cornea, but among the disulfides, diallyl disulfide is notoriously lacrimatory.

a. Houle RE: Personal communication, Nov. 1962.
b. Maugh TH II: Skunks; on the scent of a myth. *SCIENCE* 185:1146, 1974.
c. Stevens PG: American musk. III. The scent of common skunk. *J AM CHEM SOC* 67:407–408, 1945.

Slag, basic, a substance sometimes used as fertilizer, is said to contain calcium hydroxide and to have caused caustic injuries of the eye.[46] (See *Calcium hydroxide*.)

Slate, in the form of a slate pencil, proved to be an inert intraorbital foreign body for 39 years after it entered a child's orbit through the inferior cul-de-sac.[a] (However, apparently the eye was blind from the time of the accident.)

a. Mawas ME, Tremoulet O, Desbordes J: Account of an intraorbital slate pencil. *BULL SOC OPHTALMOL FRANCE* 71:528–532, 1971. (French)

Smog, a form of artificial pollution of the atmosphere, produces atmospheric haze and irritation of the eyes and respiratory tract. Irritation of the eyes has received much attention because the irritation is an unpleasant nuisance and it is the effect most commonly experienced by human beings. It is often objectionable at concentrations below those causing respiratory disturbances.[c,l] The smog of Los Angeles has received particular attention because of its notorious irritancy to the eyes, causing stinging discomfort, associated with lacrimation and conjunctival hyperemia, but no injury. The intensity of eye irritation tended to parallel a rise in concentration of oxidizing substances in the air, both reaching a maximum in the middle of the day. However, later in the day the concentration of oxidants was found to decrease more rapidly than the irritation. The irritation has seemed not to be caused by the oxidants themselves.[j,w,x,za]

Considerable information has been obtained from detailed analyses of smog atmosphere and extensive testing of synthetic smogs on human volunteers. The opinion has been widely held that the eye irritation is caused by products of a reaction promoted by sunlight, involving oxides of nitrogen and unsaturated hydrocarbons in the atmosphere.[j,w,x] The hydrocarbons are believed to come mainly from automobile exhaust.

Among the products of the reaction that have been recognized are ozone, aldehydes, and organic peroxides. The formation of ozone accounts for most of the increase in oxidizing capacity of Los Angeles smog, but the concentration of ozone does not become great enough to cause irritation of the eyes. It was at one time suspected that the ocular discomfort was caused mainly by formaldehyde, acrolein, and peroxyacetyl nitrate, because these were the first substances found which, when tested in pure form in concentrations such as found in smog, produced eye irritation of the same type and intensity as natural smog.

Sulfur dioxide and sulfur trioxide have been identified in Los Angeles smog, but only at concentrations too low to be lacrimatory (always less than 0.3 ppm).[j] Sulfur dioxide has been implicated in formation of aerosols which account for some of the optical haze of smog. However, sulfur dioxide added experimentally at a concentration of 0.1 ppm to artificial photochemical smog mixtures was found by Doyle and associates actually to reduce the eye irritancies slightly.[h]

The possibility has also been investigated that adsorption of irritant products of the photochemical reaction on dust particles or condensation in aerosols might enhance irritant effects on the eye.[e,g] Experiments have provided varying results, and opinions differ on their significance, but the majority opinion has seemed to discount the role of particles or aerosols in ocular irritation by smog.[e,j]

Several systematic and comprehensive studies have been made of statistical relationships among the many components of automobile exhaust, the products of reaction in irradiated atmospheres and the degree of irritation to eyes of human volunteers.[d,l,m,r,110] Although no single factor, no single compound, has yet been identified as mainly responsible, according to Jaffe (1968) the total oxidant concentrations of the atmosphere correlates well with the degree of eye irritation from natural smog,[l] and studies by Heuss and Glasson have shown that the chemical structure of hydrocarbons involved in the formation of smog is particularly important in producing eye irritation.[110] They have found that benzylic hydrocarbons and aromatic olefins in the photochemical reaction that produces smog are particularly likely to produce eye irritant substances, yielding particularly peroxybenzoyl nitrate, which is reported to be two hundred times more effective than formaldehyde as a lacrimator.[110]

In the investigation by Heuss and Glasson of the degree of eye irritancy produced by exposing a series of hydrocarbons to photo-oxidation in vapor form in the presence of ozone and nitrogen dioxide, they found that the most irritating products were obtained from reaction of styrene, methylstyrene, allylbenzene, 1,3-butadiene, n-butylbenzene, isobutylbenzene, n-propylbenzene, and toluene.[110] Special studies of the photochemical reaction of *toluene* and *xylene* and the intensity of eye irritation produced by their products have been made by Altshuller and associates.[a] They have concluded that these compounds as well as propylene and trimethylbenzene are important potential contributors to eye irritancy of smog. However, subsequent studies make it seem unlikely that substituted peroxybenzoyl nitrates, such as from trimethyl benzene, do contribute significantly.[zb]

Apart from observations on peroxybenzoyl and peroxyacetyl nitrates, much attention has been given to aldehydes as components of smog with known irritant effects on the eyes. A review has been published particularly on the effects of acetaldehyde, acrolein, and formaldehyde.[f] Most investigators seem to have concluded that aldehydes may contribute only a minor portion of the irritating effectiveness of smog.[l,p,110] However, Schuck and associates investigating the responses of human eyes to low concentrations of formaldehyde in air found that most people experience the same sensation of eye irritation at a concentration of 0.05 ppm as at 0.5 ppm, and some sensed irritation at concentrations as low as 0.01 ppm, suggesting that the very low concentration found in natural smog might be enough to contribute significantly to the unpleasant sensation.[t,u]

The sensation of eye irritation produced by substances in smog is so subjective and variable and so readily affected by incidental factors such as rate of blinking, eye movement, and probably many other factors that quantitation of the irritant effect has been difficult[n,o,u] and has caused several investigators to attempt to find some kind of change in the cornea that could be correlated with irritancy to human eyes, but could be more objectively measured. It has been recognized that if some objectively measurable change in the cornea could be correlated with irritancy in human eyes, it would potentially have the additional advantage of allowing more meaningful use of experimental animals in place of human volunteers. A series of studies by Mettier, Hine, Boyer, and McEwen have been performed on rabbit eyes in this connection.[114,172,173] Testing specifically acrolein, nitrogen dioxide, ozone, and sulfur dioxide, as well as artifical smog and gasoline engine exhaust, they found that concentrations that produced obvious sensation of irritation of the eyes of the rabbits produced no discernible damage by ordinary inspection, nor any appreciable change in thickness of the cornea, rate of repair of standard artifical wounds of the corneal epithelium, or activity of several enzymes of the corneal epithelium (G6-PDH, 6-PGDH, LDH, MDH). While no damage to the eye from smog has been shown, two changes, besides familiar increased tearing, hyperemia, and blinking, are a reduced concentration of lysozyme in the tears,[r,s,zc,zd] and a decrease in the pH of the tears.[zc,zd]

Actual disease or injury of the eye has almost never been attributed to city smog. However, in one report it was claimed that a policeman had follicular conjunctivitis and recurrent keratitis caused by fumes from automobile traffic, and that when he was removed from these surroundings he was cured.[v]

Smoke in some respects resembles smog, containing unidentified substances which may cause intense discomfort of the eyes and lacrimation, but these substances may either be more toxic or more concentrated than the irritants in smog, because occasionally smoke or fumes from fires cause superficial transitory keratitis.[i,o]

Medical treatment of ocular irritation from city smog is nonspecific and unsatisfactory. Topical vasoconstrictors and corticosteroids have been employed with some relief of conjunctival hyperemia and discomfort, but not without risk of inducing other problems. In treatment of patients having acute irritation from smog, smoke, or fumes, it is strongly advisable that repeated use of local anesthetics and corticosteroids be avoided. (See *Anesthetics, local* and *Corticosteroids.*) The most logical approach has been to attempt to prevent smog by reducing the air pollution which causes it.

a. Altshuller AP, Kopczynski SL, et al: Photochemical reactivities of aromatic hydrocarbon-nitrogen oxide and related systems. *ENVIRON SCI TECHNOL* 4:44–49, 1970.
c. Battigelli MC: Effects of diesel exhaust. *ARCH ENVIRON HEALTH* 10:165–167, 1965.
d. Buchberg H, Wilson KW, et al: Interacting atmospheric variables and eye irritation thresholds. *AIR WATER POLLUTION* 7:257–280, 1963.
e. Cadle RD, Magill BL: Study of eye irritation caused by Los Angeles smog. *ARCH INDUST HYG* 4:74, 1951.
f. Community Air Quality Guides: Aldehydes. *AM IND HYG ASSOC J* 29:505–512, 1968.
g. Dautrebande L, Shaver J, et al: Influence of particulate matter on the eye irritation produced by volatile irritants and importance of particle size in connection with atmospheric pollution. *ARCH INTERN PHARMACODYN* 84:1–47, 1950.
h. Doyle GJ, Endow N, Jones JL: Sulfur dioxide role in eye irritation. *ARCH ENVIRON HEALTH* 3:657–666, 1961.
i. Glees M: Clinical picture of smoke damage to the eye. *KLIN MONATSBL AUGEN-HEILKD* 113:43–44, 1948.
j. Haagen-Smit AJ: Atmospheric reactions of air pollutants. *IND ENG CHEM* 48:65A–70A, 1958.
l. Jaffe LS: Photochemical air pollutants and their effects on men and animals. *ARCH ENVIRON HEALTH* 16:241–255, 1968.
m. Nicksic SW, Harkins J, Painter LJ: Statistical survey data relating to hydrocarbon and oxides of nitrogen relations in photochemical smog. *AIR WATER POLLUTION* 10:15–23, 1966.
n. Orcutt JA: The quantal response in environmental toxicology. *J AM OSTEOPATH ASSOC* 66:1376–1383, 1967.

o. Orcutt JA: The quantal response in environmental toxicology. *J AM OSTEOPATH ASSOC* 66:1383–1385, 1967.

p. Renzatti NA, Bryan RJ: Atmospheric sampling for aldehydes and eye irritation in Los Angeles smog-1960. *J AIR POLLUT CONTROL ASSOC* 11:421–427, 1961.

r. Sapse AT, Bonavida B, et al: Human tear Lysozyme III. Preliminary study on lysozyme levels in subjects with smog eye irritation. *AM J OPHTHALMOL* 66:76–80, 1968.

s. Sapse AT, Bonavida B, et al: Smog eye irritation: effect of air pollution on the tear protein pattern. *OPHTHALMOLOGICA ADDIT AD* 158:421–427, 1969.

t. Schuck EA, Cranz FW, et al: Eye irritation in photo-oxidized mixtures of olefins and oxide of nitrogen. *AM CHEM SOC DIV WATER WASTE CHEM PREPRINTS,* 1963, pp. 299–306.

u. Schuck EA, Stephens ER, Middleton JT: Eye irritation response at low concentrations of irritants. *ARCH ENVIRON HEALTH* 13:570–575, 1966.

v. Sedan J, Sedan Bauby S: Conjunctival reactions from combustion products of gas and oil emitted by trucks on public ways. *ANN OCULIST* (*Paris*) 184:168, 1951. (French)

w. Shortridge RW, Morriss FV, et al: Studies on smog produced in irradiated reaction chambers. *AM IND HYG ASSOC J* 19:213–217, 1958.

x. Wayne LG, Orcutt JA: Common organic solvents as precursors of eye irritants in urban atmospheres. *J OCCUP MED* 2:383–388, 1960.

za. Basu PK: Air pollution and the eye. *SURV OPHTHALMOL* 17:78–93, 1972.

zb. Glasson WA, Heuss JM: Synthesis and evaluation of potential atmospheric eye irritants. *EVNIRON SCI TECHNOL* 11:395–398, 1977.

zc. Okawada N, Iwamura Y, et al: Effects of photochemical smog on the human eye. *FOLIA OPHTHALMOL JPN* 28:561, 1977. (English summary)

zd. Shimizu K, Ishikawa S, et al: Effects of photochemical smog on the human eye. *JPN J OPHTHALMOL* 23:174–184, 1979.

Snake venon from spitting cobras causes injury through external contact with the eyes, while venoms injected by poisonous snake bites cause eye disturbances through systemic absorption.

Effects of external contact will be summarized first. The black-necked spitting cobra, *Naja nigricollis,* has been described in a number of reports, mostly from West Africa, of being capable of squirting venom at the eyes of an intruder, not uncommonly over a distance of 2 or 3 meters.[c,g,j,p,s,u,y] When the venon strikes the eye it causes immediate pain, blepharospasm, and watering of the eyes. Typically when the patient is first examined there is conjunctival hyperemia and corneal edema, and there may be loss of corneal epithelium.[c] The severity of injury presumably relates to the amount of venon that strikes the eye, but case reports suggest that the outcome may also be affected by complicating factors, such as secondary infection. There is no evidence of systemic poisoning. Most accounts indicate that with simple treatment, commonly with antibiotic eyedrops, the eyes may recover in 2 or 3 days, but sometimes may take a week or two if corneal edema is severe at the onset. However, there are a small number of cases in which corneal ulceration, hypopyon, perforation, and corneal scarring have resulted, with loss of vision.[p,y] These seem to have been cases in which the patients neglected the condition of their eye while complications were developing. Such serious consequences do not seem to have been observed in patients who were under reasonably close medical supervision until their eyes healed. There is no specific treatment, and antivenom has not been demonstrated to be effective in treatment of the eyes.[y] Whether there are species differences in vulnerability seems not to have been investigated, but one report indicates that in dogs injury from spitting cobra venom has regularly resulted in blindness.[t]

Systemic poisoning with eye involvement can be produced by the bites of three families of snakes, the *Elapidae* (elapids), the *Hydrophiidae* (sea snakes), and the *Viperidae* (vipers), according to an instructive synopsis by Campbell.[d] The eye manifestations are most commonly reversible paralysis of the extraocular muscles, less commonly transient loss of vision, and rarely retinal hemorrhage, but the tendency to produce these effects varies greatly among the different families of snakes. The characteristic reported ocular effects will be described for each of the families, elapid snakes, sea snakes, and vipers.

Elapid snakes include all the poisonous snakes of Australia and New Guinea, tiger snakes, taipans, cobras of Asia and Africa, mambas of Africa, kraits of Southern Asia, and coral snakes of America.[d] Their venom contains a neurotoxin which kills by inducing paralysis. Pre-paralysis there have been instances of temporary loss of vision for a half to two hours, of undefined mechanism.[v,w,x,y] According to Campbell's first-hand observation of poisonings by Australian snakes, signs of paralysis appear first in the extraocular muscles, with ptosis, restriction of eye movements, sometimes diplopia, and eventually complete external ophthalmoplegia.[d] This may be accompanied by paralysis of jaws, tongue, and pharynx, and, most seriously, paralysis of respiration. Similar effects have been reported from cobra bites. Typically paralysis of extraocular muscles lasts two days, and recovers over the next two to five days.[d] Treatment with antivenom is effective.[d,q]

Sea snakes of warm waters of Indian and Pacific Oceans have a very potent venom that acts on the neuromuscular system, causing pain and general paralysis of body muscles. Ptosis and restriction of eye movement are a relatively minor part of the picture.[r] Antivenom is effective, but death may occur from a combination of respiratory failure, hyperkalemia, and renal failure.[d]

Vipers include pit vipers, rattlesnakes, and berg adders, which have venoms that generally have limited paralytic effects. These may be limited to transitory internal and external ophthalmoplegia.[f,h,n,o,z] In rare instances temporary loss of vision has been reported.[b]

Blatt described how a *Viper berus* bit a woman on the foot, and one-half hour later she experienced dimming of vision, drooping of her eyelids, and severe diarrhea. At twenty-four hours she had complete paralytic ptosis of both upper lids, wide mydriasis and complete cycloplegia (without response to light or accommodation), but normal visual acuity, normal fundi, media, and eye movements. From the fourth to the sixth days there was gradual improvement; first the pupil and then accommodation recovered, then the ptosis. Recovery was complete.[b]

The viper family of snakes has apparently been the only one held responsible for retinal hemorrhages and optic neuropathy, and accounts of these have been rare.

Guttmann-Friedmann described how a young man bitten on the leg by *Vipera lebetina gray* developed extensive hemorrhagic reactions with hemoglobin dropping to 4.5 g/100 ml. Visual loss was first noted on the sixth day, reduced to finger counting. Papilledema and many hemorrhages in the fundi were observed, diagnosed as bilateral optic neuritis. Partial bilateral optic atrophy with permanently severely impaired vision resulted. The author believed this was secondary to hemorrhaging rather than due to the toxin or the antivenin that was given.[i]

Rattlesnake bite has caused retinal hemorrhage.[l] Bites of other snakes not completely identified have caused in one case bilateral branch occlusions of retinal arteries and optic atrophy,[e] and in another reduction of visual acuity with persistent concentric contraction of visual fields.[j]

Antivenin serum administered in treatment of a bite by a nonpoisonous snake has been responsible for an unusual instance of transient papillitis and clouding of the lens, ascribed to allergy.[k]

Alvaro has recounted many instances of involvement of eyes or of vision in people bitten by South American poisonous snakes. Most were in the form of personal communications from many observers and were brief and rather superficial. Also Alvaro described a series of original experiments giving various venoms to rabbits, either parenterally or locally, and observing what happened in the eyes, but they were too variegated to abstract or generalize upon. Alvaro gave no summary or organized conclusions.[a]

In one bizarre case infarction of the orbit and loss of the eye followed a bite on the eyebrow by an unidentified snake, the venom presumably having been injected into an orbital vein.[m]

a. Alvaro ME: Snake venom in ophthalmology. *AM J OPHTHALMOL* 22:1130–1146, 1939.
b. Blatt N: On the casuistry of eye disturbances in poisoning by snake bite. *Z AUGEN-HEILKD* 49:280–282, 1922. (German)
c. Brown CJ: Ocular envenomization by the West African spitting cobra. *ANN OPHTHAL-MOL* 12:868–870, 1980.
d. Campbell CH: The effects of snake venoms and their neurotoxins of the nervous system of man and animals. *CONTEMP NEUROL SER* 12:259–293, 1975.
e. Davenport RC, Budden FH: Loss of sight following snake bite. *BR J OPHTHALMOL* 37:119, 1953.
f. Ferrannini G: On a case of partial ophthalmoplegia from a viper bite. *MIN OFTALMOL* 12:62–64, 1970. (Italian)
g. Gilkes MJ: Snake venom conjunctivitis. *BR J OPHTHALMOL* 43:638–639, 1959.
h. Gomes B: External ophthalmoplegia from crotal (snake) poison. *OPHTHALMOS* 3:187–194, 1943.
i. Guttmann-Friedmann A: Blindness after snakebite. *BR J OPHTHALMOL* 40:57–59, 1956.
j. Khalil M: Snake bite. *BULL OPHTHALMOL SOC EGYPT* 51:687–695, 1958.
k. Mathur SP: Allergy to antivenine serum. *BR J OPHTHALMOL* 43:50–51, 1959.
l. McLane J: Retinal hemorrhage in case of rattlesnake bite. *J FLORIDA MED ASSOC* 30:22–25, 1943.

m. Mechain M, Rolland A: Note on a case of venomous infarction of the orbit. *REV INT TRACK* 51:43–44, 1974. (French)

n. Montgomery J: Two cases of ophthalmoplegia due to Berg adder bite. *CENTRAL AFRICA J MED* 5:173, 1959.

o. Orsini J: Ocular effects of snake venom. *ARCH OTTALMOL* 56:285, 1952. (Italian)

p. Payne T, Warrell DA: Effects of venom in eye from spitting cobra. *ARCH OPHTHALMOL* 94:1803, 1976.

q. Reid HA: Snakebite in the tropics. *BR MED J* 2:359–362, 1968.

r. Reid HA: Antivenom in sea-snake bite. *LANCET* 1:622–623, 1975.

s. Ridley H: Snake venom ophthalmia. *BR J OPHTHALMOL* 28:568, 1944.

t. Shattock FM: Injuries caused by wild animals. *LANCET* 1:412–415, 1968.

u. Sinka AK: Cobra-venon conjunctivitis. *LANCET* 1:1026, 1972.

v. Trinca JC, Graydon JJ, et al: The rough-scaled snake *Tropidechis carinatus*) a dangerously venomous Australian snake. *MED J AUST* 2:801–809, 1971.

w. Wall F: Fatal case of ophitoxaemia. *INDIAN MED GAZ* 49:253, 1914.

x. Wallace I: Effects of tiger snake bite. *VICT NAT* 70:227–228, 1954.

y. Warrell DA, Ormerod LD: Snake venom ophthalmia and blindness caused by the spitting cobra (*Naja nigricollis*) in Nigeria. *AM J TROP MED HYG* 25:525–529, 1976.

z. Zeppa R: A case of lid ptosis and mydriasis from viper bite. *ARCH OTTALMOL* 65:21–24, 1961. (Italian)

Snuff, finely powdered tobacco, when dusted in the eyes causes immediate irritation with blepharospasm and conjunctivitis, but apparently with no permanent aftereffect.[253]

Soap is usually a sodium salt of long-chain fatty acids, but soft or liquid soap may be based on potassium rather than sodium, and many other substances may be added.[171] Very few reports of injuries of human eyes by soaps have been published.[171] These injuries have been transient. Common experience with hand or household soaps in human eyes is that the stinging pain induced by contact with soap causes tearing and induces prompt efforts at cleansing the eye with water so that no lasting or significant injury results. An exception is met in commercial laundry soap having free alkali, sometimes at a pH of 12 or more. Such very strong soap, usually in gelatinous fluid form, has caused severe permanent corneal injury with opacification such as produced by sodium hydroxide.[81]

Experimental application of pure granulated white soap to rabbit eyes causes a moderately severe reaction, graded 8 on a scale of 1 to 10 after twenty-four hours.[27] However, if the rabbit is allowed to respond in a normal manner to the immediate discomfort from the soap, enough is eliminated by action of the lids, nictitating membrane, and tears so that conjunctival and corneal epithelial reaction is slight, and recovery is rapid.[81] Similarly 5% solution of soap causes transient mild conjunctival hyperemia and optical irregularity of the corneal epithelium if the exposure is brief. U.S.P. tincture of green soap tested on rabbit eyes has caused mild temporary injury, graded 5 on a scale of 1 to 10, after twenty-four hours.[27]

Comparisons of the reactions of eyes of rabbits, monkeys, and human beings to applications of a 5% soap solution have shown the effect on the human eye to be more closely paralleled by the monkey eye than by the rabbit eye.[a] The type of soap and its pH were not specified, but consistently 0.1 ml was applied to the eyes. The human volunteers were allowed to wash their eyes with water after one-half minute, but the animals were not irrigated. The human subjects showed mainly conjunctival hyperemia for six hours, and one had punctate superficial epithelial defects discernible by biomicroscope and fluorescein staining at fifteen minutes, but these disappeared by six hours. The monkeys showed loss of patches of corneal epithelium at twenty-four hours with fine stippling of the surface still present at three days. The rabbits showed only biomicroscopically visible corneal stippling at one hour and this was all gone in twenty-four hours.

In a systematic examination of the effects of coconut oil soap applied as granules or as a 10% slurry to the eyes of rabbits and monkeys W.R. Green et al judged these substances to be "corrosive" or "harmful" in most cases, but there was considerable variation among animals, and most eyes showed slight injury 21 days after exposure.[322]

A number of soaps and shampoos for human use induce corneal anesthesia in rabbits for several hours, but not in human beings.[b]

Many detergents are not true soaps, and some are much more injurious than soaps. (See INDEX for *Detergents* and *Surfactants* for further information.)

   a. Beckley JH, Russell TJ, Rubin LF: Use of the rhesus monkey for predicting human response to eye irritants. *TOXICOL APPL PHARMACOL* 15:1–9, 1969.
   b. Harris LS, Kahanowioz Y, Shimmyo M: Corneal anesthesia induced by soaps and surfactants, lack of correlation in rabbits. *OPHTHALMOLOGICA* 170:320–325, 1975.

Sodium acetate, tested on rabbit eyes as 0.1 M solution adjusted to pH 7.0 to 7.5 and made 0.46 osmolar with sodium chloride or sucrose, caused no disturbance of the cornea, though applied continuously for three hours.[209]

Sodium alginate (Alginon) is reported to have been injected into the vitreous body of rabbits and of patients with retinal detachment without notable toxic effect.[a]

   a. Mori S: Experimental study on the substitute of the vitreous body. *ACTA SOC OPHTHALMOL JPN* 71(1):22–26, 1967.

Sodium aluminate is strongly alkaline. It has caused injuries of the eyes similar to those caused by sodium hydroxide.[153,253]

Sodium azide, a salt of hydrazoic acid, inhibits respiration of bovine cornea, presumably by poisoning cytochrome exidase.[108] Applied to rabbits' eyes as 0.1 to 2% eyedrops it has caused a rise of 1 to 5 mm Hg in intraocular pressure acutely, lasting less than an hour, apparently due to increase in formation of aqueous humor, preventable by phenoxybenzamine.[c] Administered systemically to experimental animals sodium azide was noted by Noell in the 1950's to cause a rapid characteristic change in electrical potential across the retina. A review by Graymore points out that the visual cells could be destroyed by iodoacetate, despite which the electrical response to azide was preserved, and furthermore that the response to azide could be abolished by iodate without affecting the a- and b-waves of the ERG.[319] This and other evidence suggested that the site of action of azide was most likely the retinal pigment epithelium.

Experiments by Francois measuring the EOG and the c-wave of the ERG led to the same conclusion.[a] Studies on electrical activity of isolated retina have shown, however, that if the azide concentration is great enough, not only is the pigment epithelium affected, but the b-wave can be abolished,[e] and degeneration of rod cells is histologically demonstrable.[99]

Lesions also in the optic nerves and tracts have been reported in several rats surviving two or three days after being poisoned severely with azide.[b]

  a. Francois J, Jonsas C, DeRouck A: Experimental studies of the effect of sodium azide on the electroretinogram and the electrooculogram in rabbits. *AN INST BARRAQUER* 9:293–298, 1969.
  b. Hicks SP: Brain metabolism *in vivo. ARCH PATHOL* 50:535–561, 1950.
  c. Krupin T, Weiss A, et al: Increased intraocular pressure following topical azide or nitroprusside. *INVEST OPHTHALMOL VIS SCI* 16:1002–1007, 1977.
  d. Noell WK: Azide sensitive potential difference across the eye bulb. *AM J PHYSIOL* 170:217, 1952.
  e. Wundsch L, Lutzow A, Reuter JH: Effect of azide on the isolated mammalian retina. *PFLUG ARCH EUR J PHYSIOL* 356:237–244, 1975.

Sodium bicarbonate, tested on rabbit eyes by application of 0.1 M solution adjusted to pH 7.0 to 7.5 and made 0.46 osmolar with sodium chloride or sucrose, caused no disturbance of the cornea, though applied continuously for three hours.[209]

Sodium bisulfite is of interest in regard to ocular toxicity because it is present as an antioxidant in some eyedrops, and undoubtedly is one of the substances formed in association with burns of the eye from sulfur dioxide.

In a study of injury to the corneal endothelium by bisulfite-preserved epinephrine introduced into the anterior chamber, the endothelial surface of excised rabbit and monkey corneas was perfused for 3 hours with mock aqueous humor containing bisulfite, and comparisons were made with control corneas. Abnormal thickening of the corneas, endothelial cell swelling and collapse, and loss of the normal mosaic of cell borders occurred in corneas exposed to 0.1% and 0.08% solutions, but not in those exposed to 0.05%.[b]

In a study investigating the mechanism of injury of the cornea by sulfur dioxide, a 5.5 M solution of sodium bisulfite at its natural pH of 3.8 was dropped on the eyes of rabbits for 30 minutes. This caused severe conjunctival hyperemia and chemosis, grayness and irregularity of the corneal epithelium, and swelling and translucent opacity of the stroma. However, in 10 days the corneas cleared completely.[a]

(For comparative observations on *sodium sulfite* and *sulfur dioxide,* see INDEX.)

  a. Grant WM: Ocular injury due to sulfur dioxide. *ARCH OPHTHALMOL* 38:762–774, 1947.
  b. Hull DA, Chemotti MT, et al: Effect of epinephrine on the corneal endothelium. *AM J OPHTHALMOL* 79:245–250, 1975.

Sodium carbonate (soda ash, washing soda) is soluble in water, forming an alkaline solution with pH up to 11.6.[171] Such a solution is alkaline enough to injure the corneal epithelium, but if promptly washed from the eye with water it is unlikely to cause permanent damage to the corneal stroma. Application of several drops of 10% solution of sodium carbonate (pH 10.7) to a rabbit's eyes followed by irrigation with water in thirty seconds caused no injury detectable by inspection or by staining with fluorescein.[81] A 2% solution has been employed clinically in treatment of acid burns.[a]

Instances of permanent corneal opacification attributed to sodium carbonate, reported more than fifty years ago,[46] were caused not by the pure chemical at room temperature, or in aqueous solution, but by a splash of molten chemical at 820° C in one instance, and by a mixture containing calcium hydroxide, which is well known to be seriously injurious, in another instance.[253]

Dry, powdered sodium carbonate, as 25% to 75% of a mixture with dry sodium sulfate, applied to eyes of rabbits and monkeys in a systematic study by W.R. Green et al was judged "corrosive" or "harmful" to both species, whether or not followed by irrigation at two minutes after application. However, most monkey eyes exposed to 50% mixture showed little or no persistent injury 21 days after exposure.[322]

    a. Schwarz E: Observations on burns of the eye. *BEITR Z AUGENHEILK* VI;309–311, 1903. (German)

Sodium chloride at concentrations much above that in tears causes a stinging sensation on contact with the eye. Solutions up to 10% do not alter the permeability of the corneal epithelium, but solutions more dilute than 0.9% sodium chloride cause increased permeability.[c, 123] On rabbit eyes continuous irrigation for three hours with sodium chloride solutions from 0.3 to 0.6 M and pH 6.0 to 8.0 has produced no morphologic change in the corneas.[209]

Subconjunctival injection of hypertonic sodium chloride solutions has long been known to cause hyperemia and a transitory rise of intraocular pressure in rabbit and human eyes.[b]

Intracarotid injection of 2M sodium chloride solution in cats rapidly produces cataract on the same side.[d]

Many years ago it was alleged that eating too much table salt caused a variety of choroidal and retinal diseases, but this was simple speculation unsupported by scientific evidence.[a]

    a. Ewing AE: Sodium chlorid, a possible cause of some obscure diseases of the choroid and the retina. *AM J OPHTHALMOL* 31:193–198, 1914.
    b. Kollner H: On intraocular pressure in glaucoma simplex and its relationship to the circulation. *ARCH AUGENHEILK* 83:135–167, 1918.
    c. Maurice DM: Influence on corneal permeability of bathing with solutions of differing reaction and tonicity. *BR J OPHTHALMOL* 39:463–472, 1955.
    d. Chavira RA, Anguiano GL, et al: Acute experimental cataract from hypertonic saline solution. *AN SOC MEXIC OFTALMOL* 44:151–155, 1971.

Sodium chloroacetate (sodium monochloroacetate, Defolex), a chemical defoliant, has been noted in Garner's book on veterinary toxicology to be a hazard to the eye either in powder or concentrated solution,[64] reputedly causing "temporary corneal clouding and ulceration," but the origin of this information is uncertain. This suggests a similarity to sodium bromoacetate and iodoacetate, which are both toxic to the eye.

Sodium cyanurate has been tested on rabbit eyes because it is present in swimming pools in which chlorinated cyanurates are employed as disinfectants. Sodium cyanurate has been shown to cause no injury to the rabbit's eye when 0.1 ml of aqueous suspensions containing 0.8% to 8% were applied daily five days a week for three months.[a]

a. Hodge HC, Panner BJ, Downs WL, Maynard EA: Toxicity of sodium cyanurate. *TOXICOL APPL PHARMACOL* 7:667–674, 1965.

Sodium hexametaphosphate is the principal ingredient of water softeners such as *Calgon* and *Micromet.* These substances keep calcium, magnesium, and iron in solution. Tests of 0.1% and 5% solutions of *Calgon* on rabbit eyes indicate that a splash followed by irrigation with water should cause no serious injury. However, these solutions were found much too injurious to use for the purpose of removing calcium from the cornea. Irrigation of the surface of the eye for fifteen minutes after removal of the corneal epithelium caused chemosis and numerous hemorrhages in the conjunctiva and nictitating membrane, followed by corneal edema and hyperemia of the iris. The eyes generally recovered from this reaction and returned to normal within a week.[81]

Sodium hyaluronate (Etamucin; Healon; Healonid; HYVISC), an ophthalmic surgical aid, is a natural mucopolysaccharide present in vitreous humor, umbilical cord, synovial fluid, cock's comb, and many other tissues. In the eye it has been used as a replacement for vitreous humor, and has been placed in the anterior chamber as an aid to insertion of intraocular lenses. A synopsis by Balazs et al (1972) reviews the transitory ocular inflammatory reactions encountered with early preparations of relatively low molecular weight and low viscosity (e.g. Etamucin), compared with later high molecular weight, high viscosity and elasticity preparations (e.g. Healon-H from human umbilical cord, and Healon-A from rooster comb).[b] Transient inflammatory responses have been described even with the later preparations, though they have been said to be well-tolerated clinically.[f,g] In a small series of patients, more cells and blood clots were seen in the anterior chambers, and briefly higher pressures were found, in those in whom Healon was used during intraocular lens implantation.[d] In rabbit eyes the bursting strength of penetrating corneal wounds tested after 10 days was found to be unaffected by sodium hyaluronate placed in the anterior chamber.[a] In rabbit and monkey eyes, MacRae et al have found Healon to produce no corneal endothelial injury detectible by scanning or transmission electron microscopy, but it did cause a transient rise in intraocular pressure in early hours after injection into the anterior chamber.[349] In enucleated human eyes, perfusion measurements on the aqueous outflow system have shown increased resistance to outflow, which can be abolished by treatment with hyaluronidase.[c] This accounts for the considerable rises of intraocular pressure seen in patients, lasting for a day or more after introduction of sodium hyaluronate into the anterior chamber at cataract surgery, presumably due to physical obstruction of outflow rather than a toxic manifestation.[c,e]

Most of the publications on sodium hyaluronate in the ophthalmic literature are limited to descriptions of its clinical utility, rather than adverse effects, and are not included in the following bibliography.

a.   Arzeno G, Miller D: Effect of sodium hyaluronate on corneal wound healing. *ARCH OPHTHALMOL* 100:152, 1982.
b.   Balazs EA, Freeman MI, et al: Hyaluronic acid and replacement of vitreous and aqueous humor. *MOD PROBL OPHTHALMOL* 10:3–21, 1972.
c.   Berson FG, Patterson MM, Epstein DL: Obstruction of the aqueous outflow by sodium hyaluronate in enucleated human eyes. *AM J OPHTHALMOL* 95:668–672, 1983.
d.   Binkhorst CD: Inflammation and intraocular pressure after the use of Healon in intraocular lens surgery. *J AM INTRA-OCULAR INPLANT SOC* 6:340–341, 1980.
e.   Cherfan GM, Rich WJ, Wright G: Raised intraocular pressure and other problems with sodium hyaluronate and cataract surgery. *TRANS OPHTHALMOL SOC UK* 103:277–279, 1983.
f.   Constable LJ, Swann DS: Biological vitreous substitutes. *ARCH OPHTHALMOL* 88:544–548, 1972.
g.   Pruett RC, Schepens CL, Swann DA: Hyaluronic acid vitreous substitute. *ARCH OPHTHALMOL* 97:2325–2330, 1979.

Sodium hydrosulfite (sodium sulfoxylate, sodium dithionite) is employed in dyeing and for removing dyes from fabrics. A 2% aqueous solution adjusted to pH 7 tested on rabbit eyes by irrigation of the surface of the eye for ten minutes after removal of the corneal epithelium caused slight corneal edema and slower than normal healing, but the eyes recovered completely within a week.[81] See INDEX for additional testing of hydrosulfite in connection with injury of the eyes by dyes, under *Dyes, cationic.*)

Sodium hydroxide (caustic soda, lye) is a white solid that dissolves readily in water to make a very strongly alkaline solution. Sodium hydroxide, as solid or solution, is severely injurious to all tissues. It causes some of the most severe, blinding injuries of the eye. Because it may be considered public enemy number one for causing chemical burns of the eye, sodium hydroxide has been the chemical caustic most extensively studied in animal and clinical investigations. Foremost have been studies of its mechanisms of injurious action, and what has been learned has been the basis for scientific improvements in means of treatment. Sodium hydroxide has important features in common with other strong alkalies, such as ammonium hydroxide and calcium hydroxide, and it is assumed that what is learned with sodium hydroxide will be to some degree applicable to the other caustics.

Under the heading "Alkalies" (see INDEX for page number) there are descriptions and comparisons of the general effects of the various strong alkalies on the eye. In a chapter on "Treatment of Chemical Burns of the Eye" (see Table of Contents) there are descriptions and evaluations of various treatments that have been evolved. Here we will concentrate on sodium hydroxide itself, and its destructive effects.

The serious public health problem presented by sodium hydroxide and other alkalies has been succinctly and well described by Stanley (1965), emphasizing particularly the dangers of caustic household drain cleaners that contain sodium hydroxide.

The effects of splashes of sodium hydroxide on the eyes of human beings have been described clinically innumerable times. (The general character of these burns is described under *Alkalies;* see INDEX.) In particular, Girard (1970), Pfister (1983), and Reim and Schmidt-Martens (1982) have provided reviews and illustrations.

Damage of the cornea, conjunctiva, and episcleral tissues predominates. Injury of retina and choroid is rare. In a very unusual case a localized burn of the retina was noted by Reinecke (1962) after a patient allowed a particle of solid sodium hydroxide (Drano) to remain in his lower conjunctival cul-de-sac. The particle caused deep localized erosion of both bulbar and palpebral conjunctiva, but no significant damage of the cornea or disturbance of vision. Ophthalmoscopically, corresponding to the position of the localized burn on the outside of the globe, a localized whitening of the retina near the ora serrata was seen. This area began to become pigmented several weeks later. A case of the same sort was reported by Smith (1976), resulting in a localized chorioretinal scar, but normal cornea and visual acuity. In another case described by Smith (1976), a child 16 months old had a severe splash burn of the anterior segment, but by age 30 months it was possible to see patchy pigment proliferation in the fundus, and also a retinal fold.

Clinically, the worst features of burns of the eye by sodium hydroxide are the great rapidity with which extreme damage can be done to the anterior segment of the eye, and the tendency for the cornea to ulcerate and perforate in the worst burns, or to become densely vascularized and opaque, a poor candidate for keratoplasty, in burns that are not quite so severe.

A great deal of experimental work has been done, mostly on anesthetized rabbits, aiming for better treatment. In some investigations, sodium hydroxide solution has simply been dropped or swabbed on the eye so that it contacts the whole cornea and conjunctiva. More precise control of the degree and nature of injury has been obtained in other investigations by limiting the amount applied to a small measured volume, or by applying discs, rings or strips of filter paper wet with the caustic solution, or by placing cylindrical plastic wells in contact with the surface of the eye to restrict the exposure to a desired area. The duration of exposure in most studies has ranged from 15 seconds to 2 minutes, one minute being most common. (This timing favors induction of reproducible or standard types of lesions, and corresponds to the estimated time that it might take a human being to get first-aid irrigation started after a splash of sodium hydroxide on the eye.) The concentration of sodium hydroxide used in these experiments has ranged from 0.25 N to 6 N, with 1 to 2 N being most common. (1 N equals 4% solution.) The times and concentrations cited represent conditions studied in a series of 15 different published experimental programs. Examples of effects produced in the eyes of rabbits are as follows. According to Pfister (1971), drop application of 1N for 30 seconds before rinsing caused severe injury with ultimate perforation of most corneas, whereas 0.5 N for 30 seconds caused less severe damage. Exposures to 2 N for 15 to 20 seconds caused some "severe" and some "mild" injuries, according to Stein (1973). According to Reim (1982), 0.25 N for 30 seconds caused "mild" burns.

Species differences have been observed in degrees of damage and of recovery after contamination of the eye with sodium hydroxide. In comparisons made by Buehler (1964)[23], Carter (1965)[29], Green (1978)[322], and Paterson (1973) the eyes of monkeys react a little less, and recover a little better, than the eyes of rabbits. It is believed that human eyes are more like monkey eyes.

Histologically, in lye-burned rabbit eyes all the cells in areas in close contact with the alkali are killed (Brown 1969).[19] Reparative and destructive processes follow (Francois 1972). Surviving corneal cells try to replace killed cells and to replace damaged collagen. Opposed to this is inflammatory infiltration and destruction of collagen, worst when the limbal region has been involved, and least when only central cornea has been affected, or blood vessels have grown into the injured cornea (Pfister 1976; Reim 1982; Vrabec 1975, 1976).

Histologically, an increase in numbers of leucocytes in the anterior chamber appears to parallel inflammatory infiltration of alkali-injured corneal limbus (Graupner 1972). Destruction of corneal endothelium by alkali may result in formation of retrocorneal membranes, which may involve the angle of the anterior chamber and aqueous outflow system (Crabb 1978; Matsuda 1973; Renard 1978; Stein 1973). Damage of the ciliary body from penetration of sodium hydroxide through the sclera is characterized by death of ciliary body cells, inflammatory infiltration, thrombosis of vessels, hemorrhage, and atrophy (Pfister 1971; Stein 1973).

Chemically, there is loss of ground substance measured as hexosamine or mucopolysaccharide in the corneal stroma (Brown 1969[18-20]; Grant 1955[89]; Thiele 1965). In the aqueous humor, the ascorbate concentration, which normally is many times higher than in the blood, drops dramatically, presumably secondary to caustic damage to the ciliary body. Deficiency of ascorbate may interfere with regeneration of corneal collagen. The glucose content of aqueous humor and cornea may also drop. A series of studies by Obenberger and colleagues on the influence of lye burns on the metabolism of the cornea, beyond the scope of this synopsis, are to be found in *Cesk Oftalmol* and *Graefes Arch Ophthalmol* from 1972 through 1977.

Enzymatic investigations have demonstrated liberation of collagenases from surrounding corneal cells and especially from polymorphonuclear leucocytes invading alkali-injured cornea (Brown 1969[18-20]; Brown 1970; Dohlman 1969[43]; Gnadinger 1969[71]; Matsuda 1973). These collagenases have been found not to attack the collagen of normal corneas, in which the fibers of collagen are protected by a sheath of mucopolysaccharide, but after the sheath has been damaged by alkali the collagenases can cause a breakdown which is seen histologically (Francois 1972[71]). The breakdown of corneal collagen appears to be the basis for corneal ulceration or melting which is seen clinically and histologically beginning in several days after severe alkali injury and persisting for weeks or months, sometimes ending in Descemetocele and perforation.

The intraocular pressure in rabbit eyes, and to less degree in monkey eyes, may go through successive phases of elevation and depression. Immediately after a damaging concentration of sodium hydroxide (pH around 12) is dropped on a rabbit eye the pressure may rise to 60 mm Hg due to sudden shrinkage of the outer coats of the eye (Chiang 1971; Paterson 1973, 1974; Stein 1973). The same response is obtained in enucleated eyes (Grant 1955; Stein 1973). The peak is passed quickly, with return toward normal pressure in 5 to 10 minutes. A second but smaller rise and peak may develop more slowly, in about 80 minutes. This second rise has been attributed to prostaglandins which are released into the eye after alkali injury (Paterson 1973, 1974, 1975). The prostaglandin-induced rise is observed also in monkeys, but less than in rabbits (Paterson 1973). In eyes that are severely burned, with destruction of the ciliary body, instead of a pressure rise in the second phase, the eye may go into permanent hypotony (Paterson 1971, 1974; Pfister 1973). Less severely burned eyes with functioning ciliary body but injury to the angle of the anterior chamber may have chronically elevated pressure (Stein 1973).

The acute pressure response of lye-burned human eyes has not been measured, and what harm a brief high peak of pressure may do to a burned eye is not known. Thiel (1962)[241], while investigating the pH of the aqueous humor after lye-burns in rabbits, noted that the burned corneas had become grossly cloudy a minute after burning, but immediately lost some of their cloudiness when he withdrew a sample of aqueous humor. Undoubtedly part of the clouding was from high pressure, which was relieved by paracentesis, though Thiel may have been unaware of the mechanism. Whether paracentesis a minute or two after a lye burn would be of lasting benefit is untested, but anyway it seems impractical to consider in first-aid treatment of human eyes.

The influence of intraocular pressure at a later phase in rabbits' eyes burned by sodium hydroxide has been investigated by Heydenreich, concluding that subnormal intraocular pressure may increase the tendency to vascularization and degeneration in the corneal stroma, though it may slightly hasten regeneration of epithelium. However, in occasional patients who have secondary glaucomas as a result of chemical burns, Heydenreich has shown that an elevated intraocular pressure is unfavorable for the outcome of keratoplasty in eyes with opaque corneas.[112,113]

Paracentesis, to release the aqueous humor from the anterior chamber, has been of interest as a possibly beneficial early maneuver in alkali-burned eyes, not only to reduce the pressure, but to remove possibly caustic material from within the eye. In considering this, there have been the following questions to answer: (1) How much alkali reaches the anterior chamber and aqueous humor? (2) How long does penetrated alkali remain in the anterior chamber? (3) How much alkali in the aqueous humor can be tolerated by normal eyes, and by eyes with cornea and other tissues already injured? The first two questions have been investigated by measurements of the pH of the aqueous humor in experimental animals. The third question is still open.

Data relating to the first two questions have been obtained by investigators who have applied sodium hydroxide in various amounts to the eyes of rabbits and at various times have withdrawn samples of aqueous humor, and have measured the pH. Here is an outline of reported results.

Feller (1966) applied 2 N NaOH for 1 minute, and at 2 minutes found pH 10.5 in the aqueous humor.

Girard (1970) applied 0.12 N for 1 minute, and at 3 minutes found pH 9.5 to 10 [after 30 minutes the pH was essentially normal].

Graupner (1973) applied 1 N for 2 minutes, and at 10 minutes found pH 9.3 [falling by 90 minutes to pH 7.87].

Laux (1975) applied 1 N, 3 N, 6 N for 1 minute, and at 7.5 minutes found pH 9.4, pH 10.7, pH 12.7 respectively [after 0.5, 2.5, 5 hours respectively all had fallen to pH 8.5].

Orlowski (1956) applied 0.1 N for 5 minutes, and at 15 minutes found pH 10.3 [after 1.5 to 3 hours pH was normal].

Paterson (1975) applied 20, 50, and 100 μl of 2 N, and within 6 minutes found pH 10.2, pH 11.9, and pH 12 respectively [after 2 hours pH values were 8.5, 10, and 10.5 respectively].

Schmidt-Martens (1977) applied 0.25 N for 30 seconds, and at 2 minutes found pH 8 [after one hour fallen to pH 7.7].

Thiel (1962)[241] applied 2 N for 1 minute, and at 1 minute found pH 9.

Thiel (1962)[241] applied 1 N for 1 minute, and at 1 hour found pH 8.4 [after 1.5 hours pH 8.3].

In general, these data establish that exposure of the rabbit eye to amounts of sodium hydroxide that are known to be seriously damaging can cause the pH of the aqueous humor to rise to the pH 10 to 11 range in a few minutes, or higher in extreme cases, slowly falling close to normal within a couple of hours thereafter, except in extreme cases.

Additionally, Graupner (1973) and Paterson (1975) have shown that after paracentesis and removal of the primary aqueous humor the pH of the anterior chamber is reduced significantly.

(It should be kept in mind that the series of observations outlined above are concerned only with the effects of sodium hydroxide, and that the findings may be different with a more rapidly penetrating alkali, such as ammonium hydroxide, or a more slowly penetrating one, such as calcium hydroxide.) (A comparison with ammonium hydroxide has been made by Paterson (1975).)

Unfortunately, the reports on sodium hydroxide outlined above failed to include observations on the condition of the eyes, and did not evaluate whether eyes that had early paracentesis and removal of alkaline aqueous humor actually ended up in significantly different condition than comparably exposed eyes that did not have paracentesis.

However, other observations have been made that add information on effects of treatment. These are described in the chapter on "Treatment of Chemical Burns of the Eye" (see Table of Contents), but in brief Bennett (1978) has found benefit from perfusing the anterior chamber with buffer solution within 15 minutes; Laux (1975) has found prolonged irrigation of the surface of the eye with saline solution or buffer reduces the pH of the anterior chamber; Paterson (1975) found the effect of surface irrigation with saline solution on the pH of the aqueous humor after lye burn to be rather slow.

The question of how much alkali in the aqueous humor can be tolerated by normal eyes, and by eyes with the cornea and other tissues already injured, was not addressed by the experiments outlined above. However, Gonnering et al (1979), using excised rabbit and human corneas, perfused the endothelial side and examined the corneal thickness and cell morphology at various pH levels, finding that at pH 10 there was rapid corneal swelling and cell death in 15 minutes. (This suggested greater susceptibility to alkali injury than an observation by Grant (1950) that the anterior chamber of live rabbits could be irrigated with pH 10 sodium or ammonium hydroxide for several minutes without producing clinically significant injury.)

Also, see INDEX for *Treatment of Chemical Burns of the Eye.*

Bennett TO, Peyman GA, Rutgard J: Intracameral phosphate buffer in alkali burns. *CAN J OPHTHALMOL* 13:93–95, 1978.

Brown SI, Weller CA, Akiya S: Pathogenesis of ulcers of the alkali-burned cornea. *ARCH OPHTHALMOL* 83:205–208, 1970.

Chiang TS, Moorman LR, Thomas RP: Ocular hypertensive response following acid and alkali burns in rabbits. *INVEST OPHTHALMOL* 10:270–273, 1971.

Crabb CV: A light microscopic study of ground substance changes in alkali-burned corneas. *AM J OPHTHALMOL* 86:92–96, 1978.

Feller K, Graupner K: The hydrogen ion concentration in the anterior chamber of rabbit eyes after experimental burning with acid and lye. *GRAEFES ARCH OPHTHALMOL* 170:373–376, 1966. (German)

Francois J, Feher J: Collagenolysis and regeneration in corneal burnings. *OPHTHALMOLOGICA* 165:137–152, 1972.

Girard LJ, Alford WE, et al: Severe alkali burns. *TRANS AM ACAD OPHTHALMOL OTOL* 74:788–803, 1970.

Gonnering R, Edelhauser HF, et al: The pH tolerance of rabbit and human corneal endothelium. *INVEST OPHTHALMOL VIS SCI* 18:373–390, 1979.

Grant WM: Experimental investigation of paracentesis in the treatment of ocular ammonia burns. *ARCH OPHTHALMOL* 44:399–404, 1950.

Grant WM, Trotter RR: Tonographic measurements in enncleated eyes. *ARCH OPHTHALMOL* 53:191–200, 1955.

Graupner OK, Kalman EV, Le Petit GF: The significance of the buffer properties of the cornea and aqueous humor for the protection of the eye in burns. *GRAEFES ARCH OPHTHALMOL* 182:351–356, 1971. (German)

Graupner OK, Hausmann CM, Kalman EV: The leucocyte content of the aqueous humor of rabbit eyes after experimental burning with acid or alkali. *GRAEFES ARCH OPHTHALMOL* 184:202–207, 1972. (German)

Graupner OK: The effect of a drainage of the aqueous humor after burning with acid and alkali on the hydrogen ion concentration in the anterior chamber of the rabbit eye. *GRAEFES ARCH OPHTHALMOL* 186:67–72, 1973. (German)

Laux H, Roth HW, et al: The hydrogen ion concentration of the aqueous humor after alkali burns of the cornea and its responsiveness to treatment. *GRAEFES ARCH OPHTHALMOL* 195:33–40, 1975. (German)

Matsuda H, Smelser GK: Epithelium and stroma in alkali burned corneas. *ARCH OPHTHALMOL* 89:396–401, 1973.

Matsuda H, Smelser GK: Endothelial cells in alkali burned corneas: ultrastructural alterations. *ARCH OPHTHALMOL* 89:402–409, 1973.

Orlowski WJ, Wekka Z: The hydrogen ion concentration in the aqueous humor of eyes with lye burns. *OPHTHALMOLOGICA* 137:244–253, 1959 (French); and *KLIN OCZNA* 26:117–126, 1956. (English summary)

Paterson CA, Pfister RR: Ocular hypertensive response to alkali burns in the monkey. *EXP EYE RES* 17:449–453, 1973.

Paterson CA, Pfister RR: Intraocular pressure changes after alkali burns. *ARCH OPHTHALMOL* 91:211–218, 1974.

Paterson CA, Pfister RR, Levinson RA: Aqueous humor pH changes after experimental alkali burns. *AM J OPHTHALMOL* 79:414–419, 1975.

Paterson CA, Pfister RR: Prostaglandin-like activity in the aqueous humor following alkali burns. *INVEST OPHTHALMOL* 14:177–183, 1975.

Pfister RR, Friend J, Dohlman CH: The anterior segments of rabbits after alkali burns. *ARCH OPHTHALMOL* 86:189–193, 1971.

Pfister RR, McCulley JP, et al: Collagenase activity of intact corneal epithelium in peripheral alkali burns. *ARCH OPHTHALMOL* 86:309–313, 1971.

Pfister RR, Burnstein N: The alkali burned cornea. *EXP EYE RES* 23:519–535, 1976.

Pfister RR: Chemical injuries of the eye. *OPHTHALMOLOGY* 90:1246–1253, 1983.

Reim M, Schmidt-Martens FW: Treatment of burns. *KLIN MONATSBL AUGENHEILKD* 181:1–9, 1982. (German)

Reim M, Conze A, Kaszuba HJ: Adenosine phosphate and glutathione levels in the regenerated corneal epithelium after abrasion and mild alkali burns. *GRAEFES ARCH OPHTHALMOL* 218:42–45, 1982.

Reinecke R: Personal communication, 1962.

Renard G, Hirsch M, Pouliquen Y: Corneal changes due to alkali burns. *TRANS OPHTHALMOL SOC UK* 98:379–382, 1978.

Schmidt-Martens FW, Hennighauser U, Bremer HJ: Aqueous humor changes after alkali burns. *TRANS OPHTHALMOL SOC UK* 97:715–718, 1977.

Smith RE, Conway B: Alkali retinopathy. *ARCH OPHTHALMOL* 94:81–84, 1976.

Stanley JA: Strong alkali burns of the eye. *N ENGL J MED* 273:1265–1266, 1965.

Stein MR, Naidoff MA, Dawson CR: Intraocular pressure response to experimental alkali burns. *AM J OPHTHALMOL* 75:99–109, 1973.

Thiele H, Jorascky W: On the fine structure of the cornea. *KLIN MONATSBL AUGENHEILKD* 147:899–907, 1965. (German)

Vrabec F, Obenberger J, Vrabec J: Ring-shaped alkali burns of the rabbit cornea. *GRAEFES ARCH OPHTHALMOL* 197:233–240, 1975; *ibid* 198:121–128, 1976; *ibid* 199:191–196, 1976.

Sodium hypochlorite is commonly available in aqueous solution, widely employed as a bleach and antiseptic. *Household laundry bleaches* under various names such as Clorox, and Dazzle usually are approximately 5% solutions with pH close to 11. Commercial laundry bleach, known as *caustic soda bleach,* contains 15% sodium hypochlorite at a pH slightly over 11.

Very few human eye injuries have been reported, presumably because most accidental splashes in the eye have been with the weaker 5% household solutions, and recovery has been rapid and complete. As an example, a patient who accidentally splashed Clorox in her eyes washed her eyes with water several minutes later because of much burning discomfort, and when seen later the same day had only slight superficial disturbance of the corneal epithelium, which cleared completely in the next day or two without special treatment.[317] McLaughlin has also reported one instance of recovery within forty-eight hours after a splash of Clorox.[165] In a personal communication, Carl Johnson (1985) described a patient who splashed Clorox in one eye. She felt smarting, and immediately flushed her eye with water. Later the same day the corneal epithelium was seen by slit-lamp to be peppered with many fine grey dots, some of which were confluent. She had reddened lids, but only mild discomfort, easily keeping her eyes open without anesthetic. By the next day, without special treatment, she reported being essentially back to normal.

The more concentrated 15% solutions used in commercial laundries and in swimming pools as a disinfectant would naturally be expected to cause more serious injury from splash in the eye, and this is indicated in rabbit experiments. There seem to be no well-documented clinical reports, but there is one report of three eyes burned by strong sodium hypochlorite solutions, by Roth, with the actual concentration not given, which had slow recovery; one required a Denig graft.[b]

In tests on rabbit eyes, 5% solutions which had pH 11.1 to 11.6 caused immediate pain, but if washed off with water within thirty seconds, left only slight transient corneal epithelial haze and conjunctival edema, with return to normal within a day or less.[81] If this test solution is not washed from the rabbit's eye with water, the reaction is more severe, consisting of greater corneal and conjunctival edema with small hemorrhages in the conjunctiva, gradually returning to normal within a week. An interesting difference between rabbit and monkey eyes in response to exposure to 5.5% solution has been reported by Carter and Griffith, indicating that the monkey eye recovers much more rapidly, maybe more like the human.[a] On rabbit eyes Griffith et al. found 5% solution to cause "moderate irritation," clearing within 7 days.[324]

In tests of higher concentrations on rabbit eyes, one drop of 15% solution at pH 11.2 caused immediate severe pain, and if it was not promptly washed away with water it caused hemorrhages from the conjunctiva and nose, plus rapid onset of ground-glass appearance of the corneal epithelium. This was followed by moderate bluish edema of the whole cornea, chemosis and discharge for several days. Such eyes sometimes healed in two to three weeks with slight or no residual corneal damage, but they had neovascularization of the conjunctiva and distortion of the nictitating membrane by scarring.[81]

Household bleaches mixed with ammonia give off irritating vapors, described under *Hypochlorite-ammonia mixtures* (see INDEX). Similar irritating products are encountered in swimming pools from reaction between hypochlorite and ammonia, described under *Swimming pool water* (see INDEX).

a. Carter RO, Griffith JF: Assessment of eye hazard. *TOXICOL APPL PHARMACOL* 7:70–73, 1965.
b. Roth A: New mechanism of chemical burn of the eye. *BULL SOC OPHTALMOL FRANCE* 66:209, 1966. (French)

Sodium iodide applied as a saturated aqueous solution to rabbit corneas for 5 to 6 seconds after the epithelium was scraped off caused temporary flattening of the corneas, but they soon healed and reverted to normal condition, judged grossly and by histology.[a]

a. Cress J, Maurice DM: An attempt at a chemical treatment of myopia. *ARCH OPHTHAL-MOL* 86:692–693, 1971.

Sodium lactate tested on rabbit eyes by three hours of continuous application of a

0.1 M solution at pH7.0 to 7.5, adjusted to 0.46 osmolar by addition of sodium chloride or sucrose, caused no disturbance of the cornea.[209]

Sodium, metallic, is a silvery white metal which reacts violently with water, forming sodium hydroxide and hydrogen, which may ignite spontaneously. Some severe burns of the eyes which have been caused by sodium are attributable principally to the sodium hydroxide.[46,249]

Sodium N-methyldithiocarbamate (Vapam), a soil fumigant, is reported to be irritating to the eyes, skin, and mucous membranes, but no detailed information was found.[36]

Sodium nitrate (Chile saltpeter), in the only reported instance of eye disturbance from ingestion, caused transitory blindness, deafness, speechlessness, and tetanic convulsions, but gradually recovery in a girl who took 16 g.[153]

In tests on rabbit eyes, a 10% aqueous solution of sodium nitrate applied continuously for five minutes was practically innocuous to the surface of the eyes. The conjunctivae became mildly hyperemic, but the corneas remained clear, and the eyes rapidly returned completely to normal.[81] Also, no disturbance of the cornea occurred in a more prolonged test with sodium nitrate dripped continuously for three hours on rabbit eyes as a 0.1 M solution at pH 7.0 or 7.5 made up to 0.46 osmolar with sodium chloride or sucrose.[209]

Old reports of corneal clouding or conjunctivitis in animals and human beings from crude chile saltpeter employed in fertilizer were undoubtedly caused by ingredients other than sodium nitrate, since the pure chemical has been so well tolerated in tests on rabbit eyes.[96,249,253]

Sodium nitrite has been employed as a vasodilator in doses of 30 to 60 mg, and in treatment of cyanide poisoning. One patient who took 14.5 g orally described temporary darkening of the whole visual field of both eyes.[a]

Testing of sodium nitrite on rabbit corneas by application of 0.08 M solution after removal of the corneal epithelium, or by injection into the stroma, has caused no local injury.[123]

    a. Vetter J: Neurocirculatory dystonia of retinal vessels. *KLIN MONATSBL AUGENHEILKD* 118:165–171, 1951. (German)

Sodium oxybate (sodium hydroxybutyrate; Gamma-OH), a hypnotic, applied as eyedrops to rabbit eyes is reported to reduce oxygen utilization by eye tissues, and to disturb the b-wave of the ERG.[a]

    a. Zaretskaya RB, Trutneva KV, et al: The effect of sodium hydroxybutyrate solution on the oxygenation process in eye tissues and retina potentials. *METAB PEDIATR OPHTHALMOL* 4:201–204, 1980.

Sodium perborate apparently has not been involved in eye injuries, but when tested on cultures of retina *in vitro* it was found to cause selective destruction of the rod cells at a concentration of 5×10^{-5} M.[99]

Sodium perchlorate tested on rabbit eyes by application of 0.08 M solution to the cornea after removal of the epithelium, or by injection into the corneal stroma, caused very slight reaction.[123]

Sodium phosphate, tested on rabbit eyes by continuous exposure for three hours as 0.1 M solution at pH 7.0 to 7.5 made up to 0.46 osmolar with sodium chloride or sucrose, caused no disturbance of the cornea.[209]

Sodium silicate (water glass, egg preserver) is commonly employed as a 40% solution which is strongly alkaline. Accidental splashes in the eye followed promptly by washing with water have been observed to damage the corneal epithelium.[46,81]

Sodium metasilicate is used with sodium carbonate in heavy duty alkaline laundry detergents. In rabbits this type of detergent causes damage to the cornea, with opacification, proportional to the alkalinity of the preparation. Irrigation of the eye with water must be done within 60 seconds to reduce the severity of injury.[a]

   a. Scharpf LG Jr, Hill ID, Kelby RE: Relative eye injury potential of heavy duty phos-
       phate and non-phosphate laundry detergents. *FOOD COSMET TOXICOL* 10:829–837,
       1972.

Sodium sulfide contact with workmen's eyes has been noted to cause burns which may be slow healing,[165] owing presumably to strong alkalinity.

Sodium thiosulfate ("hypo") has been administered intravenously in experimental treatment of various poisonings in human beings without disturbance of the eyes or vision. Testing on rabbit eyes by application to the cornea after removal of the epithelium or by injection into the corneal stroma has shown slight reaction to 0.08 M concentration, and even less at lower concentration.[123]

   In human eyes a solution of sodium thiosulfate plus potassium ferricyanide has been injected subconjunctivally and has been applied to the surface of the corneal stroma in treatment of ocular argyrosis, with benefit and no apparent injurious effect.[81] (See *Silver* in INDEX).

Solanum plants include the potato (*Solanum tuberosum*), black or woody nightshade (*Solanum nigrum*), and bitter-sweet (*Solanum dulcamara*), which contain solanine, solanidine, and other toxic but unidentified substances.[171, 152] Rarely, ingestion of portions of these plants, such as the berries of *Solanum nigrum,* or eating potatoes which are green and sprouting, has caused severe intoxication, with mydriasis as one of the minor features.[153, 214, 246, 252]

   A purported influence on color vision seems without sound basis.[214] *Datura stramonium* and deadly nightshade (*Atropa belladonna*) which are also in this family, contain atropine, hyoscyamine, and scopolamine, which are very effective in caus-ing mydriasis and cycloplegia. (See INDEX for *Atropine, Belladonna,* and *Datura stramonium.*)

   Potato leaf, smoked as a wartime substitute for tobacco, has been reported to have caused retinal hemorrhages in five cases within one to two weeks of beginning this practice.[a]

a. Sedan J: Retinal hemorrhages in smokers of potato leaves. *OPHTHALMOLOGICA* 102:361–365, 1941. (French)

Solketal (2,2-dimethyl-1,3-dioxolane-4-methanol), a solvent and plasticizer, tested on rabbit eyes by application of 0.1 ml undiluted produced irritation and increase in corneal thickness still present after 24 hours[295], but 25% aqueous solution had little or no effect.[338]

Solvent vapors that particularly affect the eyes or vision are summarized here, but descriptions of the properties of each in greater detail can be located through the INDEX.

Solvent vapor exposures may be deliberate, as in "glue sniffing", or involuntary, as in most industrial exposures. Deliberate inhalation of solvent vapors, has been practiced by adolescents more often than by adults, seeking excitment or euphoria. They have inhaled vapors from plastic glues and cements, and from lacquer thinners, and many other household sources of solvents, including toluene, xylene, benzene, n-hexane, alcohol, acetone, and amyl acetate. The practice of "glue sniffing" has been well reviewed by Wyse.[f] Although visual and auditory hallucinations are described as common, and blurred vision and diplopia are mentioned, toxic effects on the eyes have been rare. Encephalopathy attributed particularly to *toluene* inhalation has been described by King et al, noting one patient had coarse rotary nystagmus in all directions of gaze associated with severe ataxia, presumably from cerebellar and cerebral damage.[c] In a case of encephalopathy from repeated inhalation of cement vapors that probably contained toluene, Channer and Stanley described long-persisting visual hallucinations with delayed visual evoked cortical responses.[a] Ehyai and Freemon have reported bilateral optic atrophy, hearing loss, and peripheral polyneuropathy in a patient with cerebral and cerebellar atrophy after 5 years of glue sniffing. Individuals with sickle cell disease have been known to develop erythrocytic aplastic crises after glue sniffing, and in one boy who died from this complication, the retinal arteries and veins were engorged, the retina was edematous with blurring of margins of the optic nerveheads and a macula star, but no abnormality was found in the optic nerves histologically.[d]

Shoemakers in Italy have developed shoemaker's polyneuropathy from chronic inhalation of hexacarbon solvents, especially n-hexane, in cements used to assemble pieces of leather. (At one time the polyneuropathy was thought to be attributable to tricresyl phosphate, but this proved to be wrong.) Effects on the eyes or on vision in association with shoemaker's polyneuropathy have been rather vague, with poorly documented mentions of blurred vision, optic atrophy, abnormal color vision, and macular edema. (For more details, see INDEX for *n-Hexane.*)

Solvent vapors from lacquers, furniture polishes and plastic cements have caused corneal epithelial keratopathy, or "vacuolar keratopathy." Descriptions of this condition are remarkably consistent, regularly depicting fine transparent vacuoles or bubbles in the corneal epithelium as the principal feature. These vacuoles are visible only with magnification. With the slit-lamp biomicroscope they can be seen best by retroillumination. By direct illumination, the most superficial vacuoles appear as tiny gray flecks on the surface and may stain with fluorescein, but the majority, which are located in the middle layers of the epithelium, are transparent and do not stain.

Patients may be asymptomatic or may have moderate irritation and tearing, most notable on opening the eyes after sleep. The corneas return completely to normal in a few days when exposure to the solvents is discontinued.

In several instances butyl alcohol has been the principal solvent and has been the main suspect, but in all reported instances other solvents have been present too, and in no instance has typical vacuolar keratitis been induced experimentally in animals exposed to pure butyl alcohol. (See INDEX for *n-Butanol.*)

Experimentally in cats, characteristic epithelial vacuoles have been described after exposure for several hours to near-lethal concentrations of *toluene, xylene, methyl acetate, ethyl acetate,* and *butyl acetate.*[216] Possibly the vacuolar keratitis which is seen in human beings can also be produced by several different solvents, particularly by *xylene.*

The subject has been well reviewed with comprehensive bibliography in 1957 by Schmid[216] and by Sommer.[230]

Spray painters of railway cars in Finland exposed daily for years to numerous paint solvent vapors are reported to have a higher incidence of lens abnormalities than unexposed matched controls, but a specific responsible solvent has not been identified.[e]

a. Channer KS, Stanley S: Persistent visual hallucinations secondary to chronic solvent encephalopathy. *J NEUROL NEUROSURG PSYCHIATRY* 46:83–86, 1983.

b. Ehyai A, Freemon FR: Progressive optic neuropathy and sensorineural hearing loss due to chronic glue sniffing. *J NEUROL NEUROSURG PSYCHIATRY* 46:349–351, 1983.

c. King MD, Day RE, et al: Solvent encephalopathy. *BR MED J* 283:663–665, 1981.

d. Powars D: Aplastic anemia secondary to glue sniffing. *N ENGL J MED* 273:700–702, 1965.

e. Raitta C, Husmann K, Tossavainen A: Lens changes in car painters exposed to a mixture of organic solvents. *GRAEFES ARCH OPHTHALMOL* 200:149–156, 1976.

f. Wyse DG: Deliberate inhalation of volatile hydrocarbons: a review. *CAN MED ASSOC J* 108:71–74, 1973.

Sparsomycin, a cytostatic antibiotic, has caused retinopathy in two patients who were under treatment for cancer.[a] Sparsomycin was given intravenously, and in two weeks the retinal pigment was seen to begin to gather in coarse clumps. The patients were aware of disturbance of vision, and ring scotomas were found. Both patients died two to two and one-half months after the start of treatment. Histologically it appeared probable that the primary toxic effect was in the retinal pigment epithelium, with secondary damage to contiguous rods and cones. In previous animal studies no eye toxicity had been detected.

a. McFarlane JR, Yanoff M, Scheie HG: Toxic retinopathy following sparsomycin therapy. *ARCH OPHTHALMOL* 76:532–540, 1966.

Spider venom appears rarely to have any selective toxic effect on the eye. A small number of cases are known in which stings on the lids by poorly identified spiders caused severe but usually transient reactions in the lids.[153,253] Also in one instance the juice of a squashed garden spider reportedly caused severe irritation to the eyes of a child for a week.[253] In a report from Japan swelling of the lids, conjunctival edema and subconjunctival hemorrhages have been attributed to contact of the eye with either the body or the web of a spider.[f]

The **brown recluse spider** (*Loxosceles reclusus*) may cause a localized gangrenous reaction. One case of gangrene of the lids has been described as a typical example, although the spider in this case was not positively identified. After a bite on the cheek local pain developed only after 8 to 24 hours, with considerable systemic reaction. In 6 to 7 days there was severe laryngeal edema and gangrene of the lids requiring corrective surgery. The eyes themselves remained normal.[c] Separately, evidence has been presented that systemic treatment with dapsone is helpful when serious skin lesions are starting to develop.[g]

Poisoning by the **black widow spider** (*Latrodectus mactans*) may incidentally be accompanied by edema of the eyelids, ptosis, and conjunctivitis;[h] but more important, according to Gotlieb, the pupils are constricted, and treatment by subcutaneous injections of atropine (0.3 mg repeated as needed) has relieved most of the manifestations of poisoning, including colic and pain in the muscles.[a,d,e]

The venom of the poisonous spider **Phoneutria fera** in Brazil is said to cause pain at the site of the sting, visual disturbances including blindness, and disorders of the heart and respiration. There seems to be no published information concerning the nature or duration of the visual disturbances, but their appearance is said to be one of the indications for use of a specific antiserum.[b]

Tarantula hairs, thrown off the tarantula's back by agitation of the hind legs, have been well recognized as a source of skin irritation, and in one case caused immediate pain in a patient's eye.[i] Vision was not disturbed, but in the following month foreign body sensation persisted. Infiltrates in the corneal stroma and mild iritis developed in association with fine hairs in the corneal stroma and in the anterior chamber, some protruding through Descemet's membrane. During four months under topical corticosteroid treatment the eye gradually quieted. After nine months, hair fragments were still visible in the corneal stroma and adhering to the iris. Whether a toxic factor is involved is unknown.

a. Atropine for spider bite. *LANCET* 1:1285–1286, 1965.
b. Bucherl W: Studies on dried venom of Phoneutria fera Perty 1833. In Buckley: Porges (Eds.): VENOMS. *AM ASSOC FOR THE ADVANCEMENT OF SCIENCE,* Pub. No. 44, Washington, D.C., 1956.
c. Edwards JJ, Anderson RL, Wood JR: Loxoscelism of the eyelids. *ARCH OPHTHALMOL* 98:1997–2000, 1980.
d. Gotlieb A: Spider bites. *LANCET* 1:246, 1970.
e. Gotlieb A, Fried D: *HAREFUAH* 68:223, 1965.
f. Kawashima J: Eye disease by spiderbody-or net-toxin. *J CLIN OPHTHALMOL* 15:232–233, 1961.
g. King LE Jr, Rees RS: Dapsone treatment of a brown recluse bite. *J AM MED ASSOC* 250:648, 1983.

h. Russell FE: Muscle relaxants in black widow spider poisoning. *AM J MED SCI* 243:159, 1962.
i. Stulting RD, Hooper RJ, Cavanagh HD: Ocular injury caused by tarantula hairs. *AM J OPHTHALMOL* 96:118–119, 1983.

Spiperone (spiroperidol), an anti-psychotic, has been shown to reduce the spontaneous activity of optic nerve neurons in cats in proportion to systemic dosage.[332]

Spironolactone (Aldactone), an aldosterone antagonist and diuretic, has had no adverse effect on intraocular pressure in normal or glaucomatous patients or rabbits, but may instead reduce the pressure slightly. Spironolactone has induced acute transient myopia in one case, similar apparently to the phenomenon seen as a rare idiosyncratic reaction to many other and unrelated drugs.[a] (Further discussion of this type of response see INDEX for *Myopia, acute transient.*)

a. Belci C: Transitory myopia in the course of treatment with diuretics. *BOLL OCULIST* 47:24–31, 1968. (Italian)

SQ 11290, a substituted dibenzoxazepine with psychopharmacologic properties, was found to be cataractogenic when fed to rats, mice, and dogs, but not in hamsters or monkeys.[a] In the lenses of rats the glutathione was reduced in association with formation of cataracts, and in incubated rabbit lenses the compound caused both glutathione and potassium concentrations to decrease.[b]

a. DeBaecke PJ, Kulesza JS, Poutsiaka JW: Comparative cataractogenic studies of dibenzazepines in laboratory animals. *TOXICOL APPL PHARMACOL* (Abstract 109), 25:439, 1973.
b. Wong KK, Wang GM, et al: Effect of substituted dibenzoxazepines on levels of reduced glutathione and potassium ions in lenses of rabbits invitro and of rats invivo. *J PHARM SCI* 63:854–857, 1974.

Squill has been used as a rat poison and formerly was employed medically like digitalis. Severe keratoconjunctivitis and iritis have been reported in a patient employed in grinding squill to a powder.[a] At this work for six days he had no discomfort except for violent sneezing, but in the evenings he noted colored rainbows about lights. At the end of a week he began to have tearing, photophobia, and pain in the eyes. Vision was 6/18. The surface of both corneas appeared stippled in the palpebral fissure. The corneal stromas were thickened and hazy, and the posterior surfaces were wrinkled. The pupils were miotic, and there were cells in the aqueous humor, but the tensions were normal. In the course of a week on conservative treatment, the iritis improved and the corneal edema gradually cleared.

Experiments on rabbits, carried out by applying 0.1 to 0.5 mg of powdered squill directly to the eyes, caused no evident injury at first, but after several hours the conjunctiva became inflamed and the corneal sensitivity decreased. In nine to fifteen hours the corneal epithelium became stippled and the stroma became cloudy. Inflammatory exudate appeared in the anterior chamber, and posterior synechias developed. However, within a few days the inflammation subsided spontaneously and the corneas cleared. Microscopically the corneal stroma and subconjunctival tissues were found to be infiltrated with leukocytes. Patchy defects in the corneal endothelium and inflammatory exudate in the anterior changer were found.[a] Thus it appears well established that squill powder is capable of producing a severe keratoconjunctivitis with iritis after a latent period of at least several hours. (Compare *Cardiac glycosides.*)

a. Achermann E: Kerato-iritis from squill dust. *KLIN MONATSBL AUGENHEILKD* 81:196–199, 1928. (German)

Stannic chloride (tin tetrachloride) is a fuming caustic liquid, highly irritating to the eyes and mucous membranes.[46,171] The irritation presumably is attributable to the hydrochloric acid which is generated when stannic chloride reacts with water.

Starch powder, and modified starch (Bio-Sorb), have been employed as surgical dusting powders. In six patients Bio-Sorb powder from surgical drapes entered the anterior chamber during cataract extraction, and caused post-operative inflammation, associated with discrete white specks on the vitreous face, and particulate haze in the vitreous body.[b] Aspirated aqueous humor was found to contain starch granules, with a lymphocytic reaction in cases of mild inflammation, or a PMN reaction in severe cases. With topical corticosteroid treatment the process resolved.

Tests of starch powder by Schwartz and Linn by instillation into the anterior chamber and under the superior rectus muscle in rabbits produced granulomatous reactions, but less severe than produced by talc.[f] Similar tests by Aronson, placing 0.5 ml containing 0.2 or 2 mg of Bio-Sorb in the anterior chamber or vitreous body of rabbits caused a dose-related inflammatory reaction that was maximal by the second day, and gradually cleared.[b] Histologic findings were similar to those found in patients. With the larger dose, phagocytosis was seen. However, Leonard and Watson came to a different conclusion after injecting 0.05 ml containing 3.5 mg of Bio-Sorb into the anterior chambers of rabbits, finding no more reaction than in control eyes, either by biomicroscopy, or histological examination after 21 days.[d] They noted that the Bio-Sorb gradually absorbed during 7 to 10 days. Despite the varied results of animal testing, it appears from the clinical observations of endophthalmitis, and many reports of peritonitis, that starch powders really can provoke significant inflammation.

A negative result has been reported in an experiment in rabbits in which starch-powdered nylon sutures were introduced into the cornea, but it appears that the starch was probably wiped off as the suture entered the cornea.[e]

Petechial hemorrhages in the retinas of patients after renal angiography have been suspected to be caused by particles, especially starch glove powders, contaminating solutions and needles used for injection.[g] This has not been proved. Retinal vascular changes after carotid angiography have generally been ascribed to other causes, usually to the radiopaque media or to mechanical dislodging of material from the walls of the arteries themselves.

Retinal emboli of both starch and talc have come from intravenous injections of crushed tablets by drug abusers, and have been identified histologically post mortem as well as by ophthalmoscopy in life.[a,c] Vision is not necessarily affected, although macula edema has been reported, along with pulmonary hypertension from multiple emboli of the lungs.[a] In one patient, neovascularization of disk and peripheral retina was observed clinically, but there was no way to be sure whether starch or talc, or both, shared responsibility.[c]

a. AtLee WE Jr: Talc and cornstarch emboli in eyes of drug abusers. *J AM MED ASSOC* 219:49–51, 1972.
b. Aronson SB: Starch endophthalmitis. *AM J OPHTHALMOL* 73:570–579, 1972.
c. Brucker AJ: Disk and peripheral retinal neovascularization secondary to talc and cornstarch emboli. *AM J OPHTHALMOL* 88:864–867, 1979.
d. Leonard BC, Watson AG: The effect of surgical glove powder on the anterior chamber of rabbit eyes. *CAN J OPHTHALMOL* 7:430–434, 1972.
e. Olson RJ, Wander AH: Glove powder and corneal inflammation. *ANN OPHTHALMOL* 13:725–726, 1981.
f. Schwartz FE, Linn JG Jr: The effects of glove powders on the eye. *AM J OPHTHALMOL* 34:585–592, 1951.
g. Yunis EJ, Landes RR: Hazards of glove powder in renal angiography. *J AM MED ASSOC* 193:124–125, 1965.

Steel as an intraocular foreign body can cause siderosis and the same types of ocular disturbance as iron, if the steel is of readily corrodible type. Steels vary greatly in their resistance to oxidation and corrosion. Experiments on rabbits have shown that the least reactive, stainless, steels may be tolerated in the eye without producing siderosis.[a,b] (Compare *Iron.*)

a. Dollfus MA, Borsotti I: Tolerance of stainless steels in the rabbit eye. *BULL SOC OPHTALMOL PARIS* 422–423, 1938. (French)
b. Gronvall H, Hultgren A: Ocular splinters of steel, some clinical and metalographic data. *ACTA OPHTHAL* 37:413–466, 1960.

Stramonium (Asthmador), a preparation of dried leaves and flowers of *Datura stramonium* is used as an anticholinergic and antiasthmatic agent. Stramonium contains hyoscyamine, atropine, and scopolamine. Reactions to overdosage are similar to those in atropine or belladonna poisoning. Poisoning has developed from smoking cigarettes made with stramonium and from eating powdered stramonium, most commonly the commercial preparation, Asthmador. This has occurred most frequently in teen-agers who have intentionally taken excessive amounts to induce disorientation and hallucinations.[a,g] Characteristically the pupils have become widely dilated and unreactive to light. There has been excitement and confusion, visual and auditory hallucinations, tachycardia, dry mouth, and dry flushed skin. The visual hallucinations most often have consisted of seeing insects, which the patients try repeatedly to pick up and throw away. Most of the reaction usually subsides within twenty-four hours, with the mydriasis disappearing more slowly. Blurred vision, presumably from mydriasis and cycloplegia, has been noted, and mention has been made of complaint of green lights by some patients.[b] Apparently in only one case has persistent visual disturbance been related to stramonium. This was an instance of bilateral central scotoma, suspected to have been caused by smoking stramonium in treatment of asthma.[255] However, since no other case like this has been reported, despite many instances of undoubted poisoning by stramonium, it is quite doubtful that the stramonium could be held responsible in that unique case.

Besides the poisonings from medicinal preparations of stramonium, there have been many poisonings from the plant from which stramonium is prepared. This is described under *Datura stramonium* (see INDEX).

Treatment of stramonium should theoretically be like that for systemic atropine or belladonna poisoning, but spontaneous recovery from stramonium poisoning generally is so rapid, particularly in young people, that antidotes in most cases seem not to be needed.

a. Dean ES: Self-induced stramonium intoxication. *J AM MED ASSOC* 185:168–169, 1963.
b. DiGiacomo JN: Toxic effect of stramonium simulating LSD trip. *J AM MED ASSOC* 204:265–267, 1968.
c. Gabel MC: Purposeful ingestion of belladonna for hallucinatory effects. *J PEDIATR* 72:864–866, 1968.
d. Goldsmith SR, Frank I, Ungerleider JT: Poisoning from ingestion of a stramonium-belladonna mixture. *J AM MED ASSOC* 204:169–170, 1968.
e. Koff M: Poisoning from ingestion of asthma "powders." *J AM MED ASSOC* 198:170, 1966.
f. Teitelbaum DT: Stramonium poisoning in "Teeny-Boppers." *ANN INTERN MED* 68:174, 1968.
g. Wilcox, WP Jr: (Letter to Editor.) *N ENGL J MED* 277:1209, 1967.

Streptokinase (streptococcal fibrinolysin) has caused an inflammatory reaction in two human eyes when 625 units/ml were injected into the anterior chamber.[b] Also in rabbit eyes a mixture of streptokinase (13,000 units) and streptodornase (216 units) injected into the vitreous humor has caused a considerable inflammatory reaction in the iris and retina.[14]

Systemically administered streptokinase has also been considered to have unwanted ocular effects, as in the case of a man with an acute occlusion of a central retinal vein which was treated promptly with streptokinase and heparin, but by the next day was complicated by choroidal hematoma, followed by massive vitreous hemorrhage, and later vitreous organization and retinal detachment.[a]

a. Bec P, Arne JL, et al: Choroidal and vitreous hemorrhage in the course of treatment of a thrombosis of the central retinal vein with streptokinase. *BULL SOC OPHTALMOL FRANCE* 80:607–609, 1980. (French)
b. Berger B: The effect of steptokinase irrigation on experimentally clotted blood in the anterior chamber of human eyes. *ACTA OPHTHALMOL* 40:373–378, 1962.

Streptomycin, antibacterial (tuberculostatic), can cause vestibular damage and can affect hearing, but nystagmus can be induced without impairment of hearing or vestibular disturbance, as has been observed for instance by Bucci in twenty patients who had been treated with 0.5 g per day.[e] Illusory movement of the environment on turning the head is said to be an early sign of labyrinthine involvement.[n] Even without noticeable nystagmus, a blurring of vision has been described by Bender as occuring only during walking, riding, or moving the head. It has been reported after five weeks of streptomycin treatment.[c]

Paralysis of extraocular muscles has been observed by Bucci and Masci in three out of 720 patients given 0.5 g of streptomycin daily.[e]

Acute transient muscular weakness and impairment of vision in one patient apparently due to weakness of accommodation, but dramatically relieved by administration of neostigmine and atropine as in treatment of myasthenia gravis has been ascribed by Loder and Walker to neuromuscular blocking by streptomycin.[l]

Toxic effects on vision from streptomycin have been rare, but several instances have been reported. In a few cases long-continued administration of streptomycin has caused temporary visual disturbances such as xanthopsia with central scotoma for blue,[g,t] and nerve fiber bundle scotomas.[a,q] One patient is reported having bilateral optic neuritis with central scotoma, and subsequent recovery.[p] Bilateral central scotomas also developed in a man who had been receiving both streptomycin 1 g per day and chloramphenicol 2 g per day for twenty weeks, but it could not be said for sure which drug was responsible.[r] Vision recovered in a month after both drugs were discontinued and vitamin treatment was given.

Several instances of blindness or optic atrophy have been reported following intrathecal administration of streptomycin.[d,k,m,u]

Effects on color vision from streptomycin and dihydrostreptomycin have been studied by Laroche, who has reported that total dosage of 8 to 12 g given in a short time has produced green blindness, with normal color vision slowly recovered later in most patients, but apparently recovery has not been complete in patients who had some previous abnormality of their color vision.[i,j]

Indications of potential toxicity of streptomycin to retina or retinal vessels has been obtained by intravitreal injection, which rapidly produced retinal edema and subsequent clumping of pigment with loss of cellular elements of the retina, and migration of pigment from the pigment epithelium.[h] This sort of damage to the retina was not produced by streptomycin injected subconjunctivally in animals, though this is said to have produced congestion of uveal blood vessels and some hemorrhages.[b,h] Whether streptomycin given systemically has any deleterious effect on retinal vessels is uncertain, but this is suspected in at least two reports.[b,o]

Exfoliative dermatitis has occurred in treatment of tuberculosis with both streptomycin and aminosalicylic acid associated with corneal ulceration and permanent impairment of vision in one patient and blepharitis in several others. However, the aminosalicylic acid has been the primary suspect.[132]

Contact dermatitis among those handling streptomycin has been known to involve the eyelids, presumably carried there on the fingers.[f,s]

A more detailed review-synopsis of adverse effects of streptomycin on the eyes and vision was published in 1972 by Dralands and Garin, with 52 more references than in the bibliography below, but most seem to be largely of historical interest.[301]

a. Applemans M, De Graeve A: Streptomycin in the treatment of ocular manifestations of tuberculosis. *BULL SOC BELGE OPHTALMOL* 90:593–603, 1948. (French)

b. Arkin W, Trzcinska-Dabrowska Z: Toxic effect of steptomycin on the vessels of the eye. *KLIN OCZNA* 31:343–348, 1961.

c. Bender MB: Oscillopsia. *ARCH NEUROL* 13:204–213, 1965.

d. Bethoux L, Isnel R, et al: Blindness from primary optic atrophy in the course of tuberculous meningitis treated with streptomycin. *BULL SOC MED HOP PARIS* 65:489–491, 1949. (French)

e. Bucci MG, Masci EL: Streptomycin and ocular muscle balance. *BOLL OCULIST* 40:203–215, 1961. (Italian)

f. Dufour R: Palpebral eczema due to streptomycin. *PRAXIS* 37:427–428, 1948. (French)

g. Eiselt E, Kloubeck A: Disorders of color and space perception following administration of streptomycin. *CS LEK CESK* 87:549–551, 1948. (Ref. from Duke-Elder, 1954.[46])

h. Gardiner PA, Michaelson IC, et al: Intravitreous streptomycin; its toxicity and diffusion. *BR J OPHTHALMOL* 32:449–456, 1948.

i. Laroche J, Laroche C: Effect of some antibiotics on color vision. *ANN PHARM FR* 28:333–341, 1970. (French)

j. Laroche J: Modifications of color vision in human beings under the influence of certain medicinal substances. *ANN OCULIST* (*Paris*) 200:275–286, 1967. (French)

k. Lebas H: Optic atrophy caused by streptomycin. *BULL SOC BELGE OPHTALMOL* 93:450–452, 1949.

l. Loder RE, Walker GF: Neuromuscular blocking action of streptomycin. *LANCET* 1:812–813, 1959.

m. Mejer F: On disturbances of vision in streptomycin-treatment of tuberculous meningitis. *WIEN KLIN WOCHENSCHR* 61:407–409, 1949. (German)

n. Sannella LS: An early symptom of streptomycin neurotoxicity. *ARCH OPHTHALMOL* 50:331, 1953.

o. Schulz AE: Altitudinal hemianopia during streptomycin therapy. *AM J OPHTHALMOL* 32:211–213, 1949.

p. Sykowsky P: Streptomycin in miliary choroidal tuberculosis. *AM J OPHTHALMOL* 35:414–415, 1952.

q. Thomas EB: Scotoma in conjunction with streptomycin therapy. *ARCH OPHTHALMOL* 43:729–741, 1950.

r. Walker G: Blindness during streptomycin and chloramphenicol therapy. *BR J OPHTHALMOL* 45:555–559, 1961.

s. Weekers L: An occupational disease of nurses, lid eczema due to streptomycin. *REV MED LIEGE* 5:320–322, 1950. (French)

t. Weigelin S: Xanthopsia from streptomycin poisoning. *KLIN MONATSBL AUGEN-HEILKD* 114:266–267, 1949. (German)

u. Weismann-Netter R, Gandon J, du Sorbierh: On ocular complications of intrathecal streptomycin treatment. *BULL SOC MED HOP PARIS* 65:761–766, 1949. (French)

Streptozotocin, an antineoplastic agent, produces diabetes in albino rats after a single intravenous injection, due to a specific destructive effect on beta cells of the pancreas, and causes the lenses to become opalescent in about five weeks. Dense cataracts form within four to ten months (Verheyden-1967). Von Sallman and Grimes found cataractous changes to be already visible after ten to fourteen days. They also noted transient hemorrhages in the anterior segment at this time, but did not know where they came from. The morphology of the developing cataracts and associated changes in composition of the lenses have been studies by Sasaki and Kuriyama. Cataracts have also been produced in monkeys by streptozotocin (Howard). In rats, the development of cataracts were interfered with by administering nicotinamide (White), an unsaturated fat diet (Hutton), vitamin E (Ross), or aldose-reductase inhibitors (Poulsom). However the interpretation of these observations remains uncertain.

Von Sallmann when studying development of the cataracts noted that the retinas remained normal during three months of observation, based on ophthalmoscopy and light microscopy. However, Sevenberger et al in 1971, and Sosula et al in 1972, discovered by electron microscopy that significant ultrastructural changes were taking place in the capillaries of the retina during that time. Great interest evolved in the possibility that the retinopathy associated with streptozotocin-induced diabetes in the rat might provide an animal model corresponding to the diabetic retinopathy which is such a serious problem in human beings. Leuenberger et al, and Babel and Leuenberger, have reported that the rats showed loss of retinal capillary endothelium and mural cells, variations in capillary diameter, saccular microaneurysms, and change in the basement membranes of capillaries. Increase in thickness of the basement membrane with deposition of collagen-like material has been noted (Papachristodoulou). In mice also, disappearance of retinal mural pericytes has appeared analogous to findings in human diabetic retinopathy.

Besides the morphologic changes in retinal vessels, the retinal pigment epithelium has been found to undergo a marked increase of infolding of the membrane at the basal surface of the cells, with doubling of its area, and an associated increase in penetration of fluorescein into the cells (Grimes). In Muller cells a marked increase has been reported in lysosomal enzymes, which may help eliminate debris from necrotic pericytes and digest excessive glycogen (Hori).

Fluorophotometry of the vitreous humor after intravenous administration of fluorescein to test the blood-vitreous barrier has shown that in streptozotocin-diabetic rats there is abnormal permeability (Kernell; Krupin; Vine), similar to what is found in human diabetes. The same increased permeability was found in guinea pigs, although they lack retinal vessels (Klein). In rats, both passive and facilitated transport of glucose across the blood-vitreous barrier are affected early (Di Mattio). Providing increased insulin interfered with breakdown of the barrier (Kernell; Krupin). Streptozotocin did not cause breakdown of the blood-vitreous barrier to dextran-labeled fluorescein (Krupin), or to horse-radish peroxidase (Wallow). In the first week or two, Maepea found that even before breakdown of the blood-ocular barriers, organic acids could accumulate in the vitreous body as a result of reduced outward transport.

Testing for toxicity to the retina in rabbits indicated that 0.1 mg streptozotocin per ml could be injected into the vitreous body without damage evident by light microscopy histology, or by ERG.[277]

Agren A, Rehn G, Naeser P: Morphology and enzyme activity of the retinal capillaries in streptozotocin-diabetic mice. *ACTA OPHTHALMOL* 57:1065–1069, 1979.

Babel J, Leuenberger P: A long term study on the ocular lesions in streptozotocin diabetic rats. *GRAEFES ARCH OPHTHALMOL* 189:191–201, 1974.

DiMattio J, Zadunaisky JA, Altrzuler N: Onset of changes in glucose transport across ocular barriers in streptozotocin-induced diabetes. *INVEST OPHTHALMOL VIS SCI* 25:820–826, 1984.

Grimes PA, Laties AM: Early morphological alteration of the pigment epithelium in streptozotocin-induced diabetes. *EXP EYE RES* 30:631–639, 1980.

Hori S, Nishida T, Mukai N: Ultrastructural studies on lysosomes in retinal Muller cells of streptozotocin-diabetic rats. *INVEST OPHTHALMOL VIS SCI* 19:1295–1300, 1980.

Howard Jr CF, Peterson LH: Cataract development in streptozotocin diabetic monkeys. *LAB ANIM SCI* 23:366–369, 1973.

Hutton JC, Schofield PJ, et al: The effect of an unsaturated fat diet on cataract formation in streptozotocin induced diabetic rats. *BR J NUTR* 36:161–177, 1976.

Kernell A, Arnquist H: Effect of insulin treatment on the blood-retinal barrier in rats with streptozotocin-induced diabetes. *ARCH OPHTHALMOL* 101:968–970, 1983.

Klein R, Engerman RL, Ernst T: Fluorophotometry. II. Streptozotocin-treated guinea pigs. *ARCH OPHTHALMOL* 98:2233–2234, 1980.

Krupin T, Waltman SR, et al: Fluorometric studies on the blood-retinal barrier in experimental animals. *ARCH OPHTHALMOL* 100:631–634, 1982.

Krupin T, Waltman SR, et al: Ocular fluorophotometry in streptozotocin diabetes mellitus in the rat. *INVEST OPHTHALMOL VIS SCI* 18:1185–1190, 1979.

Kuriyama H, Sasaki K, Fukuda M: Studies on diabetic cataract in rats induced by streptozotocin. *OPHTHALMIC RES* 15:191–197, 1983.

Leuenberger P, Cameron D, et al: Ocular lesions in rats rendered chronically diabetic with streptozotocin. *OPHTHALMOL RES* 2:189–204, 1971.

Maepea O, Karlsson C, Alm A: Blood-ocular and blood-brain barrier function in streptozotocin-induced diabetes in rats. *ARCH OPHTHALMOL* 102:1366–1369, 1984.

Papachristodoulon D, Heath H: Ultrastructural alteration during the development of retinopathy in sucrose-fed and streptozotocin-diabetic rats. *EXP EYE RES* 25:371–384, 1977.

Poulsom R, Boot Handford RP, Heath H: Some effects of aldose reductase inhibition upon the eyes of long-term streptozotocin-diabetic rats. *CURR EYE RES* 2:351–355, 1982–3.

Ross WW, Creighton MO, et al: Modelling cortical cataractognesis. *CAN J OPHTHALMOL* 17:61–66, 1982.

Sallmann L von, Grimes P: Eye changes in streptozotocin diabetes in rats. *AM J OPHTHALMOL* 71(1-Part 2): 312–319, 1971.

Sasaki K, Kuriyama H, et al: Studies on diabetic cataract in rats induced by streptozotocin. *OPHTHALMIC RES* 15:185–190, 1983.

Sosula L. Beaumont P, et al: Dilatation and endothelial proliferation of retinal capillaries in streptozotocin-diabetic rats. *INVEST OPHTHALMOL* 11:926–935, 1972.

Verheyden MD: Experimental cataract induced by streptozotocin. *BULL SOC BELGE OPHTALMOL* 147:479–485, 1967. (French)

Vine AK, Kisly AM, et al: Vitreous fluorophotometry in rats with streptozotocin-induced diabetes. *ARCH OPHTHALMOL* 102:1083–1085, 1984.

Strontium acetate tested on a rabbit's eye by application of 0.1 M solution for ten minutes after removal of the corneal epithelium (to facilitate penetration) caused no appreciable opacity or injury.[90]

Strontium hydroxide forms very alkaline solutions, pH about 13.5.[171] Splashed in the eye it has caused burns as serious as those caused by the other strong alkalies,[34,242] and applied experimentally to cattle and rabbit eyes it has produced corneal opacities.[a,89,137] Strontium hydroxide appears not to lead to calcification of the cornea either in patients or in rabbits.[34,81]

Strontium oxide forms strontium hydroxide when it reacts with water. It too is severely injurious to the eyes.[a]

a. Haurowitz F, Braun G: On lime burn of the cornea. *Z PHYSIOL CHEM* 123:79–89, 1922. (German)

Strychnine poisoning is characterized by painful tonic convulsions, which may be accompanied by mydriasis, proptosis, and conjugate or dissociated deviations of the eyes.[153,196,214,255] Lewin and Guillery in 1913 mentioned that persistent blindness had been observed following attempts at suicide with strychnine and *nux vomica*, but gave no references, and none were found subsequently.[153]

A thorough investigation by Schlaginweit disputed any effect of strychnine on vision or visual fields.[d] Oskarsson in 1962 showed that visual acuity in normal human beings is not affected any more by intramuscular injection of 4 mg strychnine nitrate than by injection of sodium chloride placebo.[c]

Intravitreal injection of strychnine (0.0012 M) in rabbits has had little or no effect on the ERG or light-induced optic nerve potential, but intravenous injection in cats has been reported to increase the spontaneous electrical activity of the optic nerve neurons.[b] An effect on frog retina has also been observed.[a]

a. Burkhardt DA: Effects of picrotoxin and strychnine upon electrical activity of the proximal retina. *BRAIN RES* 43:246–249, 1972.
b. Heiss WD: The protracted activity of retinal neurons under the influence of strychnine and picrotoxin. *VISION RES* 7:583–598, 1967.
c. Oskarsson V: The effect of strychnine on visual acuity. *ACTA PHARMACOL* 19:16–22, 1962.
d. Schlaginweit E: On effect of strychnine on the senses, especially on the eye. *NAUNYN- -SCHMIEDEBERG'S ARCH EXP PATH PHARMAK* 95:104–123, 1922. (German)

Stypandra imbricata is a grass-like plant, which, when eaten by sheep, goats, and rats, has caused blindness. In Western Australia it has been known as "blind grass." A review of its effects and a report on experimental work on rats have been provided by Huxtable et al. Rats on a diet containing *Stypandra imbricata* developed a paresis of the hind limbs and blindness in 2 to 5 days. Dissections at this stage of acute poisoning revealed gross swelling of optic nerves and chiasm. Ophthalmoscopy showed nothing abnormal in the ocular fundi except engorgement of retinal veins. If a normal diet was given at this time, the rats recovered, but remained blind; otherwise they soon died from respiratory paralysis. The optic nerves showed vacuolation of their myelin, axonal degeneration, and reactive changes in glial cells. During 2 to 3 months the optic nerves became completely atrophic. At the same time the retinas histologically showed loss of outer plexiform layer, outer nuclear layer, and photoreceptors, indicating that the retinas had been poisoned as well as the optic nerves. This has been reported also in sheep and goats. Huxtable et al have pointed out that the acute edema of central and peripheral myelin and axonal degeneration caused by *Stypandra imbricata* were remarkably similar to changes that can be produced by poisoning with *hexachlorophene*. The chemical basis for this had not been determined.

Huxtable CR, Dorling PR, Slatter DH: Myelin oedema, optic neuropathy and retinopathy in experimental *Stypandra imbricata* toxicosis. *NEUROPATHOL APPL NEUROBIOL* 6:221–232, 1980.

Styrene (styrol, phenylethylene, vinyl benzene) has been tested by application to rabbit eyes and found to cause moderate hyperemia of the conjunctiva and slight injury of the corneal epithelium, with rapid return to normal.[265] The reaction has been graded 4 on a scale of 1 to 10 after twenty-four hours.[27] Splash contact with human eyes has resulted in similar superficial transient disturbance, with return to normal within forty-eight hours in twenty-nine out of thirty cases.[165] In the exceptional case healing took three to ten days.

The vapor of styrene tested on rats has been found to have transient irritant effect on eyes and nose at concentrations of 200 to 400 ppm, and caused definite signs of eye and nose irritation at concentrations of 1,300 ppm. However, exposure to 1,300 ppm for seven to eight hours a day, five days a week for six months produced no permanent injury.[188]

Styrene vapor exposure of human beings to 100 ppm in air causes mild irritation of the eyes and throat in twenty minutes in some people. Even at 375 ppm not all people feel significant eye irritation in fifteen minutes, but all have nasal irritation at this concentration.[j] Concentrations of 400 and 500 ppm more consistently cause irritation of eyes and nose, but can be tolerated.[c,j,k] Irritation becomes so extreme at 1,300 ppm that it provides a safeguard against voluntary exposure to concentrations which might have narcotic effect.[e,i]

Products having high irritancy to the human eye are formed when styrene is photo-oxidized with ozone and nitrogen dioxide as in formation of smog. (See *Smog* for further details.) Also, a potent lacrimator has been formed when styrene wastes became mixed with bromine or chlorine wastes and reacted under the influence of sunlight.[a]

A suspicion that styrene might produce retrobulbar neuritis was raised by Elliot and by Pratt-Johnson in 1964, reporting a rapid decrease in visual acuity associated with centrocecal scotomas in both eyes of a man making fiberglass boats in a small room with no control over styrene or other vapor concentrations and no precautions to avoid contact of the material with his skin.[e,h] Medical investigation detected none of the known causes of retrobulbar neuritis or centrocecal scotoma. The patient avoided further exposure and was given vitamin treatment for six months. His vision recovered completely within a year from a low of 20/400. The optic nerveheads and fundi appeared normal at all times. The evidence implicating styrene was entirely circumstantial. Another patient was seen by Donaldson and Cogan with the same type of exposure before developing central scotomas, but in this case thorough study of the patient and his relatives indicated that the exposure was coincidental; the patient actually had Leber's optic atrophy and his relatives had the same trouble without exposure.[d]

A study of 345 people working in a styrene plant by Kohn in 1978 produced no evidence of optic neuropathy or other significant eye disease, despite considerable acute and chronic exposures.[f]

Experimentally, styrene given intravenously to monkeys has caused appreciable changes in the c-wave of the ERG and in the standing potential of the eye, suggesting some action on the retinal pigment epithelium, but the clinical significance is uncertain.[g]

In 1952 Barsotti and associates mentioned that three out of nine workmen who had been exposed to *ethyl benzene* vapor (0.8 to 1.2 mg/liter of air) for eighteen or more months complained of reduced vision in dim illumination. Polystyrene resin was being manufactured and presence of styrene vapor (0.8 mg/liter of air) was also mentioned, but no examination of the eyes was reported except note of hyperemia of the conjunctiva.[b] The significance of these observations relative to styrene toxicity is quite open to question.

a. Anonymous: Report of Air Pollution and Smoke Prevention Association of America. *CHEM ENG NEWS* 30:2704–2705, 1952.
b. Barsotti, M, Parmeggiani L, Sassi C: Observations of occupational pathology in a plant making polystyrene resins. *MED LAVORO* 43:418–424, 1952. (Italian)
c. Carpenter CP, Shaffer CB, et al: Studies on the inhalation of 1,3-butadiene; with a comparison of its narcotic effect with benzol, toluol and styrene, and a note of the elimination of styrene by the human. *J IND HYG* 26:69–78, 1944.
d. Donaldson DD: Personal communication, 1962.
e. Elliot AJ: Personal communication, 1962.
f. Kohn AN: Ocular toxicity of styrene. *AM J OPHTHALMOL* 85:569–570, 1978.
g. Skoog KO, Nilsson SEG: Changes in the c-wave of the electroretinogram and in the standing potential of the eye after small doses of toluene and styrene. *ACTA OPHTHALMOL* 59:71–79, 1981.
h. Pratt-Johnson JA: Retrobulbar neuritis following exposure to vinyl benzene (styrene). *CAN MED ASSOC J* 90:975–977, 1964.
i. Spencer HC, Irish DD, et al: The response of laboratory animals to monomeric styrene. *J IND HYG* 24:295–301, 1942.
j. Stewart RD, Dodd HC, et al: Human exposure to styrene vapor. *ARCH ENVIRON HEALTH* 16:656–662, 1968.
k. Wilson RH: Health hazards encountered in the manufacture of synthetic rubber. *J AM MED ASSOC* 124:701–703, 1944.

Subathizone has been employed in the treatment of tuberculosis. In one patient who received 200 mg daily for a month vision gradually became reduced to 6/24 in each eye. Ophthalmic examination was completely negative except for the decrease in visual acuity. Diagnosis of toxic amblyopia was made and the drug discontinued. Vision returned to normal in the course of several months.[a]

a. Jopling WH, Kirkwan EWO'G: Toxic amblyopia caused by TB3. *TRANS ROY SOC TROP MED HYG* 46:656–657, 1952.

Substance P, a natural peptide, is thought to be a neurotransmitter involved in a portion of the inflammatory response of the eye to antidromic sensory irritation. When injected into the rabbit's eye, it can cause strong miosis, which is a part of the inflammatory response, without breaking down the blood-aqueous barrier.[a,b]

a. Holmdahl G, Hakanson R, et al: A substance P antagonist inhibits inflammatory responses in the rabbit eye. *SCIENCE* 214:1029–1031, 1981.
b. Stjernschantz J, Sears M, Mishima H: Role of substance P in the antidromic vasodilation,

neurogenic plasma extravasation and disruption of the blood-aqueous barrier in the rabbit eye. *NAUNYN-SCHMIED ARCH PHARMACOL* 321:329–335, 1982.

Succinylcholine (suxamethonium; Anectine; Quelicin; Sucostrin; Sux-Cert), a skeletal muscle relaxant, causes transient contraction of the extraocular muscles and temporary rise of intraocular pressure. It has in rare instances caused prolonged apnea in patients whose cholinesterase had been inactivated by systemic absorption of anticholinesterase miotic eyedrops used in treatment of glaucoma[v], or from absorption of anticholinesterase insecticides.[x] Also, in rare individuals who genetically have lacked the proper cholinesterase to inactivate succinylcholine, there have been episodes of prolonged apnea.[t]

Many clinical and experimental observations have been published concerning the transitory elevation of intraocular pressure produced by parenterally administered suxamethonium as an adjunct to general anesthesia.[b–h, j–s, u, w, y–za] The subject has been reviewed by Self and Ellis.[w] Generally the increase in intraocular pressure has been attributed to contraction of the extraocular muscles. It has caused a rise of intraocular pressure usually in the range of 5 to 15 mm Hg, but this has been brief, gone in minutes, and is dangerous only if the eyeball has been opened before the muscular contraction occurs. If the globe has been opened surgically or by traumatic laceration, the contraction can cause expulsion of ocular contents, potentially seriously damaging the eye. Succinylcholine is therefore either to be avoided if the globe has already been opened, or its effect on the eye should be blocked by prior administration of gallamine or d-tubocurarine.[b, e, j, s]

Also the effect of suxamethonium on extraocular muscles and on intraocular pressure is said to be reduced by deep general anesthesia. Glaucoma is not a contraindication to use of succinylcholine, since the influence on intraocular pressure is so brief.

In vitro, human and animal extraocular muscles contract under the influence of succinylcholine.[d, i]

In anesthetized patients, duction testing has shown residual influences on extraocular muscles for a significantly longer time than would be expected from the brief elevation of intraocular pressure.[f]

Ultrasound studies have shown in patients a brief flattening of the lens and deepening of the anterior chamber, as though the ciliary muscle is paralyzed at about the same time the intraocular pressure is raised.[a]

a. Abramson DH: Anterior chamber and lens thickness changes induced by succinylcholine. *ARCH OPHTHALMOL* 86:643, 1971.
b. Cook JH: The effect of suxamethonium on intraocular pressure. *ANESTHESIA* 36:359–365, 1981.
c. Craythorne NWB, Rottenstein HS, Dripps RD: The effects of succinylcholine on intraocular pressure in adults, infants and children during general anesthesia. *ANESTHESIOLOGY* 21:59–63, 1960.
d. Dillon JB, Sabawala P, et al: Action of succinylcholine on extraocular muscles and intraocular pressure. *ANESTHESIOLOGY* 18:44–49, 1957.
e. Donlon JV Jr: Anesthesia factors affecting intraocular pressure. *ANESTHESIOL REV* 8:13–18, 1981.

f. France TD (1979): Quoted by Metz.ʳ

g. Goldsmith E. An evaluation of succinylcholine and gallamine as muscle relaxants in relation to intraocular tension. *ANESTH ANALG* 46:557–561, 1967.

h. Goldstein JH, Gupta MK, Shah MD: Comparison of intramuscular and intravenous succinylcholine on intraocular pressure. *ANN OPHTHALMOL* 13:173–174, 1981.

i. Hofmann H, Lembeck F: Pharmacologic studies on isolated human extraocular muscle. *GRAEFES ARCH OPHTHALMOL* 158:277–279, 1956. (German)

j. Katz RL, Eakins KE: Mode of action of succinylcholine on intraocular pressure. *J PHARMACOL EXP THER* 162:1–9, 1968.

k. Katz RL, Eakins KE: Actions of neuromuscular blocking agents on extraocular muscle and intraocular pressure. *PROC ROY SOC MED* 62:1217–1220, 1969.

l. Katz RL, Eakins KE, Lord CO: The effects of hexafluorenium in preventing the increase in intraocular pressure produced by succinylcholine. *ANESTHESIOLOGY* 29:70–78, 1968.

m. Kornblueth W, Jampolsky A, et al: Contraction of the oculorotary muscles and intraocular pressure. *AM J OPHTHALMOL* 49:1381–1387, 1960.

n. Lessell S, Kuwabara T, Feldman RG: Myopathy and succinylcholine sensitivity. *AM J OPHTHALMOL* 68:789–796, 1969.

o. Lincoff HA, Ellis CH, et al: The effect of succinylcholine on intraocular pressure. *AM J OPHTHALMOL* 40:501–510, 1955.

p. Lincoff HA, Breinin GM, DeVoe G: The effect of succinycholine on the extraocular muscles. *AM J OPHTHALMOL* 43:440–444, 1957.

q. Macri FJ, Grimes PA: The effects of succinylcholine on the extraocular striate muscles and on the intraocular pressure. *AM J OPHTHALMOL* 44:221–230, 1957.

r. Metz HS, Venkatesh B: Succinylcholine and intraocular pressure. *J PEDIATR OPHTHALMOL* 18:12–14, 1981.

s. Miller RD, Way WL, Hickey RF: Inhibition of succinylcholine-induced increased intraocular pressure by non-depolarizing muscle relaxants. *ANESTHESIOLOGY* 29:123–126, 1968.

t. Nelson LB, Wagner RS, Harley RD: Prolonged apnea caused by inherited cholinesterase deficiency after strabismus surgery. *AM J OPHTHALMOL* 96:392–393, 1983.

u. Pandey K, Badola RP, Kumar S: Time course of intraocular hypertension produced by suxamethonium. *BR J ANESTH* 44:191–195, 1972.

v. Pantuck EJ: Echothiophate iodide eye drops and prolonged response to suxamethonium. *BR J ANAESTH* 38:406–407, 1966.

w. Self WG, Ellis PP: The effect of general anesthetic agents on intraocular pressure. *SURV OPHTHALMOL* 21:494–500, 1977.

x. Seybold R, Brautigam KH: Prolonged succinyl-induced apnea as pointer to alkylphosphate poisoning. *DTSCH MED WOCHENSCHR* 93:1405–1506, 1968. (German)

y. Smith RB, Babinski M, Leano N: The effect of lidocaine on succinylcholine-induced rise in intraocular pressure. *CAN ANAESTH SOC J* 26:482–483, 1979.

z. Verma RA: "Self-taming" of succinylcholine-induced fasciculations and intraocular pressure. *ANESTHESIOLOGY* 50:245–247, 1979.

za. Wynands JE, Crowell DE: Intraocular tension in association with succinylcholine and endotracheal intubation. *CAN ANAESTH SOC J* 7:39–43, 1960.

Sucrose has shown no toxicity to the corneas of rabbits when applied for three to seven hours in neutral aqueous solution.[209]

In rats in which 72% of the diet consisted of sucrose both vascular and neural retinopathies developed within a year.[b] These did not develop in control rats on diets containing corn starch in place of the sucrose. Changes in the vessels were similar to those in human beings with non-proliferative diabetes and in diabetic animals. There was degeneration of the photoreceptor cells, affecting both rod and outer nuclear layers, but ganglion cells, pigmented epithelium, and choroid were undisturbed. The ERG was severely affected.[a]

 a. Cohen AM, Freund H, Auerbach E: The electroretinogram in sucrose and starch-fed rats. *METABOLISM* 19:1064, 1970.

 b. Cohen AM, Michaelson IC, Yanko L: Retinopathy in rats with disturbed carbohydrate metabolism following a high sucrose diet. *AM J OPHTHALMOL* 73:863–875, 1972.

Sulfaethoxypyridazine, a veterinary antimicrobial, has caused cataracts in rats and dogs after chronic oral administration.[a] The cataracts appeared after several months, actually after the administration of the drug had been discontinued. The cataracts were diagnosed by ophthalmoscopy, and the initial report said nothing about other parts of the eye or histological examination of the eye. This was believed to be the first report of induction of cataracts by a sulfonamide. The mechanism was not known.

 a. Ribelin WE, Owen G, et al: Development of cataracts in dogs and rats from prolonged feeding of sulfaethoxy-pyridazine. *TOXICOL APPL PHARMACOL* 10:557–564, 1967.

Sulfamic acid is widely employed industrially where a strong acid is needed. On rabbit eyes application of 0.5 cc of a 4% solution is reported to have caused moderate conjunctivitis and edema, but no serious injury.[a]

Some unusual eye injuries have occurred in personnel cleaning an evaporator with a solution of sulfamic acid containing also *diethylthiourea* (1%).[b] The people exposed worked inside a large cupronickel evaporator, removing sediment and dead fish and inspecting the job after the acid solution had been drained. Some who were exposed to the atmosphere in the evaporator developed severe eye irritation several hours later, with swelling of the lids and blepharospasm. Some loss of corneal epithelium was observed. However, recovery was complete. Most likely some substance other than sulfamic acid itself was responsible for the injuries. Some suspicion naturally falls on the *diethylthiourea* which was present in small amounts, and this suspicion is encouraged by a report of a series of patients who developed painful superficial keratitis after exposure to probable decomposition products of *diethylthiourea* in manufacture of synthetic rubber where no sulfamic acid was present. (For more details see INDEX for *Diethylthiourea.*)

 a. Ambrose AM: Studies on the physiological effects of sulfamic acid and ammonium sulfamate. *J IND HYG* 25:26–28, 1943.

 b. Hargens CW: Personal communication, 1970.

Sulfolane, an organic solvent, tested full strength on rabbit eyes was only mildly irritating, producing conjunctival reaction which lasted only a few hours, and no injury of the cornea.[a]

a. Brown VKH, Ferrigan LW, Stevenson DE: Acute toxicity and skin irritant properties of sulfolane. *BR J IND MED* 23:302–304, 1966.

Sulfonamide drugs include compounds such as *sulfacetamide, sulfadiazine, sulfanilamide, sulfapyridine,* and *sulfathiazole,* which have been employed in treatment of infections, as well as compounds such as *acetazolamide* employed principally for their inhibitory effect on carbonic anhydrase. Sulfonamide drugs have been held responsible for several types of ocular disturbance, including acute transient myopia, conjunctivitis, and keratitis associated with skin reactions, rarely disturbances of the optic nerve and retina, and temporary impairment of depth perception. Comprehensive surveys of these toxic effects were provided in 1957 by Walsh,[255] and in 1972 by Dralands and Garin, with 66 references from the period 1940–1968.[301]

The effect upon the eye which has most commonly been produced by systemically administered sulfonamide drugs is induction of acute and completely reversible myopia. More than thirty-five publications have presented original case reports and observations concerning the induction of this side effect by antibacterial sulfonamides. Several other publications have been concerned with the same effect produced by sulfonamides having primarily carbonic anhydrase-inhibiting action. Since the same type of "acute transient myopia" has been produced also by other classes of drugs, mainly diuretics, this reaction will not be described further here, but is more comprehensively described in a separate section. (See the INDEX for *Myopia, acute transient.*)

Reactions of the conjunctiva have occurred in a small proportion of patients receiving sulfonamide drugs systematically, most commonly from sulfathiazole.[v] Inflammation and chemosis of the conjunctiva have been accompanied by swelling of the lids, and in the more severe cases by photophobia, lacrimation, and discharge. The majority of conjunctival reactions have not been severe and have not produced permanent changes, but have cleared within a few days after discontinuing drugs. In the more serious cases, changes in the conjunctiva resembling pemphigus have produced symblepharon. These rare pemphigoid lesions have been associated particularly with the use of sulfadiazine[i,m,n] and sulfamerazine.[l]

The most severe combined skin and conjunctival reactions to systemic sulfonamides have been instances of the Stevens-Johnson syndrome[e] and the Lyell syndrome.[q] An extensive review of the Stevens-Johnson syndrome, with numerous references and a well-illustrated case report of this type of reaction to treatment with sulfamethoxypyridazine and streptomycin, was published by Rossi in 1966.[o]

Retinal and preretinal hemorrhages have in very rare instances been observed following administration of sulfanilamide and sulfathiazole.[b,f,j] In at least one instance the hemorrhages were associated with aplastic anemia from which the patient eventually died.[f]

Sulfhemoglobinemia showing up as a "vivid light lavender color" in the retinal arteries and veins has been graphically described by Walsh and Beehler as a side effect in a patient who had taken sulfamethizole for eight years and also chlorotrianisene for nearly as long.[w]

Visual disturbances have in a few cases been attributed to effects of sulfonamides on the optic nerve or retina.[s,v] Xanthopsia or yellow vision has been noted in single instances after taking sulfathiazole and sulfadiazine. A review of reports of toxic amblyopia in 1955 by Taub and Hollenhorst indicated that very few such cases had previously been published, but they added four new cases which had been discovered during a ten-year period at the Mayo clinic.[s] From these observations it appears that amblyopia associated with use of sulfonamides, usually from small doses, most commonly has been attributable to optic neuritis, usually with papilledema. Central scotoma has been found, but there has been strong tendency to complete recovery.[d,s]

In one case transitory ptosis and paresis of extraocular muscles has been attributed to sulfonamides. A study by Walsh and associates in 1943 on patients with normal eyes showed that orally administered sulfathiazole and sulfadiazine frequently impaired depth perception, causing tendency to exophoria at near and decrease of adduction power.[255]

Sulfonamides applied directly to the eyes have in rare cases produced side effects similar to those from systemic medication. Stevens-Johnson syndrome has been induced by topical sulfacetamide,[k,p] and also lupus erythemathosus.[a]

Conjunctival concretions from use of sulfadiazine eyedrops, several times a day for a year, have been described in one patient. These were proven analytically to be sulfadiazine crystals located within superficial cysts in the palpebral conjunctiva, or protruding from the surface. Redness and irritation of the eyes resolved when the sulfadiazine was discontinued and the concretions were removed.[c]

Sunburn of the upper lids limited to the area of application of sulfisoxazole ointment to the lid margins has been described in four patients as a phototoxic reaction.[g,h]

   a. Adams JD: Drug induced lupus erythematosus case report. *AUSTRALASIAN J DERM* 19:31–33, 1978.
   b. Baker JP JR: Sulfanilamide therapy followed by hemorrhages in fundus of eye. *VIRGINIA MED MONTHLY* 67:562–563, 1940.
   c. Boettner EA, Fralick FB, Wolter JR: Conjunctival concretions of sulfadiazine. *ARCH OPHTHALMOL* 92:446–448, 1974.
   d. Bucy PC: Toxic optic neuritis resulting from sulfanilamide. *J AM MED ASSOC* 109:1007–1008, 1937.
   e. Cameron AJ, Baron JH, Priestly BL: Erythema multiforme drugs, and ulcerative colitis. *BR J MED* 2:1174–1178, 1966.
   f. Carrot E, Oudot B: Hemorrhagic retinopathy as first sign of serious hemopathy after sulfonamide treatment. *REV OTONEUROOPHTALMOL* 21:180–189, 1949. (French)
   g. Flach A: Photosensitivity to sulfisoxazole ointment. *ARCH OPHTHALMOL* 99:609–610, 1981.
   h. Flash AJ, Peterson JS, Mathias CGT: Photosensitivity to topically applied sulfisoxazole ointment. *ARCH OPHTHALMOL* 100:1286–1287, 1982.
   i. Friedman B: Therapeutic sulfadiazine poisoning with pemphigoid lesions. *ARCH OPHTHALMOL* 38:796–805, 1947.
   j. Goar EL: Retinal hemorrhages following the ingestion of sulfathiazole. *AM J OPHTHALMOL* 25:332–333, 1942.
   k. Gottschalk HR, Stone OJ: Stevens-Johnson syndrome from ophthalmic sulfonamide. *ARCH DERMATOL* 112:513, 1976.
   l. Newell FW, Greentham JS: Pemphigus conjunctivae. *AM J OPHTHALMOL* 29:1426–1431, 1946.

m. Prado D: Strange ocular complication caused from intoxication by sulfadiazine. *ARCH BRAS OFTALMOL* 8:169–172, 1945.

n. Raffeto JF, Nichols S: A nearly fatal reaction to sulfadiazine in a 10 year old girl, involving skin, eyes and oropharynx. *J PEDIATR* 20:753, 1942.

o. Rossi A: Observations on the Stevens-Johnson syndrome. *RASS ITAL OTTALMOL* 34:3–21, 1965–1966. (Italian)

p. Rubin Z: Ophthalmic sulfonamide-induced Stevens-Johnson syndrome. *ARCH DERMATOL* 113:235–236, 1977.

q. Saraux H, Chigot PL, et al: Ocular manifestations in the course of the Lyell syndrome in relation to three cases developed after use of sulfonamides. *BULL SOC OPHTALMOL FRANCE* 65:915–919, 1965. (French)

r. Slaughter D: Sulfonamides and dark adaptation. *J LAB CLIN MED* 31:987–990, 1946.

s. Taub RG, Hollenhorst RW: Sulfonamides as a cause of toxic amblyopia. *AM J OPHTHALMOL* 40:486–490, 1955.

t. Todenhofer H: Toxic side effects of sulfadiazine used as geriatric medication for dogs. *DTSCH TIERAERZTL WOCHENSCHR* 76:14–16, 1969. (German)

u. Volini IF, Levitt RO, O'Neil HB: Cutaneous and conjunctival manifestation of sulfathiazole intoxication. *J AM MED ASSOC* 116:938–940, 1941.

v. Wagener HP: Toxic effects of sulfonamides on the eyes. *AM J MED SCI* 206:261–268, 1943.

w. Walsh TJ, Beehler C: Fundus in sulfhemoglobinemia. *ARCH INTERN MED* (Chicago), 124:377–378, 1969.

Sulfosalicylic acid, a protein precipitant, inhibits the swelling of pieces of cornea in water, and in rabbit eyes is toxic to the cornea at pH more acid than 5.5.[79,123] A neutral 0.1 M solution of *sodium sulfosalicylate* has been tested on rabbit eyes by irrigation of the surface for ten minutes after the corneal epithelium was removed mechanically to facilitate penetration.[81] A slight transient haze of the cornea and hyperemia of the iris resulted, but was followed by complete healing and return to normal. The effect of *sodium sulfosalicylate* in combating local toxic effects of beryllium has been examined and found beneficial.[90] (See INDEX for *Beryllium.*)

Sulfur as a dust has been noted to induce slight to severe irritation of the eyes.[b,d,33,81,129,249] Chemical determinations have indicated that the thresholds for amorphous and crystalline sulfur as aerosols to cause ocular irritation are 0.2 and 9 ppm respectively.[b]

The symptoms and signs are strikingly similar to those caused by hydrogen sulfide. An individual may be exposed for several hours or days to sulfur dust before beginning to develop sensation of scratchy discomfort in the eyes. This may then progress to burning and tearing, with blurring of vision. Keratitis epithelialis may be found, and there may be loss of patches of corneal epithelium with no evident abnormality of the deeper layers of the cornea.[81] Recovery is spontaneous and complete within two or three days when exposure is discontinued.

It is possible that conversion of sulfur to hydrogen sulfide is involved in the induction of ocular irritation, but this mechanism has not been investigated in the eye. There is evidence that elsewhere sulfur is reduced to hydrogen sulfide biologically, and that this may be the basis of the fungicidal action of sulfur.[a,c] (See also *Hydrogen sulfide.*)

a. Outline of information on pesticides. Part I. Agricultural fungicides. Council on Pharmacy and Chemistry. *J AM MED ASSOC* 157:237–241, 1955.
b. Magill PL, Rolston MV, Bremmer RW: Determination of free sulfur in the atmosphere. *ANAL CHEM* 21:1411, 1949.
c. Shepard HH: THE CHEMISTRY AND ACTION OF INSECTICIDES. New York, McGraw-Hill, 1951.
d. Wyers H: Some recent observations of hazards in the chemical industry. *PROC 9TH INTERN CONGR IND MED London*, 1948, 1949, pp. 900–903.

Sulfur dioxide is a colorless gas easily compressible to a liquid. Mettier in 1960 provided a review and bibliography of observations on irritant effects of gaseous sulfur dioxide on the eye under conditions such as might be encountered in industry or in smog.[172]

Sulfur dioxide gas has a strong suffocating odor, and it is irritating to the respiratory tract at lower concentrations than are irritating to the eyes. Tests of the effect of various concentrations of sulfur dioxide in air on a large number of human beings have shown that at 3 to 5 ppm a smell or taste is detectable; at 8 to 12 ppm slight irritation of the throat is definite, and smarting of the eyes and lacrimation begin; at 50 ppm there is strong irritation of the eyes, throat, and lower respiratory tract.[f] Impermeable "hard" contact lenses have been found to protect against the lacrimogenic effect of low concentration sulfur dioxide in air.[b]

Chronic irritation and inflammation of the respiratory tract and alteration of sense of smell and taste is not uncommon as a result of frequent exposure to 30 to 100 ppm. Less commonly, conjunctivitis with discomfort and lacrimation is noted.[f,h,k]

Since 1960, investigations of the effects of low concentrations of sulfur dioxide in air have been prompted mainly by an interest in smog and air pollution control. Studies on rabbits exposed for several hours daily to 6 to 11 ppm in air have shown no significant effect on the cornea, as measured by transparency, integrity of the epithelium, thickness of the cornea, rate of regeneration of artificial wounds of the epithelium, and by measurements of activity of several enzymes in the corneal epithelium.[114,172,173] Similarly, normal human beings have shown no damage of the eye detectable by ordinary clinical examination after six minutes exposure to 9 ppm in air, although in some people this caused considerable sensation of irritation.[114] Although sulfur dioxide is commonly present in smog, tests of its effects on human and animal eyes at the concentrations found in smog seem to provide very little basis for incriminating sulfur dioxide as a cause for eye irritation by smog.[d]

Actual injury of the eye from industrial exposure to sulfur dioxide in air or in gas form is extremely rare. (Essentially all injuries have been produced by liquid sulfur dioxide.) In one report an obvious mistake has been made attributing keratitis in the viscose industry to sulfur dioxide,[o] and attention was promptly called to this error in the literature.[j] The agent responsible for the type of keratitis described was actually hydrogen sulfide. (For further details see *Hydrogen sulfide.*)

The corneas of experimental animals have been damaged by exposure to sulfur dioxide gas but only at concentrations higher than human beings could tolerate on account of respiratory irritation. For instance, exposure of rabbits, guinea pigs, and mice to 400 ppm in air for four hours caused temporary clouding of the corneas, and exposure of guinea pigs to 980 ppm caused corneal clouding within an hour.[1] Exposure of mice and guinea pigs to 110 to 300 ppm for approximately three days caused corneal opacification, and exposure of guinea pigs to 10,000 ppm for fifteen minutes caused severe conjunctivitis and corneal opacity.

When the whole animal has been exposed, keratitis and corneal clouding in rabbits and guinea pigs have occurred only under conditions of time and concentration which have ultimately been lethal (460 to 490 ppm for 30 hours, or 800 to 1,000 for 24 hours.)[e] On the other hand, very severe corneal and conjunctival damage can be produced by a five-second exposure to a rapid stream of pure sulfur dioxide gas (at atmospheric pressure and room temperature) restricted to the eyes of rabbits.[e] With this type of exposure the cornea immediately became gray, and conjunctiva became chemotic within a few minutes. The cornea remained gray for several days, with the opacity mostly in the superficial layers, but extending also in a granular and laminar fashion throughout the stroma, which was thicker than normal. In ten days interstitial vascularization was evident, and in six months the corneas were extensively vascularized and moderately opaque. Histologically such eyes presented changes characteristic of severe acid burns.[e]

Severe injuries of human eyes by sulfur dioxide have been produced only by the liquefied form. Formerly this circumstance, and the fact that liquid sulfur dioxide was commonly used as a refrigerant, led to the belief that injury was attributable to freezing of the eye, but an investigation in experimental animals and comparison of the clinical characteristics of freezing and of sulfur dioxide burns have established conclusively that the ocular damage is attributable to chemical toxic effect and not to freezing.[e]

Several severe burns of the eye by liquid sulfur dioxide have been reported.[c,e,g,i,n,153,249] Other cases have been mentioned incidentally without details. In the mildest cases in which the cornea and conjunctiva have been injured superficially, the eyes have recovered and superficial clouding of the cornea has cleared.[i,153] In the most severe cases the corneas have been rendered permanently opaque and densely vascularized, sometimes accompanied by extensive symblepharon.

Typically, in severe burns of the eyes from a spray of liquid sulfur dioxide the patient may experience little discomfort at the time of exposure, and may be aware of the seriousness of his injury only in the course of several hours or days. The vision is immediately blurred, but may become progressively poorer. Discomfort is slight even with serious injury, owing to the fact that sulfur dioxide damages the corneal nerves and renders the anterior segment anesthetic.

Immediately after the eye has been sprayed with liquid sulfur dioxide, or a mixture of lubricating oil and liquid sulfur dioxide in the case of accidents with refrigerators, the corneal epithelium becomes gray and irregular, but remains adherent to the stroma, as in acid burns. Several hours later the lids become swollen. The conjunctival epithelium appears white and rather opaque. Vessels which can be inspected with a slit-lamp biomicroscope may be seen to be thrombosed.

Several days later the opaque epithelium is spontaneously lost from the cornea and conjunctiva, and this temporarily may permit an improvement in vision.

However, slit-lamp biomicroscope examination in case of severe injury reveals evidence of deeper damage, stromal edema, opacity of the corneal nerves, and grayness and irregularity of the endothelium. Subsequently in the course of several weeks and months the stroma may become infiltrated and densely vascularized, with increasing opacification and severe interference with vision. Conjunctival overgrowth of the cornea and formation of symblepharon are frequent complications.

Experimental studies attempting to find an explanation for the remarkably injurious effects of sulfur dioxide on the eye have determined that the injury has a chemical basis and is not attributable to freezing. The damage produced by low temperature in the absence of toxic substances, either in patients or experimental animals, produces a distinctly different type of injury. In rabbits, freezing by means of liquid Freon-12 for several seconds, analogous to what might result from a squirt of liquid sulfur dioxide, produces only mild and transient disturbance of the eye. Freezing for 0.5 to 1.5 minutes causes loss of corneal endothelium and edema of the stroma and epithelium, which are unlike the changes produced by sulfur dioxide.[e] Furthermore, as already mentioned, pure sulfur dioxide gas at room temperature and atmospheric pressure applied to rabbit eyes for several seconds produces injury which is the same as that caused by a squirt of sulfur dioxide in liquid form. The most injurious form of sulfur dioxide in the cornea and in biological systems in general appears to be as undissociated *sulfurous acid,* which is formed by reaction of sulfur dioxide with water, and exists in increasing concentration as the pH is lowered below pH3. The *bisulfite* and *sulfite* ions which exist at higher pH levels have been tested on rabbit corneas and found far less injurious. No significant conversion of sulfurous to sulfuric acid has been detected in the cornea.[d]

Sulfur dioxide and sulfurous acid are well known from extensive biochemical studies to denature proteins and inactivate numerous enzymes. However, sulfurous acid has not been found to have an inordinate denaturant effect on the corneal stroma, as measured by the capacity of pieces of exposed cornea to swell in water, when compared with numerous other acids. Sulfurous acid does, however, have an exceptionally great speed of penetration through corneal epithelium, presumably because of high solubility in fats, as well as in water, and high molecular mobility.[d]

In treatment of burns of the eye by liquid sulfur dioxide, no specific antidote or therapy has been discovered. Immediate irrigation is logical, especially when sulfur dioxide is mixed with oil in which it may be soluble, but sulfur dioxide by itself is so readily volatile that within seconds it is mostly gone from the surface. Nevertheless irrigation seems worthwhile in the hopes of extracting some from the cornea.

a. Clark CP: Accidental freezing of the eye by sulfur dioxide. *AM J OPHTHALMOL* 19:881–884, 1936.
b. Coe JE, Douglas RB: The effect of contact lenses on ocular responses to sulphur dioxide. *J SOC OCCUP MED* 32:92–94, 1982.
c. Culler AM: Management of burns of the cornea. *OHIO MED J* 34:873–878, 1938.
d. Doyle GJ, Endow N, Jones JL: Sulfur dioxide role in eye irritation. *ARCH ENVIRON HEALTH* 3:657–667, 1961.
e. Grant WM: Ocular injury due to sulfur dioxide. I. Report of 4 cases. II. Experimental study and comparison with ocular effects of freezing. *ARCH OPHTHALMOL* 38:755–761, 762–774, 1947.

f. Holmes JA, Franklin EC, Gold RA: Report of the Selby Smelter Commission. *BUR MINES BULL* 98:172–175, 1915.

g. Iliff CE: Beta irradiation in ophthalmology. *ARCH OPHTHALMOL* 38:415–441, 1947.

h. Kehoe RA, Machle WF, et al: On the effects of prolonged exposure to sulfur dioxide. *J IND HYG* 14:159–173, 1932.

i. Kennon BR: Report of a case of injury to skin and eyes by liquid sulphur dioxide. *J IND HYG* 9:486–487, 1927.

j. Knapp P: On the question of traumatic keratitis as a result of the action of gasses. *SCHWEIZ MED WOCHENSCHR* 4:702, 1923. (German)

k. McNally W: The use of sulfur dioxide. *IND MED SURG* 8:234, 1939.

n. Sorsby A, Symons HM: Amniotic membrane grafts in caustic burns of the eye. *BR J OPHTHALMOL* 30:337–345, 1946.

o. Strebel J: Eye injuries caused by SO$_2$. *SCHWEIZ MED WOCHENSCHR* 4:560–561, 1923. (German)

Sulfur hexafluoride is a colorless, odorless gas which is stable and inert. When injected into the anterior chamber or the vitreous cavity, a bubble of this gas remains about twice as long as a bubble of air, because of relatively low solubility in water. This greater persistence offers an advantage over air in treatment of retinal detachment. Sulfur hexafluoride has been examined for toxicity in animal experiments and in numerous operations in human beings, and so far its effects on the eye appear to be no worse than the effects of air. However, there is one important physical difference. A bubble of sulfur hexafluoride in the eye increases in volume because of diffusion of nitrogen (or nitrous oxide anesthetic) from blood and surrounding tissues into the bubble, until an equilibrium with surrounding tissues is reached.[e] With air this does not occur. Much has been published on the parameters relating amount of sulfur hexafluoride injected, the height to which the swelling bubble can raise the intraocular pressure, and the potential seriousness of this effect (e.g. optic atrophy), but it appears generally accepted that these are physical factors, rather than toxic phenomena.[a,b] In one series of cases, it has been noted that postoperative elevated intraocular pressure was particularly common in aphakic eyes with fibrin in the pupil, and it was suggested that contact of the gas with the iris might have irritated the iris, but this was simply speculation.[a]

In owl monkeys, Constable and Swann compared sulfur hexafluoride and air as substitutes for vitreous humor.[c] Both caused a faint flare in the aqueous humor, but no more than caused by injection of saline solution. Both caused a slight increase in permeation of blood proteins into the vitreous cavity, more than induced by saline solution. In the lenses, posterior subcapsular vacuoles were seen when the sulfur hexafluoride bubble was in contact with the lens, but not after the bubble was gone. Fineberg, Machemer, et al also noted posterior subcapsular vacuoles or feathery opacities when a bubble was in contact for 12 to 14 hours, but the same effect was produced by air as by sulfur hexafluoride, and in either case tended to disappear when the bubbles were gone.[d] In the retina of owl monkeys, Fineberg et al found intravitreal sulfur hexafluoride caused no significant abnormality of the ERG b-wave or threshold responses, and by light and EM examination only non-specific thickening of outer segments and a few macrophages between retina and pigment epithelium, the same as from intravitreal air. Intraocular pressures in monkeys could rise as in human eyes from swelling of bubbles of intravitreal sulfur hexafluoride.

In rabbits, Van Horn et al have described reversible changes in the corneal endothelium. Within a day after injection of the gas into the anterior chamber the corneal endothelium developed a guttate appearance visible with the slit-lamp biomicroscope where the bubble was in contact with the cornea.[g] This corresponded with a histologic appearance of small multilayered patches of endothelium, either from duplication or multiplication of these cells. Also a new layer of Descemet's membrane began to form. When the gas bubbles were gone, the biomicroscopic appearance returned to normal, and the endothelium returned to a single layered structure, with the new layer of Descemet's membrane incorporated by the old. The important features of this are not only that the process was reversible, but that the same phenomena were induced by a bubble of air in the anterior chamber. In monkeys, in preliminary experiments, these changes in the endothelium were not observed.

The essentially negative animal experiments, and extensive clinical experience, have led to an impression expressed by Sabates et al that, "if any toxicity is present, it is of a very low order." However, the same authors noted that in posterior segment surgery in which sulfur hexafluoride is used there is risk of cataract, but that it was not yet evident whether the risk was more than when air was used.[f]

One case report from Germany has described a man who had a contusion injury requiring extensive surgery with most of the vitreous twice replaced by an air-sulfur hexafluoride mixture, associated with rapid appearance of posterior subcapsular vacuoles. These persisted after the gas was gone. After a month, cataract extraction was performed. The anterior hyaloid was found intact. Scanning EM confirmed the presence of posterior subcapsular vacuoles. The authors wondered if sulfur hexafluoride was as non-toxic to the lens as previously considered.[h]

a. Abrams GW, Swanson DE, et al: The results of sulfur hexafluoride gas in vitreous surgery. *AM J OPHTHALMOL* 94:165–171, 1982.
b. Bourgeois JE, Machemer R: Results of sulfur hexafluoride gas in vitreous surgery. *AM J OPHTHALMOL* 96:405–406, 1983.
c. Constable IJ, Swann DA: Vitreous substitution with gases. *ARCH OPHTHALMOL* 93:416–419, 1975.
d. Fineberg E, Machemer R, et al: Sulfur hexafluoride in owl monkey vitreous cavity. *AM J OPHTHALMOL* 79:67–76, 1975.
e. Machemer R, Aaberg TM: VITRECTOMY, 2nd ED. New York, Grune and Stratton, 1979.
f. Sabates WI, Abrams GW, et al: The use of intraocular gases. *OPHTHALMOLOGY* 88:447–454, 1981.
g. VanHorn DL, Edelhauser HF, et al: In vivo effects of air and sulfur hexafluoride gas on rabbit corneal endothelium. *INVEST OPHTHALMOL* 11:1028–1036, 1972.
h. Werry H, Brewitt H: Cataract development after intravitreal injection of SF_6-gas. *KLIN MONATSBL AUGENHEILKD* 182:331–333, 1983. (German).

Sulfuric acid (battery acid) can cause devastating damage to the eyes. *Exploding automobile batteries* are the most common source of eye burns from sulfuric acid.[b,c] The caustic and chemical properties of concentrated sulfuric acid differ greatly from those of diluted acid. Concentrated sulfuric acid in contact with the eye or skin appears to attack the tissues chemically in a different and more destructive manner than is explainable simply on the basis of hydrogen ion concentration. This may be analogous to the well-known charring of sugar, wood, and other organic substances by concentrated sulfuric acid, which seems to be related to a great affinity for the oxygen and hydrogen of which water molecules are composed. When the acid is diluted, and the avidity for water molecules at least partially satisfied, the caustic and chemical properties become more like those of simpler acids, such as hydrochloric acid.

The literature contains many case reports of devastating injuries of the eyes with dissolution of the anterior segment of the globe from splashes of concentrated acid. Clinical descriptions of severe sulfuric acid eye burns have included glaucoma and cataract as complications.[d] There are also many reports of transient injury with complete recovery following splashes of diluted acid.[46,153] Experimentally in rabbit eyes similar results are observed: very severe injury from concentrated acid[27] but no permanent damage from 1% in water.[101] Fine sprays of sulfuric acid in the air cause acute stinging and burning of the eyes, but rapid dilution by the tears may prevent significant injury.[61]

Histologic details of the damage produced in rabbits and rats have been provided for successive intervals during several weeks after experimental application of sulfuric acid.[e,g,h] Histologic details have also been provided on the eyes of a patient who died five days after extensive burns from concentrated sulfuric acid, showing extensive damage to the cornea and conjunctiva, but not to intraocular structures.[f]

Additional information on the effects of sulfuric acid on the eyes of experimental animals is to be found in several studies in which the prime interest was in evaluating various treatments, in which sulfuric acid was employed as the agent for producing a standard burn of the eye.[30,57,92,140,241]

The rate of penetration of dilute sulfuric acid into the aqueous humor in rabbit eyes has been examined but the relationship to intraocular injury remains to be defined.[a]

Emergency treatment of splashes of sulfuric acid in the eye is the same as for practically all other splash burns, immediate and copious irrigation with water. The speed with which irrigation can be started is of the greatest importance. In the case of the concentrated acid, every second counts.

a. Feller K, Graupner K: The hydrogen ion concentration in the anterior chamber of the rabbit eye after experimental burning with acid and alkali. *GRAEFES ARCH OPHTHALMOL* 170:370–376, 1966. (German)

b. Holekamp TLR, Becker B: Ocular injuries from automobile batteries. *TRANS AM ACAD OPHTHALMOL OTOL* 83:805–810, 1977.

c. Minatoya HK: Eye injuries from exploding car batteries. *ARCH OPHTHALMOL* 96:477–481, 1978.

d. Peyresblanques J, LeGoff JR: Two new cases of eye burns by sulfuric acid in resin-tappers. *BULL SOC OPHTALMOL FRANCE* 65:986–988, 1965. (French)

e. Priani P, Falcon O, Linares H: Experimental study of acid burns of the cornea. *ARCH OFTALMOL B AIR* 38:103–106, 1963.

f. Schultz G, Henkind P, Gross EM: Acid burns of the eye. *AM J OPHTHALMOL* 66:654–657, 1968.

g. Vancea P, Niculescu A: Contribution to the anatomo-pathologic study of experimental corneal burns with sulfuric acid. *ARCH OPHTALMOL (Paris)* 29:291–298, 1969. (French)

h. Viano-Yasenetskii VV, Dumbrova NE: Ultrastructure of multilaminar fibrillary tissue developed behind Descemet's membrane following corneal burn with sulfuric acid. *OFTALMOL ZH* 26:599–603, 1971. (English summary)

Sulfur monochloride (sulfur chloride, disulfur dichloride) vapors which are corrosive and irritating to the eyes, nose, and throat, inducing tearing and affecting breathing.[56,61,171,188] Even 2 to 9 ppm in air are irritating to the eyes.[215]

Sulfur trioxide (Sulfan) reacts violently with water, fumes in air, and causes great irritation of the eyes and respiratory tract, even at concentrations as low as 1 ppm in air.[56,171] Contact with the liquid can be expected to cause devastating damage to the eye, as with concentrated sulfuric acid.

Sulfuryl chloride (SO_2Cl_2) vapors are extremely irritating to the eyes and corrosive to skin and mucous membranes.[56,171,252]

Sulindac (Clinoril), a non-steroid anti-inflammatory drug, has been the subject of a variety of suspicions reported to Fraunfelder's National Registry and to the U.S. Food and Drug Administration.[312] However, there appears to be no report of a controlled study for toxic effects on the eye. Fraunfelder in 1982 expressed the opinion that ocular effects were rare, usually transient visual disturbances, and that possibilities of macular pigmentation or perforated corneal ulcers were "only suspects."[312]

Sulpiride, an anti-depressant, was reported in one case to be associated with diplopia from a reversible oculomotor paresis when taken in conjunction with cimetidine, but only when both drugs were taken.

Malbrel PH, Woilliez M: A case of iatrogenic oculo-motor paresis. *BULL SOC OPHTALMOL FRANCE* 82:1285–1287, 1982. (French)

Sulthiame (Conadil; Opsolot; Trolone) an anticonvulsant, has infrequently caused ocular side effects. One out of a series of seventy-three patients receiving this drug developed edema of the face, hands, and feet after twenty months of treatment, and this was associated with drooping of one eyelid.[a] In another series of fifty-four patients two complained of blurring of vision and one had drooping of the lids, but no further information was given on the nature or cause of the blurring of vision.[b]

One instance of diplopia and one of papilledema have been listed.[c] The patient who had papilledema also had transient changes in color vision subjectively, but all returned to normal in two weeks after the drug was stopped, and there was no definite evidence that the drug was responsible. It has been known to cause Stevens-Johnson syndrome.[d,312]

a. Engelmeirer MP: On clinical evaluation of anti-epileptic drugs with special attention to Opsolot. DEUTSCH MED WSCHR 85:2207–2211, 1960. (German)
b. Garland H, Summer D: Sulthiame in treatment of epilepsy. *BR MED J* 1:474, 1964.
c. Liske E, Forster FM: Clinical evaluation of the anticonvulsant effects of sulthiame. *J NEW DRUGS* 3:32–36, 1963.
d. Taffe A, et al: A case of Stevens-Johnson syndrome associated with the anti-convulsants sulthiame and ethosuximide. *BR DENT J* 138:172–174, 1975.

Superphosphate fertilizer is a product of reaction of mineral calcium phosphates with either sulfuric or phosphoric acid, which renders the mineral phosphates more soluble and available for assimilation by plants. An excess of acid may sometimes be present, and occasionally burns have resulted from accidental contamination of the eyes with particles of fertilizer.[34, 46, 153] Typically the cornea has become whitened about the area of contact with the particle, and there has been superficial necrosis, but in general the eyes have healed with only localized residual opacities or no opacity. The severity of reaction appears to have been related to the amount of free acid.

Suramin (Antrypol; Moranyl), a drug used in treating onchocerciasis and trypanosomias, can cause serious reactions. A systematic ophthalmologic study of a hundred patients treated for ocular onchocerciasis with suramin, suramin plus diethylcarbamazine, or placebo was reported by Anderson et al in 1976.[a] Summarizing what seemed like adverse effects of treatment, it appeared that punctate and sclerosing keratitis could be aggravated, and that anterior uveitis could be provoked, or be seriously aggravated, and this appeared to be associated with the killing of a large number of microfilariae by the drugs. Optic atrophy occurred in both treated and untreated patients, and it was difficult to know whether suramin was simply ineffective in treating onchocerchosis of optic nerve and posterior segment, or whether it aggravated conditions in the optic nerves by a reaction secondary to killing microfilariae there. Comparative numbers after 2 years provide helpful grounds for weighing whether treatment with suramin was better or worse than no treatment. For lesions of the anterior segment the numbers were: without treatment 0% improved, 46% were unchanged, 54% were worse; whereas with treatment 55% improved, 35% were unchanged, 10% were worse. For the posterior segment, without treatment 0% improved, 10% were unchanged, 80% were worse, whereas with treatment 0% improved, 73% were unchanged, 27% were worse.

a. Anderson J. Fuglsang H, Marshall TFdeC: Effects of suramin on ocular onchocerciasis. *TROPENMED PARASITOL* 27:279–296, 1976.

Surfactants (surface active agents, detergents, wetting agents) are synthetic organic compounds having hydrophilic properties at one end of the molecule to provide tendency for water solubility, and hydrocarbon or fat-like structure at the other end of the molecule to provide affinity for oils, fats, and greases. Surfactants of various structures have in common the property of lowering the surface tension of water.

Surfactants are used in great quantity and variety industrially and domestically for cleaning, washing and scouring. In surgical patients, anti-infective scrubs containing surfactants have injured the corneal epithelium when used around the eyes.[350] Some surfactants are used in cosmetics, and some as preservatives in ophthalmic solutions. (See *Preservatives*). Many are known to be injurious in contact with the eye. Domestically, the greatest opportunity for contaminating the eyes with surfactants is presented by shampoos and liquid household detergents. Although manufacturers of shampoos have made efforts to minimize danger to the eyes in their selection of the surfactant ingredients, some trade-named preparations have been found injurious and very irritating when tested on rabbit eyes. Since the composition of trade-named preparations may be varied at any time, without notice to the consumer, the results of tests on such preparations do not seem worthwhile listing here. Only information on specific, individual, chemically identifiable surfactant compounds is to be considered.

Toxic effects of surfactants on the eyes will be described according to the nature of exposure, as follows: (1) External Surfactant Contact Injuries, (2) Anterior Chamber Surfactant Contact Injuries, and (3) Intra-Vitreous Surfactant Contact Injuries. The external contact injuries are by far the most common.

(1) External Surfactant Contact Injuries:

Surfactants can be classified chemically as cationic, anionic, and non-ionic. Testing on rabbit eyes has indicated a general but not inviolable rule that the cationic surfactants are the most damaging, the anionic are less injurious, and the nonionic are the least. Several reports give the results of testing of various of these compounds for toxicity on rabbit eyes.[a-l,o,t,107,338]

In certain instances testing has had as its object the selection of compounds to be used in low concentration to increase penetration of drugs from eyedrops into the eye.[g,j,t,351] In a few instances it has been possible, by addition of surfactants in concentrations too low to cause clinically appreciable injury, to achieve worthwhile improvement in the absorption of certain drugs which by themselves penetrate poorly from the surface of the eye. Among drugs which have been benefited in this way are carbachol, epinephrine, penicillin, sulfacetamide. The agent most commonly used in this ophthalmic pharmaceutic application has been *benzalkonium.*

Investigation of the relationship between injuriousness to the eye and the physical properties of the various types of surfactants has revealed several noteworthy facts. The cationic type excel in precipitating proteins; the anionics cause lysis of cells, the nonionics generally lack both of these properties.[l,n,107]

Cationic surfactants generally are quaternary ammonium derivatives. The following cationic compounds are among those which have been tested, and at concentrations of 0.1% to 1.0% in water have been significantly irritating or injurious to the rabbit eye:

Benzalkonium chloride (Zephiran, Roccal)[i,o,107,331]
Benzethonium chloride (Phemerol, Hyamine 1662)[l,t]
Cetrimonium chloride (CTAB; hexadecyltrimethylammonium)[d,80]
Cetylpyridinium chloride (Ceepryn)[l]
Decyltrimethylammonium bromide[80,81]
Dodecytrimethylammonium bromide[80]

Emcol E607[1]
Emulsol 607, 607M[107]
G271[1]
Hexadecyldimethylethylammonium bromide[331]
Isothan Q15[1,316]
Tetradecyltrimethylammonium bromide[80]

(See INDEX for detailed descriptions of *Benzalkonium* and *Cetrimonium*)
(*Decyltrimethylammonium bromide* at 0.1 M concentration applied to rabbit eyes for 10 minutes after removal of corneal epithelium caused severe corneal opacification; it was much more injurious than shorter-chain homologous alkyl trimethyl ammonium compounds.[81])

Anionic surfactants are usually sodium salts, or occasionally triethanolamine salts, of alkyl sulfates, aromatic sulfonates, or carboxylic acids. The oldest member of the group is soap, which is a sodium, or sometimes potassium salt of various fatty carboxylic acids, such as stearic acid. (Also see INDEX for *Soap*.)

As a generalization, the injuries of the eye resulting from splash contamination with anionic surfactants are less serious than those from cationic, but may entail more discomfort and irritation than from nonionic surfactants.

The following anionic compounds are among those which have been tested at concentrations of 0.5% to 1% in water and have been found significantly irritating or injurious to the rabbit eye, typically causing immediate discomfort, hyperemia of the conjunctiva, edema of the corneal epithelium with punctate stainability by fluorescein, but healing in a day or two, usually with no opacity:

Aerosol 05[o]	Lissapol N[j]
Aerosol OT (see Docusate)	Nacconol NRSF[g]
Alkyl sodium sulfate series[e]	Santomerse D[l]
Armour #600 KOP soap[g,1]	Sodium lauryl sulfate
	(Duponol C)[l,107,324]
Docusate sodium (Aerosol OT)[e,o,t,45]	Tergitol-4[s]
Dodecyl sodium sulfate[e,1]	Tergitol-7[g,o,107]
Duponol[351]	Tergitol-0[o]
Duponol ME[o,t]	Triethanolamine lauryl sulfate
	(Drene)[107]
Duponol WAT[l]	Triton W 30[107]
Entsufon sodium	Triton X 30[g]
Igepon AP[f]	Ultrawet 30 DS[g]
Ivory soap[l]	Ultrawet 60L[l]

Following application of 1% Armour 600 KOP soap, Ivory soap, and Ultrawet 60L, a somewhat more severe reaction with temporary clouding of the cornea has been noted.[1]

In the *alkyl sodium sulfate series* of compounds of varying molecular size from *octyl* to *octadecyl,* maximum irritation was produced by *dodecyl sodium sulfate.*[b]

Docusate has been mildly and reversibly damaging to rabbit eyes at 0.5 and 2% concentration, but severely damaging at 10%.[45]

Dodecyl sodium sulfate tested at 40% concentration on rabbit and monkey eyes was "corrosive" and almost as injurious as 1% sodium hydroxide, taking as long as 21 days to heal, with some residual scarring and vascularization.[322]

Duponol at 0.25 to 1% concentration caused severe pain when applied to the eyes of human volunteers.[351]

Duponol WAT, sometimes used in shampoos, tested at 50% concentration on rabbit eyes caused only mild injury of the corneal epithelium, with prompt healing.[u]

Entsufon sodium, the detergent component of pHisoHex scrub, has been injurious to human eyes. (See INDEX for *pHisoHex.*)

Sodium lauryl sulfate, is said to have been the commonest cause of eye irritation by commercial shampoos.[i] Rabbit eyes apparently are more irritated than human or monkey eyes.

Sodium dodecylbenzene sulfonate has been tested on rabbit and monkey eyes in a dry mixture with inorganic detergents. (See INDEX for *Detergents.*) The morphology of corneal epithelial changes produced in rabbits by 1 to 30% solutions of *sodium alkylbenzene sulfonates* has been examined by scanning and transmission electron microscopy.[m] *Alkylbenzene sulfonates* and *arylbenzene sulfonates* have usually produced only transient irritation when tested on rabbit eyes, and have appeared less irritant to dogs, and even less to monkeys and human beings.[a,r]

Tests of several of the anionic surfactants on excised beef corneas using a concentration of 0.1 M (approximately 3%) in water has shown that these substances do not loosen the corneal epithelium from the stroma, but appear to attack the epithelial cells themselves, and gradually transform the epithelium into a slimy mass, progressively from the surface to the basal layer.[107] This action on the epithelial cells may be analogous to the hemolytic action which anionic surfactants have on blood cells.

Nonionic surfactants generally are ester or ether combinations of fatty acids or fatty alcohols with polyoxyethylene or sorbitol. Certain of these compounds, for instance dodecylpolyethyleneoxide with molecular weight about 600, have been found to have local anesthetic action on the cornea[n] and may be damaging to the epithelium. (See INDEX for *Polyoxethylene dodecanol* and *Polyethyleneglycolethers.*) Also certain alkylaryl polyethylene oxide and fatty acid amine condensates have local anesthetic effects on the cornea.[162] Interestingly, a series of surfactants present in facial soaps and shampoos were found to cause corneal anesthesia in rabbits similar to 0.5% tetracaine, but not in human beings.[k] This appears to be a species dependent phenomenon, at least for some surfactants.

The following nonionic compounds are among those which have been tested on rabbit eyes and have caused little or no damage even when applied undiluted:[l]

Brij-35	Myrj-52
G1441	Polysorbate 80 (Tween 80)[h]
G1790	Renex
G7569J	Span 20, 80
Myrj-45	Tween 20, 40, 60, 65[h]

The following nonionic surfactants have caused more significant irritation or injury to rabbit eyes than those in the foregoing list:

Brij-30

G1690

G2132

G3721

Laurithyl

Tetradecylheptaethoxylate

Tridecylhexaethoxylate

Triton X155

G1690 has caused severe irritation and corneal opacity in rabbits at concentrations less than 10%.[1]

Brij-30, G2132, and *G3721* produced slight rabbit corneal opacity at concentrations of 10% to 20%.[1]

Tetradecylheptaethoxylate and *tridecylhexaethoxylate* full strength on rabbit eyes caused long-lasting or permanent damage, but 10% concentration caused damage that was reversible.[b] Monkey eyes were strikingly less vulnerable, suffering no permanent damage from full strength exposure, and clearing within 14 days.[b]

The following nonionic surfactants tested on eyes of human volunteers at 1% concentration caused no noteworthy injury:[351]

Aptet 100

Brij-35

G1045

Myrj 52, 53

Polysorbate 80 (Tween 80)[g]

Polyoxyethylene (20) oleyl ether

Spans 20, 40, 85

Tweens 20, 40, 81

Brij-58 at 10% concentration on human eyes did cause discomfort, epithelial edema, and haloes.[351] Also, *Triton X 155* at 1% concentration applied four times within 25 minutes to a human eye caused pain, photophobia and loss of corneal epithelium, but the eye healed rapidly.[g]

(2) Anterior Chamber Surfactant Contact Injuries:

Accidental introduction of surfactant-containing solutions into the anterior chamber during surgery could cause serious permanent damage to the corneal endothelium and possibly the lens.

Most information on injurious effects of surfactants in the anterior chamber come from experimental work. Green et al in isolated rabbit corneas showed that physiological and structural alterations of the endothelium are produced by concentrations of benzalkonium chloride and cetylpyridinium chloride much below what is employed as a preservative in solutions for extraocular use.[321] In excised bovine corneas electrical resistance and potassium exchange have been used to measure the effects of surfactants on epithelium and endothelium, substantiating greatest effect from cationic *cetyltrimethyl ammonium,* less by anionic *dodecyl sulfate,* and least by nonionic *Triton X-100; Ortoxynol* surfactants.[d] However, even the least active by those measurements, *Triton X-100,* when injected into the anterior chamber of a rabbit eye as 10μl of 1% solution (i.e. 0.1 mg), caused the cornea to become white and edematous, with subsequent corneal edema, marked loss of endothelium, and infiltration with inflammatory cells.[p]

(3) Intra-Vitreous Surfactant Contact Injuries:

In rabbits, cataracts have been produced by injecting into the vitreous humor 0.1 ml containing any one of the following surfactants:[375]

Cetylpyridinium chloride (0.1 mg)
Cetyltrimethylammonium bromide (0.3 mg)
Sodium lauryl sulfate (0.5-0.2 mg)
Sodium deoxycholate (0.1-0.2 mg)
Triton X-100 (octoxynol) (0.25 mg)

A cationic surfactant identified only as *alkenyldimethylethylammonium bromide* has caused inflammation and degeneration of the iris and chorioretinitis when injected into the vitreous humor in rabbits.[14]

Sodium lauryl sulfate similarly has caused severe inflammation.[14]

Oronite NIW (an alkylaryl sulfonate) has produced relatively slight disturbance.[14]

a. Beckley JH: Comparative eye testing: man vs animal. *TOXICOL APPL PHARMACOL* 7:93–101, 1965.

b. Benke GM, Brown NW, Walsh MJ: Safety testing of alkyl polyethoxylate nonionic surfactants. *FOOD COSMET TOXICOL* 15:309–318, 1977.

c. Bierbower GW, Seabaugh VM, et al: Report on toxicological tests on 152 detergents. *TOXICOL APPL PHARMACOL* 33:144 (Abstract 56), 1975.

d. Carter LM, Duncan G: Effects of detergents on the ionic balance and permeability of isolated bovine cornea. *EXP EYE RES* 17:409–416, 1973.

e. Daweke H: The irritating effect of higher alcohol sulfates on the conjunctiva of the eyes of rabbits. *ARCH KLIN EXP DERMA* 209:520–524, 1959. (*CHEM ABSTR* 54:9119, 1960)

f. Draize JH, Kelley EA: Toxicity to eye mucosa of certain cosmetic preparations containing surface-active agents. *PROC SC SECT TOILET GOODS ASSOC* 17:1–4, 1952. (*CHEM ABSTR* 46:8774.)

g. Feldman JB, DeLong P, Brown CP: Practical application of surface-active drugs in ophthalmology. *ARCH OPHTHALMOL* 40:668–679, 1948.

h. Gakenheimer WC, Ludwig KG: Physiological safety of Tween 20 and Tween 80 as cosmetic surfactants. *PARFUEM KOSMET* 54:43–44, 1973. (German)

i. Gaunt IF, Harper KH: The potential irritancy to the rabbit eye mucosa of certain commercially available shampoos. *J SOC COSMET CHEM* 15:209, 1964. (*FOOD COSMET TOXICOL* 2:514, 1964.)

j. Ginsburg M, Robson JM: Further investigations on the action of detergents on the eye. *BR J OPHTHALMOL* 33:574–579, 1949.

k. Harris LS, Kahanowicz Y, Shimmyo M: Corneal anesthesia induced by soaps and surfactants, lack of correlation in rabbits and humans. *OPHTHALMOLOGICA* 170:320–325, 1975.

l. Hazelton LW: Relation of surface-active properties to irritation of the rabbit eye. *PROC SC SECT TOILET GOODS ASSOC* 17:5–9, 1952.

m. Kambe J: Effect of surfactants on rabbit cornea. *ACTA SOC OPHTHALMOL JPN* 78:1109–1129, 1974.

n. Klingmuller V, Schroeder W: Proteins, especially of the corneal epithelium, and analgesic, nonionic wetting agents. *NAUNYN-SCHMIEDEBERG'S ARCH EXP PATH PHARMAK* 218:215–221, 1953. (*CHEM ABSTR* 47:12441, 1953.)

o. Leopold IH: Local toxic effect of detergents on ocular structures. *ARCH OPHTHALMOL* 34:99–102, 1945.

p. Meltzer DW, Drews RC, Hajek AS: Millipore filters in ophthalmic surgery. *AM INTRA-OCULAR IMPLANT SOC J* 7:143–146, 1981.

q. Montastier C: Local tolerance of some surfactants used in shampoos. *LABO-PHARMA-PROBL TECH* 24:598–602, 1976. (French)

r. Opdyke DL, Snyder FH, Rubenkoenig H: Toxicologic studies on household synthetic detergents. II. Effects on the skin and eyes. *TOXICOL APPL PHARMACOL* 6:141–146, 1964.

s. Scholz J: Tolerance of the eye for cosmetic detergents. *AESTHET MED* 12:343, 1963. (German) (*FOOD COSMET TOXICOL* 2:514–515, 1964.)

t. Swan KC: Reactivity of the ocular tissues to wetting agents. *AM J OPHTHALMOL* 27:1118–1122, 1944.

u. Weltman AS, Sparber SB, Jurtshuk T: Comparative evaluation and the influence of various factors on eye irritation scores. *TOXICOL APPL PHARMACOL* 7:308–319, 1965.

Suture materials of many different types have been compared for the amount of inflammatory reaction that may accompany their use in surgery of the eye. The observations have been made by tests on rabbit eyes and by clinical observations. The results are reported in terms of amount of inflammatory reaction seen histologically or clinically. Such observations have been published on the following materials:

Catgut[h,l], Chomic catgut,[h,j] Chromic collagen,[j] Collagen,[g] Dacron,[l] Nylon(Ethilon),[a,c,d,g,j] Polyglactin 910 (Vicryl),[e,j] Polyglycolic acid (Dexon),[b,f,i,m] Polypropylene (Prolene),[j] Rat tail tendon,[b,h] Silk.[a,b,c,g,h,j,k,l,m]

There is also a large literature, which is not included here, on clinical experiences with various suture materials, mainly concerned with physical properties, or concerned with the degradation of these materials in various locations in the eye.

a. Arsonson SB, McMaster PRB, et al: The pathogenesis of suture toxicity. *ARCH OPHTHALMOL* 84:641–644, 1970.

b. Bainkoff G, Ballereau L, Clergeau G: Synthetic absorbable sutures in ocular surgery. *ANN OCULIST* (*Paris*) 210:667–673, 1977. (French)

c. Basu PK, Hasany SM: A histochemical study on corneal suture reaction. *CAN J OPHTHALMOL* 4:328–341, 1971.

d. Ehinger B, Palm E: Experimental iris sutures in the monkey. *ACTA OPHTHALMOL* 5:853–860, 1973.

e. Harmard H, Pouliquen Y, et al: Absorbable polyglactin sutures. *ARCH OPHTALMOL* (*Paris*) 37:583–596, 1977. (French)

f. Henriquez AS, Robertson DM, Rosen DA: Tolerence of the cornea and eyelid to polyglycolic acid and rat-tail tendon sutures. *CAN J OPHTHALMOL* 9:89–103, 1974.

g. McMaster PRB, Aronson SB, Moore TE: Suture toxicity in the germfree guinea pig. *ARCH OPHTHALMOL* 84:776–782, 1970.

h. Olah Z: Experimental investigation of the tolerance of suture materials in the limbal zone of the eye. *ARCH OPHTALMOL* 37:383–390, 1977. (French)

i. Olah Z: Reaction of limbal tissue to a synthetic absorbable suture "Dexon." *J FR OPHTALMOL* 2:609–612, 1979. (French)

j. Salthouse TN, Matlaga BF, Wykoff MH: Comparative tissue response to six suture materials in rabbit cornea, sclera, and ocular muscle. *AM J OPHTHALMOL* 84:224–233, 1977.

k. Soong HK, Kenyon KR: Adverse reactions to virgin silk sutures in cataract surgery. *OPHTHALMOLOGY* 91:479–483, 1984.

l. Steinbach PD, Rockert H: Histologic studies after implantation of various suture materials. *GRAEFES ARCH OPHTHALMOL* 182:239–249, 1971. (German)

m.   Theodossiadis G, Baltatzis S, et al: Comparative studies of sutures of virgin silk and of polyglactine (Dexon) on the rabbit cornea. *J FR OPHTALMOL* 4:747–750, 1981. (French)

Swimming-pool water in prolonged contact with the eyes under some conditions causes temporary redness of the conjunctiva and burning sensation in the eyes, with appearance of colored haloes around lights, but very slight or no blurring of vision. The foremost factors responsible for these symptoms seem to be hypotonicity and excessive concentration of chloramines or nitrogen trichloride in the water.

The appearance of colored haloes around lights after swimming in fresh water is caused by edema of the corneal epithelium, which has been well described by Giardini and by Haag, based on slit-lamp examinations of people who saw haloes after pool swimming.[e,f] In addition to edema they found the corneal epithelium in practically all these people stained with fluorescein, and showed punctate or linear erosions. All returned to normal by the next day.

Simple edema of the corneal epithelium, with colored haloes around lights, can be induced by bathing the eye in pure water, a situation in which hypotonicity is the only factor to consider. Edema is prevented when 0.7% sodium chloride is added to the water. Adding chlorine at a concentration of 1 ppm at pH 7.2 to 7.8, as most commonly encountered in swimming pools, produces no more irritation to the eyes than pure water.[i] The same 1 ppm chlorine added to 0.7% sodium chloride solution is no more irritating than saline solution alone.[i]

These observations provide evidence that the hypotonicity of pool water can account for some of the corneal edema that is found in pool swimmers, but these observations do not explain why swimmers sometimes experience considerably greater irritation and discomfort. The reason is that there is an important difference in the composition of the simple solutions used in these experiments and the composition of pool water. Swimming pools accumulate nitrogen compounds from sweat and urine. When chlorine is added to pool water it reacts with these nitrogen compounds and produces chloramines. It appears that it is the chloramines that account for the special irritancy of some pool water.[b,c,d,g,h,i,j] In the experiments already mentioned, with no chloramines present, it was noted that chlorine in a concentration and at a pH ordinarily encountered in swimming pools was not irritating to the eyes. Monochloramine in pure water is distinctly irritating.[i]

Swimming-pool chemistry is complex, but there are some instructive publications that aid in understanding the problems involved in avoiding irritating conditions at the same time as ensuring sanitation. The following points seem particularly noteworthy.[a,b,g,j]

Chlorine is by far the most widely used sanitizing substance for swimming pools, supplied mostly in the form of sodium hypochlorite, calcium hypochlorite, or lithium hypochlorite for home pools, or as liquefied chlorine gas for the largest pools. Some is supplied in the form of sodium dichloro-S-triazine trione (i.e. sodium dichloriosocyanurate). Regardless of the form, each of these when added to water produces the key sanitizing agent, hypochlorous acid. Some of the hypochlorous acid is used up in destroying bacteria and algae, some is broken down by sunlight, but if there are nitrogen compounds such as ammonia, urea, and creatinine in the water, the hypochlorous acid reacts with them to form monochloramine, dichloramine, and nitrogen trichloride.[a, b, c, h, j] The higher the concentration of hypochlorous acid, the greater the degree of chlorination, and the more rapidly the products are carried off into the air. Chloramines in pool water rob the water of "active" chlorine. They are irritating to the eyes, and they cause the unpleasant odor that is often unjustly attributed to chlorine itself. However, because the chloramines, especially dichloramine and trichloramine (nitrogen trichloride), are volatile they can be useful in carrying nitrogen away from the pool into the air.

The water in swimming pools can be tested for chlorine content and pH in a number of ways. The testing is counted on to be a helpful guide to the amount of chemicals needed each day to maintain proper water sanitation. However, the results of some water tests can be misleading. Some tests do not distinguish between "free" chlorine (present as hypochlorous acid or hypochlorites) and "combined" chlorine that is present in the form of chloramines, but indiscriminately measure "total chlorine." This is important, because "free" chlorine is most valuable for sanitation, and chloramine chlorine not only is much less effective against bacteria, but also is undesirable as an eye irritant. Results from a non-discriminating test may be interpreted incorrectly as indicating that a proper amount of free chlorine is present, when in fact there may be practically no free active chlorine, and most of the chlorine may be in the form of chloramines, with the swimmers suffering from eye irritation due to the unsuspected overload of chloramines.

When swimming pool operators encounter complaints of eye irritation, they should determine whether the pH is within the desired range of 7.2 to 7.8, and they should test separately for free chlorine and for chloramine chlorine. If excessive chloramine chlorine is found, explaining eye irritation in excess of the irritation attributable to simple hypotonicity, the procedure to get rid of it is "superchlorination." This consists of adding chlorine or hypochlorite to the pool in an amount that is 3 to 5 times the ordinary daily amount, with swimmers temporarily out of the pool. This large amount of chlorine converts the chloramines predominantly to dichloramine and nitrogen trichloride, which pass away into the air. (In case of indoor pools, adequate ventilation should be provided. Otherwise asthmatic reactions may develop in people around the pool.[h]) In swimming pools used by many people, with tendency for accumulation of bodily ammonia, urea, and creatinine in the water, eye irritation may be prevented by routinely "superchlorinating" every week or two. The temporary excess of hypochlorous acid or hypochlorites produced by this procedure is not a problem, since it is rapidly broken down by sunlight. (In some pools, iso-cyanuric acid is used to protect the daily additions of chlorine from being broken down by sunlight, but this protects only a small fraction of the chlorine used in superchlorination.)

It has been mentioned above that a pH between 7.2 and 7.8 is desirable. These limits are set by the facts that at lower pH hypochlorous acid is too unstable, and that at higher pH too much of the hypochlorous acid is converted to hypochlorite, which is less effective than hypochlorous acid as an antimicrobial.

(For further information relating to swimming and the eyes, see INDEX for *Acidic lake water* and *Water.*)

a. Brown WE: Maintaining and testing pool water. *SWIMMING POOL AGE AND SPA MERCHANDISER.* June 1983, pages 13–15.

b. Buyer AS (editor): *Swimming Pool Manual.* National Association of Pool Owners, 280 Hillside Avenue, Needham, Massachusetts, 1975.

c. Crabill MB, Lyman ED: Eye irritation associated with swimming. *NEBR MED J* 48:454–455, 1963.

d. Eichelsdoerfer D, Slovak J, et al: The irritant effect of chlorine and chloramines in swimming pool water. *VOM WASSER* 45:17–28, 1975. (German)

e. Giardini A, Giardini P: Corneal disturbances in swimming pool athletes. *MIN OFTALMOL* 19:217–219, 1977. (Italian)

f. Haag JR, Gieser RG: Effects of swimming pool water on the cornea. *J AM MED ASSOC* 249:2507–2508, 1983.

g. Palin AT: Analytical control of water disinfection. *J INST WATER ENG SCI* 28:139–154, 1974.

h. Penny PT: Swimming pool wheezing. *BR MED J* 287:461–462, 1983.

i. Rylander R, Victorin K, Sorensen S: Effect of saline on the eye irritation caused by swimming-pool water. *J HYG* (London) 71:587–592, 1973.

j. White GC: The background of today's pool water chlorination methods. *SWIMMING POOL WEEKLY AND SWIMMING POOL AGE.* July 7, 1969, pages 28–30; July 14, 1969, pages 28–30; July 28, 1969, pages 34; August 4, 1969, pages 28–29.

Talc (talcum; powdered hydrous magnesium silicate), used as a dusting powder for surgeons' gloves, has induced granulomas in and about the eye.[b,g,i] Talc employed in fulling of cloth is said to have caused conjunctival inflammation resulting in symblepharon, severe enough to require surgery in some instances.[253]

Talc has been injected experimentally into the anterior chambers of eyes of rabbits and monkeys.[c,f,i] In rabbit eyes talc causes pseudohypopyon, which has been observed for two weeks, but by four weeks disappeared, and remnants of talc found later histologically in the iris and angle of the anterior chamber appeared to be producing no granulomatous reaction.[c,i] Whether talc produces a disturbance of intraocular pressure in rabbits seems not to have been established, but in monkey eyes talc in the anterior chamber has induced persistent glaucoma, useful in study of the effects of elevated intraocular pressure on ocular structures.[b]

Talc has been injected intravenously by many drug abusers, who have used tablets of psychotropic drugs in which talc is used along with starch as a filler. When tablets are crushed and injected over a long time, usually years, serious damage is done to the lungs and a characteristic retinopathy appears.[a] Atlee first described the retinopathy as consisting of numerous tiny glistening crystals concentrated mainly in small vessels about the macula. Vision could be undisturbed despite this appearance, but a series of reports have documented serious complications in some cases, e.g. peripheral retinal neovascularization, macular ischemia, vitreous hemorrhage, optic disc neovascularization, and retinal detachment. All these changes have been ascribed to the embolic effect of the talc particles, not to any toxic property of the particles. Ischemia from obstruction of small vessels, rather than any inflammatory or granulomatous reaction has been held responsible, though large numbers of eosinophils were found in the choroid of one of the first autopsied cases.[a,d,h]

Experimentally, Atlee reproduced the retinal condition by intracarotid injection of talc in rabbits.[a] The talc was identified by characteristic birefringence in the autopsy cases and the animals. Schatz and Drake similarly demonstrated talc microscopically in the retinas of monkeys after intracarotid injection.[h] In a series of studies by other investigators it was shown that after numerous intravenous injections in monkeys the typical retinopathy could be reproduced.[d,e] It was confirmed that it was essentially an ischemic retinopathy, and that the talc in retinal vessels was mainly taken up by macrophages or retinal endothelial cells, and together they obstructed the blood flow. The particles appeared to be inert, and to produce no granulomatous reaction in the eye, although they were known to do so in the lung. The ERG was undisturbed.

a. Atlee WE Jr: Talc and cornstarch emboli in eyes of drug abusers. *J AM MED ASSOC* 219:49–51, 1972.
b. Chamlin M: Effect of talc in ocular surgery. *ARCH OPHTHALMOL* 34:369–373, 1945.
c. Eggenschwyler H: Experimental studies of the actions of quartz and glass dust in the anterior chamber of the rabbit. *Z UNFALLMED BERUFSKR* 42:287–303, 1949. (German)
d. Jampol LM, Setogawa T, et al: Talc retinopathy in primates. *ARCH OPHTHALMOL* 99:1273–1280, 1981.
e. Kaga N, Tso MOM, et al: Talc retinopathy in primates. *ARCH OPHTHALMOL* 100:1644–1648; 1649–1657, 1982.
f. Kalvin NH, Hamasaki DI, Gass JDM: Experimental glaucoma in monkeys. *ARCH OPHTHALMOL* 76:94–103, 1966.
g. McCormick GL, Macaulay WL, Miller GE: Talc granulomas of the eye. *AM J OPHTHALMOL* 32:1252–1254, 1949.
h. Schatz H, Drake M: Self-injected retinal emboli. *OPHTHALMOLOGY* 86:468–483, 1979.
i. Schwartz FE, Linn JG Jr: The effects of glove powders on the eye. *AM J OPHTHALMOL* 34:585–592, 1951.
j. Zolog N, Antanescue F, Chercota G: Consequences of magnesium silicate "blockade" of the anterior chamber angle in rabbits. *OFTALMOLOGIA* (*Bucarest*) 9:297–302, 1965. (*ZBL GES OPHTHALMOL* 97:22, 1966.)

Tamoxifen citrate (Nolvadex), an anti-estrogen used in treatment of breast cancer, was reported in 1978 to have produced retinopathy in 4 women who had received 108 to 230 g during 17 to 27 months.[b] All had fine white refractile opacities superficially in their retinas, especially in the macular areas. Three had cystic macular edema and reduced visual acuity. One patient had punctate areas of depigmentation of the retinal pigment epithelium. Three had corneal opacities visible only with the slit-lamp, forming superficial subepithelial whorls or lines. Subsequently, one of these patients was observed to have an increasing number of paramacular superficial refractile opacities in the retinas, but nearly normal visual acuity when she died.[c] Histologically, lesions were found only in the nerve fiber and inner plexiform layers of the retinas. They were intracellular, and were thought most likely to represent products of axonal degeneration.

A fifth case was reported in which there was decrease of visual acuity to 20/50 with central scotomas, and retinopathy consisting of myriads of yellow-white refractile intra-retinal lesions, with bilateral cystoid macular edema.[d] These abnormalities were found after 90 g of tamoxifen had been taken during 17 months.

High dosage was thought to be an important factor in these cases of retinopathy, since a survey of patients taking 40 mg per day for 3 months to 4 years disclosed no ocular side effects.[a] However, in a separate group of 17 patients who had been receiving only 30 mg per day some evidence of retinopathy was found in 2 patients.[e] One of these had temporary impairment of visual acuity, and both had what appeared to be the characteristic multiple yellowish-white dots at the posterior pole. One of these patients had constricted visual fields and pigmentary changes in the periphery of the retinas not previously described in other cases. Four out of the 17 patients had subtle subepithelial changes in the corneas, described as brownish in 3, and as a white streak in one.

a. Beck M, Mills PV: Ocular assessment of patients treated with tamoxifen. *CANCER TREAT REP* 63:1833–1834, 1979.
b. Kaiser-Kupfer MI, Lippman ME: Tamoxifen retinopathy. *CANCER TREAT REP* 62:315–320, 1978.
c. Kaiser-Kupfer MI, Kupfer C, Rodrigues MM: Tamoxifen retinopathy. *OPHTHAL-MOLOGY* 88:89–93, 1981.
d. McKeown CA, Swartz M, et al: Tamoxifen retinopathy. *BR J OPHTHALMOL* 65:177–179, 1981.
e. Vinding T, Nielsen NV: Retinopathy caused by treatment with tamoxifen in low dosage. *ACTA OPHTHALMOL* 61:45–50, 1983.

Tannic acid (tannin), an astringent, is a precipitant of proteins. A 10% solution applied to intact conjunctiva causes slight or mild reaction, but prolonged application causes discoloration.[46] Application to corneas denuded of their epithelium has indicated that tannic acid can precipatate proteins in the stroma of rabbit corneas and can cause some injury even at neutral or slightly alkaline pH.[a,b,123] However, several studies have been made of the possibility of using tannic acid in emergency treatment of eyes contaminated with dyes, and these studies revealed no noteworthy deleterious action.

a. Friedenwald JS, Hughes WF, Hermann H: Acid-base tolerance of the cornea. *ARCH OPHTHALMOL* 31:279–283, 1944.
b. Friedenwald JS, Hughes WF, Hermann H: Acid burns of the eye. *ARCH OPHTHALMOL* 35:98–108, 1946.

Tantalum, a metal that has been considered inert in tissues, after implantation in rabbit eyes appeared completely inert and was well tolerated during observation for a year.[340] However, orbital implants of plastic partially covered with tantalum mesh have developed complications after 10 to 15 years, which suggests that this metal is not totally inert.[a]

a. Przybyla VA Jr, LaPiana FG: Complications associated with use of tantalum-mesh-covered implants. *OPHTHALMOLOGY* 89:121–123, 1982.

Tantalum fluoride (tantalum pentafluoride) in a single case of burn of the cornea listed in the literature, the patient's eye is reported to have healed within forty-eight hours.[165]

Tantalum oxide powder has been tested by application to rabbit eyes from which a portion of the corneal epithelium had been removed by curetting, and no irritative effect was found.[a]

a. Cole HG, Hughes WL: The treatment of abraded corneas of rabbits with Chloresium ointment and tantalum oxide powder. *AM J OPHTHALMOL* 36:1508–1510, 1953.

Tartaric acid, has been employed as a buffering agent in eyedrops. Dilute solutions have at times also been employed as eyewashes with the aim of counteracting the effects of alkalies in alkali burns. In tests on human eyes 0.16 M tartaric acid partially neutralized to pH 3 with sodium phosphate causes severe stinging but no injury. When adjusted to pH 4, it causes mild to moderate stinging and at pH 5 causes only slight discomfort.[317]

Sodium bitartrate 1% solution (pH 3.5) similarly causes moderate stinging and a sensation of dryness, but no injury, and when neutralized to pH 6 causes no discomfort.[317]

Guillery in 1910 recorded observations on the effects of various concentrations of tartaric acid on rabbit corneas.[96] He cauterized portions of the cornea by local application of 10% and 20% solutions, observing the corneas to become locally white and opaque in ten to twenty minutes, but during the next five days the opacity became much less. Histologically in the corneal stroma in the cauterized area, cells had disappeared and endothelial cells were partly missing. Concentrations of 0.25% and 0.5% applied as an eyebath for ten to twenty minutes also gradually produced turbidity of the cornea. The next day the corneas were clearer but still abnormal. They were more rapidly injured by reapplication of the same solution, but apparently all recovered in about six days.

Potassium bitartrate powder, which has been employed as a dusting powder on gloves, has been tested by instillation into the anterior chamber of rabbits and by placing under the superior rectus muscle, and was found to produce no significant reaction.[a] Neutral *ammonium tartrate* solution formerly was widely employed in treatment of burns of the eye by lime and other chemicals. (See INDEX for *Ammonium tartrate.*)

a. Schwartz FE, Linn JG Jr: The effects of glove powders on the eye. *AM J OPHTHALMOL* 34:585–592, 1951.

Tattooing of the cornea as a therapeutic or cosmetic procedure was the subject of a number of publications in the era before successful keratoplasties. It involved the introduction of numerous black or dark-colored materials into the cornea, including metal salts that required reduction to metallic particles within the cornea, such as gold, palladium, and platinum, also particulate carbon and various minerals.[b,d] One corneal button removed 20 years after tattooing showed platinum granules mainly in keratocytes.[a] Toxicologic aspects of the substances used are mostly described elsewhere in this book under the names of the individual substances.

Tattooing of the skin remote from the eyes generally has not involved the eyes, but an extraordinary reaction has been described in which three patients who developed granulomas in light blue tattoos of the skin, apparently owing to a delayed allergic reaction to *cobalt* in the tattoos, simultaneously developed uveitis.[b] The uveitis improved in two of the patients when the inflamed tattoos were excised. It is suggested that this association of tattoo skin granulomas and uveitis may represent a hypersensitivity syndrome.

   a. Olander K, Kanai A, Kaufman HE: An analytical electron microscopic study of a corneal tattoo. *ANN OPHTHALMOL* 15:1046–1049, 1983.
   b. Pickrell K, et al: Tattooing the cornea. *AM J SURG* 95:246–254, 1958.
   c. Rorsman H et al: Tattoo granuloma and uveitis. *LANCET* 2:27–28, 1969.
   d. Tota G: Tattoo of the cornea with palladium chloride. *BOLL OCULIST* 44:45–54, 1965. (Italian)

Tea, has not been suspected of toxicity to the eyes in recent times,[255] but at the end of the nineteenth century several authors were convinced that excessive tea-drinking caused decreased visual acuity and vitreous opacities. Tea and tea leaves have occasionally figured in folk medicine as an eye treatment applied locally. Tea leaves are said to cause moderate conjunctival reaction.[153]

Teakwood contains irritant substances known to cause dermatitis which may involve the lids.[a, b]

   a. Delor F: On occupational dermatosis from teakwood. *MED LAVORO* 37:244, 1946. (Italian)
   b. Reuscher B: Blepharitis after working with teakwood. *KLIN MONATSBL AUGEN-HEILKD* 82:802–805, 1929. (German)

Tear gas weapons and their effects on the eyes will be described here. The individual lacrimogenic chemicals are described elsewhere in greater detail, as listed in the INDEX. Also, the lacrimogenic mechanism is discussed elsewhere. (See INDEX for *Lacrimatory action.*)

Tear gas weapons can be divided into two basic categories: (*a*) *Explosive or thermal type* and (*b*) *Solvent spray type*. The older explosive or thermal type tear gas weapons include grenades, bombs, cannisters, and tear gas cartridges for pistols and tear gas pens, all of which contain the lacrimatory agent in solid form with an explosive or combustible charge to vaporize and disseminate the solid lacrimator. (There is one less common subgroup in which a liquid lacrimator is spread by an explosive charge.) The newer nonexplosive solvent spray type of tear gas weapon is exemplified by its prototype, Chemical Mace. In this type of tear gas weapon the lacrimator is dissolved in a solvent and is under pressure in a container from which it may be sprayed in a stream of droplets.

Up to 1970 all the extremely serious injuries of human eyes from tear gas were from the explosive type of tear gas weapons, and no authenticated instance of permanent eye damage had been reported from the solvent spray type, despite the fact that the same lacrimator, *alpha-chloroacetophenone,* frequently was used in both types of weapons. The great difference in danger to the eyes was that in the explosive type of tear gas cartridge or grenade the lacrimator is in the most concentrated possible form, and explosion of a weapon of this type close to the eye can drive particles of the solid chemical into the tissues.

By contrast, in the nonexplosive solvent spray type of tear gas weapon the lacrimator is in solution and is never driven in highly concentrated form into the tissues, but remains on the surface in a limited concentration. Both the nature of the exposure and the concentration of the injurious lacrimator are significantly different for the two types of weapon. A particularly clear description of the differences between the old explosive or thermal type tear gas weapons and the new solvent spray type was given by MacLeod in 1969. More details follow.

(a) Explosive Type Tear Gas Weapons. These include cartridges for pistols and tear gas guns containing gun powder and solid particles of lacrimator, grenades containing explosive charges with concentrated lacrimator, and cannisters with combustible mixtures to expel the lacrimator in clouds. Short-range injury of the eye by this type of weapon has produced a great many severe injuries of the eyes, corneal opacifications, and loss of eyes. The lacrimatory substances in these weapons at low concentrations in air cause much discomfort in the eyes and blepharospasm, usually without recognizable injury to the cornea, but at high concentrations resulting from direct blast of tear gas in the eyes from an explosive tear gas cartridge at close range the injury has been so devastating in some instances that the eye has had to be removed.

In instances of more moderate injury, tear gases have been damaging to the corneal endothelium, causing bluish corneal edema and wrinkling of the posterior surface of the cornea. This has been observed in patients by Oaks.[161] Complete recovery has been observed in cases in which the cornea was not opacified other than by transient edema.

Extensive reviews and bibliographies on injuries of the eyes by explosive tear gas weapons have been published by Hoffmann, MacLeod, and Midtbo. A series of forty-five cases in which thirty-four had corneal opacities has been presented and well-illustrated by Hoffmann. Five more were described by Laibson and Oconor. Bleckman and Sommer have described 40 cases, and have called special attention to contusion effects on the lens, iris and anterior chamber angle accompanying the burns. Keates et al described a child who required corneal transplantation.

Histologic studies on fourteen enucleated eyes by Levine and Stahl and on an excised piece of leukomatous cornea by Doden and Marquardt, all resulting from explosive type tear gas weapons, showed necrosis and evidences of vascularization and inflammatory reactions that had lasted for years after injury in some cases. There was also evidence of mechanical damage and foreign bodies as well as necrosis from chemical injury.

According to a review and tabulation of eye injuries by explosive type tear gas weapons assembled by MacLeod, the lacrimators which have been held responsible for the injuries include *chloroacetophenone* in most cases, but also *bromoethyl acetate, bromobenzyl cyanide, bromoacetone, chloroacetone,* and *bromomethylethyl ketone. Chloroacetophenone* (CN), the lacrimator most commonly identified or suspected of being the injurious chemical, was responsible in cases reported by Doden and Marquardt, Hoffmann, and Midtbo.

In some reports of severe injuries of the cornea from explosive type tear gas weapons, the specific lacrimatory chemical is not identified. This is the case in a series of descriptions by Bregeat, and by Guillaumat and Chatellier concerning injuries from explosive tear gas grenades in the 1968 Paris riots. They have described the grenades as containing a liquid tear gas which was severely injurious to the eyes when the grenades exploded very close to the face. They have described loss of corneal epithelium, severe edema of the corneal stroma with wrinkling of Descemet's membrane, and vascularization and scarring of the corneas in the most severe cases. Royer and Gainet described a series of injuries in 1973 in France which seem quite similar, and were proven to be caused by *ethyl bromoacetate*. Long periods of corneal anesthesia and slow recovery were highly characteristic. (See *ethyl bromoacetate* in INDEX for details.)

For immediate treatment, irrigation of the eye and thorough mechanical removal of particles, under local anesthesia, appears to be as good initial treatment as any available, according to Durix, Hartmann, Oaks, and Zauleck. No specific antidote has been proven to be of value.

(b) Solvent Spray Type Tear Gas Weapons. Mace (Chemical Mace, Mark IV) was the prototype of the nonexplosive, pressurized, solvent spray tear gas weapons. Chemical Mace consists of a potent lacrimator, alpha-chloroacetophenone (0.9% to 1.2%) dissolved in a mixture of trichlorotrifluoroethane (70% to 80%), 1,1,1-trichloroethane (5%), and hydrocarbons resembling kerosene (approximately 4%). The mixture is maintained under pressure in a metal container and released as a spray of small liquid droplets directed in a stream that may travel six to ten feet. Most of the solvents evaporate from the droplets, leaving the less volatile residue consisting mainly of the kerosene type hydrocarbons, a variable amount of tri-chloroethane, and the chloroacetophenone.

In this oily residue the chloroacetophenone is considerably more concentrated than the 1% in the original mixture. The droplets of oily spray very effectively wet and spread on the skin. They cause intense stinging and burning sensation in the eyes, inducing outpouring of tears and involuntary closure of the lids, also strong irritation and watering of the nose, and burning sensation of the skin. I have experimented with a droplet of the oily residue placed on the skin of the cheek below one eye and have found this to be sufficient to cause strong smarting, tearing, hyperemia of the conjunctiva, and spasm of the lids of the eye on that side, also irritation and running of the nose.

The first published authoritative description of animal testing of Chemical Mace on the eyes was a report by MacLeod in 1969, who described experiments on rabbits and monkeys. MacLeod reported that the liquid residue at atmospheric pressure obtained from spray cans of Chemical Mace, Mark IV, when dropped directly on the eyes of unanesthetized animals caused loss of corneal epilethlium and clouding of the corneal stroma, but these healed in three to ten days. If rabbits were anesthetized before the liquid was applied, the reaction was much more severe, consisting of greater stromal edema, development of corneal opacity, iridocyclitis, and hypopyon, with serious degenerative changes in the corneas in some animals. In monkeys, similarly, when the liquid was applied with the animals under general anesthesia, there was loss of cornea epithelium, severe stromal edema, corneal clouding persisting at least sixty days, and corneal vascularization. When monkeys were exposed to the spray from a distance with the lids held open, under general anesthesia, there was loss of epithelium from the cornea and edema of the conjunctiva and lids, but these eyes recovered in a few days.

The great importance of the self-protective reflexes of conscious animals was shown by experiments in which monkeys which were not anesthetized and were unrestrained were sprayed with Chemical Mace from a distance of six feet. These animals successfully protected themselves from eye lesions, except one that was prevented from turning its face away had partial loss of the corneal epithelium which healed in four days. Comparative experiments with the solvents of Chemical Mace, minus the chloroacetophenone, conclusively demonstrated that the only significantly injurious component was the chloroacetophenone. The report by MacLeod established that under conditions of greatly excessive exposure in restrained animals, and particularly in anesthetized animals incapable of self-protection, Chemical Mace was capable of doing serious damage to the eye. These results were substantiated by Thatcher et al in restrained rabbits.

As quoted by Ley, studies carried out for the manufacturer on rhesus monkeys showed that no damage to the cornea resulted from one-to five-second spraying at a distance of six feet, and that in unanesthetized albino rabbits, application of 0.1 ml of Chemical Mace liquid produced no damage detectable twenty-four to seventy-eight hours later.

Rose in 1969 reported briefly having sprayed the eyes of three rabbits with Chemical Mace from a distance of six inches, and reported that one of the rabbits developed a dense corneal scar, which was shown in a photograph as dense opacity of the whole cornea at twelve weeks, but Rose did not say whether the rabbits were under general anesthesia, or for how long they were sprayed.

Rose described twelve patients who were said to have been sprayed in the eyes with Chemical Mace, Mark IV, at a distance of six to twelve inches and had no opportunity to irrigate their eyes after exposure. Rose reported that all had injuries of the epithelium of cornea and conjunctiva demonstrable by staining with fluorescein, but that nine out of the twelve healed in seventy-two hours. The other three had more extensive epithelial injury which took fourteen to twenty-one days to heal completely, as judged by testing for staining with fluorescein. In one eye a superficial stromal opacity was described as persisting for five months, but this was superficial and located peripherally in the cornea. In two cases Rose described recurrences of punctate stainability with fluorescein three to four months after the acute episode.

Another instructive report, by Oksala and Salminen in 1975, described 5 patients who had been injured by spray-type tear-gas weapons at short range, less than a meter. The fact that 4 out of the 5 had injury to only one eye was supporting evidence that they were sprayed at short range. All had been drunk at the time of spraying, and most were not examined until 24 hours later. Then all had loss of corneal epithelium and had corneal stromal edema. Inflammatory reaction in the anterior chamber cleared rapidly, but corneal stromal edema cleared slowly (8 days to some months). All recovered useful vision, and most recovered most of their vision.

A letter to the editor by Dott in 1969, reported a case of alleged blindness from Chemical Mace, but upon critical questioning by Neuhardt, it was determined that an explosive type tear gas cartridge, not the solvent spray nonexplosive Chemical Mace, had been involved.

It appears that the solvent-spray type tear gas weapon is far less dangerous than the explosive type tear gas weapons. Used from a recommended distance of six feet or more it appears to have caused no serious eye injury, but both animal experiments and clinical observations indicate that if used at short range it can cause serious, slow-healing corneal injuries, most particularly when the subject's self-protective reflexes of closing the eye and pouring out tears are blocked by unconsciousness, as induced by general anesthesia in experimental animals.

Many imitations of the original Chemical Mace under numerous trade names have appeared, some containing CS (o-chlorobenzylidene malononitrile) instead of CN (chlorocetophenone), and probably with other changes in formulation. Therefore it is uncertain how generally the earlier experiments and clinical observations are applicable to present and future models of spray-type tear-gas weapons. In future reporting of observations it may be important to specify with care the composition of the particular spray involved. (See INDEX for additional information on *o-Chlorobenzylidene malononitrile, Chloroacetophenone, Ethyl bromoacetate*, and *Lacrimatory action.*)

Bleckmann H, Sommer C: Clinical aspects of tear gas burns of the cornea. *KLIN MONATSBL AUGENHEILKD* 178:141–144, 1981. (German)

Bregeat P: Ocular injuries by lacrimogenic agents. *BULL SOC OPHTALMOL FRANCE* 68:531–541, 1968; *ANN OCULIST(Paris)* 201:1057–1059, 1968. (French)

Doden W, Marquardt R: On clinical aspects and histopathology of congenital and tear-gas-induced corneal degenerations. *KLIN MONATSBL AUGENHEILKD* 155:855–859, 1969. (German)

Dott AB: (Correspondence.) *N ENGL J MED* 281:851; 1431, 1969.

Durix C, Gallet M: Serious ocular injuries by tear gasses. *BULL SOC FR OPHTALMOL* 69:125, 1956. (French)

Guillaumat L, Chatellier P: Delayed development of burns from tear gas. *BULL SOC OPHTALMOL FRANCE* 69:548–554, 1969. (French)

Hartman K: Addendum to the work: On injury of the cornea by tear gas pistols. *KLIN MONATSBL AUGENHEILKD* 126:760–762, 1955. (German)

Hoffman DH: Injuries of the eyes from short range discharge of tear gas weapons. *KLIN MONSTSBL AUGENHEILKD* 147:625–642, 1965. (German)

Keates RH, Billig SL, Ortiz E: Tear gas keratopathy in a child. *OPHTHALMIC SURG* 5:38–41, 1974.

Laibson PR, Oconor J: Explosive tear gas injuries of the eye. *TRANS AM ACAD OPHTHALMOL OTOL* 74:811–819, 1970.

Levine RA, Davidson KL, Nicol J: Ocular injury caused by the tear gas billy. *TRANS AM ACAD OPHTHALMOL OTOL* 78:926–932, 1974.

Levine RA, Stall CJ: Eye injury caused by tear-gas weapons. *AM J OPHTHALMOL* 65:497–508, 1968.

Ley HL Jr: Statement to Subcommittee on the consumer. *U.S. SENATE COMMERCE COMMITTEE.* MAY 21, 1969.

MacLeod IF: Chemical Mace: Ocular effects in rabbits and monkeys. *J FORENSIC SCI* 14:34–47, 1969.

Midtbo A: Eye injury from tear gas. ACTA OPHTHALMOL 42:672–679, 1964.

Neuhardt GR: (Correspondence). N ENGL J MED 281:1431, 1969.

Oaks LW, Dorman JE, Petty RW: Tear gas burns of the eye. ARCH OPHTHALMOL 63:689–706, 1960.

Oksala A, Salminen L: Eye injuries caused by tear-gas hand weapons. ACTA OPHTHALMOL 53:908–913, 1975.

Rose L: Mace, a dangerous police weapon. OPHTHALMOLOGICA ADDIT AD 158:448–454, 1969.

Royer J, Gainet F: Ocular effects of ethyl bromoacetate tear gas. BULL SOC OPHTALMOL FRANCE 73:1165–1171, 1973. (French)

Thatcher DB, Blaug SM, et al: Ocular effects of Chemical Mace in the rabbit. CLIN MED 78:11–13, 1971.

Zauleck D: Corneal damage by tear gas. KLIN MONATSBL AUGENHEILKD 126:740–742, 1955.

Tegafur, an antineoplastic related to fluorouracil, has been associated with severe blepharospasm in two patients.[a] One patient also received mitomycin, and the other was receiving cyclophosphamide and doxorubicin in addition to tegafur. These patients complained of itching of the eyes and photophobia, but ocular examinations showed no abnormality other than blepharospasm. This seems to be somewhat different from the effect of fluorouracil, which has caused blepharoconjunctivitis. (See INDEX for *Fluorouracil.*)

a. Salminen L, Jantti V, Gronross M: Blepharospasm associated with tegafur combination chemotherapy. *AM J OPHTHALMOL* 97:649–650, 1984.

Tellurium metal is unreactive except with strong acids and bases.[171] However, experimentally in cats, chronic poisoning has been induced by injection of an oily suspension of metallic tellurium subcutaneously or intramuscularly, and this has been found after three months to cause degenerative changes in the ganglion cells of the retina and in the brain.[194] Pentschew, writing in the neuro-ophthalmology textbook of Walsh and Hoyt,[256] has described that the retinal ganglion cells of cats developed honeycombed vacuolar degeneration, and that poisoning of monkeys also produced encephalopathy and changes in the retinal ganglion cells, optic nerves, optic tracts, and in the lateral geniculate bodies. No description seems to have been published on the effects on vision or on any related clinical observations.

Among the compounds of tellurium, *tellurium oxide,* which is very poorly soluble, has been employed in a shampoo under the name of Teles Suspension,[171] and has been dismissed in the literature as of no significance to the eyes.[129] *Hydrogen telluride,* on the other hand, is a highly poisonous gas,[171] but it too appears to have caused no eye disturbances.[129]

Terbium chloride, tested on rabbit eyes by application of 0.1 ml of 1:1 aqueous solution, caused immediate irritation of the eye and produced some injury of cornea and hyperemia of iris which returned to normal in forty-eight hours. The conjunctiva became ulcerated and healed slowly during eighteen days.[97] The pH of the solution was above 3, and the reaction was more severe than that induced by hydrochloric acid at pH 1. Other lanthanide or rare-earth chlorides have been injurious to the cornea only when the corneal epithelium was damaged preliminarily, allowing penetration to the corneal stroma. (See INDEX for *Rare-earth salts.*)

Terephthaloyl chloride, tested on rabbit eyes by applying 3 mg, produced moderate irritation, but apparently not severe injury.[37]

Testosterone, an androgen, when given systemically has been alleged to raise the intraocular pressure in glaucomatous patients, and in rats and rabbits, but retesting has failed to show an effect on intraocular pressure in normal or glaucomatous patients.[a] An extensive review concerning reported effects of this and other sex hormones on intraocular pressure and glaucoma was published in 1968 with numerous references.[b]

   a. Avasthi P, Luthra MC: Effect of sex hormones on intraocular pressure. *INT SURG* 48:350–355, 1967.
   b. Caramazza R, Anselmi P, Meduri R: The changes induced in the dynamics of the aqueous humor in simple glaucoma by an estrogen-progestin combination. *ANN OTTALMOL CLIN OCUL* 94:299–321, 1968. (Italian)

Tetanus toxin effect on the eye has been examined from a pharmacologic rather than a toxicologic viewpoint. In the anterior chamber it paralyses the pupillary sphincter by blocking the release of acetylcholine from the nerves of the iris, and this is not reversible by antitoxin.[a]

   a. Fedinec AA: Antitoxin's effect on tetanus toxin-induced sphincter pupillae in the rabbit. *NAUNYN-SCHMIEDEBERG'S ARCH PHARMACOL* 276:311–320, 1973.

Tetrachloroethane (1,1,2,2-tetrachloroethane; acetylene tetrachloride) has many uses as a solvent, but there appear to have been no eye injuries reported from it, and tests on rabbits indicate that it is only slightly irritating to the eye.[b] Dogs exposed to vapors of tetrachloroethane have developed no corneal injury even though they underwent repeated narcosis.[a]

   a. Steindorff K: On the effect of some chlorinated derivatives of methane, ethane, and ethylene on the cornea of the animal eye. *GRAEFES ARCH OPHTHALMOL* 109:252–264, 1922. (German)
   b. Truhaut R, et al: Toxicological study of 1,1,1,2-tetrachloroethane. *ARCH MAL PROF MED TRAV SECUR SOC* 35:593–608, 1974. (French)

Tetrachloroethylene (perchloroethylene, Perclene, Nema) is employed as a solvent in dry cleaning of clothes and in degreasing metals. Also it has been employed as an anthelmintic.[171] High concentration of vapor causes mild sensation of irritation to the eyes, but serious injury is not likely.[a] Experimental momentary spraying of rabbits eyes with tetrachloroethylene from a pressurized fire extinguisher from a distance of one foot caused immediate pain and blepharospasm. The corneal epithelium became granular and optically irregular, and patches of epithelium were lost, but the eyes recovered completely within two days.[81]

   a. Rowe VK, McCollister DD, et al: Vapor toxicity of tetrachloroethylene for laboratory animals and human subjects. *ARCH OCCUP HYG* 5:566–578, 1952.

Tetrachlorophenol has been employed as a fungicide. Its dust has been found irritating to the nose and throat, and in contact with animal eyes causes considerable irritation.[36]

Tetrachlorosilane (silicon tetrachloride) is a fuming liquid, having a suffocating odor. The vapor is irritating to the eyes and respiratory tract.[46,171] A small drop of the liquid on rabbit eyes causes severe damage.[211]

Tetracycline, an antimicrobial, has had rare but varied ocular side effects. Tetracycline in ophthalmic 1% ointment has been tested on rabbit eyes by repeated application and caused no detectable injury, as measured by corneal thickness or rate of regeneration of corneal endothelium after a standard injury.[120]

After systemic administration of tetracycline, acute transient myopia has occurred within twenty-four hours in two patients. In one patient the myopia developed on five separate occasions when she took the drug, and each time cleared again within a couple of days after stopping it.[c] The other patient had the acute myopia on only the second occasion on which she received the drug, having taken it a month previously without visual disturbance.[b] In this case the myopia cleared in eight days. The depth of the anterior chambers, the angles, and intraocular pressures were not compromized. Atropine had no appreciable antagonistic effect. The findings were quite similar to those in many other instances of acute transient myopia induced by many other drugs. (For further on this phenomenon, see INDEX for *Myopia, acute transient.*)

Benign intracranial hypertension with papilledema, occasional retinal hemorrages, and diplopia from sixth nerve palsy have become well known as complications of systemic tetracycline treatment, more frequent in infants than in adults.[d,g,k–p,386] However, among forty-two children treated for cystic fibrosis with large amounts of tetracyclines no ocular side effects were found in a special study.[f] A number of adolescents and young adults, mostly females, have developed reversible intracranial hypertension under treatment for acne.[l,o,p] Some of these patients had been receiving both tetracycline and vitamin A. Since each of these can produce intracranial hypertension, an additive adverse effect has been suspected.[o,p]

Tetracycline was listed among drugs taken during pregnancy by three mothers who had infants with congenital cataracts, but whether tetracycline was responsible is uncertain.[e] Experiments in rats have shown that the newborn can have discoloration of the lens, as well as the cornea and sclera, after administration of tetracycline to the mother during pregnancy.[h] In young rabbits, intensive direct exposure of the eyes by wearing tetracycline-impregnated hydrophilic contact lenses for several days has caused the crystalline lenses to become yellowish, with opacification, especially in the nucleus.[i] The corneas also developed yellow-brown discoloration.[j] Calf lens epithelium in culture with *rolitetracycline* tolerated 4 mg/100 ml, but higher concentrations caused degeneration with formation of lipid vacuoles.[355]

In two patients who had taken tetracycline and *minocycline* orally for several years black or brown concretions were found in small cysts of the palpebral conjunctiva, closely resembling those that are well known to be produced by topical epinephrine.[a,n] The material fluoresced like tetracycline, and was thought to be a calcium chelate of the drug. The concretions produced no symptoms.

a. Brothers DM, Hidayat AA: Conjunctival pigmentation associated with tetracycline medication. *OPHTHALMOLOGY* 88:1212–1215, 1981.

b. Capperucci G: On a case of transitory myopia from tetracycline. *ANN OTTALMOL CLIN OCUL* 90:891–900, 1964. (Italian)

c. Edwards TS: Transient myopia due to tetracycline. *J AM MED ASSOC* 186:175–176, 1963.

d. Giles CL, Soble AR: Intracranial hypertension and tetracycline therapy. *AM J OPHTHALMOL* 72:981–982, 1971.

e. Harley JD, Farrar JF, et al: Aromatic drugs and congenital cataracts. *LANCET* 1:472–473, 1964.

f. Keith CG, DeHaller J, Young WF: Side effects to antibiotic administration and to severity of pulmonary involvement. *ARCH DIS CHILD* 41:262–266, 1966.

g. Koch-Weser J, Gilmore EB: Benign intracranial hypertension in an adult after tetracycline therapy. *J AM MED ASSOC* 200:345–347, 1967.

h. Krejci L, Brettschneider I, Triska J: Eye changes due to systemic use of tetracycline in pregnancy. *OPHTHALMIC RES* 12:73–77, 1980.

i. Krejci L, Brettschneider I, Triska J: Tetracycline hydrochloride and lens changes. *OPHTHALMIC RES* 10:36–40, 1978.

j. Krejci L, Brettschneider I: Yellow-brown cornea, a complication of topical use of tetracycline. *OPHTHALMIC RES* 10:131–134, 1978.

k. O'Doherty NJ: Acute benign intracranial hypertension in infant receiving tetracycline. *DEV MED CHILD NEUROL* 7:677–680, 1965.

l. Ohlrich GD, Ohlrich JG: Papilloedema in an adolescent due to tetracycline. *MED J AUST* 1:334–335, 1977.

m. Maroon JC, Mealy J Jr: Benign intracranial hypertension sequel to tetracycline therapy in a child. *J AM MED ASSOC* 216:1479–1480, 1971.

n. Messmer E, Font RL, et al: Pigmented conjunctival cysts following tetracycline/minocycline therapy. *OPHTHALMOLOGY* 90:1462–1468, 1983.

o. Pearson MG, Littlewood SM, Bowden AN: Tetracycline and benign intracranial hypertension. *BR MED J* 282:568–569, 1981.

p. Walters BNJ, Gubbay SS: Tetracycline and benign intracranial hypertension; report of 5 cases. *BR MED J* 282:19–20, 1981.

Tetraethylammonium bromide or **chloride,** a ganglion blocking agent, can cause transient mydriasis, and ptosis.[171,252]

Tetraethylammonium hydroxide is a very strong caustic base, available only in water solution as a hydrate.[171] It is capable of causing severe permanent opacification of the cornea, similar to that produced by sodium hydroxide.[89] The injurious effect is attributable to the high alkalinity rather than to any special toxic effect of the *tetraethylammonium ion,* since dilution or neutralization to pH 11 or below largely eliminates the injurious action on the rabbit cornea even when it is applied to the bared corneal stroma.[80,89]

Tetraethyl lead (lead tetraethyl, TEL), employed as an additive to gasoline, has caused acute lethal and chronic poisoning. Poisonings have occurred during industrial contact with concentrated material, and as a result of repeated inhalation ("sniffing") of tetraethyl lead in gasoline. The foremost toxic effects are on the central nervous system, manifested by insomnia and excitement, confusion, and headache. Tremors, twitching, and spasticity have been described.[124,252] Fundamentally, the effects of tetraethyl lead are different from those of inorganic lead, but signs and symptoms of the latter have been reported after prolonged exposure to low concentrations of the tetraethyl compound.[252] Tetraethyl lead changes to triethyl lead, and then partially to inorganic lead.

The outstanding effect of accidental ingestion of pure tetraethyl lead in a patient described by Stasik in 1969 was great elevation of intracranial pressure. This patient died, but before going into coma was noted to have dilated and unreactive pupils. The retinal vessels were said to be narrowed, but no comments were made concerning vision or the appearance of the optic nerveheads, and no postmortem examination of the eye was reported, although the brain and other organs were examined. Capillary vascular lesions, particularly in the CNS, were most notable. The severity of lesions found postmortem correlated approximately with the concentration of triethyl lead found in various organs.[s]

In four cases of acute occupational poisoning by tetraethyl lead with encephalopathy reported by Beattie in 1972, there was no mention of disturbance of eyes or vision.[b]

Triethyl lead formed after absorption of tetraethyl lead is thought to be responsible for the toxic effects on the brain. Triethyl lead is retained by soft tissues (rather than by bone) and is lost from the tissues in the course of several weeks.[d] This storage of triethyl lead and slow loss provides a mechanism for developing poisoning by accumulation of small doses from chronic repeated exposures. Triethyl lead is a metabolic inhibitor, but it is not reactive with thiols, and its toxic effect is not blocked by substances such as dimercaprol. The usual antidotes for heavy metal poisoning such as edetate, dimercaprol or penicillamine are no help in acute poisoning by tetraethyl or triethyl lead, before much inorganic lead has been formed.[d,e] The experimental toxicology of these compounds was reviewed by Bolanowska in 1968.[d]

Exemplifying the possibility of cumulative poisoning, Law and Nelson in 1968 described a case of encephalopathy from daily inhalation of gasoline containing tetraethyl lead for three or four hours a day during eight months. No effects on vision and no examination of the eyes were mentioned in this case, except that cranial nerve examination was normal.[j]

Similarly, in other cases of poisoning from habitual sniffing of gasoline containing tetraethyl lead by Boeckx,[c] by Hansen,[i] by Robinson,[k] and by Young,[t] there has been organic lead encephalopathy, but little comment on eyes or vision. Robinson mentioned limitation of upward gaze in a severely poisoned child who died, and rotary nystagmus on lateral gaze. Interestingly, in the more chronic cases, with presumably more conversion and accumulation of lead in inorganic form, chelation treatment appeared to be more helpful than in acute tetraethyl lead poisoning.

Very little firsthand or detailed information appears to have been published on toxic effect of tetraethyl lead or triethyl lead on the eye. Machle mentioned "impaired vision" in nine out of a group of seventy-eight patients exposed to tetraethyl lead, but in all cases this was said to be due to "weakness of the extrinsic muscles of the eye," and no abnormality was recognized in the eye grounds. No details of visual acuity were given.[m]

A report by Baisi claimed that in chronic tetraethyl lead poisoning the eyes have shown rapidly increasing mydriasis and loss of pupillary reflex to light; also that in some cases optic neuritis has occurred, resulting in atrophy.[a] Gralek likewise ascribed bilateral optic neuritis to tetraethyl lead vapors in one case in Poland.[h]

Lillie described in detail an acute loss of vision which followed contact of the hands with gasoline containing tetraethyl lead over a period of nine months and swallowing of a mouthful of the gasoline on one occasion.[l] Vision decreased rapidly to finger counting, and absolute central scotoma was present, but the fundi remained normal. There was severe headache, but neurological examination was negative. It is noteworthy that in this case there were signs and symptoms characteristic of chronic poisoning by inorganic lead, rather than the disturbances which have characterized acute poisonings with tetraethyl lead. The patient had abdominal cramps, lead line of the gums, and lead in the urine. Under treatment for inorganic lead poisoning the vision gradually improved and the visual fields returned to normal.[l]

In yet another case, quite briefly described by Davis, inorganic lead poisoning with "severe amblyopia" but normal fundi and fields occurred in a man who daily washed the upper part of his body with gasoline.[f] Lead line in the gums and urinary lead excretion indicated lead poisoning. Under treatment with calcium edetate and dimercaprol the patient recovered.

Ermakov in 1969 mentioned disturbances of vision and hearing in a study of 400 patients believed to have tetraethyl lead poisoning. They reported abnormalities of the EEG in about one third of the patients, but no details of the nature of disturbance of vision were given in the available English abstract of the study published in Russian.[g]

According to German abstracts, Skripnichenko has reported in the Russian literature that tetraethyl lead poisoning causes functional disturbances of the eye characterized by changes of the limits of visual fields for colors, changes in adaptation, alteration of the elasticity of the eye, leading later to papillitis, retrobulbar neuritis, optic atrophy, and glaucoma.[q] It is not evident how much evidence supports these claims.

A series of articles by Skripnichenko from 1956 to 1968 have been concerned with induction of glaucoma in rabbits by tetraethyl lead.[q,r] These articles, and an earlier one on the subject by Shevalev, have been published in Russian or Hungarian. A portion of Skripnichenko's 1955 and 1956 publications have been translated into English and published by Posner in 1962.[o] There seem to be no corroborating reports from other authors concerning elevation of intraocular pressure by tetraethyl lead, either experimentally or clinically.

Concerning local effects on the eye from direct contact, there was recorded by Leake in 1926 a strange account of a contamination of the eyes from a splash of gasoline containing tetraethyl lead, after which the patient was said to have been unable to see for three-fourths of an hour, cause undetermined.[k]

Gasoline containing tetraethyl lead applied to rabbit eyes causes immediate pain and blepharospasm lasting several minutes.[81] When the application was repeated ten times in the course of five minutes under local anesthesia, it produced conjunctival hyperemia and moderate flocculent discharge, but no damage to cornea or conjunctiva.[81] However, scanning electron microscopy is said to show changes in the corneal epithelium from exposure to leaded gasoline vapor.[n]

a. Baisi AV: Ocular disturbances in chronic poisoning by tetraethyl lead vapors. *VERK 6 INTERNAT KONG UNFALL U VERUFSKRH* 784, 1931. (Ref. from Haensch P. 129)

b. Beattie AD, Moore MR, Goldberg A: Tetraethyl lead poisoning. *LANCET* 2:12–15, 1972.

c. Boeckx RL, et al: Gasoline sniffing and tetraethyl lead poisoning in children. *PEDIATRICS* 60:40–45, 1977.

d. Bolanowska W: Distribution and excretion of triethyl lead in rats. *BR J IND MED* 25:203–208, 1968.

e. Creme J: Biochemical studies on the toxicity of tetraethyl lead and other organo-lead compounds. *BR J IND MED* 16:191–199, 1959.

f. Davis PL: Lead poisoning with bladder colic and amblyopia. *J AM MED ASSOC* 175:257, 1961.

g. Ermakov EV, Murashov BF: Mechanism of action of tetraethyllead. *GIG TR PROF ZABOL* 13:53–54, 1969.

h. Gralek M, Bogorodzki B: Optic neuritis caused by contact with lead compounds. *KLIN OCZNA* 46:663–665, 1976. (English abst.)

i. Hansen KS, Sharp FR: Gasoline sniffing, lead poisoning, and myoclonus. *J AM MED ASSOC* 240:1375–1376, 1978.

j. Law WR, Nelson ER: Gasoline sniffing by an adult. *J AM MED ASSOC* 204:1002–1004, 1968.

k. Leake WP, et al: FULL REPORT OF INVESTIGATION OF HEALTH HAZARDS FROM TETRAETHYL LEAD. *U.S. Public Health Service*, #163, 1926.

l. Lillie WI: The clinical significance of retrobulbar and optic neuritis. *AM J OPHTHAL-MOL* 17:110–119, 1934.

m. Machle WF: Tetraethyl lead intoxication and poisoning by related compounds of lead. *J AM MED ASSOC* 105:578–585, 1935.

n. Niebroj TK, et al: Scanning microscopy of cornea and conjunctiva in animals chronically exposed to leaded (tetraethyl lead) gasoline vapor. *KLIN OCZNA* 44:879–881, 1974. (English abst.)

o. Posner A: Glaucoma caused by exposure to tetraethyl lead gasoline. *EYE EAR NOSE THROAT MONTHLY* 41:129–130, 1962.

p. Robinson RO: Tetraethyl lead poisoning from gasoline sniffing. *J AM MED ASSOC* 240:1373–1374, 1978.

q. Skripnichenko ZM: Experimental finding on the influence of tetraethyl lead on the regulation of intraocular pressure. *OFTAL ZH* 11:143–148, 1956; 12:372–379, 1957. (*ZBL GES OPHTHALMOL* 69:305, 1957; 74:106, 1958.)

r. Skripnichenko ZM: Toxic glaucoma from ethylbenzene and tetraethyl lead. *ACTA MED ACAD SCI HUNG* 25:175–184, 1968.

s. Stasik M, Byczkowska Z, et al: Acute tetraethyllead poisoning. *ARCH TOXIKOL* 24:283–291, 1969.

t. Young RS, et al: Recurrent cerebellar dysfunction as related to chronic gasoline sniffing in an adolescent girl. *CLIN PEDIATR* 16:706–708, 1977.

Tetraethylpyrophosphate (TEPP), a cholinesterase inhibitor, at one time was used in treatment of glaucoma, myasthenia gravis, and pediculosis of the eyelashes. It caused miosis and spasm of accommodation for near, accompanied by aching in the eye and blurring of distant vision.[a] Systemic absorption causes similar eye disturbances, but also gastrointestinal, neurological, and muscular disturbances. In two patients treated intensively with atropine for systemic TEPP poisoning, the size of the pupils appeared to correlate with the condition of the patient and responses to treatment, becoming less constricted with general improvement.[b]

  a. Grant WM: Miotic and antiglaucoma activity of tetraethyl pyrophosphate in human eyes. *ARCH OPHTHALMOL* 39:579–586, 1948; *ARCH OPHTHALMOL* 44:362–364, 1950.
  b. Reeder DH: Organic phosphate insecticide poisoning. *J OCCUP MED* 3:129–130, 1961.

2,5-Tetrahydrofurandimethanol (THF glycol) has a reputation of being highly irritating to the eyes, skin, and mucous membranes, but original observations were not found.[171]

Tetrahydrofurfuryl alcohol is irritating to human and rabbit eyes.[171] In rabbit eyes 24 hours after application of 0.1 ml there was still irritation and increased thickness of the cornea.[295,338]

Tetrahydronaphthalene (Tetralin) vapor is said to cause sensation of irritation of the eyes and respiratory tract,[70,171,252] but test application of the liquid to rabbit eyes caused no injury detectable twenty-four hours later.[225]

Administered orally to rabbits and guinea pigs, it has been found to induce cataracts even more readily than naphthalene itself,[a,b] but not in rats.[307] In guinea pigs, opacities appear in the cortex of the lens at the equator in a few days, and proceed posteriorly. Also, round gray spots develop in the fundus, and the retina has a turbid appearance.[b] (Compare *Naphthalene* and *Decahydronaphthalene*.)

  a. Basile G: The action of some products of hydrogenation of naphthalin (tetralin and decalin) on the lens and deep ocular membranes of the rabbit. *BOLL OCULIST* 18:951–957, 1939. (Italian)
  b. Badinand A, Paufique L, Rodier J: Experimental intoxication by 1,2,3,4-tetrahydro-naphthalene. *ARCH MAL PROF* 8:124–130, 1947. (*CHEM ABSTR* 42:7878.)

Tetrahydro-β-naphthylamine given to human beings orally or subcutaneously in doses from 0.075 to 0.225 g caused vomiting, headache, vertigo, and mydriasis.[252] Application of 0.5% to 1% solution to the eyes is said to have caused much pain and in ten to fifteen minutes induced mydriasis which lasted thirty to sixty minutes.[153]

Tetramethylammonium hydroxide is a strongly basic substance available in aqueous solution, having a strong ammonia-like odor.[171] On rabbit eyes it causes severe alkali burns with permanent opacification similar to burns caused by other strong alkalies.[89] Dilution or titration with acid to pH 11 or less greatly reduces the injurious effect. Such preparations do not produce opacification in rabbit corneas. In neutral solution, the *tetramethylammonium ion* is not injurious to the eye, but induces transient miosis.[80]

Tetramethyl-butanediamine (N,N,N′,N′-tetramethyl-1,3-butanediamine) has shown unusual effects on the eyes of animals and people. In rabbits, tests of 0.005 ml undiluted and 0.5 ml of 5% aqueous solution both caused severe damage to the cornea, and 1% solution caused moderate injury.[a,228] In workmen exposed to vapors a delayed effect on the corneal epithelium has been noted, causing misty vision with haloes around lights in the evening after a day of exposure at work, sometimes with photophobia, but usually little discomfort, sometimes clearing by the next morning.[a,b,40] The misty vision with haloes around lights is explained by transitory edema of the corneal epithelium. (For comparisons, see INDEX for *Amines*.)

In addition to the effect on the cornea, mydriasis and cycloplegia have been observed in workmen exposed to the vapors.[a,b,40] The mydriasis has lasted as long as a week, considerably longer than the edema of the corneal epithelium. Mydriasis has also been noted in mice exposed to the vapor.[a]

   a. Goldberg ME, Johnson HE: Autonomic ganglion activity and acute toxicologic effects of N,N,N',N'-tetramethyl-1,3-butanediamine and triethylenediamine, two foam catalyst amines. *TOXICOL APPL PHARMACOL* 4:522–545, 1962.
   b. Smagghe, G: Ocular disturbances from tetramethylbutane-diamine. *ARCH MAL PROF* 28:457–459, 1967. (French)

Tetramethyl ethylenediamine applied as a drop to rabbit eyes, without irrigation and with the lids then held closed, in 5 minutes caused corneal haze and sloughing the surface, according to Mellerio and Weale.[170] The injury was graded 8 on a scale of 10 after 24 hours.[27,223]

Tetranitromethane vapors are very irritating to the eyes, nose, and respiratory passages.[a,51,215] It has been proposed for use as an irritant war gas.[171] Animals show evidence of irritation of the eyes rather quickly at concentrations from 3.3 to 25.2 ppm in air.

   a. Hager KF: Tetranitromethane. *IND ENG CHEM* 41:2168, 1949.

Tetryl (Nitramine; 2,4,6-trinitrophenylmethylnitramine) dust stains the skin yellow and causes a sensitization-type dermatitis which may involve the eyelids.[a,176,252] Conjunctivitis, keratitis, and iridocyclitis are also said to have occurred.[a]

   a. Troup HB: Clinical effects of tetryl (CE Powder). *BR J IND MED* 3:20–23, 1946.

Thalidomide (Contergan, Distaval, Kevadon), a sedative and hypnotic, caused a large number of congenital abnormalities in babies of women who took the medication early in pregnancy. It was therefore withdrawn from the market worldwide. Agenesis of limbs was the most common fetal abnormality. The eyes were involved in 10 to 50% of cases.[o] The literature on eye involvement has been reviewed by Rafuse, Pabst, and Schmidt-Mumm.[i,j,l] The embryology of the ocular defects and the critical time of drug action have been discussed, particularly by Cullen.[b–d]

In several series of clinical and postmortem case reports the ocular malformations that have been described include anophthalmos, microphthalmos, colobomas of the iris, retina, choroid, and optic nerve, malformations of the lens, retinal dysplasia, persistence of hyaloid vessels, palsies of muscles affecting the eyes or eye movements, particularly the abducens, levator of the lid and facial muscles.[a–f,h–p] Less commonly, there have been epicanthus, three instances of uveitis, and one instance of megalocornea with no mention of glaucoma.[1] The commonest abnormalities appear to have been abnormalities of the extraocular muscles, microphthalmos, and colobomas from abnormal closures of the fetal optic cleft. Abnormalities of the crystalline lens seem to have been relatively rare.

Reports in the 1970's, mostly from examination of school-age children, include an instance of failure of the lens to separate from the ectoderm,[o] three cases of a combination of 6th nerve palsy and lacrimation associated with eating,[n] and peripheral pigmentary and atrophic retinopathy in 8 out of 19 "thalidomide children."[m]

In rabbits, administration of thalidomide during pregnancy has caused deformities of the limbs like those in human beings, and caused histologic abnormalities of extraocular muscles in about one third of the fetuses.[g] Microphthalmos with abnormalities of iris, retina and choroid was relatively rare.

a. Casanovas J, Carbonnel M: Ocular malformations in thalidomide embryopathy. *ARCH SOC OFTAL HISP-AM* 24:947–955, 1964. (Spanish)

b. Cullen JF: Ocular defects in thalidomide babies. *BR J OPHTHALMOL* 48:151–153, 1964.

c. Cullen JF: Teratogenic agents and thalidomide. *TRANS OPHTHALMOL SOC UK* 86:101–113, 1966.

d. Cullen JF: Clinical anophthalmos in a ? thalidomide child. *J PEDIAT OPHTHALMOL* 3:10–14, 1966.

e. Gilkes MJ, Strode M: Ocular anomalies in association with developmental limb abnormalities of drug origin. *LANCET* 1:1026–1027, 1963.

f. Honegger H, Pape R: Thalidomide and congenital malformations of the eyes. *BER DTSCH OPHTHALMOL GESELLSCH* 65:222–227, 1963. (German)

g. Laszczyk WA, et al: Changes in the visual system of rabbit fetuses after thalidomide administration. *OPHTHALMIC RES* 8:146–151, 1976.

h. Otto J: Contergan deformities with eye involvement. *BER DTSCH OPHTHALMOL GESELLSCH* 65:220–222, 1963. (German)

i. Papst W: Thalidomide and congenital anomalies of the eyes. *BER DTSCH OPHTHALMOL GESELLSCH* 65:209–215, 1963. (German)

j. Rafuse EV, Arstikaitis M, Brent HP: Ocular findings in thalidomide children. *CAN J OPHTHALMOL* 2:222–225, 1967.

k. Schmidt JGH: Eye muscle pareses with thalidomide-embryopathy. *BER DTSCH OPHTHALMOL GESELLSCH* 65:215–220, 1963. (German)

l. Schmidt-Mumm E: On eye malformations with the dysmelia syndrome. *KLIN MONATSBL AUGENHEILKD* 148:150–156, 1966. (German)

m. Schutte E, Klaas D, Lizin F: Serial studies in thalidomide damaged children. *BER DTSCH OPHTHALMOL GESELLSCH* 74:578–580, 1977. (German)

n. Trieschmann W: Crocodile tears in contergan embryopathy. *KLIN MONATSBL AUGENHEILKD* 162:546–550, 1973. (German)

o. Welge-Lussen L: Thalidomide embryopathy with peculiar eye changes. *KLIN MONATSBL AUGENHEILKD* 158:372–378, 1971. (German)

p. Zetterstrom B: Ocular malformations caused by thalidomide. *ACTA OPHTHALMOL* 44:391–395, 1966.

Thallium is a heavy metal used mostly in the form of soluble salts such as *thallium acetate* and *thallium sulfate,* for extermination of rodents, and formerly as a depilatory.

The literature on thallium poisoning amounts to more than 1,000 references. At least forty publications have been concerned with the effects of thallium poisoning on the eyes.

Hundreds of cases of poisoning have been reported, a few from industrial exposure, but the majority from ingestion of thallium salts given medically or with criminal intent, or from absorption from depilatories applied to the skin. Particularly notorious sources of thallium poisoning have been Zelio Paste and Thalgrain rodenticide, first introduced in Germany in 1920, and Koremlu, a depilatory cream introduced in 1931 but discontinued after a few years because of its poisonous actions.

The general effects of thallium poisoning consists of gastrointestinal disturbance, painful neuritis affecting the feet and legs, with subsequent weakness or paralysis of the legs, loss of hair, psychic disturbances, and in a small proportion of cases, death from respiratory and circulatory disturbance. The characteristics of the poisoning have been well described in reviews.[q,t,194,252]

Among the eye disturbances caused by thallium poisoning have been decrease in visual acuity and paralyses of extraocular muscles. Thallium poisoning has also been known to produce cataracts, but probably only in experimental animals.

Decrease in visual acuity attributed to optic or retrobulbar neuritis has occurred more often in chronic than in acute thallium poisoning.[24,194] Bohringer believed that in single acute poisonings, the incidence of optic nerve damage was 25%, but in repeated poisonings that optic nerve damage was the rule.[b] Most commonly the retrobulbar portion of the nerve was believed to have been affected, causing blurring of vision with central scotoma, with the optic nerveheads and fundi appearing normal. Less commonly there have been visible congestion and blurring of the nervehead. In most instances symptoms of retrobulbar neuritis have been partially reversible, but several cases of optic atrophy with blindness or permanent reduction of vision have been reported.[b,f,h,j,l–n,w,x,177,194] Moeschlin observed one patient progress from an appearance of optic neuritis with hyperemic optic discs with blurred margins to white optic atrophy.[177] Irreversible damage to the optic nerves has been observed most likely to occur in chronic poisoning, although in exceptional cases optic atrophy has been known to develop as a result of acute poisoning.[24,194]

In a case reported by Lang in 1952, bilateral retrobulbar neuritis developed five weeks after two doses of thallium sulfate had been taken orally at ten-day intervals, and resulted in optic atrophy.[l]

In 1952, from observations on nine instances of optic atrophy among twenty-four individuals poisoned by thallium, Bohringer concluded that despite partial atrophy, the vision could improve in the course of a year, but remained unchanging after that.[b]

The earliest observations of what was diagnosed as postneuritic atrophy of the optic nerve in chronic thallium poisoning appear to have been made in 1927 by Kaps and by Krauss.[h,j] The first was from criminal administration of the poison, and the other from chronic industrial exposure.

Girot and Braun described blurring of vision due to central scotomas in a man who had taken injections and inunctions of thallium acetate for four months.[f] The optic nerveheads were slightly pale, and vision improved only slightly after thallium was discontinued.

During the period 1932 to 1935 several cases of retrobulbar or optic neuritis of rather uniform sort resulted from use of a depilatory, Koremlu Cream, containing approximately 7% thallium acetate. Such cases were described by Lillie,[m] Mahoney,[n] Rudolphy,[w] and Stine.[x]

In a case of acute poisoning reported by Hennekes in 1983 the visual acuity was very low 21 days after the poison was taken, and there was severe peripheral polyneuropathy, but no optic atrophy was discernible at that time.[g] The electroretinogram showed hypernormal scotopic b-wave amplitude. Subsequently, definite optic atrophy developed. The ERG remained the same. This case seems particularly noteworthy because it not only documents the development of optic atrophy, but it provides evidence that the thallium poisoning had a direct toxic effect on the retina, most likely on the neurons of the inner retinal layers. The findings in this case suggest that the optic atrophy may have developed in an ascending manner from the retina, rather than in a descending manner from presumed retrobulbar neuritis, as generally assumed in earlier cases in the absence of ERG measurements.

The first anatomic study of the effect of systemic thallium poisoning on the human eye was reported by Manschot, who in 1968 described a case of optic atrophy.[o,p] He examined the eyes of a woman who died nineteen years after having been very severely poisoned, displaying all the characteristics of thallium alopecia, optic neuritis, polyneuritis, and psychosis. The most dramatic finding was a highly selective and complete loss of retinal ganglion cells, while the outer nuclear layer and the rods and cones appeared to be undamaged. The nerve fibers and optic nerves were almost completely atrophic. The anterior segments of the eyes were normal.[o,p] The ERG measurements reported in 1983 by Hennekes have been considered consistent with Manschot's histologic findings.[g]

Oculomotor nerves and other cranial nerves have been affected in thallium poisoning less often than the optic nerve.[194] Polyneuritis of the extremities has practically always been present in patients with neuritis of the cranial nerves. The disturbance of extraocular muscles is apparently part of a generalized neuritic process, but it may be peculiarly spotty, sometimes affecting only a single fourth nerve or a single sixth nerve.[1,194] Strabismus, ptosis, and facial paralysis have been reported.[177,194] Occasionally palsies have occurred in association with retrobulbar or optic neuritis.

In severe poisoning with external ophthalmoplegia, Cavanagh in 1974 reported finding degenerative changes in nerve fibers in the extraocular muscles.[c] In a particularly dramatic case reported by Davis in 1980 the patient had swallowed five-times the lethal dose of thallium and by the end of the same day had widespread peripheral polyneuropathy.[d] By the third day the patient had almost complete paralysis of facial and extraocular muscles. Autopsy on the ninth day showed in cranial and peripheral nerves that there was primarily axonal degeneration, with preservation of most of the overlying myelin. In this case clinically there was no indication of involvement of the optic nerves, and histologically only minor abnormalities were found in these nerves.

One quite unusual case of thallium poisoning, possibly involving iris and lens as well as optic nerve, has been described in two reports in 1927 and 1928 and has been referred to repeatedly since.[r,v] In this case, a man who suffered severe thallium poisoning from industrial exposure, had the common finding of impaired visual acuity due to bilateral central scotomas and progressive optic atrophy, but was observed also to have immature cataract, and in one eye to have posterior synechias. However, there appears to have been no evidence to show that thallium was responsible for the changes in the anterior segment. It is quite possible that the immature cataracts and posterior synechias were preexistent or unrelated to the poisoning.

Disturbance of the lens in thallium poisoning of human beings seems to be very rare. One case has been reported in which snowflake type of opacities were seen in the deeper parts of the anterior and posterior cortex, but three months later when the patient was much improved from the poisoning, the opacities seemed much less.[k] No instance of a disabling degree of cataract formation has been reported. The effect on the lens in animals appears to be significantly different from that in human beings.

In experimental poisoning of animals several effects have been observed which are different from what has been reported in human beings. In particular, cataract, keratitis, and intraocular inflammation, which have been rare or nonexistent in human poisonings, appear to have been a prominent feature of animal poisonings. Rats poisoned with thallium have repeatedly been observed to develop cataracts.[e,z,194] Thallium has been shown in mice to have a tendency to accumulate particularly in the lens.[a] Kinsey showed that rabbit lenses in culture could actually concentrate thallium, and that if a concentration of 30mM was reached in the lens, opacification developed.[i] Exchange for tissue potassium was shown to be involved in the uptake of thallium. Potts showed this exchange also provided a mechanism for accumulation of thallium in retina and optic nerve, but what relationship this may have to toxic action is not yet known.[t]

Keratitis and corneal ulcers have developed in dogs poisoned with thallium.[u,64] Dogs which were given sublethal doses by Swab in 1934 became unable to stand or walk, and developed lacrimation and purulent discharge in both eyes.[z] Within a week the corneas were said to be dull and the pupils reacted very sluggishly to light. Also, rabbits and rats poisoned by thallium developed red lids, conjunctivitis, and discharge from the eyes. Histologic examination of the eyes of these animals showed inflammatory signs consisting of cellular infiltration in all parts of the anterior segments and in the retina, but not in the choroid. Also inflammatory cell infiltration was found in the optic nerve and optic tract. However, in these acutely poisoned animals there was no evidence of cataract.[y]

Pentschew, writing in the Neuro-ophthalmology textbook of Walsh and Hoyt, has described experiments in rhesus monkeys which were given thallium sulfate intravenously repeatedly, inducing amblyopia, conjunctivitis, alopecia, with burning feet syndrome and severe cerebellar ataxia. Histologic examination showed damage in the optic nerves, optic tract, and lateral geniculate bodies, but findings in the eyes themselves were not mentioned.[256]

Experiments concerned with the local effects of thallium on the eye suggest that contact of thallium salts with the eye, such as by accidental splash contamination, is unlikely to cause serious damage, especially if promptly washed away with water. Experimentally, a rather drastic exposure of a rabbit eye for ten minutes to a neutral saturated solution of thallium chloride, with the epithelium preliminarily removed to facilitate penetration, caused moderate edema and haze in the cornea, which gradually cleared from the periphery, but left a nebulous area axially.[81,90] Splash contact with intact epithelium presumably would be even less damaging.

Treatment of thallium poisoning is in such an unsatisfactory and somewhat controversial state that no attempt will be made to cover it here. Cavanagh in 1974 provided a comprehensive review of treatments that had been tried.[c]

a. Andre T, Ulberg S, Winquist G: Accumulation and retention of thallium in tissues of the mouse. *ACTA PHARMACOL TOXICOL* 16:229–234, 1960.

b. Bohringer HR: Optic nerve injuries from thallium poisoning. *PRAXIS* 41:1092–1094, 1952. (German)

c. Cavanagh JB, Fuller NH, et al: The effects of the thallium salts, with particular reference to the nervous system changes. *Q J MED* 43:293–319, 1974.

d. Davis LE, Standefer JC, et al: Acute thallium poisoning. *ANN NEUROL* 10:38–44, 1981.

e. Ginsberg S, Buschke A: Eye changes in rats after thallium feeding. *KLIN MONATSBL AUGENHEILKD* 71:385–399, 1923. (German)

f. Girot L, Braun S: A case of optic neuritis from poisoning by thallium acetate. *REV NEUROL* 36:244–245, 1929. (French)

g. Hennekes R: Impairment of retinal function in acute thallium poisoning. *KLIN MONATSBL AUGENHEILKD* 182:334–336, 1983. (German)

h. Kaps L: Criminal lethal subacute thallium poisoning. *WIEN KLIN WOCHENSCHR* 1:967, 1927. (German)

i. Kinsey VE, McLean IW, Parker J: Studies on the crystalline lens. *INVEST OPHTHALMOL* 10:932–942, 1971.

j. Krauss: Post-neuritic atrophy of both optic nerves. *KLIN MONATSBL AUGENHEILKD* 79:829, 1927. (German)

k. Kubesooa J: Retrobulbar neuritis and cataract in thallium poisoning. *CESK OFTALMOL* 5:149–153, 1949.

l. Lange F: Bilateral optic atrophy after acute thallium poisoning. *KLIN MONATSBL AUGENHEILKD* 121:221–223, 1952. (German)

m. Lillie WI, Parker HL: Retrobulbar neuritis due to thallium poisoning. *J AM MED ASSOC* 98:1347–1349, 1932.

n. Mahoney W: Retrobulbar neuritis due to thallium poisoning from depilatory cream. *J AM MED ASSOC* 98:618–620, 1932.

o. Manschot WA: Ophthalmic pathological findings in a case of thallium poisoning. *EXCERPTA MED INT CONGR SERIES 160(III CONGR EUROP SOC OPHTHAL)* Abstr. No. 26, June 1968.

p. Manschot WA: Ophthalmic pathological findings in a case of thallium poisoning. *OPHTHALMOLOGICA ADDIT AD* 158:348–349, 1969.

q. Mathys R, Thomas F: Criminal thallium poisoning. *J FORENSIC MED* 5:111–121, 1958.

r. Meyer S: Changes in the blood as reflecting industrial damage. *J IND HYG* 10:29, 1928.

s. Passarge C, Weick HH: Thallium polyneuritis. *FORTSCHR NEUROL PSYCHIATR* 33:447, 1965. (*FOOD COSMET TOXICOL* 4:545–546, 1966.)

t. Potts AM, Au PC: Thallous ion and the eye. *INVEST OPHTHALMOL* 10:925–931, 1971.

u. Richet C: On the toxicity of thallium, and keratitis in chronic poisoning by lead or by thallium. *CR SOC BIOL* 1:252, 1899. (French)

v. Rube, Hendricks: Occupational thallium poisoning. *MED WELT* (No 20):733, 1927. (German)

w. Rudolphy JB: Optic atrophy due to thallium. *ARCH OPHTHALMOL* 13:1108–1109, 1935.

x. Stine GH: Optic neuritis and optic atrophy due to thallium poisoning following the prolonged use of Koremlu Cream. *AM J OPHTHALMOL* 15:949–952, 1932.

y. Swab CM: Ocular lesions resulting from thallium acetate poisoning as determined by experimental research. *ARCH OPHTHALMOL* 12:547–561, 1934.

z. vonSallmann L, Grimes P, Collins E: Triparanol induced cataract in rats. *ARCH OPHTHALMOL* 70:522–529, 1963.

Thiabendazole (Tiabendazole, Mintezol), an anthelmintic and fungicide, has been alleged to cause disturbance of color vision occasionally, but original observations documenting the nature of this disturbance were not located.[174]

A mother and daughter developed keratitis sicca syndrome two or three weeks after taking thiabendazole.[a] These patients suffered dry eyes, dry mouth and cholestatic jaundice, but eventually recovered. Diffuse desquamation of corneal epithelium and abnormalities of the tears caused several months of discomfort. It was suspected that the drug may have induced production of autoantibodies in these patients.

External contact tests on rabbit eyes by application of 4% thiabendazole in ointment or 10% in suspension in saline for five to ten minutes caused no irritation.[b]

a. Fink AI, MacKay CJ, Cutler SS: Sicca complex and cholestatic jaundice in two members of a family caused by thiabendazole. *TRANS AM OPHTHALMOL SOC* 76:108–115, 1978.

b. Robinson HJ, Stoerk HC, Graessle O: Studies on the toxicologic and pharmacologic properties of thiabendazole. *TOXICOL APPL PHARMACOL* 7:53–63, 1965.

Thiacetazone (Amithiozone, Conteben, Tibione) has been used in treatment of tuberculosis, leprosy, and lupus vulgaris.[171] Among its many side effects are occasional instances of a sensation of burning and pain in the eyes, and photophobia.[252] (Compare *Nicothiazone*, a related drug which has caused discomfort and photophobia from corneal disturbance.)

In one instance a central scotoma for colors and irreversible decrease of visual acuity to 5/20 has been associated with the use of thiacetazone in combination with aminosalicylic acid.[a] (Compare *Subathizone*, a related drug which has caused toxic amblyopia with very slow recovery.)

a. Steiner C: Poisoning by PAS and analogous substances. *ANN OCULIST* (*Paris*) 184:637, 1951. (French)

Thiamphenicol (Thiomycetin), an antibacterial, differs chemically from *chloramphenicol* only in having *methylsulfonylphenyl* in place of *nitrophenyl*. In one instance a child being treated with thiamphenicol for meningitis became blind from bilateral optic neuritis in ten days.[a] After the drug was stopped the vision improved partially, but temporal pallor of the discs developed, and the VER became abnormal.

(Compare optic neuropathy induced by *Chloramphenicol*.)

a. Malbrel C, Talmud M, et al: Concerning a new case of optic neuritis from chlorampenicol in a child. *BULL SOC OPHTALMOL FRANCE* 77:999–1001, 1977. (French)

Thimerosal (Thiomersal; Merthiolate), a topical mercurial anti-infective, and a preservative in eyedrops, has been tested in several ways to evaluate toxicity to the cornea, yielding varied results related to the type of exposure and the sensitivity of the tests. Ancill reported 0.5% solution applied repeatedly to eyes of guinea pigs and rats produced no corneal opacities.[6] Gasset found no damage to the corneas of rabbits by clinical, histologic, or endothelial microscope examination after 2% solution was applied twice a day for a week.[314] Burton found no change in corneal epithelial oxygen uptake in rabbits after their eyes were exposed to 1% solution for 1 minute.[c] However, according to Burnstein, excised rabbit corneas exposed to 0.0004% solution of thimerosal had great decrease in electrical resistance associated with disruption of surface epithelial cell layers.[285] Takahashi reported the temperature-reversal effect in rabbit corneas was eliminated by immersing whole excised rabbit eyes in 0.003% solution, but not in 0.001%.[383]

In experiments in which the endothelial surface of corneas was exposed to 0.0005 to 0.1% thimerosal solutions, swelling of the corneas and ultrastructural changes in endothelial cells were reported by Van Horn, increasing markedly in severity with increase in concentration.[e] Even at commonly used antibacterial concentrations of 0.001 to 0.005% there was enough functional and structural damage to advise against use of thimerosal during intraocular surgery or for preserving excised corneas.[e]

Because of the mercury content of thimerosal, and the mercurial discoloration of the lens produced by phenylmercuric salts, there has been interest in possible effects of thimerosal on the lens. Abrams looked for mercurialentis and found none in twenty-one patients who had been using pilocarpine eyedrops containing thimerosal two to four times a day for four to ten years.[a] Subsequently chemical assays for mercury in the lens of rats to which eyedrops containing mercurial preservatives had been applied repeatedly for as long as twenty-one weeks showed a higher uptake of mercury in the lens, also in the retina, ciliary body, and blood, from eyedrops containing 0.5% thimerosal than from drops containing 0.167% phenylmercuric acetate. Differences in the stability and nature of the mercury binding and reversibility of reaction with the lens have been proposed as possible explanations for a smaller tendency of thimerosal to induce mercurialentis.[a,b,6]

In clinical use as an antibacterial agent in eyedrops and solutions for use with contact lenses, thimerosal appears not to have been injurious to the eye except when hypersensitivity has developed; then there is irritation, and Wilson has described a reversible epithelial keratopathy.[f]

Testing for teratogenicity in rats and rabbits from thimerosal administered to the eyes or given systemically has been negative.[d]

a. Abrams JD: Mercurial preservatives in eye drops. *BR J OPHTHALMOL* 49:146–147, 1965.

b. Ancill RJ, Richens ER, Norton DA: Aspects of the penetration and the distribution of organic mercurials within the eye. In Pigott, PV (Ed.): *EVALUATION OF DRUG EFFECTS ON THE EYE.* London, FJ Parsons, 1968.

c. Burton GD, Hill RM: Aerobic responses of the cornea to ophthalmic preservatives, measured in vivo. *INVEST OPHTHALMOL VIS SCI* 21:842–845, 1981.

d. Gasset AR, Itoi M, et al: Teratogenicities of ophthalmic drugs. *ARCH OPHTHALMOL* 93:52–55, 1975.

e. Van Horn DL, Edelhauser HF, et al: Effect of the ophthalmic preservative thimerosal on rabbit and human corneal endothelium. *INVEST OPHTHALMOL VIS SCI* 16:273–280, 1977.

f. Wilson LA, McNatt J, Reitschel R: Delayed hypersensitivity to thimerosal in soft contact lens wearers. *OPHTHALMOLOGY* 88:804–809, 1981.

Thiodiglycol (2,2'-thiodiethanol; Kromfax Solvent) applied to rabbit eyes causes pain, but one or two drops cause only conjunctival hyperemia without corneal damage.[27,123] A single splash is not dangerous, although it is painful. Intracorneal injection or irrigation of the surface of the eye with thiodiglycol for five minutes does, however, cause moderately severe reaction, graded 45 to 62 on a scale of 0 to 100.[123]

Reaction of thiodiglycol with hydrochloric acid or with thionyl chloride produces severely toxic and injurious products, principally mustard gas.

Thioformaldehyde has been said to cause sore eyes in the artificial silk industry when present in concentration of 8 ppm or more in air,[176] but insufficient information has been given to assess the validity of this observation. Many investigations have pointed to *hydrogen sulfide* as the cause of eye irritation in the viscose silk industry. No publications were found concerning tests of thioformaldehyde for toxicity to the eye. (Compare *Hydrogen sulfide*.)

Thioglycolates are *salts of thioglycolic acid,* most commonly encountered as sodium or ammonium thioglycolates, which are employed principally in the cold-waving of hair. Such preparations are generally safe when used as directed, but occasional individuals develop dermatitis from repeated contact, usually from prolonged occupational contact. An extensive dermatologic and medical investigation of patients exposed to cold-wave preparations, and particularly *ammonium thioglycolate,* indicated that these substances have a low level of irritative effect and give no evidence of systemic intoxication despite frequent exposure.[a]

A survey of the literature in 1965 concluded that any toxic effects from ingestion of hair-waving solutions containing thioglycolate were most likely attributable to the high alkalinity of the preparation or to hydrogen sulfide formed by decomposition.[d]

In rare instances toxic effects on the eyes have been alleged. In one case a young woman developed mydriasis, cycloplegia, and loss of convergence several hours after a cold hair wave. Medical history and examination were negative. There was no history of exposure to atropine. The pupils did not respond to eserine, and it was postulated that there was a mesencephalic neurologic disturbance. The eyes returned almost to normal within four days and eventually were completely normal. There was actually no good evidence to inculpate thioglycolate.[b]

In another report a mother and daughter who did not live together both developed bilateral optic neuritis. One thing that they had in common was the use of a cold-wave lotion. No cause for the optic neuritis was found, but thioglycolate in the permanent-wave preparations was blamed.[e] Extreme scepticism has been expressed about this by Walsh and Hoyt and others.[f,256]

In another case, equally speculative, a cosmetician is reported to have complained of dizziness and irritation of the eyes when working with cold-wave solutions, and this has been interpreted as an effect of thioglycolates.[g,56]

Local action of thioglycolates on the eye has been investigated in rabbits and has been found to be influenced by pH. A 10% solution of thioglycolic acid neutralized to pH 7 by addition of ammonia and dropped continuously for fifteen seconds on eyes of rabbits caused no damage.[81] The same exposure at pH 9 caused small hemorrhages in the nictitating membrane and loss of small patches of epithelium from the cornea, but the eyes returned to normal within two days. Similarly, application of two drops of a popular commercial cold-waving lotion having pH 9.4 to 9.5, but of undetermined thioglycolate content, caused tiny hemorrhages in the nictitating membrane and conjunctiva, but was not significantly injurious to the cornea.[81]

Ocular injuries in patients have been attributed in one case to a splash of *ammoniacal thioglycolate,* and in another case to *thioglycolic acid* itself. In the first case a cold-wave preparation was accidentally splashed in a patient's eye, causing a brief burning sensation, but no disturbance of vision until the next day, when vision seemed obstructed as by a veil. On the following day the cornea was found to be stippled with fine round dots and the conjunctiva was hyperemic. On the third following day turbidity of the cornea became progressively deeper and denser despite disappearance of conjunctival inflammation, and in three weeks the vision was reduced to 5/15 in bright light and 5/6 in dim light. Eight months later the cornea still had diffuse clouding of the central layers of the stroma, but vision was improved to 5/7 in daylight and 5/5 in dim light.[c]

Test application of the same cold wave preparation to rabbit eyes caused no significant injury at the dilution employed on the patient, but when applied undiluted, it caused corneal epithelial erosion and progressive opacification of the stroma in following weeks, despite healing of the epithelium.[c] Neither the pH nor the thioglycolate content was specified, but the preparation was referred to as "ammoniacal thioglycolate." However, the reaction evoked in both patient and rabbit eye is so unlike the mild transient disturbance produced by a simple solution of ammonium thioglycolate in the pH range 7 to 9.5 that it seems probable the peculiar corneal injury caused by this particular cold-wave preparation is to be attributed to something other than thioglycolate, possibly to free thioglycolic acid or to some wetting agent. The injury appears most closely to have resembled that caused by free thioglycolic acid. (See *Thioglycolic acid* for further discussion and description of the second case.) (Also see INDEX for *Hair-waving preparations.*)

a. Behrman HT, Combes FC, et al: The cold permanent hair waving process. *J AM MED ASSOC* 140:1208–1209, 1949.

b. Halbron P: Bilateral internal ophthalmoplegia poisoning by ammonium thioglycolate. *BULL SOC OPHTALMOL FRANCE* 49:748–750, 1949. (*ARCH OPHTALMOL* 9:618, 1949. *ANN OCULIST* [Paris] 184:166, 1951.) (French)

c. Kuster A: Eye injury from thioglycolic acid in the performance of the so-called "cold wave." *KLIN MONATSBL AUGENHEILKD* 119:616–618, 1951. (German)

d. Norris JA: Toxicity of home permanent waving and neutralizer solutions. *FOOD COSMET TOXICOL* 3:93–97, 1965.

e. Robson JT, Cameron W: Optic neuritis from cold permanent wave. *NORTHWEST MED J* 48:701, 1949.

f. Robson JT, Cameron W: Optic neuritis from cold permanent wave. *BR J IND MED* 7:94, 1950.

g. Van der Burg APJ: Toxicity of cold wave solutions. *NEDERL T GENEESK* 93:3400, 1949. (Reference from Fairhall L.[15])

Thioglycolic acid (thioglycollic acid, mercaptoacetic acid) testing on rabbit eyes by application of 2 drops of a fresh 10% solution at pH 1.6, with no subsequent irrigation, caused immediate pain, and the epithelium turned gray within seconds. Half an hour later the corneas were clearer, although the epithelium maintained a ground-glass texture. The conjunctivae were edematous, but the blood vessels appeared normal. Two days later the deeper portions of the corneas were diffusely opaque. The conjunctivae were hyperemic and there was moderate discharge. In the course of six weeks the corneal clouding gradually, but not completely, cleared.[81] (This type of injury is fundamentally different from the reaction caused by neutral or mildly alkaline *thioglycolate salts* in rabbits.)

One accident has been reported in which a bottle of concentrated thioglycolic acid was dropped and splashed onto the eyes, face, legs, and arms, causing second degree burns of the skin. Within an hour or two the cornea of one eye was so clouded that a view of the anterior chamber with the slit-lamp was scarcely possible, but in the other eye the cornea was only superficially slightly clouded. The vision was 2/20 and 5/10, respectively. The conjunctivae were edematous and in the worse eye appeared bloodless.

The less injured eye returned to normal rapidly. In the other, although the conjunctiva became necrotic, the cornea cleared partially by the third day, but soon again clouded, reaching its greatest opacification at about 10 days. After two weeks the cornea slowly began to clear, and the necrotic conjunctiva regenerated and vascularized. By three weeks the cornea retained only a very delicate opacity in its lower portion in middle stromal layers, and seven months after the accident the vision was 5/4 in that eye, and 5/5 in the other.[a] The injuries in this case correspond to those produced experimentally in rabbits with pure thioglycolic acid solution.

In widely available commercial cold-wave preparations for waving the hair there is no free thioglycolic acid. Instead these preparations contain ammonium, sodium, or calcium thioglycolate at mildly alkaline pH, commonly pH 9.5, and are far less dangerous to the eye than is free thioglycolic acid.[b] (Compare *Thioglycolates* and *Hair-waving preparations.*)

a. Butscher P: Contribution on the treatment of eye injuries from thioglycolic acid in the performance of so-called cold waves. *KLIN MONATSBL AUGENHEILKD* 122:349–350, 1953. (German)

b. McCord CP: Toxicity of thioglycolic acid used in "cold permanent wave" process. *J AM MED ASSOC* 131:776, 1946.

Thionaphthenequinone tested in 0.05 M solution by application to the rabbit cornea after removal of the epithelium caused slight reaction, graded 12 on a scale of 0 to 100.[123]

Thionyl chloride is a colorless fuming liquid, having an irritating suffocating odor. Its vapors are very irritating to the eye, and the liquid is corrosive to the skin.[56,61,171] (No reports of burns of the eye from liquid thionyl chloride were found, but one would expect an injury comparable to that caused by concentrated hydrochloric acid.)

Thiopental (Pentothal), an anesthetic, caused cortical blindness in one case in which there was a period of apnea.[255] The cerebral damage was presumably due to asphyxia rather than to a toxic action of the drug. (Compare *Barbiturates* and *Anesthesia, general.*)

Thioridazine hydrochloride (Mellaril), an anti-psychotic, used mainly in treatment of schizophrenia, is one of the very few phenothiazine derivatives that are known to cause pigmentary retinopathy and decrease in vision. This toxic effect is related to excessive dosage.

An analysis of 39 cases of thioridazine pigmentary retinopathy has been carried out, examining the maximum and average daily dosage, the duration of treatment, and the total amount of drug consumed. (These were cases reported by Ardouin (1969), Bonaccorsi (1967), Brunold (1959), Cameron (1972), Connell (1964), Curtin (1978), Daumail (1964), Davidorf (1973), de Margerie (1962), Finn (1964), Grutzner (1969), Hagopian (1966), Heshe (1961), Leinfelder (1964), Meredith (1978), Miller (1982), Potts (1966), Reboton (1962), Scott (1963), Sidall (1966–68), and Weekley (1960). In nearly all cases either the maximum daily dose or the average daily dose exceeded 1,000 mg per day. Four cases may be exceptions. Concerning two cases reported by Ardouin and Grutzner, we have information only for the average daily dose and do not know how high the maximum dosage may have been.[b,95] The single cases reported by Heshe and by Reboton with maximum daily doses of 700 and 750 mg may be genuine instances of retinopathy at exceptionally low dosage.[s,za] In Heshe's and Ardouin's cases both the length of time and the total dosage were greater than in most cases.[b,s]

The only instance found in which pigmentary retinopathy has been attributed to thioridazine used at a maximum daily dosage definitely below 700 mg per day was a case reported by Brunold, with retinal pigmentation, but no visual loss, in a patient receiving 150 mg per day for a long period.[d] However, additional information on this case obtained from Jenny, the consulting ophthalmologist, and reported as a personal communication by Scott, established that, despite the report that the retina showed fine granular pigmentation after several months of treatment at this dosage, this pigmentation subsequently disappeared completely, and visual acuity remained unchanged while the patient continued to receive thioridazine at the same rate for four more years, to a total dose greater than 200 g.[zc]

Not included in the cases of pigmentary retinopathy, but involving a complaint of difficulty in reading and loss of dark adaptation is a case reported by Morrison in which a patient had been given an average daily dose of 400 mg for two and a half months, but the basis for the complaint and the relationship to retinopathy seems uncertain.[x]

Surveys of a series of patients in whom no pigmentary retinopathy has been found have indicated that a dosage up to 600 mg per day has proved safe.[a,d,l,n,q,r,ze] The range between 600 and 800 mg per day seems to be a dose range of some uncertainty, but very rarely suspect. It appears that if over 600 mg per day are administered, periodic ophthalmoscopic examinations and measurements of visual acuity should be made.

Rarely blindness or very severe loss of vision has been reported from excessive and prolonged administration of thioridazine. A twelve-year-old child described by Bonaccorsi developed optic atrophy and bilateral chorioretinal pigmentary degeneration after treatment for a year at doses ranging from 100 mg per day up to 1,600 mg per day during at least 1.5 months.[c] A patient described by Siddall became completely blind after receiving from 1,600 to 4,000 mg per day for thirty-eight days.[zd]

More often pigmentary retinopathy has been discovered with minor disturbance of vision, and in several cases visual acuity has improved significantly or returned to normal after medication was discontinued.[d,g,t,z,zc]

The pigmentary retinopathy appears as a coarse black pigmentary stippling, mostly in the central portion of the fundi, but tending to spare the papillomacula area and extending peripherally. The granular dots of pigment may appear no larger than the diameter of the major retinal vessels at first, but later may form large plaques with contiguous areas of depigmentation. Typically there is no bone corpuscle type of pigment. Several good photographic illustrations of thioridazine pigmentary retinopathy have been published.[g,l,q,r,z,zc,zd,95]

The pigmentation may be evident while visual acuity is normal, but in acute cases from large dosage with rapid onset the first complaint may be blurred vision with reduced visual acuity, and at that time no pigmentation may be seen. Retinal edema has been described at this stage. In acute cases, after several days retinal pigmentation may become visible. In some cases it has developed and become more conspicuous after thioridazine has been stopped. Early it was noted that there is a tendency for vision to improve and in some cases for pigment to become less conspicuous after thioridazine had been stopped. However, later long-term follow-ups of several cases established the important fact that in some cases the retinopathy can become worse for years after thioridazine has been stopped. Davidorf in a 6-year follow-up of a patient found progression of retinal pigmentary degeneration and visual field loss, but visual acuity remained near normal.[k] Large accumulations of pigment corresponded to areas of visual field loss. Davidorf suggested that the choriocapillaris was injured first, and that the retinal changes resulted. Meredith in a study of late complications in three patients described nummular areas of loss of retinal pigment epithelium with associated loss of choriocapillaris.[u] Progressive atrophy of remaining retinal pigment epithelium was found to go on for years after thioridazine was stopped, though visual acuity could remain relatively good. An autopsy study by Miller on a patient who developed severe thioridazine retinopathy 18 years earlier showed similar nummular areas of hypopigmentation and choroidal atrophy.[v] Also, the photoreceptor outer segments were found atrophic and disorganized. It was suggested that loss of retinal pigment and choriocapillaris followed the degneration of the photoreceptors.

Standard EOG and ERG measurements in Davidorf's case were normal, but the macular ERG amplitude was subnormal.[k] In Meredith's cases in late stages the dark adaptation, EOG and ERG were abnormal.[u] In a severe case of thioridazine retinopathy examined by Tamai, the scotopic ERG was subnormal, and the results were interpreted as indicating good cone function, but impairment of the rod system including the retinal pigment epithelial cells.[zf] Miyata and Cholibutr from studies of patients and rats reported the O_2 wavelet of the oscillatory potentials to be particularly sensitive to thioridazine, even in eyes without evidence of retinopathy.[f,w]

Deposits in the cornea and lens such as produced by chlorpromazine are believed not to be produced in human beings by thioridazine.[n] However, Satanove observed that fluorescence could be elicited with proper irradiation in the corneas of people who had taken both chlorpromazine and thioridazine, and thought this was particularly related to dosage of thioridazine above 400 mg per day.[zb]

Experimental studies in animals and *in vitro* have demonstrated that thioridazine has an affinity for melanin granules and tends to accumulate in close association with uveal pigment.[166,203] Investigation of the oxidation of retinol in homogenized cattle retinas by Muirhead has revealed no difference in the effects of thioridazine and chlorpromazine, and therefore no obvious correlation with retinotoxicity, since *in vivo* only thioridazine definitely produces retinopathy.[y]

Meier-Ruge and Werthemann in their monograph on drug retinopathy in 1967 included studies on the effects of thioridazine on retinal enzymes *in vitro* and observations on experimental induction of retinopathy in cats, comparing the effects of thioridazine and piperidylchlorophenothiazine, the latter being shown to have the greater toxicity.[167]

The metabolic products of thioridazine, *thioridazine sulfoxide* and *thioridazine sulfone,* were found by Meier-Ruge and Werthemann to have relatively slight effect on retinal enzymes *in vivo* and no evident toxic effect on the retina in cats.[167] Gauron and Rowley in 1967 found that they could make rats photophobic by repeated intramuscular injection of *thioridazine sulfoxide.* However, no examination of the eyes of these animals seems to have been reported.[j]

Unrelated to retinopathy, transitory unilateral internuclear ophthalmoplegia has been reported by Cook in a patient who was comatose from large overdosage of thioridazine.[h]

a. Appelbaum A: An ophthalmoscopic study of patients under treatment with thioridazine. *ARCH OPHTHALMOL* 69:578–580, 1963.

b. Ardouin M, Feuvrier YM, Delattre A: Ocular manifestations in the course of treatment by phenothiazine derivatives. *BULL SOC OPHTALMOL FRANCE* 69:395–401, 1969. (French)

c. Bonaccorsi MT: Optic atrophy and systemic disturbance. *LAVAL MED* 38:84–88, 1967. (French)

d. Brunold H: Experiences with a new phenothiazine derivative (Melleril, Sandoz). *THER UMSCH* 16:90–92, 1959. (German)

e. Cameron ME, Lawrence JM, Olrich JG: Thioridazine (Melleril) retinopathy. *BR J OPHTHALMOL* 56:131–134, 1972.

f. Chotibutr S, Miyata M, et al: Change in oscillatory potential by thioridazine. *OPHTHALMOLOGICA* 178:220–225, 1979.

g. Connell MM, Poley BJ, McFarlane JR: Chorioretinopathy associated with thioridazine therapy. *ARCH OPHTHALMOL* 71:816–821, 1964.

h. Cook FF, Davis RG, Russo LS Jr: Internuclear ophthalmoplegia caused by phenothiazine intoxication. *ARCH NEUROL* 38:465–466, 1981.

i. Curtin DM, Mooney D: Thioridazine retinopathy. *IRISH J MED SCI* 147:255, 1978.

j. Daumail J, Lauxerois G, Peyronnaud G: Appearance of a retinitis with pigment migration in the course of treatment with thioridazine. *BULL SOC OPHTALMOL FRANCE* 64:473–475, 1964. (French)

k. Davidorf FH: Thioridazine pigmentary retinopathy. *ARCH OPHTHALMOL* 90:251–255, 1973.

l. de Margerie J: Ocular changes produced by a phenothiazine drug, thioridazine. *TRANS CAN OPHTHALMOL SOC* 25:160–175, 1964.

m. Finn R: Pigmentary retinopathy associated with thioridazine. *AM J PSYCHIATRY* 120:913, 1964.

n. Forrest FM, Snow HL: Prognosis of eye complications caused by phenothiazines. *DIS NERV SYST* 29:26–28, 1968.

o. Gauron FE, Rowley VN: Some effects of thioridazine sulfoxide in the laboratory rat. *TOXICOL APPL PHARMACOL* 10:375–377, 1967.

p. Grutzner P.[95].

q. Hagopian V, Stratton DB: Five cases of pigmentary retinopathy associated with thioridazine administration. *AM J PSYCHIATRY* 123:97–100, 1966.

r. Hagopian V: Pigmentary retinopathy due to thioridazine or Mellaril. *KRESGE EYE INST BULL* 10:33–39, 1966.

s. Heshe J, Engelstoft FH, Kirk L: Retinal injury developing under thioridazine treatment. *NORD PSYKIATR TIDSSKR* 15:442–447, 1961.

t. Leinfelder PJ, Burian HM: Mellaril intoxication of retina with full restitution of function. *INVEST OPHTHALMOL* 3:446, 1964.

u. Meredith TA, Aaberg TM, Willerson WD: Progressive chorioretinopathy after receiving thioridazine. *ARCH OPHTHALMOL* 96:1172–1176, 1978.

v. Miller FS III, Bunt-Milam AH, Kalina RE: Clinical-ultrastructural study of thioridazine retinopathy. *OPHTHALMOLOGY* 89:1478–1488, 1982.

w. Miyata M, Imai H, et al: Changes in human electroretinography associated with thioridazine administration. *OPHTHALMOLOGICA* 181:175–180, 1980.

x. Morrison SB: Transient visual symptoms associated with Mellaril medication. *AM J PSYCHIATRY* 116:1032, 1960.

y. Muirhead JF: Drug effects on retinol oxidation, retinal alcohol: NAD + oxidoreductase. *INVEST OPHTHALMOL* 6:635–641, 1967.

z. Potts AM: Drug induced macular disease. *TRANS AM ACAD OPHTHALMOL OTOLARYNGOL* 70:1054, 1966.

za. Reboton J Jr, Weakley RD, et al: Pigmentary retinopathy and iridocycloplegia in psychiatric patients. *J NEUROPSYCHIATRY* 3:311–316, 1962.

zb. Satanove A, McIntosh JS: Photoxic reactions induced by high doses of chlorpromazine and thioridazine. *J AM MED ASSOC* 200:209–212, 1967.

zc. Scott AW: Retinal pigmentation in a patient receiving thioridazine. *ARCH OPHTHALMOL* 70:775–778, 1963.

zd. Siddell JR: Ocular toxic changes associated with chlorpromazine and thioridazine. *CAN J OPHTHALMOL* 1:190–198, 1966.

ze. Siddall JR: Ocular complications related to phenothiazines. *DIS NERV SYST* 29:10–13, 1968.

zf. Tamai A, Holland MG: Electrophysiological studies on a case of thioridazine pigmentary retinopathy. *ACTA SOC OPHTHALMOL JPN* 80:113–116, 1976. (English abstract)

zg. Weekley RD, Potts AM, et al: Pigmentary retinopathy in patients receiving high doses of a new phenothiazine. *ARCH OPHTHALMOL* 64:65–74, 1960.

Thiotepa (triethylenethiophosphoramide), an antineoplastic, apparently has rarely if ever caused ocular complications when administered systemically to patients. Its main ophthalmologic interest has been in local therapeutic application for prevention of corneal vascularization and prevention of recurrence of pterygium.

From systemic use one case of bilateral plastic acute fibrinous uveitis was described by Himelfarb in 1963 as having developed three weeks after a patient had mastectomy for carcinoma of the breast and was treated with thiotepa.[h]

Application of thiotepa to the eye in experimental animals was reported in 1960 by Langham to inhibit or suppress vascularization of the cornea after chemical burns of the eye.[l] Since then this treatment has been reinvestigated several times with varying conclusions about its overall effectiveness. Ahuja, Ey, and Lavergne confirmed that repeated application of thiotepa suppressed vascularization of corneas of rabbits that had been injured with sodium hydroxide or alloxan.[2,54,145–147] Others found that although vascularization was retarded initially, the long term results of treatment of experimentally burned animal eyes was not improved by thiotepa. Specifically, Burns found that retardation of vascularization of guinea pig corneas in response to carrageenin was temporary.[c] Paul concluded that the treatment was of doubtful value because in thermally burned animal eyes, though it retarded new vessel growth, it also delayed wound healing.[q] Rock reported the end results to be no better in those treated with thiotepa than in controls when corneal transplants were performed on eyes with vascularization from injection of alloxan into the anterior chamber, and furthermore that wound healing was retarded by the treatment.[t] Finally, Lavergne in a comprehensive study of treatments for preventing corneal vascularization reported that in four out of twenty-eight rabbit eyes burned with sodium hydroxide and treated with 1% thiotepa in oil, though vascularization was inhibited, there was ulceration and descemetocele, and that no such complication occurred in identically burned eyes not treated with thiotepa.[145]

Relatively few evaluations have been reported of use of thiotepa on human eyes to prevent corneal vascularization after chemical burns or keratoplasty, but Lavergne described one patient who was treated with topical thiotepa starting on the fourth day after sodium hydroxide burn at a time when there was severe opacity and edema with beginning vascularization. The vascularization in this eye appeared to be retarded during two five-day periods of treatment, but when the treatment was stopped, the cornea became completely vascularized. Lavergne also described treatment of a patient's eye that had been burned with calcium hydroxide, in which the treatment was stopped when the cornea became ulcerated. In a third patient's eye which had been injured with plastic glue, vascularization had begun, but appeared to be prevented by treatment with thiotepa.[145] Varying clinical results in conjunction with corneal transplantation in human beings have been expressed by discussors of a clinical report by Zehetbauer.[u]

The postoperative treatment of pterygium with thiotepa appears to have produced clinical observations of effectiveness and success when a sufficiently low concentration, such as 1:2,000 dilution, has been used.[d,e,k,n,o,r] This solution, applied several times a day for six weeks to three months after operation, generally has produced no signs of irritation and appeared to reduce recurrences during follow-ups of one to three years. When a higher concentration (1 : 100 dilution in oil) was tried for the same purpose by Cooper, it produced excessive irritation of the eyes, and in two cases caused obstruction of the lacrimo-nasal duct.[e]

Untoward side effects of thiotepa eyedrops have consisted of contact allergic reactions, depigmentation of the eyelids and eyelashes, and possibly a case of keratitis. Contact allergic reactions of the skin of lids and face have subsided when the treatment was discontinued.[m,145] Depigmentation of the eyelids and lashes in one case developed in six months after a 1% solution in peanut oil had been used for three weeks.[b] In several other cases depigmentation has developed after 1 : 2000 aqueous solution has been used in the usual way to prevent recurrence of pterygium, usually appearing many months later,[a,i,j] but in one case six years later.[i] Depigmentation has been most notable in people with dark complexions, and may be precipitated by sunbathing.[a] In one case specific note has been made of the fact that the iris was not affected.[b]

In a patient described by Nelson a considerable keratitis with edema and clouding of the cornea, wrinkling of Descemet's membrane, and loss of epithelium occurred within four days after operation for pterygium and application of 1 : 2000 thiotepa eyedrops twelve times a day.[p] The explanation for this extraordinary occurrence is unknown.

Weanling rats treated with 1:445 or 1:1000 thiotepa eyedrops during six weeks have developed corneal vascularization and cataract, but no comparable effect has been seen in human beings.[s]

Intravitreal injection of thiotepa in rabbits in a concentration of 8 mg/ml has been reported to be tolerated without excessive inflammation or alteration of the ERG, but to ensure "non-toxic" infusion fluid for lens extraction and vitrectomy the concentration was limited to 8 μg/ml.[277]

a. Asregadoo E: Surgery, thio-tepa and corticosteroids in the treatment of pterygium. *AM J OPHTHALMOL* 74:960–963, 1972.
b. Berkow JW, Gills JP, Wise JB: Depigmentation of eyelids after topically administered thiotepa. *ARCH OPHTHALMOL* 82:415–420, 1969.
c. Burns RP, Beighle R: Effects of triethylenethiophosphoramide on the carrageenin granuloma of the guinea pig cornea. *INVEST OPHTHALMOL* 1:666–671, 1962.
d. Cassady JR: The inhibition of pterygium recurrence by Thiotepa. *AM J OPHTHALMOL* 61:886–888, 1966.
e. Cooper JC: Pterygium: Prevention of recurrence by excision and post-operative thiotepa. *EYE EAR NOSE THROAT MONTHLY* 45:59–61, 1966.
f. Ericson L, Karlerg B, Rosengren BH: Trials of intravitreal injections of chemotherapeutics agents in rabbits. *ACTA OPHTHALMOL* 42:721–726, 1964.
g. Foster JB: Thio-tepa drops for corneal vascularization: a clinical trial. *TRANS OPHTHALMOL SOC AUST* 24:104–107, 1965.
h. Himelfarb HM: Personal communication, 1963.
i. Hornblass A, Adler RI, et al: A delayed side effect of topical thiotepa. *ANN OPHTHALMOL* 6:1155–1157, 1974.

j. Howitt D, Karp EJ: Side-effect of topical thio-tepa. *AM J OPHTHALMOL* 68:473–474, 1969.

k. Joselson GA, Muller P: Incidence of pterygium recurrence. *AM J OPHTHALMOL* 61:891–895, 1966.

l. Langham M: The inhibition of corneal vascularization by triethylene thiophosphoramide. *AM J OPHTHALMOL* 49:1111–1117, 1960.

m. Lenkevich MM, Gundorova RA: Combined surgicomedicamentous treatment of recurrent and cicatrical pterygiums. *VESTN OFTAL* 77:58–61, 1964. (English summary)

n. Liddy BS, Morgan JF: Triethylene thiophosphoramide (thio-tepa) and pterygium. *AM J OPHTHALMOL* 61:888–890, 1966.

o. Meacham CT: Triethylene thiophosphoramide in the prevention of pterygium recurrence. *AM J OPHTHALMOL* 54:751–753, 1962.

p. Nelson J: Personal communication, 1969.

q. Paul SD, Batra DV: Effect of thio-tepa on corneal vascularization. *ORIENT ARCH OPHTHALMOL* 4:96–103, 1966.

r. Rabinovitz E, Flores J: Thio-tepa in prevention of recurrence of pterygium. *ANAL SOC MEXICANA OFTALMOL* 41:31–36, 1968. (Spanish)

s. Robertson DM, Creasman JP: Effects of topical thio TEPA on rat eyes. *AM J OPHTHALMOL* 73:73–77, 1972.

t. Rock RL: Inhibition of corneal vascularization by triethylene thiophosphoramide (thio-tepa). *ARCH OPHTHALMOL* 69:330–334, 1963.

u. Zehetbauer G: The influence of triethylene-thiophosphoramide on vascularization of corneal transplants. *ZBL OPHTHALMOL* 97:13, 1966. (German)

Thiothixene (Navane), an anti-psychotic, has been said by the manufacturer to have produced "fine lenticular pigmentation" in a small number of patients treated for prolonged periods. Very slight and nonspecific visual complaints have been noted transiently in the first days of treatment, but ophthalmologic examinations revealed no significant toxic effects.[a] No serious eye effects have been reported.[353]

a. Haase HJ, Bergener M, Sauerland L: Cliniconeuroleptic study of tiotixene. *ARZNEIMIT-TELFORSCHUNG* 17:1043–1047, 1967. (German)

Thiouracil (Deracil; 2-mercapto-4-hydroxypyrimidine) and the derivatives *methyl thiouracil* and *propyl thiouracil* have been used in treatment of hyperthyroidism and angina pectoris. They appear to have no selective toxicity to the eye, but in one instance administration of *methyl thiouracil* was associated with nystagmus and visual illusion of movement of the environment, accompanying severe vertigo. The nystagmus persisted for several months after the drug was discontinued and the vertigo relieved.[a]

Chronic experimental administration of *propyl thiouracil* to rats has been shown to induce exophthalmos.[b]

a. Prowse CB: A toxic effect of thiouracil hitherto undescribed. *BR MED J* 2:1312, 1950.

b. Sellers EA, Ferguson JKW: Exophthalmos in rats after prolonged administration of propylthiouracil. *ENDOCRINOLOGY* 45:345–346, 1949.

Thiourea, formerly used as an antithyroid agent, was tested by Sorsby by administration to rabbits because of a chemical relationship to dithizone, but thiourea, unlike dithizone, did not damage the retina or affect the blood sugar.[233] Screening tests on rabbit corneas have shown moderate toxicity when thiourea was introduced into the corneal stroma.[123]

Thiram (bis [dimethylthiocarbamoyl] disulfide, tetramethyl thiuramdisulfide) as a dust or spray is irritating to the eyes and respiratory tract and may cause allergic skin reactions.[5, 171]

Thistle bracts or prickles (from *Cirsium lanceolatum*) appeared to have no toxic effect on the eye in a case in which they were driven into the cornea and protruded into the anterior chamber for 2 days before removal.[a] They behaved as inert foreign bodies.

   a.   Bhargava SK: Penetrating thistle bracts injury. *BR J OPHTHALMOL* 55:421–423, 1971.

Thorium chloride as a 0.1 M solution at pH 2 was tested by dropping on a rabbit's eye for ten minutes after removal of the corneal epithelium. This caused no immediate opacity, but in subsequent days the eye developed a severe iritis and permanent patchy opacification and vascularization of the cornea. This reaction appeared to be at least partially attributable to the toxicity of thorium rather than to the moderate acidity of pH 2. The same type of exposure carried out after neutralization of the solution to pH 5 by addition of ammonium hydroxide caused a similar, but milder, irregular nebulous opacification and vascularization of the cornea.[81, 90]

Thulium chloride, tested on rabbit eyes by application of 0.1 ml of 1 : 1 aqueous solution at about pH 3.5, caused irritation and small spots of ulceration of the conjunctiva, which healed within four days. No effect on the cornea was noted.[97]

Thymoxamine hydrochloride (moxisylyte; Opilon), an alpha-adrenergic blocking agent, has been the subject of numerous reports concerning its pharmacologic properties.[c] It has had no known toxic effects on the eyes except transient stinging and conjunctival hyperemia after topical application. At 5% concentration the irritation is too much for clinical use.[b] At 1% and 0.5% the stinging sensation is tolerable.[a, c] Application of 1% eyedrops daily to 100 patients for at least a year had "no untoward effect."[a]

   a.   Mapstone R: Safe mydriasis. *BR J OPHTHALMOL* 54:690–692, 1970.
   b.   Pau H: Sympathicolysis from local conjunctival application of Opilon to the eye. *KLIN MONATSBL AUGENHEILKD* 126:171–176, 1955. (German)
   c.   Wand M, Grant WM: Thymoxamine hydrochloride. *SURVEY OPHTHALMOL* 25:75–84, 1980.

Thyroidin was a dried extract of thyroid that is of some historical interest because between 1900 and 1916 it was suspected of having caused eleven cases of bilateral retrobulbar neuritis with central scotoma, which were at least partially reversible when thyroidin was stopped. In most cases thyroidin had been taken for weight reduction. A review of five published cases, plus 3 original cases, and bibliography, was published by Standish in 1916.[a] Apparently no cases have been seriously suspected since then.

Experimentally, in 1905 Birch-Hirschfeld and Inoue reported in 3 out of 4 dogs having produced temporal pallor of the optic nerve heads, with histologic abnormalities of the retinal ganglion cells and diffuse degeneration of the nerve fibers, by feeding large amounts of thyroidin.

   a. Standish M: Retrobulbar neuritis with central scotoma from toxic action of thyroidin. *TRANS AM OPHTHALMOL SOC* 14:608–613, 1916.

Thyrotropin releasing hormone has caused acute severe but transient loss of vision and headache in two patients with pituitary tumors, possibly due to acute swelling of the gland.[a,b]

   a. Cimino A, et al: Transient amaurosis in patient with pituitary macroadenoma after intravenous gonadotropin and thyrotropin releasing hormones. *LANCET* 2:95, 1981.
   b. Drury PL, Belchetz PE, et al: Transient amaurosis and headache after thyrotropin releasing hormone. *LANCET* 1:218–219, 1982.

Thyroxine, an amino acid, is reported to have caused cataracts in fetuses when administered to young pregnant rats from the ninth to the twentieth days of pregnancy.[a]

   a. Giroud A, Martinet M: Changes in the epithelium and the fibers of the crystalline lens after thyroxine. *ARCH OPHTALMOL* (Paris), 14:247–258, 1954. (French)

Tilbroquinol and **Tiliquinol,** derivatives of 8-quinolinol, analogous to clioquinol, have been suspected in one case of having produced a condition similar to SMON (subacute myelo-optic neuropathy) after being taken for four years as a combination preparation, Intetrix. The eye manifestations of bilateral papilledema, color vision disturbance, and scotoma in one eye developed after onset of peripheral sensory neuritis, and persisted after the latter improved following discontinuance of the medication.[a]

   a. Soffer M, Basdevant A, et al: Oxyquinoline toxicity. *LANCET* 1:709, 1983.

Tilorone hydrochloride, an antiviral and antineoplastic, can produce intracytoplasmic inclusions in cornea, conjunctiva, and retina resembling the lipidosis produced by amiodarone, chloroquine and several other drugs.[a] Kaufman found that when tilorone was applied to the eyes of volunteers it caused the corneal epithelium to change in appearance to resemble slight edema after 10 days, due to drug storage in the epithelium. Visual acuity remained normal despite subjective blur and halos around lights. The condition cleared in 2 months after tilorone application was discontinued.[b] In rats fed the drug for 6 months, Larson and Gibson found intracytoplasmic inclusion bodies not only in the cornea and in lymphocytes, but also in retinal ganglion cells.[c]

Among patients undergoing prolonged oral treatment with tilorone, Weiss found 5 who developed a dose-related diffuse clouding of the corneal epithelium, with fine white epithelial and subepithelial opacities, which formed whorl-like patterns at more advanced stages.[c] Histologically there was cloudy swelling of the corneal epithelium and cytoplasmic inclusions, with myelinoid bodies. The patients were asymptomatic except for slight subjective blur and blue halos around lights. Two of the five patients also had evidence of retinopathy.[e] They showed fine pigment mottling of the macula areas and arterial narrowing, though slight or no impairment of visual acuity. Both had constriction of peripheral visual fields, and had color vision deficiencies. The EOG was attenuated in both, and in the patient with the greater field constriction the photopic ERG response was absent. When tilorone was discontinued, the corneas cleared, and the visual fields expanded to normal in one of the patients.[d,e] (Also see INDEX for *Lipidosis.*)

a. D'Amico DJ, and Kenyon KR: Drug-induced lipidoses of the cornea and conjunctiva. *OPHTHALMOLOGY* 4:67–76, 1981.
b. Kaufman HE, Centifanto YM, et al: Tilorone hydrochloride. *PROC SOC EXP BIOL MED* 137:357, 1971.
c. Larson EJ, Gibson JP: Six month oral toxicity study with tilorone hydrochloride in rats. *MERRELL-NATIONAL LABORATORIES,* July 1978, as quoted by Weiss JN, et al.[e]
d. Weiss JN, Weinberg RS, Regelson W: Keratopathy after oral administration of tilorone hydrochloride. *AM J OPHTHALMOL* 89:46–53, 1980.
e. Weiss JN, Ochs AL, et al: Retinopathy after tilorone hydrochloride. *AM J OPHTHALMOL* 90:846–853, 1980.

Timolol maleate (Timoptic; Timoptol; Timacar; Blocadren), a beta-receptor-blocking anti-adrenergic drug, has been widely used in eyedrops (e.g. Timoptic) in treating glaucoma, and has been administered orally (e.g. Blocadren) in treatment of systemic hypertension and coronary disease. When administered systemically, timolol has commonly reduced the intraocular pressure, and has had practically no adverse ocular effects (Zimmerman). However, when administered in eyedrops timolol has produced systemic reactions, as well as unwanted ocular effects. Comprehensive reviews of the systemic and local side effects of timolol eyedrops are available (Fraunfelder; Kats; McMahon; Van Buskirk). Van Buskirk's survey in 1980 has been one of the most instructive, providing an analysis of more than 500 notifications of adverse reactions to timolol eyedrops received by Fraunfelder's National Registry. Approximately half were concerned with systemic reactions, some of them life-threatening. Because of the importance of the systemic reactions induced by timolol eyedrops, we will consider these first, then the ocular side effects of the eyedrops.

Numerous case reports and clinical studies have clearly shown that patients with obstructive pulmonary disease and patients with cardiovascular disease are at special risk from use of timolol eyedrops (Ahmad; Altus; Charan; Corbel; Holtmann; Jones; Scharrer; Schoene; Van Buskirk; Vonwil; and several others). Aggravation of asthma with bronchospasm, and congestive heart failure have resulted. Often patients who have a history of pulmonary disease or heart disease have been well compensated before starting to take timolol eyedrops, but after starting to take the drops for periods varying from days to months have developed bronchospasm or cardiac decompensation. When the drops have been stopped, there usually has been distinct improvement. In patients with chronic obstructive pulmonary disease timolol eyedrops can cause a distinct decrease in forced expiratory volume at one second (Charan; Schoene), and it has been suggested that spirometry be utilized before and after a trial administration of timolol eyedrops to identify those prone to develop broncho-spasm (Schoene).

Special aspects of pulmonary or cardiac adverse effects that have been noted include apneic spells in a neonate (Olson), and life-threatening bradycardia and respiratory distress in a child with congenital heart defects (Burnstine; Williams). Caprioli and Sears reported a case of acute sinus bradycardia and fall of blood pressure apparently attributable to timolol eyedrops in a patient being prepared for operation for glaucoma. Ros and Dake have noted that in patients who have no adverse cardiac effects and have little or no slowing of the heart while taking timolol eyedrops, if the drops are abruptly stopped there may be an increase in pulse rate of 10 beats per minute, which might be of significance to patients with arrythmias.

A review of systemic side effects from systemically administered timolol provided by Zimmerman provides a frame of reference when evaluating suspected systemic effects of timolol eyedrops. Depression, anxiety and confusion reported by McMahon and Van Buskirk from the eyedrops are not unlike occasional effects of systemic medication, but more evidence seems needed relating to the aggravation of diabetes reported by Angelo-Nielsen, or aggravation of myasthenia gravis reported from timolol eyedrops by Shaivitz and by Coppeto.

There is uncertainty over the safety of timolol during pregnancy due to lack of information. Blaul reported that one woman who started using timolol eyedrops in the third month of pregnancy produced a normal infant, and that the baby's development while on mother's milk was normal.

The local ocular side effects of timolol eyedrops have been summarised by Fraunfelder and Van Buskirk, and characterized as mostly of nuisance variety. They have included simple local discomfort without evident lesions, and occasional local allergic reaction. Superficial punctate keratopathy, mostly asymptomatic, with and without corneal anesthesia has been seen. Case reports and studies of asymptomatic corneal anesthesia have been published by Calissendorff and by Van Buskirk. In normal people Draeger et al found a local corneal anesthetic effect lasting only a few minutes after drop application, while Kitazawa found no abnormality of corneal sensitivity or of tear production during chronic timolol eyedrop administration. Review of the literature and further clinical experiments by Strasser and Grabner disclosed 10 publications reporting transitory reduced tear flow, but they found no evidence for a long persisting decrease or change in composition of the tears from timolol eyedrops. It appears that reduction of tearing early after the start of treat-ment does not require discontinuing timolol because of the transitory nature of the reduction (Nielsen; Strasser).

Investigations in rabbits have shown a slowing of corneal epithelial wound closure by Timoptic drops applied five times a day, but this was thought to be attributable to the vehicle (containing benzalkonium), rather than to timolol (O'Brien). Wound closure was not altered by application at eight hour intervals (Nork). However, in monkeys the initial fast phase of epithelial healing was slowed (Nork). In rabbits, applying timolol drops in combination with wearing of gas-permeable contact lenses caused ultrastructural changes in both the corneal epithelium and the endothelium, and this occurred in the absence of preservatives (Arthur). However, bovine corneal endothelium in culture was found by Staatz et al not to be lethally affected by pure timolol maleate at a concentration used in eyedrops, though the cells were rapidly killed by the benzalkonium-containing vehicle. In human beings, Brubaker et al have shown that clinical use of timolol eyedrops does not affect the permeability of the corneal endothelium.

Disturbances of vision in patients using timolol eyedrops have been noted by several observers, generally with little explanation (Fraunfelder; McMahon; Van Buskirk). When a miotic eyedrop is discontinued at the same time timolol is started, adverse effects on visual acuity and on accommodation could be attributed to loss of the effects of the miotic on the pupil and on the ciliary muscle. However, some of the visual complaints are not this easily explained. Reversible decrease in central vision not improved by refraction, and reversible myopia, have been unexplained and have raised conjecture about possible effects on the retina. In cultured retinas timolol has been shown to inhibit phagocytic activity of the retinal pigment epithelium, but whether this has any relevance to the clinical visual complaints is unknown (Matsuda).

Ahmad S: Cardiopulmonary effects of timolol eyedrops. *LANCET* 2:1028, 1979.

Altus P: Timolol-induced congestive heart failure. *SOUTH MED J* 74:88, 1981.

Angelo-Nielsen K: Timolol topically and diabetes mellitus. *J AM MED ASSOC* 244:2263, 1980.

Arthur BW, Hay GW, et al: Ultrastructural effects of topical timolol on the rabbit cornea. *ARCH OPHTHALMOL* 101:1607–1610, 1983.

Blaul G: Local beta-blocker during pregnancy. *KLIN MONATSBL AUGENHEILKD* 179:128–129, 1981. (German)

Brubaker RF, Coakes RL, Bourne WM: Effect of timolol on the permeability of the corneal endothelium. *OPHTHALMOLOGY* 86:108–111, 1979.

Burnstine RA, Felton JL, Ginther WH: Cardio-respiratory reaction to timolol maleate in a pediatric patient. *ANN OPHTHALMOL* 14:905–906, 1982.

Calissendorff B: Corneal anesthesia after topical treatment with timolol maleate. *ACTA OPHTHALMOL* 59:347–349, 1981.

Caprioli J, Sears M:: Caution on the preoperative use of topical timolol. *AM J OPHTHALMOL* 95:561–562, 1983.

Charan NB, Lakshminarayan S: Pulmonary effects of topical timolol. *ARCH INTERN MED* 120:843–844, 1980.

Coppeto JR: Timolol-associated myasthenia gravis. *AM J OPHTHALMOL* 98:244–245, 1984.

Corbel M: Additional note on the use of timolol in asthmatics. *BULL SOC OPHTALMOL FRANCE* 82:235–236, 1982. (French)

Draeger J, Schneider B, Winter R: The local anesthetic effect of metipranolol in comparison with timolol. *KLIN MONATSBL AUGENHEILKD* 182:210–213, 1983. (German)

Fraunfelder FT: Drug-related complications. Timolol maleate ocular side effects. *OPHTHALMIC FORUM* 1:57, 1983.

Holtmann HW, Holle JP, Glanzer K: Alteration of bronchial flow resistance due to timolol 0.25% eyedrops in bronchial asthma. *KLIN MONATSBL AUGENHEILKD* 176:441–444, 1980. (German)

Jones FL Jr, Ekberg NL: Exacerbation of obstructive airway disease by timolol. *J AM MED ASSOC* 244:2730, 1980.

Katz IM, Kasdin SL: Safety and tolerability of timolol maleate ophthalmic solution in perspective. *J OCULAR THER SURG* 1:76–80, 1981.

Kitazawa Y, Tsuchisaka H: Effects of timolol on corneal sensitivity and tear production. *INT OPHTHALMOL* 3:25–29, 1981.

Matsuda H, Yoshimura N: The retinal toxicity of befunolol and other adrenergic beta-blocking agents. *ACTA OPHTHALMOL* 61:343–352, 1983.

McMahon CD, Shaffer RN, et al: Adverse effects experienced by patients taking timolol. *AM J OPHTHALMOL* 88:736–738, 1979.

Nielsen NV, Prause JV, Eriksen JS: Lysozyme, alfa-1-antitrypsin and serum albumin in tear fluid of timolol treated glaucoma patients. *ACTA OPHTHALMOL* 59:503–509, 1981.

Nork TM, Holly FJ, et al: Timolol inhibits corneal wound healing in rabbits and monkeys. *ARCH OPHTHALMOL* 102:1224–1228, 1984.

O'Brien WJ, DeCarlo JD, et al: Effects of Timoptic on corneal reepithelialization. *ARCH OPHTHALMOL* 100:1331–1333, 1982.

Olson RJ, Bromberg BB, Zimmerman TJ: Apneic spells associated with timolol therapy in a neonate. *AM J OPHTHALMOL* 88:120–122, 1979.

Ros FE, Dake CL: Timolol eye drops; bradycardia or tachycardia? DOC OPHTHALMOL 48:283–289, 1980.

Scharrer A, Ober M: Cardiovascular and pulmonary effects in local beta-blocking treatment. *KLIN MONATSBL AUGENHEILKD* 179:362–363, 1981. (German)

Schoene RB, Martin TR, et al: Timolol-induced bronchospasm in asthmatic bronchitis. *J AM MED ASSOC* 245:1460–1461, 1981.

Schoene RB, Abuan T, et al: Effects of topical betaxolol, timolol, and placebo on pulmonary function in asthmatic bronchitis. *AM J OPHTHALMOL* 97:86–92, 1984.

Shaivitz SA: Timolol and myasthemia gravis. *J AM MED ASSOC* 242:1611–1612, 1979.

Staatz WD, Radius RL, et al: Effects of timolol on bovine corneal endothelial cultures. *ARCH OPHTHALMOL* 99:660–663, 1981.

Strasser G, Grabner G: The influence of long-term treatment with timolol on human tear lysozyme and albumin content. *GRAEFES ARCH OPHTHALMOL* 218:93–95, 1982.

Van Buskirk EM: Corneal anesthesia after timolol maleate therapy. *AM J OPHTHALMOL* 88:739–743, 1979.

Van Buskirk EM: Adverse reactions from timolol administration. *OPHTHALMOLOGY* 87:447–450, 1980.

Van Buskirk EM, Fraunfelder FT: Ocular beta-blockers and systemic effects. *AM J OPHTHALMOL* 98:623–624, 1984.

Vonwil A, Landolt M, et al: Bronchoconstrictive side effect of timolol eyedrops in patients with obstructive lung disease. *SCHWEIZ MED WOCHENSCHR* 111:665–669, 1981. (German)

Williams T, Ginther WH: Hazards of ophthalmic timolol. *N ENGL J MED* 306:1485–1486, 1982.

Zimmerman TJ, Leader BJ, Golof DS: Potential side effects of timolol therapy in the treatment of glaucoma. *ANN OPHTHALMOL* 13:683–689, 1981.

Tin implanted as a particle of metal in the vitreous body of rabbits has been well tolerated for at least a year.[340]

Titanium implanted as a particle of metal in the vitreous body of rabbits has been well tolerated for at least a year.[340]

Titanium dioxide, a white pigment, has been introduced by tatooing into the cornea of rabbits and patients having corneal scars, and has caused permanent white coloration, but no irritation.[199]

Titanium iodides (*titanium tetraiodide* and *diiodide*) particles applied to eyes of rabbits under anesthesia caused immediate whitening and surface coagulation of cornea and conjunctiva in the areas of contact, and this was attended by release of small amount of white fumes. Opacification of the corneas was dense and white for several days, and the corneas became vascularized. In the course of six weeks considerable clearing occurred, leaving permanent scars only in those portions of the cornea where the iodide particles originally had been in direct contact.[81]

In a laboratory accident a young woman was exposed to a blast of hot vapors of a mixture of iodine, titanium diiodide, and titanium tetraiodide when a reaction vessel being heated in an electric furnace exploded close to her face. The eyes were immediately irrigated with water. When examined three hours later, both corneas were lusterless from irregular loss of epithelium, and the anterior stroma of one cornea was irregularly gray. The conjunctivae were edematous, but the blood vessels appeared normal. The skin of the lids and face was red, as though from sunburn, and somewhat tender and swollen.

Local cortisone and sulfacetamide were employed in treatment of the eyes. The corneal epithelium regenerated in three days, and the superficial stromal grayness gradually cleared, but hypesthesia of the corneas persisted for about two weeks. Many small subconjunctival hemorrhages appeared at about five days, but reabsorbed without complication. The eyes were essentially normal within three weeks.[81]

Titanium tetrachloride reacts vigorously with water, and its vapors react with moisture in air to form dense white fumes of titanium dioxide and hydrochloric acid. Titanium tetrachloride has caused serious burns of the skin and permanent damage of the eyes.[a] Rats exposed to a heavy concentration of fumes of titanium tetrachloride developed white corneas. Damage to the corneas occurred in five human beings who had been severely exposed to these fumes, with particularly severe effects on the cornea in a patient who died from the exposure.[a]

In emergency treatment of a splash in the eye, it has been recommended that the eyelids and face should be immediately wiped with a dry cloth, and then the eyes should be copiously irrigated with water.[a] The preliminary wiping has been recommended with the aim of minimizing the liberation of heat and acid from reaction of water with titanium tetrachloride, but the wiping should be performed as quickly as possible in order to get irrigation of the eyes started as rapidly as possible.

a. Lawson JJ: Toxicity of titanium tetrachloride. *J OCCUP MED* 3:8–12, 1961.

Toad poisons are secreted by glands in the skin of the toad as a protection for the animal. In contact with the eyes this secretion has caused a variety of toxic effects. In 1964 Peyresblanques published a comprehensive survey of the literature on the composition, properties, and case reports of effects of toad poison on the eye.[e] Active constituents of toad poisons have been investigated chemically and pharmacologically.

At least one of the constituents, *bufotalin,* is irritating to the eye when applied in aqueous solution.[d, 153]

Among several case reports from the nineteenth century reviewed in 1913 by Wagenmann were the original observations by Carron du Villiards that certain toads have glands from which they can eject a poison which is irritating to the eyes, causing much swelling of the lids, conjunctivitis, and phlyctenular reaction.[253] He had seen several cases of this sort, and experimentally in rabbits found he could cause marked inflammation of the eyes with the secretion from these glands.

It was subsequently disputed that toads have glands which can actually eject a poison. Possibly the apparent ejection was caused by squeezing the animal, as in a case investigated in 1888 by Staderini.[g] A woman grasped or squeezed a toad with a pair of shears and felt something squirt into her eye. She developed mild corneal clouding and paresis of the eye muscles with ptosis lasting two days. Staderini experimented with dried toad poison, which maintained its activity even when kept for months, and he found that in experimental animals the undiluted material caused marked inflammation and clouding of the cornea lasting for weeks, but that when diluted to 1% and tested on human eyes it caused corneal and conjunctival anesthesia with lowering of the intraocular pressure. The action was thought to be like that of erythrophleine. On the other hand, the venon from some species of toads is said to contain 2% to 5% epinephrine and norepinephrine, which should be considered in connection with lowering of the intraocular pressure.[a]

Another instance of corneal clouding, anesthesia, and lowering of intraocular pressure was described in 1965 by Collier.[b] In this case a man who was believed to have contaminated one eye with some unidentified fluid from a toad, possibly its urine, next day had reduced visual acuity associated with central nebula in the cornea in the contaminated eye. The cornea was anesthetic and there was no pain. The eye was hypotonic. The pupil was small but reactive and accommodation was normal. By slit-lamp examination the corneal epithelium was normal, but the stroma was edematous and there were folds and breaks in Descemet's membrane. By ophthalmoscopy, central retinal edema and many whitish dots on the front of the retina in the posterior vitreous were described in the affected eye while the other eye was found normal. The fundus changes were said to have been similar to those in a similar case reported in 1900 by Simi.[f] Unfortunately there was no follow-up examination to determine the outcome.

In 1964 Peyresblanques described a patient who was said to have been sprayed by a toad and three hours later was found to have superficial clouding of the cornea, hyperemia of the conjunctiva, but normal iris, and complete healing in two days.[e] In 1966 Tosti and Renna described a patient said to have been spat in the eye by a toad, and who had immediate burning and pain, with conjunctivitis, keratitis, and iritis, with vision reduced to 3/10, but complete recovery in two days.[h]

A different sort of reaction was reported in 1900 by Simi, who described maximal mydriasis and edema of the retina with reduced vision for twelve hours after contamination of one eye with three or four drops of fluid from the skin glands of a toad, but observed only slight redness of the conjunctiva and no injury of the cornea.[f] It is not evident whether the toads were of different types.

From these various reports it appears that the fluids from toads, whether they squirt or otherwise reach the eyes, have varied local toxic effects among which the transitory edema and clouding of the cornea, the anesthesia of the cornea, and the hyperemia of the conjunctiva seem to have been the most common.

a. Chen KK, Kovarikova A: Pharmacology and toxicology of toad venom. *J PHARM SCI* 56:1535–1541, 1967.
b. Collier M: Ocular disturbances from toad venom. *BULL SOC OPHTALMOL FRANCE* 65:129–131, 1965. (French)
c. Epstein D: Effect of toad venom on the eye. *S AFR MED J* 6:403–404, 1932.
d. Gallo A, Toledo C: Ophthalmia from frog poison. *OPHTHALMOS* 2:393–401, 1941. (*AM J OPHTHALMOL* 25:901, 1942.)
e. Peyresblanques J: Ocular disturbance by toad poison. *BULL SOC OPHTALMOL FRANCE* 64:493–502, 1964. (French)
f. Simi A: Toad ophthalmia. *BOLL OCULIST* 20:9, 1900. (Italian)
g. Staderini C: On toad venom. *ANN OTTALMOL CLIN OCUL* 18:424–438, 1888. (Italian)
h. Tosli E, Renna V: On three ocular injuries by an unusual mechanism. *BOLL OCULIST* 45:389–393, 1966. (Italian)

Tobacco smoke external effect on the eyes is principally irritation, felt as itching and burning. Questionnaires and blink rates have been used to evaluate irritation, and under experimental conditions the concentration of carbon monoxide in the air has been used as a measure of air pollution by cigarette smoke, though carbon monoxide is not itself irritant.[c–f] One study found the concentration of *acrolein* in air containing cigarette smoke correlated with eye irritation in a suggestive manner.[d] Another study found eye irritation was reduced if the *particulate components* of the smoke were filtered out.[f]

The break-up time of the tear film in volunteers has been found significantly shortened by cigarette smoke, presumably due to increase in the watery component and decrease in mucus and lipid in the film.[a] In hamsters, scanning electron microscopy of the conjunctiva has shown that cigarette smoke causes distortion of conjunctival cells and loss of microvilli.[b]

a. Basu PK, Pimm PE, et al: The effect of cigarette smoke on the human tear film. *CAN J OPHTHALMOL* 13:22–26, 1976.
b. Basrur PK, Bam PK: Effect of cigarette smoke of the surface structure of the conjunctival epithelium. *CAN J OPHTHALMOL* 15:20–23, 1980.
c. Speer F: Tobacco and the non-smoker. *ARCH ENVIRON HEALTH* 16:443–446, 1968.
d. Weber A, Jermini C, Grandjean E: Irritating effects on man of air pollution due to cigarette smoke. *AM J PUBLIC HEALTH* 66:672–676, 1976.
e. Weber A, Fischer T, Grandjean E: Passive smoking in experimental and field conditions. *ENVIRON RES* 20:205–216, 1979.
f. Weber A, Fischer T, Grandjean E: Passive smoking. *ARCH OCCUP ENVIRON HEALTH* 43:183–193, 1979.

Tobacco smoking has been suspected to have effects on vision for at least 150 years. "Tobacco amaurosis" was a diagnosis not uncommonly made in a period when causes of blindness could not be as accurately determined as today. No longer is there a reason to suspect that tobacco causes blindness. "Tobacco amblyopia" is a less extreme diagnosis, which is still made, and is still actively disputed. Today even this diagnosis is rarely made in some parts of the world, but in 1913 it had sufficient importance to occupy thirty nine pages of Lewin and Guillery's text on drugs and poisons affecting the eye.[153] By 1954 it merited only five pages in Duke-Elder's text.[46] Practically from the beginning it was generally assumed that some toxic substance in tobacco smoke attacked the optic nerves, and at times suspicions have been directed particularly at *nicotine,* at *carbon monoxide,* and currently at *cyanide.* Long ago a suspicion arose that abuse of alcohol and malnutrition were important associated factors, giving rise to commonly used terms "tobacco-alcohol" or "alcohol-tobacco" amblyopia. There has long been controversy over the question of whether tobacco amblyopia and alcohol amblyopia are separate entities, and over the question of whether a distinct tobacco amblyopia actually exists.

A comprehensive survey of the long historical background of this controversy and the development of different points of view was published by Dunphy in 1969, and Potts in 1973 published a scholarly review of the history, together with a critical analysis of evidence for existence of tobacco amblyopia and evidence for a possible nutritional basis instead of a toxin from tobacco. Potts seriously questioned the existence of a true toxic tobacco amblyopia. In the published discussion of his paper, Harrington, Phillips, and Foulds defended their belief in such an entity. Harrington was convinced that he had seen at least a dozen cases in forty years, and Foulds said he had studied more than 100 cases. Geographically, apparently there has been particular familiarity with the condition in Scotland and England. Bronte-Stewart remarked that tobacco was responsible for the commonest toxic optic neuropathy in Glasgow.

Those discussing tobacco amblyopia in recent years seem to have accepted a clinical characterization first offered by Traquair in which there is bilateral reduction of visual acuity associated with cecocentral scotomas, particularly for red. Foveal sensitivity to red is said to be reduced (Bhargava). Harrington substantiated that the scotomas had sloping margins with islands of increased density between fixation and blind spot, and that the peripheral fields were normal. In most cases vision recovered when smoking was stopped or vitamin treatments were given. Harrington regarded alcohol amblyopia as being different, not on a toxic basis but on a nutritional deficiency basis, with central scotomas having maximum density at fixation and relatively steep slope at the margins. Generally nothing abnormal was to be seen in the fundi, except occasional temporal pallor of the nerve heads. Harrington advised that the term "tobacco-alcohol amblyopia" should be eliminated.

To the contrary, Victor and Dreyfus believed tobacco amblyopia and alcohol amblyopia were the same entity, based on nutritional deficiency and not a manifestation of a toxic action. They accordingly suggested the condition should be called nutritional retrobulbar neuropathy. They supported their view with a very small number of cases having definite clinical evidence of nutritional deficiency corrected by administration of thiamine and by histologic demonstration of retrobulbar degeneration in the optic nerves in the papillomacula portion.

The term "tobacco amblyopia" has been most prominently used since the 1960's by a number of investigators in Great Britain who have considered this to be a toxic optic neuropathy and have particularly suspected cyanide in tobacco smoke as its cause. They have at the same time given attention to the possibilities that tobacco smoking and cyanide or other toxic component might be aggravating factors in development of optic neuropathies in pernicious anemia and in Leber's hereditary optic atrophy.

The findings which suggested that cyanide might be responsible were principally the following observations. The plasma thiocyanate was reported to be elevated by tobacco smoking, indicating appreciable absorption of cyanide (Foulds). The optic neuropathies of tobacco smoking, pernicious anemia, and Leber's hereditary optic atrophy all appeared to be benefited by treatment with hydroxocobalamin, which could bind and presumably detoxicate cyanide, forming cyanocobalamin. Poor absorption of vitamin B_{12} and low serum levels have been found in patients with tobacco amblyopia, suggesting in accord with the cyanide hypothesis that those people not protected from the supposedly toxic effects of cyanide by adequate hydroxocobalamin detoxicating mechanism may be most likely to develop the optic neuropathy (Chisholm; Watson-Williams).

Several instances have been reported in which patients recovered from tobacco amblyopia when treated with hydroxocobalamin, although they kept on smoking (Bronte-Stewart; Smith).

Tobacco smoking in relation to the retrobulbar neuritis of pernicious anemia has been considered in detail by Freeman and Heaton, who reviewed the available evidence and concluded that the optic neuropathies of pernicious anemia and tobacco smoking were the same, that both were associated with low vitamin B_{12} in the serum, and that the toxic effects of tobacco were responsible for precipitating the optic neuropathy in patients with pernicious anemia. They found no reports of retrobulbar neuritis in patients with pernicious anemia who were nonsmokers. In 1969 Foulds and associates called attention to this relationship from another aspect, noting that among patients presenting with tobacco amblyopia the incidence of pernicious anemia was remarkably high. However, questions have been raised by deCrousaz in 1969, reporting four cases of bilateral optic neuropathy with central scotomas associated with pernicious anemia and subnormal vitamin B_{12}, but pointing out that three of these patients were nonsmokers, and raising serious doubts about the relationship to tobacco smoking postulated by the other authors.

More recently, as outlined by Bronte-Stewart et al, a belief has grown that in tobacco amblyopia there may be a disturbance of sulfur metabolism and a deficiency of sulfur needed to detoxify cyanide by conversion to thiocyanate. This belief has been based on a finding that in some patients with tobacco amblyopia the blood thiocyanate has been lower than expected. Furthermore in such patients the red blood cell glutathione has been subnormal (Pettigrew). Hydroxocobolamin treatment raised the glutathione and improved vision.

The possibility that zinc might have a role has been suggested by reports of subnormal blood concentrations in association with tobacco amblyopia by Bechetoille; Grignolo; and Saraux. (Bechetoille reported simultaneous elevation of lead concentration.) Grignolo observed that the zinc level improved as the vision improved. Bechetoille administered a high dosage of zinc sulfate for a month, and noted improvement in the central $5°$ of vision.

Efforts to study tobacco amblyopia by electrophysiologic means have shown no significant abnormalities in the ERG unless special efforts were made to increase the sensitivity of measurement, as by Hennekes. The EOG in normal people immediately after cigarette smoking is reported by Haase to be undisturbed, and by Schmidt to be slightly but significantly depressed. In patients diagnosed as having tobacco amblyopia, the VER with checkerboard pattern has been reported by Franck as detecting abnormality at an early stage when the only abnormality of vision was defective color vision. Kupersmith et al in more advanced cases reported gross abnormalities in the VER, but with characteristics pointing away from demyelination of the optic nerves and away from vitamin B_{12} deficiency as a cause of tobacco amblyopia.

Effects other than tobacco amblyopia that have been reported from tobacco smoking include a slight but significant impairment of dark adaptation (Calissendorff), and a suggestion of a possible relationship to senile disciform macular degeneration (Paethkau), but no difference in average visual acuity or intraocular pressure between chronic smokers and non-smokers (Shephard). (Effects of tobacco smoke externally on the eye are described under *Tobacco smoke external effects.*) (For more on *alcohol, carbon monoxide, cyanide, nicotine,* and *zinc,* see the INDEX.)

Bechetoille A, Allain P, et al: Changes in the blood concentrations of zinc, lead and the activity of ALA-dehydratase in the course of alcohol-tobacco optic neuropathies. *J FR OPHTALMOL* 6:231–235, 1983. (French)

Bechetoille A, Ebran JM, et al: Therapeutic effect of zinc sulfate on the central scotoma of alcohol-tobacco optic neuropathies. *J FR OPHTALMOL* 6:237–242, 1983. (French)

Bhargava SK, Phillips CI: Foveal spectral threshold in tobacco amblyopia. *ACTA OPHTHALMOL* 52:66–72, 1974.

Bronte-Stewart J, Pettigrew AR, Foulds WS: Toxic optic neuropathy and its experimental production. *TRANS OPHTHALMOL SOC UK* 96:355–358, 1976.

Calissendorff B: Effects of repeated smoking on dark adaptation. *ACTA OPHTHALMOL* 55:261–268, 1977.

Chisholm IA: Serum cobalamin and folate in the optic neuropathy associated with tobacco smoking. *CAN J OPHTHALMOL* 13:105–109, 1978.

de Crousaz G: Ocular symptoms and signs in vitamin B_{12} deficiency. *OPHTHALMOLOGICA* 159:295–306, 1969.

Dunphy EB: Alcohol and tobacco amblyopia. *AM J OPHTHALMOL* 68:569–578, 1969.

Foulds WS, Bronte-Stewart J, Chisholm IA: Serum thiocyanate concentrations in tobacco amblyopia. *NATURE* 218:586, 1968.

Foulds WS, Chisholm IA, et al: The optic neuropathy of pernicious anemia. *ARCH OPHTHALMOL* 82:427–432, 1969.

Franck H, Meyer F, Bronner A: Visual evoked potentials in the early diagnosis of alcohol-tobacco optic neuritis. *BULL SOC OPHTALMOL FRANCE* 80:1067–1070, 1980. (French)

Freeman AC, Heaton JM: The aetiology of retrobulbar neuritis in Addisonian pernicious anemia. *LANCET* 1:908–911, 1961.

Grignolo FM, La Rosa G, et al: Measurement of plasma zinc in retrobulbar optic neuritides. *BOLL OCULIST* 59:801–811, 1980.

Haase E, Muller W: Is there measurable influence on the EOG by cigarette smoking? *KLIN MONATSBL AUGENHEILKD* 158:677–681, 1971.

Harrington DO: Amblyopia due to tobacco, alcohol and nutritional deficiency. *AM J OPHTHALMOL* 53:967–973, 1962.

Hennekes R: Clinical ERG findings in tobacco-alcohol amblyopia. *GRAEFES ARCH OPHTHALMOL* 219:38–39, 1982.

Kupersmith MJ, Weiss PA, Carr RE: The visual-evoked potential in tobacco-alcohol and nutritional amblyopia. *AM J OPHTHALMOL* 95:307–314, 1983.

Paetkau ME, Boyd TAS, et al: Senile disciform macular degeneration and smoking. *CAN J OPHTHALMOL* 13:67–71, 1978.

Pettigrew AR, Fell GS, Chisholm IA: Red cell glutathione in tobacco amblyopia. *EXP EYE RES* 14:87–90, 1972.

Potts AM: Tobacco amblyopia. *SURVEY OPHTHALMOL* 17:313–339, 1973.

Saraux H, Bechetoille A, et al: The diminution of the level of serum zinc during some toxic optic neuritis cases. *ANN OCULIST* 208:29–31, 1975.

Schmidt B: Influence of cigarette smoking on the EOG. *KLIN MONATSBL AUGEN-HEILKD* 156:523–531, 1970. (German)

Shephard RJ, Ponsford E, et al: Effects of cigarette smoking on intraocular pressure and vision. *BR J OPHTHALMOL* 62:682–687, 1978.

Smith ADM, Duckett S: Cyanide, vitamin B_{12} experimental demyelination and tobacco amblyopia. *BR J EXP PATHOL* 46:612–622, 1965.

Victor M, Dreyfus PM: Tobacco-alcohol amblyopia. *ARCH OPHTHALMOL* 74:649–657, 1965.

Watson-Williams EJ, Bottomley AC, Ainsley RG: Absorption of vitamin B_{12} in tobacco amblyopia. *BR J OPHTHALMOL* 53:549–552, 1969.

Tobramycin (Tobrex) or **Tobramycin sulfate** (Nebcin), an antibacterial, applied as 5% eyedrops to rabbit eyes caused only mild conjunctival erythema,[b] and as 0.3% ointment to human eyes caused slight local reaction in 2.5% of patients, compared to 23.4% of patients treated with gentamicin sulfate.[c] However, 0.3% tobramycin eyedrops interfered with healing of rabbit corneal endothelium.[382] Injected subconjunctivally in rabbits, 8 to 12 mg tobramycin sulfate caused moderate transitory conjunctival reaction, and no disturbance of the cornea.[a,b] In rabbits, 0.5 mg injected into the anterior chamber caused definite damage of the corneal endothelium.[271] After vitrectomy in rabbits, infusion fluid containing 50 μg/ml caused histologic abnormality in all layers of the retina and extinguished the ERG, but 10 μg/ml had no toxic effect on the retina.[380] In owl monkeys, intravitreal injection of 2 mg caused retinal degeneration, extinguished the ERG photopic response, induced minute opacities of the posterior lens capsule and clouding of the vitreous body, but 0.5 mg was not appreciably damaging.[280]

a. Belfort R Jr, Smolin G, et al: Nebcin in treatment of experimental Pseudomonas keratitis. *BR J OPHTHALMOL* 59:725–729, 1975.
b. Purnell WD, McPherson SD Jr: The effect of tobramycin on rabbit eyes. *AM J OPHTHALMOL* 77:578–582, 1974.
c. Stewart RH, Smith RE, et al: Tobramycin in the treatment of external ocular infections. *J OCULAR THER SURG* 1:72–78, 1982.

Tolazoline hydrochloride (Priscol, Priscoline), a peripheral vasodilator, has caused elevations of intraocular pressure in human eyes after subconjunctival injections.[a,e-j] The rise of intraocular pressure may be greater in glaucomatous eyes, and this has been used as a provocative test for glaucoma.

Intravenous injection of tolazoline generally has had no influence on intraocular pressure, according to Fanta.[b] Zahn in 1966 in testing 10 mg given subcutaneously to patients with systemic hypertension found no rise, but rather an insignificant fall of intraocular pressure.[266] Newell and associates in 1951 found no reduction of intraocular pressure in glaucoma by intravenous administration.[d]

In treatment of chemical burns of the eye topical tolazoline has not been found significantly beneficial in controlled trials. This has been reviewed and discussed particularly by Brancato and Campana in 1965[17] and by Castren and Mustakallio in 1964.[30]

a. Di Tizio A, Cameo D: Clinical contribution to the early diagnosis of glaucoma with the priscol test. *ANN OTTALMOL CLIN OCUL* 93:1502–1511, 1967. (Italian)
b. Fanta H: The effect of Priscol on healthy and diseased eyes. *GRAEFES ARCH OPHTHALMOL* 149:199–219, 1949. (German)
c. Leydhecker W: The Priscol test in glaucoma. *KLIN MONATSBL AUGENHEILKD* 125:57–61, 1954. (German)
d. Newell FW, Ridgway WL, Zeller RW: The treatment of glaucoma with dibenamine. *AM J OPHTHALMOL* 34:527–535, 1951.
e. Norskov K: Priscol provative test. *ACTA OPHTHALMOL* 44:828–836, 1966.
f. Primrose J: Priscol provocative test. *BR J OPHTHALMOL* 46:129–137, 1962.
g. Rethy I: Diagnosis of carotid thrombosis by vasotonometry. *KLIN MONATSBL AUGEN-HEILKD* 146:819–825, 1965. (German)
h. Stepanik J: The effect of Priscol on the episcleral venous pressure. *GRAEFES ARCH OPHTHALMOL* 160:411–413, 1958.
i. Sugar HS: The priscoline provocative test. *AM J OPHTHALMOL* 40:510–514, 1955.
j. Swanljung H, Blodi FC: Tonography in some provocative tests for glaucoma. *AM J OPHTHALMOL* 41:187, 196, 1956.

Tolbutamide (Orinase), an antidiabetic, has had no proven toxic effect on the eyes of patients, but in one case was thought possibly to have caused bilateral retrobulbar neuritis.[a] The severe diabetes from which the patient was suffering could itself have been the cause rather than the tolbutamide.

Occasional slight transitory changes in refraction four or five days after starting treatment are presumed due to variation in water content of the crystalline lens.[a,b] Experimentally, lifelong administration of tolbutamide to rats at dosage levels five to forty times those employed in human beings has caused opacification of the lens and cornea, vascularization of the cornea, and posterior synechias, usually observable at eight to twenty-four months.[b] Carbutamide and chlorpropamide have had this same toxic effect, but insulin has not.[c]

a. Catros, Vivien, et al: Bilateral axial optic neuritis in the course of treatment with D860. *REV OTONEUROPATHOL* 30:253–257, 1958. (French)
b. Kapetansky FM: Refractive changes with tolbutamide. *OHIO STATE MED J* 59:275, 1963.
c. Wright HN: Corneal and lenticular opacities in eyes of rats following long-term administration of sulfonylurea derivatives. *DIABETES* 12:550–554, 1963.

Tolnaftate (Actate, Tinactin), an antifungal, tested as a 2% suspension on rabbit eyes has caused no damage.[a]

a. Hashimoto Y, Nogushi T, Kitagawa H, Ohta G: Toxicologic and pharmacologic properties of tolnaftate. *TOXICOL APPL PHARMACOL* 8:380–385, 1966.

Toluene (toluol, methyl benzene) vapor causes noticeable sensation of irritation to human eyes at 300 to 400 ppm in air, but even at 800 ppm irritation is slight.[d,183] In human volunteers exposed to concentrations as high as 800 ppm there has been described a dilation of the pupils and impairment of reaction in association with fatigue at the end of eight hours, also slight pallor of the fundi.[d] Whether related or not, small doses of toluene intraveously in monkeys has caused changes in the c-wave of the ERG and in the standing potential of the eye, suggestive of an influence on the retinal pigment epithelium.[c]

Exposure of cats to vapor concentrations which were just sublethal caused the appearance of fine vacuoles in the corneal epithelium within six hours, but after exposure was discontinued these were gone by the next day.[216]

Toluene tested by drop application to rabbit eyes has been reported by one experimenter to cause slight transient conjunctival irritation with no corneal damage detectable by fluorescein staining,[265] but another experimenter has reported moderate injury.[27] Difference in duration of contact may explain the variation. Injury of human eyes from liquid toluene has so far not been serious.

Two patients accidentally splashed with toluene are reported to have suffered transient superficial disturbance of the eyes, with healing complete within forty-eight hours.[165] Another patient splashed with a solution of stearic acid in toluene similarly experienced only transient epithelial injury.[81] In this last case the patient felt immediate, severe, burning pain, and had involuntary blepharospasm. Although no irrigation was carried out for four or five minutes, only moderate conjunctival hyperemia and corneal epithelial edema resulted, with complete return to normal within two days.

Toluene vapor was one of the principal substances inhaled in the "glue sniffing" fad of the 1960's. Inhalation of vapors to produce inebriation, popular among young people at that period, in rare instances produced ocular disturbances. One patient who ultimately developed encephalopathy noted at times "reddening of vision" acutely and briefly after inhaling toluene, but never developed other disturbance of vision or visual field.[a] One patient developed aplastic anemia after glue sniffing likely involving exposure to other solvents besides toluene, possibly benzene, and developed blurring of the optic disc margins, engorgement of the retinal veins and arteries, and a macular star. The influence on vision was not described. At autopsy, after death from subarachnoid hemorrhage, the optic nerves were found to be normal.[b]

(Concerning glue sniffing and related problems, also see INDEX for *Solvent vapors.*)

a. Knox JW, Nelson JR: Permanent encephalopathy from toluene inhalation. *N ENGL J MED* 275:1494–1496, 1966.

b. Powars D: Aplastic anemia secondary to glue sniffing. *N ENGL J MED* 273:700–702, 1965.

c. Skoog KO, Nilsson SEG: Changes in the c-wave and in the standing potential of the eye after small doses of toluene and styrene. *ACTA OPHTHALMOL* 59:71–79, 1981.

d. vonOettingen WF, Neal PA, Donahue DD: The toxicity and potential dangers of toluene. *J AM MED ASSOC* 118:579–584, 1942.

Toluenediamine (toluylene diamine) exists as several isomers, of which *2,5-diaminotoluene* and *2,4-diaminotoluene* appear to be the most important. The 2,5-diamino compound, in which the amino groups are in *para* positions, resembles paraphenylenediamine. Both of these p-diamino compounds readily become oxidized in neutral or alkaline solution to form dark products, and both induce contact sensitization and dermatitis. Toluenediamine used as a dye on the eyelashes is reported in one instance to have caused keratoconjunctivitis and blepharitis with opacities of the cornea which gradually cleared in the course of several weeks.[a,215,252] This is the same type of injurious action for which paraphenylenediamine is notorious in hypersensitive individuals.

The toluenediamines appear not to be primary irritants, according to tests on rabbit eyes in which 0.02 M solutions of each of the isomers all at pH 6.5 were tested by dropping on rabbit eyes for ten minutes after mechanical removal of the corneal epithelium to permit penetration. The eyes healed and returned to normal within two to four days without evidence of chemical injury.[81]

a. Haurowitz F: Damage from hair dyes. *SAMML VERGIFTUNGSF* 7:A59, 1936.

Toluene diisocyanates (TDI, Desmodur-T) and other polyisocyanates are used in the manufacture of *polyurethane foams* by reaction with polyalcohols in the presence of amines. The amines act as catalysts and cross-linking agents. During the foam-forming reaction there has been described release of vapors which are irritating to the eyes, respiratory tract, and skin, and may induce sensitization.[g,h,252] Finished *polyurethane foam* plastic appears to be free from these irritating materials.[h]

Exposure of volunteers to vapors of toluene diisocyanate have shown that eye and nose irritations begin at concentrations of 0.05 to 0.1 ppm in the air, and that irritation is definite in all instances at 0.5 ppm.[c]

Luckenback and Kielar have described disturbances of the corneal epithelium experienced by 9 workers employed in polyurethane foam production and exposed to high vapor concentrations of toluene diisocyanates. They all developed microcystic corneal epithelial edema with subjective impression of foggy or smoky vision, but no discomfort. Exposure for one day was sufficient to produce this disturbance. Visual acuity was usually reduced only one line on the Snellen chart, but slit-lamp examination showed clearly the microcystic changes in the corneal epithelium. The corneas were otherwise unaffected. The condition was spontaneously reversible in all cases, within 12 to 48 hours after one day's exposure, or within several days after repeated daily exposure. There was no persistent disturbance from chronic exposure.[d]

Although these findings were attributed to toluene diisocyanates in this report, there are good reasons to suspect that the amines used in manufacture of polyurethane foam were more likely responsible. The transient corneal epithelial edema and haziness of vision are characteristic of amines, and were attributed by Dernehl[40] in 1966 to commonly used *substituted morpholines* and *triethylene diamine*. The symptoms from corneal epithelial edema were attributed by Belin and associates more specifically to *N-methylmorpholine*.[a] Belin pointed out that earlier analytical methods for determining small amounts of amines in the work atmosphere were of low sensitivity compared to present methods, and allowed the role of amines to be overlooked. Belin described 20 polyurethane workers with the characteristic "blue haze" symptoms from amines. (For more on these symptoms, see INDEX for *Amines*.)

Accidental splash of toluene diisocyanate in the eyes of workmen has caused keratitis and conjunctivitis. One case report describes "an unusual amount of photophobia and blepharospasm," but gives no details, or information on the course of recovery.[e] A second case, involved severe iridocyclitis and secondary glaucoma.[f] In this case a workman gave a history of splashing the chemical in one eye. He was seen six days later with many clumps of inflammatory cells all over the posterior surface of the cornea, and the intraocular pressure was elevated. Epithelial edema was present, but whether this was due to the glaucoma or the initial splash injury was uncertain. The eye responded well to standard treatment for iridocyclitis and secondary glaucoma. It is very difficult to be sure in such cases of the cause of such a severe reaction. There has been no other indication to suggest that this could be due to any peculiar toxic property of toluene diisocyanate.[f]

Test application of a drop of meta and para toluenediisocyanates on rabbit eyes caused immediate pain, lacrimation, swelling of the lids, and conjunctival reaction. However, the corneal epithelium was only mildly damaged, and the amount of damage could be reduced by prompt flushing with water.[g,h]

a. Belin L, Wass V, et al: Amines: possible causative agents in the development of bronchial hyperreactivity in workers manufacturing polyurethanes from isocyanates. *BR J IND MED* 40:251–257, 1983.

b. Brugsch HG, Elkins HB: Toluene di-isocyanate (TDI) toxicity. *N ENGL J MED* 268:353–357, 1963.

c. Henschler D, Assmann W, Meyer K: On the toxicology of toluene diisocyanate. *ARCH TOXIKOL* 19:364–387, 1962. (German)

d. Luckenbach M, Kielar R: Toxic corneal epithelial edema from exposure to high atmospheric concentration of toluene diisocyanates. *AM J OPHTHALMOL* 90:682–686, 1980.

e. Munn A: Experiences with diisocyanates. *TRANS ANN INDUSTR MED OFFICERS* (*London*) 9:134–138, 1960.

f. Padfield EG: Personal communication, 1963.

g. Schrenk HH: Industrial hygiene. *IND ENGIN CHEM* 47:107A–108A, 1955.

h. Zapp JA Jr: Hazards of isocyanates in polyurethane foam plastic production. *ARCH IND HEALTH* 15:324–330, 1957.

o-Toluidine applied full strength to rabbit eyes was injurious to the corneal epithelium, graded 8 on a scale of 1 to 10,[228] but when applied as a 0.02 M solution at pH 6 for ten minutes after removal of the epithelium, it was innocuous to the rabbit cornea.[81]

Tomatine, an antifungal agent from tomato plants, tested in rabbits by applying a 5% ointment to the eye, made the lids edematous. However, the eyes recovered completely in a few days.[a]

a. Wilson RH, Poley GW, DeEds F: Some pharmacologic and toxicologic properties of tomatine and its derivatives. *TOXICOL APPL PHARMACOL* 3:39–48, 1961.

Toxaphene, an insecticide, is reported to have caused acute poisoning in goats, with apparent blindness.[a] However, no examination of the eyes has been published, and it has been stated that although the animals performed as though blind, they might actually have been able to see.

a. Radcleff RD: Toxaphene poisoning; symptomatology and pathology. *VET MED* 44:436–442, 1949.

Toxotoxin, from Toxoplasma, injected intraperitoneally in rabbits, has caused changes in retinal nuclear layer and retinal pigment epithelium.[a]

a. Pecori-Giraldi J, Pivetti-Pezzi P, et al: Effects on the eyes from intraperitoneal injection of toxotoxin in the rabbit. *BOLL OCULIST* 50:407–417, 1971. (Italian)

Tranexamic acid (Amstat), hemostatic, antifibrinolytic, is reported to have had retinotoxic effects in dogs in unpublished studies in the laboratories of two drug companies. Theil described these unpublished studies as having disclosed focal retinal atrophy, mostly either macular or peripheral, after a year of feeding 800 to 1600 mg/kg/day, but said no thromboses were found in intraocular blood vessels.[d] Theil carried out a thorough ophthalmologic examination of 14 patients who had received tranexamic acid for an average of 6 years and found no evidence of a toxic action.[d] Johnson et al similarly looked for evidence of ocular toxicity in rabbits, but found no change in retinal ultrastructure or ERG after 0.5g/day for up to 10 months.[b]

In non-glaucomatous and glaucomatous patients tranexamic acid orally has had no influence on intraocular pressure.[a] Transexamic acid orally caused a slight temporary decrease in central corneal thickness, but had no adverse effects.[a,d]

a. Bramsen T: A double-blind study on the influence of tranexamic acid on the intraocular pressure. *ACTA OPHTHALMOL* 56:998–1005, 1978.
b. Johnson NF, McKecknie N, Forrester JV: An investigation of retinal function and structure in rabbits treated long-term with tranexamic acid. *TOXICOL APPL PHARMACOL* 40:59–63, 1977.
c. Olsen T, Ehlers N, Bramsen T: Influence of tranexamic acid and acetylsalicylic acid on the thickness of the normal cornea. *ACTA OPHTHALMOL* 58:767–772, 1980.
d. Theil PL: Ophthalmological examination of patients in long-term treatment with tranexamic acid. *ACTA OPHTHALMOL* 59:237–241, 1981.

Tranylcypromine sulfate (Parnate), a monoamine oxidase inhibitor antidepressant, has exhibited no ocular toxic effect in usual dosage of 20 mg per day, but large overdosage may possibly have resulted in ocular and visual disturbances in two cases.

A manic depressive patient attempted suicide by taking 300 mg tranylcypromine and 30 mg trifluoperazine dihydrochloride. Twenty days later the patient's eyes were examined because of complaints of reduced visual acuity, phosphenes, and headaches. Vision with glasses was 5/10 and 4/10; central visual fields were abnormal with red test objects; ERGs were subnormal. There was no obvious cause for the abnormal visual findings apart from the history of poisoning. Within seven months the central visual fields became normal, but the ERG did not improve.[b]

A schizophrenic patient attempted suicide by taking 250 mg tranylcypromine plus 25 mg trifluoperazine dihydrochloride. The patient required intensive medical treatment for three weeks. He was then found to have anterior uveitis and corneal stromal band opacities in the palpebral fissures, with vision much reduced, and ERGs abnormal. Tensions remained normal. Whether either drug was to blame remained obscure, and seems unlikely.[a] Trifluoperazine has been given separately to many patients in dosage from 4 to 20 mg per day without producing disturbances such as described above. (See INDEX for *Trifluoperazine.*)

Single cases have been registered by Davidson[298] of mydriasis with angle-closure glaucoma, and of sixth nerve palsy, but these could well have been coincidental.

   a. Alfieri G, Ramusino MC: Ocular manifestations in a case of acute intoxication by a phenothiazine derivative. *RASS ITAL OTTALMOL* 34:283–289, 1965–1966. (Italian)
   b. Liuzzi L, Diversi A: Campimetric and electroretinographic aspects of a case of intoxication by trifluoperazine. *RASS ITAL OTTALMOL* 35:219–226, 1967. (Italian)

Tretamine (triethylenemelamine, TEM), an antineoplastic, has been shown to induce cataracts in mice when administered parenterally.[a–c]

Effects of injection of tretamine into the anterior chamber in cats have been investigated by Betrix.[283] Injection of 0.05 to 0.1 mg/kg causes severe bullous keratopathy and anterior chamber reaction with destruction of corneal endothelial cells and lens epithelium. Much less damage is done by 0.025 mg, and almost none by 0.01 mg/kg. The cat's corneal endothelium and lens epithelium were found to be capable of much regeneration.

In clinical use of tretamine, patients seem to have escaped eye injuries.

   a. Christenberry KW, Conklin JW, et al: Induction of cataracts in mice by 4-(p-dimethylaminostyryl) quinoline. *ARCH OPHTHALMOL* 70:250–252, 1963.
   b. Conklin JW, Upton AC, et al: Comparative late somatic effects of some radiomimetic agents and x-rays. *RADIAT RES* 19:156, 1963.
   c. vonSallmann L, Grimes P: The effect of triethylene melamine on DNA synthesis and mitosis in the lens epithelium. *DOCUM OPHTHALMOL* 20:1–12, 1966.

Tretinoin (Retin-A, retinoic acid, vitamin A acid), a keratolytic, has been applied in vegetable oil as 0.1% eyedrops in rabbits in therapeutic tests, without adverse effects, and has been similarly applied to patients with corneal xerophthalmia.[a,b] In these patients application up to 3 times a day was beneficial, but 5 times a day caused "conjunctival injection and increased corneal vascularization and scarring."[a] (Compare *Isotretinoin.*)

   a. Sommer A: Treatment of corneal xerophthalmia with topical retinoic acid. *AM J OPHTHALMOL* 95:349–352, 1983.
   b. Smolin G, Okumoto M, Friedlaender M: Tretinoin and corneal epithelial wound healing. *ARCH OPHTHALMOL* 97:545–546, 1979.

Triacetin (glyceryltriacetate), an antifungal, tested on rabbit eyes has been found to cause no injury.[123,275,295,338] However, commercial triacetin may contain diacetin, as well as monoacetin, and when applied to animal or human eyes causes burning pain and much redness of the conjunctiva, but no injury.[a,45] Diacetin causes considerably more discomfort than pure triacetin.[a]

> a. Gomer JJ: Corneal clouding from pure acetone. *GRAEFES ARCH OPHTHALMOL* 150:622–644, 1950. (German)

Triamterene (Dyrenium), a diuretic agent, has been tested for influence on intraocular pressure in glaucoma. It has caused no elevation of pressure and little if any reduction.[192] Given intravenously to rabbits it has caused a 40% increase in the b-wave of the ERG.[a]

> a. Tota G, Cavallacci G: The electroretinogram after administration of triamterene. *ANN OTTALMOL CLIN OCUL* 97:143–153, 1971.

Triaziquone (Trenimon), an antineoplastic, has been used systemically and locally.

A superficial papillomatous growth spreading over half of the cornea was treated by triaziquone (1:100,000 dilution) by subconjunctival injection and as eyedrops, with satisfactory result except for pain lasting three months and transitory secondary glaucoma.[g] In a case of precancerous melanosis of the conjunctiva, triaziquone (0.33 mg/ml) was injected repeatedly into the area of the tumor and appeared to be effective and tolerated satisfactorily.[e] Caution is needed to keep the concentration or the volume down, so that excessive inflammation and damage is avoided. In rabbits a single subconjunctival injection of 0.1 mg/ml caused violent local reaction and extensive necrosis of the conjunctiva.[e]

Intracarotid injections of nearly LD_{50} doses in rabbits produced ipsilateral retinal edema, visible ophthalmoscopically as a clouding of the retina, affecting particularly the area around the optic nerve. In the next few days, progressive chorioretinal atrophy and pigment dispersion were seen. The choroid and all layers of the retina were involved. Also atrophy of the iris developed and histologically both the iris and ciliary body showed inflammatory reaction. There was total opacification of the lens in three months.[a–d,f]

> a. Apponi-Battini G, Lamberti O, Loffredo A: Histologic study of alterations induced in the iris, ciliary body and lens by Trenimon (Bayer) given intracarotid. *ARCH OTTALMOL* 67:395–406, 1963. (Italian)
>
> b. Apponi-Battini G, Loffredo A, Lamberti O: Histologic study of the changes induced in rabbit retina by Trenimon (Bayer) given intracarotid. *ARCH OTTALMOL* 67:385–393, 1963. (Italian)
>
> c. Apponi G, Rinaldi E, De Simone S: Monolateral cataract after intracarotid injection of Trenimon (Bayer). *ANN OTTALMOL CLIN OCUL* 90:224–229, 1964. (Italian)
>
> d. Apponi G, Tieri O, Rinaldi E: The retinotoxic action of Trenimon. *ACTA OPHTHALMOL* 42:64–67, 1964.
>
> e. Frezzotti R, Guerra R: Illustrated notes on local treatment with an alkylating agent in a case of precancerous melanosis of the conjunctiva. *BOLL OCULIST* 47:265–267, 1968. (Italian)
>
> f. Rinaldi E, Apponi G: Action of some antimitotic substances given intracarotid. *ANN OTTALMOL CLIN OCUL* 90:177–182, 1964. (Italian)

g. Van Den Heuvel JEA: Papilloma conjunctivae et corneae treated with Trenimon. *OPHTHALMOLOGICA* 152:537, 1966.

Trichlorfon (Chlorofos, Dipterex), a phosphonate cholinesterase inhibitor insecticide and anthelmintic, when applied to the eyes of rabbits has short-lasting miotic effect and produces little or no irritation.[a]

a. Kadin M: Studies on the toxicity and effect of Dipterex in rabbits. *AM J OPHTHALMOL* 53:512–517, 1962.

Trichlormethiazide, a diuretic and antihypertensive, has induced acute transient myopia, the same as numerous other drugs, especially diuretics.[a] (Also see INDEX for *Myopia, acute transient.*)

a. Beasley FJ: Transient myopia during trichlormethiazide. *ANN OPHTHALMOL* 12:705–706, 1980.

Trichloroacetic acid has been used in 10% to 25% aqueous solution to cauterize the surface of the cornea in treatment of recurrent erosion and bullous keratopathy. When such solutions are applied to the corneal epithelium, it becomes white and coagulated.[184] If the epithelium is first scraped off with a knife and the solution is applied with a cotton swab directly to the surface of the corneal stroma for fifteen seconds, only very slight grayness results. If the surface of the eye is then flushed with water or saline, the cornea heals and retains a slight diffuse stromal haze. The regenerated epithelium adheres well and appears to have a reduced tendency to form bullae or to come loose.[a, b]

A saturated solution of trichloroacetic acid has been used successfully to cauterize unwanted postoperative filtering blebs of the conjunctiva by carefully localized application, but in one patient some of the acid ran on to half of the cornea, turning it immediately white. Although this was immediately irrigated thoroughly with sodium chloride solution, the eye remained hyperemic and uncomfortable for several days and it took several weeks for the epithelium to heal in the cauterized area, but the cornea regained normal clarity.[a]

Experiments on rabbits eyes were performed in 1910 by Guillery, who described the appearance of the cornea after intensive applications of trichloroacetic acid.[96]

Epithelial implantation cysts of the anterior chamber have been treated in human beings by injection of 10% trichloroacetic acid.[c, d] This was allowed to remain from 30 to 120 seconds before it was withdrawn. This has been reported to have cured two very large cysts which had intact walls, but appeared to be suitable only for cataractous or aphakic eyes. In cases in which spread of the acid into adjacent corneal tissue could not be prevented, the treatment caused protracted inflammation and dense local opacity of the cornea.[c] This appears to be a procedure to be used with great caution in special cases.

Tests of partially neutralized trichloroacetic acid on rabbit corneas after removal of the epithelium or by injection into the stroma have shown no injurious effect from trichloroacetate when the pH is above 3.[123]

a. Chandler PA: Personal communication.
b. Chandler PA: Recurrent erosion of the cornea. *TRANS AM OPHTHALMOL SOC*, 42:355–371, 1944.
c. Csapody I: Chemical abolition of a large iris cyst. *KLIN MONATSBL AUGENHEILKD* 139:674–676, 1961. (German)
d. Lindner K: Operated iris cyst. *Z AUGENHEILKD* 93:96–97, 1937. (German)

Trichloroacetonitrile (Tritox) is a volatile liquid with vapors that are intensely irritating to the eyes and respiratory tract, causing lacrimation, closure of the lids, and escape if possible. The compound is very toxic, and can be damaging to the respiratory tract.[a, 181]

Testing of trichloroacetonitrile by application to rabbit eyes indicated severe injurious effect, graded 10 on a scale of 1 to 10.[228]

a. Treon JF, Kitzmiller KV, et al: The physiological response of animals to trichloroacetonitrile administered orally, applied on the skin, or inhaled as a vapor in air. *J IND HYG TOXICOL* 31:235–249, 1949.

Trichlorobenzene (1,2,3-trichlorobenzene) vapors are said to be irritating to the eyes and respiratory tract.[70, 171] Solid *1,2,4-trichlorobenzene* also is irritating and causes severe pain on contact with the eyes.[a]

a. Brown VK, Muir C, Thorpe E: Acute toxicity and skin irritant properties of 1,2,4-trichlorobenzene. *ANN OCCUP HYG* 12:209–212, 1969.

Trichloroethane (1,1,1-trichloroethane; methyl chloroform; Chlorothene) tested by drop application to rabbit eyes caused slight conjunctival irritation and no corneal damage.[a, 276, 352] By splash or spray on the human eye its injurious effect has been superficial and transient.[165] By inhalation it appears to be one of the least toxic chlorinated aliphatic hydrocarbon solvents, and to have no known systemic toxic effect on the eye.[b, c]

a. Tarkelson T, Oyen F, et al: Toxicity of 1,1,1-trichloroethane as determined on laboratory animals and human subjects. *AM IND HYG ASSOC J* 19:353, 1958.
b. Stewart R: Toxicology of 1,1,1-trichloroethane. *ANN OCCUP HYG* 11:71–79, 1968.
c. Stewart R, et al: Experimental human exposure to methyl chloroform vapor. *ARCH ENVIRON HEALTH* 19:467–472, 1969.

Trichloroethylene (Chlorylen) is a volatile liquid used in great quantities for degreasing and dry cleaning. Medically, trichloroethylene has been employed as an inhalation analgesic and anesthetic in many thousands of patients. However, it can decompose to form toxic products under the influence of heat and light, in the presence of moisture, or in contact with strong alkalies or finely divided metal catalysts.

Inhalation of trichloroethylene vapors can induce deep narcosis, and this in several industrial accidents has resulted in death, but there appears to be no report of injury of cranial or other nerves by undoubtedly pure trichloroethylene that has not been subjected to decomposition (Mitchell). However, trichloroethylene which has been subjected to decomposition has produced numerous cases of trigeminal and oculomotor nerve paralyses, optic or retrobulbar neuritis, and optic atrophy.

Extensive reviews of the general toxicology of trichloroethylene without special attention to the eye have been published by Smith in 1966, and by Waters et al in 1977.

We will review the ophthalmic aspects of trichloroethylene toxicology as follows: (a) *trigeminal and oculomotor cranial nerve disturbances, (b) disturbances of vision, (c) decomposition products, (d) experimental administration, (e) local actions of trichloroethylene on the eye from direct contamination with vapor or liquid.*

(a) Reports of trigeminal or extraocular muscle palsies from trichloroethylene:

Between 1916 and 1927 at least ten instances of loss of sensation in the distribution of the trigeminal nerve on one or both sides from trichloroethylene were reported following industrial exposure (Kalinowsky; Plessner; Stuber). All were the result of acute exposures rather than chronic intoxication. These cases were occasionally complicated by corneal epithelial ulceration, which did not cause discomfort because of the corneal anesthesia due to paralysis of the sensory nerve. Oculomotor paralysis accompanied the trigeminal palsies in a few of these cases, but early observers were most impressed with what seemed to be a selective paralytic effect on the trigeminal nerve, and this led to the medical use of inhalations of trichloroethylene for the treatment of trigeminal neuralgia or tic douloureux. This proved somewhat disappointing because the purified trichloroethylene prescribed for patients produced only non-specific analgesia such as might be obtained with chloroform.

In the 1940's, nineteen instances of cranial nerve palsies, most of which were trigeminal sensory palsies, were recorded as a complication of improper procedure in use of trichloroethylene for general anesthesia (Carden; Enderby; Humphrey; McAuley; McClelland). The histories were remarkably uniform. Cranial nerve injury was noted only when trichloroethylene was used with a soda-lime carbon dioxide absorber, never when administered by means of an "open circuit." Typically patients were asymptomatic for 24 to 48 hours, but then began to complain of increasing numbness of the face in the distribution of the fifth nerve. Lacrimation was reduced and corneal sensation absent. Keratitis developed in at least one instance (Enderby). In one instance the facial nerve was also affected, and in two cases oculomotor palsies were mentioned (Enderby; Carden). Spontaneous improvement usually took place in the course of several months.

In 1952 Heuner and Petzold reported three additional cases in which poisoning affecting the cranial nerves resulted from inhalation of trichloroethylene vapor exposed to alkali. In addition to trigeminal, abducens, and facial paralysis, one patient developed optic atrophy with severe loss of vision.

In 1967 Buxton and Hayward described a particularly informative case, establishing a central site for the injury of cranial nerves from acute exposure to decomposing trichloroethylene. They observed at autopsy severe damage in the brain stem, affecting particularly the nuclei and tracts of the fifth and sixth nerves, in a patient who had trigeminal paralysis, limitation of eye movements with diplopia, and facial paralysis with ptosis before he died from respiratory infection. In 1967, 1969 and 1970, Feldman, reporting a case of involvement of vision as well as involvement of several cranial nerves, considered that neurotoxicity from trichloroethylene was due to an effect on the nerves themselves, possibly through action on the myelin.

Episodes of poisoning of crews of space capsules and nuclear submarines have been reported by Saunders in 1967, attributed to decomposition of trichloroethylene and possibly methylchloroform by air-purifying apparatus used in these enclosed spaces. Henschler and associates in 1970 described the poisoning of two workmen cleaning out a tank car. Trigeminal palsies and herpes of the lips developed in the victims of both these episodes. One workman described by Henschler developed palsies of eye movement. (These reports are described in more detail under the heading *Dichloroacetylene.* See INDEX.)

(b) Reports of disturbances of vision from trichloroethylene:

In 1916 Plessner, incidental to describing cases of trigeminal paralysis from trichloroethylene, mentioned two cases of disturbance of color vision.

In 1927 Baader listed three cases in which loss of vision had occurred in degreasing metal with trichloroethylene. Baader himself had seen only one of these patients, a man who had become addicted to inhaling the vapors. This patient was stated to have developed severe irreversible retrobulbar neuritis, but no details of ocular examination or visual fields were given. The second case listed by Baader was relayed from a verbal report from Zangger and was merely described as a case of blindness. The third case listed by Baader as a case of blinding by trichloroethylene was also heard of indirectly, with details entirely lacking.

In 1929 Meyer described two cases in which the relationship of visual disturbance to trichloroethylene was extremely vague.

In 1935 Kunz and Isenschmid relayed the information that Teleky had observed in one patient a decrease of visual acuities to 6/10 and 4/10, associated with temporal pallor of the optic nerveheads, after nine months' occupational exposure to trichloroethylene, and improvement had been slight after exposure was discontinued.

Kunz and Isenchmid reported an original case which they considered to be the fifth case of visual impairment from trichloroethylene in the literature. They described a man who had been exposed for several months to vapors of trichloroethylene at his work, complaining of burning sensation in his eyes during that time. His vision had gradually failed to 0.1 in both eyes, but the fundi appeared normal. After about a year at the same work, temporal pallor appeared in both discs, and vision decreased to counting fingers at 0.5 meter in one eye, but remained 0.1 in the other. He was found to have central and paracentral scotomas breaking through to the periphery. A diagnosis of retrobulbar neuritis and polyneuritis was made. It was also postulated that there was a disturbance in the oculomotor nuclei because the pupils were abnormal.

In 1937 McNally presented brief reports on two patients, one of whom he had not seen but had been described to him. This patient had been exposed to trichloroethylene in dry cleaning of clothes much of the time during fourteen months, and had complained of decrease in vision for six weeks. Vision was reported to be 20/100 and 4/200 due to central scotoma in each eye. Subsequently, visual loss was said to have progressed to complete blindness, but apart from the above-mentioned measurements of vision, no information was furnished concerning examination of the eyes.

The second patient, who was actually observed by McNally, worked over a degreasing tank for five days, then went home feeling sick, and slept for two days.

He had headache and was found to have nystagmus, reduced visual acuity, and enlarged blind spot. No further details of the eye examination were given, but he recovered sufficiently to return to work at a different job.

In 1952 Heuner and Petzold described in excellent detail an accidental poisoning of three coal miners by trichloroethylene subjected to decomposition in closed circuit oxygen respirators. The accident was caused by an estimated 2 to 3 g of trichloroethylene which remained in oxygen cylinders after they had been washed out with this solvent prior to filling with oxygen. Cannisters of alkali in the rebreathing system for removing carbon dioxide were known to become as hot as 120° C while the men worked. The first signs of poisoning developed four to six hours after work had ended, consisting of headache, faintness and vomiting, numb feeling in the face, much salivation, and difficulty in eating and swallowing. Vision was affected, first noted as diplopia. Trigeminal anesthesia was found and paralysis of the oculomotor, abducens, facial, vestibular, glossopharyngeal, and hypoglossal nerves. Later, also peripheral ulnar and peroneal nerve injuries were noted in one case.

Each patient complained of dimness of vision and diplopia during the first day. There was paralysis of accommodation in all, and limitation of eye movements plus nystagmus in one case. The optic nerveheads were hyperemic and edematous in two of the patients, but in only one was there severe and permanent optic nerve injury and visual loss. This particular patient on the first day of acute symptoms had severe hyperemia and edema of his optic nerveheads, with small peripapillary hemorrhages in both eyes, but no gross field defect. He had horizontal nystagmus and slight cerebellar ataxia. By the third day his vision became poorer, and the optic nerveheads appeared relatively pale. The cerebrospinal fluid pressure was found to be elevated. By the fourth day vision was worse and the visual fields were beginning to become constricted. Headache and signs of meningismus became acutely but transiently worse, and the visual fields became further constricted. During the first month after onset, optic atrophy became increasingly evident in both eyes. The peripapillary hemorrhages absorbed. At 3.5 months after onset the corrected visual acuity was 5/36 and 5/24, with visual fields severely constricted. The fundi showed postneuritic optic atrophy with severe narrowing of the retinal arteries. About 1.5 years after the acute poisoning the vision in the right eye had decreased to less than 5/60, the left to 5/30. Extreme constriction of the fields persisted. The optic nerveheads were porcelain white from severe atrophy. Heuner and Petzold clearly pointed out that the toxic effects in these cases were not such as one would expect from trichloroethylene itself, but presumably were attributable to products of decomposition of trichloroethylene by hot alkali, and they mentioned that such products were known to include *glycolic acid, dichloroacetylene,* and *hexachlorobenzol,* but they did not know which of the decomposition products to blame.

In 1955 Luvoni and Penzani carried out an ophthalmologic examination of fourteen people who had been exposed to trichloroethylene vapor for periods ranging from four months to twelve years in degreasing procedures. All appeared to be in good health. No significant abnormality of visual acuity was found, but pallor of the temporal portion of the papilla was suspected in seven. The visual fields were said to be 5° to 20° less than normal especially temporally. However, no control unexposed group was included for actual comparison.

In 1966 Tabacchi and associates described a girl who had severe loss of central vision due to central scotomas, and gradually developed temporal atrophy of the optic nerveheads after working eight to nine hours a day for fifteen months using a mixture containing mostly trichloroethylene, but also 8% dichloroethane and 0.5% benzene. Extensive neurologic study was negative for any other cause of optic nerve abnormality.

In 1967, 1969 and 1970, Feldman and associates described a man who was exposed for 1.5 hours to vapors inhaled through a mask and chemical-containing cannister from a degreasing machine containing hot trichloroethylene, and who became ill ten to twelve hours later, with reduced vision in both eyes and partial palsies of cranial nerves III, V, VI, and VII. Visual acuity was 20/40, but the fields were constricted. Eye movements and fields recovered in ten months. The fundi were normal. Inequality of the pupils and sluggish reactivity were noted early and were still present after eighteen months.

In 1967 Buxton and Hayward described two patients who had cranial nerve injuries, one of whom had visual disturbance after acute exposure to trichloroethylene and possible degradation products while working for several hours cleaning the inside of tanks containing residues of water and deteriorating aluminum paint. Both developed trigeminal paresthesias and hypesthesia, facial palsies with ptosis, and extraocular motor palsies with diplopia. One of these patients complained of photophobia and pain on movement of the eyes. The fundi appeared normal. Central fields were said to be constricted. Paracentral scotoma was found in one eye and enlargement of the blind spot in the other.

In 1968 Djerassi and Lumbroso described a worker exposed to vapors containing trichloroethylene (64%), carbon tetrachloride (10%), and carbon disulfide (26%), for two days in fumigating grain in silos, a day or two before blurring of vision, xanthopsia and confusion. Visual acuity was normal. Visual fields were slightly contracted early but were normal in three weeks, and ocular fundi remained normal. The carbon disulfide in the mixture was thought more likely to responsible for the intoxication than the trichloroethylene or carbon tetrachloride.

In 1969 Mitchell and Parsons-Smith mentioned a 4° enlargement of the blind spot in the right eye compared to the left in a man who had trigeminal paresthesias and reduced sensation on the right after working at metal degreasing, but there was no stronger evidence of eye involvement.

In summary, it appears clear that decomposition products of trichloroethylene can produce acute illness after a latent period of a few hours or more. The cranial nerves are affected, most typically the trigeminal, with paresthesias and anesthesia developing in its distribution, often followed by development of oral herpes. The oculomotor nerves and the facial nerves are also attacked and paralyzed, though less commonly. Anatomic evidence indicates that the site of toxic action may be within the CNS. Optic neuritis and optic atrophy, with impaired visual acuity and constriction of visual fields, also occur and may be associated with palsies of other cranial nerves, but disturbances of vision have been relatively infrequent compared to trigeminal, oculomotor, and facial palsies.

(c) Decomposition products from trichloroethylene.

(c) Decomposition products from trichloroethylene. Repeatedly suspicions have been expressed that the injuries of cranial nerves have been caused by products

of decomposition or by impurities, rather than by trichloroethylene itself. The strongest support of this hypothesis is found in the instances of cranial nerve palsies resulting from the use of pure trichloroethylene in conjunction with soda lime in the anesthesia accidents already described.

Dichloroacetylene has long been a primary suspect, since it is known to be produced from trichloroethylene by the action of hot alkalies such as soda-lime (Carden), and in the investigations reported by Saunders and Henschler both *dichloroacetylene* and *monochloroacetylene* were shown to be present in the air where the intoxications developed. (See INDEX for *Dichloroacetylene.*)

The normal products of trichloroethylene metabolism, in particular *chloral hydrate, trichloroethanol* and *trichloroacetate*, have no known toxic effect on cranial nerves.

(d) Experimental administration. Feldman and Lessel, attempting to imitate conditions of some of the accidental poisonings have described exposing a cat to vapors of "trichloroethylene mixed with soda-lime in a closed container at 80° to 90°F" for four hours, then finding facial hypalgesia and reduced corneal reflexes, but no histologic abnormalities in the eyes, optic nerves, or CNS when the animal was killed twenty-seven days later.

Meyer in 1929 attempted to induce toxic effects in the eyes of five dogs by repeatedly anesthetizing them with trichloroethylene by inhalation or by subcutaneous injections, performing as many as twenty-five anesthesias on one dog, but he did not succeed in producing any abnormality recognizable clinically in the fundus or cornea, or by histological examination in the retina or optic nerve.

In Savic's rabbit experiments with trichloroethylene a total of 9 ml/kg injected intramuscularly in divided doses in the course of three weeks reduced the ATP content of the retina and reduced the activity of several enzymes in the lens, but produced no morphologic or clinically detectable evidence of damage to the lens or retina. There has been no suspicion of lens changes in patients exposed to trichloroethylene.

Inhalation of pure trichloroethylene vapor up to 1,000 ppm in air by normal people has had no selective effect on vision or visual pathways, though causing some alteration in depth perception and opticokinetic nystagmus (Kylin;Vernon).

(e) Local actions on the eye. Direct external contact of trichloroethylene vapor or liquid with the eye has caused solvent-type burns of the lids, conjunctiva, and cornea in several instances. In most cases injury has resulted from splash of the liquid onto the eye or from exposure of an unconscious individual to a high concentration of vapor. A splash of a drop on the eye causes smarting pain, and injures corneal epithelium in a manner similar to chloroform. Complete spontaneous recovery is usual. The same effect is produced in rabbits. Epithelium may be lost, but rapidly regenerates.

Most severe exposure has occurred in patients who have inhaled trichloroethylene vapors, have become unconscious, and have fallen and remained exposed to high concentrations of vapor or to liquid. In such cases solvent burns of the skin may result from the defatting action of trichloroethylene. The corneal epithelium may be lost and the corneas become slightly turbid. The lids and conjunctivae become hyperemic and edematous. In cases of this sort so far observed, the eyes have recovered spontaneously (Grant[81]; Maloof). Irritation of the eyes is not a common feature of industrial exposure when the concentration in the air is maintained below 100 to 200 ppm and there is no decomposition. Exposure of three albino rabbits and three guinea pigs to concentrations of trichloroethylene in air increasing from 300 ppm to 500 ppm during six weeks produced no signs or symptoms of irritation of the eyes, grossly, by slit-lamp biomicroscopy, or by fluorescein test.[81]

Atkinson RS: Trichloroethylene anesthesia. *ANESTHESIOLOGY* 21:64–66, 1960.

Baader EW: Progress report of the division for occupational illness of the Empress August-Victoria hospital. *ZBL GEWERBEHYG* 4:385–393, 1927. (German)

Buxton PH, Hayward M: Polyneuritis cranialis associated with industrial trichloroethylene poisoning. *J NEUROL NEUROSURG PSYCHIATR* 30:511–518, 1967.

Carden S: Hazards in the use of closed circuit technique for Trilene anesthesia. *BR MED J* 1:319–320, 1944.

Djerassi LS, Lumbroso R: Carbon disulphide poisoning with increased ethereal sulphate excretion. *BR J IND MED* 25:220–222, 1968.

Eichert H: Trichloroethylene intoxication. *J AM MED ASSOC* 106:1652–1653, 1936.

Enderby GEH: The use and abuse of trichloroethylene. *BR MED J* 1:300–302, 1944.

Feldman RG, Lessel S: Neuro-ophthalmic aspects of trichloroethylene intoxication. In Brunette J, Barbeau A (Eds.): *PROGRESS IN NEURO-OPHTHALMOLOGY.* Amsterdam, Excerpta Med. Foundation, 1969.

Feldman RG, Mayer RRF: Studies of trichloroethylene intoxication in man. *NEUROLOGY* 18:309, 1968.

Feldman RG, Mayer RM, Taub A: Evidence for peripheral neurotoxic effect of trichloroethylene. *NEUROLOGY* 20:599–606, 1970.

Henschler D, Broser F, Hopf HC: "Polyneuritis cranialis" from poisoning by chlorinated acetylenes. *ARCH TOXIKOL* 26:62–75, 1970. (German)

Heuner W, Petzold E: Severe poisonings from an oxygen breathing apparatus (from trichloroethylene?) *ZBL ARBEITSMED* 2:4–11, 1952. (German)

Humphrey JH, McClelland M: Cranial nerve palsies with herpes following general anesthesia. *BR MED J* 1:315–318, 1944.

Kalinowsky L: Industrial sensory paralyses of the trigeminal. *Z GES NEUROL PSYCHIATR* 110:245–256, 1927.

Kung E, Isenschmid R: On the toxic action of trichloroethylene on the eye. *KLIN MONATSBL AUGENHEILKD* 94:577–585, 1935. (German)

Kylin B, Axell K, et al: Effect of inhaled trichloroethylene on the CNS as measured by optokinetic nystagmus. *ARCH ENVIRON HEALTH* 15:48–52, 1967.

Lachnit V, Rankl W: Chronic trichloroethylene poisoning. *Z UNFALLMED BERUFSKR* 43:334–341, 1950. (German)

Luvoni R, Penzani B: Toxic action of trichloroethylene on the organ of vision. *RASS MED IND* 24:27–40, 1955. (Italian)

McAuley JD: Trichloroethylene and trigeminal anesthesia. *BR MED J* 11:713, 1943.

McClelland M: Some toxic effects following Trilene decomposition. *PROC ROY SOC MED* 37:526–528, 1944.

McNally WD: A case of phosgene poisoning due to the inhalation of decomposition products of trichloroethylene. *IND MED* 6:539–544, 1937.

Maloof CC: Burns of the skin produced by trichloroethylene vapors at room temperature. *J IND HYG* 31:295–296, 1949.

Matruchot D: The role of impurities in trichloroethylene poisoning. *ZBL GEWERBEHYG* 27:112, 1940. (*CHEM ABSTR* 36:3548.)

Meyer H: Investigations on the poisonous action of trichlorothylene, especially on the eye. *KLIN MONATSBL AUGENHEILKD* 83:309–317, 1929. (German)

Mitchell ABS, Parsons-Smith BG: Trichloroethylene neuropathy. *BR MED J* 1:422–423, 1969.

Plessner: On trigeminal injury from trichloroethylene poisoning. *BERLIN KLIN WOCHENSCHR* 53:25, 1916. (German)

Rohrschneider W: The influence on corneal sensitivity by trichloroethylene (Chlorylen). *ZBL AUGENHEILKD* 58:12, 1925. (German)

Saunders RA: A new hazard in closed environmental atmospheres. *ARCH ENVIRON HEALTH* 14:380–384, 1967.

Savic S, Baaske J, Hockwin O: Biochemical changes in the rabbit eye in poisoning by trichloroethylene. *GRAEFES ARCH OPHTHALMOL* 175:1–6, 1968. (German)

Savic S, Hockwin O: Biochemical changes in the rabbits eye in poisoning by organic solvents. *OPHTHALMOLOGICA ADDIT AD* 158:359–363, 1969. (German)

Smith GF: Trichloroethylene: a review. *BR J IND MED* 23:249–262, 1966.

Stuber K: Health disturbances in industrial use of trichloroethylene. *ARCH GEWER-BEPATH GEWERBEHYG* 2:398–456, 1931. (German)

Tabacchi G, Corsico R, Gallenelli R: Retrobulbar neuritis from suspected chronic poisoning by trichloroethylene. *ANN OTTALMOL CLIN OCUL* 92:787–792, 1977. (Italian)

Vernon RJ, Ferguson RK: Effects of trichloroethylene on visual motor performance. *ARCH ENVIRON HEALTH* 18:894–900, 1969.

Waters EM, Gerstner HB, Huff JE: Trichloroethylene. *J TOXICOL ENVIRON HEALTH* 2:671–707, 1977.

Trichlorofluoromethane (Freon 11), a liquid used mainly as a refrigerant, has no known systemic toxic effect on the eye. It is reported to have produced no harmful effects on rabbit eyes when nine applications of 0.1 ml were made during an eleven-day period.[a] Also, exposing the eyes of rabbits to five-second bursts of the propellant from a distance of 20 cm from the cornea five days a week for a month is said to have produced nothing more than hyperemia of the eye lasting several hours, and mild inflammation of the eyelids.[b]

   a. Trichlorofluoromethane (Fluorotrichloromethane, Trichloromonofluoromethane, Fluorocarbon No. 11) Hygienic guide series. *AM IND HYG ASSOC J* 29:517–520, 1968.
   b. Quevauviller A: Hygiene and safety of propellants for medicated aerosols. *PRODUITS PHARM* 20:14, 1965. (Abstr: *FOOD COSMET TOXICOL* 4:467, 1966.)

Trichloromethane sulfonyl chloride has tear gas properties that have been of military interest.[155]

Trichloromethanethiol (perchloromethyl mercaptan) is a stink and tear gas that has been of military interest.[155,227] It is also irritating to the respiratory tract.[227]

Trichlorophenol (2,4,6-trichlorophenol), a fungicide, in contact with the eye is said to cause severe irritation and lacrimation.[36,46,215] Dust or fumes from heating the material are also said to cause pain and irritation of the eyes and nose, but not to cause significant injury.[a]

> a. McCollister DD, Lockwood DT, Rowe VK: Toxicological information on 2,4,5-trichlorophenol. *TOXICOL APPL PHARMACOL* 3:63–70, 1961.

2,4,6-Trichloropyrimidine volatilizes readily with heat, and has been described as a lacrimatory, lung irritant and vesicant substance, but cases of injury of the eye appear not to have been reported.[73]

1,1,3-Trichlorotrifluoroacetone has been described by Deichmann and Gerarde as a liquid that is irritant to the skin and volatilizes to give vapors that are lacrimogenic and irritant to the lungs.[37]

Trifluorotrichloroethane (1,1,2-trichloro-1,2,2-trifluoroethane) applied to rabbit eyes is reported to be innocuous or nearly so.[a, b]

> a. 1,1,2-Trichloro-1,2,2-trifluoroethane. *AM IND HYG ASSOC J* 29:521–525, 1968.
> b. Deprat P, Delsuat L, Gradiski D: Irritant power of the principal aliphatic chlorinated solvents. *EUR J TOXICOL ENVIRON HYG* 9:171–177, 1976.

Tricresyl phosphate (tri-*ortho*-cresyl phosphate, tri-o-cresyl phosphate, tritolyl phosphate) has caused thousands of poisonings, almost all from ingestion of adulterated food oils, Jamaica ginger, apiol, or "phospho-creosote." In a few instances, poisoning has occurred without known ingestion, likely by absorption through the skin.[f] Of the three isomers of tricresyl phosphate, the *ortho* isomer is by far the most toxic, and it is much more toxic than *triphenyl phosphate*. Unlike organophosphorus cholinesterase inhibitors, the tricresyl phosphates do not cause miosis.

The characteristics of tricresyl phosphate poisoning, whether from acute or chronic absorption, consist of an initial upset of the gastrointestinal tract; then in about ten days discomfort begins in the distal portions of the arms and legs, usually soreness, aching, and feeling of numbness, but little sensory involvement. In another ten days this is followed by paralyses of arms and legs, mostly peripheral to the elbows and knees.[f] Usually there is some improvement subsequently, but many victims have been disabled permanently. Autopsy examinations have shown, in addition to damage of peripheral motor nerves, damage of anterior horn cells and pyramidal tract.[l] The paralysis is commonly known as *jake* or *ginger paralysis*. It has been reproduced and studied in animals.[f]

In typical tricresyl phosphate poisoning there is no disturbance of vision or eye complication.[b,c,f,l] In rare cases ocular disturbances have been attributed to tricresyl phosphate, but so far without conclusive evidence.

The question of ocular involvement was raised by Werden in 1932 as a result of a survey of fifty patients who had peripheral motor palsies and were thought to have been poisoned by tricresyl phosphate.[j] He was of the opinion that irregularity or inequality of the pupils and poorer reaction to light than to accommodation were common in this group, and that temporal pallor of the discs and blurring of the nasal margins were frequently present. These findings could be explained by the fact that the patients were chronic alcoholics, and in many instances were syphilitic. In two patients definite optic atrophy was found, but was thought probably to have been caused by syphilis.[i] Measurements of vision or visual fields were not reported.

A patient, described in 1950 by Michaud, developed symptoms of polyneuritis and muscular weakness which were thought to be attributable to chronic poisoning by tricresyl phosphate in varnish with which he worked. He also developed central scotoma and optic neuritis in one eye, and when he died five years later (of pneumonia) was found to have demyelinization (atrophy) in both optic nerves, as well as in the sciatic and other peripheral nerves. The author thought it possible that the patient had had methanol poisoning as well as poisoning by tricresyl phosphate.[g]

In shoe-makers in Italy tricresyl phosphate in the adhesive was initially thought to be the cause of headache, vertigo, loss of appetite, parethesias and decrease in strength of the arms and legs.[d] Eye examinations in eleven patients showed no disturbance of accommodation or oculomotion, but did reveal visual disturbances in three of the patients. The visual acuities in each eye of these patients ranged from 2/50 to 6/10. The visual fields showed no significant peripheral abnormality, but did reveal multiple pericentral scotomas in all eyes of the three patients, mostly within 20° of fixation, tending to be most dense in the centrocecal region. Ophthalmoscopy showed only temporal pallor of the optic nerveheads, consistent with the finding of central scotomas and suggestive of optic neuritis. However, subsequently it was shown that there was not enough tricresyl phosphate to cause significant poisoning. Also, there was evidence to implicate paraffin hydrocarbons, particularly *n-hexane*.[a]

Staehelin has been quoted as reporting that 10 per cent of patients with paralysis of legs or hands from tri-o-cresyl phosphate poisoning had temporary paralysis of accommodation.[f]

Strong evidence against ocular involvement in triaryl phosphate poisoning has been provided in an authoritative survey published by Albertini, Gross, and Zinn in 1968 concerning an epidemic of 10,000 cases of serious flaccid and spastic paralysis from contaminated cooking oils which occurred in Morocco in 1959. From this study it was concluded that "cranial nerves appear to have remained immune." Ophthalmoscopic examination "showed no indication of damage to the optic nerves." Also, they stated, "the nerves of the eye muscles had also remained normal." However, in one locality in Morocco a few cases of trigeminal nerve sensory disturbance with corneal anesthesia were observed in this survey.[b]

A long-term follow-up by Morgan in 1978 of eleven patients poisoned and paralyzed to varying degrees by tricresyl phosphate in 1930 disclosed no cranial nerve involvement.[i]

Experimentally, degeneration of motor nerve cells and peripheral nerves has been induced in animals by means of triorthocresyl phosphate, tricresyl phosphite, and triphenyl phosphate, and lesions have been observed histologically in the nuclei of the nerves of the extraocular muscles of animals.[g] However, no abnormality of oculomotion seems to have been noted in animals or patients.

A single accidental splash contact of tricresyl phosphate with a patient's eye has been briefly mentioned and noted not to have produced a burn of the eye.[e] (For comparison with other organophosphorus neurotoxins, see INDEX for *Organophosphorus compounds.*)

a. Abbritti G, Siracusa A, et al: Shoe-makers polyneuropathy in Italy. *BR J IND MED* 33:92, 1976.

b. Albertini A, Gross D, Zinn WM (Eds): TRIARYL-PHOSPHATE POISONING IN MOROCCO 1959. Stuttgart, Georg Thieme Verlag, 1968.

c. Aring CD: The systemic nervous affinity of triorthocresyl phosphate (Jamaica ginger palsy). *BRAIN* 65:34–47, 1942.

d. Battistini A: Disturbances of the visual apparatus in an epidemic of motor polyneuritis from poisoning. *ARCH OTTALMOL* 62:53–65, 1958. (Italian)

e. Calhoun JA: Tricresyl Phosphate. *J AM MED ASSOC* 178:1123, 1961.

f. Hunter D, Perry KMA, Evans RB: Toxic polyneuritis arising during the manufacture of tricresyl phosphate. *BR J IND MED* 1:227–231, 1944.

g. Lillie RD, Smith MI: The histopathology of some neurotoxic phenol esters. *NAT INST HEALTH BULL* 160:54–62, 1932.

h. Michaud L: Poisoning by triorthocresyl phosphate. *BULL SCHWEIZ AKAD MED WISS* 6:125–129, 1950. (French)

i. Morgan JP, Penovich P: Jamaica ginger paralysis. *ARCH NEUROL* 35:530–532, 1978.

j. Staehelin R: On triorthocresyl phosphate poisoning. *SCHWEIZ MED WOCHENSCHR* 7:1–5, 1941. (Cited by Albertini.[b])

k. Werden DH: Ascending paralysis resulting from the drinking of Jamaica ginger. *ANN INTERN MED* 5:1257–1266, 1932.

l. Zeligs MA: Upper motor neuron sequelae in "Jake" paralysis. *J NERV MENT DIS* 87:464–470, 1938.

Triethanolamine is a moderately strong base. Tested by application of a drop to rabbit eyes, according to one test it caused moderate, presumably transient injury, graded 5 on a scale of 1 to 10 after twenty-four hours,[27] and in another test caused negligible irritation.[324]

Triethylamine is strongly alkaline, and when a drop is applied to a rabbit's eye, causes severe injury, graded 9 on a scale of 1 to 10 after twenty-four hours.[225] Tests of aqueous solutions on rabbit eyes at pH 10 and pH 11 indicate the injuriousness is related principally to the degree of alkalinity.[89] Chronic exposure of rabbits to triethylamine vapors at concentrations as low as 50 ppm in air causes multiple erosions of the cornea and conjunctiva, and injuries of the lungs in the course of six weeks.[a]

a. Brieger H, Hodes WA: Toxic effects of exposure to vapors of aliphatic amines. *ARCH IND HYG* 3:287–291, 1951.

Triethylenediamine, a catalyst used in making polyurethane foams, can cause corneal disturbance in workers exposed to the vapor. It is reported to have induced fine corneal epithelial edema and to have caused people to see haloes around lights several hours after exposure. This seems to be similar to the effects of several other volatile amines.[a] (See INDEX for *Amines.*)

Aqueous solutions tested on rabbit eyes by applying 0.5 ml of a 5% solution caused corneal injury which was considered "minor," but 25% solutions caused more severe injury.[b]

a. Dernehl CU: Health hazards associated with polyurethane foams. *J OCCUP MED* 8:59–62, 1966.

b. Goldberg ME, Johnson HE: Autonomic ganglion activity and acute toxicologic effects of N,N,N',N'-tetramethyl-1,3-butanediamine and triethylenediamine. *TOXICOL APPL PHARMACOL* 4:522–545, 1962.

Triethylene glycol applied to rabbit eyes causes immediate pain, but no injury detectable twenty-four hours later.[27] Splash contamination in man likewise causes acute smarting, and this may be followed by transitory disturbance of the corneal epithelium with gradually diminishing sensation and signs of irritation, but no persistent injury is to be expected.[27]

Triethyl tin causes edema of the brain in human beings and animals. A large number of cases of accidental poisoning which occurred in 1954 in France provided the first extensive documentation of the toxic effects of triethyl tin and other organo-tin compounds on human beings, particularly on the eye and vision. Prior to that, according to Flury and Zernik, ethyl tin and methyl tin compounds, especially tetraethyl tin, had been reputed to be toxic to the nervous system, particularly to the optic nerve and retina, but information on the effects on human beings was fragmentary.[61]

The mass poisoning which has furnished most of our information occurred when a proprietary medicine containing tin alkyl compounds, known as Stalinon, was sold for treatment of furuncolosis and other staphylococcal infections in France. At least 1,000 people are believed to have taken the medicine; 217 are known to have been poisoned, and 100 to 110 died.[c, 194] Stalinon is said to have been composed principally of *diethyl tin*, plus smaller amounts of *triethyl tin*. Animal experiments have indicated the latter to be especially toxic.

Symptoms of poisoning after taking Stalinon usually started in about four days. The most frequent symptom was headache, which was present in almost all patients, sometimes extremely severe. Psychic disturbances were common, especially clouding of consciousness. Convulsions occurred occasionally. Coma or loss of consciousness apparently occurred only in those who died, or who had severe aftereffects.[a] Transitory paralyses of one or more extremities, lasting a few hours, were not unusual,[a] but permanent disabilities were uncommon.[b]

During acute poisoning the most frequent visual complaint was photophobia, which occurred in about one-third of the cases. Compared to headache, photophobia was a minor complaint, but in some cases was sufficient for patients to wear dark glasses. Other visual disturbances occurred relatively uncommonly, but included occasional amblyopia or transitory blindness, and disturbances of extraocular muscles.[a]

In a study of 111 cases of poisoning, examination showed the fundi to be normal in two-thirds despite severe headache and undoubted cerebral edema. Even among forty-eight patients who died, the fundi remained normal in thirty-eight, but there was congestion or slight edema of the optic nervehead in sixteen cases, definite edema in thirteen cases, stasis in five, and partial or complete optic atrophy in four.[a]

The eyes may have been affected particularly severely in children.[h] A twelve-year old boy who had signs of encephalitis, but no disturbance of vision, was found to have enormous papilledema with hemorrhages and dilated veins; he died in a few days. A nine-year-old girl similarly had symptoms of encephalitis and developed enormous bilateral papilledema with numerous hemorrhages about the disc, but suffered no reduction of visual acuity. Her edema decreased gradually and was completely gone in six weeks. The edema of the nervehead improved at the same time as the symptoms of encephalitis. A sixteen-year-old girl having symptoms of encephalitis also developed bilateral papilledema, but, in addition, her vision began to decrease, reaching a low of 2/10 in the course of two weeks, then gradually improved despite persistence of edema. This girl's vision and fundi returned completely to normal in six weeks. (In the last two cases it was thought that treatment with dimercaprol may have helped the recovery.[h])

Permanent impairment of vision, mostly apparently from optic atrophy, has been uncommon, occurring in six patients in a series of 210 cases of poisoning.[a] One extraordinary patient became bilaterally permanently blind in twenty-four hours.[a]

In one noteworthy case a woman took Stalinon for five days, then began to have very severe headaches, accompanied on the eighth day by blindness which lasted for about fifteen minutes. At that time she was found to have slight papilledema without congestion. She became completely foggy mentally for three to four weeks. Surgical exploration showed extensive diffuse edema of the brain, which caused the ventricles to be abnormally small. In the course of a year the patient gradually improved, although still complaining of frequent headaches and continuing to have psychic disturbance. She then had a rapid decrease in visual acuity again, accompanied by bilateral papilledema. Ventriculography at that time showed no abnormality. The optochiasmatic region was explored surgically, and although not described in detail, was said to have shown arachnoiditis. Subsequently vision recovered, but headaches and psychic disturbances continued.[i,j]

Disturbance of the extraocular muscles has occurred in rare instances.[a,e] Strabismus from sixth nerve paralysis was presumably attributable to increased intracranial pressure.

The cause of the headaches, papilledema, disturbance of vision, and extraocular muscle palsy has been attributed to cerebral edema of a special type (status spongiosus), associated with elevated cerebrospinal fluid pressure. The edema appears to be principally interstitial in the white matter of the brain, and has tended to compress, rather than enlarge, the ventricles. The edematous character of the brain has been established both at surgery and at autopsy. Surgical decompression of the cranium has been carried out in several cases, and at times appeared to be a lifesaving measure.[a,c,d,55]

Experimental administration of Stalinon to mice, rabbits, and monkeys was reported by Alajouanine and associates in 1958 to produce changes in the central nervous system almost exactly the same anatomically (cerebral medullary edema) and symptomatically as had been observed in human beings.[a]

The same characteristic toxic effects that were observed with Stalinon have been repeatedly produced by administration of triethyl tin to animals. *Diethyl tin*, the other component of Stalinon, does not cause cerebral edema. *Tetra-alkyl tin* compounds in animal experiments have produced convulsive movements, closure of the eyelids, photophobia, weakness, paralysis, and respiratory failure, but owe their toxicity to conversion to trialkyl tin compounds.

Triethyl tin and other trialkyl tin compounds have been reported by Barnes and Stoner to have a selective inhibitory effect on oxygen uptake by brain slices, and to inhibit oxidative phosphorylation by mitochondria.[b,c]

In investigation of the relationship of cerebral edema to optic nerve disturbances in animals, Scheinberg and associates in 1966 reported that poisoning of rabbits with triethyl tin sulfate caused edema of the optic nerves in their proximal portions like tracts of cerebral white matter rather than like peripheral nerves.[k] Cranial nerves other than the optic nerves and the peripheral nerves of the rabbits did not become edematous. In an extensive study of papilledema produced experimentally in animals, Hedges and Zaren reported in 1969 that triethyl tin acetate raised the intracranial pressure in both cats and monkeys, but that only in the monkeys was this associated with swelling of the orbital portions of the optic nerves.[l] The swelling in monkeys was most at the chiasm, moderate in the orbital portions of the optic nerves, and least in compact regions adjacent to the lamina cribrosa of the sclera or the bony foramen of the orbit. Hedges and Zaren postulated that differences in anatomy of the venous arrangements at the optic nervehead could explain the facts that human beings and primates developed papilledema from swelling of the retrobulbar portion of the optic nerve, but that the lower animals such as cats and rabbits did not develop papilledema. The same investigators showed also, by means of fluorescein angiography and fluorescein microscopy, that there was no defect of the blood-brain barrier and no leakage from vessels in the edematous nerveheads of the monkeys. Vision seemed not to be affected in either the poisoned monkeys or the cats, although their pupils became large and sluggish.[l] This seems to correspond fairly well to the findings in the numerous cases of poisoning of human beings by Stalinon, in which vision usually was not affected unless secondary optic atrophy developed.

In experiments carried out by Pecori-Giraldi et al in rabbits with a prime interest in effects on intraocular pressure, it was found that triethyl tin injected intra-peritoneally or into the vitreous body had little influence, but when injected into the anterior chamber it caused a rise in intraocular pressure of 12 to 30 mm Hg, beginning within 24 hours and lasting a week or longer.[g] This was associated with fibrinous exudate into the anterior and posterior chambers, hemorrhages in the iris and ciliary processes, and synechias in the angle of the anterior chamber.

External contact of triethyl tin with the eyes or with the skin would presumably cause much irritation and injury, since trialkyl tin compounds and also dialkyl tin compounds commonly have vesicant and lacrimatory effects, most notable in the series from methyl to butyl derivatives.[f] Specific information on contact toxicity of organo-tin compounds is to be found elsewhere in this volume under the headings *Dibutyl tin dichloride, Dibutyl tin dilaurate, Bis(tri-n-butyl tin) oxide,* and *Triphenyl tin hydroxide.* (See INDEX.) (For comparison with neurotoxins having similar effects, see *Status spongiosus* in the INDEX.)

a. Alajouanine T, Derobert L, Thieffry S: Comprehensive clinical study of 210 cases of poisoning by organic salts of tin. *REV NEUROL* 98:85–96, 1958. (French)

b. Barnes JM, Stoner HB: Toxic properties of some dialkyl and trialkyl tin salts. *BR J IND MED* 15:15–22, 1958.

c. Barnes JM, Stoner HB: Toxicology of tin compounds. *PHARMACOL REV* 11:211–231, 1959.

d. Drault-Toufesco N: Concerning two cases of serious poisoning by stalinon. *BULL SOC OPHTALMOL PARIS* 54–58, 1958. (French)

e. Gayral L, Lazorthes G, Planque J: Hypertensive meningo-encephalitis from poisoning by stalinon, recovered. *REV NEUROL* 98:143–144, 1958.

f. Ingham RK, Rosenberg SD, Gilman H: Organotin compounds. *CHEM REV* 60:459–439, 1960.

g. Pecori-Giraldi J, Pelegrino N, et al: Experimental triethyltin ocular hypertension. *KLIN MONATSBL AUGENHEILKD* 170:579–586, 1977. (German)

h. Pesme P: Ocular complications observed in four children poisoned by "Stalinon." *ARCH FR PEDIATR* 12:327–328, 1955. (French)

i. Rouzaud M, Lutier J: Subacute cerebromeningeal edema due to a poisoning of current interest. *PRESSE MED* 62:1075, 1954. (French)

j. Rouzaud M: Poisoning by stalinon. *REV NEUROL* 98:140–142, 1958.

k. Scheinberg LC, Taylor JM, et al: Optic and peripheral nerve response to triethyltin intoxication in the rabbit: biochemical and ultrastructural studies. *J NEUROPATH EXP NEUROL* 25:202–213, 1966.

l. Hedges TR, Zaren HA: Experimental papilledema: A study of cats and monkeys intoxicated with triethyl tin acetate. *NEUROLOGY* 19:359–366, 1969.

Triethyltrithiophosphite is a very toxic substance. A 0.1 M solution instilled into the conjunctival sacs of rabbits caused death in some animals within a week. It also caused corneal opacity. In animals which survived, the corneas cleared in the course of a month. Flushing the eye with water or 1% silver nitrate solution gave no demonstrable improvement, and in some instances appeared to cause worse opacification. A related compound, *trimethyltrithiophosphite*, also caused corneal opacities, but less severe and more readily reversible than from the triethyl compound.[a]

a. Rockhold WT, Wright HA, et al: Toxicological studies on trimethyl and triethyltrithiophosphites. *ARCH IND HEALTH* 12:483–493, 1955.

Trifluoperazine hydrochloride (Stelazine), a phenothiazine derivative antipsychotic, can induce extrapyramidal side effects resembling parkinsonism. It can also produce oculogyric crises.[e] Blurring of vision has been mentioned occasionally, associated with dryness of the mouth, which suggests that the blurring might be due to anticholinergic mydriasis and cycloplegia. However, pupillography in schizophrenic patients taking trifluoperazine has shown no significant influence on the pupil. Disturbance of vision appears to be rare during use of trifluoperazine, as exemplified in a report of no complaints regarding vision in one series of sixty-eight patients receiving this drug.[d]

Because certain phenothiazine drugs, in particular *thioridazine*, have been known to have caused pigmentary retinopathy, all other phenothiazine derivatives, including trifluoperazine, have come under suspicion, but in the case of trifluoperazine there seems to be a report of only one patient representing a possible instance of induced pigmentary retinopathy, which was noted in 1962 after a mean dose of 50 mg per day was taken for 153 days.[h] Another patient was mentioned in 1968 by Wheeler and colleagues as having "ocular pigmentation," but subsequently Wheeler made clear that there was no *retinal* pigmentation.[i,j]

Because *chlorpromazine,* another phenothiazine drug, has produced pigmented deposits on the front of the lens and in the cornea, all phenothiazine derivatives, including trifluoperazine have been watched for similar side effects, but because most schizophrenic patients have been treated with several phenothiazine derivatives, usually including chlorpromazine, it has been difficult to establish which of these drugs may produce these anterior segment pigment deposits. There have been suspicions,[f,9] but no conclusive evidence that trifluoperazine produces deposits in lens or cornea.[b] A study by Prien et al in 1970, with follow-up by Crane et al in 1971, led to a conclusion that 80 mg/day for 1.5 to 2 years produced no different ocular findings than placebo medication in controls.[a,g]

Chronic administration of chlorpromazine to dogs produced accumulations of granules in their corneas, but trifluoperazine produced no such abnormality.[278]

a. Crane GE, Johnson AW, Buffaloe WJ: Long-term treatment with neuroleptic drugs and eye opacities. *AM J PSYCHIATR* 127:1045–1054, 1971.

b. DeLong SL: Incidence and significance of chlorpromazine-induced eye changes. *DIS NERV SYS* 29:19–22, 1968.

c. Dundee JW, Moore J, et al: Drugs given before anesthesia. *BR J ANAESTH* 37:332–353, 1965.

d. Honigfeld G, Rosenblum M, et al: Behavioral improvement in the older schizophrenic patient. *J AM GERIAT SOC* 8:57–72, 1965.

e. Lee SH, Knopp W: Pupillary reactivity in medical students, schizophrenics without phenothiazines and schizophrenics treated with trifluoperazine. *EYE EAR NOSE THROAT MONTHLY* 47:55–61, 1968.

f. Margolis LH, Goble JL: Lenticular opacities with prolonged phenothiazine therapy. *J AM MED ASSOC* 193:95–97, 1965.

g. Prien RF, DeLong SL, et al: Ocular changes occurring with prolonged high dose chlorpromazine therapy. *ARCH GEN PSYCHIATR* 23:464–468, 1970.

h. Reboton J Jr, Weakley RD, et al: Pigmentary retinopathy and iridocycloplegia in psychiatric patients. *J NEUROPSYCHIATR* 3:311–316, 1962.

i. Wheeler RH, Bhalerao VR, Gilkes MJ: Ocular pigmentation, extrapyramidal symptoms and phenothiazine dosage. *BR J PSYCHIATR* 115:687–690, 1968.

j. Wheeler RH: Personal communication, January 1977.

dl-(p-Trifluoromethylphenyl) isopropylamine hydrochloride (P-1727) causes retinopathy in rats and dogs when given at very high doses orally.[a] In rats no ophthalmoscopic changes were induced, but disappearance of rods and cones, degeneration in other layers, and in some areas complete atrophy of the retina were found histologically after feeding for three months. In dogs the same dosage given orally caused constriction of the retinal vessels which could be seen in about one-half hour, followed by an appearance of hyperemia of the fundi. In five months the dogs were blind, and the fundi had a slight peppery pigment disturbance recognizable ophthalmoscopically, also persistent constriction of the vessels and ischemia of the retina. Histologically at this stage the rods and cones had disappeared and pigment had migrated into what remained of the retina. The endothelial cells had disappeared from the walls of the retinal capillaries and melanin was found in the walls of the veins. It was postulated that constriction of the vessels, ischemia, and anoxia in both retina and choroid were responsible for the damage.

  a. Delahunt CS, O'Connor RA, et al: Toxic retinopathy following prolonged treatment with dl-(p-trifluoromethylphenyl) isopropylamine hydrochloride (P-1727) in experimental animals. *TOXICOL APPL PHARMACOL* 5:298–305, 1963.

Trifluperidol (Triperidol), an antipyschotic butyrophenone derivative, has been suspected as a cause of cataract in Japan. Okamoto and Fujiwara described a 34-year-old patient who had been treated with Triperidol and chlorpromazine for schizophrenia, and had developed bilateral cataracts with complete opacity, water clefts, and some swelling of both lenses.[b] The corneas and anterior chambers were normal. In support of their suspicion, they cited single cases of cataracts associated with use of Triperidol that had been reported by Honda,[a] by Setogawa,[c] and by Yamamoto.[d] (These are quoted below as cited.)

  a. Honda S, et al: Drug-induced cataract in mentally ill subjects. *JPN J CLIN OPHTHAL-MOL* 28:521–526, 1974.
  b. Okamoto S, Fujiwara H: Total cataract formation after Triperidol therapy. *ACTA SOC OPHTHALMOL JPN* 82:415–417, 1978.
  c. Setogawa T: Lens changes associated with long-term psychotropica therapy. *YONAGO ACTA MEDICA* 19:103, 1975.
  d. Yamamoto K, et al: *JAPANESE REVIEW OF CLINICAL OPHTHALMOLOGY* 71:401–405, 1977.

Trifluridine (trifluorothymidine, Viroptic), an ophthalmic antiviral, does not retard healing of corneal epithelial wounds in rabbits when applied as in clinical use, though histologically the epithelial cells may appear abnormal, and development of stromal wound strength may be delayed.[308, 315] In patients, no ocular toxicity has been associated with short-term use of 1% eyedrops, but prolonged treatment of herpes simplex keratitis has caused corneal epithelial dysplasia, with ground glass appearance, and conceivably precancerous potentiality.[a]

  a. Maudgal PC, Van Damme B, Misotten L: Corneal epithelial dysplasia after trifluridine use. *GRAEFES ARCH OPHTHALMOL* 220:6–12, 1983.

Trihexyphenidyl hydrochloride (Antitrem, Artane, Benzhexol, Pipanol, Tremin), anticholinergic and antiparkinsonian, given systemically may cause mydriasis, blurring of vision from cycloplegia, and dry mouth. One report describes three cases of angle-closure glaucoma attributed to this drug.[b] As described elsewhere under *Anticholinergics,* this is a risk in eyes that are anatomically prone to angle-closure because of small, shallow anterior chamber and narrow angle.

Testing for cataract formation by feeding to chicks was negative.[a]

  a. Cunningham RW, et al. *J PHARMACOL EXP THER* 96:151–165, 1949.
  b. Friedman Z, Neumann E: Benzhexol induced blindness in Parkinson's disease. *BR MED J* 1:605, 1972.

Trimethadione (Tridione), an anticonvulsant, causes an altered sensitivity of the eyes to light, commonly in adult or adolescent patients, but rarely in young children. The most common symptom is glare in bright light with fading of colors.[c] Adaptation to changes in light intensity appears to be much delayed, and unpleasant dazzling whiteness is experienced particularly on stepping from a building or other shelter into the sunlight. The experience is similar to that of the normal eye but exaggerated and greatly prolonged. When the patient is constantly in subdued illumination, the vision is essentially normal. When the drug is discontinued, the symptoms gradually disappear, and there seems to be no evidence of permanent damage or morphologic change in the eyes of human beings.[b,i,46,255] Sloane and Gilger established that the functional disturbance occurs at the retinal level.[h] Siegel and Arden pointed out that in human beings the action is specifically and entirely on the cone mechanism, leaving rod sensitivity unimpaired.[g]

Acute poisoning with trimethadione in rabbits has caused reduction of the b-wave in four to five days. The a-wave became extinguished after five to seven days. Luizzi and Franchino concluded that this acute poisoning had permanent effect on the first and second neurons in the rabbit retina.[e]

A severe toxic reaction of skin and mucous membranes with involvement of the conjunctival sac, as in Stevens-Johnson syndrome, has been described in a child receiving both trimethadione and Protactyl.[a]

In another rare case a ten-year-old girl under treatment for epilepsy developed what appeared to be myasthenia gravis with diplopia and ptosis at about the same time she developed proteinuria which was attributed to trimethadione. The proteinurea cleared when the drug was stopped, and the myasthenia responded to pyridostigmine.[f]

A *fetal trimethadione syndrome* has been described affecting the offspring of epileptic mothers receiving this medication during pregnancy. The eye involvement consists of V-shaped eyebrows and epicanthus, more rarely myopia and strabismus, associated with a number of non-ocular congenital anomalies.

a. Budde E: Hyperplastic conjunctival proliferation after several months of administration of an anti-epileptic (Tridione). *KLIN MONATSBL AUGENHEILKD* 146:262–266, 1965. (German)

b. Capello H: Visual effects of tridione. *ARCH BRAS OFTALMOL* 11:78–79, 1948. (*EXCERPTA MED* 3:1910.)

c. Dekking HM: Visual disturbances due to Tridione. *ACTA CONG OPHTHALMOL* 1:465–467, 1950.

d. Lennox W: The petit mal epilepsies. Their treatment with tridione. *J AM MED ASSOC* 129:1069, 1945.

e. Liuzzi L, Franchino M: Electroretinographic findings in acute poisoning from Tridione in the rabbit. *RASS ITAL OTTALMOL* 35:325–328, 1967. (Italian)

f. Peterson H. deC: Association of trimethadione therapy and myasthenia gravis. *N ENGL J MED* 274:506–507, 1966.

g. Siegel EM, Arden GB: The effect of drugs on colour vision. In Herxheimer (Ed): DRUGS AND SENSORY FUNCTIONS. Boston, Little, 1968, pp. 210–228.

h. Sloane LL, Gilger AP: Visual effects of tridione. *AM J OPHTHALMOL* 30:1387–1405, 1947.

i. Vail D: Tridione and the eye. *AM J OPHTHALMOL* 29:606–607, 1946.

j. Zackai EH, Mellman WJ, et al: The fetal trimethadione syndrome. *J PEDIATR* 87:280–284, 1975.

Trimethylamine

Trimethylamine is a gas, having an unpleasant fishy ammoniacal odor. Tests of single drops of aqueous solutions applied to animal eyes have shown that 1% solution causes severe irritation, 5% causes hemorrhagic conjunctivitis, and 16.5% causes severe reaction with conjunctival hemorrhages, corneal edema, and opacities, followed by some clearing but much vascularization.[63]

In an accident a student placed a glass ampule of liquified trimethylamine in dry ice and was attempting to open it when it exploded. The student was wearing glasses, but a blast of vapor struck one eye. There were no mechanical injuries, but it was very soon observed that the epithelium had been lost from the cornea. The epithelium healed promptly. There was no edema of the corneal stroma, and the eye was entirely normal within four or five days.[a] This certainly was a much milder reaction than would have been produced by trimethylamine in liquid form.

a. Dunphy EB: Personal communication, 1968.

3,3,5-Trimethylcyclohexanol-1

3,3,5-Trimethylcyclohexanol-1 has been tested on rabbit eyes and found to cause severe injury, graded 9 on a scale of 1 to 10 after twenty-four hours.[27,224] This is a surprising degree of injury from an apparently simple compound, except that it may be noted that this substance is not greatly different in structure from *menthol*, which is also surprisingly injurious to the cornea.

Trimethyl tin

Trimethyl tin (trimethytin chloride) has been relatively little studied compared to *triethyl tin*, but it is known to produce irreversible damage to the brain in rats and marmosets. The eyes of marmosets have been examined after acute poisoning and showed many pyknotic nuclei in the inner and outer nuclear layers of the retina.[a] All layers of retinal neurons are affected in rats.[b] Visual evoked responses from the visual cortex and optic tract in poisoned rats have shown alterations also suggestive of retinal changes.[c]

a. Aldridge WN, Brown AW, et al: Brain damage due to trimethyltin compounds. *LANCET* 2:692–693, 1981.
b. Bouldin TW, Goines ND, Krigman MR: Trimethyltin retinopathy. *J NEUROPATHOL EXP NEUROL* 43:162–174, 1984.
c. Dyer RS, Howell WE, Wonderlin WF: Visual system dysfunction following acute trimethyltin exposure in rats. *NEUROBEHAV TOXICOL TERATOL* 4:191–195, 1982.

Trimipramine maleate

Trimipramine maleate (Surmontil), an antidepressant, has been suspected in two cases of being responsible for glaucoma in patients with narrow angles or shallow anterior chambers, though the evidence seems to have been rather inconclusive.[210] The fact that trimipramine has been reported to cause dryness of the mouth and blurred vision suggestive of anticholinergic side effects, makes it reasonable to suppose that in patients with anatomically predisposed, very narrow angles, slight mydriasis from the medication could induce angle-closure glaucoma.[a]

a. Today's Drugs: Trimipramine. *BR MED J* 1:98, 1967.

Trinitrobenzene (trinitrobenzol) is alleged to have caused optic neuritis and amblyopia.[77] Chronic intoxication also is said to have caused yellowing of the conjunctiva or sclera. These reports of intoxication and ocular disturbances have come from the munitions industry where commonly there is exposure to a variety of substances, and it is difficult to be sure of the individual substance responsible. (Compare *Chlorodinitrobenzene, Dinitrobenzene, Dinitrotoluene*, and *Trinitrotoluene.*)

Trinitrotoluene (trinitroltoluol, TNT) may cause irritation of the eyes and skin among munitions workers exposed to its dust or vapor. Toxic effects upon the optic nerve have been reported rarely. Cataracts have been diagnosed in a considerable proportion of chronically exposed workers.

Reis in 1922 reported retrobulbar neuritis in two patients.[k] One worked for four years with pure TNT, and in the course of the fourth year noticed gradual diminution of vision. He then had bilateral central scotomas for red and green and slight temporal pallor of the discs. Vision was 20/100 in both eyes. No cause was found other than exposure to TNT.[f] The other patient worked with TNT for two years, then had diminution of vision to blindness in both eyes overnight. The pupils were dilated and unreactive to light. The optic nerveheads were blurred and hyperemic. Vision improved gradually, but at least a year later was still much subnormal, with definite central scotomas and white optic nerveheads. The man was said not to be alcoholic and not to have been exposed to methanol.

Aiello in 1946, reporting on a patient who had reduction of vision after working with TNT for four years, described different findings. This patient noted diminished vision in the lower field of one eye, and was found to have punctate and flame-shaped retinal hemorrhages with mild papillitis. Four months later this patient had hemorrhage into the vitreous body in the same eye. This patient was also exposed to dinitrophenol and dinitro-o-cresol, but gave no indication of systemic illness.[a]

While the rarity of these cases occasions some skepticism about the relationship to TNT, optic neuritis has been ascribed to several related aromatic nitro compounds such as *chlorodinitrobenzene, dinitrobenzene, dinitrotoluene,* and *trinitrobenzene,* which makes it seem more credible that the optic neuropathy could have been due to the TNT.

A report from the Soviet Union, which is difficult to evaluate, mentions 18 patients with constriction of visual fields by a special method of examination after working with TNT, and describes obtaining marked improvement by oxygen therapy.[i]

Cataracts in people working with TNT have been described in several reports from the Soviet Union since 1953,[b,d,e,f,h,i,l] and more recently from Bulgaria,[m] and Finland.[c,g] In 1953 Glecerov reported that industrial exposure to TNT had been known in the Soviet Union since 1932 to produce lens opacities both in the pupil and at the equator.[b] Drawings were furnished by Tyukina in 1967.[l] Later publications have stressed that the characteristic cataract is an equatorial ring.

Kroll and Kolevatykh in 1965 agreed that TNT produced a special type of lens opacity, occurring at any age after exposure for three or more years and, according to them, consisting at first of opacities at the equator of the lens which did not interfere with vision and could be detected only with the pupil widely dilated. The cataract was said to be gradually progressive, but to be arrested if contact with TNT was discontinued. The cataract was not reversible.[f] Both these authors and Manoilova, who reported in 1968 on 163 people with cataract attributed to TNT, concluded that the cataracts were caused by direct action of TNT on the lens rather than by an indirect effect of systemic poisoning.[f,h]

Hassman and Juran in 1968 detected a remarkably high incidence of cataract in people handling TNT. They reported that twenty-six out of sixty-one people having had average exposure of 8.4 years showed the characteristic peripheral cataract, and that most had no other indications of adverse effect of TNT.[d]

Harkonen and associates reported in 1983 from Finland the results of examination of twelve workers chronically exposed to TNT, finding bilateral peripheral, equatorial cataracts in six.[c] The opacities were of the type described by Hassman and others,[d,e] not affecting visual acuity, and not detectable unless the pupils were very widely dilated. (Photographs were published.) Makitie and Harkonen in 1984 reported on detecting the opacities by coaxial retroillumination.[g] Comparing the workers with these special lens opacities and those without, there was no significant difference in length of exposure to TNT, but the mean age of those with opacities was significantly greater, 43.8 years compared to 35.2 years.[c] None had abnormality of blood glucose or deficiency of glucose-6-phosphate. Zlateva et al have reported from Bulgaria that ring cataracts developed in guinea pigs after months of application of TNT to the skin.[m] Histologic abnormalities were seen in retina and choroid.

a. Aiello G: Poisoning by trinitrotoluene and ocular diseases. *ANN OTTALMOL CLIN OCUL* 72:17–21, 1946. (Italian)

b. Glezerov CY: Cataracts from trinitrotoluene. *VESTN OFTALMOL* 32:21–32, 1953. (English summary)

c. Harkonen H, Karki M, et al: Early equatorial cataracts in workers exposed to trinitrotoluene. *AM J OPHTHALMOL* 95:807–810, 1983.

d. Hassman P, Juran J: Cataract in people working with trinitrololuene. *ARCH GEWER-BEPATH GEWERBEHYG* 24:310–318, 1968.

e. Hassman P: Health state of workers after long lasting contact with trinitrotoluene. *SB VED PR LEK FAK KARL UNIV* 22:1, 1979. (Ref. from Harkonen.)

f. Kroll DS, Kolevatykh VP: Ringlike cataract in chronic intoxication with trinitrotoluene. *OFTALMOL ZH* 20:180–183, 1965. (English summary)

g. Makitie J, Harkonen H, et al: Trinitroluene induced lens opacities and the use of retroillumination photography. *ACTA OPHTHALMOL* (Suppl) 164:40, 1984.

h. Manoilova IK: On the pathogenesis of the crystalline lens involvement following trinitrotoluene action on the human organism. *VESTN OFTALMOL* 4:76–81, 1968. (English summary)

i. Manoilova IK: Injury of the eyes under the long-term effect of trinitrotoluene. *SB NAUCH TR KUIBYSHEV NAUCH–ISSLED INST GIG* 7:170–172, 1972. (English abst)

j. Nemiseev GI, Smolianinova NS: Oxygenotherapy of toxic neuropathies of neurooptic pathway in persons working in contact with nitroderivatives of toluol. *OFTALMOL ZH* 31:352–355, 1976. (English summary)

k. Reis: Optic nerve disease from trinitrotoluene. *Z AUGENHEILKD* 47:199–208, 1022. (German)

l. Tyukina GA: Some features specific to the clinical picture of trinitrotoluene induced cataracts. *VESTN OFTALMOL* 80:43–47, 1967. (English summary)

m.   Zlateva V, Krustev L, Donchev N: Experimental and morphological study of the eyes and liver after trinitrotoluene treatment. *OFTALMOLOGIA (Sofia)* 25:135–141, 1977. (English abstract)

Trioxsalen (Trimethyl psoralen, Trisoralen), a pigmentation agent, given orally, has been tested in rabbits and dogs by daily administration orally for two weeks, and the animals were also exposed daily to longwave ultraviolet. No ocular damage was discoverable by ophthalmoscopy, slit-lamp biomicroscopic, or histologic examinations.[a] (For information on ocular effects of other psoralen derivatives, see *Methoxsalen*.)

a.   Becker SW Jr, West B: Detection of photosensitizers in tissue. *ARCH DERM* 92:457–460, 1965.

Triparanol (MER-29) formerly was used medically to interfere with formation of cholesterol, but was withdrawn after about two years. The principal reason for withdrawal was production of cataracts in less than 1% of patients. The cataracts were first recognized by Kirby in 1961.[c,j,l] In 1967 a summation of clinical and experimental observations on triparanol cataracts was published by Kirby.[k]

The cataracts typically developed only in those who had severe side effects involving the skin and hair, and often the eyelids. Characteristically these patients had taken triparanol for months, and then developed icthyosis, bleaching and loss of hair (sometimes including eyebrows and eyelashes), reddening and thickening of the lid margins. Some patients had slight disturbances of corneal and conjunctival epithelium associated with the skin disturbance and blepharitis, but with no obvious correlation with the induction of cataracts.[o,q,r] Stippled crystalline deposits in the corneal epithelium have been mentioned but not regularly seen.[v]

In some cases the medication was stopped because of the changes in the skin and hair while the vision was still normal and the lenses still clear, and only some months later was gradual decrease in visual acuity noted. Lens opacities were then evident. At their onset the cataracts were described as consisting of both posterior and anterior subcapsular opacities, the posterior having the amber or brassy granular character of cataracta complicata, and the anterior appearing as fine white lacy branching opacities. These were accompanied by peripheral cortical opacities and lines of opacity extending from the equator. It was supposed that if the equator of the lens could be seen as readily as the axial portion, the abnormalities might be seen to develop first there and then to spread to the posterior and anterior subcapsular regions.[b]

Cataracts in patients characteristically developed rapidly to a stage requiring surgical extraction in several months. The surgical results apparently were no different from those of other types of cataracts.

Cataracts in animals were first produced in dogs by feeding very high doses, and at first the cataracts were thought to be reversible, because the opaque appearance disappeared and the fundi became visible again, but Cogan discovered that this clearing was due to spontaneous absorption of opaque lens substance rather than reversal of opacification.[d]

Unsuccessful attempts have been made to induce cataracts with triparanol in rabbits[k] and monkeys.[n]

In rats most investigators have succeeded in inducing cataracts by feeding high dosage of triparanol,[a,f,k,u] but failure to induce cataracts has also been reported.[e] The histologic character of the developing cataracts in rats have been studied and described.[a,k,u] In 1969 Harris and Gruber reported that the triparanol-induced cataracts in rats were slowly reversible when the rats were returned to a normal diet; this was followed by a series of studies aimed at elucidating the mechanism of induction and reversal.[g,h,i,p,s,t] In development of the cataracts there was increased permeability, disturbed cation transport, with a large increase in sodium and water content, but a relatively small decrease in potassium.[g,h,k] As the cataracts cleared these values returned toward normal.[g,h] The cataractous lenses were smaller and had less protein than the normal.[i] Desmosterol, which accumulated when triparanol blocked its conversion to cholesterol, was found to constitute 10% of the sterol in the cataractous lenses, compared to 1% in normals, yet clearing lenses had approximately the same desmosterol content as the cataractous lenses.[p] No increase in desmosterol was reported in lenses that remained clear despite administration of triparanol.[e] The glutathione content decreased with development of cataract, but not as much as in most cataracts, and the content returned toward normal as the lenses cleared.[s]

In experiments on drug-induced retinal lipidosis, Drenckhahn and Lullmann-Rauch fed large amounts of triparanol to rats for several weeks and found lipidosis-like changes in the retinal pigment epithelium and Muller cells.[304]

a. Balazs T, Ohtake S, Noble JF: Changes in the lens of aging rats. *TOXICOL APPL PHARMACOL* 14:634, abstr #54, 1969.

b. Bellows JG: Lens opacities produced by cataractogenic agents. *AM J OPHTHALMOL* 55:537–541, 1963.

c. Cogan DG: Triparanol and medical reporting. *ARCH OPHTHALMOL* 67:397–398, 1962.

d. Cogan DG: Discussion of von Sallman (1963).[u]

e. Feldman GL: The lipids in pathology of the eye. *J AM OIL CHEM SOC* 44:615–622, 1967.

f. Gordon S, Balazs T: Cataractogenicity of various drugs in rats. *TOXICOL APPL PHARMACOL* 10:393, abstr. #41, 1967.

g. Harris JE, Gruger L: The reversal of triparanol induced cataracts in the rat. *DOC OPHTHALMOL* 26:324–333, 1969.

h. Harris JE, Gruber L: The reversal of triparanol induced cataracts in the rat. *INVEST OPHTHALMOL* 11:608–616, 1972.

i. Harris JE, Gruber L: The reversal of triparanol induced cataracts in the rat. *INVEST OPHTHALMOL* 12:385–388, 1973.

j. Kirby TJ Jr: Cataracts as possible complications of treatment with triparanol. *ARCH OPHTHALMOL* 67:543–544, 1962.

k. Kirby TJ: Cataracts produced by triparanol (MER/29). *TRANS AM OPHTHALMOL SOC* 65:493–543, 1967.

l. Kirby TJ, Anchor RWP, et al: Cataract formation after triparanol therapy. *ARCH OPHTHALMOL* 68:486–489, 1962.

m. Laughlin RC, Carey TF: Cataracts in patients treated with triparanol. *J AM MED ASSOC* 181:339–340, 1962.

n. McMaster RH: Personal communication quoted by Bellows, 1963.[b]

o. Minton LR, Bounds GW: Ectodermal side-effects of MER/29. *AM J OPHTHALMOL* 55:787–791, 1963.

p. Mizuno G, Ellison E, et al: Lipids of the triparanol cataract in the rat. *OPTHALMIC RES* 6:206–215, 1974.

q. Perdriel MG: Cataract and triparanol. *BULL SOC OPHTALMOL FRANCE* 64:699–701, 1964. (French)

r. Perry HO, Winkelmann RK, et al: Side effects of triparanol therapy. *AM J MED SCI* 244:556–563, 1962.

s. Rathbun WG, Harris JE, et al: The reversal of triparanol-induced cataract in the rat. *INVEST OPHTHALMOL* 12:388–390, 1973.

t. Rathbun WB, Hough M, et al: The reversal of triparanol-induced cataract in the rat. *INTERDISCIP TOP GERONTOL* 12:132–140, 1978.

u. VonSallman L, Grimes P, Collins E: Triparanol-induced cataract in rats. *TRANS AM OPHTHALMOL SOC* 61:49–58, 1963. (*ARCH OPHTHALMOL* 70:522–529, 1963.)

v. Winkelmann RK: Cutaneous syndromes produced as side effects of triparanol therapy. *ARCH DERM* 87:372–377, 1963.

Tripelennamine (Pyribenzamine), an antihistaminic, has no special injurious effect topically.[91] In cases of overdosage, isolated instances of nystagmus and strabismus have been noted, and the pupils may be dilated and poorly responsive to light.[171,252]

Triphenyl tin hydroxide (Vancide KS), a fungicide, has been tested on the eyes of animals and found to be extremely irritating, even if the eyes are irrigated two seconds after application. Although this compound is said to be extremely insoluble, it has produced corneal opacities in all test animals.[a]

a. Marks MJ, Winek CL, Shanor SP: Toxicity of triphenyltin hydroxide (Vancide KS). *TOXICOL APPL PHARMACOL* 14:627, abstr #37, 1969.

Trisodium phosphate (sodium phosphate tribasic, Oakite) forms strongly alkaline solutions. The pH ranges from 11.5 to 11.9 for solutions of 0.1% to 1% concentration, and sometimes in technical grades additional alkali is present.[171] Splash of aqueous solution on human eyes has been known in one case to cause slight transient injury.[165] In two other cases it has caused moderate permanent corneal opacification and vascularization, similar to sodium hydroxide.[81] In one of the latter cases the solution was hot, and this undoubtedly increased its injurious effect.

Tromantadine, an antiviral, tested in an ointment on rabbit eyes, retarded regeneration of corneal epithelium more than did idoxuridine, and tromantadine caused more histologic changes in the corneal stroma and Descemet's membrane.

Kilp H, Walzer P, Hardke W: Influence on the speed of epithelialisation in the rabbit eye by IDU—and tromantadine eye ointments. *KLIN MONATSBL AUGENHEILKD* 168:354–361, 1976. (German)

Tromethamine (trometamol; tris (hydroxymethyl) aminomethane; THAM; Tris Amino), an alkalizer and buffer particularly effective in the pH range 7 to 9, has been used medically in correction of metabolic acidosis, and has been investigated for initial treatment of acid burns of the eye, also as an osmotic agent for reduction of intraocular pressure.

In experimental acid burns of the eyes of rabbits Feller and Graupner in 1966 reported that irrigation with a solution of tromethamine was more effective as an initial treatment than were the more common irrigating solutions.[58] Graupner and Hausmann in 1968 and 1970 showed after application of nitric acid to the cornea that there was less change in the pH of the aqueous humor if the eyes were irrigated with tromethamine ascorbate solution than if irrigated with unbuffered solutions.[92,93] The irrigations were started thirty to sixty seconds after 0.01 ml of concentrated nitric acid was applied. In these tests there was no demonstration that the very small alterations of pH of the aqueous humor of the rabbit's eye was in itself a factor in determining degree of injury of the eye, but presumably the amount of change of pH of the aqueous humor could be utilized as an indirect indicator of changes of pH in the cornea, which no doubt were much greater.

Oral administration of tromethamine to normal and glaucomatous patients, and to dogs, has had no adverse effect on the eyes.[a,b,c]

   a. Leopold IH, Kirschner RJ, Praeger D: Evaluation of the influence of THAM on intraocular pressure. *TRANS AM OPHTHALMOL SOC* 60:335–345, 1962.
   b. Trevor-Roper PD: Use of oral glycerol in glaucoma. *PROC ROY SOC MED* 57:37–38, 1964.
   c. Trevor-Roper PD: Experience with the use of glycerol and other hypotensive agents in glaucoma. *EYE EAR NOSE THROAT MONTHLY* 44:74–76, 1965.

Tropicamide (Mydriacyl), an ophthalmic anticholinergic, is used in concentrations of 0.5% and 1% in mydriatic-cycloplegic eyedrops which are notable for their brief action. Tropicamide has been investigated for influence on intraocular pressure. Application to normal human eyes has seldom caused a rise of pressure as great as 3 mm Hg.[a–e,g] Tonographic facility of outflow in normal eyes also generally has been unaffected. One long-term study on school children has shown that daily application of 0.5% solution for fifty-seven months had no adverse effect on intraocular pressure.[i]

In open-angle glaucomatous eyes, application of tropicamide causes occasional greater rise of intraocular pressure and decrease of facility of outflow than in normal eyes.[d,e,g]

In eyes with shallow anterior chambers and abnormally narrow angles, tropicamide can induce angle-closure glaucoma in the same manner as other mydriatics.[c,d] (Also see *Anticholinergics*.)

Tests for topical toxicity in the eyes of young dogs have been made by applying tropicamide (0.5% twice daily for 1 year); this produced no abnormality detectable histologically.[i]

Systemic toxicity from absorption of tropicamide eyedrops is not likely to be encountered in a chronic form, since this drug is usually employed only for inducing mydriasis and cycloplegia for purposes of examination. One acute transient reaction was reported by Wahl in 1969 in an apparently healthy ten-year-old boy who fell to the floor unconscious "immediately following one drop of 0.5% tropicamide in each eye." He had transitory muscular rigidity and cyanosis, but without special treatment relaxed and regained consciousness, being essentially normal again within an hour.[h] Because of the suddeness of onset the explanation for this episode remains obscure.

Tropicamide has often been used in combination with phenylephrine with the aim of obtaining greater mydriasis. Danger of possible systemic hypertension from absorption of phenylephrine has been recognized, and the concentration of phenylephrine accordingly has been reduced in common practice, especially in low weight and premature infants. Observations on a small number of infants suggest that use of 0.5% tropicamide alone might be safer and almost as effective.[f]

a. Armaly MF, Jepson NC: Accommodation and the dynamics of the steady-state intraocular pressure. *INVEST OPHTHALMOL* 1:480–483, 1962.

b. Hollwich F, Ulmer E: Testing of tropicamide on normal eyes of volunteers. *KLIN MONATSBL AUGENHEILKD* 129:685–687, 1956. (German)

c. Kimura R: Clinical studies on glaucoma. *ACTA SOC OPHTHALMOL JPN* 71:1993–1999, 1967.

d. Makabe R: Tonography under mydriasis. *KLIN MONATSBL AUGENHEILKD* 152:37–45, 1968. (German)

e. Makabe R: Comparative testing of the influence of different mydriatics on tonography. *KLIN MONATSBL AUGENHEILKD* 154:217–220, 1969. (German)

f. Rosales T, Isenberg S, et al: Systemic effects of mydriatics in low weight infants. *J PEDIATR OPHTHALMOL* 18:42–44, 1981.

g. Ternes T: Comparison between the action of tropicamide and of homatropine. *OPHTHALMOLOGICA* 136:78–82, 1958. (German)

h. Wahl JW: Systemic reaction to tropicamide. *ARCH OPHTHALMOL* 82:320–321, 1969; *ARCH OPHTHALMOL* 83:383, 1970.

i. Yamaji R, et al: Study on pseudomyopia. *ACTA SOC OPHTHALMOL JPN* 72:2083–2150, 1968.

Trypan blue is an anionic, acid dye, which like anionic dyes in general appears to have little toxicity to the cornea. It has been tested by addition to the aqueous humor of excised, incubated rabbit and cat eyes, and has been found to cause no increase in uptake of water by the cornea under conditions in which a variety of metabolic inhibitors and cationic dyes do cause corneal swelling.[198] An extensive series of clinical observations have been made by Norn, filling the anterior chamber of patients with dye solution at the time of cataract extraction, washing it out, and examining in particular the corneal endothelium.[b,e,f] In preliminary observations, 1% trypan blue did not cause injury, but a mixture of 0.25% trypan blue with 0.25% Rose Bengal caused corneal edema in 7 out of 9 eyes.[d] Subsequent clinical studies with 0.1% trypan blue filling of the anterior chamber showed no significant increase in corneal thickness, and therefor no disturbance of corneal function.[e] An eight-year follow-up revealed no late adverse effects.[f]

Trypan blue and closely related *Evans blue* have been employed to color the blood to make changes in diameter of the blood vessels of the eye more conspicuous. Intravenous administration of *Evans blue* to human beings has caused blue staining of the sclera and skin,[171] but has not injured the eyes. Trypan blue has been observed in animals to pass through the walls of the vessels of iris and choroid, but not through the walls of retinal vessels.[c]

Teratogenic effects of purified trypan blue have been shown in rats, appearing as deformities of the eyes and other malformations.[a, b] Anophthalmia and microphthalmia were the main anomalies induced by intraperitoneal injection of trypan blue on day 9 of pregnancy.

a. Amels D, Checiu M, Sandor S: Contributions to the study of bisazo dyes induced eye anomalies in rats. *REV ROUM MEP SER MORPHOL* 23:93–101, 1977. (English abstract)

b. Beck F, Lloyd JB: The preparation and teratogenic properties of pure trypan blue and its common contaminants. *J EMBRYOL EXP MORPH* 11:175–184, 1963.

c. Cunha-Vaz JG, Shakib M, Ashton N: Studies on the permeability of the blood-retinal barrier. *BR J OPHTHALMOL* 50:441–453, 1966.

d. Norn MS: Vital staining of corneal endothelium in cataract extraction. *ACTA OPHTHALMOL* 49:725–733, 1971.

e. Norn MS: Pachometric study on the influence of corneal endothelial vital staining. *ACTA OPHTHALMOL* 51:679–686, 1973.

f. Norn MS: Per-operative trypan blue vital staining of corneal endothelium. *ACTA OPHTHALMOL* 58:550–555, 1980.

Tryparsamide (sodium N-(carbamoylmethyl) arsanilate), formerly used in treating syphilis and African trypanosomiasis, was notorious as a cause of optic neuritis, and optic atrophy. The disturbance was characterized by constriction of visual fields and impairment of vision 24 to 48 hours after one of the first ten injections. For detection of early eye involvement, reliance was placed primarily on the visual fields rather than appearance of the fundi, which might not be significantly altered until late.[a, d, e]

Experimental administration of tryparsamide to monkeys has induced lesions in the optic tracts.[b] In rabbits it has caused hemorrhages in the chiasm and brain substance, and in one rabbit it induced peripapillary edema and degeneration of retinal ganglion cells.[c] In cultures of animal retina, tryparsamide has caused rod cell degeneration, but only at concentrations of 0.05 M or greater. Other arsenicals have been damaging at much lower concentrations.[99]

Testing of tryparsamide on the rabbit cornea by injection of 0.04 M solution into the stroma or by dropping on the surface after removal of the epithelium caused no reaction.[123] (For information on related compounds see INDEX for *Arsenicals, organic.*)

a. Buley HM, Albers ED: Tryparsamide therapy and impairment of the optic nerve. *ILLINOIS MED J* 81:477, 1942.

b. Hurst EW: The lesions produced in the central nervous system by certain organic arsenical compounds. *J PATH BACT* 77:523–534, 1959.

c. Lazar NK: Effect of tryparsamide on the eye. *ARCH OPHTHALMOL* 11:240–253, 1934.

d. Potter W: Visual impairment during tryparsamide therapy. *ARCH OPHTHALMOL* 30:669–687, 1943.

e. Sloan LL, Woods AC: Effect of tryparsamide on the eye. *AM J SYPH* 20:583–613, 1936.

Trypsin (Tryptar), a proteolytic enzyme, has been used topically for debriding necrotic tissues. Experiments on excised beef corneas showed that 5 to 10 mg injected into the stroma caused loosening of the epithelium in four hours.[107] Subsequently, an eye bath or eye drops of trypsin, and subconjunctival or intramuscular injection, was reported to give good therapeutic results in patients with dendritic keratitis, and to cause no notable damaging effect.[a, e] However, some observers have considered direct application of trypsin to the eye to be damaging and have recommended against its use.[d,e,171]

A rapid destruction of the cornea and loss of the eye has been reported after subconjunctival administration of trypsin in two cases of severe burns of the eye.[f]

Experimentally in rabbits the effect of treatment with trypsin after injury of the cornea with a thermocautery has been compared with results from no special treatment. Miller and Brini found that powdered trypsin could be applied to rabbit eyes without producing injury if the epithelium was intact, but if the epithelium was first injured by a hot cautery, the enzyme had very destructive effect on the corneal stroma.[d] The investigators concluded that trypsin should not be used topically in treatment of corneal injuries. On the other hand, they considered the enzyme to be of value in the absence of corneal wounds for removing necrotic conjunctival tissue, especially in preparation for grafting.[b,c]

Intravitreal injection of 200μg of trypsin in rabbit eyes has caused chorioretinitis, retinal degeneration, and cataract.[14]

a. Liegel O: Trypsin treatment in ophthalmology. *KLIN MONATSBL AUGENHEILKD* 132:486–497, 1968. (German)
b. Miller HA: Burns of the eye. *BULL SOC OPHTALMOL FRANCE* (Suppl 4) 1–174, 1958. (French)
c. Miller HA, Brini A, Gaud F: Trypsin in burns of the cornea. *BULL SOC OPHTALMOL FRANCE* 294–312, 1958. (French)
d. Miller HA, Brini A: Experimental works on the effect of trypsin on the cornea of the rabbit. *TRANS OPHTHALMOL SOC UK* 81:17–22, 1961.
e. Szeghy G, Kenyeres B: On the heparin-trypsin treatment of herpes simplex keratitis. *KLIN MONATSBL AUGENHEILKD* 153:827–830, 1968. (German)
f. Thomas C, Cordier B, et al: Must one make use of trypsin in serious burns of the anterior segment? *BULL SOC OPHTALMOL FRANCE* 458–461, 1957. (French)

Tungsten metal has been implanted in the vitreous body of rabbit eyes and found by Lauring and Wergeland to be well tolerated for at least a year.[340]

Tungstic acid is insoluble in water, but with alkali metals it forms soluble tungstate salts. Experiments on rabbit eyes have shown tungstate ion to be toxic in the range of pH 7 to 9 when applied directly to the corneal stroma without the protection of the epithelium. Practically, neither tungstic acid nor the tungstates appear to present much hazard to the eye.[a,123]

a. Friedenwald JS, Hughes WF, Herrmann H: Acid burns of the eye. *ARCH OPHTHALMOL* 35:98–108, 1946.

Turpentine vapor causes irritation of the human eye, perceptible at 175 ppm in air, and unpleasant at 720 to 1,100 ppm.[183] Cats give evidence of irritation of the eyes and respiratory tract at 540 to 720 ppm.[61,188]

Contact of the liquid with the eye causes immediate severe pain and blepharospasm. This may be followed by much conjunctival hyperemia and slight transient injury of the corneal epithelium. In severe cases temporary erosion of the epithelium may occur, but no damage of the corneal stroma has been noted in patients or rabbits after splash contact.[c, 153]

Subconjunctival injection of turpentine causes a much more severe reaction, and in one case caused phthisis bulbi.[a] Injection into the anterior chamber of animals causes a fibrinopurulent inflammation with corneal opacification from endothelial injury and infiltration of leukocytes.[150] The cornea has also been rendered opaque in rabbits by injection of turpentine into the corneal stroma. Within two days after the injection the amount of hexosamine in the cornea has been found to be considerably diminished.[b]

a. Liebermann Lv: A phthisis bulbi caused by subconjunctival injection of turpentine. *SZEMESZET* 56:6–7, 1922. (*ZBL GES OPHTHALMOL* 8:316, 1923.) (German abstract)

b. Hughes WF: Alkali burns of the eye. *ARCH OPHTHALMOL* 35:423–449, 1946.

c. Wollenberg A: Superficial eye burns from shoe polish containing turpentine. *KLIN MONATSBL AUGENHEILKD* 78:410–411, 1927.

Tyrosine, a naturally occurring amino acid, causes keratitis in young rats when added in sufficient amount to their diet. Also, in human beings an abnormally high concentration of tyrosine in the blood, caused by an inborn defect in metabolism of dietary tyrosine, can be associated with development of a special type of keratitis at an early age. Comprehensive synopsis-reviews of both conditions have been published (Bardelli 1977; Godde-Jolly 1979; Jaeger 1978). Most important, the keratitis in human beings can be dramatically relieved by changing to a diet with a specially low tyrosine content.

In the rat experiments, it has been known since 1932 that when L-tyrosine was added equivalent to 1 to 20% of the diet it caused within a week or two an exudative blepharitis and ulcerative keratitis, with corneal infiltration by inflammatory cells, accompanied by swelling and redness of the toes and legs, and at high doses usually early death (Lillie 1932; Sullivan 1932; Hueper 1943; Schweizer 1947). More recent experiments with diets limited to 5% have kept rats alive longer, and permitted closer study (Rich 1973; Beard 1974; Gipson 1975, 1977; Landolfo 1976). Under these conditions, within 24 hours the corneal endothelium begins to become edematous. During the first week the corneas become infiltrated with leukocytes, and appear opaque. Subsequently a remarkable spontaneous clearing of the corneas is possible, despite continuation on the same diet (Beard 1974; Schweizer 1947). Electron and polarizing microscopy of early corneal epithelial lesions have shown crystals, probably tyrosine crystals, that extend from one cell to another, disrupting the membranes of the cells and their nuclei (Gipson 1975). It appears likely that tyrosine crystals form within epithelial cells, disrupting their lysosomes and cell membranes, releasing lysosomal enzymes and leading to a leukocytic inflammatory reaction (Gipson 1977).

In human beings there are four or more systemic diseases involving excessive tyrosine (tyrosinosis or tyrosinemia), but apparently only one of these diseases affects the eyes. The Richner-Hanhart syndrome, first described in 1938 consists of bilateral pseudo-dendritic keratitis, hyperkeratotic lesions of the palms and soles, and usually some mental retardation. From the first month of life the patient may have photophobia and painful eyes with branching corneal lesions resembling dentritic figures, limited to the epithelium in some cases, but involving anterior stroma in others. The figures stain less with fluorescein than do real herpes simplex ulcers, and they are unresponsive to antiviral and antimicrobial treatments. Circumscribed round areas of keratosis develop on the palms and soles, and these are tender, and may make walking uncomfortable.

A relationship of the Richner-Hanhart syndrome to tyrosinemia was apparently not appreciated until around 1970, but then a series of clinical studies were published providing evidence for an important connection (Holston 1971; Kennaway 1971; Burns 1972; Goldsmith 1973; Zaleski 1973; Billson 1975, 1976; Sandberg 1975; Bienfang 1976; Goldsmith 1976; Bardelli 1977; Godde-Jolly 1979; Charlton 1981). One of the most persuasive observations, made in a number of cases, was that when the patient's diet was changed from ordinary to special low-tyrosine, the plasma tyrosine dropped rapidly, the keratitis cleared and the dermatokeratosis improved dramatically, with elimination of all painful symptoms. In some cases, trial doses of tyrosine given to patients who had been relieved of their symptoms by low-tyrosine diet caused a striking transient return of symptoms (Billson 1975, 1976).

Study of the basis for high plasma tyrosine levels in patients with corneal ulcers demonstrated that they had a hereditary lack of a liver enzyme, soluble tyrosine aminotransferase, which normally is important in the metabolism of tyrosine (Kennaway 1971; Burns 1972).

A conjunctival biopsy from a patient with tyrosinemia and Richner-Hanhart syndrome showed needle-like crystals, presumably tyrosine, but no inflammation (Bienfang 1976).

Comparison of the case reports indicates that the bilateral pseudo-dendritic keratopathy with pain and photophobia may be the most typical eye involvement associated with tyrosinemia in human beings, but in some cases there has been broader corneal ulceration (as pointed out by Bienfang 1976). Occasional patients have had nystagmus or strabismus. One patient had cataracts without keratitis at age 17 years (Wadman 1968), and one 23 year-old has been reported to have both Wilson's hepatolenticular degeneration with Kayser-Fleischer rings and Richner-Hanhart syndrome (Thiel 1983).

Comparison of the eyes of rats fed tyrosine and human beings with the tyrosine aminotransferase deficiency syndrome shows considerable differences in the histopathology, as already mentioned, the rats going through a phase of inflammation involving the whole cornea, while the human eyes generally have their corneal abnormality limited to the epithelium, with relatively little inflammatory reaction. However, in both rat and human eyes the corneas can spontaneously clear considerably with age, even though maintained on constant diets.

Bardelli AM, Borgoni P, et al: Familial tyrosinemia with eye and skin lesions. *OPHTHALMOLOGICA* 175:5–9, 1977.

Beard ME, Burns RP, et al: Histopathology of keratopathy in the tyrosine-fed rat. *INVEST OPHTHALMOL* 13:1037–1041, 1974.

Bienfang DC, Kuwabara T, Pueschel SM: The Richner-Hanhart syndrome. *ARCH OPHTHALMOL* 94:1133–1137, 1976.

Billson FA, Danks DM: Corneal and skin changes in tyrosinaemia. *AUST J OPHTHALMOL* 3:112–115, 1975; *BR J OPHTHALMOL* 60:600, 1976.

Burns RP: Soluble tyrosine aminotransferase deficiency: an unusual cause of corneal ulcers. *AM J OPHTHALMOL* 73:400–402, 1972.

Charlton KH, Binder PS, et al: Pseudodendritic keratitis and systemic tyrosinemia. *OPHTHALMOLOGY* 88:355–360, 1981.

Gipson IK, Burns RP, Wolfe-Lande JD: Crystals in corneal epithelial lesions of tyrosine-fed rats. *INVEST OPHTHALMOL* 14:937–941, 1975.

Gipson IK, Anderson RA: Response of the lysosomal system of the corneal epithelium to tyrosine-induced cell injury. *J HISTOCHEM CYTOCHEM* 25:1351–1362, 1977.

Godde-Jolly D, Larregue M, et al: A case of Richner-Hanhart syndrome (Tyrosinosis with ocular, skin and mental manifestations). *J FR OPHTALMOL* 2:23–28, 1979. (French)

Goldsmith LA, Kang E, et al: Tyrosinaemia with plantar and palmar keratosis and keratitis. *J PEDIATR* 83:798–805, 1973.

Goldsmith LA, Read J: Tyrosine-induced eye and skin lesions. *J AM MED ASSOC* 236:382–384, 1967.

Heuper WC, Martin GJ: Tyrosine poisoning in rats. *ARCH PATHOL* 35:685–694, 1943.

Holston JL Jr, Levy HL, et al: Tyrosinosis: a patient without liver or renal disease. *PEDIATRICS* 48:393–400, 1971.

Jaeger W, Gallasch G, et al: Tyrosinemia as cause of a bilateral herpetiform corneal epithelial dystrophy (Richner-Hanhart syndrome). *KLIN MONATSBL AUGENHEILKD* 173:506–515, 1978. (German)

Kennaway NG, Buist NRM: Metabolic studies in a patient with hepatic cytosol tyrosine aminotransferase deficiency. *PEDIATR RES* 5:287–297, 1971.

Landolfo A, Albini L, Savastano S: Toxicity of tyrosine and of phenylalanine for the eye of the albino rat. *ANN OTTALMOL CLIN OCUL* 102:135–144, 1976. (Italian)

Lillie RD: Histopathologic changes produced in rats by the addition to the diet of various amino-acids. *PUBLIC HEALTH REP* 47:83–90, 1912.

Rich LF, Beard ME, Burns RP: Excess dietary tyrosine and corneal lesions. *EXP EYE RES* 17:87–97, 1973.

Sandberg HO: Bilateral keratopathy and tyrosinosis. *ACTA OPHTHALMOL* 53:760–764, 1975.

Schweizer W: Studies on the effect of L-tyrosine on the white rat. *J PHYSIOL* 106:167–176, 1947.

Sullivan MX, Hess WC, Sebrell WH: Studies on the biochemistry of sulfur. *PUBLIC HEALTH REP* 47:75–82, 1932.

Thiel HJ, Weidle E: Tyrosinosis and hepatolenticular degeneration (Wilson's disease). *KLIN MONATSBL AUGENHEILKD* 182:232–234, 1983. (German)

Wadman SK, Van Sprang FJ, et al: An exceptional case of tyrosinosis. *J MENT DEFIC RES* 12:269–281, 1968.

Westmore R, Billson FA: Pseudo-herpetic keratitis. *BR J OPHTHALMOL* 57:654–656, 1973.

Zaleski WA, Hill A, Murray RG: Corneal erosions in tyrosinosis. *CAN J OPHTHALMOL* 8:556–559, 1973.

Undecylenic acid (component of Cruex, Desenex, Fulvidex), an antifungal, has been reported in the course of dermatologic treatment to have caused conjunctivitis and more rarely keratoconjunctivitis.[a]

a. Belz Ollyvier, Darbon, Raymond: Bilateral keratoconjunctivitis in the course of dermatologic treatment with undecylenic acid. *ANN OCULIST* (*Paris*) 183:68, 1950. (French)

Uranium compounds are highly toxic. Several uranium compounds tested by dropping on the eyes of rabbits, guinea pigs, and rats have caused severe eye damage as well as systemic poisoning. The following compounds caused injury to the eyes: *uranium pentachloride, uranium tetrachloride, uranyl nitrate, uranyl fluoride, sodium diurinate, uranium tetrafluoride, ammonium diurinate, uranium trioxide, uranium dioxide* and *uranium peroxide.*[a]

Application of 1 mg of solid *uranium pentachloride* to the eyes of rabbits caused the most severe necrosis of conjunctivae and lids, and perforating ulceration of the cornea. The other *chlorides* and the *nitrate* were also severely damaging. The mildest damage was caused by the various *uranium oxides.*

a. Orcutt JA: The toxicology of compounds of uranium following application to the eye. In Voegtlin C, Hodge HC (Eds): PHARMACOLOGY AND TOXICOLOGY OF URANIUM COMPOUNDS. New York, McGraw-Hill, 1949.

Urea contact with the eye is damaging only at high concentrations or with extended exposure. Soaking beef corneas in 1 M solution for one hour loosens the epithelium from the stroma,[107] with attendant slow decrease of electric resistance of the cornea.[184] On rabbit eyes saturated urea solution causes loss of epithelium from the cornea after five minutes contact, and produces moderate grayness of the stroma, with subsequent slow regeneration of the epithelium.[81] A rabbit's cornea can return to normal in several weeks after exposure for an hour to 40% urea solution.[81] In patients with squamous cell carcinoma of palpebral and bulbar conjunctiva, repeated applications of urea powder have been made to eradicate the malignant growth.[b] Powdered urea has been applied repeatedly and 10% solution has been injected subconjunctivally and applied as eyedrops. No irritation or discomfort developed from the 10% solution used several times a day for a year. When urea powder has been used, an attempt has been made to protect the cornea. When this has been impossible, the cornea has developed opacity, which has cleared completely several weeks after the end of treatment.

Therapeutic use of urea intravenously or orally for reduction of intraocular pressure in glaucoma has caused rare adverse ocular side effects. So called rebound glaucoma, a physical rather than a toxic phenomenon, has been described.[a,c]

Intravenous urea in monkeys has not damaged the ciliary epithelium, supporting a belief that reduction of intraocular pressure in glaucomatous patients is accomplished by an osmotic, rather than a toxic mechanism.[i] However, *intracarotid* injection of concentrated urea in monkeys has done dramatic damage to the retina[f] and the ciliary body.[d,e,g,h,i] Retinal pigment epithelial cells are affected and blood-retina barrier broken down.[f] The blood-aqueous barrier is broken down secondary to changes in the capillaries and selective damage to the ciliary body epithelium.[d,e,g,h,i] Intraocular pressure is strikingly reduced and the aqueous outflow system rapidly shows swelling of the connective tissue of the inner wall of Schlemm's canal, and then edema of the trabecular meshwork. However, in several weeks there is general return to normal, except for failure of pigmented ciliary epithelium to regenerate.[d,e]

Intravitreal injection of 0.2 ml 10 M urea in rabbits has caused inflammation, chorioretinitis, and degeneration of the retina.[14]

a. Bonnet M: Pupillary block in an aphake after infusion of urea. *BULL SOC OPHTALMOL FRANCE* 67:472–482, 1967. (French)

b. Danopoulos ED, Danopoulou IE, et al: Effects of urea treatment in malignancies of the conjunctiva and cornea. *OPHTHALMOLOGICA* 178:198–203, 1979.

c. Hill K, Whitney JB, Trotter RR: Intravenous hypertonic urea in the management of acute angle-closure glaucoma. *ARCH OPHTHALMOL* 65:497–502, 1961.

d. Okisaka S, Kuwabara T, Rapoport SI: Selective destruction of the pigmented epithelium in the ciliary body of the eye. *SCIENCE* 184:1298–1299, 1974.

e. Okisaka S, Kuwabara T, Rapoport SI: Effect of hyperosmotic agents on the ciliary epithelium and trabecular meshwork. *INVEST OPHTHALMOL* 15:617–625, 1976.

f. Okinami S, Okhuma M, et al: Disruption of blood-retinal barrier at the retinal pigment epithelium after systemic urea injection. *ACTA OPHTHALMOL* 56:27–39, 1978.

g. Rapoport SI: Effect of concentrated solutions on blood-brain barrier. *AM J PHYSIOL* 223:323, 1970.

h. Rapoport SI, Bachman DS, Thompson HK: Chronic effects of opening of the blood-brain barrier in the monkey. *SCIENCE* 176:1243, 1972.

i. Shabo AL, Maxwell DS, Kreiger AE: Structural alterations in the ciliary process and the blood-aqueous barrier of the monkey after systemic urea injections. *AM J OPHTHALMOL* 81:162–172, 1976.

Urea-formaldehyde resins have been employed as finishing agents on cloth for crease-resistance, and under certain conditions of temperature and humidity these have been known to release formaldehyde, causing nose and eye irritation. Urea-formaldehyde resin used for gluing wood caused five cases of corneal disturbance with intense photophobia and blepharospasm.[a] The dust of dry glue was believed to get in the air during machining operations, and a great many fine refractile foreign bodies of varying color were found in the corneal epithelium by slit-lamp examination; the particles were surrounded by a small white halo of reaction. All became asymptomatic, but 6 months later fine refractile particles could still be seen beneath the corneal epithelium. Dermatosis of the face and hands was caused by the same material.

a. Sedan J: Keratitis caused by wood glue utilized in aeronautic construction. *BULL SOC OPHTALMOL (Paris)* 449–450, 1951. (French)

Urethane (urethan, ethyl carbamate), an antineoplastic and veterinary anesthetic, causes toxic retinopathy when given by repeated subcutaneous injection to young rats. Neoplasms and melanotic lesions in the iris, ciliary body and choroid have also been induced.[f,j] Kendry and Roe described generalized fundus pigmentary abnormalities.[f] Retinal pigment clumping, and some loss of retinal pigment gave a typical ophthalmoscopic appearance of interspersed areas of hypo- and hyperpigmentation.[e,h] Tamaki and Amemiya described degeneration of the retina and severe alteration of the ERG.[a,b,l] Belhorn et al showed that repeated injections caused degeneration of the photoreceptors and derangement of the retinal pigment epithelium with ingrowth of fenestrated vessels within the pigment epithelium.[e] Kritzinger et al demonstrated fluorescein leakage from these vessels.[h] Korte et al have studied the break-down of the blood-retinal barrier using horseradish peroxidase as an ultrastructural probe.[g]

Dark adaptation is retarded in monkeys given an anesthetic dose of urethane.[387]

An appearance of crystals in the cornea was described in a patient under treatment with urethane for multiple myeloma, but the occurrence of similar appearance in patients with this illness not treated by urethane made it likely the corneal abnormality represented a deposit of a paraprotein from the disease, rather than an effect of the drug.[c,i]

Cysts of the ciliary body were described by Slansky in 1966 in four patients who had had treatment with urethane, considering the possibility that the urethane might have been responsible for the development of the cysts, but Ashton in 1967 pointed out that he had found cysts of the ciliary body and pars plana in patients with multiple myelomatosis who had not received urethane.[k,d]

Study of the ciliary processes in rabbits by Wegner in 1967 showed that when animals were killed by an overdose of either urethane or pentobarbital, this caused edema of the ciliary epithelium and stroma.[m] This observation raised a question of the possibility that smaller doses employed as a general anesthetic in animals might also affect the ciliary body and the formation of aqueous humor.

a. Amemiya T: Electron microscopic study of the retina of rats repeatedly treated with urethan. *ACTA SOC OPHTHALMOL JPN* 72:293–298, 1968.

b. Amemiya T: Fine structure of Bruch's membrane in vitamin A deficiency and urethan intoxication. *ACTA SOC OPHTHALMOL JPN* 73:1008–1015, 1969.

c. Aronson SB, Shaw R: Corneal crystals in multiple myeloma. *ARCH OPHTHALMOL* 61:541–546, 1959.

d. Ashton N: Cystic changes and urethan. *ARCH OPHTHALMOL* 78:416, 1967.

e. Belhorn RW, Bellhorn M, et al: Urethan-induced retinopathy in pigmented rats. *INVEST OPHTHALMOL* 12:65–76, 1973.

f. Kendry G, Roe FJC: Melanotic lesions of the eye in August hooded rats induced by urethane or N-hydroxyurethane. *J NAT CANCER INST* 43:749–762, 1969.

g. Korte GE, Bellhorn RN, Burns MS: Urethane-induced rat retinopathy. *INVEST OPHTHALMOL VIS SCI* 25:1027–1034, 1984.

h. Kritzinger EE, Bellhorn RW: Permeability of blood-retinal barriers in urethane-induced rat retinopathy. *BR J OPHTHALMOL* 66:630–635, 1982.

i. Markoff N: On crystal formation in the cornea during urethane treatment of multiple myeloma. *SCHWEIZ MED WOCHENSCHR* 78:987–988, 1948. (German)

j. Roe FJC, Millican D, Mallett JM: Induction of melanotic lesions of the iris in rats by urethane. *NATURE* 199:1201, 1963.

k. Slansky HH, Bronstein M, Gartner S: Ciliary body cysts in multiple myeloma. *ARCH OPHTHALMOL* 76:686–689, 1966.

l. Tamaki S: Electroretinographic studies on the experimental hypervitaminosis A and vitamin A deficiency. *ACTA SOC OPHTHALMOL JPN* 71:2095–2102, 1967.

m. Wegner K: Regional differences in ultrastructure of the rabbit ciliary processes. *INVEST OPHTHALMOL* 6:177–191, 1967.

Uric acid has been tested in rabbit eyes by introduction of crystals into the cornea, the anterior chamber, and the vitreous body.[150] In the cornea it caused practically no reaction except for a small number of leukocytes which wandered in to phagocytose the particles. In the anterior chamber also it caused no inflammation, except that where crystals rested against the endothelium of the lower portion of the cornea, they caused local corneal edema and vascularization, probably from mechanical injury of the endothelium. In the vitreous humor the crystals were absorbed without inflammatory reaction.

In gout, urate crystals have been identified electronmicroscopically in the corneal epithelium by Slansky and Kuwabara, with no evidence of toxicity, either microscopically or clinically.[a]

a. Slansky HH, Kuwabara T: Intranuclear urate crystals in corneal epithelium. *ARCH OPHTHALMOL* 80:338–344, 1968.

Urokinase (Abbokinase, Breokinase), a plasminogen activator, has been of clinical ophthalmic interest in treatment of hemorrhage in the anterior chamber and in the vitreous body.

Irrigation of the anterior chamber to dissolve blood clots was reported in several patients by Pierse, using 1000 units/ml, and finding the treatment effective and well tolerated. However, in rabbit experiments Horven found 2500 to 5000 units/ml caused considerable reaction of the iris, protein in the anterior chamber, and clouding of the cornea. Podos found 7000 units/ml caused opacification of the rabbit cornea.

Intravitreal injection of 25000 units in 0.5 ml in 3 patients with vitreous hemorrhage was reported by Dugmore to be effective and well tolerated, but in a brief review of other clinical experiences Textorius has directed attention to reactions that include transient hypopyon, uveitis, and secondary glaucoma noted by several observers after intravitreal injection of 1000 to 55000 units (Chapman-Smith; Cleary; Forrester; Holmes Sellors), as well as folds in Descemet's membrane (Chapman-Smith), and temporary thickening of the cornea (Bramsen). A decrease of the b-wave of the ERG which gradually recovered was reported by Cleary.

Intravitreal injection of urokinase in monkeys has caused changes in the retina when the dose approached 2500 units (Koziol). In rabbits an acute uveitis followed intravitreal injection of 10000 units (Pandolfi; Textorius). Also, retinal hemorrhages, vitreous opacities, cataracts, and reduced ERG b-wave followed (Textorius).

Experiments with urokinase directly on rabbit corneas have also been carried out. Specular microscopy has shown no change in the endothelium of excised corneas after perfusion for 3 hours with 1000 to 5000 units/ml (Hull). In vivo intracorneal injection of urokinase 2 mm from the limbus has stimulated growth of vessels into the cornea, but the vehicle or inactivated enzyme did not (Berman).

Berman M, Winthrop S, et al: Plasminogen activator (urokinase) causes vascularization of the cornea. *INVEST OPHTHALMOL VIS SCI* 22:191–199, 1982.

Bramsen T: The effect of urokinase on central corneal thickness and vitreous hemorrhage. *ACTA OPHTHALMOL* 56:1006–1012, 1978.

Chapman-Smith JS, Crock GW: Urokinase in the management of vitreous haemorrhage. *BR J OPHTHALMOL* 61:500–505, 1977.

Cleary PE, Davies EWG, et al: Intravitreal urokinase in the treatment of vitreous haemorrhage. *TRANS OPHTHALMOL SOC UK* 94:587–590, 1974.

Dugmore WN, Raichand M: Intravitreal urokinase in the treatment of vitreous hemorrhage. *AM J OPHTHALMOL* 75:779–781, 1973.

Forrester JV, Williamson J: Lytic therapy in vitreous haemorrhage. *TRANS OPHTHAL-MOL SOC UK* 94:583–586, 1974.

Holmes Sellors PJ, Kanski JJ, Watson DM: Intravitreal urokinase in the management of vitreous haemorrhage. *TRANS OPHTHALMOL SOC UK* 94:591–598, 1974.

Horven I, Opsahl R: Fibrinolysis and hyphema. *ACTA OPHTHALMOL* 42:957–961, 1964.

Hull DS, Green K: Effect of urokinase on corneal endothelium. *ARCH OPHTHALMOL* 98:1285–1286, 1980.

Koziol J, Peyman GA, et al: Urokinase in experimental vitreous hemorrhage. *OPHTHALMIC SURG* 6:79–82, 1975.

Pandolfi M: Stimulation of fibrinolysis in the vitreous body. *BIBL ANAT* 18:292–297, 1979.

Pierse D: The use of urokinase in the anterior chamber. *TRANS OPHTHALMOL SOC UK* 84:271–274, 1964.

Podos S, Liebman S, Pollen A: Treatment of experimental total hyphemas with intraocular fibrinolytic agents. *ARCH OPHTHALMOL* 71:537–541, 1964.

Textorius O, Stenkula S: Toxic ocular effects of two fibrinolytic drugs. *ACTA OPHTHAL-MOL* 61:322–331, 1983.

Vaccinium uliginosum L is a shrub having dark berries with colorless juice. In rare cases reported from northern Europe ingestion of large quantities of the berries has caused mydriasis and abnormality of color vision. White objects are said to assume a blue and green-yellow appearance for a few hours.[252]

Vacor Rat-Killer (PNU; pyriminyl), a rodenticide, has caused numerous severe, sometimes fatal, poisonings after accidental or suicidal ingestion. It has induced diabetes, and caused disturbances of the autonomic, peripheral and central nervous systems, but involvement of the eyes generally has been limited to miosis with asymmetrical and sluggishly reactive pupils, sometimes ptosis of the lids, and occasionally nystagmus.[a] In one extraordinary case a patient was found to have homonymous hemianopia, presumably from occipital infarct after intestinal perforation, hemorrhaging, and emergency surgery.[b] This patient, like most patients with Vacor poisoning, had low blood pressure with persistent severe disabling orthostatic hypotension. For treatment of this hypotension, 2.5 years after the initial poisoning the patient was given 42 mg of ergotamine tartrate orally during a period of 3 weeks. Subjectively the patient developed distortion and blurring of vision, without objective decrease in visual acuity or change in visual fields, but there was slight macular edema, decreased vascularity of the optic discs, thread-like retinal arterioles, and extinguished ERG's. Since the fundi had been normal earlier after the Vacor poisoning, these new findings appeared to be attributable to the action of high-dosage ergotamine superimposed on the after-effects of Vacor poisoning, but to what degree there was an interaction was uncertain.[b] (For further comparison, see the INDEX for *Ergotamine*.)

a. LeWitt PA: The neurotoxicity of the rat poison Vacor. *N ENGL J MED* 302:73–77, 1980.
b. Mindel JS, Rubenstein AE, Franklin B: Ocular ergotamine tartrate toxicity during treatment of Vacor-induced orthostatic hypotension. *AM J OPHTHALMOL* 92:492–496, 1981.

Valinomycin, an ionophore antibiotic, can cause an increase in lens sodium and decrease in lens potassium, and can cause cataract in incubated mouse and rabbit lenses without increase in water content, when added to the culture medium.[a] Accumulation of calcium in the lens appears to be the primary cause of the opacification.[b]

 a. Iwata S, Horiuchi M: Studies on experimental cataracts induced by ionophores. *EXP EYE RES* 31:543–551, 1980.
 b. Hightower KR, Harrison SE: Valinomycin cataract. EXP EYE RES 34:941–943, 1982.

Vanadate salts (e.g. sodium vanadate) have been of pharmacologic and physiologic interest since they were found to inhibit membrane NaK-ATPase, an enzyme important in sodium-potassium pumps. Becker has reported that when 0.5 to 1% vanadate is applied to the eyes of rabbits the rate of formation of aqueous humor is reduced, apparently due to inhibition of this enzyme in the ciliary body epithelium, and he has cautioned that theoretically the lens epithelium and corneal epithelium, as well as the ciliary epithelium, might be adversely affected, but did not actually note toxic side effects on the eyes.[a] Candia and Podos have shown in excised corneas of bullfrogs that vanadate can inhibit sodium and chloride transport by the epithelium, but the significance with respect to ocular toxicity remains a question.[b]

 a. Becker B: Vanadate and aqueous humor dynamics. *INVEST OPHTHALMOL VIS SCI* 19:1156–1165, 1980.
 b. Candia OA, Podos SM: Inhibition of active transport of chloride and sodium by vanadate in the cornea. *INVEST OPHTHALMOL VIS SCI* 20:733–737, 1981.

Vanadium pentoxide appears to be the only vanadium compound for which ocular disturbances have been reported. The dust causes a sensation of burning and irritation of the eyes, and signs of conjunctivitis, accompanied by irritation of the nose and throat. The respiratory irritation occurs at lower concentration than does the ocular irritation.[b–e]

Inhalation of large amounts of the pentoxide dust was alleged in one case in 1911 to have caused neuroretinitis and amaurosis,[a] but it seems likely that something other than vanadium may have been to blame for the neuroretinal disease.

 a. Dutton WF: Vanadiumism. *J AM MED ASSOC* 56:1648, 1911.
 b. Lewis CA: Biological effects of vanadium. *ARCH IND HEALTH* 19:497–503, 1959.
 c. Sjoberg S: Health hazards in the production and handling of vanadium pentoxide. *ARCH IND HYG* 33:631–646, 1962.
 d. Zenz C, Bartlett JP, Thiede WH: Acute vanadium pentoxide intoxication. *ARCH ENVIRON HEALTH* 5:542–546, 1962.
 e. Zenz C, Berg B: Human responses to controlled vanadium pentoxide exposure. *ARCH ENVIRON HEALTH* 14:709–712, 1967.

Vancide-TH (hexahydro-1,3,5-triethyl-S-triazine), an industrial bacteriostatic and fungistatic, caused permanent corneal opacity when applied undiluted to rabbit eyes.[a]

 a. Winek CL, Fochtman FW, et al: Acute and subacute toxicology and safety evaluation of hexahydro-1,3,5-triethyl-S-triazine. *DRUG CHEM TOXICOL* 1:1–18, 1978.

Vancomycin hydrochloride (Vancocin hydrochloride), an antibacterial, when given by intravitreal injection in a volume of 0.1 ml in rabbit eyes more than 10 mg caused complete retinal destruction, 5 mg caused localized damage and temporary whitish reaction in the vitreous body, but 1 mg or less caused no change in transparency of the media and no abnormality in the ERG.[a]

a. Homer P, Peyman GA, et al: Intravitreal injection of vancomycin in experimental staphylococcal endophthalmitis. *ACTA OPHTHALMOL* 53:311–320, 1975.

Vasodilator drugs are of interest in ophthalmic toxicology principally in relation to intraocular pressure. A review of this subject has been published giving references to most of the relevant literature to 1968.[83]

Some authorities in the latter part of the nineteenth century and early twentieth century supposed that dilation of blood vessels within the eye caused vitreous body, lens, and iris to move forward to close the angle and induce acute glaucoma. This concept developed prior to the introduction of gonioscopy into general clinical use, and at a time when glaucomas of different types were characterized according to symptoms and external appearances. The term "congestive" was widely used in describing eyes that appeared hyperemic with obviously dilated superficial vessels in association with high intraocular pressure. The concept of vasodilation as a cause of glaucoma was based mainly on the clinical appearance of vascular congestion and on histologic findings of dilated vessels in eyes that had been enucleated because of intractable angle-closure glaucoma. The concept seemed to be supported by animal experiments in which ligation of vortex veins induced engorgement of intraocular vessels, shallowing of the anterior chamber, and transitory glaucoma. Also, clinical observations utilizing the Valsalva phenomenon showed that venous congestion could cause a transient rise of intraocular pressure, even in normal eyes. Accordingly, anything with a vasodilating action was thought to be dangerous to eyes subject to glaucoma.

In more recent years, particularly with the experience gained in wide-spread use of gonioscopy, a different interpretation of the earlier clinical and histologic observations can be made. It is now evident that in many cases of glaucoma the angle of the anterior chamber is open at all times, and in cases in which glaucoma is attributable to closure of the angle, the closing is in most instances caused by accumulation of aqueous humor behind the iris causing the periphery of the iris to bulge forward. Vessels become visibly dilated after the intraocular pressure has become elevated from closure of the angle, rather than before. Examination at the onset of angle-closure glaucoma and gonioscopy immediately after iridectomy early in the course of an attack of angle-closure glaucoma typically reveal no evidence of vasodilation or vascular engorgement of the ciliary processes sufficient to have closed the angle. It appears now that vascular "congestion" of the eye is not a common cause of angle-closure glaucoma. (Hemorrhages and abnormal accumulation of fluid in the choroid or behind the anterior vitreous in special cases (e.g. after central retinal vein occlusion) may push vitreous, lens, and iris forward to close the angle, but this is something other than vasodilation.)

Present ideas about the relationship of ocular blood vessels to intraocular pressure in eyes with glaucoma of the open-angle type lead one to expect that dilation of intraocular blood vessels should cause a rise of intraocular pressure, but that this would be a transient rise with its duration dependent upon the ease with which a compensatory equal volume of aqueous humor could be expelled from the eye. It is currently postulated that a vasomotor mechanism would cause sustained change in intraocular pressure only if it raised orbital or episcleral venous pressure, or if it altered the rate of formation of aqueous humor or the facility of aqueous outflow, in some way as yet undemonstrated.

Search of the literature for evidence concerning the influence of vasodilator drugs on intraocular pressure in human eyes provides a number of demonstrations that subconjunctival injection, and occasionally retrobulbar injection, of powerful vasodilators can cause transient elevation of intraocular pressure, especially in glaucomatous eyes, but the search has so far failed to disclose evidence that vasodilator drugs administered orally, intramuscularly, or intravenously have adverse effects on intraocular pressure or on vision in patients with open-angle glaucoma or in patients with anatomic predisposition to angle-closure glaucoma. There appears to be no adequately documented instance of closure of the angle, even by subconjunctival injection of the powerful vasodilators that transiently raise the pressure in the eye.

The following vasodilator drugs and their influences on intraocular pressure are described elsewhere (see INDEX) under their individual names: *Amyl nitrite, Bamethan, Buphenine, Carbon dioxide, Cyclandelate, Dipyridamole, Hydralazine, Isosorbide dinitrate, Isoxsuprine, Nicotinic acid, Nitroglycerin, Pentaerithrityl tetranitrate,* and *Tolazoline.*

Verapamil hydrochloride (Calan, Isaptin), anti-anginal, cardiac depressant, and calcium blocker, has been reported when given in toxic doses (60 mg/kg) to cause cataracts in some groups of beagle dogs, but not in others, and not to cause cataracts in rats, rabbits or baboons.[a,b,c] In rats, verapamil did not enhance cataractogenesis from x-ray exposure, galactose, or tryptophane-free diet.[b] In incubated pieces of bovine lens the relationship of lens epithelium to lens capsule was alterable by verapamil, but only at concentrations 100 to 1000 times greater than encountered clinically.[c]

Intraocular pressure in normal people, according to Beatty et al,[279] is not affected by 80 mg orally, and is transiently raised less than 2 mm Hg by 2% eyedrops, but in rabbits 5% eyedrops cause nearly a 10 mm Hg transitory rise, probably due to increase in intraocular blood volume.

    a. Goke N: Investigations of the influence of oral verapamil administration on the development of Roentgen-cataract in rats. *DISS BONN* (1975) (German); reference from Rattke.[c]

    b. Hockwin O: Influence of verapamil on development of experimental cataracts in rats. Page 104 in FRAUNFELDER (1979).[311]

    c. Rattke W, Glasser D: Effects of verapamil on bovine lens epithelium in primary culture. *OPHTHALMIC RES* 10:162–167, 1978.

Veratridine, a veratrum alkaloid, has toxic effects on excised rabbit retina shown by alteration of the ERG, and enhancement of the retinal toxicity of aspartate.[a]

    a. Honda Y: The mode of action of veratridine on the electrical activity of the mammalian retina. *ACTA SOC OPHTHALMOL JPN* 81:135–143, 1977. (English abstract)

Veratrine (veratrin), a very poisonous mixture of alkaloids which formerly was used on the skin as a counterirritant. Small amounts in contact with the eye cause much irritation, lacrimation, and inflammation of the conjunctiva. The dust causes violent sneezing.[153,171,214,246]

Veratrum californicum is a plant that has been found to be teratogenic in sheep in the state of Idaho, causing cyclopian malformations when eaten by ewes during the second and third weeks of pregnancy.[a,b] The teratogenic components have been identified as *cyclopamine, cycloposine,* and *jervine.*[c]

  a. Babbott FL, Binns W, Ingalls TH: Field studies of cyclopian malformations in sheep. *ARCH ENVIRON HEALTH* 5:109–113, 1962.
  b. Binns W, James LF, et al: Cyclopian-type malformation in lambs. *ARCH ENVIRON HEALTH* 5:106–108, 1962.
  c. Mulvihill JJ: Congenital and genetic disease in domestic animals. *SCIENCE* 176:132–137, 1972.

Vick's Vapo Rub, an aromatic household remedy used for upper respiratory congestion and sometimes for headache, was tested on two rabbit eyes by applying it to the upper limbus after inducing local anesthesia with proparacaine eyedrops. These eyes showed no injury detectable by slit-lamp biomicroscopy at any time after the exposure.[a]

Of possible historical interest, a modified form, "Stainless" Vicks VapoRub, was a greaseless gel preparation which was marketed on a trial basis until Dahl in 1969 found that it caused a characteristic keratoconjunctivitis.[a] In place of petrolatum it had a greaseless vehicle of secret composition. When patients applied the greaseless gel preparation to the nose and temples they noticed blurring of vision four to twelve hours later, usually without discomfort at the onset of blurring, but with pain developing two to twenty-four hours later. Visual acuity was reduced by edema of the cornea and irregularity of the epithelium. In some patients the corneal epithelium was partially lost. Some had edema of the stroma of the cornea and wrinkles in Descemet's membrane. In most patients there were no signs of iritis. All patients recovered, usually within two or three days.

Tests on rabbit and human eyes confirmed that the greaseless gel preparation was injurious to the cornea, and provided evidence that the injury was caused by the secret greaseless gel base, not by the volatile constituents. The material apparently spread from the surrounding skin to the eyes.

  a. Dahl AA, Grant WM: Unusual keratitis from a household remedy. *AM J OPHTHALMOL* 68:858–862, 1969.

Vidarabine (Vira-A, Ara-A), an antiviral, has been used as a 3% ophthalmic ointment in treatment of herpes simplex keratitis. It has also been used as a 5% suspension injected subconjunctivally.[c] Although literature from the manufacturer of the ointment says, "Lacrimation, irritation, pain, and photophobia are among the reactions which been reported," published series of patients, as well as experiments in rabbits, indicate very little toxicity to the eye.[a,c,d,e] In one series of more than 100 patients only 3 reported mild itching or irritation, and one had moderate redness of the conjunctiva with temporary punctate keratitis, and none had punctal occlusion.[e] In rabbits, healing of experimental corneal epithelial defects was not retarded and histology was normal, but the strength of healed penetrating stromal wounds was subnormal.[c, d]

One report in the eye literature of testing for teratogenic effects in rabbits after systemic administration was negative,[b] but manufacturer's literature warns of teratogenic, mutagenic, and oncogenic effects detected in experimental animals.

(Also, see *Vidarabine phosphate.*)

a. Chin GN: Treatment of herpes simplex keratitis with idoxuridine and vidarabine. *ANN OPHTHALMOL* 10:1171–1174, 1978.
b. Gasset AR, Akaboski T: Teratogenicity of adenine arabinoside (Ara-A). *INVEST OPHTHALMOL* 15:556–558, 1976.
c. Kaufman HE, Ellison ED, Townsend WM: The chemotherapy of herpes iritis with adenine arabinoside and cytarabine. *ARCH OPHTHALMOL* 84:783–787, 1970.
d. Langston RHS, Pavan-Langston D, Dohlman CH: Antiviral medication and corneal wound healing. *ARCH OPHTHALMOL* 92:509–513, 1974.
e. Pavan-Langston D: Clinical evaluation of adenine arabinonide and idoxuridine in the treatment of ocular herpes simplex. *AM J OPHTHALMOL* 80:495–502, 1975.

Vidarabine phosphate (ara AMP), an antiviral, is more soluble than plain vidarabine, which was discussed above. Although non-toxic to normal rabbit eyes, a 3% solution applied to rabbit eyes with surgically produced corneal epithelial defects has been shown by Foster and Pavan-Langston to retard healing and to produce histologic evidence of toxicity to the regenerating epithelium.[308] Excised rabbit corneas perfused with concentrations of the drug more than a thousand times what might be attained in the aqueous humor clinically showed no functional or ultrastructural disturbance of the endothelium.[a]

a. Hull DS, Bowman K, Green K: Effect of vidarabine and related compounds on corneal endothelium. *INVEST OPHTHALMOL VIS SCI* 16:545–549, 1977.

Vinblastine sulfate (Vincaleukoblastine sulfate, Velban, Velbe), an antineoplastic from *Vinca rosea,* is of ophthalmic interest mainly because of toxicity to the cornea in accidental splash injuries, and because of toxicity to intraocular structures after experimental intraocular injection. Vinblastine is related to *vincristine,* which is notoriously neurotoxic, but neurotoxic involvement of the eye from vinblastine has been uncommon; two patients treated with vinblastine were reported by Albert to have developed extraocular muscle palsies and lagophthalmos.[a]

Four cases have been reported in which contamination of eyes from accidental squirt or spray of vinblastine intravenous-solution caused a fairly consistent type of keratopathy with a latent period, slow evolution and slow clearing.[e, i, j, 346] In the first case, reported by Morci in 1967, a physician accidentally squirted vinblastine solution from a broken syringe in one eye. Mosci did not say how long it was before symptoms developed and he saw the patient, but by then there was epiphora, photophobia, and reduction of vision to distinguishing hand movements. The cornea was not grossly opacified or roughened, but there was so much optical irregularity that no fundus details could be distinguished ophthalmoscopically.

This appeared to be associated with diffuse keratitis epithelialis, which appeared as gray specks by slit-lamp biomicroscopy and stained with fluorescein. Later some of the superficial gray areas became confluent, but all cleared within two months, and vision returned to normal with correcting lens. Astigmatism of 0.75 diopter developed as a result of the injury. Early in this case there was temporary corneal anesthesia.

Cordier described a nurse who sought attention six days after squirting vinblastine solution in one eye, having developed by this time photophobia, pain, tearing, and redness of the eye, with vision reduced to 1/10. Microcystic edema involved the entire corneal epithelium, and in the following days the epithelium ulcerated and came off in small sheets. Healing from the periphery toward the center began 2 weeks after the accident, and in 3.5 weeks the eye returned to normal.[e]

In a case described by Lisch a physician had sprayed the solution into both eyes, and 2 days later began to see rainbows from microcystic edema of the corneal epithelium.[346] At that stage there was little staining by fluorescein, but in following days staining became pronounced and larger epithelial cysts formed. Recovery was slow. The corneas appeared normal only after 2.5 weeks.

McLendon and Bron described a physician who sprayed the solution in both eyes.[i] Symptoms developed only after a latent period of 24 hours. Then there were haloes around lights and conjunctival redness. Cystic epithelial keratopathy and punctate epithelial keratopathy and erosions developed. During the next 8 days there were increasing blepharospasm, photophobia, and epiphora, decrease of vision to 6/60 in the worse eye, with development of epithelial bullous patches and a mild reaction in the anterior chamber. Corneal sensation was reported normal throughout. By 6 weeks the corneas were much better. There was no scarring, but a persistent dryness of one eye.

In 3 of the 4 cases the intraocular pressures were reported, and appeared to be normal.

Cordier and independently McLendon and Bron showed that a similar toxic effect on the cornea could be produced experimentally with topical vinblastine in rabbits.[e,i]

Unrelated to these experiments, Betrix found that vinblastine, 0.005 to 0.020 mg/kg, injected into the anterior chamber of rabbits produced small anterior polar cataracts and vascularization of the cornea, although the endothelium did not appear to be injured.[283]

Vinblastine has been utilized as an experimental tool in a series of studies of retinal function and ultrastructure.[b,c,d,h] By injection into the vitreous body it has been used to disrupt the microtubules of retinal ganglion cells and block rapid axonal transport from ganglion cells to superior colliculus.

Intraocular injection of vinblastine sulfate has also been reported to cause recoverable loss of corneal sensation and function of the sphincter pupillae muscle.[g]

Vinblastine has been shown to be teratogenic in hamsters, producing microphthalmia, anophthalmia, and other malformations.[f]

a. Albert DM, Wong V, Henderson ES: Ocular complications of vincristine therapy. *ARCH OPHTHALMOL* 78:709–713, 1967.
b. Bunt AH: Effects of vinblastine on microtubule structure and axonal transport in ganglion cells of the rabbit retina. *INVEST OPHTHALMOL* 12:579–590, 1973.

c. Bunt AH: Paracrystalline inclusions in optic nerve terminals following intraocular injection of vinblastine. *BRAIN RES* 53:29–39, 1973.

d. Chihara E, Sakugawa M, Entani S: Recovery of fast axonal transport and retinal protein synthesis in rabbits after intraocular administration of vinblastine. *BRAIN RES* 241:179–181, 1982.

e. Cordier J, Mendelsohn P: Corneal ulceration from an antimitotic. *BULL SOC OPHTAL-MOL FRANCE* 70:116–122, 1970. (French)

f. Ferm VH: Congenital malformations in hamster embryos after treatment with vinblastine and vincristine. *SCIENCE* 141:126, 1963.

g. Hahnenberger RW: Influence of intraocular colchicine and vinblastine on the cat iris. *ACTA PHYSIOL SCAND* 98:425–432, 1976.

h. Hansson HA: Retinal changes induced by treatment with vincristine and vinblastine. *DOCUM OPHTHALMOL* 31:65–68, 1972.

i. McLendon BF, Bron AJ: Corneal toxicity from vinblastine solution. *BR J OPHTHAL-MOL* 62:97–99, 1978.

j. Mosci L: Astigmatism against the rule in a case of burning of the cornea by vincaleuko-blastine. *ANN OTTALMOL CLIN OCUL* 93:94–100, 1967. (Italian)

Vincristine sulfate (Oncovin), an antineoplastic from *Vinca rosea*, is related to vinblastine, but has greater neurotoxicity. Vincristine in therapeutic use commonly causes sensory and motor peripheral neuropathy, cranial nerve neuropathy including optic nerve neuropathy, and injury to the retina. In experimental animals, injury to the retina can be produced by intravenous administration, and especially severe damage by intravitreal injection. Cataract can be induced in cultured lenses.

Cranial nerve involvement in one series of 50 patients caused facial paralysis, ptosis, or diplopia in 32% of the group (Sandler). In another series, among 18 patients who had ocular muscle complications from vincristine 14 had ptosis, 13 had paresis of rectus and oblique muscles, 6 had facial nerve palsy, and 2 had corneal hypesthesia (Albert). These conditions usually improved with reduction of dosage. Experimentally in mice, ultrastructural changes have been found in the fibers of the eye muscles themselves (Kaczmarski).

Optic neuropathy from systemic administration of vincristine (with nitrogen mustard and procarbazine) was suspected in 1976 in a patient whose vision dropped to 20/40 in each eye with mild pallor of the optic discs (Sanderson). At autopsy there was loss of retinal ganglion cells and diminution of nerve fibers in the retina, behind the lamina cribrosa, at the chiasm, and in the optic tracts. The lesions were non-inflammatory, necrotic, with demyelinating nerve bundles and lipid-laden macrophages in the chiasm and optic tracts. Subsequently, Norton described two children with severe unilateral retrobulbar pain and reduced vision, with much improvement after vincristine was discontinued. One of these children had an appearance of papillitis (Norton). Another child has been described as having reversible bilateral centro-cecal scotomas and dyschromatopsia (Caramazza).

In a patient who became night-blind after treatment with vincristine and other antineoplastic drugs, extensive functional studies by Ripps et al showed the a-wave potentials of the ERG to be normal, but the b-wave to be much depressed. It was speculated that synaptic transmission between photoreceptors and second-order neurons had been affected by vincristine (Ripps).

Cases of permanent loss of vision from vincristine have been reported by Fishman and Awidi. In Fishman's two cases the clinical and histological characteristics were more indicative of radiation-necrosis of optic nerve tissue than of purely toxic effect (Fishman). Awidi's patient had permanent bilateral blindness with optic atrophy, also severe peripheral and cranial nerve neuropathies (Awidi).

Transient cortical blindness has occurred in three children as a complication of vincristine therapy (Bryd).

Observation of ERG changes in patients led to experiments in rabbits, which showed that intravenous vincristine could cause an increase in the amplitude of the b-wave (Rix). Microscopic examination showed dose-related cell destruction in all layers of the retina, but some proved to be reversible (Koniszewski). Chronic administration to rabbits produced changes particularly in the outer plexiform layer of the retina (Haas).

Intravitreal injection of vincristine sulfate in rabbits was shown by Vrabec in 1968 to be rapidly injurious to the retina, producing histologic changes within 24 hours (Vrabec). To avoid morphologic change or alteration of the ERG the injected dose had to be kept to 1 mcg, or 0.4 mcg/ml.[277,369] In rats, intravitreal vincristine caused rapid appearance of ultrastructural abnormalities in retinal neurons and the inner segments of photoreceptor cells (Hansson). In monkeys, intravitreal injection of 0.1 to 10 mcg produced extreme atrophy of all layers of the retina and optic nerve (Green).

Posterior subcapsular cataract has been induced in cultured rat lenses by addition of vincristine sulfate to the medium (Mikuni).

Albert DM, Wong VG, Henderson ES: Ocular complications of vincristine therapy. *ARCH OPHTHALMOL* 78:709–713, 1967.

Awidi AS: Blindness and vincristine. *ANN INTERN MED* 93:781, 1980.

Byrd RL, Rohrbaugh TM, et al: Transient cortical blindness secondary to vincristine therapy in childhood malignancies. *CANCER* 47:37–40, 1981.

Caramazza R, Cellini M: Optic neuritis in the course of treatment with vincristine. *BOLL OCULIST* 60:579–590, 1981. (Italian)

Fishman ML, Bean SC, Cogan DG: Optic atrophy following prophylactic chemotherapy and cranial radiation for acute lymphocytic leukemia. *AM J OPHTHALMOL* 82:571–576, 1976.

Green WR: Retinal and optic nerve atrophy induced by intra-vitreous vincristine in the primate. *TRANS AM OPHTHALMOL SOC* 73:389–416, 1975.

Haas K, Koniszewski G, Rix R: Changes in the outer plexiform layer of the rabbit retina after long-term application of vincristine. *GRAEFES ARCH OPHTHALMOL* 211:23–33, 1979. (German)

Hansson HA: Retinal changes induced by treatment with vincristine and vinblastine. *DOCUM OPHTHALMOL* 31:65–88, 1972.

Kaczmarski F, Dabros W: Ultrastructural alterations in extrinsic eye muscles induced by vincristine. *FOLIA HISTOCHEM CYTOCHEM* 17:85–91, 1979.

Koniszewski G, Rix R, Brunner P: A histological and electron microscopic study of the rabbit retina after application of vincristine. *GRAEFES ARCH OPHTHALMOL* 199:147–156, 1976.

Mikuni I: Vincristine sulfate-induced cataract in vitro. *JPN J OPHTHALMOL* 24:232–240, 1980.

Mikuni I: Histological comparison of senile posterior subcapsular cortical cataract and experimental posterior subcapsular cortical cataract induced by vincristine sulfate. *TOKAI J EXP CLIN MED* 5:243–250, 1980.

Norton SW, Stockman JA: Unilateral optic neuropathy following vincristine chemotherapy. *J PEDIATR OPHTHALMOL* 16:190–193, 1979.

Ripps H, Carr RE, et al: Functional abnormalities in vincristine-induced night blindness. *INVEST OPHTHALMOL VIS SCI* 25:787–794, 1984.

Rix R, Mieckley W: The electroretinogram of the rabbit under vincristine. *BER DTSCH OPHTHALMOL GESELLSCH* 73:175–176, 1975.

Sanderson PA, Kuwabara T, Cogan DG: Optic neuropathy presumably caused by vincristine therapy. *AM J OPHTHALMOL* 81:146–150, 1976.

Sandler SG, Tobin W, Henderson ES: Vincristine-induced neuropathy. *NEUROLOGY* 19:367–374, 1969.

Vrabec F, Obenberger J, Bolkova A: Effect of intravitreous vincristine sulfate on the rabbit retina. *AM J OPHTHALMOL* 66:199–204, 1968.

Vinyl acetate, Vinyl chloride, and **Vinyl ethyl ether** have each been listed in single instances of injury of the human cornea, with return to normal in 48 hours.[165]

Vinyl propionate tested as 10% solution in propylene glycol by application of a drop to rabbit eyes caused only slight conjunctival hyperemia and edema lasting twenty-four hours.[a]

a. Ambrose AM: Toxicological studies of compounds investigated for use as inhibitors of biological process. I. Toxicity of vinyl propionate. *ARCH IND HYG* 2:582, 1950.

Vinyl toluene has been tested by application of a drop to rabbit eyes and found to cause slight transient conjunctival irritation, but no injury of the cornea demonstrable by staining with fluorescein.[265]

Vitamin A (retinol) in large overdosage causes elevated intracranial pressure with papilledema (Gelpke; Morrice; Parent; Pasquariello; Smith; Van Dyk;[386] Van Oye), and in some cases peripapillary hemorrhages (Smith). Adverse effects of excessive vitamin A have been well reviewed by Van Oye. Diplopia has been the presenting symptom in several cases, secondary to increased intracranial pressure (Morrice; Oliver; Turtz; Van Oye). Vision and visual fields generally have been little, if at all, affected. Ocular manifestations most commonly appear after many months of overdosage, and characteristically are accompanied by headache, nausea and vomiting, somnolence, pains in the bones, and fissuring of the angles of the mouth (Morrice). Skin changes may be associated with loss of hair, including eyelashes and eyebrows (Di Benedetto; Oliver; Stimson; Van Oye). Acute poisoning can also occur. Instances of acute rise of cerebrospinal fluid pressure from single very large doses have been observed in infants. A similar acute rise is thought to have occurred in adults from eating shark or polar bear liver, which contain large amounts of vitamin A (Oliver). It is possible that a specific retinol-binding protein normally protects from the toxic effects of free retinol, but when the amount of the vitamin exceeds the amount of the specific protein, poisoning occurs (Smith).

Exophthalmos has been induced in animals by large doses of vitamin A (Josephs;

Maddock), but in human beings increased prominence of the eyes has been reported only in exceptional cases (Stimson).

Discontinuance of vitamin A has usually caused rapid reduction of symptoms. Blurring of the margins of the optic nerveheads may be gone in days (Smith), or may take months to resolve (Oliver).

An investigation of the effect of vitamin A on intraocular pressure was carried out to see whether this pressure might be raised like the intracranial pressure, but in rabbits and normal human beings it was found instead to be appreciably reduced. In five cases of primary open-angle glaucoma no significant effect was found (Hartmann).

In rats, experimental hypervitaminosis A has been shown to damage the retina, mainly the outer segments and pigment epithelium according to electron microscopy (Amemiya). The ERG of poisoned rats was altered, but returned to normal when the rats were allowed to recover (Tamaki). No change in appearance of the fundi was observed during the poisoning. *In vitro,* release and activation of lysosomal enzymes has been found, raising the speculation that if this occurs *in vivo* it might explain the retinal disturbances detected by histology and ERG (Vento).

Deficiency of vitamin A is a notorious factor in keratomalacia. However, excessive vitamin A intake does not seem to affect the cornea by clinical standards. Experimentally in rabbits an effect is found when very large doses are given intravenously. This has reduced the mucoid content of the cornea and the number of conjunctival goblet cells, at the same time causing a somewhat analogous collapse of ear cartilage (Akinosko).

Ocular teratogenic effects from excessive vitamin A have been reported in various animals, though not yet demonstrated in human beings. Effects in rats, mice, rabbits and chickens summarized by Van Oye have included anophthalmos, microphthalmos, and cataract (Van Oye). Subsequently reports have appeared of abnormalities induced during pregnancy in the lenses and retinas of rats (Kalter), anophthalmos in rats (Barbuta), coloboma in hamsters (Geeraets), and exophthalmos in hamsters and guinea pigs secondary to shallow orbits (Robens).

Akinosho EA, Basu PK: Ocular mucoid depletion in hypervitaminosis A. *CAN J OPHTHALMOL* 6:143–147, 1971.

Amemiya T: Cytochemical and electron microscopic examination of the retina of rats with hypervitaminosis A. *ACTA SOC OPHALMOL JPN* 71:2236–2251, 1967.

Barbuta R, Apostol S, et al: Experimental congenital malformations induced by hypervitaminosis A. MORFOL NORM PATHOL 17:337–343, 1972.

Di Benedette RJ: Chronic hypervitaminosis A in an adult. *J AM MED ASSOC* 201:700–702, 1967.

Geeraets R: Experimentally induced colobomas in the golden hamster. *MED COLL VA QUART* 8:278–282, 1972.

Gelpke PM: Vitamin A intoxication. *CAN MED ASSOC J* 104:533, 1971.

Hartmann E, Saraux H: Hypervitaminosis A and ocular tension. *BULL SOC FR OPHTALMOL* 70:446, 1957. (French)

Josephs: Hypervitaminosis A. *KLIN WOCHENSCHR* 12:1732, 1933.

Kalter H: Teratogenically induced congenital aphakia. *EXP EYE RES* 3:228–229, 1964.

Maddock CL, Wolbach SB, Maddock S: Hypervitaminosis A in the dog. *J NUTRITION* 39:117, 1949.

Morrice G, Havener WH, Kapetansky F: Vitamin A intoxication as a cause of pseudotumor cerebri. *J AM MED ASSOC* 173:1802–1805, 1960.

Oliver TK, Havener WH: Eye manifestations of chronic vitamin A intoxication. *ARCH OPHTHALMOL* 60:19–22, 1958.

Parent G: Hypervitaminosis A and papilledema. *BULL SOC BELGE OPHTALMOL* 152:596–603, 1969.

Pasquariello PS Jr: Benign increased intracranial hypertension due to chronic vitamin A overdosage in a 26-month-old child. *CLIN PEDIATR* 16:379–382, 1977.

Robens JF: Teratogenic effects of hypervitaminosis A in the hamster and in the guinea pig. *TOXICOL APPL PHARMACOL* 16:88–99, 1970.

Smith FR, Goodman DS: Vitamin A transport in human vitamin A toxicity. *N ENGL J MED* 294:805–808, 1976.

Stimson WH: Vitamin A intoxication in adults. *N ENGL J MED* 265:369–373, 1961.

Tamaki S: Electroretinographic studies on experimental hypervitaminosis A. *ACTA SOC OPHTHALMOL JPN* 72:156–163, 1968.

Turtz CA, Turtz AI: Vitamin A intoxication. *AM J OPHTHALMOL* 50:165–166, 1960.

Van Oye R: THE VITAMINS. Chapter 16 in Michiels (1972).[359]

Vento R, Cacioppo F: The effect of retinol on the lysosomal enzymes of bovine retina and pigment epithelium. *EXP EYE RES* 15:43–49, 1973.

Vitamin D in excess can cause calcification in the cornea and conjunctiva in the form of band keratopathy.[a, c-f] The opacity is superficial, just beneath the epithelium of the cornea, close to the limbus in the palpebral fissure, but actually separated from the limbus by a narrow clear interval. The opacity tends to fade out toward the center of the cornea. Often the keratopathy is accompanied by white flecks and crystal-like opacities in the bulbar conjunctiva.[a]

Experimentally in rabbits, administration of large amounts of vitamin D has produced band keratopathy, but only after uveitis was induced by injection of egg albumin into the vitreous body, and only when the animals were allowed to keep their eyes open, permitting evaporation. This was believed to be an example of calciphylaxis, in which calcification was produced by a combination of tissue alteration (by uveitis) and a calcium mobilizing agent (vitamin D).[b] Possibly this is related to development of calcific band keratopathy that occurs in some human beings who have chronic uveitis.

Calcific band keratopathy from vitamin D poisoning can gradually disappear after the poisoning is stopped, or it can be removed surgically by scraping the cornea, or it can be dissolved in ten to twenty minutes by application of 0.01 to 0.05 M sodium edetate (EDTA) at physiologic pH after removal of the epithelium from the cornea.[c]

a. Cogan DG, Albright F, Bartter FC: Hypercalcemia and band keratopathy. *ARCH OPHTHALMOL* 40:624–638, 1948.

b. Doughman DJ, Olson GA, Nolan S, Hajny RG: Experimental band keratopathy. *ARCH OPHTHALMOL* 81:264–271, 1969.

c. Grant WM: A new treatment for calcific corneal opacities. *ARCH OPHTHALMOL* 48:681–685, 1952.

d. Leira H: Hypercalcemia and band keratopathy. *ACTA OPHTHALMOL* 32:605–614, 1954.

e. Walsh FB, Howard JE: Conjunctival and corneal lesions in hypercalcemia. *J CLIN ENDOCRINOL* 7:644–652, 1947.

f. Severin M, Bulla M: Corneal deposits in children on dialysis and vitamin D_3 and 1,25 DHCC. *KLIN MONATSBL AUGENHEILKD* 175:670–676, 1979.

Volcanic ash from eruptions of Mount St. Helens in the state of Washington in 1980 caused sensations of eye irritation and conjunctival hyperemia in many people exposed to the ash in the form of dust in the air. An extensive ophthalmologic survey concluded that the irritation was attributable to the physical properties of the dust particles, and no evidence of chemical or toxic action was found.[a]

a. Fraunfelder FT, Kalina RE, et al: Ocular effects following the volcanic eruptions of Mt St Helens. *ARCH OPHTHALMOL* 101:376–378, 1983.

Warfarin (Coumadin) has been used as a rodenticide and as an anticoagulant in human beings. One of its well-known adverse side effects is production of hemorrhages. In rare instances it has produced hemorrhages in the retina,[b,d] and hyphema.[c]

Teratogenesis affecting the eyes of offspring of mothers who have taken warfarin or other anticoagulants early in pregnancy has been documented. Disaia described one instance of bilateral optic atrophy.[a] A review of the literature by Shaul and Hall disclosed that 5 out of 14 infants with abnormalities associated with use of anticoagulants during pregnancy had eye abnormalities, including optic atrophy, microphthalmos, lens opacity, and large eyes.[e]

a. Disaia PJ: Pregnancy and delivery of a patient with a Starr-Edwards mitral valve prothesis. *OBSTET GYNECOL* 28:469–472, 1966.

b. Gordon DM, Mead J: Retinal hemorrhage with visual loss during anticoagulant therapy. *J AM GERIAT SOC* 16:99–100, 1968.

c. Koehler MP, Sholiton DB: Spontaneous hyphema resulting from warfarin. *ANN OPHTHALMOL* 15:858–859, 1983.

d. Markson VI: Long-term anticoagulant therapy as an office procedure. *ANGIOLOGY* 15:51–56, 1964.

e. Shaul WL, Hall JG: Multiple congenital anomalies associated with oral anticoagulants. *AM J OBSTET GYNECOL* 127:191–198, 1977.

Wasp stings appear to be more painful and cause more reaction than stings of bees. (See INDEX for *Bee stings*.) Swelling of the lids and inflammation is more persistent. The seriousness of wasp sting of the cornea has long been known.[153] The cornea rapidly becomes opaque about the site of injury. This may be accompanied by iritis with hypopyon and much pain. Secondary glaucoma and cataract have followed in some instances. The inflammatory reaction usually subsides in two or three weeks, but bullous keratitis has been known to persist for many months.[a,d,g,h] After the acute reaction to wasp venom, the wasp's stinger may remain in the eye as an inert foreign body. A case has been described in which a wasp sting was seen to be sticking from the front of the lens 28 years after it had penetrated through the cornea and had caused an acute transient reaction. Vision was 6/9, due to a tiny corneal scar and small anterior polar lens opacity.[c]

A very unusual reaction to penetration of the cornea by the sting of a mud-dauber wasp was described by Landers in 1967.[f] The same day after the stinging occurred, the patient noted enlargement of the pupil and loss of perception of light in the injured eye. Four days later when the eye was first examined, the patient was unable to discern the direction of light with the eye. In the cornea around the tract of the sting was a 3 mm hazy zone, but the eye did not appear inflamed, and the aqueous, vitreous, and fundus appeared normal. Under systemic treatment with corticosteroids the vision and the pupil gradually returned to normal. Landers postulated that a paralytic agent in the venom had acted upon the sphincter muscle of the iris and also upon the optic nerve or retina, or both.[f]

A case of retrobulbar neuritis has been reported by Konstas and Nicolinacos, who described reduction of vision to 5/10 a week after a man had been stung by a wasp on the edge of the upper eyelid. Within a few weeks the visual acuity had improved nearly to normal, but a small paracentral scotoma persisted. Since the fundi had appeared normal at each examination, it was postulated that the venom had caused retrobulbar neuritis.[e]

Myasthenia gravis with ptosis of the lids, and a positive edrophonium test, followed wasp stings on the finger in a most unusual case.[b]

a. Bar C: Cataract after sting of wasp. *KLIN MONATSBL AUGENHEILKD* 51:314–315, 1913. (German)
b. Brumlik J: Myasthemia gravis associated with wasp sting. *J AM MED ASSOC* 235:2120–2121, 1976.
c. Gilboa M, Gdal-on M, Zonis S: Bee and wasp stings of the eye. *BR J OPHTHALMOL* 61:662–664, 1977.
d. Johnson MC: Wasp sting of the cornea. *J AM MED ASSOC* 99:2025–2026, 1932.
e. Konstas P, Nicolinacos G: Retrobulbar neuritis following wasp sting. *ARCH SOC OPHTAL GREECE NORD* 14:144–147, 1965. (*EXCERPTA MED* (SECT 12), 21:1186, 1967.)
f. Landers PH: Mud dauber wasp venom in anterior chamber. *AM J OPHTHALMOL* 64:1168, 1967.
g. Norris S: A wasp sting. *BR J OPHTHALMOL* 28:139, 1944.
h. Zahn K: Wasp sting injury of the cornea. *CESK OFTALMOL* 217–220, 1950.

Water might scarcely be considered a toxic substance, and its effects on the eye are mainly physical, yet applied to the eye without sufficient dissolved substances to provide physiologic tonicity, it does cause edema of the corneal stroma and epithelium, and if applied to the endothelium can cause injury.[b, 123] Bathing the eyes with water for 20 minutes causes primarily corneal epithelial edema, which increases sensitivity to glare and may cause appearance of halos around lights, but the effect is promptly reversible.[a] First-aid irrigation of chemically burned eyes likewise can cause transient epithelial edema, but no persistent harm has been shown, and it appears safe and proper to use water for this purpose without wasting time in seeking some more physiologic solution.

While bathing the eyes with distilled water may produce transient corneal epithelial edema without discomfort, other hypotonic but less pure waters may cause notable irritation and discomfort. (For further on this, see INDEX for *Swimming pool water,* and *Acidic lake water.*)

a. Carney LG, Jacobs RJ: Mechanisms of visual loss in corneal edema. *ARCH OPHTHAL-MOL* 102:1068–1071, 1984.

b. Cogan DG: Applied anatomy and physiology of the cornea. *TRANS AM ACAD OPHTHALMOL OTOL* 329–355, 1951.

Witch hazel (*Hamamelis virginiana*) alcoholic extract splashed into the eyes causes immediate pain and conjunctival hyperemia, but no serious injury, and recovery has been rapid.[249]

Wood dusts, particularly from tropical woods, have frequently caused irritation of the skin and inflammation of the eyes, with hyperemia of the conjunctiva; swelling of the lids, discomfort, lacrimation, and occasionally keratitis epithelialis.[a-c] Usually the dusts have been carried to the eyes in the air or on the fingers of workmen sawing and sanding the woods.

Woods that have been identified as causing ocular irritation include *boxwood*,[46] *cedar*,[215] *Khaya anthoteca*,[b] *Machaerium scleroxylon*,[b] *Makare, Monsonia altissima*,[a] *Mimusops toxisperma*,[a] *Moule wood*,[c] *Pau d'arco*,[a] *satinwood*,[46] and *teakwood*, but there are many others.[d] (Additional concerning *Makare, Manchineal*, and *Teakwood* is to be found under separate listings in the INDEX.)

Some European woods, including *beech, fir, larch*, and *oak*, have been tested in rabbit eyes and found not to be particularly irritating, whereas some of the tropical woods mentioned above caused definite irritation and injury to the corneal epithelium in rabbits.[a]

a. Kubena K, Kadlec K, Hanslian C: Professional eye diseases caused by timber dust. *KLIN OCZNA* 38:53–55, 1968.

b. Morgan JWW, Orsler RJ, Wilkinson DS: Dermatitis due to the wood dusts of *Khaya anthotheca* and *Machaerium scleroxylon*. *BR J IND MED* 25:119–125, 1968.

c. Piorkowski FO: Woodworker's dermatitis in East Africa. *E AFR MED J* 21:60–64, 1944.

d. Peyresblanques J: Blepharo-conjunctivitis from the dusts of "colonial" woods. *BULL SOC OPHTALMOL FRANCE* 77:177–178, 1977. (French)

Wood foreign bodies cause problems both outside and inside the globe, and, because of their radio-transparency, they present difficulties in detection and identification.

Extraocular wood foreign bodies, in the lids or orbit, typically cause swelling and suppuration with a chronically draining fistula, not relieved by antibiotics, only partially helped by corticosteroids, and only cured by removal of the wood. In exceptional cases in which there appears to be no secondary infection a foreign-body granuloma with draining fistula is characteristic, nevertheless, suggesting some toxic effect of wood on surrounding tissues. As a rule clinical descriptions of wood foreign bodies in the lids or orbit do not mention the kind of wood involved, nor do they discuss mechanisms by which wood may incite its inflammatory and granulomatous effects.[a,e,f,k]

Intraocular wood foreign bodies, from being struck in the eye by tree branches, wood chips, or wooden arrows, characteristically cause intraocular inflammation with abcess and granulomatous reaction, with foreign body giant cells, in the anterior chamber[b,c,l,m] or vitreous body.[g,l,m] The reaction in some cases is prompt and acute, possibly involving bacterial infection, or may be delayed for weeks or months if there is fungal infection.[h] In some cases fragments of wood have become surrounded by granulomas in the iris[b,c,d,j] or angle of the anterior chamber,[i] and have remained quiet for years. However, after years of quiescence an acute inflammatory reaction has developed in some cases,[c,i,l] and sympathetic uveitis in at least one.[l]

In most reports the kind of wood has not been mentioned, though mention has been made of *pine bark*[b] and *oak wood*[g] in one case each, without implying any special properties. In cases in which bacterial or fungal infection is obvious there is no reason to speculate on toxicity of wood. However, in several cases there appears to have been no secondary infection,[b,c,g,i] and in other cases only saprophytic fungi have been identified, apparently not having an active role in inflammation.[h] The cases in which no infection has been detected, but in which wooden foreign bodies have caused characteristic intraocular inflammation and granulomatous reactions raise the question of toxic effect of wood on ocular tissues. Wolter[m] has speculated concerning wood foreign bodies that, "Irritation can be due to a reaction that results from the dissolution of these substances by tissue fluids or phagocytes and it can also be caused by toxic oxidation products."

a. Brock L, Tanenbaum HL: Retention of wooden foreign bodies in the orbit. *CAN J OPHTHALMOL* 15:70–72, 1980.

b. Cornand G, Brisou B, et al: Iris granuloma from a foreign body. *ANN OCULIST (Paris)* 208:227–232, 1975. (French)

c. Eagle RC, Shields JA, et al: Intraocular wooden foreign body clinically resembling a pearl cyst. *ARCH OPHTHALMOL* 95:835–836, 1977.

d. Fox SA: Intraocular foreign body of wood. *AM J OPHTHALMOL* 25:1105–1107, 1942.

e. Legras M, Lecoq PJ: Orbital wounds with retention of foreign bodies (radio-transparent). *ARCH OPHTALMOL (Paris)* 30:57–60, 1970.

f. Macreae JA: Diagnosis and management of a wooden orbital foreign body. *BR J OPHTHALMOL* 63:848–851, 1979.

g. Meyer Rf, Ritchey CL: Migration of a wooden foreign body into the lens. *CAN J OPHTHALMOL* 10:408–411, 1975.

h. Meyer RF, Hood CI: Fungus implantation with wooden intraocular foreign bodies. *ANN OPHTHALMOL* 9:271–278, 1977.

i. Onishi: A case of an old injury by a piece of bamboo enclosed in the chamber angle for 13 years. *KLIN MONATSBL AUGENHEILKD* 51:742, 1913. (German)

j. Pickard R: Implantation tumour of the iris containing wood fibers. *TRANS OPHTHALMOL SOC UK* 26:62–66, 1906.

k. Wesley RE, Wahl JW, et al: Management of wooden foreign bodies in the orbit. *SOUTH MED J* 75:924–932, 1982.

l. Wilder HC: Intraocular foreign bodies in soldiers. *AM J OPHTHALMOL* 31:57–64, 1948.

m. Wolter JR: The lens as a barrier against foreign body reaction. *OPHTHALMIC SURG* 12:42–45, 1981.

Xenon gas injected into rabbit eyes to replace part of the vitreous humor was absorbed within several hours without clinically evident toxic effects.[345]

Xylene (xylol, dimethylbenzene) vapor causes sensation of irritation of the eyes in some individuals at 200 ppm in air. For day-long working conditions most experimentally exposed subjects have selected 100 ppm as the highest tolerable concentration.[b, 183]

Foggy vision was described by Lewin and Guillery in 1913 in one patient after exposure to xylene vapors of unknown concentration for several weeks, but the nature of the visual disturbance was not established.[153] Conceivably this patient's fogging of vision was due to vacuolar epithelial keratopathy such as reported by Matthaus in 1964 in several workers a few days after beginning all-day exposure to high vapor concentration of "practically pure" xylene, said to be accompanied by negligible amounts of benzene or toluene.[c] The vacuolar keratopathy in these patients appeared to be the same as that which has been produced by n-butanol. (This is described under *n-Butanol* and under *Solvent vapors; see INDEX.*) The workmen recovered spontaneously when exposure to xylene vapor was reduced.

By exposing cats for several hours to concentrations of xylene vapor which were just sublethal, Schmid in 1957 succeeded in producing vacuoles in the corneal epithelium which appeared to be analogous to those in vacuolar keratopathy occurring in workmen from exposure to solvent vapors.[216] Matthaus in 1964 also succeeded in causing some corneal epithelial damage in rabbits by exposure to xylene vapors, but noted no vacuoles in these animals.[c] (There may well be species differences in propensity to formation of corneal epithelial vacuoles.)

Liquid xylene dropped on rabbits' eyes causes immediate discomfort and blepharospasm, followed by hyperemia of the conjunctiva and very slight transient injury of the corneal epithelium, demonstrable by staining with fluorescein.[35, 46, 81, 265] Accidental splash in the human eyes similarly causes only transient superficial damage, with rapid recovery.

Injection of xylene into the vitreous body in animals has, as might be expected, been damaging to the retina.[a]

a. Adachi J: Experimental studies on the effect of some hemolytic agents on the eyes. *ACTA SOC OPHTHALMOL JPN* 39:2332–2345, 1935.
b. Clinton M: Xylene. *AM PETROL INST TOXIC REV,* March 1948.
c. Matthaus W: Contribution concerning the corneal disturbance of finish-workers in the furniture industry. *KLIN MONATSBL AUGENHEILKD* 144:713–717, 1964. (German)

Xylose has been among the sugars studied for cataract production in animals. It has been shown to produce cataracts in weanling rats, but older rats are resistant to this effect.[a-d] The cataract produced by xylose consists of an opacification of the lens which is transient. The influence of age of the rats appears to be due to differences in metabolism and differences in concentrations of xylose that are attained in the blood. vanHeyningen has shown that the development of the opacity is associated with accumulation of polyols (*xylitol* and *sorbitol*) and that the clearing of the opacity is correlated with the disappearance of these polyols.

In incubated rat lenses, Obazawa et al have shown rapid development of opacity due to accumulation of *xylitol,* electrolytes and water when D-xylose is added to the medium. Addition of an aldose reductase inhibitor prevents these effects of xylose, demonstrating the primary role of this enzyme in the cataractogenic process, similar to its role in experimental galactose cataracts.

    a. Obazawa H, Merola LO, Kimoshita JH: The effects of xylose on the isolated lens. *INVEST OPHTHALMOL* 13:204–209, 1974.

    b. Patterson JW, Bunting KW: Sugar cataracts, polyol levels and lens swelling. *DOCUM OPHTHALMOL* 20:64–72, 1966.

    c. Schrader KE: Morphology and pathogenesis of experimental xylose cataract. *GRAEFES ARCH OPHTHALMOL* 163:422–443, 1961. (German)

    d. Van Heyningen R: Xylose cataract; A comparison between the weanling and the older rat. *EXP EYE RES* 8:379–385, 1969.

Xylyl bromides and **chlorides** (including o-, m-, and p-isomers) are strongly lacrimatory.[171]

(See also Bromoxylene.)

Ytterbium chloride tested on rabbit eyes by applying 0.1 ml of 1 : 1 aqueous solution at pH 3.05 to 3.78, caused "conjunctival irritation" and ulceration which healed in ninety-six hours.[97]

Yttrium chloride applied to rabbit eyes as a 0.1 M solution (pH 5.4) for ten minutes caused no injury, but similar exposure of eyes from which the corneal epithelium had been removed to facilitate penetration of the yttrium chloride resulted in immediate slight haziness of the cornea, with subsequent increasing opacity in the next several days. Finally the corneas became completely opaque and vascularized. Exposure to 0.01 M solution after removal of the epithelium resulted in slight to mild permanent opacification.

    Treatment by irrigation with neutral 0.01 to 0.1 M sodium edetate (EDTA) solutions for fifteen minutes immediately after exposure to yttrium chloride solution prevented much of the opacification and vascularization. Similar treatment with sodium chloride solution was without appreciable effect.[88] (Compare *Rare-earth salts; see INDEX.*)

Zinc chloride and **zinc sulfate** are described together because they have strong similarities in their properties, though injuries of the cornea have been more commonly related to the chloride than to the sulfate, and most animal experiments have been carried out with the chloride. Both salts are white, odorless solids, very soluble in water (1 g in 0.5 or 0.6 ml of water, forming slightly acid solutions, pH 4 or 4.5). Zinc chloride is used in high concentration in soldering fluxes, galvanizing baths, sometimes in golf balls, and in "chemosurgery" of skin cancer. Dilute solutions (0.2% to 1%) have long been used as astringent eyedrops without difficulty, but concentrated solutions and pastes such as encountered industrially have caused very severe injuries of the cornea in numerous cases of accidental splash in the eye.

    The following description is organized to present information on the toxic effects in the following order: (a) human eye injuries from concentrated zinc chloride,

(b) eye injuries from concentrated zinc sulfate, (c) animal experiments with zinc chloride, and (d) clinical experience with dilute zinc salt solutions.

Human eye injuries from concentrated zinc chloride. These have been reported several times since 1903. Lewin and Guillery and Wagenmann summarized what had been reported to 1913.[153,253] Tillot, according to Wagenmann, reported the first case of corneal ulceration and iritis, but eventual partial recovery, after accidental splash of a concentrated zinc salt in 1903.

Zur Nedden reported in detail concerning a workman who splashed a zinc chloride solution of unstated concentration in one eye, causing at first only some redness, and persistent discomfort, but within six days leading to a discrete stromal opacity in the lower part of the cornea with irregularity of the overlying epithelium.[268] The opacity was grayish, located in the anterior layers of the stroma. During the next month, while some portions cleared, the remainder became dense white, and was thought to be a zinc encrustation. A discrete white opacity covered by epithelium remained, and because it was in the lower part of the cornea did not affect vision. Strader also reported a case of partial irreversible corneal opacification from zinc chloride burn.[n]

Van Lint described a workman who had splashed in one eye a liquid composed of zinc chloride, ammonium chloride, iron chloride, and hydrochloric acid, producing a burn of the cornea, and subsequently white spots in the front of the lens.[o] At six weeks after the injury the cornea still had stromal infiltration. The lens showed a great many white spots of varied shape beneath the anterior capsule, smaller than initially. From 2.5 to 6 months after injury the vision recovered only from 1/10 to 1/6, with a correcting spectacle. The impairment of vision was due to abnormality of the cornea rather than to the anterior subcapsular lens changes. The deeper parts of the lens remained normal.

Rzehulka described in detail a patient who had an eye accidentally burned by instillation of one drop of 50% zinc chloride solution.[m] There was immediate severe pain, which persisted despite immediate irrigation with water. The corneal epithelium became eroded. Large folds developed in Descemet's membrane, and the corneal stroma was turbid. This was accompanied by severe iritis with small hemorrhages in the iris. Deep and superficial vascularization of the cornea followed. The eye was treated with mydriatic and cortisone eyedrops and 5% neutral ammonium tartrate eye bath. In four months the cornea cleared sufficiently to permit 6/8 vision.

De Rose described a workman who splashed a reaction mixture of zinc and hydrochloric acid in one eye, causing great pain.[a] After irrigation of the surface, the cornea was found to have lost its epithelium but the stroma appeared transparent. Two days later most of the cornea was transparent, but for the first time small opacities appeared in the anterior cortical layers of the lens. Vision was reduced to 1/12 and the intraocular pressure was subnormal. At six days the anterior cortical lens opacity was more diffuse and the aqueous turbid. At ten days the surface of the cornea was almost healed, but the lens opacity and turbidity of the aqueous were more accentuated, and much pigment became deposited on the posterior surface of the cornea. The intraocular pressure remained low, and treatment with mydriatics and local corticosteroid was continued. At twenty days the patient had acute glaucoma with pain, corneal edema, and tension of 50 mm Hg, responding to treatment with oral acetazolamide during several days, but at about thirty days from the injury the glaucoma and pain returned. The cornea was diffusely clouded by edema and much pigment on the posterior surface. A scleral staphyloma developed. Vision was so low and pain so great that the eye was enucleated. Histologic examination confirmed extensive dissemination of pigment on the back surface of the cornea and in the trabecular meshwork. Also, iridocorneal synechias were present irregularly. The iris was mostly degenerated, with nearly complete loss of pigment. The lens had become cataractous. It was believed that these extensive injuries were attributable to the action of zinc chloride. The glaucoma was believed to have been due to infiltration of the trabecular meshwork with pigment.

Houle and Pavan-Langston have reported on two patients who had severe damage to their eyes from concentrated zinc chloride.[e, k] One of these patients had zinc chloride solder-flux paste splashed into one eye. The other patient had his eyes accidentally drenched by concentrated zinc chloride solution used in galvanizing steel. Both patients within the next day or two developed changes in the appearance of their eyes that was remarkably similar to the appearance of eyes that have very recently undergone severe acute attacks of angle-closure glaucoma. These eyes had extensive corneal edema, with wrinkling of the posterior surface, cells in the aqueous humor, and small discrete spots of gray opacity on the front of the lens, exactly like Glaukomflecken. Both patients took many months for subsidence of their corneal edema and for recovery of useful vision. Glaucoma was not a problem in these patients, but acetazolamide was given with the hope of making the intraocular pressure lower than normal. Corticosteroids given systemically seemed to help relieve discomfort and photophobia that developed after the corneal epithelium (and presumably the corneal nerves) regenerated. In these cases, as in those previously described in the literature, the spots in the lenses that were evident within the first few days after injury not only looked like Glaukomflecken, but also subsequently behaved like Glaukomflecken, persisting, but tending to become smaller, and causing no significant trouble. The corneas were the great problem.

In treatment of cancer of the eyelid and closely neighboring skin, Mohs has used a saturated solution of zinc chloride made into a paste by addition of powdered stibnite (antimony trisulfide) and sanguinaria powder.[g, h] Fortunately, injury to the eye has not occurred. This may be explained by the fact that the paste has been applied to the outer surface of the eyelid, and care has been taken not to bring the paste into direct contact with the eye.

Human eye injuries from concentrated zinc sulfate solutions. These seem all to have been reported in the 1950's as a complication of use of 20% zinc sulfate solution for treatment of dendritic keratitis, recurrent erosion, and ulcus serpens. Prior to 1955 the application of 20% zinc sulfate solution on a swab directly to such ulcers was considered to be fairly safe, and though some cursory mention had been made of occasional delicate branching opacities which had developed under the anterior lens capsule, such complications were considered to be rare.[c, i] Pillat presented the first detailed description of cases of white flecks induced in the lens after cauterization of the cornea with 20% zinc sulfate, having the characteristic appearance of the "Glaukomflecken" of Vogt, such as typically are associated with acute attacks of glaucoma, but Pillat established that in these cases there were no elevations of intraocular pressure.[1]

Filipovic reported that in three cases cauterization of herpetic dendritic keratitis with 20% zinc sulfate solution caused Glaukomflecken to appear by the next day.[b] The corneas became gray, but cleared while the flecks in the lenses remained. The same author noted that he had used 10% zinc sulfate solution in treating dendritic keratitis in three children, and that this had cured the keratitis and had caused no lens opacities. (All reports of Glaukomflecken had involved use of more concentrated solution in adult patients.)

Animal experiments with zinc chloride solutions. Experiments probably were undertaken before 1885, according to Hoffman, who mentioned that application of zinc chloride to frogs' eyes had been reported to cause purulent keratitis,[d] but the first significant observations from experiments appear to have been made by Zur Nedden, who experimented on enucleated pig eyes.[268] He found that he could produce a grayish, but not a white, opacity of the cornea by applying zinc salts, and this could be done easier with zinc chloride than zinc sulfate. His experiments led him to believe that the opacifications were due to formation of a zinc-mucoid precipitate, not due to a zinc-collagen combination, and he concluded that there was little or no formation of zinc carbonate.

Guillery found that when he applied 50% zinc chloride solution repeatedly to one eye of an albino rabbit, it caused opacity of the cornea, and that six days later the eye had become very hard, with extensive hemorrhage in the anterior segment, and that there was much infiltration with inflammatory cells, loss of corneal endothelium, and clouding of the anterior portion of the lens.[96]

Johnstone and Sullivan investigated whether using sodium edetate (EDTA) in first aid treatment of eyes contaminated with zinc chloride might be beneficial.[f] They measured the turgescence properties of pieces of bovine cornea in water and obtained evidence that denaturation or fixation occurred when cornea was brought into contact with zinc chloride solution. When pieces of cornea were exposed to 50% zinc chloride solution and were subsequently placed in water they were found to have lost 85% of their normal capacity to swell, and only about 5 per cent of their normal swelling capacity could be restored by treatment with edetate. When cornea was exposed to only 1.36% (0.1M) zinc chloride solution, the swelling in water was similarly inhibited, but by treatment with edetate about half of the swelling capacity was restored.

Johnstone and Sullivan exposed the eyes of rabbits to 50% zinc chloride solution in a standard manner for one minute. When the eyes were irrigated with 0.05 M sodium edetate, starting one minute after termination of exposure to zinc chloride, the corneas developed during the next four days a degree of opacification similar to that of the corneas irrigated with sodium chloride, but then they showed progressive improvement, and by two weeks had relatively slight residual opacity. The edetate-treated eyes became strikingly better than those irrigated with sodium chloride. Unfortunately, if the interval from termination of exposure to beginning of irrigation with edetate solution was increased to five minutes, the treatment gave no evident benefit, and at two weeks the corneas were densely opaque. It was concluded from these experiments that irrigation with neutral sodium edetate solution would be worthwhile in immediate or first aid treatment of patients who had splashed zinc chloride into their eyes, but that it would have to be started very quickly to be of benefit.

Clinical experience with dilute zinc salt solutions. As already mentioned, solutions up to 1% concentration appear almost never to have caused injury, but Paul reported a single case in which a patient's cornea developed an intense white precipitate in one small portion of an ulcerated area that had been treated repeatedly over a long time with 0.5% to 1% solution of zinc salt, probably zinc sulfate. He considered this to be a zinc encrustation rather than a burn.[j]

a. DeRosa C: On a case of severe ocular caustic action of a zinc salt. *RASS ITAL OTTALMOL* 28:280–290, 1959. (Italian)

b. Filipovic A: On prevention of Vogt's acute subepithelial disseminated cataract after zinc burn of the cornea. *KLIN MONATSBL AUGENHEILKD* 133:268–269, 1958. (German)

c. Fleischanderl A: On treatment of recurrent erosion. *KLIN MONATSBL AUGENHEILKD* 125:747–748, 1954. (German)

d. Hoffman FW: On keratitis and the development of hypopyon. *BER OPHTHALMOL GESELLSCH HEIDELBERG* 17:67–80, 1885. (German)

e. Houle RE, Grant WM: Zinc chloride keratopathy and cataracts. *AM J OPHTHALMOL* 75:992–996, 1973.

f. Johnstone MA, Sullivan WR, Grant WM: Experimental zinc chloride ocular injury and treatment with disodium edetate. *AM J OPHTHALMOL* 76:137–142, 1973.

g. Mohs FE: Chemosurgical treatment of cancer of the eyelid. *ARCH OPHTHALMOL* 39:43–59, 1948.

h. Mohs FE: Chemosurgery. *NEW YORK J MED,* Apr 1, 1968, pp. 871–876.

i. Nemetz U: On the question of acute glaucomatous cataract. *KLIN MONATSBL AUGENHEILKD* 115:417–421, 1949. (German)

j. Paul L: On corneal ulcerations from diplobacilli. *KLIN MONATSBL AUGENHEILKD* 43:154–184, 1905. (German)

k. Pavan-Langston D: Personal communication, 1970.

l. Pillat A: On the development of Vogt's acute anterior subepithelial disseminated cataract after zinc burn of the cornea. *KLIN MONATSBL AUGENHEILKD* 126:561–568, 1955. (German)

m. Rzehulka G: On burns of the eye with zinc chloride. *KLIN MONATSBL AUGENHEILKD* 130:539–544, 1957. (German)

n. Strader: *COLORADO OPHTHALMOL SOC* 21, 1908. (Reference from Guillery, 1910.[96])

o. Van Lint M: Vogt's subepithelial disseminated cataract of traumatic origin. *BULL SOC BELGE OPHTALMOL* 72:62–65, 1936. (French)

Zinc phenosulfonate (zinc sulfocarbolate) has been used as an astringent, and insecticide.[171] A single instance has been reported in which use of a 3% solution in eye compresses resulted in complete necrosis of both corneas of an infant.[a] Experimental application of this solution eight times to the eye of a rabbit caused the cornea to become completely opaque in seven days.

a. Velhagen K: A disastrous iatrogenic eye injury. *KLIN MONATSBL AUGENHEILKD* 126:580–585, 1955.

Zinc pyrithione (zinc pyridinethione; zinc omadine; zinc-2-pyridinethion-1-oxide; the zinc chelate of pyrithione) is an antifungal, antibacterial compound that has been used as an antidandruff agent in shampoo formulations, such as Head and Shoulders Shampoo. When tested on rabbit and monkey eyes by application of 0.5% to 2% suspensions as used in shampoos, it was found not to be injurious,[b,c] although 1% in dimethyl sulfoxide caused irritation comparable to 70% isopropyl alcohol.[352]

Systemic administration of zinc pyrithione, and also pyrithione itself, has demonstrated interesting species differences in toxic effects. When zinc pyrithione has been administered systemically to dogs, it has produced blindness, associated with detachment of the retina. This same effect was produced by pyrithione without zinc. However, no such effects on the retina were produced in rats, rabbits, or monkeys.[a,c,d] In cats, orally administered zinc pyrithione has caused tapetal degeneration and atrophy, but not the severe reaction seen in dogs, which have shown not only degeneration of tapetal cells but also tapetal and retinal inflammation with intraretinal hemorrhage, and subretinal edema leading to retinal detachment and blindness.[a]

It has been of particular interest that normal beagle dogs which have a tapetum lucidum show this reaction, while another variety of beagle dog which lacks a tapetum lucidum does not show injury. This corresponds to lack of reaction in monkeys, human beings, rats and rabbits which also do not have this structure.

It is of interest, as pointed out by Cloyd et al, that the tapetum lucidum is rich in zinc, and that certain metal chelating agents (dithizone and diethyldithiocarbamate) injure the normal dog's eye in the same manner as pyrithione and zinc pyrithione.[a] However, they also point out that ethambutol and related compounds that can chelate the zinc of the tapetum lucidum only cause a loss of color of the tapetum which is reversible, and do not cause inflammatory and degenerative changes. Cloyd et al have suggested that zinc pyrithione (as well pyrithione, dithizone, and diethyldithiocarbamate) may not only chelate some of the zinc of the tapetum but may also react with sulfhydryl groups that are necessary for important metabolic processes in that region. (See INDEX for *Pyrithione, Dithizone,* and *Diethyldithiocarbamate.*)

a. Cloyd GG, Wyman M, et al: Ocular toxicity studies with zinc pyridinethione. *TOXICOL APPL PHARMACOL* 45:771–782, 1978.
b. Opdyke DL, Burnett CM, Brauer EW: Antiseborrheic qualities of zinc pyrithione in a cream vehicle. II. Safety evaluation. *FOOD COSMET TOXICOL* 5:321–326, 1967.
c. Snyder FH, Buehler EV, Winak CL: Safety evaluation of zinc 2-pyridinethiol-1-oxide in a shampoo formulation. *TOXICOL APPL PHARMACOL* 7:425–437, 1965.
d. Winek CL, Buehler EV: Intravenous toxicity of zinc pyridinethione and several zinc salts. *TOXICOL APPL PHARMACOL* 9:269–273, 1966.

Zinc sulfide, a pigment, has been identified in the tissues of the conjunctivae and lids of two children who were accidentally squirted with material from the liquid center of golf balls. The zinc sulfide, as well as barium sulfate which was similarly encountered, produced only slight macrophage reaction and negligible tissue damage.[a]

a. Johnson FB, Zimmerman LE: Barium sulfate and zinc sulfide deposits resulting from golf-ball injury to the conjunctiva and eyelid. *AM J CLIN PATH* 44:533–538, 1965.

Zinc systemic levels, particularly the concentrations measured in the plasma or serum, are found to be subnormal in certain diseases and some toxic conditions. Reviews of the biochemistry and physiology of zinc make clear that zinc has many important natural functions in the eye, but adverse effects on the eyes that may result from deficiencies of zinc are much less well defined.[i,p]

The following are some of the clinical correlations that have been made in which no toxic substances were involved and ocular effects were believed to be secondary to reduction of systemic zinc levels by systemic diseases. In chronic liver disease, such as alcoholic cirrhosis, dark adaptation has been impaired,[i,j,m] and in some patients dark adaptation improved when zinc was administered; in these patients treatment with vitamin A had failed.[m] Similarly in a patient who had abnormal dark adaptation associated with Crohn's disease and low serum zinc, there was improvement of the dark adaptation when zinc was administered.[l] Another patient with Crohn's disease, and very low serum zinc following parenteral administration of nutrition, had paracentral scotomas which disappeared when the zinc deficiency was corrected.[h] In rats, severe diet-induced zinc deficiency has caused accumulation of osmiophilic inclusion bodies in the retinal pigment epithelium and degeneration of outer segments of photoreceptors.[k] Patients with dietary zinc deficiency, or failure to absorb zinc, as in acrodermatitis enteropathica, may have serious general effects without visual symptoms.

When exposure to toxic substances is associated with low zinc levels, it is difficult to assess the role of the deficiency of zinc in adverse effects on the eyes. The following are circumstances involving toxic substances and adverse effects on the optic nerves with decrease of vision, sometimes optic atrophy, associated with subnormal plasma or serum zinc.

In 1975 Saraux and colleagues[n] followed up earlier reports of effects of ethambutol on zinc in experimental animals (see INDEX for *Ethambutol*), and reported that a single serum zinc measurement in each of 3 patients with retrobulbar neuritis and central scotoma from ethambutol (plus ioniazid in 2 of the patients) showed subnormal zinc levels averaging 0.75 mg/l compared to normal controls of 1.09 mg/l. Also they reported that one patient with optic neuropathy from disulfiram (see INDEX for *Disulfiram*) had 0.95 mg/l. Furthermore, they found that out of 7 patients with alcohol-tobacco retrobulbar neuritis, 3 had zinc levels as low as 0.75, while the other 4 were in the range of 0.90 to 1.00.[n] However, subsequent measurements before and after varying periods of treatment with ethambutol (for tuberculosis) did not show a reduction of zinc levels.[c,d,e] It was then suggested that when pre-treatment zinc levels were low this increased the risks of retrobulbar neuritis.[d,e] This was supported by an observation that of 108 patients with pre-treatment plasma zinc above 0.8 mg/l none had any visual disturbance, but that 7 out of 20 with zinc below 0.8 mg/l had decreased visual acuity with central scotoma; 3 of these appeared to have macular degeneration.[e]

The relationship of *alcohol-tobacco amblyopia* and systemic zinc, after the report by Saraux,[n] were studied further by Gerhard in 1982,[f] finding in half the cases serum zinc ranged from 0.45 to 0.85 mg/l, compared to normal values of 1.0 to 1.2 mg/l. These patients had evidence of alcoholic cirrhosis which might account for the abnormal zinc levels. In another 52 cases of alcohol-tobacco optic neuropathy, Bechetoille and colleagues found significant subnormality of systemic zinc levels, slight subnormality of magnesium, normal copper, and lead above normal.[a] Eight patients with central scotomas attributed to alcohol and tobacco were given 400 mg of zinc sulfate per day, and nine others were given a placebo. (No vitamins were given, but alcohol intake and smoking were reduced during the trial.) After a month the visual acuity and color vision were improved in both groups, but not significantly more in the treated than in the control group. Only by special examination of the central 5° of visual field with the Friedmann analyzer was there evidence of some superiority in those with the zinc treatment.[b]

In another group of 10 patients with alcohol-tobacco retrobulbar neuritis, Grignolo found serum zinc significantly lower than in 10 controls. Then, after 60 days of medical treatment (not described), 6 of 10 had improvements in visual acuity, visual field or chromatic sense, and these patients showed increase in their zinc levels.[g]

Iodoquinol (diiodohydroxyquin) formerly was used in treatment of acrodermatitis enteropathica, an inherited disease with failure of zinc absorption, which now is more effectively treated by administering zinc. (See INDEX for *Iodoquinol.*) The old treatment with iodoquinol may have aided absorption of zinc, but in a small number of cases the treatment led to optic atrophy. Acrodermatitis enteropathica is generally lethal when untreated, but, since it is not known to cause optic neuropathy, some have considered that the optic atrophy associated with iodoquinol treatment to be a toxic effect of the drug. Others have proposed that the optic neuropathy might be attributable to severe zinc deficiency, and that the iodoquinol merely helped the patients to survive long enough to manifest the optic neuropathy from the deficiency.[o,p]

If any conclusion is warranted, it seems to be that the relationship of zinc deficiency to optic neuropathy is in need of further study.

a. Bechetoille A, Allain P, et al: Modifications of blood concentrations of zinc and lead and the activity of ALA-dehydratase in the course of alcohol-tobacco optic neuropathies. *J FR OPHTALMOL* 6:231–235, 1983. (French)
b. Bechetoille A, Ebran JM, et al: Therapeutic effect of zinc sulfate on the central scotoma of alcohol-tobacco optic neuropathies. *J FR OPHTALMOL* 6:237–242, 1983. (French)
c. Campbell IA, et al: Ethambutol and the eye; zinc and copper. *LANCET* 2:711, 1975.
d. Deloux E, Moreau Y, et al: Prevention of ocular toxicity of ethambutol. *J FR OPHTALMOL* 1:191–196, 1978. (French)
e. Fioretti F, Minervino M: Zincemia as a clue to the ocular toxicity of ethambutol. *ANN OTTALMOL CLIN OCUL* 106:543–548, 1980. (Italian)
f. Gerhard JP: On an advance concerning ocular zinc. *BULL SOC OPHTALMOL FRANCE* 82:1125–1127, 1982. (French)
g. Grignolo FM, La Rosa G, et al: Evaluation of plasma zinc in retrobulbar optic neuropathies. *BOLL OCULIST* 59:801–821, 1980. (Italian)
h. Haas J: Acute zinc deficiency syndrome. *AKTUEL NEUROL* 9:55–57, 1982. (German)
i. Karcioglu ZA: Zinc in the eye. *SURVEY OPHTHALMOL* 27:114–122, 1982.
j. Keeling PWN, O'Day J, et al: Zinc deficiency and photoreceptor function in chronic liver disease. *CLIN SCI* 62:109–111, 1982.

k. Leure-duPree AE, Mc Clain CJ: The effect of severe zinc deficiency on the morphology of the rat pigment epithelium. *INVEST OPHTHALMOL VIS SCI* 23:425–434, 1982.

l. Mc Clain CJ, Su LC, et al: Zinc-deficiency-induced retinal dysfunction in Crohn's disease. *DIG DIS SCI* 28:85–87, 1983.

m. Morrison SA, Russell RM, et al: Zinc deficiency: A cause of abnormal dark adaptation in cirrhotics. *AM J CLIN NUTR* 31:276–281, 1978.

n. Saraux H, Bechetoille A, et al: The diminution of the level of serum zinc during some toxic optic neuritis cases. *ANN OCULIST* 208:29–31, 1975. (French)

o. Sturtevant FM: Zinc deficiency, acrodermatitis enteropathica, optic atrophy, subacute myelo-optic-neuropathy, and 5,7-dihalo-8-quinolinols. *PEDIATRICS* 65:610–613, 1980.

p. Wong EK Jr, Leopold IH: Zinc deficiency and visual dysfunction. *METAB PEDIATR OPHTHALMOL* 3:1–4, 1979.

Zyklon A, a fumigant mixture of 90% methyl cyanocarbonate and 10% methyl chlorocarbonate, was inhaled and caused acute poisoning in a man who survived collapse and convulsions, but then had reduced visual acuity with macula edema. In subsequent weeks the visual acuity returned essentially to normal, but many pigment flecks developed in the fundi, particularly in the neighborhood of the foveas. The patient died with nephrosis 2 months after poisoning.

a. Illig KM: Retinal injury by cyanide poisoning. *KLIN MONATSBL AUGENHEILKD* 120:310–312, 1952. (German)

Chapter III

TREATMENT OF CHEMICAL BURNS
OF THE EYES

Steps in Treatment

1. Immediate or "first aid" decontamination.

2. Specific emergency treatments or antidotes for specific types of chemicals.

3. Further medical and surgical treatments, early and during healing.

4. Attempts to repair lasting damage.

Generally it seems to have been agreed that step 1 consists of irrigation of the eye as quickly as possible. The list of step 2 specific emergency antidotes is meager. Truly proven additions to the list are infrequently made. Step 3 has received the greatest attention, to judge from the bulk of the literature.

1. Immediate or "first aid" decontamination should be carried out with the most speed possible. Human experience and animal experiment repeatedly show that if started within seconds, flooding the eye with water can have the greatest value. Practically, the importance of time so outweighs other considerations that the first water, or innocuous watery solution, at hand should be used. Time should not be wasted in looking for some special irrigation fluid. Special treatment, if indicated, can come later, after irrigation with water has been started.

For continuing irrigation, ordinary tap water has served well in a great many cases. For the patient's comfort in performing prolonged irrigation, a drop of local anesthetic and slightly warmed water are helpful. After irrigation has been started with the first available water, if sterile saline or other more physiologic solutions are available in quantity, they may be better for continuing irrigation.

How long irrigation should be continued depends upon the nature of the chemical, also on the concentration and quantity involved. Common practice has been to advise irrigation for 20 to 30 minutes to be sure of thorough cleansing. However, if the nature of the contaminant is definitely known, it seems sensible to regulate the length of irrigation according to what is known of the properties of the contaminant. For severe alkali and acid burns, clinical comparisons of results have led Saari et al (1984) to recommend continuing irrigation for 1 to 2 hours. Based on pH measurements on the aqueous humor in alkali-burned and externally irrigated rabbit eyes, Laux (1975) found that more than 2 hours of irrigation might be needed before the aqueous humor came down to a desirable level.

Prolonged irrigation is most appropriate after contamination of the eye with strong alkalies, since in this particular case it is possible to demonstrate that the pH of the conjunctival sac may take many minutes to return to the normal range.

Testing of the conjunctival sac with wide-range pH test paper, such as *pHydrion* paper (pH 1 to 11), every five to ten minutes in the course of irrigation can be used to obtain a measure of the rate at which the pH is returning to a tolerable value, such as pH 8 or 8.5. (It should not be expected to come to pH 7.)

In acid burns it may be observed that the pH of the conjunctival sac returns to normal range during irrigation in fewer minutes than in alkali burns.

In solvent burns of the eyes, involving substances such as alcohols, ketones, and chlorinated hydrocarbons, which are not chemically reactive with the tissues, but which have injurious physical (solvent or protein-denaturing) properties, it may be expected that decontamination can be accomplished very rapidly by irrigation with water in most cases. Clinical experience indicates that prompt brief irrigation is usually sufficient for solvents which are chemically unreactive and are not uncommonly viscous or oily.

Whenever there is uncertainty about the nature of the substance, it is safer to err on the side of irrigating longer than may actually be necessary, rather than to irrigate inadequately.

Whenever there is any possibility of contamination of the eye with solid particles, it is of the greatest importance that a search be made of the whole conjunctival sac, completely everting the lids, and removing these particles mechanically as quickly as possible, continuing irrigation while this is done. A drop of local anesthetic can make the cleansing procedure much easier, and more comfortable for the patient, but proper cleansing should not be delayed for lack of local anesthetic. In the case of materials containing calcium hydroxide (such as mortar and plaster) use of a solution of sodium edetate (EDTA) is helpful in loosening and removing deposits. Swabs of cotton tightly wrapped around a match stick or toothpick should be used if particles are adherent. Toothless forceps may be needed to remove particles buried in the conjunctiva, especially white phosphorus from incendiary bombs.

Use of fluorescein to stain and reveal epithelial damage on the cornea or conjunctiva is unnecessary in the hands of a physician skilled in examination of the eye with slit-lamp biomicroscope and ophthalmoscope. These instruments reveal much more than does the staining procedure. However, when the necessary instruments and skills are unavailable, it has been a very common and widespread practice to rely upon a drop of sodium fluoresceinate solution to demonstrate injury of the surface. The one great danger in this practice is that solutions of fluorescein may harbor the pyocyaneus organism *Pseudomonas aeruginosa*, which is devastatingly infectious and damaging to the cornea. If fluorescein is to be used, the greatest attention should be given to its sterility, making use either of individual sterile paper strips impregnated with the dye, or individual sterile, sealed containers of solution to be used once and discarded.

Staining of the cornea by fluorescein serves merely to indicate that the surface has been injured. It does not provide the detailed information which is obtainable by examination with slit-lamp biomicroscope and ophthalmoscope. It merely warns that further attention is needed. Testing with fluorescein can not be depended upon to rule out injury, since in certain cases there may be a latent period of several hours after exposure before the signs and symptoms of damage become evident. A latent period of this sort is encountered most commonly after exposure to gases, vapors, and fumes, but can also occur after contact with certain liquids and solids.

(See Chapter I for an outline of delayed or latent injurious effects on the cornea.)

To neutralize chemical contaminants of the eye, a great variety of reagents have been proposed, in most instances based merely upon the principle of neutralizing alkalies with acids, and vice versa. Laux (1975) found that the pH of the aqueous humor of alkali-burned rabbit eyes came down faster when the surface was irrigated with a buffer solution. Despite theoretical advantage, this type of neutralization has seldom been shown to provide a significant improvement over immediate irrigation with water or saline, which is usually much more readily available for first aid treatment. The few instances in which specific chemical antidotes do offer an advantage when added to immediate irrigation are listed under step 2.

2. Specific emergency treatments or antidotes for specific types of chemicals are at present disappointingly few, but the number presumably will grow in time. Those listed represent a start in this direction. (See the INDEX for more specific details.)

Contaminant	Treatment
Ammonia	? Paracentesis (see discussion below)
Ammonium hydroxide	? Paracentesis (see discussion below)
Benzenethiol	0.5% Silver nitrate solution effective in rabbits
Beryllium salts	2.5% Sodium sulfosalicylate solution effective in rabbits
Calcium hydroxide	0.05 M sodium edetate (EDTA)* helps in removing particles
Dyes, cationic or basic	10% Tannic acid within three minutes effective in rabbits
Lanthanum salts	0.01 M neutral sodium EDTA* effective on rabbits
Lewisite	Dimercaprol
Mercury fulminate	2% Sodium thiosulfate solution
Phenol	30% to 50% solution polyethylene-glycol-400 for eye decontamination
Phosphorus, white	3% Copper sulfate solution
Potassium permanganate	10% Ascorbate and neutral EDTA* solution
Saponins	Cholesterol (lanolin) ointment
Silver	Sodium thiosulfate and potassium ferricyanide solution
Sodium hydroxide	? Paracentesis (see discussion below)
Yttrium salts	0.01 M neutral sodium EDTA* effective on rabbits

| Zinc chloride | 0.05 M neutral sodium edetate EDTA* helpful in rabbits only within first few minutes |

---

*A 0.05 M (1.86%) neutral solution of EDTA (disodium edetate) can be prepared by diluting a 20 ml ampule of Endrate disodium (150 mg/ml) (Abbott Laboratories) with 180 ml of sterile 0.9% sodium chloride solution. (Higher concentrations of EDTA have been used, but with greater risk of undesirable effects on the cornea.) (For removing lime particles, Glasmacher has made a case for using EDTA at pH 4.7.[69])

Paracentesis (surgical evacuation of the anterior chamber) as a special treatment in alkali burns theoretically might have good effect, because it can quickly release alkali from the anterior chamber. From experiments on rabbit eyes there is good evidence that strong alkalies, such as ammonium hydroxide and sodium hydroxide, can within minutes penetrate the cornea and raise the pH of the aqueous humor. Spontaneous return toward normal pH is relatively slow, taking many minutes, or hours in severe cases. (This is described in detail in Chapter II under *Alkalies, Ammonia,* and *Sodium hydroxide;* see INDEX.) Undoubtedly paracentesis, especially if followed by irrigation of the anterior chamber, can bring the pH of the anterior chamber to normal more rapidly than the pH can spontaneously normalize, or than pH can be normalized by irrigating the outer surface. This fact raises hopes that the procedure would be beneficial. Some authors have advised in favor, particularly Paterson, Pfister and Levinson (1975), Bennett, Peyman and Rutgard (1978), and Pfister (1983). Paterson et al (1975) based their advice on measurements of the pH of the aqueous humor, finding the pH after severe exposures to sodium hydroxide could remain above pH 11 for an hour or more unless paracentesis was performed early. They did not compare the resulting degrees of injury. Bennett et al (1978) based their advice on observations in rabbits that after 0.5 N sodium hydroxide was applied to the cornea for 40 seconds with an 8 mm paper disc the end results were improved by irrigating the anterior chamber for 10 minutes with pH 7.25 phosphate buffer solution, beginning within 15 minutes.

Earlier, Grant (1955) had concluded from experiments in rabbits with less severe exposures to ammonium hydroxide that paracentesis was ineffective. However, no tests were done after ammonium hydroxide exposures severe enough to damage the iris and lens.

Very little clinical experience with paracentesis in treatment of alkali burns is available as yet. Burns (1979) has reported one desperate case in which it was impossible to discern benefit from paracentesis and irrigation of the anterior chamber with buffer.

More controlled appraisals of paracentesis in animals, with and without irrigation of the anterior chamber, is needed to define better the circumstances under which it may be beneficial. Particularly from a practical standpoint more information is needed on how critical the time after exposure may be during which some benefit could be expected, since it usually takes some time for victims of severe splash injuries to arrive where there is the expertise necessary to perform paracentesis safely.

There is no reason to consider paracentesis in treatment of chemical burns of less severity than those from strong alkalies or acids, especially those which affect mainly the corneal epithelium, or have reasonably good prognosis without paracentesis.

Possible future specific treatments for substances with a latent period before onset require more exploration for their development. In Chapter I and in the INDEX more than 40 substances have been characterized as causing "Corneal injury with delayed onset, from local action," and some of their possible mechanisms of action have been discussed in Chapter II. (Among the better known of these substances are cardiac glycosides, colchicine, dimethyl sulfate, emetine, hydrogen sulfide, mustard gas, osmic acid, and vinblastine.)

Despite what is known of the mechanism of toxic action of some of these, treatment of eyes exposed to chemicals that have a latent period before onset of obvious biological derangement is at present almost entirely nonspecific, consisting of ordinary first aid irrigation with water. However, it seems reasonable to expect that in time when the biochemical mechanisms become better understood, the latent or delayed type of toxic action should offer the best opportunity for specific and logically designed protective or corrective treatment. If it is valid to assume that there is initially a rapid chemical reaction, usually with binding of the toxic substance to components of the cell, and that it takes time before this seriously deranges the whole economy of the cell, there should be opportunity in that latent period to undo or remove the denaturing effect of the substance bound to the cell. This has been attempted, so far unsuccessfully, in the case of mustard gas. It would be analogous in a general sense to the treatment of arsenic poisoning with dimercaprol, the relief of metal poisonings by chelating agents, and the reactivation of cholinesterase by substances such as pralidoxime. An interception or abortion of toxic manifestations from the rare-earth salts lanthanum chloride and yttrium chloride in the cornea by timely treatment with sodium edetate has at least partially restored physical properties (swelling capacity) of the cornea and its viability in experiments in rabbits. It seems reasonable to expect that specific antagonists or antidotes should in time be found for most of the toxic agents that have a latent period or delay before onset of obvious biological derangement.

3. Further medical and surgical management, early and during healing. After proper irrigation has been completed and after any specifically indicated antidote has been applied, burns of slight or mild degree usually do well if secondary infection is prevented and nothing is done to interfere with healing. This usually involves nothing more than applying an antibiotic ointment and keeping the patient's eyes closed and quiet, for his comfort as well as to facilitate regeneration of epithelium. Discomfort in the eye may be reduced by applying a mydriatic-cyloplegic drug such as atropine, scopolamine, or homatropine, but local anesthetics should not be used as a part of the treatment. It is safer for the eye to rely upon systemic medication for discomfort, utilizing aspirin, codeine, and related drugs.

In case of severe burns, usually from strong alkalies or acids, a long course of treatment may be required, and despite all efforts the damage may prove irreparable. During many days or weeks a variety of treatments may be tried, as will be described below. During that period, Ralph and Slansky (1974) have described the advantages of providing continuing irrigation of the surface of the eye and conjunctival sac, utilizing various devices, which they describe, for the comfort and convenience of the patient. Connection of a small portable pump by fine flexible tubing to an in-lying catheter in the conjunctival sac or via a special contact lens facilitates administration of antibiotics and medications intended to favor healing. Ralph and Slansky (1974) in their review have also provided careful authoritative advice on maneuvers to prevent symblepharon and to care for Descemetoceles and perforated corneas. These matters are of such importance that the interested reader should consult their original text.

Since the early 1970's a great deal of research has been carried on with the goal of improving medical treatment of severely burned eyes, especially alkali-burned eyes, which present some of the worst problems. New treatments have evolved from what has been learned about mechanisms of injury. Reviews of developments in this area that are particularly noteworthy have been published by Francois and Feher (1972), Pfister (1983), Ralph and Slansky (1974), and Wright (1982).

Various plans of treatment that have evolved, as well as older procedures that still have some support, are listed and described below. (Measures that seem to offer little more than historical interest will be mentioned only briefly.)

a. *Collagenase inhibitors* have been utilized in treatment of alkali burns because of much evidence that collagenases released from leukocytes and other cells at the site of injury can cause breakdown of the corneal stroma. A description of the sequence of changes in the cornea has been given under *Sodium hydroxide* in Chapter II, much as presented in the reviews of Francois and Feher (1972), Ralph and Slansky (1974), Pfister (1983), and Wright (1982). In brief, in severe alkali burns it appears that all corneal cells that are exposed to a sufficiently high pH are quickly killed, and the stromal collagen and acid mucopolysaccharide are greatly affected, with loss of much of the latter. In a week or two, infiltration with leukocytes occurs, and these inflammatory cells, as well as epithelial and other cells of the cornea, release collagenases which attack the stromal collagen, opposing regenerative or repair mechanisms that may have been undertaken by fibroblasts. Ulceration results, and may lead to perforation some weeks after the initial burn occurred. Several inhibitors of collagenases have been evaluated as a secondary treatment in rabbit eyes, started 2 to 7 days after burning with sodium hydroxide. Significant reduction of the incidence of ulceration and perforation have been obtained, varying somewhat with the severity of burning. Slansky (1970) found cysteine and acetylcysteine effective. Anderson (1971), after potassium hydroxide burn, found ulceration inhibited by sodium edetate and cysteine, but the ulcerative process became reactivated if treatment was stopped too soon. Francois (1972) also reported cysteine to be effective in preventing ulceration, but noted that the treated corneas were no less opaque than the untreated controls. Francois (1973) reported penicillamine to provide particularly effective protection. It was evident that all these agents were chelating agents, and it seemed likely that interaction with the zinc of the zinc-dependent collagenases was the basis for their favorable action.

In later comparisons with ascorbate and citrate treatment to prevent ulceration it appeared that the first group of collagenase inhibitors might be at least partially superceded.

It is to be kept in mind that the aim of these secondary treatments of severe alkali burns has primarily been to save the eye from destruction, and possibly permit keratoplasty sometime in the future.

b. Ascorbate (ascorbic acid) treatment is rationalized by the fact that the concentration of ascorbate in the anterior segment of the eye is reduced when the ciliary body is damaged in an alkali burn, and by the fact that ascorbate is needed for formation of collagen. Scorbutic conditions in the cornea secondary to alkali burns appeared to interfere with the reparative process, and to favor breakdown of the stroma. After alkali burns that were not excessively severe the incidence of ulceration and perforation of rabbit corneas was reduced by ascorbate administered subcutaneously in large dosage (Levison 1976; Pfister 1976, 1977), and also by repeated topical application of 10% sodium ascorbate eyedrops (Pfister 1978). With more severe burns and greater damage to the ciliary body, systemic administration proved less effective than topical treatment (Pfister 1980, 1980). In still more severely alkali-burned eyes, which with or without treatment ultimately became phthisical, topical ascorbate had little effect, similar to treatment with acetyl cysteine, and worse than treatment with topical sodium citrate (Pfister 1981, 1982).

In the less severe alkali burns in which systemic ascorbate treatment reduced the incidence of ulceration, there appeared to be no effect on corneal epithelial healing (Reim 1982). Rabbit eyes burned with hydrochloric acid responded to systemic ascorbate treatment with reduced incidence of ulceration as in the moderately severe alkali burns (Wishard 1980).

Clinical observations by Wright (1982) in treatment of moderately severe alkali burns gave the impression that oral administration and frequent application of 10% ascorbate eyedrops for several weeks improved the outcome.

Another mechanism for therapeutic action by ascorbate has been proposed. It may act as a scavenger of superoxide radicals released by polymorphonuclear leukocytes infiltrating a burn (Nirankari 1981). Experiments in rabbits showed that administration of superoxide dismutase reduced the incidence of ulcerations and perforations, presumably by replacing naturally occurring enzyme lost in the burn process. Ascorbate was also effective, maybe also compensating for the loss of superoxide dismutase.

An *adverse effect of ascorbate* has been shown in experiments with thermal burns of the cornea in rabbits. Thermally burned eyes, unlike alkali-burned eyes, retain normal ascorbate levels, are not scorbutic and not in need of added ascorbate. When rabbits with thermally-burned corneas have been given large amounts of ascorbate locally and systemically, inflammatory infiltration with neutrophils was increased, ulceration was accelerated, and the incidence of perforation was much increased (Phan 1985). This adverse effect suggests that intensive ascorbate treatment should be used only in severe alkali and acid burns, and not be used in other burns of the eye in which there has been no evidence of severe damage to the ciliary body, nor evidence of serious secondary deficiency of ascorbate in the eye.

   c. Citrate treatment, in the form of 10% sodium citrate eyedrops administered for weeks, was found by Pfister and colleagues (1981, 1983) to reduce the incidence of corneal ulcers and perforations in rabbit eyes that had been so severely burned by sodium hydroxide that acetyl cysteine and ascorbate treatment had essentially no beneficial effect. Subsequently, clinical trials were undertaken to make a systematic comparison of citrate, ascorbate, and unmedicated vehicle. Pfister (1983) obtained experimental evidence that citrate probably acted through chelation of calcium to interfere with harmful effects of polymorphonuclear leukocyte infiltrates in alkali burns, including release of proteolytic enzymes and superoxide free radicals, and phagocytosis.

   d. Corticosteroid treatment in chemical burns of the eye has a long and confusing history. As described in more detail in the 2nd edition of this book, animal experiments in the 1960's indicated that inflammatory reaction could be reduced by corticosteroids, and that under certain circumstances vascularization of burned corneas was less under treatment, but that the incidence of ulceration and perforation might be increased by use of topical corticosteroids on eyes burned with sodium hydroxide.

   Some of the same ambiguity, but still greater caution has been expressed in the early 1980's. Wright (1982) has referred to this as an area of controversy, and has suggested that topical corticosteroid be used to help suppress inflammatory cell infiltration after severe alkali burns of the cornea, but only before signs of melting of the stroma appear, and then to change to a collagenase inhibitor, possibly to sodium citrate. Ralph and Slansky (1974) have advised that if the epithelium has not covered surface defects by the fifth to seventh days, the corticosteroids should be stopped. Experiments by Donshik et al (1978) in rabbits with corneas burned by sodium hydroxide indicated that at certain phases in the response to burning the effect of topical corticosteroid could be good, but at another phase could be harmful. In particular, intensive corticosteroid treatment was not harmful during the first week, but during the second and third week this treatment could increase the severity of ulceration, probably by interfering with repair processes, rather than by raising collagenase activity. Then in a third phase, in the fourth and fifth weeks, corticosteroids could be used again without evident harm.

   What has been said above applies only to severe burns. There are a great many minor chemical burns that heal rapidly and completely without special treatment. It would seem superfluous to use corticosteroid treatment in such cases. Clinical impression of benefit in a series in which all patients are treated, with no untreated controls for comparison, and no controlled experimental animal studies, is scientifically inconclusive (Plain 1979).

   e. Medroxyprogesterone acetate treatment is experimental, based on a progestin that was shown *in vitro* to suppress formation of collagenases in injured tissue. Topical or parenteral administration to rabbits with eyes burned by sodium hydroxide resulted in perforation of the cornea in only 8 out of 87, whereas perforation occurred in 49 out of 85 controls (Newsome 1977). However, the treatment was not found to retard ulceration (Lass 1981).

f. Immunosuppression experimentally with cyclophosphamide or specific antiserum in guinea pigs with alkali-burned eyes caused reduction in the number of neutrophils infiltrating the burned area, and resulted in a significant reduction in the proportion of corneas that underwent ulceration (Foster 1982).

g. Autohemotherapy, the injection of the patient's, or the animal's, own blood under the conjunctiva has been the subject of many old claims of beneficial effect in acid and alkali burns, not so much in preventing corneal opacification as in preventing symblepharon. It acquired the name "Novosibirsk method" after hundreds of patients were treated by this method in that Siberian city in the 1950's. It still has its supporters, who testify to its value particularly in treatment of patients with lime burns (Pezzi 1972). Ribas Montobio (1974) published results of comparison of autohemotherapy in rabbits, and concluded that this treatment was superior for sulfuric acid burns, but not as good as EDTA for alkali burns.

h. Corneal tissue preparations in the form of hydrolysates or homogenates have been claimed to promote healing and reduce scarring when applied to alkali-burned corneas in exploratory experiments (Moczar 1973; Niebrof 1975).

i. Hypertonic ointment treatment of rabbit eyes burned with sodium hydroxide, utilizing 40% glucose or 5% sodium chloride three times a day for 6 weeks is reported by Korey and colleagues (1977) to have resulted in less corneal neovascularization and corneal ulceration than in untreated controls. Glucose appeared to have no advantage over sodium chloride.

j. Vasodilators and vasoconstrictors for a long time were the subject of many articles, mostly claiming benefits in treatment of chemical burns of the eye, but in recent times there appears to have been widespread loss of faith in these claims. Brancato and Campana (1965)[16,17] particularly deserve credit for a careful objective evaluation of the claims. In experiments on rabbits, Bozac (1974) has confirmed lack of value of tolazoline in acid and alkali burns.

k. Passow operation, consisting of peritomy and undermining of the conjunctiva early after a chemical burn, was supposed to release hypothetical toxic material from the tissues (Passow 1955). Clinically it was enthusiastically used, and apparently still has its clinical supporters. It was given an enthusiastic review by Hollwich and Huismans (1968). Since then there appear to have been no definitive controlled studies in its support. In rabbits, Bozac (1974) found no evident benefit from the Passow operation after acid or alkali burns.

l. Other old treatments are numerous and varied. Many were formerly enthusiastically recommended on the basis of simple clinical impression, with no attempt at controlled clinical comparisons, nor evaluation in experimental animals. Some were dropped when scientific comparisons were made and revealed the illusory nature of the supposed benefit. An occasional treatment had merit for a very special purpose, but unfortunately came to be used inappropriately for the wrong purposes, with resulting disappointment and condemnation. Others just went out of favor when initial apparent clinical success gave way to disappointment on further use. Maybe some did have value and should not have been dropped without more thorough testing. In any case, the following old treatments for chemical burns apparently are no longer promoted and used as they once were: calsulfhydryl (Hydrosulphosol), cocaine denuding of the cornea, heparin subconjunctivally, irradiation, neutral ammonium tartrate, oxygen subconjunctivally, thiotepa, trypsin, vasoconstrictors, vasodilators.

4. Attempts to repair lasting damage. After the initial reaction of the eye to a chemical burn and its subsequent healing, extensive damage may remain in spite of the best available treatment at every stage. Symblepharon, or scarring and adhesion of the conjunctiva of the lids and the globe may require surgical correction. Corneal opacification and vascularization may present a need for corneal transplantation. These and other important surgical steps for repair of lasting damage are beyond the scope of toxicology, but Ralph and Slansky (1974) have provided a knowledgeable guide, which should be consulted.

Anderson RE, Kuns MD, Dresden MH: Collagenase activity in alkali-burned cornea. *ANN OPHTHALMOL* 3:619–621, 1971.

Bennett TO, Peyman GA, Rutgard J: Intracameral phosphate buffer in alkali burns. *CAN J OPHTHALMOL* 13:93–95, 1978.

Bozac E, Simu G: Histochemical aspects in experimental corneal burns. *ANN OCULIST (Paris)* 207:103–114, 1974. (French)

Brown SI, Weller CA: Collagenase inhibitors in prevention of ulcers of alkali-burned cornea. *ARCH OPHTHALMOL* 83:352–353, 1970.

Brown SI, Tragakis MP, Pearce DB: Treatment of alkali-burned cornea. *AM J OPHTHALMOL* 74:316–320, 1972.

Burns RP, Hikes CE: Irrigation of the anterior chamber for the treatment of alkali burns. *AM J OPHTHALMOL* 88:119–120, 1979.

Donshik PC, Berman MB, et al: Effect of topical corticosteroids on ulceration in alkali-burned corneas. *ARCH OPHTHALMOL* 96:2117–2120, 1978.

Foster CS, Zelt RP, et al: Immunosuppression and selective inflammatory cell depletion. *ARCH OPHTHALMOL* 100:1820–1824, 1982.

Francois J, Cambie E: Collagenase and the collagenase inhibitors in torpid ulcers of the cornea. *OPHTHALMIC RES* 3:143–159, 1972.

Francois J, Feher J: Collagenolysis and regeneration in corneal burnings. *OPHTHALMOLOGICA* 165:137–152, 1972.

Francois J, Cambie E, et al: Collagenase inhibitors (penicillamine.) *ANN OPHTHALMOL* 5:391–408, 1973.

Francois J: Penicillamine in the treatment of alkali-burned corneas. *OPHTHALMIC RES* 4:223–236, 1972–1973.

Hollwich F, Huismans H: On early Passow operation in lime burn. *KLIN MONATSBL AUGENHEILKD* 153:233–238, 1968. (German)

Korey M, Peyman GA, Berkowitz R: The effect of hypertonic ointments on corneal alkali burns. *ANN OPHTHALMOL* 9:1383–1387, 1977.

Lass JH, Campbell RC, et al: Medroxyprogesterone on corneal ulceration. *ARCH OPHTHALMOL* 99:673–676, 1981.

Laux U, Roth HW et al: The hydrogen ion concentration of the aqueous humor after alkali burns of the cornea and its responsiveness to treatment. *GRAEFES ARCH OPHTHALMOL* 195:33–40, 1975. (German)

Levinson RA, Paterson CA, Pfister RR: Ascorbic acid prevents corneal ulceration and perforation following experimental alkali burns. *INVEST OPHTHALMOL* 15:986–993, 1976.

Moczar E, Moczar M, et al: Action of hydrolysates of corneal stroma on the enzymes of corneal ulcers. *ANN OCULIST (Paris)* 206:287–295, 1973. (French)

Newsome DA, Gross J: Prevention by medroxyprogesterone of perforation in the alkali-burned rabbit cornea. *INVEST OPHTHALMOL VIS SCI* 16:21–31, 1977.

Niebroj TK, Gierek A: Scanning microscope observation of alkali-burned rabbit cornea treated with embryonic corneal homomogenates. *OPHTHALMOLOGICA* 170:64–71, 1975.

Nirankari VS, Varma SA, et al: Superoxide radical scavenging agents in treatment of alkali burns. *ARCH OPHTHALMOL* 99:886–887, 1981.

Passow A: Early ambulatory operation on the eye for treatment and prevention of corneal opacities. *KLIN MONATSBL AUGENHEILKD* 127:129–142, 1955. (German)

Pezzi PP, Grenga R: Subconjunctival autohemotherapy in corneo-conjunctival burns from lime. *BOLL OCULIST* 51:153–158, 1972. (Italian)

Pfister RR, Paterson CA: Additional clinical and morphological observations on the favorable effect of ascorbate in experimental ocular alkali burns. *INVEST OPHTHALMOL VIS SCI* 16:478–487, 1977.

Pfister RR, Paterson CA, Hayes SA: Topical ascorbate decreases the incidence of corneal ulceration after experimental alkali burns. *INVEST OPHTHALMOL VIS SCI* 17:1019–1024, 1978.

Pfister RR, Paterson CA, et al: The efficacy of ascorbate treatment after severe experimental alkali burns depends upon the route of administration. *INVEST OPHTHALMOL VIS SCI* 19:1526–1529, 1980.

Pfister RR, Paterson CA: Ascorbic acid in the treatment of alkali burns of the eye. *OPHTHALMOLOGY* 87:1050–1057, 1980.

Pfister RR, Nicolaro ML, Paterson CA: Sodium citrate reduces the incidence of corneal ulcerations and perforations in extreme alkali-burned eyes; acetylcysteine and ascorbate have no favorable effect. *INVEST OPHTHALMOL VIS SCI* 21:486–490, 1981.

Pfister RR, Paterson CA, Hayes SA: Effect of topical 10% ascorbate solution on established corneal ulcers after severe alkali burns. *INVEST OPHTHALMOL VIS SCI* 22:382–385, 1982.

Pfister RR: Chemical injuries of the eye. *OPHTHALMOLOGY* 90:1246–1253, 1983.

Phan TMM, Zelt RP, et al: Ascorbic acid therapy in a thermal burn model of corneal ulceration in rabbits. *AM J OPHTHALMOL* 99:74–82, 1985.

Plain IH, Hein HF: Subconjunctival steroid injections for the treatment of chemically burned eyes. *ANN OPHTHALMOL* 11:329–332, 1979.

Ralph RA, Slansky HH: Therapy of chemical burns. *INT OPHTHALMOL CLIN* 14:171–191, 1974.

Reim M, Beil KH, et al: Influence of systemic ascorbic acid treatment on metabolite levels after regeneration of the corneal epithelium following mild alkali burns. *GRAEFES ARCH OPHTHALMOL* 218:99–102, 1982.

Ribas Montobbio JB: Treatment of corneoconjunctival chemical burns. *ARCH SOC ESP OFTALMOL* 34:487–528, 755–774, 1974. (Spanish)

Saari KM, Leinonen J, Aine E: Management of chemical eye injuries with prolonged irrigation. *ACTA OPHTHALMOL SUPPL* 161:52–59, 1984.

Slansky HH, Berman MB, et al: Cysteine and acetylcysteine in the prevention of corneal ulcerations. *ANN OPHTHALMOL* 2:488–491, 1970.

Wishard P, Paterson CA: The effect of ascorbic acid on experimental acid burns of the rabbit cornea. *INVEST OPHTHALMOL VIS SCI* 19:564–566, 1980.

Wright P: The chemically injured eye. *TRANS OPHTHALMOL SOC UK* 102:85–87, 1982.

Chapter IV

TESTING METHODS, AND SPECIES SPECIFICITY

While a small monograph could be written on test methods that may be in use or in prospect for evaluating ocular toxicity, this area is still in such a state of evolution that only a brief synopsis is warranted here.

TESTING METHODS FOR THE EYE

1. External testing for injury and discomfort

2. Testing for cataractogenesis or other effects on the lens

3. Detection of effects on retina and choroid

4. Testing for influences on intraocular pressure

---

1. External Testing for Injury and Discomfort of the Eye

a. Gases, Vapors, and Smog, External Testing on the Eye

Many of the early studies of the general toxic effects of gases and vapors consisted of exposure of small animals in exposure chambers to regulated concentrations in air and included observations on the behavior of the animal that might suggest irritation of the eyes, such as blinking or keeping the eyes closed, and occasionally included descriptions of the appearance of cornea, conjunctiva, and iris after exposure. The concentration and time required to produce various effects on the eye have often been described. Information more directly applicable to human beings has sometimes come from similar studies on human beings, but more often from observations under industrial conditions where symptoms, and occasionally signs of eye irritation, have been correlated with concentrations of gases and vapors determined by analysis of the atmosphere in which the individuals were working. Such information on irritating or injurious effects on the eyes have been the basis for official recommendations concerning allowable concentrations and times for exposure to numerous gases and vapors.[372] A complicating problem in trying to apply data from animal exposures to standards for human beings is the inevitable difference in responses of different species. Even when the testing is done in human beings, it

1007

must take into account the fact that some disturbances of the eye, particularly of the cornea, may develop after a latent period of several hours, during which time the eyes have been asymptomatic. (See INDEX for *Corneal epithelial edema, or injury, with delayed onset.*) Some disturbances develop only after repeated exposure. It is obviously difficult to set up standard predictive or anticipatory testing methods to cover all these variables, even for controllable industrial chemicals.

b. Liquids and Solids, External Testing on the Eye

There seem to be three main reasons for testing liquid and solid substances externally on the eye. The *first* is to establish how damaging and dangerous a substance is, so that those who may need to use it *industrially* can be forewarned of the precautions that they should take, and also so that those responsible for treating and taking care of accidental contaminations of the eye will have an idea of the potential severity, how much treatment may be needed and what the prognosis may be in cases of accidental contamination of the eyes by chemicals or drugs. The *second* main purpose in external eye testing of liquids and solids seems to be to detect and identify those that may present significant hazard in *household use,* requiring warning or avoidance. The *third* purpose of testing is in the evaluation of drugs for ophthalmic therapeutic use to provide a basis for weighing the undesirable aspects against the desirable therapeutic actions. Each of these purposes requires a different approach. These may be outlined as follows.

The *first* of the aims in testing and rating severity of injuriousness to the eye mentioned above (which is to provide a guide to people handling chemicals industrially, as well as to provide a guide and prognostic indicator for medical people responsible for treating chemical splash contamination of the eye) has been achieved to a considerable extent by systematized application to rabbit eyes and systematized rating of injury on a numerical scale at specified times thereafter. A practical scheme for screening industrial chemicals for injurious potentiality has been used by Smyth, Carpenter, and their associates since 1938, with results published periodically from 1944 to 1974,[27,222,228,288] covering hundreds of chemicals. For many of the substances that they have screened for injurious action there is no other information in the public literature concerning effects on the eye. In order to make their findings more easily available to concerned people, the results that they have published have been included in the INDEX of this book.

The following is a summary of the method used by Carpenter and Smyth.[27] They applied the test chemical to the center of the cornea of the rabbit eye, with the lids kept retracted for a minute. Then 18 to 24 hours later the eyes were inspected, utilizing fluorescein staining to help evaluate degree of injury. In their first step for screening a chemical they applied 0.005 ml undiluted. Then, judging from the result at 24 hours, if little or no injury was detected, a larger volume, up to 0.5 ml, was applied to another rabbit eye, or, if severe injury was produced by the first 0.005 ml, subsequent rabbits were tested with dilutions of the chemical in propylene glycol, water, or deodorized kerosine. They rated results on a scale of 1 to 10, based on a numerical rating of injury, reflecting mainly degree of injury to the cornea, which is taken into consideration along with the volume and the concentration required to produce that degree of injury. For examples, injury grade 1 would be essentially no injury from 0.5 ml; grade 5 would be severe corneal injury from 0.005 ml undiluted; and grade 10 would be severe corneal injury from 0.5 ml diluted to 1%. Details for all ratings are given in the original publication. Descriptive adjectives which may parallel the 0 to 10 ratings for the danger of a chemical in contact with the eye could be 1 to 2 "undeterminate", 3 to 4 "minor", 4 to 6 "moderate", 6 to 8 "serious", 8 to 10 "severe".[g] As a screening method for chemicals, Carpenter and Smyth pointed out that the validity of their numerical scoring of eye injury at 24 hours was supported by longer observations in which they followed healing, and found the time for repair and the area of terminal corneal scar were roughly proportional to the initial scores.[27]

Another testing system for evaluating injuriousness of various substances in contact with the eye was described in detail in 1944 by Draize, Woodard, and Calvery.[45] This was based on numerical scoring of degrees of disturbances of cornea, conjunctiva, and iris at intervals of 24 hours to 7 days. This test was widely used, with an aim to answer the question whether a substance has sufficient injurious potential for the human eye that it had best be kept out of the household, or should at least bear a warning label. For the purpose of deciding whether a substance is safe enough for human beings to use in their shampoos, cosmetics, and a great variety of household items that might come in contact with their eyes, the testing problem is difficult, and is yet to be satisfactorily solved. One difficulty is in suspected differences between human beings and animals in the response of their eyes to contact with the chemicals.[316] The practical problem is that rabbits are plentiful, convenient, and not too expensive to use for testing, while monkeys are less convenient, less abundant, and much more expensive, but have the advantage of probably giving results more like those obtained in human beings.[b] Guinea pigs and rats are less satisfactory than rabbits. Cats and dogs have been relatively little evaluated or used in systematic external testing of effects on the eyes, and also lack a good basis for comparison with the human eye.

As the result of an investigation by Griffith et al (1980) in which the aim was to identify conditions in which responses of rabbit eyes would more closely resemble reported responses of human eyes, it has been recommended that 0.01 ml, rather than the 0.1 ml used in the original Draize test, should be the test dose applied to rabbit corneas.[324]

A series of publications have pointed out that the system of testing and grading on rabbit eyes described by Draize did not meet requirements for making the subtle distinctions between substances that were just a little too hazardous to use around the eyes, or in the household, and substances which human beings might use without undue risk. McDonald and Shadduck in 1977 published a comprehensive treatise on developments in topical ocular testing since 1944, with detailed description of recent adaptations and improvements in procedures.[e] Also in 1977, Reim provided a comprehensive synopsis of anatomy, physiology, biochemistry, and pathology relating to methods of topical corneal and conjunctival toxicologic testing.[b] The scope of these two works is too great to try to abstract here. Interested investigators are referred to the originals, with their extensive bibliographies. A comparable study of various topical ocular testing procedures in France has been published in

1982 by Guillot and associates.[325] It is clear from all reports that much technical experience and meticulous attention to details are required to obtain reproducible results, and results that are comparable from one group of testers to another.

Green and colleagues in 1978 produced a monumental volume reporting in the greatest detail the results of comparisons of reactions of rabbit and monkey eyes to injurious chemicals, with numerical scoring and extensive photographic and histopathologic documentation.[322] The principal conclusions from their work were as follows. The rabbit eye is more sensitive than the monkey eye to many, but not all chemicals. (An exception was 5% sulfuric acid.) Slit-lamp biomicroscopy is better than gross external observation. Histopathologic examination can confirm and further elucidatae injurious effects. Washing the eyes 2 minutes after exposure generally had little effect on the outcome. (More prompt irrigation apparently would be required to reduce the amount of the injury.) For some substances, observations have to be extended to 3 weeks for proper prediction of end results.

Buehler and Newmann have shown that if in the rabbit the contact of the test substance is limited to the cornea by means of a suction applicator cup, the lesions are more like those produced by exposure of the whole external surface of the monkey eye, and therefore presumably more like responses of the human eye.[23]

An effort has been made to utilize measurement of change in corneal thickness as an objective indicator of degree of corneal injury, and a favorable opinion has been expressed by Burton (1972)[c] and Conquet (1977).[295] Also, swelling in response to injury has been evaluated by determination of water content by weighing tissues before and after drying (Lailier 1976).[338]

For the future, effort is being made to avoid testing of injurious chemicals and drugs on animal eyes, and to substitute something like a tissue culture or a lower organism. One can speculate upon the great difficulties posed, yet imagine the potential advantages. Unfortunately, for such innovative tests, as well as for current tests utilizing animal eyes, there remains the frequently-cited problem of lack of quantitative data on human eyes for comparison.

For investigators who may be facing this problem, a survey has been made of the *Human eye burns* that are described in this book, trying to identify reasonably well-characterized examples of chemical and drug injuries that may be useful in making comparisons. The substances are listed in the INDEX under *Human eye burns, well-characterized.*

A small proportion of the substances listed have been intentionally tested on human eyes. Most of the substances have contacted the eye accidentally. The nature and the severity of the reactions have in most instances been well enough described to be potentially useful for comparison. Some of the substances have been involved in series of accidents, which can help in assessing their effects.

2. Testing for Cataractogenesis or Other Effects on the Lens

New drugs are tested for adverse effects on the lens by administering them to several different species of animals in doses much larger than are intended to be used clinically, with the hope that this will reveal any tendency to produce cataracts before human beings are exposed. Methods of examination of animals have been described by Barnett and Noel.[8] In essence, very sensitive methods for detection of abnormality of transparency or disturbance of refractive properties of the lens are available in clinical ophthalmoscopy and slit-lamp biomicroscopy. In animal testing, experience has shown that there are often enough real differences in susceptibility to cataract formation by different drugs in different species to make it highly desirable to include a number of species in the testing. Also, studies of cataractogenesis in animals have shown that very young animals tend to have greater susceptibility to cataractogenic effects of drugs and chemicals than the lenses of older animals. In part this may be due to differences in penetrability of drugs from the bloodstream through the blood-aqueous barrier into the eye, but it is also in part due to innate differences in the susceptibility of the lens itself at different ages.

Studies on the biochemical and physiological processes in the crystalline lenses of animals have been considerably aided by development and progressive improvement of methods of maintaining the lens in culture *in vitro*, where not only its transparency, but its water content, cation transport system, permeability, and highly specific metabolic and enzymatic processes can be studied quantitatively and in great detail. These techniques have been used particularly in study of galactose cataracts and in the study of the effects of miotics on the lens. (References to these methods are included under *Galactose* and *Miotics*.)

3. Detection of Effects on Retina and Choroid

If one looks in Chapter I of this book at the portion that surveys toxic effects on the posterior segment of the eye and reads the descriptions in Chapter II of the individual drugs and chemicals that have had damaging effects on the retina and choroid of animals and human beings, it becomes evident that a great variety of methods of testing and examination have been involved, and that no simple standard testing method could have been expected to detect all the toxic effects that have been discovered. Furthermore there are many instances of species differences in sensitivity to toxic effects on retina and choroid.

In animal studies, detection of toxic effects on retina and choroid have been based principally on ophthalmoscopic examination for changes in appearance of the ocular fundus, and also have been based on electrophysiologic studies, particularly electroretinography, upon histologic studies by light and electron microscopy, and upon metabolic studies.

In human beings the methods have included the same ophthalmoscopy and electrophysiologic types of examination (ERG, EOG, VER), as in animals, but in human beings evaluations of visual acuity, visual fields, and other physiologic visual parameters, such as examination of color vision and light adaptation, have had a much larger role. On the other hand, in human beings the opportunity for histologic examination naturally has been much less common than in animals.

A review of toxicologic testing of medications on the retina was published by Meier-Ruge in 1977[357] and in 1982 Koch and colleagues described an extensive testing of visual functions that could be carried out in evaluation of drugs in human beings, but could not be done in animals.[d]

4. Testing for Influences on Intraocular Pressure

Adverse influences on intraocular pressure have occasionally been tested for in human beings by tonometry before and after administration of drugs either externally or systemically, but most testing has been done looking for potentially therapeutic, pressure-lowering effects rather than to detect pressure-elevating actions. There has so far been little correlation between pressure-elevating influences in animals and in human beings. Very few drugs have been reliably shown to raise the pressure in human eyes. More have been claimed to raise the pressure in animals. Corticosteroids, which have been the best studied in human beings, and which have been shown to be prone to produce glaucoma, appear seldom to raise the pressure in animal eyes.

If a valid demonstration is obtained of an elevation of intraocular pressure from the action of a drug, it is important to try to distinguish whether it is a rapid, transient change such as might merely reflect a change in blood pressure or in the volume of the intraocular vascular bed, or whether it is a sustained change in intraocular pressure that might be attributed to a fundamental change in rate of formation of aqueous humor or resistance to aqueous outflow. The ultimate significance, especially with respect to the human being and to glaucoma, is quite different in the two cases. The sustained influences which establish a new steady state are of prime importance clinically.

Most sustained elevations of intraocular pressure that have been achieved in animal eyes have been produced by introducing toxic chemicals, or injecting viscous or particulate substances into the eye with the intention of inducing glaucoma. The artificial glaucoma can be utilized for evaluating the effectiveness of pressure-lowering drugs.

An instructive chapter on using applanation tonometry for evaluation of effects of toxic substances on intraocular pressure in animals was published by Ballantyne and colleagues in 1977.[a] This includes a background of relevant anatomy and physiology, and provides examples of pressure rises induced by topical irritants.

SPECIES SPECIFICITY

Scattered through Chapter II of this book, in which drugs, chemicals, plants and venoms, and their effects on the eye are described, there are many instances of differences in responses in human beings and in various species of animals. These differences are sometimes explainable on the basis of anatomical peculiarities, but in most instances explanations are yet to be found. Rather than reiterate the observations on species specifities here, a list is provided in the INDEX under *Species differences in toxic ocular effects,* for investigators wishing to explore the subject.

Potentially helpful to study of this subject, Barnett and Noel have well described and illustrated normal characteristics and normal species differences among rats, rabbits, cats, dogs, pigs, and baboons, with greatest attention to their ocular fundi and lenses.[8]

a. Ballantyne B, Gazzard MF, Swanston DW: Applanation tonometry in ophthalmic toxicology. Chapter 13 (Pages 158–192) in Ballantyne.[276]

b. Beckley JH, Russell TJ, Rubin KF: Use of the rhesus monkey for predicting human response to eye irritants. *TOXICOL APPL PHARMACOL* 15:1-9, 1969.
c. Burton ABG: A method for the objective assessment of eye irritation. *FOOD COSMET TOXICOL* 10:209-217, 1972.
d. Koch HR, Kremer F, et al: Evaluation of possible drug side effects on the eye in human volunteers. *KLIN MONATSBL AUGENHEILKD* 180:70-74, 1982.
e. McDonald TO, Shadduck JA: Eye irritation. *ADV MOD TOXICOL* 4(Dermatotoxicol Pharmacol):139-191, 1977. Edited by FW Marzulli and HI Maibach. Hemisphere, Washington DC
f. Reim M: Toxicological testing on cornea, conjunctiva, and tears. *ARZNEIMITTEL-NEBENWIRKUNGEN AM AUGE* 1977, 216-258. Edited by Hockwin O and Koch HR. Gustav Fischer, Stuttgart-New York. (German)
g. Salomons N: Personal communication, 1983.

INDEX

Asterisks (*) preceding entries in this INDEX signify that substances so identified are not described elsewhere in this book, but that they have been tested externally on the eyes of rabbits, and, according to the degree of injury observed after 24 hours, have been rated on a scale of 1 to 10. The most severely injurious substances have been rated 10. The ratings, and the literature sources of the information, are listed in the INDEX. Methods for determining the ratings are outlined on pages 1008 to 1010.

Following the INDEX is a related Bibliography of Numbered References.

Acridine red   *see page* 375
Acridine yellow   *see page* 375
Acriflavine   *see page* 49
Acriquine   *see* Quinacrine
Acrolein   *see page* 49
Acrylamide   *see page* 50
Acrylic acid   *see page* 51
*Acrylic acid, 2-butoxyethoxy ester rated 2 on rabbit eyes.[228]
*Acrylic acid, butyl ester rated 2 on rabbit eyes.[288]
*Acrylic acid, 1,3-butylene glycol diester rated 9 on rabbit eyes.[288]
*Acrylic acid, 2(2-cyanoethoxy)ethyl ester rated 5 on rabbit eyes.[228]
*Acrylic acid, 2-cyanoethyl ester rated 8 on rabbit eyes.[228]
*Acrylic acid, cyclohexyl ester rated 2 on rabbit eyes.[288]
*Acrylic acid, decyl ester, mixed isomers rated 1 on rabbit eyes.[228]
*Acrylic acid, dicyclopentadienyl ester rated 1 on rabbit eyes.[288]
*Acrylic acid, N,N-diethylamino ethyl ester rated 9 on rabbit eyes.[228]
*Acrylic acid, 2,2-dimethyl-1,3-propane diol diester rated 4 on rabbit eyes.[288]
*Acrylic acid, 2,3-epoxypropyl ester rated 10 on rabbit eyes.[228]
*Acrylic acid, 2-ethoxyethanol ester rated 5 on rabbit eyes.[226]
*Acrylic acid, 2-ethoxyethanol diester rated 9 on rabbit eyes.[288]
*Acrylic acid, ethylene glycol diester rated 8 on rabbit eyes.[288]
*Acrylic acid, 2-ethylhexyl ester rated 1 on rabbit eyes.[288]
*Acrylic acid, 2-(5′ethyl-pyrid-2′-yl) ethyl ester rated 2 on rabbit eyes.[228]
*Acrylic acid, hexyl ester rated 1 on rabbit eyes.[228]
*Acrylic acid, 2-hydroxypropyl ester rated 7 on rabbit eyes.[228]
*Acrylic acid, isobutyl ester rated 2 on rabbit eyes.[288]
*Acrylic acid, 2-methoxyethoxy ester rated 5 on rabbit eyes.[228]
*Acrylic acid, 2-methyl-thioethyl ester rated 4 on rabbit eyes.[228]
*Acrylic acid, 5-norbornen-2-methyl ester rated 1 on rabbit eyes.[288]
*Acrylic acid, 2-norbornyl ester rated 2 on rabbit eyes.[228]
*Acrylic acid, pentaerythritol triester rated 10 on rabbit eyes.[288]
*Acrylic acid, tridecyl ester rated 2 on rabbit eyes.[228]
*Acrylic acid, 1,1,1-trihydroxymethyl-propane triester rated 9 on rabbit eyes.[288]
Acrylonitrile   *see page* 51
*2-Acryloxyethyl dimethylsulfonium methyl sulfate rated 5 on rabbit eyes.[228]
Actaea rubra   *see page* 51
Actase   *see* Fibrinolysin, *page* 431
Actate   *see* Tolnaftate
Actinomycin D   *see page* 51
Actinopya agassizi   *see* Sea Cucumber
Acyclovir   *see page* 52
Adalat   *see* Nifedipne
Adaline   *see* Carbromal, *page* 189
Adamsite   *see* Phenarsazine chloride
Adanon   *see* Methadone
Adaptinol   *see* Helenien
Adder venom   *see* Snake venoms
Adenosine triphosphate   *in 2nd edition*
*Adipic acid, 3-cyclohexenylmethanol diester rated 1 on rabbit eyes.[288]

*Adipic acid, di(decyl) ester (mixed isomers) rated 1 on rabbit eyes.[228]
*Adipic acid, di(2-(2-ethylbutoxy)ethyl ester rated 1 on rabbit eyes.[226]
*Adipic acid, di(2-ethylbutyl) ester rated 1 on rabbit eyes.[226]
*Adipic acid, di(2-propynyl) ester rated 2 on rabbit eyes.[228]
*Adipic acid, 6-methyl-3-cyclohexenyl-methanol diester rated 1 on rabbit eyes.[288]
*Adipimide rated 4 on rabbit eyes.[288]
Adrenaline   *see* Epinephrine, *page* 394
Adriamycin   *see* Doxorubicin
Adrucil   *see* Fluorouracil
Aerosol   *see* Smog, *page* 821
Aerosol OS   *see* Anionic surfactants, *page* 871
Aerosol OT   *see* Docusate sodium, *page* 871
Aerosol sprays   *see* Hair sprays, *page* 472
AETT   *see* Acetyl ethyl tetramethyl tetralin
Agene   *see* Nitrogen trichloride, *page* 666
Agrostemma githago   *see page* 52
Agrostemmin   *see page* 52
Agrostemma seed   *see page* 52
Air   *see page* 52
Air pollution   *see*
   Ozone, *page* 693
   Smog, *page* 821
AIV solution   *see* Formic acid
Akineton   *see* Biperiden
Alba   *see* Monobenzone
Albomycin   *see* Grisein
Alcian blue   *see page* 375
Alcohol   *see pages* 53–59
Alcoholic essences and extracts,   *see page* 60
Alcoholism   *see page* 53
Alcohol-Tobacco amblyopia   *see* Tobacco smoking, *page* 921
Alcuronium   *in 2nd edition*
Aldactone A   *see* Spironolactone, *page* 845
*Aldol rated 4 on rabbit eyes.[224]
Aldomet   *see* Methyl dopa, *page* 615
Aldrin   *see page* 60
Aleudrine   *see* Isoproterenol
Alginon   *see* Sodium alginate, *page* 828
Alizarin red S   *see pages* 376, 384
Alkali disease   *see* Selenium, *page* 806
Alkalies   *see page* 60
Alkali violet   *see page* 376
Alkylation reaction   *see* Mustard gas, *page* 643
Alkylchloroacetylenes   *see* Dichloroacetylene, *page* 319
Alkyl mercury compounds   *see*
   Ethyl mercury compounds, *page* 424
   Methyl mercury compounds, *page* 621
Alkyl sodium sulfates   *see* Anionic surfactants, *page* 871
Allopurinol   *see page* 64
Allosan   *see* 2,6-Dichloro-4-nitroaniline, *page* 327
Alloxan   *see page* 65
*Allyl acetate rated 4 on rabbit eyes.[224]
Allyl alcohol   *see page* 68
Allyl amines   *see page* 69
Allyl bromide   *see page* 69
3-Allyl catechol   *see page* 69
4-Allyl catechol   *see page* 69
Allyl chloride   *see page* 69
Allyl cyanide   *see page* 69
Allyl dibromide   *see page* 69
*Allyl ether of propylene glycol rated 7 on rabbit eyes.[224]
Allyl glycerol ether   *see page* 70
Allyl glycidyl ether   *see page* 70

Biomet   *see* Bis(tri-n-butyltin) oxide, *page* 149
Biomycin   *see* Chlortetracycline
Biperiden *in 2nd edition*
*4,4'-Biphenyldiol rated 3 on rabbit eyes.[288]
Biphenyls   *see* Polychlorinated biphenyls, *page* 750
*Bis(2-acetoxyethyl)sulfone rated 2 on rabbit eyes.[228]
1,4-Bis(aminoethyl)cyclohexane   *see page* 383
*Bis(2-aminoethyl)fumarate dihydrochloride rated 8 on rabbit eyes.[288]
1,5-Bis(*p*-aminophenoxy)pentane   *see* Aminophenoxy alkanes, *page* 78
*Bis(3-aminopropyl)amine rated 8 on rabbit eyes.[228]
*N,N-Bis(3-aminopropyl)methylamine rated 8 on rabbit eyes.[228]
*9,9-Bis(2'-carbethoxyethyl)fluorene rated 3 on rabbit eyes.[288]
*9,9-Bis(2'-carboxyethyl)fluorene sulfate, sodium salt (50 % aqueous) rated 1 on rabbit eyes.[288]
Bis(2-chloroethyl)ether   *see* Dichloroethyl ether, *page* 326
*Bis(2-chloroethyl)phosphite rated 3 on rabbit eyes.[228]
Bis(2-chloroethyl) sulfide   *see* Mustard gas, *page* 643
Bis(chloromethyl)anthracene *in 2nd edition*
Bis(chloromethyl)benzene *in 2nd edition*
Bis(chloromethyl)diphenylmethane *in 2nd edition*
Bis(chloromethyl)ether   *see* Dichloromethyl ether
Bis(chloromethyl)naphthalene *in 2nd edition*
Bis(chloromethyl)xylene *in 2nd edition*
*Bis(1,2-dichloroethyl)sulfone rated 9 on rabbit eyes.[228]
Bis(diethylthiocarbamoyl)disulfide   *see* Disulfiram
Bis(dimethoxythiophosphoryl)disulfide   *see page* 147
*Bis(2-dimethylaminoethoxy)ethane rated 8 on rabbit eyes.[228]
*Bis(2-dimethylaminoethyl)ether rated 9 on rabbit eyes.[228]
1,3-Bis(dimethylamino)-2-propanol   *see page* 383
1,3-Bis(dimethylamino)-2-propanol bis methiodide   *see* Prolonium iodide
Bis(dimethylthiocarbamoyl)disulfide   *see* Thiram
*Bis(2,5-endomethylene-cyclohexylmethyl)amine rated 9 on rabbit eyes.[228]
*Bis(3,4-epoxybutyl)ether rated 7 on rabbit eyes.[228]
*Bis(3,4-epoxy cyclohexylmethyl)adipate rated 1 on rabbit eyes.[228]
*Bis(2,3-epoxycyclopenyl)ether rated 3 on rabbit eyes.[228]
*2,3-Bis(2,3-epoxypropoxy)-1,4-dioxane rated 7 on rabbit eyes.[228]
*N,N-Bis(2,3-epoxypropyl)aniline rated 1 on rabbit eyes.[228]
Bis(2,3-epoxypropyl)ether   *see* Diglycidol ether, *page* 343
Bis(2-ethylhexyl)hydrogenphosphite   *see page* 147
1,2-Bis(ethylsulfonyl)-1,2-dichloroethylene   *see page* 147
Bishydroxycoumarin   *see* Dicumarol, *page* 330
*Bis(2-isocyanatoethyl)carbonate rated 9 on rabbit eyes.[228]
*Bis(2-isocyanatoethyl)-4-cyclohexene-1,2-dicarboxylate rated 5 on rabbit eyes.[228]
*Bis(2-isocyanatoethyl)-5-norbornene-2,3-dicarboxylate rated 5 on rabbit eyes.[228]
Bismarck brown   *see page* 376
*N,N-Bis(1-methylpropylidene)-1,6-hexanediamine rated 9 on rabbit eyes.[288]
Bismuth compounds   *see page* 147
Bismuth pentafluoride   *see page* 148
Bismuth subnitrate   *see* Bismuth compounds
Bismuth trinitrate   *see* Bismuth compounds
Bis(*m*-nitrophenyl)disulfide   *see* Nitrophenide, *page* 669
Bisphenol A   *see page* 148
1,4-Bis-(phenylisopropyl)-piperazine   *see page* 148
1,4-Bis-(3-phenylprop-2-yl)piperazine   *see page* 148
Bis(tri-*n*-butyltin) oxide   *see page* 149

*2,2-Bis(2,2,2-trimethyl)oxirane rated 1 on rabbit eyes.[228]
*Bis(triphenylsilyl)chromate rated 3 on rabbit eyes.[288]
Black Leaf 40 *in 2nd edition*
Black Widow Spider   *see* Spider venom, *page* 844
Blackberry thorn   *see page* 149
Blaes-M   *see* Blasticidin-S, *page* 149
Blasticidin-S   *see page* 149
Bleach   *see* Sodium hypochlorite
Bleach and ammonia   *see* Hypochlorite and Ammonia mixtures, *page* 504
Bleaching powder   *see* Calcium hypochlorite
Blenoxane   *see* Bleomycin sulfate
Bleomycin sulfate   *see page* 150
Blind staggers   *see*
  Locoweed, *page* 567
  Selenium, *page* 806
Blistering beetle   *see* Cantharides, *page* 174
Blood cholinesterase depression   *see* Miotics, *page* 636
Bloodroot   *see* Sanguinarine, *page* 797
Borate salts   *see* Boric acid, *page* 150
Boric acid   *see page* 150
Boric anhydride   *see* Boron oxide, 150
Boron hydride disulfide   *see page* 150
Boron oxide   *see page* 150
Boron tribromide   *see page* 151
Boron trioxide   *see* Boron oxide, *page* 150
Botran   *see* 2,6-Dichloro-4-nitroaniline, *page* 327
Botulinus toxin   *see page* 153
Botulism   *see page* 151
Bouffant *in 2nd edition*
Boxwood   *see* Wood Dusts, *page* 983
Bracken fern   *see page* 154
Bradykinin   *see page* 154
Brake fluid, automobile   *see page* 155
Brass   *see* Copper, *page* 260
Brayera   *see page* 155
Bretylium tosylate *in 2nd edition*
Brick   *in 2nd edition*
Bright blindness   *see* Bracken fern, *page* 154
Brij-30   *see* Nonionic surfactants, *page* 873
Brij-35   *see* Nonionic surfactants, *page* 872, 873
Brilliant cresyl blue   *see page* 377
Brilliantfirnblau   *see page* 377
Brilliant green   *see pages* 155, 377
Brilliant green disulfonic acid   *see page* 377
Brilliant phosphin 5G   *see page* 377
Brilliant Victoria blue RB   *see page* 377
Brilliant yellow   *see page* 377
Brinolase   *see page* 155
Bristles   *see* Burdock burs, *page* 160
British anti-lewisite   *see* Lewisite, *page* 560
Bromacil   *see* Isocil, *page* 536
Bromate   *see page* 155
Bromcresol green   *see page* 377
Bromides   *see page* 156
Brominated xylol   *see* Bromo-xylene, *page* 159
Bromine cyanide   *see* Cyanogen chloride
Bromisoval   *see page* 156
Bromisovalum   *see page* 156
p-Bromoacetanilide *in 2nd edition*
Bromoacetate   *see page* 157
Bromoacetic acid methyl ester   *see* Methyl bromoacetate, *page* 610
Bromoacetone   *see page* 157
2-Bromoacetophenone   *see page* 157
Bromoacetylbromide *in 2nd edition*
Bromoantifebrin *in 2nd edition*
α-Bromobenzylcyanide   *see page* 157

Calcium hydroxide   *see pages* 60, 167
Calcium hypochlorite   *see page* 172
Calcium nitrate   *in 2nd edition*
Calcium oleate   *see* Oleic acid, *page* 675
Calcium oxalate   *see page* 172
Calcium oxide   *see page* 173
Calcium phosphate   *see* Calcium superphosphate
Calcium sulfate   *see page* 173
Calcium superphosphate   *see page* 173
Calcium thioglycolate   *see* Depilatories, *page* 309
Calotropis gigantea   *see* Crownflower, *page* 285
Calsulfhydryl   *in 2nd edition*
Camoquin   *see* Amodiaquine, *page* 94
Camphor   *see page* 173
Candelabra cactus   *see* Euphorbia, *page* 427
Cannabis   *see page* 174
Cantharides   *see page* 174
Cantharidin   *see* Cantharides, *page* 174
Cantharis vesicatoria   *see* Cantharides, *page* 174
Cantharone   *see* Cantharides, *page* 174
Canthaxanthin   *see page* 175
Capoten   *see* Captopril
Capreomycin   *see page* 175
*Caproic acid rated 8 on rabbit eyes.[27,222]
*e-Caprolactam rated 7 on rabbit eyes.[228]
Caprylic alcohol   *see* Octanol, *page* 872
Capsaicin   *see page* 175
Capsicum   *see* Capsaicin, *page* 175
Captax   *see* 2-Mercaptobenzothiazole, *page* 579
Captopril   *see page* 176
Caramiphen   *see* Anticholinergic drugs
Carbachol   *see page* 176
Carbamazepine   *see* Diethylcarbamazine, *page* 334
N-Carbamylarsanilic acid   *see* Carbarsone, *page* 177
Carbarsone   *see page* 177
Carbaryl   *see page* 177
Carbenoxolone   *see page* 177
*(2-Carboxyethyl)diethoxy(methyl)silane rated 1 on rabbit eyes.[228]
*(2-Carbethoxypropyl)diethoxy(methyl)silane rated 5 on rabbit eyes.[228]
Carbinol   *see* Methanol, *page* 591
Carbitol   *see* Diethylene glycol monoethyl ether, *page* 335
Carbitol acetate   *see* Diethyleneglycol monoethyl ether acetate, *page* 336
Carbodiimide   *see* Cyanamide, *page* 286
*(1,2-Carbo(2-ethyl)hexyloxycyclohexane rated 1 on rabbit eyes.[226]
Carbolic acid   *see* Phenol, *page* 720
Carbolochronosis   *see* Phenol, *page* 720
Carbon   *see page* 178
Carbon bisulfide   *see* Carbon disulfide, *page* 179
Carbon black   *see* Carbon, *page* 178
Carbon dioxide   *see page* 179
Carbon disulfide   *see page* 179
Carbonic acid   *see* Carbon dioxide, *page* 179
*Carbonic acid, cyclic ethylene ester rated 4 on rabbit eyes.[226]
*Carbonic acid, cyclic propylene ester rated 4 on rabbit eyes.[226]
Carbonic anhydrase inhibitors   *see*
 Acetazolamide, *page* 33
 Dichlorphenamide, *page* 328
 Ethoxolamide, *page* 411
Carbon monoxide   *see page* 183
Carbon tetrachloride   *see page* 187
Carbonyl chloride   *see* Phosgene, *page* 733

Carbowaxes   *see* Polyethyleneglycols, *page* 751
Carboxide   *in 2nd edition*
*(2-Carboxyethyl)triethoxysilane rated 1 on rabbit eyes.[228]
*(3-Carboxypropyl)diethoxy(methyl)silane rated 5 on rabbit eyes.[228]
Carbromal   *see page* 189
Carbutamide   *see page* 190
Cardiac glycosides   *see page* 190
Cardiazol   *see* Pentylenetetrazol, *page* 708
Cardrase   *see* Ethoxolamide, *page* 411
Carolina yellow jessamine   *see* Gelsemium sempervirens, *page* 456
β,β-Carotene-4,4'-dione   *see* Canthaxanthin
Carrageenan   *see page* 191
Cashew nut shell oil   *see page* 192
Cassaine   *see* Erythrophleum alkaloids, *page* 405
Cassava   *see page* 192
Cassava eating   *see* Cyanides, *page* 287
Castor beans   *see page* 192
Castor oil   *see* Castor beans, *page* 192
Castor oil seeds   *see* Ricin, *page* 793
Catalase   *see*
 Hydrogen peroxide, *page* 492
 Hydroxyamine, *page* 502
Catalin   *see* Naphthalene, *page* 650
Catapres   *see* Clonidine
Cataract (Opacity of lens substance), from systemic drugs or chemicals, *see Discussion*, *pages* 12–15
 Acetaminophen (A)
 Allopurinol ? (H)
 Alloxan (A)
 Allyl cyanide (A)
 Aminotriazole (A)
 Arabinose (A)
 5-Aziridino-2,4-dinitrobenzamide (A)
 Bis-(phenylisopropyl)-piperidine & UVA (H)
 Bleomycin (A)
 Boron hydride disulfide (A)
 Bromodeoxyuridine (reversible) (A)
 Busulfan (A,H)
 Capreomycin ?? (A)
 Carbromal ?? (H)
 Carbutamide (A)
 Chlorphentermine (A)
 Chlorophenylalanine (A)
 Chlorpropamide (A)
 Clomiphene (A)
 Cobalt chloride (A)
 Contraceptive hormones ?? (H)
 Corticosteroids (H)
 Cyanate ? (A,H)
 Decahydronaphthalene (A)
 Defroxamine ? (H)
 Diazacholesterol (A)
 Diazoxide (reversible) (A)
 Dibromomannitol ?? (H)
 Dichlorisone (A)
 Dichloroacetate (reversible) (A)
 2,6-Dichloro-4-nitroaniline & UV? (A)
 Diethylaminoethoxyandrostenone (A)
 4-(*p*-Dimethylaminostyryl)quinoline (A)
 Dimethylnitroquinoline (A)
 Dimethylterephthalate (A)
 Dinitrocresol (A,H)
 Dinitrophenol (A,H)
 Diquat (A)
 Disophenol (A)

Contergan *see* Thalidomide, *page* 895
Contraceptive hormones *see page* 252
Copper acetoarsenite *see pages* 115, 260
Copper carbonate *see page 260*
Copper chloride *see page 260*
Copper compounds, external contact, *see page 260*
Copper cyanide *see page 260*
Copper Metal Foreign Body *see pages* 260–268
Copper sulfate *see page 260*
Copper, Systemic *see page 268*
Copying pencils *see* Pencils, Indelible, *page* 702
Coral snakes *see* Elapid snakes, *page 835*
Cordarone *see* Amiodarone, *page 82*
Cordite *in 2nd edition*
Coriphosphine *see page* 377
Corn cockle seed *see* Agrostemma seed, *page* 52
Corneal, Conjunctival Inflammation, sometimes with Dermatitis, **from Systemic Substances,** *see Introduction, page* 11, *and see:*
　Allyl cyanide (rats)
　Aminosalicylic acid
　Arsenic (inorganic)
　Arsphenamine
　Barbiturates
　Bromide
　Chloral hydrate
　Chlorambucil
　Chlorpropamide
　Cyclophosphamide
　Cytarabine
　Dixyrazine
　Ethylphenylhydantoin
　Gold
　Hexachlorobenzene
　Hypericum
　Isotretinoin
　Lantana (animals)
　Methotrexate
　Methyldopa
　Noramidopyrine
　Novobiocin
　Oxprenolol
　Penicillamine
　Phenazone
　Phenolphthalein
　Phenazopyridine (dogs)
　Phensuximide
　Phenylbutazone
　Phenytoin
　Phthalofyne
　Practolol
　Sulfadiazine
　Sulfamerazine
　Sulfarsphenamine
　Sulfathiazole
Corneal (Epithelial) Deposits, in human beings, **from Systemic Drugs,** *see*
Introduction, page 10, *and see:*
　Amiodarone
　Amodiaquine
　Bismuth subnitrate
　Chloroquine
　Chlorpromazine
　Clofazimine
　Fluphenazine
　Gold
　Hydroxychloroquine
　Isotretinoin

Mepacrine
Monobenzone
Perhexiline
Tilorone
Triparanol
Corneal Epithelial Edema (painless), with delayed onset of haloes, from Local Action, *see Introduction, pages* 7–8, and *see:*
　Allyl alcohol
　Diethylamine
　Diethyl diglycolate
　Diisopropylamine
　Dimethylamine
　Dimethylaminopropylamine
　Dimethyl diglycolate
　Ethylenediamine
　N-Ethylmorpholine
　N-Ethylpiperidine
　N-Methylmorpholine
　Morpholine
　Nitronaphthalene ?
　tert-Octylamine
　Tetramethylbutanediamine
　Tetramethylethylenediamine
　Triethylenediamine
Corneal Epithelial Injury (painful), with delayed onset, from Local Action, *see Introduction, pages* 8–9, and *see:*
　Allyl alcohol
　p-Anisyl chloride
　Butyl amine
　Cardiac glycosides
　Colchicine
　Diazomethane
　Dichlorobutenes
　Diethylamine
　Diethylthiourea ??
　Digitalis glycosides
　Diisopropylamine
　Dimethylaminopropylamine
　Dimethylphosphorochloridothionate
　Dimethyl sulfate
　Diphenylcyanoarsine
　Diving Mask Defogger
　Dyes (cationic)
　Emetine
　Erythrophleine
　Ethyl amine
　Ethylene oxide
　Ethylenimine
　Euphorbias
　Fish (decomposing)
　Formaldehyde
　Hydrogen sulfide
　Hypochlorite-ammonia mixtures
　Ipecac
　Manchineel
　Methyl bromide
　Methyl chloroacrylate
　Methyl dichloropropionate
　Methyl fluorosulfate
　Methyl silicate
　Mustard gas
　Mustard oil
　Nitrosomethyl urethane
　Osmic acid
　Oxalyl chloride
　Podophyllum

*3-Cyclohexene-1-carbonitrile rated 2 on rabbit eyes.[226]
*4-Cyclohexene-1-carboxaldehyde rated 8 on rabbit eyes.[226]
*3-Cyclohexene-1-carboxylic acid rated 9 on rabbit eyes.[226]
*Cyclohexenyl-4-phenol rated 9 on rabbit eyes.[228]
*2-Cyclohexenylmethyl-3-cyclohexene carboxylate rated 1 on rabbit eyes.[288]
*3-(3-Cyclohexen-1-yl-2,4-dioxaspiro)-5,5-undec-8-ene rated 1 on rabbit eyes.[288]
*2-(4-Cyclohexenyl)-bicyclo-(2.2.1)-hept-5-ene rated 2 on rabbit eyes.[228]
Cyclohexylamine   see page 297
Cyclomandol   see Cyclandelate, page 294
Cyclomydril   see Cyclopentolate, page 297
Cycloocta-1,5-diene   see page 297
Cyclopentadiene   in 2nd edition
*Cyclopentene rated 5 on rabbit eyes.[228]
*2-Cyclopentene-1-ol rated 5 on rabbit eyes.[228]
Cyclopentolate   see page 297
*Cyclopentyl ether rated 2 on rabbit eyes.[228]
Cyclophosphamide   see page 299
Cycloplegia   see Anticholinergic Drugs, page 109
Cycloserine   see page 300
Cyclospasmol   see Cyclandelate, page 294
Cyclyme   in 2nd edition
Cycrimine   see Anticholinergic Drugs
Cyprex   see Dodine, page 372
Cyproheptadine   see Anticholinergic Drugs
Cysteine   see page 300, also see Collagenase inhibitors, page 1000
Cystic fibrosis   see Chloramphenicol
Cytarabine   see page 301
Cytisine   see page 302
Cytisus laburnum   see Cytisine
Cytosine arabinoside   see Cytarabine
Cytoxan   see Cyclophosphamide
2,4-D   see 2,4-Dichloroacetic acid
D-1514   see Octamoxin
Dactinomycin   see Actinomycin D, page 51
Dalapon   see 2,2-Dichloropropionate
Dalzic   see Practolol
DAM   see Diacetylmonoxime, page 312
Dapsone   see page 304
Daranide   see Dichlorphenamide
Daraprim   see Pyrimethamine
Darenthin   see Bretylium tosylate
Dark Adaptation Altered, in human beings, by Systemic Substances, see:
    Carbon dioxide
    Carbon disulfide
    Carbon monoxide
    Deferoxamine
    Digitalis
    Digitoxin
    Halothane
    Indomethacin
    Piperidylchlorophenothiazine
Darvocet, Darvon   see Propoxyphene
Dolene, Doloxene   see Propoxyphene
Datura arborea   see Datura stramonium, page 304
Datura cornigera   see page 305
Datura stramonium   see pages 304, 844
Dayblindness   see Furmethonol
DBI   see Phenformin, page 717
DC 200   see Silicones, page 810
o,p-DDD   see Mitotane
DD Mixture   in 2nd edition
DDT   see page 305
Debinyl   see Phenformin, page 717

Decahydronaphthalene   see page 306
Decahydronitronaphthalene   see page 306
Decalin   see Decahydronaphthalene, page 306
Decalol   see under 2-Naphthol
Decamethylenebis(trimethyl ammonium bromide)   see Decamethonium, page 307
Decamethonium   see page 307
*Decamethylcyclopentasiloxane rated 1 on rabbit eyes.[288]
*1-Decanal (mixed isomers) rated 1 on rabbit eyes.[228]
n-Decane   see Petroleum products, page 715
*Decanoic acid (mixed isomers) rated 9 on rabbit eyes.[228]
*Decanoic acid, vinyl ester (mixed isomers) rated 1 on rabbit eyes.[228]
Decanol   see Decyl alcohol
*Decyl alcohol rated 2 on rabbit eyes.[225]
*Decyl amine rated 9 on rabbit eyes.[228]
*Decyl chloride rated 1 on rabbit eyes.[228]
Decyltrimethyl ammonium bromide   see page 870
Deet   see N,N-Diethyl-m-toluamide, page 337
Deferoxamine   see page 307
Defolex   see Sodium chloroacetate, page 830
Delnay   in 2nd edition
m-Delphene   see N,N-Diethyl-m-toluamide, page 337
Delphine blue conc.   see page 377
Delvex   see Dithiazanine iodide, page 368
Demerol   see Pethidine, page 713
Dendrid   see Idoxuridine
Deobase   see Kerosene, page 545, 714
2-Deoxyglucose   in 2nd edition
2'-Deoxy-5-iodouridine   see Idoxuridine, page 573
Depen   see Penicillamine
Depigmentation of eyelashes   see page 28
Depilatories   see page 309
Deracil   see Thiouracil, page 912
Derris   see page 309
Deserpidine   in 2nd edition
Desethylchloroquine   in 2nd edition
Desferal   see Deferoxamine, page 307
Desferioxamine   see Deferoxamine, page 307
Desferol   see Deferoxamine, page 307
Desipramine   see page 309
Desmethylimipramine   see Desipramine
Desmodur-T   see Toluene diisocyanate, page 928
Desoxycortone   see page 309
Desoxyn   see Dexamphetamine, page 310
DETA   see Diethylenetriamine, page 336
Detamide   see N,N-Diethyl-m-toluamide, page 337
Detergents   see pages 5, 310
Devryl   see Clomacran
Dexamphetamine   see page 310
Dexbrompheniramine   in 2nd edition
Dexedrine   see Dexamphetamine, page 310
Dextran   see page 311
Dextran sulfate   see page 311
Dextroamphetamine   see Dexamphetamine, page 310
Dextromoramide   in 2nd edition
Dextrose   see Glucose, page 460
DFP   see Diisopropyl fluorophosphate
DHE-45   see Dihydroergotamine, page 345
Diabinese   see Chlorpropamide, page 232
Diacetin   see page 312
*Diacetone alcohol rated 5 on rabbit eyes.[223]
1,8-Diacetoxy-9-anthranol   see Dithranol triacetate, page 370
*1,1-Diacetoxy-2,3-dichloropropane rated 10 on rabbit eyes.[228]
1,1-Diacetoxyethane   in 2nd edition

β,β'-Dichloethyl sulfide   *see* Mustard gas, *page* 643
Dichloroethyne   *see* Dichloroacetylene, *page* 319
Dichloroformoxime   *see page* 326
*2,2'-Dichloroisopropyl ether rated 2 on rabbit eyes.[225]
Dichloromethane   *see* Methylene chloride, *page* 616
Dichloromethyl ether   *see page* 327
*2,3-Dichloro-2-methyl-propionaldehyde rated 8 on rabbit eyes.[228]
2,6-Dichloro-4-nitroaniline   *see page* 327
1,1-Dichloro-1-nitroethane   *see page* 327
2,3-Dichlorophenolindophenol   *in 2nd edition*
2,4-Dichlorophenoxyacetic acid   *see pages* 328, 478
*2,4-Dichlorophenoxyethanediol rated 10 on rabbit eyes.[225]
2,4-Dichlorophenoxypropionic acid   *see* Herbatox
2,4-Dichlorophenyl-p-nitrophenyl ether   *see page* 328
1,2-Dichloropropane   *see page* 328
*1,1-Dichloropropane rated 2 on rabbit eyes.[226]
*1,3-Dichloro-2-propanol rated 8 on rabbit eyes.[228]
*2,3-Dichloropropanol-1 rated 5 on rabbit eyes.[27,223]
1,3-Dichloropropropene   *see page* 328
*2,3-Dichloro-1-propene rated 5 on rabbit eyes.[70,228]
*α,β-Dichloropropionaldehyde rated 10 on rabbit eyes.[225]
2,2-Dichloropropionate   *in 2nd edition*
*2,3-Dichloropropionic acid rated 9 on rabbit eyes.[228]
*Dichlorostyrene rated 5 on rabbit eyes.[223]
*3,4-Dichlorotetrahydrothiophene-1,1-dioxide rated 4 on rabbit eyes.[288]
*2,6-Dichloro-9-thiabicyclo(3.3.1)nonane rated 1 on rabbit eyes.[288]
α,α-Dichlorotoluene   *see page* 328
*1,11-Dichloro-3,6,9-trioxaundecane rated 1 on rabbit eyes.[288]
Dichlorphenamide   *see page* 328
2,6-Dichlorthiobenzamide   *see page* 329
Dichromates   *see page* 329
Diclofenamide   *see* Dichlorphenamide
Dicoumarin   *see* Dicumarol, *page* 330
Dicoumarol   *see* Dicumarol
Dicumarol   *see page* 330
Dicumenylmethane   *in 2nd edition*
Di(2-cyanoethyl)amine   *see* Iminodipropionitrile
*Di(2-cyanoethyl)sulfide rated 1 on rabbit eyes.[27,224]
Dicyclomine   *see page* 330
*Dicyclopentadiene rated 2 on rabbit eyes.[228]
Dicycloverine   *see* Dicyclonine, *page* 330
*Di-(decanoyl)triethyleneglycol ester rated 1 on rabbit eyes.[228]
Dieffenbachia exotica   *see page* 331
Dieffenbachia picta   *see page* 331
Dieffenbachia plants   *see page* 331
Dieldrin   *see page* 332
Deltamid   *see* N,N-Diethyl-m-toluamide, *page* 337
Diepoxybutane   *see page* 333
*2,5-Di-(1,2-epoxyethyl tetrahydro)-2H-pyran rated 8 on rabbit eyes.[288]
*1,2,8,9-Diepoxylimonene rated 3 on rabbit eyes.[228]
*1,2,7,8-Diepoxyoctane rated 7 on rabbit eyes.[228]
*2,6-Di-(2,3-epoxypropyl)phenyl-2,3-epoxypropyl ether rated 5 on rabbit eyes.[288]
Diesel exhaust   *in 2nd edition*
Diethanolamine   *see page* 333
*2,2-Diethoxyacetophenone rated 1 on rabbit eyes.[288]
*Diethoxydimethylsilane rated 1 on rabbit eyes.[211]
*Diethoxytetraethylene glycol rated 2 on rabbit eyes.[228]
*2-(Diethoxyphosphinyl)ethyltriethoxysilane rated 5 on rabbit eyes.[288]
Diethylamine   *see pages* 75, 333

Diethylamine acetarsol   *see* Acetarsol
*N,N-Diethylaminoacetonitrile rated 8 on rabbit eyes.[225]
3-β-(β-Diethylaminoethoxy)androst-5-en-17-one methoxime hydrochloride   *see page* 333
Diethylaminoethoxyhexestrol   *see page* 334
*N,N-Diethylaminoethyl chloride rated 7 on rabbit eyes.[225]
2-Diethylaminopropiophenone   *see* Diethylpropion, *page* 337
*(3-Diethylaminopropyl)amine rated 9 on rabbit eyes.[228]
*Diethylazobisisobutyrate rated 1 on rabbit eyes.[288]
*Diethylbenzene rated 1 on rabbit eyes.[265]
Diethylcarbamazine   *see page* 334
Diethyl-2-chloroethylamine   *see* Nitrogen mustards, *page* 665
*Diethylcyclohexane rated 1 on rabbit eyes.[228]
Diethyl diglycolate   *see page* 334
Diethyldithiocarbamate   *see page* 335
Diethylenediamine   *see* Piperazine, *page* 741
Diethylene glycol   *see page* 335
*Diethylene glycol diacetate rated 2 on rabbit eyes.[27]
*Diethylene glycol diethyl ether rated 3 to 4 on rabbit eyes.[27]
*Diethylene glycol divinyl ether rated 1 on rabbit eyes.[228]
*Diethylene glycol ethyl vinyl ether rated 1 on rabbit eyes.[228]
Diethylene glycol monoalkoxymethyl ethers   *see page* 335
*Diethylene glycol mono-2-cyanoethyl ether rated 1 on rabbit eyes.[228]
Diethylene glycol monoethyl ether   *see page* 335
Diethylene glycol monoethyl ether acetate   *see page* 336
*Diethylene glycol mono-2-methylpentyl ether rated 6 on rabbit eyes.[228]
Diethylenetriamine   *see pages* 75, 336, 720
Diethylethanolamine   *see page* 337
*N,N-Diethylethylenediamine rated 10 on rabbit eyes.[226]
*Di-(2-ethylhexoxy)-di(ethylbutoxy)silane rated 1 on rabbit eyes.[228]
*Di(2-ethylhexyl)adipate rated 1 on rabbit eyes.[225]
*Di(2-ethylhexyl)amine rated 8 on rabbit eyes.[27,224]
*2-Di(2-ethylhexyl)aminoethanol rated 1 on rabbit eyes.[226]
*O,O'-Di(2-ethylhexyl)dithiophosphoric acid rated 8 on rabbit eyes.[228]
*Di(2-ethylhexyl)ether rated 1 on rabbit eyes.[226]
*Di(2-ethylhexyl)maleate rated 1 on rabbit eyes.[224]
*Di(2-ethylhexyl)phosphoric acid rated 9 on rabbit eyes.[228]
*Di(2-ethylhexyl)phthalate rated 1 on rabbit eyes.[27]
*Diethyl maleate rated 2 on rabbit eyes.[224]
Diethyl mercury   *see* Ethyl Mercury Compounds, *page* 424
Diethyl-p-nitrophenylthiophosphate   *see* Parathion, *page* 700
N,N-Diethyl-p-phenylenediamine   *see under* Paraphenylenediamine, *page* 696
*Diethyl phosphite rated 5 on rabbit eyes.[228]
*2,2-Diethylpropanediol-1,3 rated 5 on rabbit eyes.[226]
Diethylpropion   *see page* 337
*N,N-Diethyl-1-propynylamine rated 5 on rabbit eyes.[288]
*N,N-Diethyl-2-propynylamine rated 8 on rabbit eyes.[288]
*Diethylsuccinate rated 1 on rabbit eyes.[225]
*Diethyl sulfate rated 5 to 7 on rabbit eyes.[27,224]
1,3-Diethylthiourea   *see page* 337
N,N-Diethyl-m-toluamide   *see page* 337
Difluoro   *see page* 338
Digitalin crystalline   *see* Digitoxin, *page* 341
Digitalis   *see page* 338
Digitalis purpurea   *see* Digitalis, *page* 338

N,N-Dimethyl-p-phenylenediamine   *see*
  Paraphenylenediamine, *page 696*
*2,4-Dimethylphenyl maleimide rated 8 on rabbit
  eyes.[228]
Dimethyl phosphorochloridothionate   *see page 349*
Dimethyl phthalate   *see page 349*
*2,5-Dimethylpiperazine rated 9 on rabbit eyes.[225]
*3,4-Dimethylpyrrolidine-ethanol rated 9 on rabbit eyes.[226]
N,N-Dimethylserotonin   *see* Bufotenine, *page 159*
Dimethyl sulfate   *see page 349*
Dimethyl sulfoxide   *see page 352*
Dimethylterphthalate *in 2nd edition*
*Dimethyl tetrahydrophthalate rated 1 on rabbit eyes.[27,224]
*Dimethyltetrahydropyrone rated 8 on rabbit eyes.[224]
3,5-Dimethyltetrahydro-1,3,5-2H-thiadiazine-2-thione   *see
  page 355*
*3,5-Dimethyl-1-(trichloromethylmercapto)-pyrazole rated
  10 on rabbit eyes.[228]
N,N-Dimethyltryptamine *in 2nd edition*
*2,3-Dimethyl valeraldehyde rated 2 on rabbit eyes.[228]
Dimidium bromide   *see page 355*
2,4-Dinitro-6-aminophenol   *see page 361*
2,4-Dinitro-anisole   *see page 361*
Dinitrobenzene   *see page 355*
4,6-Dinitro-2-sec-butylphenol   *see page 356*
Dinitrochlorobenzene   *see page 357*
Dinitro-o-cresol   *see page 357*
4,6-Dinitro-o-cresol   *see* Dinitro-o-cresol, *page 357*
2,4-Dinitrofluorobenzene   *see page 358*
Dinitrogen monoxide   *see* Nitrous oxide, *page 670*
Dinitronaphthalene   *see page 358*
2,4-Dinitrophenetole   *see page 361*
2,4-Dinitrophenol   *see page 358*
2,6-Dinitrophenol   *see page 361*
Dinitrotoluene   *see page 362*
Dinoprost   *see page 362*
Dioctyl sulfosuccinate sodium   *see* Docusate sodium
*Dioctyl tetrahydrophthalate rated 5 on rabbit eyes.[27]
Diodone   *see page 363*
Diodoquin   *see* Iodoquinol, *page 524*
Diodrast   *see* Diodone, *page 363*
Dioform   *see* 1,2-Dichloroethylene, *page 325*
Dionin   *see* Ethylmorphine hydrochloride, *page 424*
*Dioxane rated 4 on rabbit eyes.[27]
*4,10-Dioxatetracyclo(5.4.0$^{3.5}$.0$^{1.7}$.0$^{9.11}$)undecane rated 7
  on rabbit eyes.[288]
*Dioxolane rated 8 on rabbit eyes.[224]
Diphenazine   *see* 1,4-Bis-(phenylisopropyl)-piperazine,
  page 148
Diphenhydramine   *see pages 112, 363*
Diphenine   *see* Phenytoin, *page 730*
Diphenyl   *see* Dowtherm-A, *page 372*
Diphenylaminechloroarsine   *see* Phenarsazine, *page 716*
Diphenylarsenic acid *in 2nd edition*
Diphenylarsinecyanide   *see* Diphenylcyanoarsine, *page
  364*
Diphenyl blue   *see page 377*
Diphenylcarbazone   *see page 363*
Diphenylchloroarsine   *see page 364*
Diphenylcyanoarsine   *see page 364*
Diphenyl guanidine   *see page 364*
Diphenylhydantoin sodium   *see* Phenytoin, *page 730*
Diphenylolpropane *in 2nd edition*
Diphenyloxide   *see* Dowtherm-A, *page 372*
Diphenylthiocarbazide   *see page 364*
Diphenylthiocarbazone   *see* Dithizone, *page 368*
Diphenylthiourea   *see page 364*
Diphtheria toxin   *see page 364*

Dipivalyl epinephrine   *see* Dipivefrin
Dipivefrin   *see page 365*
*Dipropylamine rated 9 on rabbit eyes.[228]
*Dipropylene glycol rated 1 on rabbit eyes.[27]
Dipropylene glycol monomethyl ether   *see page 365*
*Dipropylenetriamine rated 8 on rabbit eyes.[288]
Dipterex   *see* Trichlorfon, *page 933*
Dipyridamole   *see page 365*
Diquat   *see page 365*
Direct black   *see page 378*
Disipal   *see* Orphenadrine
Disoderm   *see* Dichlorisone, *page 318*
Disodium cromoglycate   *see* Cromolyn sodium
Disodium edetate   *see* Edetate, *page 389*
Disophenol   *see page 366*
Disopyramide   *see* Anticholinergic drugs
Distaval   *see* Thalidomide, *page 895*
Disulfiram   *see page 367*
Disulfur dichloride   *see* Sulfur monochloride, *page 868*
Dithiazanine iodide   *see page 368*
2,2'-Dithiobis(benzothiazole)   *see page 368*
Dithiocarb   *see* Diethyldithiocarbamate, *page 335*
Dithizone   *see page 368*
Dithranol   *see page 370*
Dithranol triacetate   *see page 370*
Ditolylmethane *in 2nd edition*
*Di-(tridecyl)amine rated 1 on rabbit eyes.[228]
Diving Mask Defogger   *see page 371*
Divinyl sulfone   *see page 371*
*2,5-Divinyltetrahydro-2H-pyran rated 2 on rabbit eyes.[288]
*3,9-Divinyl-2,4,8,10-tetraoxaspiro(5,5)undecane rated 2 on
  rabbit eyes.[228]
Dixarit   *see* Clonidine
Dixyrazine   *see page 372*
DM   *see* Phenarsazine chloride, *page 716*
DMP   *see* Dimethyl phthalate, *page 349*
DMPCT   *see* Dimethyl phosphorochloridothionate,
  page 349
DMSO   *see* Dimsthyl sulfoxide, *page 352*
DMT   *see* N,N-Dimethyltryptamine
DNCB   *see* Dinitrochlorobenzene, *page 357*
DNFB   *see* Dinitrofluorobenzene, *page 358*
DNP   *see* 2,4-Dinitrophenol, *page 358*
Docosahexenoic acid   *see page 711*
Docusate sodium   *see page 871*
Dodecylguanidine acetate   *see* Dodine, *page 372*
tert-Dodecyl mercaptan *in 2nd edition*
*Dodecylphenol rated 2 on rabbit eyes.[228]
Dodecylpolyethyleneoxide   *see under* Nonionic Surfactants,
  page 872
Dodecyl sodium sulfate   *see page 871*
Dodecyltrimethylammonium bromide   *see page 870*
Dodine   *see page 372*
Dolophine   *see* Methadone, *page 590*
DL-Dopa *in 2nd edition*
L-Dopa   *see* Levodopa
Dopamine   *see page 372*
Dopar   *see* Levodopa
Dopream   *see* Doxapram, *page 373*
Doriden   *see* Glutethimide, *page 462*
Dormison   *see* Methylpentynol
Dowicide G   *see* Pentachlorophenol, *page 706*
Down's Syndrome   *see under* Atropine, *pages 127–128*
Dowtherm-A   *see page 372*
Doxapram   *see page 373*
Doxepine *in 2nd edition*
Doxorubicin   *see page 373*
Dramamine   *see* Diphenhydramine theoclate, *page 363*

Endrate   *see* Edetate, *page* 389, 998
Endrin *in 2nd edition*
Entero-Vioform   *see* Clioquinol
Entodon   *see* Prolonium
Entsufon   *see pages* 732, 871
Enzyme-Detergent *in 2nd edition*
Eosin   *see page* 378
Eosin Y   *see pages* 378, 387
Epanutin   *see* Phenytoin, *page* 730
Ephedrine *in 2nd edition*
Epichlorohydrin   *see page* 394
Epidemic dropsy   *see* Sanguinarine, *page* 797
Epinephrine   *see page* 394
Epithelial Implantation Cysts, Treatment   *see*
    Iodine, *page* 519
    Trichloroacetic acid, *page* 933
*2,3-Epithiopropyl methoxy ether rated 2 on rabbit
    eyes.[828]
Epon 562   *see* Diglycidol resorcinol, *page* 343
1,2-Epoxy-3-allyloxypropane   *see* Allyl glycidyl ether, *page*
    70
*1,2-Epoxybutane rated 4 on rabbit eyes.[228]
1,2-Epoxy-3-butoxy propane   *see* Butyl glycidyl ether
*2,3-Epoxybutyric acid, butyl ester rated 2 on rabbit
    eyes.[228]
*1,2-Epoxy cyclohexane rated 8 on rabbit eyes.[228]
*3,4-Epoxycyclohexane carbonitrile rated 5 on rabbit
    eyes.[228]
*4,5-Epoxycyclohexane-1,2-dicarboxylic acid, di(decyl) ester
    rated 2 on rabbit eyes.[228]
*4,5-Epoxycyclohexane-1,2-dicarboxylic acid, di(2-ethylhexyl)
    ester rated 1 on rabbit eyes.[288]
*2(3,4-Epoxycyclohexyl)ethyl trimethoxy silane rated 1 on
    rabbit eyes.[228]
*3,4-Epoxy-2,5-endomethylenecyclohexane-carboxylic acid,
    ethyl ester rated 2 on rabbit eyes.[228]
1,2-Epoxyethane   *see* Ethylene oxide, *page* 419
*Epoxyethylbenzene rated 2 on rabbit eyes.[226]
*2-(a,b-Epoxyethyl)-5,6-epoxybenzene rated 7 on rabbit
    eyes.[228]
*2,3-Epoxy-2-ethylhexanol rated 5 on rabbit eyes.[228]
*2,3-Epoxy-p-menthane rated 2 on rabbit eyes.[288]
*3,4-Epoxy-6-methylcyclohexanecarboxylic acid, allyl ester
    rated 1 on rabbit eyes.[228]
*3,4-Epoxy-6-methylcyclohexanecarboxylic acid, 3,4-epoxy-
    6-methylcyclohexylmethyl ester rated 1 on rabbit eyes.[228]
*4,5-Epoxy-2-pentenal rated 10 on rabbit eyes.[288]
1,2-Epoxypropanol   *see* Glycidol, *page* 465
*3(2,3-Epoxypropoxy)propyl trimethoxy silane rated 2 on
    rabbit eyes.[228]
*2,3-Epoxypropyl butyl ether rated 5 on rabbit eyes.[228]
*N-(2,3-Epoxypropyl) diethylamine rated 9 on rabbit
    eyes.[228]
*2,3-Epoxypropyl methacrylate rated 4 on rabbit eyes.[228]
*9,10-Epoxystearic acid, allyl ester rated 1 on rabbit eyes.[228]
*9,10-Epoxystearic acid, 2-ethylhexyl ester rated 1 on
    rabbit eyes.[228]
*1,2-Epoxy-4-vinylcyclohexane rated 5 on rabbit eyes.[228]
Epsicapron   *see* Aminocaproic acid, *page* 77
Epsilon aminocaproic acid   *see* Aminocaproic acid, *page*
    77
Equanil   *see* Meprobamate, *page* 577
Equanitrate   *see* Pentaerythrityl tetranitrate, *page* 507
Eraldin   *see* Practolol
Erbium chloride *in 2nd edition*
Ergomar   *see* Ergotamine tartrate
Ergostate   *see* Ergotamine tartrate
Ergot   *see page* 402

Ergotamine tartrate   *see page* 403
Erioglaucin A   *see page* 378
Erioviolet   *see page* 378
Erythritol anhydride   *see* Diepoxybutane, *page* 333
Erythrophleine   *see* Erythrophleum alkaloids
Erythrophleum alkaloids   *see page* 405
Erythrosin   *see page* 378
Erythrosin bluish   *see pages* 378, 387
Eserine   *see* Physostigmine, *page* 736
Esidrix   *see* Hydrochlorothiazide, *page* 490
Esperal   *see* Disulfiram, *page* 367
3,17-Estradiol stearate *in 2nd edition*
Estrogens *in 2nd edition*
Estrone acetate *in 2nd edition*
Esucos   *see* Dixyrazine
Esyntin   *see* Anticholinergic drugs
Etamucin   *see* Sodium hyaluronate
Ethacrynic acid *in 2nd edition*
Ethambutol   *see page* 405
Ethamide   *see* Ethoxolamide, *page* 411
Ethanedinitrile   *see* Cyanogen, *page* 293
Ethanethiol *in 2nd edition*
Ethanol   *see* Alcohol, *page* 53
Ethanolamine   *see page* 410
*Ethanolamine hydrochloride non-injurious on
    rabbit and human eyes (personal observation)
Ethanolamine oleate   *see page* 410
Ethchlorvynol   *see page* 410
Ether   *see page* 411
Ethionamide   *see page* 411
Ethionine *in 2nd edition*
Ethizone   *see* Subathizone, *page* 855
Ethopropazine   *see page* 411
Ethotoin   *see page* 411
Ethoxolamide   *see page* 411
Ethoxyacetylene *in 2nd edition*
*2-Ethoxy-3,4-dihydro-1,2-pyran rated 5 on rabbit
    eyes.[228]
2-Ethoxyethanol   *see page* 412
*3-(2-Ethoxyethoxy)propanol rated 3 on rabbit eyes.[226]
*2-Ethoxyethylacetate rated 3 on rabbit eyes.[27,230]
*2-Ethoxy-4-methyl-3,4-dihydropyran rated 2 on rabbit
    eyes.[226,228]
*2-Ethoxy-4-methyl-tetrahydropyran rated 3 on rabbit
    eyes.[228]
*3-Ethoxy-1-propanol rated 5 on rabbit eyes.[228]
*Ethoxypropionaldehyde rated 7 on rabbit eyes.[223]
*Ethoxypropionic acid rated 9 on rabbit eyes.[223]
*Ethoxytriethylene glycol rated 1 on rabbit eyes.[225]
*Ethoxytriglycol rated 1 on rabbit eyes.[27]
Ethoxytrimethyl silane   *see page* 412
Ethyl acetate   *see page* 412
*Ethylacetoacetate rated 4 on rabbit eyes.[27,224]
*N-Ethylacetoacetamide rated 5 on rabbit eyes.[228]
Ethyl acetone   *see* Methylpropylketone, *page* 626
Ethyl acrylate   *see page* 412
Ethyl alcohol   *see* Alcohol, *page* 53
Ethylamine   *see pages* 75, 412
*2-Ethylaminoethanol rated 9 on rabbit eyes.[226]
*2-(1-Ethylamyloxy)ethanol rated 9 on rabbit eyes.[226]
*2-(2-(1-Ethylamyloxy)ethoxy)ethanol rated 9 on rabbit
    eyes.[226]
Ethylarsine dichloride   *see page* 413
Ethylbenzene   *see page* 413
*Ethyl borate rated 5 on rabbit eyes.[27]
Ethyl bromide *in 2nd edition*
Ethylbromoacetate   *see page* 413
*2-Ethylbutanol-1 rated 9 on rabbit eyes.[226]

Hashish   *see* Cannabis, *page* 174
Healon   *see* Sodium hyaluronate
Healonide   *see* Sodium hyaluronate
Hectin   *see page* 118
Hectograph ink   *in 2nd edition*
Helenien   *in 2nd edition*
Helenium autumnale   *see* Helenien
Helianthin G   *see page* 378
Helichrysum   *see page* 474
Helvella esculenta   *see page* 475
Helvellic acid   *in 2nd edition*
Hematoporphyrin   *see page* 475
Hemicholinium   *in 2nd edition*
Hemin   *see* Hematoporphyrin, *page* 475
Hemisulfur mustard   *in 2nd edition*
Hemoglobin   *see page* 475
Hemosiderin   *see page* 476
Henbane   *see* Hyoscyamus niger, *page* 504
Henna   *see pages* 378, 477
Heparin   *see page* 477
Heptachlor   *see page* 478
*Heptadecanol rated 1 on rabbit eyes.[228]
2-Heptadecyl-2-imidazoline   *see page* 478
1,7-Heptanedioic acid   *see* Pimelic acid, *page* 740
n-Heptanol   *see page* 478
*2-Heptanol rated 9 on rabbit eyes.[226]
*3-Heptanol rated 5 on rabbit eyes.[225]
*2-Heptanone rated 2 on rabbit eyes.[228]
*4-Heptanone rated 2 on rabbit eyes.[288]
n-Heptyl alcohol   *see* n-Heptanol, *page* 478
Heptyl cyanoacrylate   *see* 2-Cyanoacrylic acid esters
Heptyltrimethylammonium bromide   *in 2nd edition*
Herbatox   *see page* 478
Heroin   *see page* 478
Herplex   *see* Idoxuridine
Hetrazan   *see* Diethylcarbamazine, *page* 334
Hexachlorobenzene   *see page* 479
Hexachlorocyclohexane   *see* Lindane, *page* 561
Hexachlorocyclopentadiene   *see page* 479
*1,1,1,3,3,3-Hexachloro-2,2-difluoropropane rated 2 on rabbit eyes.[228]
Hexachloroethane   *see page* 479
Hexachloronaphthalene   *see page* 479
Hexachlorophane   *see* Hexachlorophene, *page* 479
Hexachlorophene   *see page* 479
Hexadecyltrimethylammonium bromide   *see* Cetrimonium bromide, *pages* 199, 871
*Hexa-2,4-dienal rated 8 on rabbit eyes.[226]
*2,4-Hexadien-1-ol rated 8 on rabbit eyes.[288]
*2,4-Hexadienoxypropionitrile rated 1 on rabbit eyes.[288]
*2-(2,4-Hexadienyloxy)ethanol rated 5 on rabbit eyes.[288]
Hexaethyl benzene   *in 2nd edition*
*Hexaethylene glycol rated 1 on rabbit eyes.[27]
Hexaethyl tetraphosphate   *in 2nd edition*
Hexafluoroisopropanol   *see page* 482
*Hexahydro-1,4-diazepine rated 9 on rabbit eyes.[228]
Hexahydropyridine   *see* Piperidine, *page* 741
Hexamethonium   *see page* 482
Hexamethoxydisiloxane   *see page* 628
Hexamethyldisiloxane   *in 2nd edition*
Hexamethylenediamine adipate   *in 2nd edition*
*1,6-Hexamethylene diisocyanate rated 9 on rabbit eyes.[228]
*Hexanal rated 5 on rabbit eyes.[228]
n-Hexane   *see pages* 482, 715
1,6-Hexanediamine   *in 2nd edition*
*1,6-Hexanediol rated 3 on rabbit eyes.[288]
*Hexanediol-2,5 rated 3 on rabbit eyes.[223]

2,5-Hexanedione   *see page* 483
Hexanethiol   *in 2nd edition*
*1,2,6-Hexanetriol rated 1 on rabbit eyes.[226]
*Hexanoic acid rated 8 to 9 on rabbit eyes.[226,228]
*Hexanoic acid, e-lactone rated 8 on rabbit eyes.[226]
*Hexanoic acid, vinyl ester rated 1 on rabbit eyes.[228]
1-Hexanol   *see page* 484
2-Hexanol   *see page* 484
n-Hexanol   *see* 1-Hexanol, *page* 484
2-Hexanone   *see page* 484
*3-Hexanone rated 2 on rabbit eyes.[288]
*4-Hexene-1-yne-3-one rated 10 on rabbit eyes.[228]
Hexesterol   *in 2nd edition*
Hexocyclium   *see* Anticholinergic drugs
Hexosamine of the cornea   *see* Alkalies, *page* 61
*n-Hexoxyethanol rated 8 on rabbit eyes.[225]
*Hexylamine rated 8 on rabbit eyes.[226]
*n-Hexyl benzoate rated 1 on rabbit eyes.[225]
Hexylcaine   *see page* 101
Hexyl cyanoacrylate   *see* 2-Cyanoacrylic acid esters, *page* 291
*Hexylene glycol rated 4 on rabbit eyes.[223]
*Hexyl ether rated 1 on rabbit eyes.[226]
*2-Hexyloxy-2-ethoxyethyl ether rated 5 on rabbit eyes.[228]
Hexylresorcinol   *see page* 485
*n-Hexyl vinyl sulfone rated 5 on rabbit eyes.[228]
HF   *see* Hydrofluoric acid, *page* 490
HFIP   *see* Hexafluoroisopropanol, *page* 482
Hippomane mancinella   *see* Manchineel, *page* 575
Hirudin   *see page* 485
Histamine   *see page* 485
Hollicide   *see* Bis(tri-n-butyltin) oxide, *page* 149
Holmium chloride   *in 2nd edition*
Holothurin   *see* Sea Cucumber, *page* 805
Homacridine yellow   *see page* 378
Homatropine   *see page* 486
Honeysuckles   *see* Lonicera plants, *page* 569
Hops   *in 2nd edition*
Human Eye Burns, well-characterized, *Discussion   see* pages 1008 to 1010, and *see:*
　　Acetone
　　Alcohol
　　Ammonia
　　Benzalkonium chloride
　　Benzene
　　Brake fluid
　　(Brilliant green)
　　Calcium hydroxide
　　Castor beans (ricin)
　　α-Chloroacetophenone
　　o-Chlorobenzylidene malononitrile
　　Chlorobromomethane
　　Chlorobutanol
　　2-Chloroethanol
　　Chloroform
　　Chrysarobin (chrysophanic acid)
　　Clove oil
　　Croton oil
　　Crystal violet
　　2-Cyanoacrylic acid esters
　　Cytarabine
　　Dibenzoxazepine
　　Dibutyl phthalate
　　Dieffenbachia juice
　　Digitoxin
　　Digoxin
　　Dimethyl phthalate
　　Dimethyl sulfate

*2-Mercaptoethyl trimethoxy silane rated 2 on rabbit eyes.[228]

2-Mercapto-1-hydroxypyrimidine   see Thiouracil, page 912

*3-Mercaptopropyl trimethoxy silane rated 2 on rabbit eyes.[228]

Mercurial diuretics   see page 579

Mercurialentis   see Mercury (inorganic) Poisoning, page 582

Mercuric chloride   see page 579

Mercuric iodide   see page 580

Mercuric oxide (yellow)   see page 580

Mercuric oxycyanide   see page 581

Mercuric sulfide   see page 581

Mercurous chloride   see page 581

Mercurous iodide   see page 582

Mercury alkyl compounds   see
  Ethyl mercury compounds, page 424
  Methyl mercury compounds, page 621

Mercury aryl compounds   see
  p-Chloromercuribenzoate
  p-Chloromercuribenzene sulfonate
  Hydrargaphen
  Phenylmercuric salts
  Thimerosal

Mercury fulminate   see page 582

Mercury (inorganic) poisoning   see page 582

Mercury metal (liquid)   see page 586

Merthiolate   see Thimerosal, page 902

Mesaconic acid   see page 588

Mesantoin   see Mephenytoin, page 577

Mescaline   see page 588

Mesidine   see page 588

Mesityl oxide   see page 589

Mesoridazine   see page 589

Mesquite thorn   see page 589

Mesuximide in 2nd edition

Meta-Delphene   see N,N-Diethyl-m-toluamide, page 337

Metalcaptase   see Penicillamine, page 703

Metal chelators and cataracts   see page 15

Metaldehyde   see page 589

Metanil yellow   see page 379

Metaphosphate   see Acids, page 46

Metaphosphoric acid   see Phosphoric acid, page 733

Metaraminol in 2nd edition

Metarsenobenzol in 2nd edition

Metcaraphen in 2nd edition

*Methacrylaldehyde rated 9 on rabbit eyes.[224]

*Methacrylaldehyde(O-methylcarbamoyl) oxime rated 5 on rabbit eyes.[288]

*Methacrylic acid, ally ester rated 2 on rabbit eyes.[228]

*Methacrylic acid, butyl ester rated 1 on rabbit eyes.[228]

*Methacrylic acid, 2-butyloctyl ester rated 1 on rabbit eyes.[226]

*Methacrylic acid, 1,1,1-trihydroxymethyl propane triester rated 2 on rabbit eyes.[288]

Methacrylonitrile   see page 590

Methacycline   see page 590

Methadone   see page 590

Methamphetamine   see page 591

Methanol   see pages 42, 591

Methantheline bromide   see Anticholinergic drugs

Methaqualone   see page 598

Methazolamide   see page 598

Methicillin   see page 599

Methidate   see Methylphenidate

Methixene   see page 599

Methocarbamol   see page 600

Methocel   see Methyl cellulose, page 611

Methotrexate   see page 600

Methotrimeprazine   see page 601

Methoxamine hydrochloride in 2nd edition

Methoxa Dome   see Methoxsalen

Methoxsalen   see page 601

*Methoxyacetone rated 3 on rabbit eyes.[288]

p-Methoxybenzyl chloride   see p-Anisyl chloride, page 109

*1-Methoxy-1,3-butadiene rated 2 on rabbit eyes.[228]

*3-Methoxy butyraldehyde rated 8 on rabbit eyes.[228]

*Methoxybutyric acid rated 8 on rabbit eyes.[226]

7-Methoxychlorpromazine   see page 229

2-Methoxyethanol   see Methyl Cellosolve, page 611

Methoxyethyl mercuric acetate in 2nd edition

*2(Methoxyethylthio)ethanol rated 5 on rabbit eyes.[228]

Methoxyflurane   see page 605

*2-(Methoxymethoxy)ethanol rated 2 on rabbit eyes.[226]

2-Methoxy-4-methyl phenol   see Cresols, page 284

2-Methoxy-6-n-pentyl-p-benzoquinone   see Primula, page 763

Methoxy-m-phenylenediamine   see page 605

*3-Methoxy-1-propanol rated 5 on rabbit eyes.[228]

*2-Methoxypropene rated 1 on rabbit eyes.[228]

*3-Methoxypropionitrile rated 5 on rabbit eyes.[228]

8-Methoxypsoralen   see Methoxsalen, page 601

2-Methoxy-1,2,3,4-tetrahydronaphthalene   see Naphthalene

*Methoxy triethylene glycol vinyl ether rated 3 on rabbit eyes.[228]

Methyl acetate   see page 605

*Methyl acetoacetate rated 7 on rabbit eyes.[27,223]

*Methyl acetylricinoleate rated 1 on rabbit eyes.[27]

*Methyl acrylate rated 4 on rabbit eyes.[27,223]

β-Methylacrylic acid   see Crotonic acid, page 285

Methylal   see page 606

Methyl alcohol   see Methanol, pages 42, 591

1-α-Methylallylthiocarbamoyl-2-methylthiocarbamoyl-hydrazine   see page 606

Methyl amine   see pages 75, 606

*2-Methylaminoethanol rated 9 on rabbit eyes.[226]

Methylamyl acetate   see page 607

Methyl arsine dichloride   see page 607

Methyl atropine nitrate   see page 607

Methylazoxymethanol acetate   see pages 294, 607

Methyl benzene   see Toluene, page 927

*α-Methyl benzylamine rated 9 on rabbit eyes.[225]

*α-Methyl benzylamine, N-hydroxyethyl rated 8 on rabbit eyes.[225]

*Methyl benzyl Cellosolve rated 3 on rabbit eyes.[27,223]

*α-Methylbenzyl ether rated 1 on rabbit eyes.[228]

Methyl blue   see page 379

*Methyl borate rated 2 to 3 on rabbit eyes.[27,228]

Methyl bromide   see page 607

Methyl bromoacetate   see page 610

*2-Methyl-1,4-butanediol rated 5 on rabbit eyes.[225]

*2-Methylbutanol rated 8 on rabbit eyes.[228]

*3-Methyl-2-butanone rated 3 on rabbit eyes.[288]

*2-Methyl-1-butene-3-one rated 10 on rabbit eyes.[225]

*3-Methyl-2-butenoic acid rated 9 on rabbit eyes.[288]

*3-Methyl-3-butenonitrile rated 2 on rabbit eyes.[228]

*N-Methyl(butyl)amine rated 9 on rabbit eyes.[228]

Methyl n-butyl ketone   see 2-Hexanone, page 484

*2-Methylbutyraldehyde rated 3 on rabbit eyes.[288]

*3-Methylbutyraldehyde rated 4 on rabbit eyes.[288]

*N-Methyl-e-caprolactam rated 5 on rabbit eyes.[228]

*Methyl-e-caprolactone rated 5 on rabbit eyes.[228]

*Methylcarbamylethyl acrylate rated 7 on rabbit eyes.[288]

*Methyl Carbitol rated 2 on rabbit eyes.[27,129]

*Methyl Carbitol acetate ester rated 4 on rabbit eyes.[27]

*Methyl Carbitol formal rated 1 on rabbit eyes.[27]

*4-Methyl valeraldehyde rated 3 on rabbit eyes.[228]
*b-Methyl-delta-valerolactone rated 4 on rabbit eyes.[228]
*N-Methyl-N-vinylacetamide rated 7 on rabbit eyes.[228]
Methyl vinyl carbinol   *see page* 629
Methyl vinyl ketone   *see page* 629
*2-Methyl-5-vinylpyridine rated 8 on rabbit eyes.[228]
*Methylvinyloxyethyl sulfide rated 2 on rabbit eyes.[228]
*Methylvinyl sulfone rated 5 on rabbit eyes.[228]
Methyl violet   *see pages* 379, 385, 458, 628
Methyl viologen   *see* Paraquat, *page* 699
β-Methylxylocholine   *see page* 629
Methysergide   *see page* 629
Metiapine   *see page* 630
Metoclopramide   *see page* 630
Metrazol   *see* Pentylenetetrazol, *page* 708
Metrizamide   *see page* 786
Mevinphos   *see page* 679
Mexoform   *see* Clioquinol
Miconazole   *see* page 630
Milk bush   *see* Euphorbia, *page* 427
Millipore Filters   *see page* 630
Miltown   *see* Meprobamate, *page* 577
Mimosa   *see pages* 380, 630
Mimosa pudica   *see* Mimosine, *page* 630
Mimosine   *see page* 630
Mimusops toxisperma   *see* Wood Dusts, *page* 983
Minamata Disease   *see* Methyl Mercury Compounds, *page* 621
Minipress   *see* Prazosin
Minocycline   *see page* 631
Minocyn   *see* Minocycline
Minoxidil   *see page* 631
Miochol   *see* Acetylcholine chloride, *page* 43
Miostat   *see* Carbachol, *page* 176
Miotics   *see page* 631
Mirex   *see page* 638
Mitomycin C   *see page* 638
Mitotane   *see page* 639
Modaline   *see* Anticholinergic drugs
Molybdenum metal   *see page* 639
Monase   *see* Monoamine oxidase inhibitors, *page* 639
Monkey pistol   *see*
   Euphorbia, *page* 427
   Hura crepitans, *page* 486
Monoallyl amine   *see* Allyl amines, *page* 69
Monoamine oxidase inhibitors   *see page* 639
Monochloramine   *see pages* 505, 876
Monochloroacetic acid   *see page* 640
Monoethanolamine   *see* Ethanolamine, *page* 410
*Monoisopropanol amine rated 9 on rabbit eyes.[224]
Monoisopropenylacetylene   *see* Diisopropenylacetylene
Monomethylhydrazine   *see* Methylhydrazine, *page* 619
Monosodium cyanurate   *see* Cyanuric acid, *page* 293
Monosodium glutamate   *see* Glutamate, *page* 460
Moon Flower   *see page* 640
Moranyl   *see* Suramin
Morel   *see page* 640
Morning Glory   *see page* 640
Morphine   *see page* 640
Morpholine   *see pages* 75, 642
*N-Morpholine ethanol rated 5 on rabbit eyes.[27,223]
Mortar   *see pages* 167, 642
Moths   *see page* 642
Motrin   *see* Ibuprofen
Moule wood   *see* Wood Dusts, *page* 983
Moxalactam disodium   *see page* 642
Moxam   *see* Moxalactam, *page* 642
Moxisylyte   *see* Thymoxamine, *page* 913

MPTP   *see page* 626
Mucomyst   *see* Acetylcysteine, *page* 45
Mucunain   *see* Mucuna pruriens, *page* 642
Mucuna pruriens   *see page* 642
Muriatic acid   *see* Hydrochloric acid
Muscarine *in 2nd edition*
Muscimol   *see* Amanita muscaria, *page* 74
Mushrooms   *see page* 643
Mustard Gas   *see page* 643
Mustard oil   *see pages* 70, 646
Myambutol   *see* Ethambutol, *page* 405
Myanesin   *see* Mephenesin, *page* 577
Mycotoxins   *see page* 646
Mydriacyl   *see* Tropicamide, *page* 958
Mydriatics   *see page* 647
Myelobromol   *see* Dibromomannitol, *page* 317
Mylepsin   *see* Primidone, *page* 763
Myleran   *see* Busulfan, *page* 160
Mylone   *see* 3,5-Dimethyltetrahydro-1,3,5,2H-thiadiazine-2-thione, *page* 355
Myopia, Acute Transient, from Systemic Drugs, in human beings (without cyclotonia or miosis),   *see Discussion, pages* 15–17, *and see:*
   Acetazolamide
   Aminophenazone
   Arsphenamine
   Aspirin ? ?
   Bendrofluazide
   Chlorothiazide
   Chlorthalidone
   Clofenamide
   Codeine ?
   Dichlorphenamide
   Ethoxolamide
   Hydrochlorothiazide
   Isotretinoin
   Neoarsphenamine
   Phenformin
   Polythiazide
   Prochlorperazine
   Promethazine
   Quinine
   Spironolactone
   Sulfonamides
   Tetracycline
   Trichlormethiazide
Myristica   *see* Nutmeg, *page* 671
Myristyl alcohol *in 2nd edition*
Myrj 45   *see page* 872
Myrj 52   *see page* 872, 873
Myrj 53   *see page* 873
Mysoline   *see* Primidone, *page* 763
Nacconol NRSF   *see page* 871
Nafoxidine hydrochloride   *see page* 648
Nail Hardener   *see page* 648
Nail Polish   *see page* 648
Nail Polish Remover   *see page* 648
Nalidixic acid   *see page* 649
Nalidixin   *see* Nalidixic acid, *page* 649
Nalline   *see* Nalorphine, *page* 650
Nalorphine   *see page* 650
Naloxone   *see page* 650
Naphazoline   *see page* 650
Naphtha   *see* Petroleum products, *page* 714
Naphthalane   *see* Decshydronaphthalene, *page* 306
Naphthalene   *see page* 650
Naphthalenebutylsulfonate   *see page* 655
Naphthalenediol   *see* Naphthalene, *page* 650

Optic Nerve Atrophy (*continued*)

Chenopodium ? ? (H)
Chloramphenicol (H)
Clioquinol (H)
Cortex granati (H)
Cyanide (A)(H?)
Dapsone (H)
Dinitrobenzene (H)
Dinitrochlorobenzene (H)
Dinitrotoluene ? (H)
Dynamite ? (H)
Ergot ? (H)
Ergotin ? (H)
Ethambutol (H)
Ethylene glycol ? ? (H)
Ethyl hydrocuprein (H)
Ethylmercuritoluenesulfonanilide (H)
Eucupine (H)
Finger cherries (H)
Formic acid (A)
Glibenclamide ? (H)
Halquinols (H)
Hexachlorophene (A)(H)
Hexamethonium (H)
n-Hexane ? ?
Iodoform (H)
Iodoquinol (H)
Isoniazid (H)
Lead (H)
Linamarin ? (H)
Lindane ? (H)
Methanol (A)(H)
Methyl acetate ? (H)
Methyl bromide ? (H)
Minoxidil ? (H)
Octamoxin (H)
Orsudan ? (H)
Phenazone ? ? (H)
Pheniprazine (H)
Plasmocid (H)
Quinine (H)
Solvent sniffing (H)
Sulfonamides ? ? (H)
Thallium (H)
Thioridazine ? (H)
Trichloroethylene decomp. (H)
Triethyl tin (H)
Tryparsamide (H)
Vincristine (H)

Optic Neuropathy, from systemic substances, in animals (A) and humans (H), *see **Introduction**, page 22, and see:*

Acetarsone (H)
Acetylarsan (H)
Acrylamide (A)
Amyl acetate ? ? (H)
Antirabies vaccine (H)
Arsacetin (H)
Arsanilic acid (A)(H)
Aspidium (H)
Bee sting (H)
Benzene ? ? (H)
Botulism (H)
Bromisoval ? (H)
Broxyquinoline ? (H)
Caramiphen ? (H)
Carbon disulfide (H)
Carbon monoxide ? (H)

Carbon tetrachloride ? (H)
Carbromal ? (H)
Cassava (H)
Chloramphenicol (H)
Chlorpropamide ? (H)
Cisplatin (A)(H?)
Clioquinol (A)(H)
Clomiphene ?(H)
Contraceptive hormones ?(H)
Cyanide (A)(H??)
Cyanoacetic acid (A)
DDT ?(H)
Deferoxamine (H)
Dichloroacetylene ??(H)
Dinitrobenzene (H)
Dinitrochlorobenzene (H)
Dinitrotoluene (H)
Disulfiram (H)
Ethambutol (A)(H)
Ethchlorvynol (H)
Ethionine ??(H)
Ethylene glycol (H)
Filicin (A)
Fluoride ??(H)
Fusidic acid ? ? (H)
G 1047 ??(H)
Glutamate (A)
Helichrysum (A)
Hexachlorophene (H)
Iminodipropionitrile (A)
Indarsol (A)
Iodoform (H)
Isoniazid (H)
Lead (A)(H)
Linamarin ?(H)
Mepacrine ??(H)
Mercuric chloride ?(H)
Methanol (H)
Methyl bromide ?(H)
Minoxidil ?(H)
Octamoxin (H)
Orsudan ?(H)
Penicillamine (H)
Perhexiline maleate (H)
Phenazone ??(H)
m-Phenylenediamine ?(H)
p-Phenylenediamine ?(H)
Phosphorus (H)
Plasmocid (H)
Snake venoms ?(H)
Sodium azide (A)
Streptomycin (H)
Stypandra imbricata (A)
Sulfonamides (H)
Tellurium (A)
Tetraethyl lead ?(H)
Thallium (H)
Thiamphenicol ?(H)
Tiliquinol ?(H)
Tobacco smoking ?(H)
Tolbutamide (H)
Trichloroethylene decomp. (H)
Triethyl tin (A)
Trinitrobenzene ?(H)
Trinitrotoluene (H)
Tryparsamide (H)
Vincristine (H)

Opticrom collyrium *see* Cromolyn sodium

Tridihexethyl   *see* Anticholinergic drugs
Tridione   *see* Trimethadione, *page* 951
Triethanolamine   *see page* 944
Triethanolamine lauryl sulfate   *see page* 871
*1,1,3-Triethoxybutane rated 3 on rabbit eyes.[228]
*1,1,3-Triethoxyhexane rated 2 on rabbit eyes.[228]
*1,3,3-Triethoxypropane rated 8 on rabbit eyes.[225]
*1,3,3-Triethoxy-1-propene rated 5 on rabbit eyes.[225]
Triethylamine   *see page* 944
Triethylenediamine   *see page* 944
Triethylene glycol   *see page* 945
*Triethyleneglycol dichloride rated 4 on rabbit eyes.[27]
*Triethyleneglycol monobutyl ether rated 5 on rabbit eyes.[228]
*Triethyleneglycol monomethyl ether rated 1 on rabbit eyes.[228]
Triethylenemelamine   *see* Tretamine, *page* 931
*Triethylenetetramine rated 5 on rabbit eyes.[224]
Triethylenethiophosphoramide   *see* Thiotepa, *page* 910
*Tri(2-ethylhexyl)phosphate rated 1 on rabbit eyes.[27]
Triethyl lead   *see under* Tetraethyl lead, *page* 891
Triethyl tin   *see page* 945
Triethyltrithiophosphite   *see page* 948
Trifluoperazine   *see page* 948
dl-(p-Trifluoromethylphenyl)isopropylamine   *see page* 949
Trifluorothymidine   *see page* 950
Trifluorotrichloroethane   *see page* 942
Trifluperidol   *see page* 950
Trifluridine   *see page* 950
Trihexyphenidyl   *see page* 950
Triiodothyronine *in 2nd edition*
*Tri-isobutenylsuccinic anhydride rated 7 on rabbit eyes.[228]
*Tri-isooctylamine rated 1 on rabbit eyes.[228]
*Tri-isooctyl phosphine rated 1 on rabbit eyes.[228]
*Tri-isopropanolamine rated 6 on rabbit eyes.[27,222]
*Tri-isopropyl phenyl phosphate rated 1 on rabbit eyes.[27]
Trilafon   *see* Perphenazine, *page* 712
Trilene   *see* Trichloroethylene
Trimethadione   *see page* 951
*1,1,3-Trimethoxybutane rated 2 on rabbit eyes.[226]
*Tri-(2-methoxyethanol)phosphate rated 1 on rabbit eyes.[288]
3,4,5-Trimethoxyphenethylamine   *see* Mescaline, *page* 588
Trimethoxysilane   *see* Methyl silicate, *page* 628
*Trimethyl adipic acid rated 8 on rabbit eyes.[27]
Trimethylamine   *see page* 952
2,4,6-Trimethylaniline   *see* Mesidine, *page* 588
*Trimethyl-e-caprolactone rated 5 on rabbit eyes.[228]
*3,3,5-Trimethylcyclohexancarboxaldehyde rated 2 on rabbit eyes.[226]
3,3,5-Trimethylcyclohexanol-1   *see page* 952
*2,6,8-Trimethylnonanol-4 rated 1 on rabbit eyes.[226]
*Trimethylnonanone rated 1 on rabbit eyes.[21,27]
*Trimethyl phosphate rated 2 on rabbit eyes.[228]
Trimethyl psoralen   *see* Trioxsalen, *page* 955
Trimethyl tin   *see page* 952
Trimethyltrithiophosphite   *see page* 948
Trimethyl vinyl ammonium hydroxide   *see* Neurine, *page* 660
Trimipramine   *see page* 952
Trinitrobenzene   *see page* 953
Trinitrobenzol   *see* Trinitrobenzene
Trinitrophenol   *see* Picric acid, *page* 737
Trinitrotoluene   *see page* 953
Trinitrotoluol   *see* Trinitrotoluene
Tri-ortho-cresl phosphate   *see* Tricresyl phosphate
Trioxsalen   *see page* 955

Trioxysalen   *see* Trioxsalen
Triparanol   *see page* 955
Tripelennamine   *see page* 957
Triperidol   *see* Trifluperidol, *page* 950
Triphenyl phosphate   *see under* Tricresyl phosphate
*Triphenylphosphine rated 3 on rabbit eyes.[288]
Triphenyl tin hydroxide   *see page* 957
Triptil   *see* Protriptyline, *page* 773
*Tripropylamine rated 1 on rabbit eyes.[228]
TRIS   *see* Tromethamine, *page* 957
*N,N',N''-Tris(dimethylaminopropyl)hexahydrotriazene (85% aqueous) rated 7 on rabbit eyes.[288]
*1,2-Tris(dimethylaminosilyl) ethane rated 2 on rabbit eyes.[288]
*Tris(dipropylene glycol) phosphine rated 1 on rabbit eyes.[228]
*Tris(dipropylene glycol) phosphonate rated 1 on rabbit eyes.[228]
Tris(hydroxymethyl) aminomethane   *see* Tromethamine
Trisodium phosphate   *see page* 957
Trisoralen   *see* Trioxsalen, *page* 955
*Tris(2,4-pentanedionato)chromium rated 2 on rabbit eyes.[288]
*Tris(tridecyl)amine rated 1 on rabbit eyes.[288]
*Tris(triethylene glycol) phosphate rated 1 on rabbit eyes.[288]
*3,4,5-Trithiatricyclo(5.2.1.0$^{2.6}$)decane rated 2 on rabbit eyes.[288]
Tritolyl phosphate   *see* Tricresyl phosphate, *page* 942
Triton   *see* pHisoHex, *page* 732
Triton W30   *see page* 871
Triton X30   *see page* 871
Triton X100   *see pages* 873, 874; *also see* Millipore filters, *page* 630
Triton X155   *see page* 873
Tritox   *see* Trichloroacetonitrile, *page* 934
Trolone   *see* Sulthiame
Tromantadine   *see page* 957
Trometamol   *see* Tromethamine, *page* 957
Tromethamine   *see page* 957
Tropicamide   *see page* 958
Tropilidene   *see* 1,3,5-Cycloheptatriene, *page* 295
T-Stoff   *see* Bromo-xylene, *page* 159
Trypan blue   *see pages* 382, 958
Tryparsamide   *see pages* 118, 960
Trypsin   *see page* 960
Tryptar   *see* Trypsin, *page* 960
Tubocurarine   *see* Curare, *page* 285
Tungstate   *see* Acids, *page* 46
Tungsten metal   *see page* 961
Tungstic acid   *see page* 961
Turpentine   *see page* 961
Tween 20, 40, 60, or 65   *see pages* 872, 873
Tween 80   *see* Polysorbate 80, *pages* 753, 872
Tyramine *in 2nd edition*
Tyrosine   *see page* 962
UCC-974   *see* 3,5-Dimethyltetrahydro-1,3,5,2H-thiadiazine-2-thione, *page* 355
UDMH   *see* Dimethylhydrazine, *page* 349
Ultrawet 30DS   *see page* 871
Ultrawet 60L   *see page* 871
*Undecanol rated 3 on rabbit eyes.[27,222]
Undecylenic acid   *see page* 964
Uranium compounds   *see page* 965
Urea   *see page* 965
Urea-formaldehyde resins   *see page* 966
Urethane   *see page* 966

BIBLIOGRAPHY OF NUMBERED REFERENCES

These are sources of information that have been referred to three or more times at various places in the text. They have been identified by number superscripts in the text, to distinguish them from the references given at the end of each of the numerous synopses, which are identified in the text by superscript letters. Numbered references that are new in this *third edition* start with number 270.

1. (No number "1" reference has been used, to avoid confusion with letter "l" references within the text.)

2. Ahuja OP, Nema HV: Experimental corneal vascularization and its management. AM J OPHTHALMOL 62:707–710, 1966.

3. Alberth B: *Surgical Treatment of Caustic Injuries of the Eye.* Budapest, Akademiai Kaido, 1968.

4. AMA Council on Drugs: *New Drugs,* American Medical Association, Chicago, 1965 and 1967.

5. AMA Council on Pharmacy and Chemistry: Outlines of information on pesticides. J AM MED ASSOC 157:237–241, 1955.

6. Ancill RJ, Richens ER, Norton DA: The reactions of organic mercurials on the cornea. TRANS OPHTHALMOL SOC UK 89:863–866, 1969.

7. Barkman R, Germanis M, Karpe G, Malmborg AS: Preservatives in drops. ACTA OPHTHALMOL 47:461–475, 1969.

8. Barnett KC, Noel PRB: The eye in general toxicity studies. In Piggott PV (Ed.): *Evaluation of Drug Effects on the Eye.* London, F.J. Parsons, Ltd., 1968.

9. Barsa JA, Newton JS, Saunders J: Lenticular and corneal opacities during phenothiazine therapy. J AM MED ASSOC 193:98–100, 1965.

10. Berggren L: Effect of composition of medium and of metabolic inhibitors on secretion *in vitro* by ciliary processes of the rabbit eye. INVEST OPHTHALMOL 4:83–90, 1965.

11. Berggren L: Comparison of ocular effects of pilocarpine, pilocarpidine, and pilosine. ACTA OPHTHALMOL 45:238–246, 1967.

12. Bernat R, Bombicki K: Changes in the concentration of glutathione, ascorbic acid, and sulfhydryl amino acids in experimental cataracts. ACTA PHYSIOL POL 19:205–215, 1968. (CHEM ABSTR 69:9445, 1968.)

13. Bidstrup PL: *Toxicity of Mercury and Its Compounds.* New York, Elsevier, 1964.

14. Boyer HK, Suran AA, Hogan MJ, McEwen WK: Studies on simulated vitreous hemorrhages. ARCH OPHTHALMOL 59:333–336, 1958.

15. Bozac E, Brief G, Margesco F, Munteanu H: Heparin in the treatment of ocular burns by alkalies. ANN OCULIST (PARIS) 200:693–700, 1967. (French)

16. Brancato R, Campana G: Comparative research on the action of vasodilators and vasoconstrictors on ocular burns by lime in the rabbit. ANN OTTALMOL CLIN OCUL 91:1020–1030, 1965. (Italian)

17. Brancato R, Campana G: Comparative histology in experimental ocular burns by lime treated with vasodilators and vasoconstrictors. ANN OTTALMOL CLIN OCUL 91:1273–1286, 1965. (Italian)

18. Brown SI, Akiya S, Weller CA: Prevention of the ulcers of the alkali-burned cornea. ARCH OPHTHALMOL 82:95–97, 1969.

19. Brown SI, Wassermann HE, Dunn MW: Alkali burns of the cornea. ARCH OPHTHALMOL 82:91–94, 1969.

20. Brown SI, Weller CA, Wassermann HE: Collagenolytic activity of alkali burned corneas. ARCH OPHTHALMOL 81:370–373, 1969.

21. Browning E: *Toxicity and Metabolism of Industrial Solvents.* Amsterdam, Elsevier, 1965.

22. Bucci MG: On the action of xanthopterin. BOLL OCULIST 42:638–653, 1963. (Italian)

23. Buehler EV, Newmann EA: A comparison of eye irritation in monkeys and rabbits. TOXICOL APPL PHARMACOL 6:701–710, 1964.

24. Bumke O, Krapf E: Vergiftungen durch anorganische und organische sowie durch pflanzliche, tierische und bakterielle Gift. Bumke O, Foerster O (Eds.): *Handbuche der Neurologie.* Berlin, Springer, 1936, vol 13, pp694–827.

25. Caldeira JAF: Influence of tranquilizers on intraocular pressure of rabbit. ARQ BRASIL OFTALMOL 28:79–148, 1965. (Portuguese)

26. Carlson VR: Individual pupillary reactions to certain centrally acting drugs in man. J PHARMACOL EXP THER 121:501–506, 1957.

27.* Carpenter CP, Smyth HF: Chemical burns of the rabbit cornea. AM J OPHTHAL-MOL 29:1363–1372, 1946.

28. Carroll FD: Toxic amblyopia. TRANS AM ACAD OPHTHALMOL OTO-LARYNG 60:74–82, 1956.

29. Carter RO, Griffith JF: Assessment of eye hazard. TOXICOL APPL PHARMA-COL 7:70–73, 1965.

30. Castren JA, Mustakallio A: Conservative treatment of experimental chemical burns of the eye. ANN MED EXP MED FENN 42:4–6, 1964.

31. Chandler PA, Grant WM: *Lectures on Glaucoma.* Philadelphia, Lea & Febiger, 1965.

32. Community Air Quality Guides: Aldehydes. AM IND HYG J 29:505–512, 1968.

33. Coutela C: *L'Oeil et les Maladies Professionnelles.* Paris, Masson, 1939.

34. Cramer E: Die Veratzungen. In Schieck F, Bruckner A (Eds.): *Kurzes Handbuch der Ophthalmologie.* Berlin, Springer, 1930, vol 4, pp525–543.

35. D'Asaro Biondo M: Lesions of the eye from fossil coal tar and its derivatives. RASS ITAL OTTALMOL 2:259–33, 1933. (Italian)

36. Davis EF, Tuma BL, Lee LL: Fungicides. In Dittmer DS (Ed.): *Handbook of Toxicology.* Philadelphia, Saunders, 1959, vol 5.

37. Deichmann WB, Gerarde HW: *Toxicology of Drugs and Chemicals.* New York, Academic, 1969.

38. Deichmann WB, Keplinger ML, Lanier GE: Acute effects of nitroolefins upon experimental animals. ARCH IND HEALTH 18:312–319, 1958.

39. Deichmann WB, MacDonald WE, Lampe KF, Dressler I, Anderson WAD: Nitro-olefins as potential carcinogens in air pollution. IND MED SURG 34:800–807, 1965.

40. Dernehl CU: Health hazards associated with polyurethane foams. J OCCUP MED 8:59–62, 1966.

41. deSchweinitz GE: *Toxic Amblyopias.* Philadelphia, Lea Brothers, 1896.

42. Dixon M, Needham DM: Biochemical research on chemical warfare agents. NATURE 158:432–438, 1946.

43. Dohlman CH, Slansky HH, Laibson PR, Gnadinger MC, Rose J: Artificial corneal epithelium in acute alkali burns. ANN OPHTHALMOL 1:357–361, 1969.

---

*See page 1008 for method of testing and rating on rabbit eyes.

44. Doughman DJ, Watzke RC: Experimental retinal detachment following intravitreal injection of sulfate polymers. AM J OPHTHALMOL 64:893–902, 1967.

45. Draize JH, Woodward G, Calvery HO: Methods for the study of irritation and toxicity of substances applied topically to skin and mucous membrane. J PHARMACOL EXP THER 82:377–390, 1944.

46. Duke-Elder S: *Chemical Injuries. Textbook of Ophthalmology.* St. Louis, Mosby, 1954, vol 6, ch 71.

47. Duncalf D, Rhodes Jr DH: *Anesthesia in Clinical Ophthalmology.* Baltimore, Williams & Wilkins, 1963.

48. Eerden AAJJ: Changes in corneal epithelium due to local anesthetics. OPHTHALMOLOGICA 143:154–162, 1962.

49. Efron DH (Ed.): *Ethnopharmacologic Search for Psychoactive Drugs.* Symposium, San Francisco, Jan 28–30, 1967. US Public Health Publication No. 1645.

50. Egorov YL, Andrianov LA: Toxicity of heptyl, nonyl, and decyl alcohols. UCH ZAP MOSK NAUCHN–ISSLED INST GIGIENY 1961, 47–49. (CHEM ABSTR 60:12576, 1964.)

51. Elkins HB: *The Chemistry of Industrial Toxicology,* 2nd ed. New York, Wiley, 1958.

52. Ellis PP, Smith DL: *Handbook of Ocular Therapeutics and Pharmacology,* 2nd ed. St. Louis, Mosby, 1966.

53. Estable JJ: The ocular effect of several irritant drugs applied directly to the conjunctiva. AM J OPHTHALMOL 31:837–844, 1948.

54. Ey RC, Hughes WF, Bloome MA, Tallman CB: Prevention of corneal vascularization. AM J OPHTHALMOL 66:1118–1131, 1968.

55. Fairchild EJ, Stokinger HE: Toxicologic studies on organic sulfur compounds. AM IND HYG ASSOC J 19:171–189, 1958.

56. Fairhall LT: *Industrial Toxicology,* 2nd ed. Baltimore, Williams & Wilkins, 1957.

57. Feller K, Graupner K: On the suitability of THAM for the treatment of experimental acid burns of rabbit eyes. MED PHARMACOL EXP (Basel) 14:125–126, 1966. (German)

58. Feller K, Graupner K: The hydrogen ion concentration in the anterior chamber of the rabbit eye after experimental burning with calcium hydroxide and its modification by various buffer substances. GRAEFES ARCH OPHTHALMOL 173:71–77, 1967. (German)

59. Floyd EP, Stokinger HE: Toxicity studies of certain organic peroxides and hydroperoxides. AM IND HYG ASSOC J 19:205–212, 1958.

60. Flury F, Zangger H: *Lehrbuch der Toxikologie fur Studium und Praxis.* Berlin, Springer, 1928.

61. Flury F, Zernik K: *Schadliche Gase.* Berlin, Springer, 1931.

62. Fraunfelder FT, Burns RP: Effect of lid closure in drug-induced experimental cataracts. ARCH OPHTHALMOL 76:599–601, 1966.

63. Friemann W, Overhoff W: Keratitis as an occupational illness in oil-herring fishing. KLIN MONATSBL AUGENHEILKD 128:425–438, 1956. (German)

64. Garner RJ: *Veterinary Toxicology.* Baltimore, Williams & Wilkins, 1961.

65. Geeraets WJ, Aaron SD, Guerry D III: Alkali burns of the cornea and neutral ammonium tartrate. VIRGINIA MED MONTHLY 91:493–496, 1964.

66. Gettler AO: The significance of some toxicologic procedures in the medicolegal autopsy. AM J CLIN PATHOL 13:169, 1943.

67. Giesecke H, Lohse H: Experimental studies with EDTA on the rabbit eye after lime-burn. MEDICAMENTUM (BERLIN) 9:112–114, 1968. ZENTRALBL GES OPHTHALMOL 100:443, 1968. (German)

68. Gilson M: The effects of various sympathomimetic amines (Adrianol, Effortil, isopropylnoradrianol) on ocular tension. BULL SOC BELGE OPHTALMOL 128:229–236, 1961.

69. Glasmacher H: Experimental investigations on lime burn of the cornea and its treatment. GRAEFES ARCH OPHTHALMOL 162:493–500, 1960. (German)

70. Gleason MN, Gosselin RE, Hodge HC, Smith RP: *Clinical Toxicology of Commercial Products* 3rd ed. Baltimore, Williams & Wilkins, 1969.

71. Gnadinger MC, Itoi M, Slansky HH, Dohlmann CH: The role of collagenase in the alkali-burned cornea. AM J OPHTHALMOL 68:478–483, 1969.

72. Goldblatt MW: The investigation of toxic hazards. BR J IND MED 1:20–30, 1944.

73. Goldblatt MW: Vesication and some vesicants. BR J IND MED 2:183–201, 1945.

74. Golubev AA: Changes in the diameter of the rabbit pupil under the action of some industrial poisons producing irritation. GIG TR PROF ZABOL 13:58–59, 1969.

75. Gordon S, Balazs T: Cataractogenicity of various drugs in rats. TOXICOL APPL PHARMACOL 10:393, abstr #41, 1967.

76. Gorska W, Zukowski L: The influence of sodium versenate on eye burns produced by calcium hydroxide. KLIN OCZNA 39:25–29, 1968.

77. Gottstein A:, Schlossmann A, Teleky L, (Eds.): *Handbuch der sozialen Hygiene und Gesundheitsfursorge. Gewerbehygiene und Gewerbekrankheiten.* Berlin, Springer, 1926, vol 2.

78. Graeflin: Experimental investigations concerning the injurious effect of aniline dyes in powder form on the mucous membrane of rabbit eyes. Z AUGENHEILKD 10:193, 1903. (German)

79. Grant WM: Ocular injury due to sulfur dioxide. II. Experimental study and comparison with ocular effects of freezing. ARCH OPHTHALMOL 38:762–774, 1947.

80. Grant WM: A study of the actions of quaternary ammonium compounds on the eye. TRANS AM OPHTHALMOL SOC 54:417–446, 1956.

81. Grant WM: *Toxicology of the Eye,* 1st ed. Springfield, Thomas, 1962.

82. Grant WM: Experimental aqueous perfusion in enucleated human eyes. ARCH OPHTHALMOL 69:783–801, 1963.

83. Grant WM: Systemic drugs and adverse influences on ocular pressure. In Leopold I (Ed.): *Ocular Therapy, Complications and Management.* St. Louis, Mosby, 1968, vol 3, pp57–73.

84. Grant WM: Ocular complications of drugs. J AM MED ASSOC 207:2089–2091, 1969.

85. Grant WM: Action of drugs on movement of ocular fluids. ANN REV PHARMACOL 9:85–94, 1969.

86. Grant WM: Drug induced disturbances of vision that may affect driving. In Keeney AH, (Ed.): *Proceedings of the Eleventh Annual Meeting of the American Association for Automotive Medicine.* Springfield, Thomas, 1970, pp192–200.

87. Grant WM: Drug intoxications and chemical injuries of the eye. In Sorsby A (Ed.): *Modern Ophthalmology. Systemic Aspects.* London, Butterworths, 1963, vol 2.

88. Grant WM, Kern HL: Corneal bonding of rare earths and other cations. In Kyker GC, Anderson EB (Eds.): *Conference on Rare Earths in Biochemical and Medical Research.* Oak Ridge Institute of Nuclear Studies, 1955. (ORINS 12:346–355, 1956.)

89. Grant WM, Kern HL: Action of alkalies on the corneal stroma. ARCH OPHTHALMOL 54:931–939, 1955.

90. Grant WM, Kern HL: Cations and the cornea. AM J OPHTHALMOL 42:167–181, 1956.

91. Grant WM, Loeb DR: Effect of locally applied antihistamine drugs on normal eyes. ARCH OPHTHALMOL 39:553–554, 1948.

92. Graupner OK, Hausmann CM: The alteration of the pH in the anterior chamber of the rabbits eye burned with the smallest volumes of concentrated acid and base. GRAEFES ARCH OPHTHALMOL 176:48–53, 1968.

93. Graupner OK, Hausmann CM: The alteration of the pH in the anterior chamber of the rabbit eye after burning with the smallest volumes of acid and alkali in ordinarily used concentrations. GRAEFES ARCH OPHTHALMOL 180:60–71, 1970. (German)

94. Grignolo A: Rhodopsin cycle and fine structure of rabbit retina in experimental degeneration induced by retinotoxic agents. EXP EYE RES 8:254, 1969.

95. Grutzner P: Acquired color vision defects secondary to retinal drug toxicity. OPHTHALMOLOGICA ADDIT AD 158:592–604, 1969.

96. Guillery H: On the significance of corneal mucoid for the development of the primary burn opacity. ARCH AUGENHEILKD 66:252–271, 1910. (German)

97. Haley TJ, Komesu N, Flesher Am, Mavis L, Cawthorne J, Upham HC: Pharmacology and toxicology of terbium, thulium, and ytterbium chlorides. TOXICOL APPL PHARMACOL 5:427–436, 1963.

98. Haley TJ, Koste L, Komesu N, Efros M, Upham HC: Pharmacology and toxicology of dysprosium, holmium and erbium chlorides. TOXICOL APPL PHARMACOL 8:37–43, 1966.

99. Hansson HA: Selective effects of metabolic inhibitors on retinal cultures. EXP EYE RES 5:335–354, 1966.

100. Hapke HJ: Effects of drugs on the eye. DTSCH TIERARZTL WOCHENSCHR 74:312–313, 368–372, 1967. (German)

101. Harley RD: An experimental study on the evaluation of Hydrosulphosol in the treatment of ocular injuries due to chemical burns. AM J OPHTHALMOL 35:1653–1675, 1952.

102. Harris LS: Cycloplegic-induced intraocular pressure elevations. ARCH OPHTHALMOL 79:242–246, 1968.

103. Havener HA: *Ocular Pharmacology.* St. Louis, Mosby, 1966.

104. Heinc A: The burned eye and keratoplasty. KLIN MONATSBL AUGENHEILKD (Suppl 52):1–87, 1969. (German)

105. Heiss W-D, Heilig P, Hoyer J: The effect of psychopharmaceuticals on the activity of retinal neurons. VISION RES 9:493–506, 1969. (German)

106. Heiss W-D, Hoyer J, Heilig P: The effect of psychopharmaceuticals on the visual evoked potentials of the cat. VISION RES 9:507–513, 1969. (German)

107. Herrmann H, Hickman FH: The adhesion of epithelium to stroma in the cornea. BULL JOHNS HOPKINS HOSP 82:182–207, 1948.

108. Herrmann H, Moses G, Friedenwald JS: Influence of Pontocaine hydrochloride and chlorobutanol on respiration and glycolysis of cornea. ARCH OPHTHALMOL 28:652–660, 1942.

109. Herxheimer A: A comparison of some atropine-like drugs in man, with particular reference to their end-organ specificity. BR J PHARMACOL 13:184–192, 1958.

110. Heuss JM, Glasson WA: Hydrocarbon reactivity and eye irritation. ENVIRON SCI TECHNOL 2:1109–1116, 1968.

111. Heydenreich A: Corticosteroids in burns of the eye. KLIN MONATSBL AUGENHEILKD 141:726–736, 1962. (German)

112. Heydenreich A: Secondary glaucoma in association with burns. KLIN MONATSBL AUGENHEILKD 146:382–390, 1965. (German)

113. Heydenreich A: Regeneration of the cornea and intraocular pressure. KLIN MONATSBL AUGENHEILKD 148:500–509, 1966. (German)

114. Hine CH, Hogan MJ, McEwen WK, Meyers FH, Mettier SR, Boyer HK: Eye irritation from air pollution. J AIR POLLUT CONTR ASSOC 10:17–20, 1960.

115. Hine CH, Kodama JK, Wellington JS, Dunlop MK, Anderson HH: The toxicology of glycidol and some glycidyl ethers. ARCH IND HEALTH 14:250–264, 1956.

116. Hine CH, Leob P, Anderson HH: Comparative toxicity of 5 glycerol ethers. ARCH IND HYG 2:574, 1950.

117. Hirano J: Experimental study of the effect of subconjunctival oxygen on the corneal vascularization. JPN J CLIN OPHTHALMOL 23:811–816, 1969.

118. Hoffer A, Osmond H: *The Hallucinogens.* New York, Academic, 1967.

119. Hommer K: The effects of quinine, chloroquine, iodoacetate and chlorodiazepoxide on the ERG of the isolated rabbit retina. GRAEFES ARCH OPHTHALMOL 175:111–120, 1968.

120. Honegger H: The effect of externally applied medications on the corneal endothelium. GRAEFES ARCH OPHTHALMOL 168:594–598, 1965. (German)

121. Honegger H, Genee E: Disturbances of accommodation in association with treatment with tuberculostatics. KLIN MONATSBL AUGENHEILKD 155:371–380, 1969. (German)

122. Houle RE, Grant WM: Alcohol, vasopressin, and intraocular pressure. INVEST OPHTHALMOL 6:145–154, 1967.

123. Hughes WF Jr: The tolerance of rabbit cornea for various chemical substances. Appendix I. BULL JOHNS HOPKINS HOSP 82:338–349, 1948.

124. Hunter D: Industrial toxicology. QUART J MED 12:185–258, 1943.

125. Igersheimer J: On the effect of Atoxyl on the eye. GRAEFES ARCH OPHTHALMOL 71:379–428, 1909. (German)

126. Ikemoto F, Iwata S, Narita F: Effects of cataractogenic compounds, fatty acids and related compounds on cation transport of the incubated lens. OSAKA CITY MED J 17:1–18, 1971.

127. Imre G, Bogi J: New possibility of prevention of corneal vascularization. ACTA MED ACAD SCI HUNG 22:155–160, 1966. (EXCERPTA MED (SECT.12) 21:642, 1967.)

128. Itoi M, Gnadinger MC, Slansky HH, Dohlman CH: Prevention of ulcers of the corneal stroma thanks to the use of a calcium salt of EDTA. ARCH OPHTALMOL (PARIS) 29:389–392, 1969. (French)

129. Jaensch PA: *Augenschadigungen in Industrie und Gewerbe.* Stuttgart. Wissenschaftliche Verlagsgesellschaft M.B.H., 1958.

130. Jancso N, Jancso-Gabor A, Szolcsanyi J: The role of sensory nerve endings in neurogenic inflammation induced in human skin and in the eye and paw of the rat. BR J PHARMACOL 33:32–41, 1968

131. Jess A: The dangers of chemotherapy for the eye, especially concerning a component of quinine and its derivatives seriously injurious to the organ of sight. GRAEFES ARCH OPHTHALMOL 104:48–74, 1921. (German)

132. Kalinowski SZ, Lloyd TW, Moyes EN: Complications in the chemotherapy of tuberculosis. AM REV RESP DIS 83:359–371, 1961.

133. Karli P: Spontaneous and experimental retinal degenerations in animals. FORTSCHR AUGENHEILKD 14:51–89, 1963. (French)

134. Kern HL, Grant WM: Interaction of acidic and basic dyes and beef corneal stroma. J HISTOCHEM CYTOCHEM 9:380–384, 1961.

135. Kleifeld O, Hockwin O: The effect of dinitrophenol (DNP), ethylenediamine tetraacetic acid, diamox and butazolidin on the metabolism of the lens. GRAEFES ARCH OPHTHALMOL 158:54–63, 1956.

136. Knave B: Electroretinography in eyes with retained intraocular metallic foreign bodies. ACTA OPHTHALMOL (Suppl 100), 1969.

137. Kornblueth W, Ben-Shlomo E: Glucose utilization of the retina. ARCH OPHTHALMOL 55:813–817, 1956.

138. Kotsuka N: Experimental studies on lamellar keratoplasty for alkali burns. ACTA SOC OPHTHALMOL JPN 71:454–462, 1967.

139. Kozlova LP: Effects of industrial hazards on the ophthalmotone. VESTN OFTALMOL 79:57–60, 1966.

140. Krejci L, Obenberger J, Kloucek F, Lehky B, Jansa J: Experiences with a new neutralizing agent, DETA, in acid burns of the eye. CESK OFTALMOL 20:314–320, 1964. (ZENTRALBL GES OPHTHALMOL 95:84, 1965.)

141. Kuwahara: Experimental and clinical observations on the action of aniline dyes on the eye. ARCH AUGENHEILKD 49:157, 1903. (German)

142. Lampe KF, Fagerstrom R: *Plant Toxicity and Dermatitis.* Baltimore, Williams & Wilkins, 1968.

143. Lampe KF, Mende TJ, Deichmann WB, Eye MG, Palmer LF: Evaluation of conjugated nitro-olefins as eye irritants in air pollution. IND MED 27:375–377, 1958.

144. Laroche J: Modification of color vision by certain medications. ANN OCULIST 200:275–286, 1967.

145. Lavergne G: Experimental and clinical studies of the influence of triethylene-thiophosphoramide on vascularization of the cornea. BULL SOC FRANC OPHTALMOL 80:146–155, 1967. (French)

146. Lavergne G, Colmant IA: Comparative study of the action of thiotepa and triamcinolone on corneal vascularization in rabbits. BR J OPHTHALMOL 48:416–422, 1964.

147. Lavergne G, Colmant IA: Inhibition of corneal vascularization by triethylene-thiophosphoramide. BULL SOC BELGE OPHTALMOL 133–135:498–504, 1963. (French)

148. Lazenby GW, Reed JW, Grant WM: Short-term test of anticholinergic medication in open-angle glaucoma. ARCH OPHTHALMOL 80:443–448, 1968. Anticholinergic medication in open-angle glaucoma, long-term tests. ARCH OPHTHALMOL 84:719–723, 1970.

149. Leach EH, Lloyd JPF: Experimental ocular hypertension in animals. TRANS OPHTHALMOL SOC UK 76:453–459, 1956.

150. Leber T: *Die Entstehung der Entzundung und die Wirkung der entzundung-erregenden Schadlichkeiten: Nach vorzugsweise am Auge angestellten Untersuchungen.* Leipzig, Wilhelm Englemann, 1891.

151. Lehmann and Flury: *Toxicology and Hygiene of Industrial Solvents.* King and Smyth Translation. Baltimore, Williams & Wilkins, 1943.

152. Leopold IH, Comroe JH Jr: Effect of intramuscular administration of morphine, atropine, scopolamine and neostigmine on the human eye. ARCH OPHTHALMOL 40:285–290, 1948.

153. Lewin L, Guillery H: *Die Wirkungen von Arzneimitteln und Giften auf das Auge*, 2nd ed. Berlin, August Hirschwald, 1913.

154. Lewis E: Toxicology of organometallic compounds. J OCCUP MED 2:183–187; 225–228, 1960.

155. Lohs K: *Synthetische Gifte*. Berlin, Deutscher Militarverlag, 1967.

156. Lohse H, Giesecke H: Animal experimental investigation with EDTA and its therapeutic use in lime burns of the eye. DTSCH GESUNDHEITSWES 23:420–423, 1968. (German) (ZENTRALBL GES OPHTHALMOL 100:345, 1968.)

157. Lucas DR, Newhouse JP: Action of metabolic poisons on the isolated retina. BR J OPHTHALMOL 43:147–158, 1959.

158. Lutzow Av, Hommer K: Influences of some drugs on the ERG of the isolated rabbit retina. OPHTHALMOLOGICA ADDIT AD 158:647–652, 1969.

159. Mach DI, Isaacs S, Greenberg: Influence of opiates and antipyretics on vision. PROC SOC EXP BIOL MED 15:46–48, 1917–1918.

160. Mackworth JF: The inhibition of thiol enzymes by lachrymators. BIOCHEM J 42:82–90, 1948.

161. Mann I, Pirie A, Pullinger BD: An experimental and clinical study of the reaction of the anterior segment of the eye to chemical injury, with special reference to chemical warfare agents. BR J OPHTHALMOL (MONOGR SUPPL XIII) 1–171, 1948.

162. Martin G, Draize JH, Kelley EA: Local anesthesia in eye mucosa produced by surfactants in cosmetic formulations. PROC SCI SECT TOILET GOODS ASSOC 37:2–3, 1962. (CHEM ABSTR 57:7560, 1962.)

163. Martin WR: Opioid antagonists. PHARMACOL REV 19:463–506, 1967.

164. Mastromatteo E: Heterocyclic amine exposure with urethane foams. J OCCUP MED 7:507, 1965.

165. McLaughlin RS: Chemical burns of the human cornea. AM J OPHTHALMOL 29:1355–1362, 1946.

166. Meier-Ruge W, Kalberer F, Cerletti A: Microhistoautoradiographic investigations of the distribution of tritium-labeled phenothiazine derivatives in the eye. EXPERIENTIA 22:153–155, 1966. (CHEM ABSTR 64:16466, 1966.)

167. Meier-Ruge W, Werthemann A: *Medikamentose Retinopathie*. Stuttgart, George Thieme Verlag, 1967.

168. Meier-Ruge W: The pathophysiological morphology of the pigment epithelium and its importance for retinal structures and functions. MOD PROBL OPHTHALMOL 8:32–48, 1968.

169. Meier-Ruge W: Drug induced retinopathy. OPHTHALMOLOGICA ADDIT AD 158:561–573, 1969.

170. Mellerio H, Weale RA: Hazy vision in amine plant operatives. BR J IND MED 23:153–154, 1966.

171. *The Merck Index of Chemicals and Drugs*, 7th and 8th eds. Rahway, N.Y., Merck, 1960, 1968.

172. Mettier SR Jr, Boyer HK, Hine CH, McEwen WK: Study of the effects of air pollutants on the eye. ARCH IND HEALTH 21:1–6, 1960.

173. Mettier SR Jr, Boyer HK, McEwen WK, Ivanhoe F, Meyers FH, Hine CH: Effects of air pollutant mixtures on the eye. ARCH ENVIRON HEALTH 4:103–107, 1962.

174. Meyler L, Herxheimer A, (Eds.): *Side Effects of Drugs*. Baltimore, Williams & Wilkins and Excerpta Med Foundation, 1968, vol 6.

175. Miller HA: Burns of the ocular globe. BULL SOC OPHTALMOL FRANCE 4(Suppl.):1–174, 1958.

176. Minton J: *Occupational Eye Diseases and Injuries.* New York, Grune, 1949.

177. Moeschlin S: *Klinik und Therapie der Vergiftungen.* Stuttgart, George Thieme Verlag, 1964.

178. Moller J, Rosen A: Comparative studies on intramuscular and oral effective doses of some anticholinergic drugs. ACTA MED SCAND 184:201–209, 1968.

179. Nakajima A: The effect of the inhibitors of carbohydrate metabolism on the rabbit electroretinogram. OPHTHALMOLOGICA 136:99–107, 1958.

180. Nau CA, Neal J, Thornton M: C_9-C_{12} fractions obtained from petroleum distillates. An evaluation of their potential toxicity. ARCH ENVIRON HEALTH 12:382–383, 1966.

181. Negherbon WO: *Insecticides. Handbook of Toxicology.* Philadelphia, Saunders, 1959, vol 3.

182. Nelken E, Nelken D: Inhibition of corneal neovascularization by vitamin A palmitate. ISRAEL J MED SCI 1:243, 1965. (EXCERPTA MED (SECT 12):20, 1708, 1966.)

183. Nelson KW, Ege JF, Ross M, Woodman LE, Silverman L: Sensory response to certain industrial solvent vapors. J IND HYG 25:282–285, 1943.

184. Oksala A: Experimental studies on the effect of some chemical caustics on the ohmic resistance of corneal epithelium. ACTA OPHTHALMOL 38:170–177, 1960.

185. Oosterhuis JA: Treatment of calcium deposits in the cornea by irrigation and by application of EDTA. OPHTHALMOLOGICA 145:161–174, 1963.

186. Passmore JA, King JH: Vital staining of conjunctiva and cornea: Review of literature and critical study of certain dyes. ARCH OPHTHALMOL 53:568–574, 1955.

187. Passow A: On eye symptoms in association with internal use of medications acting on the parasympathetic nervous system. ARCH AUGENHEILKD 97:432–459, 1926.

188. Patty EA: *Industrial Hygiene and Toxicology.* New York, Interscience, 1949.

189. Pau H: Histologic findings in connection with a foreign body remaining in a human eye. OPHTHALMOLOGICA 157:206–222, 1969. (German)

190. Peczon JD, Grant WM: Sedatives, stimulants and intraocular pressure in glaucoma. ARCH OPHTHALMOL 72:178–188, 1964.

191. Peczon JD, Grant WM: Glaucoma, alcohol and intraocular pressure. ARCH OPHTHALMOL 73:495–501, 1965.

192. Peczon JD, Grant WM: Diuretic drugs in glaucoma. AM J OPHTHALMOL 66:680–683, 1968.

193. Peczon JD, Grant WM, Lambert B: Systemic vasodilators, intraocular pressure and chamber depth in glaucoma. AM J OPHTHALMOL 72:74–78, 1971.

194. Pentschew A: Intoxikationen. Handbuch der speziellen pathologischen Anatomie und Histologie. In Lubarsch O, Henke F, Rossle R (Eds.): *Erkrankungen des zentralen Nervensystems.* Berlin, Springer, 1958, vol 12, pp1907–2502.

195. Peters RA: *Biochemical Lesions and Lethal Systhesis.* New York, Macmillan, 1963.

196. Peterson F, Haines WS, Webster RW: *Legal Medicine and Toxicology by Many Specialists,* 2nd ed. Philadelphia, Saunders, 1923.

197. Philipszoon AJ: Drugs inhibiting motion sickness; some electronystagmographic studies of the effect of drugs upon the labyrinth. In Herxheimer A (Ed.): *Drugs and Sensory Functions.* Boston, Little, 1968, pp 175–196.

198. Philpot FJ: Factors affecting the hydration of the rabbit cornea. J PHYSIOL 128:504–510, 1955.

199. Pickrell KL, Clark EH: Tatooing of the corneal scars with insoluble pigments. PLAST RECONSTR SURG 2:44–59, 1947.

200. Pigott PV, (Ed.): *Evaluation of Drug Effects on the Eye.* London, F.J. Parsons, 1968.

201. Potts AM: The concentration of phenothiazines in the eye of experimental animals. INVEST OPHTHALMOL 1:523–530, 1962.

202. Potts AM: Uveal pigment and phenothiazine compounds. TRANS AM OPH-THALMOL SOC 60:517–551, 1962.

203. Potts AM: The reaction of uveal pigment *in vitro* with polycyclic compounds. INVEST OPHTHALMOL 3:405–416, 1964.

204. Punte C, Ballard TA, Weimer JT: Inhalation studies with chloroacetophenone, diphenylaminochloroarsine and pelargonic morpholide. I. Animal exposures. AM IND HYG ASSOC J 23:194–198, 1962.

205. Punte CL, Gutentag PJ, Owens EJ, Gongiver LE: Inhalation studies with chloroacetophenone, diphenylaminochloroarsine and pelargonic morpholide. II. Human exposures. AM IND HYG ASSOC J 23:199–202, 1962.

206. Quaranta CA, Vozza R: Comparative histological study of chorioretinal altera-tions from dithizone, sodium iodate, and sodium iodoacetate. BOLL OCULIST 38:665–682, 1959. (Italian)

207. Reading HW, Sorsby A: Retinal toxicity and tissue -SH levels. BIOCHEM PHARMACOL 15:1389–1393, 1966.

208. Richter S: Animal experimental investigations into the effect of glucocorticoids in alkali burns of the eye. KLIN MONATSBL AUGENHEILKD 143:351–355, 1963. (German)

209. Rizzo AA: Rabbit corneal irrigation as a model system for studies on the relative toxicity of bacterial products implicated in periodontal disease. The toxicity of neutralized ammonia solutions. J PERIODONT 38:491–499, 1967.

210. Rosselet E, Faggioni R: Glaucoma and psychotropic drugs. OPHTHAL-MOLOGICA ADDIT AD 158:462–468, 1969. (French)

211. Rowe VK, Spencer HC, Bass SL: Toxicological studies of certain commercial silicones and hydrolyzable silane intermediates. J IND HYG 30:332–352, 1948.

212. Russell FE: Comparative pharmacology of some animal toxins. FED PROC 26:1206–1224, 1967.

213. Sallai S, Valu L, Feher J, Podhoranyi G: Experimental decontaminating trials with intralamellar corneal injections in caustic burns. GRAEFES ARCH OPHTHALMOL 171:367–371, 1967. (German)

214. Sattler CH: Augenveranderungen bei Intoxikationen. In *Kurzes Handbuch der Ophthalmologie.* Berlin, Springer, 1932, vol 7, pp229–290.

215. Sax NI: *Dangerous Properties of Industrial Materials.* New York, Reinhold, 1957.

216. Schmid E: On the corneal disturbance of furniture polishers. KLIN MONATSBL AUGEHNEILKD 130:110–115, 1957. (German)

217. Silverman L, Schulte HF, First MW: Further studies on sensory response to certain industrial solvent vapors. J IND HYG 28:262, 1946.

218. Sim VM, Pattle RE: Effect of possible smog irritants on human subjects. J AM MED ASSOC 165:1908–1913, 1957.

219. Smart JV, Sneddon JM, Turner P: A comparison of the effects of chlorphenter-mine, diethylpropion, and phenmetrazine on critical flicker frequency. BR J PHARMACOL 30:307–316, 1967.

220. Smith JL, Mickatavage RC: The ocular effects of topical digitalis. AM J OPHTHALMOL 56:889–894, 1963.

221. Smolin G, Keates RH: Retardation of corneal vascularization. AM J OPHTHALMOL 61:321–327, 1966.

222.* Smyth HF Jr, Carpenter CP: The place of the range-finding test in the industrial toxicology laboratory. J IND HYG 26:269–273, 1944.

223.* Smyth HF Jr, Carpenter CP: Further experience with the range-finding test in the industrial toxicology laboratory. J IND HYG 30:63–68, 1948.

224.* Smyth HF Jr, Carpenter CP, Weil CS: Range-finding toxicity data, List III. J IND HYG 31:60–62, 1949.

225.* Smyth HF Jr, Carpenter CP, Weil CS: Range-finding toxicity data, List IV. ARCH IND HYG 4:119–122, 1951.

226.* Smyth HF Jr, Carpenter CP, Weil CS, Pozzani UC: Range-finding toxicity data. ARCH IND HYG 10:61–68, 1954.

227.* Smyth HF Jr: Hygienic standards for daily inhalation. AM IND HYG ASSOC QUART, June 1956, pp129–185.

228.* Smyth HF Jr, Carpenter CP, Weil CS, Pozzani UC, Striegel JA: Range-finding toxicity data: List VI. AM IND HYG ASSOC J 23:95–107, 1962. List VII. AM IND HYG ASSOC J 30:470–476, 1969.

229. Sneddon JM, Turner P: Structure activity relation of some sympathomimetic amines in the guanethidine-treated human eye. J PHYSIOL 192:23P–26P, 1967.

230. Sommer S: Animal experimental studies on the effect of some technical solvents on the eye. KLIN MONATSBL AUGENHEILKD 130:105–109, 1957. (German)

231. Sorsby A, Newhouse JP, Lucas DR: Experimental degeneration of the retina. I. Thiol reactors as inducing agents. BR J OPHTHALMOL 41:309–312, 1957.

232. Sorsby A, Nakajima A: Experimental degeneration of the retina. III. Inhibitors of glycolysis and of respiration as inducing agents. BR J OPHTHALMOL 42:558–562, 1958.

233. Sorsby A, Harding R: Experimental degeneration of the retina—VIII Dithizone retinopathy: Its independence of the diabetogenic effect. VISION RES 2:149–155, 1962.

234. Sorsby A, Harding R: Oxidizing agents as potentiators of the retinotoxic action of sodium fluoride, sodium iodate and sodium iodoacetate. NATURE 210:997–998, 1966.

235. Stagni S: Emergency treatment in burns of the eye by lime. RASS ITAL OTTALMOL 28:438–447, 1959. (Italian)

236. Standish M: A compilation of thirty two cases of glaucoma reported to the New England Ophthalmological Society since its foundation. The danger of mydriasis. OPHTHALMIC RECORD 11:243–255, 1902.

237. Szeghy G, Szlamka K: Crystal elimination in the lime-burned cornea after treatment with disodium ethylenediaminetetraacetate, Komplexon III. KLIN MONATSBL AUGENHEILKD 139:667–669, 1961. (German)

238. Tartakovskaya AI: Apilac in the treatment of trophic corneal disturbances during evolution of the burn process. VESTN OFTALMOL 79(1):59–61, 1966.

239. Teleky L: *Gewerbliche Vergiftungen.* Berlin, Springer, 1955.

240. Theodore FH: Corneal complications after cataract surgery. INT OPHTHALMOL CLIN 4:913–948, 1964.

---

*See page 1008 for method of testing and rating on rabbit eyes.

241. Thiel H–L: Experimental and clinical studies of burns of the eye. GRAEFES ARCH OPHTHALMOL 164:362–373, 1962. (German)

242. Thies O: On eye injuries in the chemical industry. ZENTRALBL GES OPH-THALMOL 20:631–633, 1929. (German)

243. Thorpe HE: Foreign bodies in the anterior chamber angle, their management with the aid of gonioscopy. AM J OPHTHALMOL 61:1339–1343, 1966.

244. Tolle R, Porksen N: Thymoleptic mydriasis in the course of treatment. INT PHARMACOPSYCHIAT 2:86–98, 1969.

245. Tsuchida Y: Effects of intravitreous injection of several chemicals on the ERG and light-induced optic nerve potential in the albino rabbit. ACTA SOC OPHTHALMOL JPN 72:2151–2161, 1968.

246. Uhthoff W: Augenstrorungen bei Vergiftungen. *Graefe-Saemisch, Handbuch der Augenheilkunde,* 2nd ed. Leipzig, Wilhelm Englemann, 1901, vol 2, ch 22, part 2.

247. Uhthoff W, Metzer E: Poisons of sight and pharmacological modification of vision. HANDB NORM PATH PHYSIOL 12:812–833, 1931. (German)

248. Vaughan DG, Riegelman S: Management of corneal ulcers. In Kimura SJ, Goodner EK (Eds.): *Ocular Pharmacology and Therapeutics and the Problems of Medical Management.* Philadelphia, F.A. Davis, 1963, pp129–135.

249. Villard H: Chemical burns of the eye. ARCH OPHTALMOL (PARIS) 44:21–40; 93–111; 167–177; 222–223, 1927. (French)

250. Vogt A: Further experimental and clinical studies of the injurious influence of synthetic aniline dyes on the eye. Z AUGENHEILKD 13:117–144; 226–242, 1905. (German)

251. Vogt A: Experimental studies on the significance of the chemical properties of basic aniline dyes for their injurious action on the mucous membrane of the eye. Z AUGENHEILKD 15:58–72, 1906. (German)

252. vonOettingen WF: *Poisoning,* 2nd ed. Philadelphia, Saunders, 1958.

253. Wagenmann A: Injuries of the eye from chemical action. In *Graefe-Saemisch, Handbuch der Augenheilkunde.* Leipzig, Wilhelm Englemann, 1913, vol 9, part 5, ch 2, pp1531–1636. (German)

254. Wakayama S: Influence of some medical agents on the corneal vascularization after injury. SHIKOKU IGAKU ZASSHI (Suppl 16):868–879, 1960. (CHEM ABSTR 61:4838, 1964.)

255. Walsh FB: *Clinical Neuro-Ophthalmology.* Baltimore, Williams & Wilkins, 1957.

256. Walsh FB, Hoyt WF: *Clinical Neuro-Ophthalmology,* 3rd ed. Baltimore, Williams & Wilkins, 1969.

257. Waser PG: The Pharmacology of *Amanita muscaria.* In Efron DH (Ed.): *Ethno-pharmacologic Search for Psychoactive Drugs.* Symposium, San Francisco, Jan 28–30, 1967. U.S. Public Health Service Publication No. 1645, pp419–439.

258. Watrous RM: Health hazards of the pharmaceutical industry. BR J IND MED 4:111–125, 1947.

259. Watzke RC: Experimental retinal detachment. TRANS AM OPHTHALMOL SOC 66:1022–1059, 1968.

260. Weekers R, Collignon-Brach J: Comparative study of the effects of various sympathicomimetic amines on the eye. ACTA OPHTALMOL 44:762–777, 1966. (French)

261. Weinstock M, Marshall AS: The influence of the sympathetic nervous system on the action of drugs on the lens. J PHARMACOL EXP THER 166:8–13, 1969.

262. Wieland T: Poisonous principles of mushrooms of the genus *Amanita.* SCIENCE 159:946–952, 1968.

263. Whitworth CG, Grant WM: Use of nitrate and nitrite vasodilators by glaucomatous patients. ARCH OPHTHALMOL 71:492–496, 1964.

264. Wilbrand H, Saenger A: *Neuritis optica bei Intoxikationen. Neurologie des Auges.* Wiesbaden, Bergmann, 1913, vol 5.

265. Wolf MA, Rowe VK, McCollister DD, Hollingsworth RL, Oyen F: Toxicological studies of certain alkylated benzenes and benzene. ARCH IND HEALTH 14:387–397, 1956.

266. Zahn K: The effect of vasoactive drugs on the retinal circulation. TRANS OPHTHALMOL SOC UK 86:529–536, 1966.

267. Zeller EA, Shoch D, Andujar E: On the enzymology of the refractory media of the eye. AM J OPHTHALMOL 61:1364–1371, 1966.

268. Zur Nedden M: On injury of the cornea through the action of lime, as well as from soluble lead-, silver-, copper-, aluminum-, and mercury preparations, together with therapeutic observations, on the grounds of experimental clinical and chemical investigations. GRAEFES ARCH OPHTHALMOL 63:319–387, 1906. (German)

270. Adenis JP, Leboutet MJ, Loubet A, Loubet R, Robin A: Ultrastructural and experimental study of the ocular toxicity of antibiotics and antifungals on the corneal endothelium. J FR OPHTALMOL 4:205–212, 1981. (French)

271. Adenis JP, Loubet A: Ultrastructural study of the toxicity of certain antimicrobials on the corneal endothelium. BULL SOC OPHTALMOL FRANCE 81:787–790, 1981. (French)

272. Albert DM, Puliafito CA: Choroidal melanoma: possible exposure to industrial toxins. N ENGL J MED 296:634, 1977.

273. Argov Z, Mastaglia FL: Drug-induced peripheral neuropathies. BR MED J 1:663–666, 1979.

274. Armstrong D, Hiramitsu T, Gutteridge J, Nilsson SE: Studies on experimentally induced retinal degeneration. I. Effect of lipid peroxides on electroretinographic activity in the albino rabbit. EXP EYE RES 35:157–171, 1982.

275. Ballantyne B, Gazzard MF, Swanston DW: Effects of solvents and irritants on intraocular tension in the rabbit. J PHYSIOL 226:12–14, 1972.

276. Ballantyne B, Gazzard MF, Swanston DW: Applanation tonometry in ophthalmic toxicology. Chapter 13 in *Current Approaches in Toxicology,* edited by B. Ballantyne. Bristol, John Wright and Sons, 1977.

277. Barrada A, Peyman GA, Greenberg D, Stelmack T, Fiscella R: Toxicity of antineoplastic drugs in vitrectomy infusion fluids. OPHTHALMIC SURG 14:845–847, 1983.

278. Barron CN, Murchison TE, Rubin LF, et al: Chlorpromazine and the eye of the dog. VI. A comparison of phenothiazine tranquilizers. EXP MOLEC PATHOL 16:172–179, 1972.

279. Beatty JF, Krupin F, Nichols PF, Becker B: Elevation of intraocular pressure by calcium channel blockers. ARCH OPHTHALMOL 102:1072–1076, 1984.

280. Bennett TO, Peyman GA: Toxicity of intravitreal aminoglycosides in primates. CAN J OPHTHALMOL 9:475–478, 1974.

281. Bernstein HN: Some iatrogenic ocular diseases from systemically administered drugs. INT OPHTHALMOL CLIN 10:553–619, 1970.

282. Bernstein HN: Ocular side-effects of drugs. Chapter 10 in *Drugs and Ocular Tissues,* (Meet Int Soc Eye Res), edited by S. Dikstein. Basel, Karger, 1977.

283. Betrix AF: Tolerance to antimitotics introduced into the anterior chamber of the cat's eye. GRAEFES ARCH OPHTHALMOL 189:265–279; 281–296, 1974. (French)

284. Bito LZ, Nichols RR, Baroody RA: A comparison of the miotic and inflammatory effects of biologically active polypeptides and prostaglandin E_2 on the rabbit eye. EXP EYE RES 34:325–337, 1982.

285. Burstein NL, Klyce SD: Electrophysiologic and morphologic effects of ophthalmic preparations on rabbit corneal epithelium. INVEST OPHTHALMOL VIS SCI 16:899–911, 1977.

286. Burstein NL: Corneal cytotoxicity of topically applied drugs, vehicles and preservatives. SURV OPHTHALMOL 25:15–30, 1980.

287. Caprino L, Togna G, Mazzei M: Toxicological studies of photosensitizer agents and photodegradable polyolefins. EUR J TOXICOL ENVIRON HYG 9:99–103, 1976.

288.* Carpenter CP, Weil CS, Smyth Jr HF: Range-finding toxicity data: List VIII. TOXICOL APPL PHARMACOL 28:313–319, 1974.

289. Carricaburu P, Lacroix R, Lacroix J: Comparative electroretinographic study of ocular effects of pesticides in mice. J PHARM BELGE 34:308–311, 1979. (French)

290. Carricaburu P, Lacroix R, Lacroix J: Study of the effect of chemically similar organochloride pesticides on the electrical ocular response of the white mouse. CR SEANCES SOC BIOL SES FIL 173:1055–1060, 1979. (French)

291. Chandler PA, Grant WM: *Glaucoma*. Philadelphia, Lea and Febiger, 1979.

292. Cole DF: Site of breakdown of the blood-aqueous barrier under the influence of vasodilator drugs. EXP EYE RES 19:591–607, 1974.

293. Coles WH: Effects of antibiotics on the in vitro rabbit corneal endothelium. INVEST OPHTHALMOL 14:246–250, 1975.

294. Committee on drugs: Blindness and neuropathy from diiodohydroxyquin-like drugs. PEDIATRICS 54:378–379, 1974.

295. Conquet P, Durand G, Laillier J, Plazonnet B: Evaluation of ocular irritation in the rabbit. Objective versus subjective assessment. TOXICOL APPL PHARMACOL 39:129–139, 1977.

296. Coon RA, Jones RA, Jenkins Jr LJ, Siegel J: Animal inhalation studies on ammonia, ethylene glycol, formaldehyde, dimethylamine, and ethanol. TOXICOL APPL PHARMACOL 16:646–655, 1970.

297. Cotlier E, Apple D: Cataracts induced by the polypeptide antibiotic polymyxin B sulfate. EXP EYE RES 16:69–77, 1973.

298. Davidson SI: Reports of ocular adverse reactions. TRANS OPHTHALMOL SOC UK 93:495–510, 1973.

299. Dikstein S (editor): *Drugs and Ocular Tissues*. (Meet Int Soc Eye Res, 1976), Basel, Karger, 1977.

300. Dormans JAMA, van Logten MJ: The effect of ophthalmic preservatives on corneal epithelium of the rabbit: A scanning electron microscopical study. TOXICOL APPL PHARMACOL 62:251–261, 1982.

301. Dralands L, Garin P: Anti-infective medicaments. Chapter 17 in *The Injurious Effect of Systemic Medications on the Visual Apparatus*, edited by J. Michiels. BULL SOC BELGE OPHTALMOL 160:326–446, 1972. (French)

302. Dralands L: Cytostatics. Chapter 18 in *The Injurious Effects of Systemic Medications on the Visual Apparatus*, edited by J. Michiels. BULL SOC BELGE OPHTALMOL 160:447–463, 1972. (French)

303. Drenckhahn D, Lullmann-Rauch R: Lens opacities associated with lipidosis-like ultrastructural alterations in rats treated with chloroquine, chlorphentermine, or iprindole. EXP EYE RES 24:621–632, 1977.

---

*See page 1008 for method of testing and rating on rabbit eyes.

304. Drenckhahn D, Lullmann-Rauch R: Drug-induced retinal lipidosis: differential susceptibilities of pigment epithelium and neuroretina toward several amphiphilic cationic drugs. EXP MOL PATHOL 28:360–371, 1978.

305. Duncan AJ, Wilson WS: Some preservatives in eyedrop preparations hasten the formation of dryspots in the rabbit cornea. BR J PHARMACOL 56:359P–360P, 1976.

306. Ellis PP: Local anesthetics. Chapter 3 in *Symposium on Ocular Therapy,* 8:17–24, 1976. Edited by I.H. Leopold and R.P. Burns, New York, John Wiley and Sons.

307. Fitzhugh OG, Buschke WH: Production of cataract in rats by betatetralol and other derivatives of naphthalene. ARCH OPHTHALMOL 41:572–582, 1949.

308. Foster CS, Pavan-Langston D: Corneal wound healing and antiviral medication. ARCH OPHTHALMOL 95:2062–2067, 1977.

309. Foster CS, Lass JH, Moran-Wallace K, Giovanoni R: Ocular toxicity of topical antifungal agents. ARCH OPHTHALMOL 99:1081–1084, 1981.

310. Francois J, DeRouck A, Cambie E, Zanen A: Electrodiagnosis of retinal diseases. BULL SOC BELGE OPHTALMOL 166:1–494, 1974. (French)

311. Fraunfelder FT, Hanna C, Meyer M: Drug-induced ocular side effects. Chapter 10 in *Symposium on Ocular Therapy,* 11:97–119, 1979. Edited by I.H. Leopold and R.P. Burns, New York, John Wiley and Sons.

312. Fraunfelder FT, Meyer SM: *Drug-Induced Ocular Side Effects and Drug Interactions,* 2nd ed., Philadelphia, Lea and Febiger, 1982.

313. Fraunfelder FT, Meyer SM: Ocular toxicity of antineoplastic agents. OPHTHALMOLOGY 90:1–3, 1983.

314. Gasset AR, Ishii Y, Kaufman HE, Miller T: Cytotoxicity of ophthalmic preservatives. AM J OPHTHALMOL 78:98–105, 1974.

315. Gasset AR, Katzin D: Antiviral drugs and corneal wound healing. INVEST OPHTHALMOL 14:628–630, 1975.

316. Gershbein LL, McDonald JE: Evaluation of the corneal irritancy of test shampoos and detergents in various animal species. FOOD COSMET TOXICOL 15:131–134, 1977.

317. Grant WM: *Toxicology of the Eye,* 2nd ed., Springfield, Thomas, 1974.

318. Grant WM: The peripheral visual system as a target. Chapter 6 in *Experimental and Clinical Neurotoxicology,* edited by P.S. Spencer and H.H. Schaumburg. Baltimore, Williams and Wilkins, 1980.

319. Graymore CN (ed.): *Biochemistry of the Eye.* London/New York, Academic Press, 1970.

320. Green K, Tonjum A: Influence of various agents on corneal permeability. AM J OPHTHALMOL 72:897–905, 1971.

321. Green K, Hull DS, Vaughn ED, Malizia Jr AA, Bowman K: Rabbit endothelial response to ophthalmic preservatives. ARCH OPHTHALMOL 95:2218–2221, 1977.

322. Green WR, Sullivan JB, Hehir RM, Scharpf LG, Dickinson AW: *A Systematic Comparison of Chemically Induced Eye Injury in the Albino Rabbit and Rhesus Monkey.* Soap and Detergent Association, 475 Park Avenue South, New York, 1978.

323. Greenblatt DJ, Shader RI, DiMascio A: Extrapyramidal effects. Chapter 11 in *Psychotropic Drug Side Effects,* edited by R.I. Shader and A. DiMascio. Baltimore, Williams and Wilkins, 1970.

324. Griffith JF, Nixon JA, Bruce RD, Reer PJ, Bannan EA: Dose-response studies with chemical irritants in the albino rabbit eye as a basis for selecting optimum testing conditions for predicting hazard to the human eye. TOXICOL APPL PHARMACOL 55:501–513, 1980.

325. Guillot JP, Gonnet JF, Clement C, Caillard L, Truhaut R: Evaluation of the ocular-irritation potential of 56 compounds. FOOD CHEM TOXICOL 20:573–582, 1982.

326. Hanna C, Boozman F, Wallace TR: Ocular irritation from preservative agents. Pages 103–104 in *Symposium on Ocular Therapy*, edited by I.H. Leopold and R.P. Burns, New York, John Wiley and Sons, 1979.

327. Henkes HE, Deutman AF: Electrodiagnostic procedures in drug-induced ocular diseases. DOC OPHTHALMOL 34:209–219, 1973.

328. Hermans G: Psychotropic drugs. Chapter 1 in *Harmful Effects of Systemic Medications on the Visual Apparatus*. Edited by J. Michiels. BULL SOC BELGE OPHTALMOL 160:15–88, 1972. (French)

329. Hirst LW, Kenyon KR, Fogle J, Stark WJ: Corneal epithelial adhesion studies. AUST J OPHTHALMOL 9:103–111, 1981.

330. Hood CI, Gasset AR, Ellison ED, Kaufman HE: Corneal reaction to selected chemical agents in the rabbit and squirrel monkey. AM J OPHTHALMOL 71:1009–1017, 1971.

331. Hopper SS, Hulpieu HR, Cole VV: Some toxicological properties of surface-active agents. J AM PHARM ASSOC 38:428–432, 1949.

332. Hoyer J: Electrophysiologic investigations into damage due to drugs. KLIN MONATSBL AUGENHEILKD 162:643–648, 1973. (German)

333. Johnson DR, Burns RP: Blepharoconjunctivitis associated with cancer therapy. TRANS PAC COAST OTO–OPHTHALMOL SOC 46:43–49, 1965.

334. Jones WT, Kipling MD: Glaucopsia—blue-grey vision. BR J IND MED 29:460–461, 1972.

335. Kagan JM, Leopold IH: Drug-induced retinopathies. Chapter 11 in *Symposium on Ocular Therapy*, 7:116–126, 1974. Edited by I.H. Leopold. St. Louis, C.V. Mosby, 1974.

336. Kaufman HE: Chemical blepharitis following drug treatment. AM J OPHTHALMOL 95:703, 1983.

337. Krejci L, Harrison R: Antiglaucoma drug effects on corneal epithelium. ARCH OPHTHALMOL 84:766–769, 1970.

338. Laillier J, Plazonnet B, LeDouarec JC, Gonin MJ: Evaluation of ocular irritation in the rabbit: development of an objective method of studying eye irritation. PROC EUR SOC TOXICOL 17:336–350, 1976.

339. Laroche J, Laroche C: Effect of some antibiotics on color vision. ANN PHARM FR 28:333–341, 1970. (French)

340. Lauring L, Wergeland FL Jr: Ocular toxicity of newer industrial metals. MIL MED 135:1171–1174, 1970.

341. Lavine JB, Binder PS, Wickham MG: Antimicrobials and the corneal endothelium. ANN OPHTHALMOL 11:1517–1528, 1979.

342. Leopold IH: Problems in the use of antibiotics in ophthalmology. In *Symposium on Ocular Therapy*, 4:90–126, 1969. Edited by I.H. Leopold. St. Louis, C.V. Mosby.

343. Leopold IH, Lieberman TW: Chemical injuries of the cornea. FED PROC, FED AM SOC EXP BIOL 30:92–95, 1971.

344. Lessell S: Toxic and deficiency optic neuropathies. Chapter 4 in *Neuro-Ophthalmology Symposium of the University of Miami and Bascom Palmer Eye Institute*, edited by J.L. Smith and J.S. Glaser. Saint Louis, C.V. Mosby, Vol 7, 1973.

345. Lincoff A, Lincoff H, Solorzano C, Iwamoto T: Selection of xenon gas for rapidly disappearing retinal tamponade. ARCH OPHTHALMOL 100:996–997, 1982.

346. Lisch K: Ophthalmic-pharmacologic complications. KLIN MONATSBL AUGEN-HEILKD 169:129–133, 1976.

347. Lloyd GK, Liggett MP, Kynoch SR, Davies RE: Assessment of the acute toxicity and potential irritancy of hair dye constituents. FOOD COSMET TOXICOL 15:607–610, 1977.

348. Lullmann-Rauch R: Retinal lipidosis in albino rats treated with chlorpentermine and with tricyclic antidepressants. ACTA NEUROPATH (BERLIN) 35:55–67, 1976.

349. MacRae SM, Edelhauser HF, Hyndiuk RA, Burd EM, Schultz RO: The effects of sodium hyaluronate, chondroitin sulfate, and methylcellulose on the corneal endothelium and intraocular pressure. AM J OPHTHALMOL 95:332–341, 1983.

350. Mac Rae SM, Brown B, Edelhauser HF: The corneal toxicity of presurgical skin antiseptics. AM J OPHTHALMOL 97:221–232, 1984.

351. Marsh RJ, Maurice DM: Influence of nonionic detergents and other surfactants on human corneal permeability. EXP EYE RES 11:43–48, 1971.

352. Marzulli FN, Ruggles DI: Rabbit eye irritation test: collaborative study. J ASSOC OFF ANAL CHEM 56:905–914, 1973.

353. Mason CG: Ocular accumulation and toxicity of certain systemically administered drugs. J TOXICOL ENVIRON HEALTH 2:977–995, 1977.

354. Maudgal PC, Cornelis H, Missotten L: Effects of commercial ophthalmic drugs on rabbit corneal epithelium. GRAEFES ARCH OPHTHALMOL 216:191–203, 1981.

355. Mayer U. Lang GE: Morphologic alterations from addition of various antibiotics to cultures of lens epithelium. KLIN MONATSBL AUGENHEILKD 181:263–265, 1982. (German)

356. Meier-Ruge W: Etiology and pathogenesis of toxic side-effects of drugs on the retina. KLIN MONATSBL AUGENHEILKD 163:155–172, 1973. (German)

357. Meier-Ruge W: Toxicological testing on the retina. Pages 300–323 in *Arzneimittelnebenwirkungen am Auge.* Edited by O. Hockwin and H.R. Koch. Stuttgart-Hohenheim, Germany, Fischer, 1977. (German)

358. Merigan WH, Weiss B (Editors): *Neurotoxicity of the Visual System.* New York, Raven Press, 1980.

359. Michiels J (Editor): Noxious effects of systemic medications on the visual apparatus. BULL SOC BELGE OPHTALMOL 160:5–516, 1972. (French)

360. Michiels J: Cataract of toxic origin. BULL SOC BELGE OPHTALMOL 181:21–37, 1978. (French)

361. Morgan BS, Larson B, Peyman GA, West CS: Toxicity of antibiotic combinations for vitrectomy infusion fluid. OPHTHALMIC SURG 10:74–77, 1979.

362. Moro F, Sparatore F, Piccinini R: On the phacotoxic action of α,β-unsaturated carbonyl compounds and of β-naphthyl derivatives. ANN OTTALMOL CLIN OCUL 95:935–944, 1969. (Italian)

363. Munn A: Health hazards in the chemical industry. TRANS SOC OCCUP MED 17:8–14, 1967.

364. Neubauer H, Ruessmann W, Kilp H (Editors): *Intraokularer Fremdkorper und Metallose,* Int Symp Dtsch Ophthalmol Ges 1976 (Pub 1976). Munich, Germany, J.F. Bergmann-Verlag.

365. Okawada N, Mizoguchi I, Ishiguro T: Effects of photochemical air pollution on the human eye: concerning eye irritation, tear lysozyme and tear pH. NAGOYA J MED SCI 41:9–20, 1979. (English)

366. Olson RJ, Kolodner H, Riddle P, Escapini H Jr: Commonly used intraocular medications and the corneal endothelium. ARCH OPHTHALMOL 98:2224–2226, 1980.

367. Palmer EA: Drug toxicity in pediatric ophthalmology. J TOXICOL CUTANEOUS OCUL TOXICOL 1:181–210, 1982.

368. Petroutsos G, Guimaraes R, Giraud J, Pouliquen Y: Antibiotics and corneal epithelial wound healing. ARCH OPHTHALMOL 101:1775–1778, 1983.

369. Peyman GA, Greenberg D, Fishman GA, Fiscella R, Thomas A: Evaluation of toxicity of intravitreal antineoplastic drugs. OPHTHALMIC SURG 15:411–413, 1984.

370. Pfister RR, Burstein N: The effects of ophthalmic drugs, vehicles, and preservatives on corneal epithelium, a scanning electron microscope study. INVEST OPHTHALMOL 15:246–259, 1976.

371. Potts AM, Gonasun LM: Toxicology of the eye. Chapter 13 in *Toxicology: The Basic Science of Poisons,* edited by L.J. Casarett and J. Doull. New York, MacMillan, 1975.

372. Proctor NH, Hughes JP: *Chemical Hazards of the Workplace.* Philadelphia, J.B. Lippincott, 1978.

373. Riddell RH (Editor): *Pathology of Drug-Induced and Toxic Diseases.* New York, Churchill Livingstone, 1982.

374. von Sallmann L: On the deposition of some metals in the human cornea. GRAEFES ARCH OPHTHALMOL 128:245–264, 1932. (German)

375. Sanders D, Cotlier E, Wyhinny G, Millman L: Cataracts induced by surface active agents. EXP EYE RES 19:35–42, 1974.

376. Seiler KU, Thiel HJ, Wassermann HO: Chloroquine keratopathy as an example of drug induced phospholipidosis. KLIN MONATSBL AUGENHEILKD 170:64–73, 1977. (German)

377. Slem G, Ayan Y, Baykal E: Experimental study on the effects of insecticides on the rabbit eye. ANN OPHTHALMOL 4:874–875, 1972.

378. Spencer PS, Schaumburg HH (Editors): *Experimental and Clinical Neurotoxicology.* Baltimore/London, Williams and Wilkins, 1980.

379. Srinivasan BD, Kulkarni PS: The effect of steroidal and non steroidal anti-inflammatory agents on corneal epithelialization. INVEST OPHTHALMOL VIS SCI 20:688–691, 1981.

380. Stainer GA, Peyman GA, Meisels H, Fishman G: Toxicity of selected antibiotics in vitreous replacement fluid. ANN OPHTHALMOL 9:615–618, 1977.

381. Sternlieb I, Goldfischer S: Heavy metals and lysosomes. FRONT BIOL 45:185–200, 1976.

382. Stern GA, Schemmer GB, Farber RD, Gorovoy MS: Effect of topical antibiotic solutions on corneal epithelial wound healing. ARCH OPHTHALMOL 101:644–647, 1983.

383. Takahashi N: The influence of several disinfectants on the temperature effect of the cornea. ACTA SOC OPHTHALMOL JPN 74:684–686, 1970. (English abstract)

384. Tateishi J: Comparative study of neurotoxicity of clioquinol, ethambutol, isoniazid and chloramphenicol in dogs. FOLIA PSYCHIATR NEUROL JPN 28:11–17, 1974. (English)

385. Treon JF, Crutchfield Jr WE, Kitzmiller KV: The physiological response of animals to cyclohexane, methylcyclohexane and certain derivatives of these compounds. J IND HYG 25:323–346, 1943.

386. Van Dyk HJL, Swan KC: Drug-induced pseudotumor cerebri. In: *Symposium on Ocular Therapy*, 4:71–77, 1969. Edited by I.H. Leopold. St. Louis, C.V. Mosby.

387. Van Norren D, Padmos P: Influence of anesthetics, ethyl alcohol, and Freon on dark adaptation of monkey cone ERG. INVEST OPHTHALMOL VIS SCI 16:80–83, 1977.

388. Wilson FM II: Adverse external ocular effects of topical ophthalmic therapy: an epidemiologic, laboratory, and clinical study. TRANS AM OPHTHALMOL SOC 81:854–965, 1983.

389. Zinn KN, Marmor MF: Toxicology of the human retinal pigment epithelium. Chapter 22 in: *The Retinal Pigment Epithelium*, edited by K.M. Zinn and M.F. Marmor. Cambridge, Harvard University Press, 1979.